ENDOCRINE SURGERY

A South Asian Perspective

Editor-In-Chief

Anand Kumar Mishra, MBBS, MS, PDCC, MCh, FACS

Professor and Head, Department of Endocrine Surgery,
King George's Medical University, Lucknow

Co-editors

Amit Agarwal, MBBS, MS, FRCS

Professor and Head, Department of Endocrine Surgery,
Sanjay Gandhi Post Graduate Institute of Medical Sciences, Lucknow

Rajeev Parameswaran, BSc, MBBS, FRCS, MPhil, FRCS

Assistant Professor, Senior Consultant and Head, Division of Endocrine Surgery
Program Director, Surgery in General, National University Health System, Singapore

Kul Ranjan Singh, MBBS, MS, MCh, FACS, FICS

Associate Professor, Department of Endocrine Surgery,
King George's Medical University, Lucknow

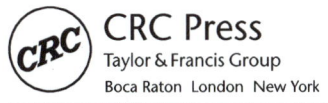

CRC Press is an imprint of the
Taylor & Francis Group, an **informa** business

First edition published 2022
by CRC Press
6000 Broken Sound Parkway NW, Suite 300, Boca Raton, FL 33487-2742

and by CRC Press
2 Park Square, Milton Park, Abingdon, Oxon, OX14 4RN

© 2022 Taylor & Francis Group, LLC

CRC Press is an imprint of Taylor & Francis Group, LLC

This book contains information obtained from authentic and highly regarded sources. While all reasonable efforts have been made to publish reliable data and information, neither the author[s] nor the publisher can accept any legal responsibility or liability for any errors or omissions that may be made. The publishers wish to make clear that any views or opinions expressed in this book by individual editors, authors or contributors are personal to them and do not necessarily reflect the views/opinions of the publishers. The information or guidance contained in this book is intended for use by medical, scientific or health-care professionals and is provided strictly as a supplement to the medical or other professional's own judgement, their knowledge of the patient's medical history, relevant manufacturer's instructions and the appropriate best practice guidelines. Because of the rapid advances in medical science, any information or advice on dosages, procedures or diagnoses should be independently verified. The reader is strongly urged to consult the relevant national drug formulary and the drug companies' and device or material manufacturers' printed instructions, and their websites, before administering or utilizing any of the drugs, devices or materials mentioned in this book. This book does not indicate whether a particular treatment is appropriate or suitable for a particular individual. Ultimately it is the sole responsibility of the medical professional to make his or her own professional judgements, so as to advise and treat patients appropriately. The authors and publishers have also attempted to trace the copyright holders of all material reproduced in this publication and apologize to copyright holders if permission to publish in this form has not been obtained. If any copyright material has not been acknowledged please write and let us know so we may rectify in any future reprint.

Except as permitted under U.S. Copyright Law, no part of this book may be reprinted, reproduced, transmitted, or utilized in any form by any electronic, mechanical, or other means, now known or hereafter invented, including photocopying, microfilming, and recording, or in any information storage or retrieval system, without written permission from the publishers.

For permission to photocopy or use material electronically from this work, access www.copyright.com or contact the Copyright Clearance Center, Inc. (CCC), 222 Rosewood Drive, Danvers, MA 01923, 978-750-8400. For works that are not available on CCC please contact mpkbookspermissions@tandf.co.uk

Trademark notice: Product or corporate names may be trademarks or registered trademarks and are used only for identification and explanation without intent to infringe.

ISBN: 9780367186388 (hbk)
ISBN: 9781032136509 (pbk)
ISBN: 9780429197338 (ebk)

DOI: 10.1201/9780429197338

Typeset in Warnock Pro
by KnowledgeWorks Global Ltd.

Access the [companion website/Support Material]: www.routledge.com/9781032136509

ENDOCRINE SURGERY

This Book is dedicated to my late mother, Vimla Mishra and papa,
Shri Suresh Prasad Mishra, who are my life-time heroes and role models.

To all lives lost in the COVID pandemic.

This book is a culmination of the medical experiences and blessings bestowed upon me by my patients.

CONTENTS

Foreword by Dr. Nair x
Foreword by Dr. Mishra xi
Foreword by Dr. Vittal xii
Preface xiii
Acknowledgments xiv
About the Editors xv
List of Contributors xvi

1. History of Thyroid Surgery 1
   Surabhi Garg, Shreyamsa M and Anand Kumar Mishra

2. Thyroid Physiology 2
   Shivendu Bhardwaj and Subhash Yadav

3. Embryology and Surgical Anatomy: Thyroid and Parathyroid Glands 10
   Dinesh Kumar Srinivasan, Krishnan Jayabharathi, Muthukrishnan Chandrika, S. Thameem Dheen, Boon Huat Bay and Rajeev Parameswaran

4. Investigations in Thyroid Diseases: Imaging 17
   Alka Ashmita Singhal

5. Investigation in Thyroid Diseases: Pathology 36
   Chanchal Rana

6. Inflammatory Diseases of Thyroid 43
   Shivendra Verma and Manisha Gupta

7. Hypothyroidism 50
   Madhukar Mittal, Parul Gupta and M K Garg

8. Hyperthyroidism: Surgeon's Perspective 58
   Sasi Mouli, PV Pradeep and Anand Kumar Mishra

9. Approach to Thyroid Nodules 71
   Chiaw-Ling Chng

10. Nonsurgical Management of Thyroid Nodules 80
    Anand Kumar Mishra

11. Management of Non-Endemic Goiters 84
    Anand Kumar Mishra

12. Management of Endemic Goiter 90
    Ranil Fernando

13. Molecular Pathways of Thyroid Carcinogenesis 96
    Chue Koy Min and Rajeev Parameswaran

14. Differentiated Thyroid Carcinoma 104
    Anand Kumar Mishra

15. Papillary Microcarcinoma of Thyroid 117
    K.M.M. Vishvak Chanthar and Sabaretnam Mayilvaganan

16. Medullary Thyroid Carcinoma 123
    Mithun Raam and Deepak Thomas Abraham

Contents

17. **Poorly Differentiated Thyroid Carcinoma** 130
    Shreyamsa M, Anand Kumar Mishra and Kul Ranjan Singh

18. **Anaplastic Thyroid Carcinoma** 137
    Sasi Mouli, Anand Kumar Mishra and Kul Ranjan Singh

19. **Rare Tumors of the Thyroid** 149
    Murat Ozdemir and Özer Makay

20. **Childhood Thyroid Cancers** 155
    Emre Divarci and Ahmet Çelik

21. **Thyroid Surgery in South Asia** 163
    *Anand Kumar Mishra, Amit Agarwal, Rajeev Parameswaran, Soe Tin, Ranil Fernando, Khalid Alhajri,
    Ali Korairi, Marya Al Suhaibani and Özer Makay*

22. **Thyroidectomy** 170
    Anand Kumar Mishra and Kul Ranjan Singh

23. **Postthyroidectomy Hypocalcemia** 184
    Loreno E. Enny, Faraz Ahmad, Kul Ranjan Singh and Anand Kumar Mishra

24. **Neck Dissections in Thyroid Cancer** 190
    Chintamani

25. **Extent Of Surgery in Thyroid Cancer** 197
    Anand Kumar Mishra and Kul Ranjan Singh

26. **Adjuvant Treatment and Follow-Up of Thyroid Cancers** 204
    Hian Liang Huang, Kelvin Loke Siu Hoong, Sumbul Zaheer and David Ng Chee Eng

27. **Recurrent Goiter** 211
    Surabhi Garg, Kul Ranjan Singh and Anand Kumar Mishra

28. **Retrosternal Goiter** 216
    Kul Ranjan Singh, Anand Kumar Mishra and Pooja Ramakant

29. **History of Parathyroid Surgery** 221
    Poongkodi Karunakaran

30. **Anatomy and Pathology of the Parathyroid Gland** 222
    Rajeev Parameswaran and Sheeja Sainulabdeen

31. **Symptoms and Natural History of Primary Hyperparathyroidism** 230
    K.M.M. Vishvak Chanthar and Gaurav Agarwal

32. **Localization Studies in Parathyroid Diseases** 240
    Alka Ashmita Singhal

33. **Familial Hyperparathyroidism** 265
    S. Dhalapathy and Smitha Rao

34. **Secondary and Tertiary Hyperparathyroidism** 271
    Lee Kai Yin and Rajeev Parameswaran

35. **Normocalcemic Hyperparathyroidism** 279
    Mayur Agrawal and Subhash Yadav

36. **Surgical Approaches in Parathyroid Diseases** 283
    Dhritiman Maitra, Chitresh Kumar and Anurag Srivastava

37. **Remote Access Thyroid and Parathyroid Surgery** 290
    Hyeong Won Yu and June Young Choi

38. **Intraoperative Adjuncts in Thyroid and Parathyroid Surgery** 297
    Sunnel Mattoo, Shreyamsa M, Roma Pradhan and Amit Agarwal

39. **Parathyroid Carcinoma** 305
    Pooja Ramakant, Chanchal Rana, Kul Ranjan Singh and Anand Kumar Mishra

40. **Management of Recurrent Primary Hyperparathyroidism** 309
    Loreno E. Enny, Kul Ranjan Singh and Anand Kumar Mishra

41. **Anesthesia for Thyroid and Parathyroid Surgery** 315
    Reetu Verma and Yogita Dwivedi

42. **History of Adrenal Surgery** 320
    Asuri Krishna, Mayank Jain, Shardool Vikram Gupta and Subodh Kumar

43. **Adrenal Gland: Embryology and Anatomy** 321
    Asuri Krishna and Mayank Jain

44. **Physiology of the Adrenal Gland** 324
    Sandeep Bhattacharya

45. **Biochemical Evaluation of an Adrenal Mass** 329
    Manish Gutch, Sukriti Kumar, Maghvendra Kumar and Manjari Dwivedi

46. **Imaging of Adrenal Masses** 334
    Jyoti Arora, Kulbir Ahlawat and Alka Ashmita Singhal

47. **Pathology of Adrenal Lesions** 345
    Preeti Agarwal

48. **Pheochromocytoma** 353
    M J Paul

49. **Cushing's Syndrome** 359
    Anand Kumar Mishra

50. **Hyperaldosteronism** 369
    Troy H Puar and Meifen Zhang

51. **Adrenal Myelolipoma** 378
    Himagirish K Rao

52. **Adrenal Surgical Diseases in Children** 384
    Ahmet Çelik and Emre Divarci

53. **Anesthetic Management for Pheochromocytoma** 396
    Divya Srivastava and Bhavya Naithani

54. **Operative Approach to the Adrenal Gland Pathology** 403
    Sendhil Rajan and Bharadhwaj Ravindhran

55. **Pancreas: Embryology, Anatomy and Endocrine Physiology** 410
    Rahul, Puneet and Sanjeev Kumar

56. **Insulinoma** 417
    Anand Kumar Mishra

Contents

57. Gastrinoma 424
Anand Kumar Mishra

58. Rare Pancreatic Endocrine Tumors 425
Anand Kumar Mishra

59. Carcinoid Tumors of the Gastrointestinal Tract 433
Linu Oommen Mathew, Sheeja Sainulabdeen and Rajeev Parameswaran

60. Carcinoid Syndrome 445
Anand Kumar Mishra

61. Gastroenteropancreatic Neuroendocrine Tumors in Children 446
Orkan Ergün

62. Multiple Endocrine Neoplasia 449
Anand Kumar Mishra

63. Non-Men Endocrine Syndromes 457
Kushagra Gaurav, Akshay Agarwal and Kul Ranjan Singh

64. Endocrine Emergencies 463
VNSSVAMS Mahalakshmi D, Sabaretnam Mayilvaganan, Kul Ranjan Singh and Anand Kumar Mishra

Index 468

FOREWORD BY DR. NAIR

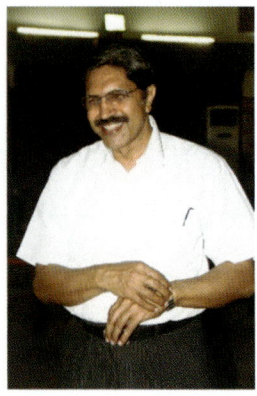

I am pleased to write this foreword for *Endocrine Surgery: A South Asian Perspective* under publication by CRC Press / Taylor & Francis Group, London.

Endocrine Surgery is a nascent specialty in the developing nations of South Asia. As a specialty, it is in constant evolution with newer imaging techniques, biochemical tests, molecular pathology, genetic testing, newer surgical techniques in minimal invasive and robotics, being added to the already available array of investigation and surgical techniques. Most of the available textbooks on Endocrine Surgery are from the west and give a different perspective compared to the prevailing entities in the South Asian countries like endemic goiters, thyroiditis, massive thyroid swellings, late presentation of endocrine disorders, vitamin D deficiency to name a few.

In creating this multiauthored textbook of Endocrine Surgery, the editorial team headed by Dr. Anand Mishra, Professor and Head of Endocrine Surgery, King George's Medical University, Lucknow, has approached knowledgeable, enthusiastic mix of young and experienced faculty in Endocrine Surgery from South Asian countries.

This textbook presents a definite insight to Endocrine Surgery, highlighting the South Asian perspective. The various chapters comprehensively cover the entire spectrum of Endocrine Surgery with equal importance to the thyroid gland, parathyroid, adrenal and endocrine disorders of the gastrointestinal tract: embryology, anatomy, physiology, biochemical investigations, imaging modalities, histopathology, operative techniques, complications and recent advances.

I enjoyed going through the topics, and I am sure general surgery residents, endocrine surgery residents, general and endocrine surgeons all around the world will find this book simple, easily readable and very informative.

I am sure the readers will enjoy reading this book and above all appreciate the South Asian perspective.

HAPPY READING
Best wishes,

Dr. Aravindan Nair, MS, MNAMS
Chief of Medical Services and
Consultant General and Endocrine Surgeon
Naruvi Hospitals
Former Professor and Head of Endocrine Surgery
Christian Medical College and Hospital
Vellore, India

FOREWORD BY DR. MISHRA

I consider it as a privilege to write the foreword for the Book titled *Endocrine Surgery: A South Asian Perspective*. Prof. Anand Kumar Mishra who is the Chief Editor of the book has roped in a number of contributors for the book from across the Asian countries. Over last three decades, the endocrine surgical discipline has been developing as a distinct subspecialty of surgery attracting young surgeons to choose it as a career. Though the surgery on endocrine glands is been practiced by various other specialty surgeons, general surgeons are getting more and more fascinated with the science and art of endocrine surgery. Dedicated departments/units are coming up in medical schools and corporate healthcare also feel the need of these specialized surgeons. As more and more academic endocrine surgeons build up knowledge base through research publications, review articles the need for compiled information resources felt. Initial texts were in the form of monograms, short textbooks. Standard textbooks on the subject of endocrine surgery were published only in last decade and half. Not many books have been published from Asia on this subject though we have a number of books published from North America and Europe. This book has focused on South Asian perspective of endocrine surgical disease presentation and management. The readers will find some unique features relating to epidemiology, clinical manifestation and natural course of endocrine surgical diseases while the management remains almost same as in other parts of the world. Some of the differences observed in this part of the globe can be explained with socioeconomic situation and nutritional status of South Asian population. The textbook will find acceptance by Endocrine Surgery residents, postgraduate residents from diverse disciplines like General Surgery, Head and Neck Surgery, Surgical Oncology and Otolaryngology.

Prof. S K Mishra, MS, DNB, FAMS, FACS
Former Head, Department of Endocrine Surgery
Sanjay Gandhi Postgraduate Institute of Medical Sciences
Lucknow, India

FOREWORD BY DR. VITTAL

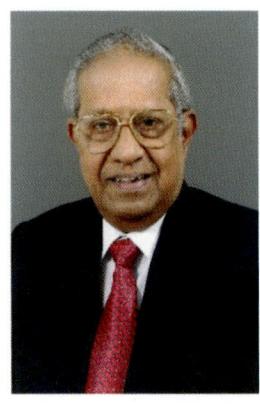

It gives me great pleasure to write a forward for this book authored by Dr. Anand Mishra and his erudite team. I am delighted that Dr. Anand Mishra (Professor, KGMU) a renowned Endocrine Surgeon hailing from Lucknow, India has taken the initiative to conceive a book titled *Endocrine Surgery: A South Asian Perspective* with him as a Chief Editor along with Dr. Amit Agarwal (Professor, SGPGIMS), Dr. Rajeev Parmeshwaran (NSU, Singapore) and Dr. Kul Ranjan Singh (Associate Professor, KGMU) as the other editors. With Endocrine Surgery getting recognition as a distinct specialty worldwide, this book will be an important and useful guide especially in the context of South Asia and South East Asia.

Dr. Anand Mishra and the other editors have to be congratulated for assembling authors from all over South and South East Asia and beyond to give the reader a flair of the disease patterns in this region. The multiple authors chosen are experts in their field with excellent academic background. I can say with certainty that having known most of them, the reader will benefit from their thorough knowledge and experience in the chapters authored by them. The standout feature of this book will be the differences highlighted in presentation and therapeutic approach of endocrine conditions between South and South East Asia and the West.

Endocrine Surgery as a distinct specialty took shape in the late 1970s and early 1980s. I am taken down memory lane when in 1983 a book on Surgical Endocrinology with Prof. R Sarathchandra and myself as Editors was published which was a multiauthor initiative as well. Advances in understanding of the disease, diagnostic modalities and therapeutic options have led to many textbooks of Endocrine Surgery being published over the years. However, as I mentioned earlier, this book gives the flavor of the endocrine disorders in South and South East Asia.

I would once again like to congratulate Dr. Anand Mishra and the entire team for their enthusiasm, commitment and hard work for bringing out this book, and I do hope it is in the bookshelf of all practicing Endocrine Surgeons and postgraduate students of Endocrine Surgery.

Prof. S Vittal
Padma Shri Awardee
Dr. B C Roy Awardee
Founder President, Indian Association of Endocrine Surgeons
Past President, Association of Surgeons of India
Past President and Past Trustee International
College of Surgeons, Indian Section

PREFACE

Some of the greatest names in the history of surgery who were general surgeons including Kocher, Halsted, Lahey, Mayo, Crile and Cope have left their mark on the development of endocrine surgery. Endocrine surgery was recognized as a separate subspeciality of general surgery in late 8th and 9th decade of last century. Endocrine surgeon requires not only technical expertise in the operating room but ensures proper preoperative preparation, postoperative care and long-term follow-up, and this requires a thorough understanding of physiology, embryology and pathology of the endocrine system. As endocrine surgery is a burgeoning specialty in Asian region edging its way out of infancy into adolescence and with growing recognition and maturation in last two decades, it was realized the scarcity of literature on various aspects of our own presentations. Most of the textbooks which are available here are by Western authors with little contribution from Asian clinicians. There is a clear requirement of a dedicated book which details the management of diseases of the thyroid, parathyroid and adrenal glands, as well as neuroendocrine tumors of the pancreas and GI tract for not only teaching, training and certification of trainee surgeons but for also practicing surgeons with interest in this specialty.

Having the distinction of becoming the first MCh, Endocrine Surgery in India and being involved in teaching, training of endocrine surgery for more than a decade and half, I have always felt a void for a reliable text of endocrine surgery that is in tune with the needs of south Asian subcontinent. And after many deliberations with seniors and colleagues, I decided to set the stage for compiling a text that would cover the specialty comprehensively and keep the south Asian focus at its core. The first edition of *Endocrine Surgery: A South Asian Perspective* is a concise and informative resource covering clinical features, diagnosis and treatment of diseases. This book departs from all other textbooks in respect of format, contents, flow charts and dedicated section titled "South Asian Perspective" highlighting our own presentation before conclusion.

We got on board distinguished experts from all the countries of the Asian subcontinent. Hence, the book stands out not only as a comprehensive guide but also as an updated compendium, keeping pace with ever-evolving knowledge and paraphernalia needed by the aspirants engaged in the pursuit of art of Endocrine Surgery. Endocrine Surgery is practiced not only by dedicated endocrine surgeons, but also by general surgeons, surgical oncologist and otolaryngologists. This book intends to fill the prevailing voids felt by all stake holders irrespective of their specialty and looks forward to become a reference textbook for trainees in India and all over world. The editorial board is immensely grateful to all the authors for their contribution to the making of this text and thanks the publishers for all their help at every stage of the publication.

Anand Kumar Mishra
Editor-in-chief
Professor and Head
Department of Endocrine Surgery
King George's Medical University, Lucknow
21st June 2021

ACKNOWLEDGMENTS

All the authors have done a tremendous job of writing the chapters very comprehensively in spite of having their involvement with duties in Covid pandemic. I profoundly feel indebted and grateful to all the contributing authors. I would like to thank my colleague and co-editor Kul Ranjan for providing rock solid support during the editorial journey. I would also like to thank my mentor and guiding force Amit Agrawal for his guidance and unconditional blessings. I acknowledge and thank the singular contribution of Dr. Rajeev for helping me in getting many lead authors on board.

This book would have not been possible without the collective support and blessing of my parents, elders of the family, colleagues, batchmates and friends. My late mother always inspired me to see the word differently, and father has always been supportive in all my academic endeavors. They both are my role models in life. I am blessed to have Anjana as my wife. She is always there as an angel when going gets tough. I appreciate her for continued care and support during this project. I owe a deep debt to God and bow before Him in reverence for bestowing on me a couple of jewels – son and daughter christened as Aditya and Gauri. Both helped me in finishing this project indirectly by asking the question on their holidays that "When your book will finish?" I also feel obliged to all my patients for giving me learning opportunities. For bestowing on me the creative imagination to write a book of this sort, I avowedly feel the benevolence of Almighty God incessantly. I pray to Him with all my sincerity at my command to continue his blessings as well.

I would like to thank Shivangi Pramanik and Himani Dwivedi for their tireless efforts, extension of deadline, constant reminders and for putting us through editorial process. Finally, I am immensely indebted to CRC Press of Taylor & Francis Group for bringing out this book.

Anand Kumar Mishra
Editor-in-chief
Professor and Head
Department of Endocrine Surgery
King George's Medical University, Lucknow
21st June 2021

ABOUT THE EDITORS

Dr. Anand Kumar Mishra, MBBS, MS, PDCC, MCh, FACS is Professor and Head, Department of Endocrine Surgery, King George's Medical University, Lucknow, India.

Dr. Amit Agarwal, MBBS, MS, FRCS is Professor and Head, Department of Endocrine Surgery, Sanjay Gandhi Post Graduate Institute of Medical Sciences, Lucknow, India.

Dr. Rajeev Parameswaran, BSc, MBBS, FRCS, MPhil, FRCS is Assistant Professor, Senior Consultant and Head, Division of Endocrine Surgery and Program Director, Surgery in General, National University Health System, Singapore.

Dr. Kul Ranjan Singh, MBBS, MS, MCh, FACS, FICS is Associate Professor, Department of Endocrine Surgery, King George's Medical University, Lucknow, India.

LIST OF CONTRIBUTORS

Deepak Thomas Abraham
Department of Endocrine Surgery
Christian Medical College
Vellore, India

Akshay Agarwal
Department of General Surgery
King George's Medical University
Lucknow, India

Amit Agarwal
Department of Endocrine Surgery
Sanjay Gandhi Post Graduate Institute of Medical Sciences
Lucknow, India

Gaurav Agarwal
Department of Endocrine Surgery
Sanjay Gandhi Post Graduate Institute of Medical Sciences
Lucknow, India

Preeti Agarwal
Department of Pathology
King George's Medical University
Lucknow, India

Mayur Agrawal
Department of Endocrinology
Sanjay Gandhi Post Graduate Institute of Medical Sciences
Lucknow, India

Kulbir Ahlawat
Medanta Division of Radiology and Nuclear Medicine
Medanta Medicity Hospital
Gurugram, India

Faraz Ahmad
Department of Surgery
King George's Medical University
Lucknow, India

Khalid Alhajri
Department of Surgery building
Riyadh, Kingdom of Saudi Arabia

Jyoti Arora
Medanta Division of Radiology and Nuclear Medicine
Medanta Medicity Hospital
Gurugram, India

Boon Huat Bay
Department of Anatomy
Yong Loo Lin School of Medicine
National University of Singapore
Singapore

Shivendu Bhardwaj
Department of Endocrinology
Sanjay Gandhi Post Graduate Institute of Medical Sciences
Lucknow, India

Sandeep Bhattacharya
Department of Anesthesia
King George's Medical University
Lucknow, India

Ahmet Çelik
Ege University Faculty of Medicine
Department of Pediatric Surgery
İzmir, Turkey

Muthukrishnan Chandrika
Department of Anatomy, Yong Loo Lin School of Medicine
National University of Singapore
Singapore

K.M.M. Vishvak Chanthar
Department of Endocrine surgery
Sanjay Gandhi Post Graduate Institute of Medical Sciences
Lucknow, India

David Ng Chee Eng
Department of Nuclear Medicine and Molecular Imaging
Singapore General Hospital and Duke-NUS Medical School
Singapore

Chintamani
Department of General Surgery
Vardhman Mahavir Medical College and Safdarjung Hospital
New Delhi, India

Chiaw-Ling Chng
Department of Endocrinology
Singapore General Hospital
Oculoplastic Department
Singapore National Eye Centre
Duke-NUS Medical School
Singapore

June Young Choi
Seoul National University Bundang Hospital
Seongnam-si, South Korea

S. Dhalapathy
Department of Endocrine Surgery
Madras Medical College
Chennai, India

S. Thameem Dheen
Department of Anatomy, Yong Loo Lin School of Medicine
National University of Singapore
Singapore

Emre Divarci
Ege University Faculty of Medicine
Department of Pediatric Surgery
İzmir, Turkey

Manjari Dwivedi
Department of Endocrinology and Diabetes
Medanta Hospital
Lucknow, India

Yogita Dwivedi
Department of Anesthesia
Government Medical College
Azamgarh, India

Loreno E. Enny
Department of Endocrine Surgery
King George's Medical University
Lucknow, India

Orkan Ergün
Ege University Faculty of Medicine
Department of Pediatric Surgery
İzmir, Turkey

Ranil Fernando
Faculty of Medicine,
University of Kelaniya
Sri Lanka

M K Garg
Department of Medicine and Endocrinology
All India Institute of Medical Sciences,
Jodhpur, India

Surabhi Garg
Department of Endocrine Surgery
King George's Medical University
Lucknow, India

Kushagra Gaurav
Department of General Surgery
King George's Medical University
Lucknow, India

Manisha Gupta
Department of Endocrinology
Regency Hospital Pvt. Ltd.
Kanpur, India

List of Contributors

Parul Gupta
Department of Endocrinology and Metabolism
All India Institute of Medical Sciences,
Jodhpur, India

Shardool Vikram Gupta
All India Institute of Medical Sciences
New Delhi, India

Manish Gutch
Department of Endocrinology and Diabetes
Medanta Hospital
Lucknow, India

Kelvin Loke Siu Hoong
Department of Nuclear Medicine and Molecular Imaging
Singapore General Hospital and Duke-NUS Medical School
Singapore

Hian Liang Huang
Department of Nuclear Medicine and Molecular Imaging
Singapore General Hospital and Duke-NUS Medical School
Singapore

Mayank Jain
Department of Surgical Disciplines
All India Institute of Medical Sciences
New Delhi, India

Krishnan Jayabharathi
Department of Anatomy, Yong Loo Lin School of Medicine
National University of Singapore
Singapore

Poongkodi Karunakaran
Government Mohan Kumaramangalam Medical College
SKS Hospital and Post Graduate Institute
Salem, India

Ali Korairi
Prince Sultan Military Medical City
Riyadh, Kingdom of Saudi Arabia

Asuri Krishna
Department of Surgical Disciplines
All India Institute of Medical Sciences
New Delhi, India

Chitresh Kumar
Department of Surgical Oncology
All India Institute of Medical Sciences
Bilaspur, India

Maghvendra Kumar
Department of Endocrinology and Diabetes
Medanta Hospital
Lucknow, India

Sanjeev Kumar
King George's Medical University
Lucknow, India

Subodh Kumar
Department of Surgical Disciplines
All India Institute of Medical Sciences
New Delhi, India

Sukriti Kumar
Department of Radiology
King George's Medical University
Lucknow, India

Shreyamsa M
Department of Endocrine Surgery
King George's Medical University
Lucknow, India

VNSSVAMS Mahalakshmi D
Department of Endocrine Surgery
Sanjay Gandhi Post Graduate Institute of Medical Sciences
Lucknow, India

Dhritiman Maitra
Department of Surgery
Medical College Kolkata
Kolkata, India

Özer Makay
Ege University Hospital
Department of General Surgery, Division of Endocrine Surgery
Izmir, Turkey

Linu Oommen Mathew
Lincoln General Hospital
Lincoln, United Kingdom

Sunnel Mattoo
Sanjay Gandhi Post Graduate Institute of Medical Sciences
Lucknow, India

Sabaretnam Mayilvaganan
Department of Endocrine Surgery
Sanjay Gandhi Post Graduate Institute of Medical Sciences
Lucknow, India

Chue Koy Min
Endocrine Surgery
National University Hospital
Singapore

Anand Kumar Mishra
Department of Endocrine Surgery
King George's Medical University
Lucknow, India

Madhukar Mittal
Department of Endocrinology and Metabolism
All India Institute of Medical Sciences
Jodhpur, India

Sasi Mouli
Department of Endocrine Surgery
King George's Medical University
Lucknow, India

Bhavya Naithani
Department of Plastic and Reconstructive Surgery
King George's Medical University
Lucknow, India

Murat Ozdemir
Ege University Hospital
Department of General Surgery, Division of Endocrine Surgery
Izmir, Turkey

Rajeev Parameswaran
National University Hospital Singapore
National Cancer Institute of Singapore
Alexandra Hospital
Singapore

M J Paul
Department of Endocrine Surgery
Christian Medical College
Vellore, India

PV Pradeep
Baby Memorial Hospital
Kozhikode, India

Roma Pradhan
Department of Endocrine Surgery
RML Institute of Medical Sciences
Lucknow, India

Troy H Puar
Changi General Hospital
Singapore

Puneet
Institute of Medical Sciences
Banaras Hindu University
Varanasi, India

Mithun Raam
Department of General Surgery
Department of Endocrine Surgery
Christian Medical College
Vellore, India

Rahul
Department of Surgical Gastroenterology
Sanjay Gandhi Post Graduate Institute of Medical Sciences
Lucknow, India

Sendhil Rajan
Department of Surgery
Aberdeen Royal Infirmary
Aberdeen, United Kingdom

Pooja Ramakant
Department of Endocrine Surgery
King George's Medical University
Lucknow, India

Chanchal Rana
Department of Pathology
King George's Medical University
Lucknow, India

Himagirish K Rao
Department of Surgery
St. John's Medical College Hospital
Bengaluru, India

Smitha Rao
Tata Memorial Hospital
Mumbai, India

Bharadhwaj Ravindhran
Guy's Hospital
London, United Kingdom

Sheeja Sainulabdeen
Department of Pathology
Medical College Kottayam
Kerala, India

Kul Ranjan Singh
Department of Endocrine Surgery
King George's Medical University
Lucknow, India

Alka Ashmita Singhal
Medanta Division of Radilogy and Nuclear Medicine
Medanta Medicity Hospital
Gurugram, India

Dinesh Kumar Srinivasan
Department of Anatomy, Yong Loo Lin School of Medicine
National University of Singapore
Singapore

Anurag Srivastava
Department of Surgical Disciplines
All India Institute of Medical Sciences
New Delhi, India

Divya Srivastava
Department of Anesthesia
Sanjay Gandhi Post Graduate Institute of Medical Sciences
Lucknow, India

Marya Al Suhaibani
Princess Nourah bint Abdulrahman University
Riyadh, Kingdom of Saudi Arabia

Soe Tin
University of Medicine 1, Yangon
Victoria Hospital
Yangon, Myanmar

Reetu Verma
Department of Anesthesia
King George's Medical University
Lucknow, India

Shivendra Verma
Department of Medicine
GSVM Medical College
Kanpur, India

Subhash Yadav
Department of Endocrinology
Sanjay Gandhi Post Graduate Institute of Medical Sciences
Lucknow, India

Lee Kai Yin
Endocrine Surgery
National University Hospital
Singapore

Hyeong Won Yu
Division of Endocrine Surgery
Department of Surgery
Seoul National University Bundang Hospital
Seongnam-si, South Korea

Sumbul Zaheer
Department of Nuclear Medicine and Molecular Imaging
Singapore General Hospital and Duke-NUS Medical School
Singapore

Meifen Zhang
Department of Endocrinology
Changi General Hospital
Singapore

1

HISTORY OF THYROID SURGERY

Surabhi Garg, Shreyamsa M and Anand Kumar Mishra

The text of this chapter is available online at www.routledge.com/9781032136509.

2

THYROID PHYSIOLOGY

Shivendu Bhardwaj and Subhash Yadav

Introduction

The thyroid gland produces two hormones, thyroxine (T4) and tri-iodothyronine (T3). Thyroid hormones perform several important roles in growth, differentiation and metabolism. Several thyroid disorders are associated with hormone excess (hyperthyroidism) and hormone deficiency (hypothyroidism) involving multiple organ systems. Understanding of thyroid physiology and testing is important for diagnosis and management of thyroid disorders.

Basic of thyroid anatomy and development

The thyroid gland derives its name from the Greek word *thyreos* meaning shield. It consists of two lateral lobes connected by an isthmus. It is located anterior to the trachea between the cricoid cartilage and the suprasternal notch. The normal thyroid is 12–20 g in weight, highly vascular and soft in consistency. Each lobe is approximately 4 cm in length, 2 cm in width and 2–3 cm in thickness. The isthmus measures about 2 cm in width, 2 cm in height and 2–6 mm in thickness. Four parathyroid glands are located posterior to each pole of the thyroid. The recurrent laryngeal nerves traverse the lateral borders of the thyroid gland and it is important to identify it during thyroid surgery to avoid injury and vocal cord paralysis (1, 2).

The thyroid gland develops from the floor of the primitive pharynx during the third week of gestation. The developing gland migrates along the thyroglossal duct to reach its final location in the neck. The development of thyroid explains the rare ectopic location of thyroid tissue at the base of the tongue (lingual thyroid) as well as the occurrence of thyroglossal duct cysts along this developmental tract. The thyroid may descend into mediastinum leading to its retrosternal location (1).

The gland produces thyroid hormones and calcitonin in two distinct cell types. The thyroid follicle cells, the most numerous cell population in the gland, form the thyroid follicles, spherical structures serving as storage and controlled release of thyroid hormones. The C cells are scattered in the interfollicular space, mostly in a parafollicular position. The two diverse cell types, responsible for the dual endocrine function of the gland, originate from two different embryological structures: the thyroid anlage is the site of origin of the thyroid follicular cells (TFCs) whereas the ultimobranchial bodies are the source of C cells. The ultimobranchial bodies are a pair of transient embryonic structures derived from the fourth pharyngeal pouch and located symmetrically on the sides of the developing neck. The C-cell precursors migrate from the neural crest bilaterally to the fourth pharyngeal pouches and become localized in the ultimobranchial bodies. Thyroid hormone synthesis normally begins at about 11 weeks of gestation. Calcitonin plays a minimal role in calcium homeostasis in humans, but the C cells are important because of their involvement in medullary thyroid cancer (3, 4).

Molecular aspect of thyroid development

During embryogenesis, the development of thyroid gland depends on coordinated expression of several developmental transcription factors. Thyroid transcription factor-1 (TTF-1), TTF-2, NKX2-1 and paired homeobox-8 (PAX-8) are the most important transcription factors involved. In combination, they dictate thyroid cell development and the induction of thyroid-specific genes such as thyroglobulin (Tg), thyroid peroxidase (TPO), the sodium iodide symporter (Na^+/I^-, NIS) and the thyroid-stimulating hormone receptor (TSH-R). Mutations in these developmental transcription factors or their downstream target genes are rare causes of thyroid agenesis or dyshormonogenesis. Transplacental passage of maternal thyroid hormone occurs before the fetal thyroid gland begins to function and provides significant hormone support to a fetus with congenital hypothyroidism (5–7).

Vascular supply of thyroid gland

The thyroid is supplied by superior and inferior thyroid arteries. Superior, middle and inferior thyroid veins form the venous system of thyroid gland (1).

Histology of thyroid gland

The thyroid gland is divided into lobules; each lobule consists of numerous spherical follicles composed of thyroid follicular cells that surround secreted colloid, a proteinaceous fluid containing large amounts of thyroglobulin, the protein precursor of thyroid hormones. The thyroid follicular cells are polarized—the basolateral surface is opposing to the bloodstream and an apical surface faces the follicular lumen (4).

Regulation of thyroid axis

Accurate regulation of thyroid hormones (triiodothyronine [T3] and thyroxine [T4]) is essential as they play a pivotal role in various metabolic process, thermogenesis, physical and mental development. TSH is the prime stimulator of thyroid hormones and the most useful physiologic marker of thyroid axis. The thyroid axis is the classic example of a hormone feedback cycle. TSH is in turn under stimulatory influence of hypothalamic hormone TRH, inhibitory influence of neurotransmitters, dopamine and somatostatin and negative feedback by thyroid hormones (T3 and T4). The dose-dependent and time-varying interplay among these regulates 24-hour TSH secretory patterns (Figure 2.1).

Thyrotropin-releasing hormone (TRH)

TRH is a tripeptide hormone secreted by paraventricular cells of hypothalamus. TRH acts via its G protein-coupled receptor on

Thyroid Physiology

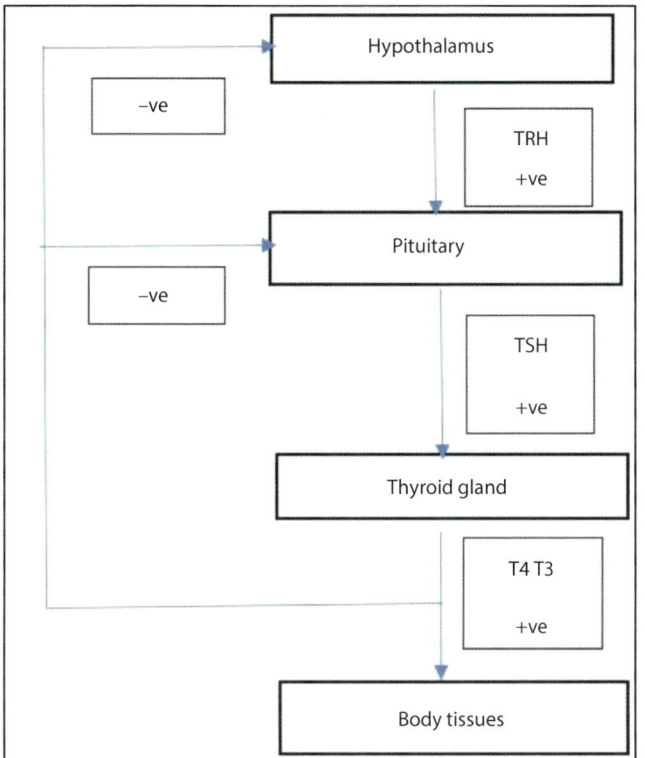

FIGURE 2.1 Hypothalamic-pituitary-thyroid axis.

thyrotropes, resulting in increase in cAMP production and subsequent TSH secretion. Other hormone signals, including dopamine, somatostatin and leptin, also modulate TSH secretion, thus having a role in central regulation of thyroid axis (8).

Thyroid-stimulating hormone (TSH)

TSH is secreted by the thyrotrope cells of the anterior pituitary. TSH is a 31-kDa hormone composed of α and β subunits; the α subunit is common to the other glycoprotein hormones (luteinizing hormone, follicle-stimulating hormone, human chorionic gonadotropin [hCG]), whereas the TSH β subunit is unique to TSH (9).

TSH is the major regulator of thyroid function. TSH mediates its effect on thyroid proliferation, differentiation and function through cAMP-mediated pathway via GTP-binding protein Gsa (10). TSH-like another pituitary hormone is secreted in pulsatile manner and exhibits diurnal variation with the highest levels at night. TSH has a long half-life of 50 min resulting in only modest excursions in TSH levels throughout the day. This property makes single measurement of TSH useful to assess adequate circulating levels (9).

Thyroid hormone synthesis, metabolism and action

Thyroid hormones are derived from thyroglobulin (Tg), and synthesis mainly involves three steps: iodide uptake, iodide oxidation and organification and hormone secretion (Figure 2.2).

Iodide uptake

Iodine plays a critical role in thyroid hormone synthesis. Adequate iodine levels are required to maintain sufficient levels of thyroid hormones. Iodine uptake occurs via sodium/iodide transporter (NIS), located on the basolateral surface of thyroid follicle against electrochemical gradient into thyroid follicles. NIS belongs to solute family carrier 5A (SLC5A). NIS is also present in low levels in salivary glands, gastric mucosa, lactating breasts and placenta. The energy required is provided by ouabain-sensitive Na/K-ATPase. From the cells, iodide is passively transported into

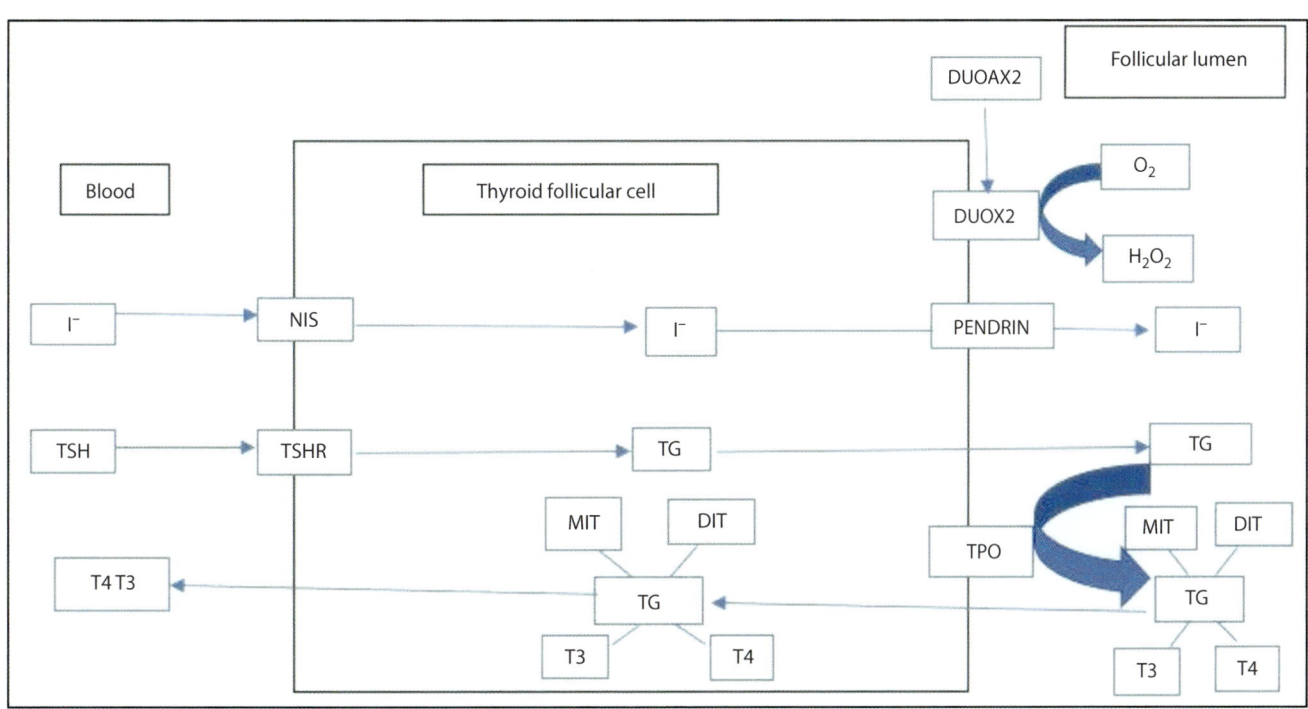

FIGURE 2.2 Thyroid hormone synthesis.

the lumen by a specialized channel present on apical surface of thyroid follicles (pendrin). Mutation in NIS and pendrin are rare causes of congenital hypothyroidism. Pendrin mutation is known to cause autosomal recessive disorder, Pendred syndrome characterized by defective organification, sensorineural deafness and goiter (10).

The iodide uptake process is a highly regulated process. TSH positively regulates iodine uptake mediated by sodium/iodide transporter via cAMP pathway. Dietary iodine intake plays a vital role in expression of NIS transporter with low iodine levels associated upregulation of NIS and subsequent increase uptake, and vice versa. High iodide levels can acutely block organification of iodide via Wolff-Chaikoff effect. Several in vivo and in vitro studies have shown that decreased expression of NIS as the underlying mechanism for this effect (11).

Organification and coupling

Organification is the process of oxidation of iodide and incorporation of resulting intermediate into the hormonally inactive iodotyrosines, monoiodotyrosine (MIT) and diiodotyrosine (DIT). At the apical surface of the thyrocyte, the enzymes thyroperoxidase (TPO) and hydrogen peroxide oxidize iodide and attach it to tyrosyl residues on thyroglobulin to produce MIT and DIT. Hydrogen peroxide required is generated by the calcium-dependent DUOX1 and DUOX2. TPO then catalyzes the coupling of the phenyl groups of the iodotyrosines through a diether bridge to form the thyroid hormones. Fusion of two DIT molecules produces T4, and fusion of MIT and DIT produces T3. Iodine comprises 65 and 59% of the weights of T4 and T3, respectively (12, 13).

In the thyroid, mature thyroglobulin (Tg), containing 0.1–1.0% of its weight as iodine, is stored extracellularly in the luminal colloid of the thyroid follicle. For release of thyroid hormones, first step is endocytosis of the colloid from the luminal colloid via macropinocytosis and micropinocytosis, this is a TSH-dependent process. After endocytosis, endosomal and lysosomal proteases digest Tg and release T4 and T3 into the circulation. Uncoupled MIT and DIT are deiodinated by enzyme dehalogenase, thereby recycling iodide not converted into thyroid hormones (Table 2.1) (14, 15).

Thyroid hormone transport and metabolism

Serum-binding proteins

Thyroid hormones circulate in blood mostly bound to a set of plasma proteins with varying affinity and concentration. The major thyroid hormone proteins are thyroxine-binding globulin (TBG), transthyretin (also called thyroxine-binding prealbumin TBPA) and albumin. 99.98% T4 and 99.7% T3 are present in bound form. Normally about 70% of T4 is bound to TBG, 10–20% to albumin and remainder to transthyretin. The plasma protein binding increases pool of hormone concentration and delay its clearance. T3 is less tightly bound to plasma proteins as compared to T4. Although the majority of thyroid hormone are protein bound, the various hormone actions, including thyroid axis regulation, is a function of free hormone concentration. Minor of circulating T4 is bound to lipoproteins although its significance (16, 17).

Thyroxine-binding globulin

TBG is a single polypeptide chain globulin, with a molecular weight of about 54 kDa encoded by a gene located on X-chromosome. Although its concentration is significantly lower than albumin and transthyretin, the majority of thyroid hormone is bound to it because of its high affinity for them. The glycosylation of TBG influences its clearance from the plasma and its behavior during isoelectric focusing.

Abnormalities in TBG can be inherited or acquired. Congenital X-linked deficiency of TBG has been described, which can be partial or complete. It is associated with extremely low levels of total T4 and T3. However, it is important to recognize this condition as it is associated with normal TSH and free hormone levels, and patient is euthyroid. Various physiological, pathological condition and medication are associated with acquired abnormalities in TBG. Acquired causes of excess TBG is the commonest cause of euthyroid hyperthyroxinemia (biochemical hyperthyroxinemia without thyrotoxicosis). Pregnancy or estrogen-containing OCPs are associated with increased hepatic production of TB leading to increase in total T4 and T3 levels. Diagnosis of euthyroid hyperthyroxinemia can be made in presence of normal levels of TSH and unbound hormones. Androgen, anabolic steroids, glucocorticoids, L-asparaginase and thyroid hormone excess are associated with decreased TBG levels (Table 2.2) (17).

Albumin

Albumin is 66-kDa protein with high capacity, low binding affinity for thyroid hormones.

Albumin normally carries 10–20% of circulating T4. Euthyroid hyperthyroxinemia can result from an inherent variant albumin associated with increased affinity for T4 (albumin concentration remains unchanged). In this autosomal dominant disorder known as familial dysalbuminemic hyperthyroxinemia, total T4

TABLE 2.1: Thyroid Hormone Properties

Hormone Property	T4	T3
Serum concentration		
Total concentration	8 µg/dl	0.14 µg/dl
Fraction of total hormone in unbound form	0.02%	0.3%
Serum half-life (day)	7	2
Fraction directly from thyroid (%)	100	20
Production rate, including peripheral conversion (µg/day)	90	32
Relative metabolic potency	0.3	1
Intracellular concentration (%)	20	70

TABLE 2.2: Acquired Causes of Increase in TBG Concentration

Physiologic
Pregnancy
New born

Non-thyroidal illness
Liver disease
Acute intermittent porphyria
Hydatidiform mole
Lymphosarcoma

Drug induced
Oral contraceptive pills
Exogenous estrogen
Clofibrate
5-Fluorouracil
Heroin and methadone

levels are increased with normal total T3, unbound T3 and T4, TSH levels are normal (16).

Transthyretin
Transthyretin (previously known as prealbumin) is a 55-kDa protein synthesized by liver.

Inherent variant of transthyretin with increased affinity for T4 is associated with mild increase in total T4 levels (16).

Iodotyrosines deiodination
Major product of the thyroid gland is thyroxine (T4) that is secreted at a rate of 10-fold that of T3. T4 is a prohormone and must be converted peripherally to T3 to mediate its action in various tissues in the body. Deiodinase enzymes take part in conversion of T4–T3. There are three types of deiodinase enzymes: D1, D2 and D3. D1 is the major source of circulating T3, while D2 provides nuclear receptor bound hormone. D3 selenodeiodinases inactivates T3 and T4 by removal of inner ring iodine. D3 is an important source of reverse T3 (rT3).

All three deiodinase have certain features in common. One is that all are integral membrane proteins, although are expressed in different locations. D1 is found in the plasma membrane and D2 in the endoplasmic reticulum (both having their active centers in the cytosol, thus allowing access to cytosolic thiol cofactors). Although precise location of D3 is more difficult to discern, with the likely location being the plasma membrane (18–20).

Selenium is essential for all the three deiodinases. Defects in SECISBP2, which is required for the synthesis of selenoproteins, have been associated with abnormal thyroid hormone metabolism (elevated T4, low T3, elevated rT3 and slightly elevated TSH). However, the benefit of selenium is not known (Figure 2.3) (20).

Thyroid hormone action

Thyroid hormone transporters
Genomic effects of thyroid hormones are mediated via nuclear receptors. Translocation of hormones across plasma membrane occurs by passive diffusion and via specific transporters such as monocarboxylate transporter (MCT 8), MCT 10 and organic anion transporting protein 1C1 (OATP1C1) (21).

MCT8 is expressed in the hypothalamus, a major site of integration of thyroid hormone feedback and gene regulation. Inactivating mutations of MCT8 transporter is associated with Allan-Herndon-Dudley syndrome, a severe form of X-linked mental retardation characterized by truncal hypotonia, poor head control and later spasticity. Thyroid profiles reveal elevated T3, low T4 and rT3, slightly elevated TSH (20).

Thyroid nuclear receptors
Many of the actions of thyroid hormones are mediated by family of high nuclear receptors (TRs). TRs belong to large family of nuclear receptors, including steroid hormones, vitamin derivatives such as vitamin D, retinoic acid, fatty acid, cholesterol metabolites and xenobiotics (22).

TRα and TRβ are the two TR genes in variable expression in different tissues. TRα has one T3-binding splice product TRα1 and two non-T3-binding slice products TRα2 and TRα3. TRα1 is predominantly expressed in brain, heart and skeletal muscles. TRβ has three T3-binding splice products—TRβ1, TRβ2 and TRβ3. TRβ1 is widely expressed, TRβ2 is primarily expressed in brain, retina and inner ear. TRβ3 is expressed in kidney, liver and lung. Various factors influence of thyroid hormone receptors, including local ligand availability, thyroid hormone transporters such as monocarboxylate transporter 8, relative expression of TR isoforms, presence of nuclear receptor coactivators and

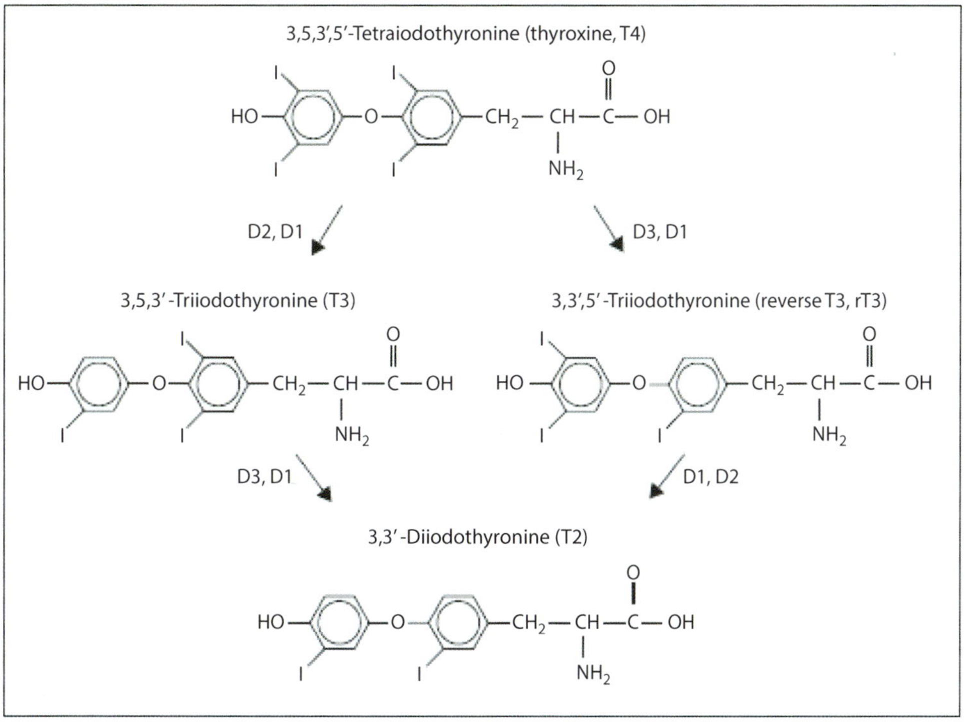

FIGURE 2.3 Thyroid hormone deiodination.

corepressors and finally thyroid response elements (TREs). Certain non-genomic actions are performed by thyroid hormone not requiring direct involvement of TR nuclear receptors. Membrane receptors like specific integrin αv/β3 for thyroid hormone have been identified at multiple sites, including blood vessels and heart (Figure 2.4) (20).

TRs likely other nuclear receptors have central DNA-binding domain and ligand-binding domain. TR recognizes specific sequence AGGTCA sequence (thyroid response elements) and binds to it as a monomer. This sequence also serves as a half-site for TR homodimers as well as heterodimers with retinoid X receptor (RXR). Both thyroid hormones (T3 and T4) have a similar affinity for TRα and TRβ receptors. Although T4 concentration is more than T3, T3 has more affinity than T4 for TRs. Thyroid hormones act as a switch between repressed and activated states on TRE-containing target gene. Thus, genes are actively repressed in the absence of thyroid hormones. Corepressors bind to C-terminal ligand-binding domain to silence the genes in the absence of thyroid hormones. Therefore, the repressive actions of the unliganded receptor have a greater physiologic action than having no receptor at all (20).

Thyroid hormone binding induces a conformational change that destabilizes corepressor binding and that favors binding of transcriptional coactivators. Apart from upregulation of genes, thyroid hormones also downregulate numerous genes. The most important physiological effect is the negative regulation of thyroid axis via suppression of pituitary TSH gene expression (22).

Thyroid function

Thyroid hormones are key regulators of metabolism and development. Thyroid hormones have various pleiotropic effects in many different organs (23).

Thyroid hormones and lipid metabolism

Thyroid hormones have stimulatory effects on adipogenesis, lipogenesis and lipolysis. These actions depend on expression of specific thyroid receptors (TRs) isoform and local activity of deiodinase. Thyroid receptor α 1 (TRα1) isoform plays an important role in adipogenesis. Thyroid hormones stimulate adipogenesis via regulation of key lipogenic genes. Although exact mechanism for lipolysis stimulation not known, certainly cross talk between thyroid hormones and catecholamines play a role (24).

Thyroid hormones and bone

Thyroid hormones regulate skeletal development, peak bone mass and adult bone remodeling. The majority of actions are mediated by thyroid receptor α (TRα). Thyroid hormone actions result in anabolic effects during childhood and catabolic effects in adulthood. Euthyroid status is essential for normal bone development

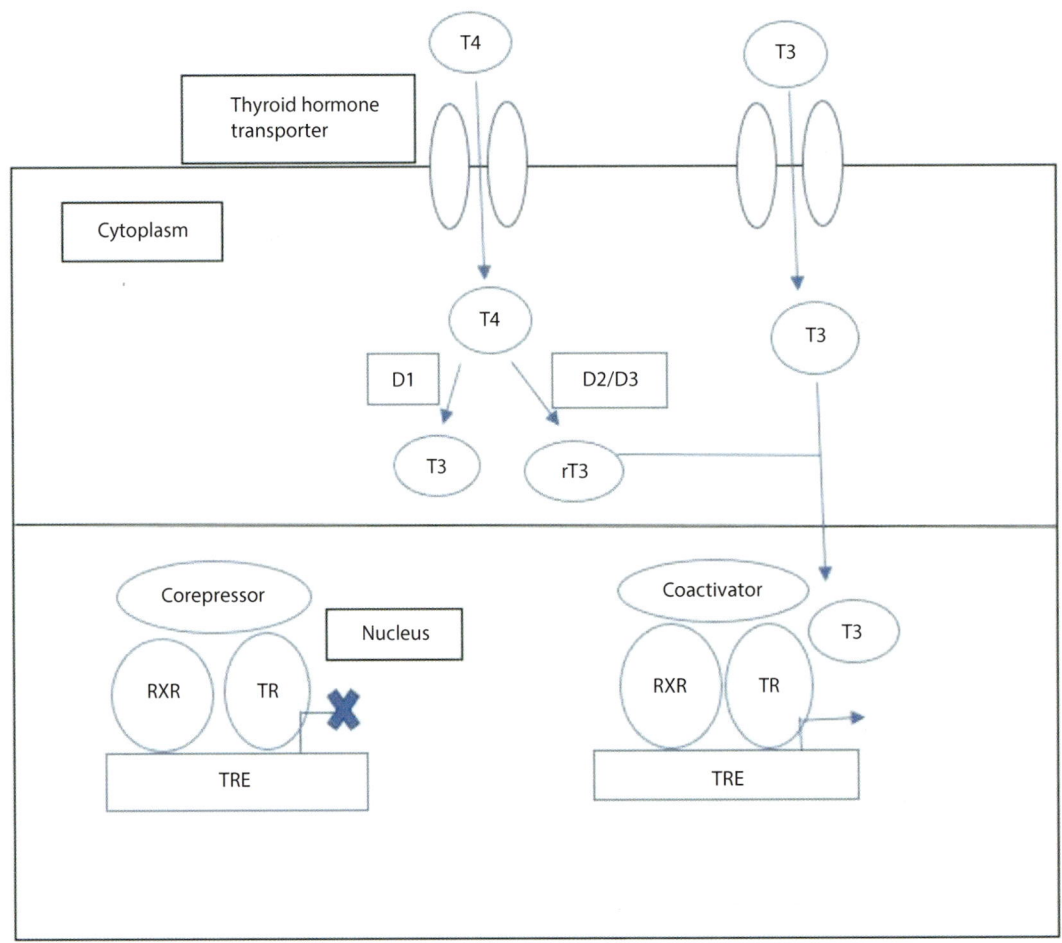

FIGURE 2.4 Thyroid hormone action.

Thyroid Physiology

and maintenance. Type 2 deiodinase controls local supply of thyroid hormones.

In children, hypothyroidism is associated with linear growth cessation, delayed bone age and epiphyseal dysgenesis. In contrast, childhood thyrotoxicosis results in premature fusion of the growth plates and short stature. In adults, thyrotoxicosis leads to increased bone turnover resulting in osteoporosis and an increased risk of fragility fracture, whereas, hypothyroidism is associated with reduced bone turnover and prolongation of remodeling cycle. Abnormal thyroid status during childhood disrupts bone maturation and linear growth, while in adulthood it results in altered bone remodeling and an increased risk of fracture (25, 26).

Thyroid and basal metabolic rate

Thyroid hormones play a determinant role in overall energy expenditure and basal metabolic rate (resting energy expenditure). All components of total energy expenditure (resting, exercise and non-exercise-related thermogenesis and adaptive thermogenesis) are modulated by thyroid hormones. Thyroid hormones regulate resting energy expenditure by regulating various metabolic cycles such as lipogenesis/lipolysis, glycogenolysis/gluconeogenesis and, thus, promoting ATP utilization. Adaptive thermogenesis is regulated by thyroid hormones via upregulation of uncoupling proteins (UCP-1), predominantly expressed in brown and beige fat. Mostly of the actions are permissive. Local modulation of thyroid signaling plays a major role rather than change in concentration of circulating hormone levels.

Dramatic effects of thyroid dysfunction on energy expenditure are well known, as seen in state of thyroid hormone excess (hyperthyroidism) or deficiency (hypothyroidism). Heat intolerance and cold intolerance are hallmark features of hyperthyroidism and hypothyroidism, respectively (8, 27, 28).

Thyroid and skeletal muscle

Thyroid hormone plays a vital role in skeletal muscle contractility, regeneration, metabolism and glucose disposal. Thyroid hormone stimulates transition to fast-twitch fibers and as well as transition to a faster myosin heavy chain (MHC) form. Skeletal muscle plays a major role in glucose disposal and muscle GLUT-4 expression is T3 dependent. D2 deiodinase plays a crucial role in local availability of T3 (29, 30).

Thyroid and carbohydrate metabolism

Thyroid hormone effects on skeletal muscle, liver, white adipose tissue and pancreas influence plasma glucose levels, insulin sensitivity and carbohydrate metabolism. Key rate-limiting enzyme, phosphoenolpyruvate carboxykinase (PEPCK) involved in hepatic gluconeogenesis, is known to be regulated by TRβ (8).

Thyroid disease has a well-documented effect on carbohydrate metabolism. In patients with thyrotoxicosis, there is increased hepatic gluconeogenesis with increased circulating free fatty acids and enhanced fatty acid uptake in muscle contributing to a state of insulin resistance and hyperglycemia. Decreased glucose uptake in muscle has been observed in animal models of hypothyroidism (31).

Thyroid physiology during pregnancy

Normal pregnancy is associated with complex changes in thyroid physiology. Various factors contribute to these changes: pregnancy being a high estrogen state is associated with increased hepatic TBG synthesis and prolongation of TBG half-life owing to estrogen-induced sialylation. This contributes to an elevation of total T4 and total T3 levels during early gestation. Levels are stabilized around mid-gestation and are maintained until term.

Serum hCG levels rise during the early gestation, with peak at 10 weeks and plateau by 20 weeks. Serum hCG shares similarities with alpha subunit of TSH. Rise in serum hCG levels is associated with reciprocal fall in TSH. Conversely, there is a positive relationship with hCG levels and free thyroxine (FT4) during early gestation. hCG-induced changes can result in transient state of thyrotoxicosis, gestational transient thyrotoxicosis. Supportive treatment is required for this condition. Graves needs to distinguish from this condition as treatment differs.

Maternal glomerular filtration rate increases in pregnancy resulting in increased renal clearance of iodide.

Later in gestation, transplacental passage of iodide to the fetus and placental metabolism of iodothyronines further contributes to relative maternal iodine deprivation. Because of the increased iodine demands in pregnancy, all pregnant women should ingest a minimum of 250 μg/day daily. Normative values of thyroid function values differ in healthy pregnant women compared to nonpregnant women. Because of this, trimester-specific reference values should use for assessment of thyroid status (32, 33).

Laboratory evaluation

Thyroid disorders are common in our population and clinicians often deal with these disorders in their routine practice. Assessment of thyroid disorders includes test for assessment of thyroid function, tests for etiology for thyroid disorders, uptake studies and imaging modalities.

Test for assessment of thyroid function

TSH is the most sensitive marker of thyroid gland. TSH follows a log-linear relationship with thyroid hormone (T4 and T3), such that a small changes in thyroid hormones results in a large change in TSH levels. A logical approach is to first measure TSH levels for assessment of suspected thyroid disease before proceeding for further tests. Highly specific and sensitive immunochemiluminometric assays (ICMAs) are available for TSH assessment. A normal TSH values indicates a normal functioning thyroid gland with few exceptions. Certain thyroid conditions such as central hypothyroidism, TSH-secreting pituitary adenomas, resistance to thyroid hormones and presence of heterophile antibodies can have normal TSH values, despite the presence of thyroid dysfunction.

The presence of abnormal elevated or suppressed levels of TSH points toward thyroid gland dysfunction. Further assessment requires measurement of thyroid hormones (T4 and T3) to diagnose hyperthyroidism or hypothyroidism. Both total or unbound thyroid hormone concentration can be measured. Total T4 and T3 being protein bound, levels can be affected by various factors such as illnesses, medications, genetic factors. One should be aware about such factors and should assess fT4 and fT3 levels if any of these factors are present. Free hormones levels can be measured by ultracentrifugation or equilibrium dialysis. Variability in accuracy of assays for free hormone measured should be kept in mind (Table 2.3) (2, 34).

One should be cautious while interpretation of thyroid tests during illness/in hospitalized patients. TSH levels could be low during illness or elevated in recovery phase despite normal functioning thyroid (non-thyroid illness/sick euthyroid syndrome).

TABLE 2.3: Interpretations of Thyroid Function Tests

TSH Levels	T4 and T3 Levels	Diagnosis
↔	↔	Euthyroidism
↑	↔	Subclinical hypothyroidism
↑	↓	Overt hypothyroidism
↓	↔	Subclinical hyperthyroidism
↓	↑	Overt hyperthyroidism

Keeping this in mind, thyroid test should be ordered in hospitalized patients only when suspicion is high.

Tests to determine the etiology of thyroid dysfunction

Autoimmune thyroid disorders (Hashimoto's thyroiditis, Graves' disease) are common causes of thyroid dysfunction. Diagnosis of these disorders can be confirmed by the presence of various autoantibodies. Three main thyroid autoantibodies can be measured: anti-TPO (tissue peroxidase, anti-Tg (thyroglobulin) and anti-TSHR antibodies.

TPO antibodies are commonly used for diagnosis of autoimmune thyroid disorders. ELISA assays are available for the measurement. Almost all patients with autoimmune hypothyroidism and up to 80% of those with Graves' disease have TPO antibodies. The presence in euthyroid individuals confers the risk of autoimmune thyroid disease in future.

Anti-TSH receptor (anti-TSHR) antibodies are present in 90% of the patients with Graves' disease and 10% of those with autoimmune hypothyroidism. Radioimmunoassay (commonly used) and bioassay are available for estimation. Remission of Graves' disease can be predicted by disappearance of anti-TSHR antibodies at the end of the antithyroid treatment. They can be used for prediction of neonatal thyrotoxicosis in a woman known to have Graves' disease and distinguish postpartum thyroiditis from Graves' disease in postpartum thyrotoxicosis. Serum Tg levels are increased in all types of thyrotoxicosis except in thyrotoxicosis factitia. The main role for Tg measurement is in the follow-up of thyroid cancer patients (35, 36).

Thyroid ultrasound

Thyroid ultrasound is easily available, noninvasive and cost-effective tool for assessment of thyroid enlargement and thyroid nodules. The main disadvantage is that it is operator dependent. Thyroid ultrasound assessment of thyroid nodule feature can help in stratification of nodules in terms of risk of malignancy and need for fine needle aspiration biopsy (37).

Radioiodine uptake studies

Radioiodine uptake scan is a functional scan of thyroid gland utilizing its ability of iodine concentration. Normal thyroid uptake among normal population varies according to iodine intake. Main utility is to differentiate hot and cold nodules during assessment of a nodular thyroid lesion, hot nodules are rare malignant. Thyroid scan can help to distinguish Graves' disease (increased uptake) from subacute thyroiditis (decreased uptake) in the case of acute onset thyrotoxicosis. Various radioiodine tracers can be used for treatment in case of Graves' disease and thyroid malignancy (38, 39).

Conclusion

The abovementioned knowledge of thyroid physiology and function will help to have a better understanding of thyroid disorders and their clinical manifestations. Interpretation of thyroid function test should be done keeping in mind changes in physiology in various thyroid disorders. Ultrasound is inexpensive noninvasive modality for assessment of thyroid nodules.

References

1. Ellis H. Anatomy of the thyroid and parathyroid glands. Surgery. 2007;25(11):467–468.
2. Larry Jameson J, Fauci AS, Kasper DL, Hauser SL, Longo JL DL. Harrison's Principles of Internal Medicine, 20e | AccessMedicine | McGraw-Hill Medical [Internet]. [cited 2020 Jul 24]. Available from: https://accessmedicine.mhmedical.com/book.aspx?bookid=2129
3. Le Douarin N, Fontaine J, Le Lièvre C. New studies on the neural crest origin of the avian ultimobranchial glandular cells–interspecific combinations and cytochemical characterization of C cells based on the uptake of biogenic amine precursors. Histochemistry. 1974 Mar;38(4):297–305.
4. Bedford FK, Ashworth A, Enver T, Wiedemann LM. HEX: a novel homeobox gene expressed during haematopoiesis and conserved between mouse and human. Nucleic Acids Res. 1993 Mar;21(5):1245–1249.
5. Civitareale D, Lonigro R, Sinclair AJ, Di Lauro R. A thyroid-specific nuclear protein essential for tissue-specific expression of the thyroglobulin promoter. EMBO J. 1989;8(9):2537–2542.
6. Bingle CD. Thyroid transcription factor-1. Int J Biochem Cell Biol. 1997;29(12):1471–1473.
7. Guazzi S, Lonigro R, Pintonello L, Boncinelli E, Di Lauro R, Mavilio F. The thyroid transcription factor-1 gene is a candidate target for regulation by Hox proteins. EMBO J [Internet]. 1994 Jul 15 [cited 2020 Jul 24];13(14):3339–3347. Available from: http://www.ncbi.nlm.nih.gov/pubmed/7913891
8. Mullur R, Liu YY, Brent GA. Thyroid hormone regulation of metabolism. Physiol Rev. 2014;94(2):355–382.
9. Jameson LJ. Harrison's Principles of Internal Medicine. 12th ed. (Vol.1 & Vol.2). In: J. Larry Jameson, A. S. Fauci, D. L. Kasper, S. L. Hauser, D. L. Longo, J. Loscalzo. Google Books. 2018.
10. Bizhanova A, Kopp P. Minireview: the sodium-iodide symporter NIS and pendrin in iodide homeostasis of the thyroid. Endocrinology. 2009;150(3):1084–1090.
11. Eng PHK, Cardona GR, Fang SL, Previti M, Alex S, Carrasco N, et al. Escape from the acute Wolff-Chaikoff effect is associated with a decrease in thyroid sodium/iodide symporter messenger ribonucleic acid and protein. Endocrinology [Internet]. 1999 [cited 2020 Jul 26];140(8):3404–3410. Available from: https://pubmed.ncbi.nlm.nih.gov/10433193/
12. Rosenberg IN, Athans JC, Behar A. Effect of thyrotropin on the release of iodide from the thyroid. Endocrinology [Internet]. 1960 Feb [cited 2020 Jul 26];66:185–199. Available from: http://www.ncbi.nlm.nih.gov/pubmed/14438952
13. Hildebrandt JD, Scranton JR, Halmi NS. Intrathyroidally generated iodide: its measurement and origins. Endocrinology [Internet]. 1979 [cited 2020 Jul 26];105(3):618–626. Available from: https://pubmed.ncbi.nlm.nih.gov/223828/
14. Rosenberg IN, Athans JC, Ahn CS, Behar A. Thyrotropin-induced release of iodide from the thyroid. Endocrinology [Internet]. 1961 [cited 2020 Jul 26];69:438–455. Available from: https://pubmed.ncbi.nlm.nih.gov/13743391/
15. Nagataki S, Uchimura H, Masuyama Y, Nakao K. Thyrotropin and thyroidal peroxidase activity. Endocrinology [Internet]. 1973 Feb [cited 2020 Jul 26];92(2):363–71. Available from: http://www.ncbi.nlm.nih.gov/pubmed/4345530
16. Schussler GC. The thyroxine-binding proteins. Thyroid [Internet]. 2000 Feb [cited 2020 Feb 13];10(2):141–149. Available from: http://www.ncbi.nlm.nih.gov/pubmed/10718550
17. Bartalena L, Robbins J. Thyroid hormone transport proteins. Clin Lab Med [Internet]. 1993 Sep [cited 2020 Jul 26];13(3):583–598. Available from: http://www.ncbi.nlm.nih.gov/pubmed/8222576
18. Orozco A, Valverde RC, Olvera A, García GC. Iodothyronine deiodinases: a functional and evolutionary perspective. J Endocrinol. 2012;215(2):207–219.
19. Larsen PR, Zavacki AM. Role of the iodothyronine deiodinases in the physiology and pathophysiology of thyroid hormone action. Eur Thyroid J. 2012;(4):232–242.
20. Brent GA. Science in medicine mechanisms of thyroid hormone action. J Clin Invest. 2012;122(9):3035–3043.
21. Visser WE, Friesema ECH, Visser TJ. Minireview: thyroid hormone transporters: the knowns and the unknowns. Mol Endocrinol. 2011;25(1):1–14.
22. Lazar MA. Thyroid hormone action: a binding contract. J Clin Invest. 2003;112(4):497–499.
23. Boelaert K, Franklyn JA. Thyroid hormone in health and disease. J Endocrinol. 2005;187(1):1–15.
24. Carmean CM, Cohen RN, Brady MJ. Systemic regulation of adipose metabolism. Biochim Biophys Acta—Mol Basis Dis. 2014;1842(3):424–430.
25. Bassett JHD, Williams GR. Role of thyroid hormones in skeletal development and bone maintenance. Endocr Rev. 2016 Apr;37(2):135–187.
26. Williams GR, Bassett JHD. Thyroid diseases and bone health. J Endocrinol Invest. 2018 Jan;41(1):99–109.
27. Kim B. Thyroid hormone as a determinant of energy expenditure and the basal metabolic rate. Thyroid. 2008;18(2):141–144.

28. Yavuz S, Salgado Nunez del Prado S, Celi FS. Thyroid hormone action and energy expenditure. J Endocr Soc. 2019;3(7):1345–1356.
29. Bloise FF, Cordeiro A, Ortiga-Carvalho TM. Role of thyroid hormone in skeletal muscle physiology. J Endocrinol. 2018 Jan;236(1):R57–R68.
30. Salvatore D, Simonides WS, Dentice M, Zavacki AM, Larsen PR. Thyroid hormones and skeletal muscle—new insights and potential implications. Nat Rev Endocrinol. 2014 Apr;10(4):206–214.
31. Salvatore D, Pansini V, Simonides WS, Dentice M, Pansini V, Zavacki AM, et al. Thyroid hormones and skeletal muscle—new insights and potential implications. Nat Rev Endocrinol. 2014;10(4):206–214.
32. Krassas GE, Poppe K, Glinoer D. Thyroid function and human reproductive health. Endocr Rev. 2010;31(5):702–755.
33. Nathan N, Sullivan SD. Thyroid disorders during pregnancy. Endocrinol Metab Clin North Am. 2014;43(2):573–597.
34. Sheehan MT. Biochemical testing of the thyroid: TSH is the best and, oftentimes, only test needed—a review for primary care. Clin Med Res. 2016;14(2):83–92.
35. Fröhlich E, Wahl R. Thyroid autoimmunity: role of anti-thyroid antibodies in thyroid and extra-thyroidal diseases. Front Immunol. 2017;8(MAY):521
36. Sinclair D. Clinical and laboratory aspects of thyroid autoantibodies. Ann Clin Biochem. 2006;43(3):173–183.
37. Vitti P, Rago T. Thyroid ultrasound as a predicator of thyroid disease [Internet]. J Endocrinol Invest. Editrice Kurtis s.r.l.; 2003 [cited 2020 Jul 25]; Vol. 26:p. 686–9. Available from: https://pubmed.ncbi.nlm.nih.gov/14594124/
38. Intenzo CM, Dam HQ, Manzone TA, Kim SM. Imaging of the thyroid in benign and malignant disease [Internet]. In: Vol. 42, Seminars in Nuclear Medicine. W.B. Saunders; 2012 [cited 2020 Jul 25]. p. 49–61. Available from: https://pubmed.ncbi.nlm.nih.gov/22117813/
39. Broome MR. Thyroid scintigraphy in hyperthyroidism. Clin Tech Small Anim Pract [Internet]. 2006 Feb [cited 2020 Jul 25];21(1):10–16. Available from: https://pubmed.ncbi.nlm.nih.gov/16584025/

3

EMBRYOLOGY AND SURGICAL ANATOMY
Thyroid and Parathyroid Glands

Dinesh Kumar Srinivasan, Krishnan Jayabharathi, Muthukrishnan Chandrika, S. Thameem Dheen, Boon Huat Bay and Rajeev Parameswaran

Introduction

The existence of the thyroid gland in humans has been known for centuries, but the exact function of the gland was undetermined at that time. The term "thyroid" (derived from the Greek term "thyreos"), which means shield, was actually named after the thyroid cartilage. Enlargement of the thyroid gland or goiter has been recognized eons ago, but there was a scarcity of medical knowledge in terms of a cure for the condition, until the 19th century. The first description of the anatomy of the gland was made in the 16th century, following cadaveric human dissections, and Leonardo da Vinci, the great Renaissance artist, was the first to illustrate the thyroid gland. Andreas Vesalius further described the gland with his pictorial illustration in the Fabrica Humanis (1). Thomas Wharton coined the term "thyroid" in his book Adenographia in 1656 (2). Vater was the first to describe the thyroglossal duct in 1723, which he named the "ductus salivalis in lingua" (the salivary duct in the tongue). Based on Wilhelm His's description, the duct was subsequently renamed as the thyroglossal duct of His (3). Current advances in thyroid surgery are based on the foundations laid by the "magnificent seven surgeons" in the mid-20th century (4).

A clear understanding of the embryology, anatomy, physiology and surgical pathology enables the surgeon to have a better insight of how thyroid nodules and tumors develop. This ultimately aids in developing surgical strategies for managing surgical conditions where indicated. The thyroid glands may be removed, partially or totally, depending on the pathology. Whilst the glands are removed, the parathyroid glands and the laryngeal nerves which are in close proximity may be injured, resulting in morbidity for the patients. Understanding the physiology is crucial in dealing with hyper- and hypothyroidism, so that appropriate medical therapy or replacement of thyroxine for patients who require them can be instituted.

Anatomy of the thyroid and parathyroid glands

The thyroid gland is situated in the anterior triangle of the neck, lies inferior to the larynx and is shaped like a butterfly. It has two lobes joined by the isthmus at the level of the second and fourth tracheal rings (Figure 3.1(a)) (5). The thyroid is bordered by the trachea and esophagus medially, the carotid sheath laterally and anterolaterally by the strap muscles. The superior pole of the thyroid lobe extends up to the oblique line of thyroid cartilage. The strap muscles are innervated by the ansa cervicalis, formed from the fibers of C1, C2 and C3. *The ansa cervicalis may be used for anastomosis to the recurrent laryngeal nerve (RLN) following a transection injury of the RLN (6).* The clinical importance of the bilateral lobes is the fact that cancers may occur in either one or both the lobes and this determines the extent of surgery along with other factors, namely, extrathyroidal extension and nodal involvement. Thyroid nodules, which are situated more posteriorly in the thyroid gland, are rarely palpable on clinical examination.

The presence of the pyramidal lobe can be variable, either existing as a thick band and extending for a variable distance from the isthmus to the hyoid bone or is just represented as a fibrous band. There is a slight tendency for the pyramidal lobe to be longer in women and arising more frequently from the left lobe of the thyroid gland (7). *The clinical significance of the lobe is that if it is not excised during thyroidectomy, the disease can recur with an incidence of 23% for benign conditions such as nodular goiter (8), and 30–45% for thyroid cancers (9, 10),* as observed on radioiodine scans. The pretracheal fascia is condensed to form the posterior suspensory ligament (Berry's ligament) enclosing the thyroid gland, which lies close to the cricoid cartilage and upper tracheal rings.

At the posterior surface of the thyroid glands and situated close to the thyroid capsule are the parathyroid glands. The superior pair of parathyroid glands is situated on the middle third of the posterolateral border of the thyroid gland, and the inferior pair along the inferior pole of the thyroid gland (Figure 3.1(a)). However, the positions of the glands vary due to aberrations in their embryological descent. It is also not uncommon to see supernumerary parathyroid glands in individuals. The parathyroid glands and the RLN are the two key structures seen in relation to the thyroid capsule (Figure 3.1(b)) (5). Recognition of the presence of these structures is important during surgery, because of the necessity to preserve both the parathyroid glands and RLN. Thyroid cancers may breach the capsule into the surrounding tissues affecting staging, prognosis and management (11, 12).

Blood supply

The thyroid gland is supplied by the paired arteries: superior thyroid artery (STA), a branch of the external carotid artery (ECA) and accompanied by the superior laryngeal nerve (SLN), and inferior thyroid artery (ITA) that arises from the thyrocervical trunk and runs parallel to the RLN. Occasionally, a branch from the thyrocervical trunk, the thyroidea ima (also known as thyroid ima) artery may supply the gland.

STA is the original artery to the primitive thyroid bud and is the primary arterial supply to the thyroid gland. It is the first branch of the ECA and supplies the thyroid gland and other structures such as the larynx and sternocleidomastoid muscle. The artery descends along the lateral border of the thyrohyoid to the superior pole of the gland and during its course accompanies

Embryology and Surgical Anatomy

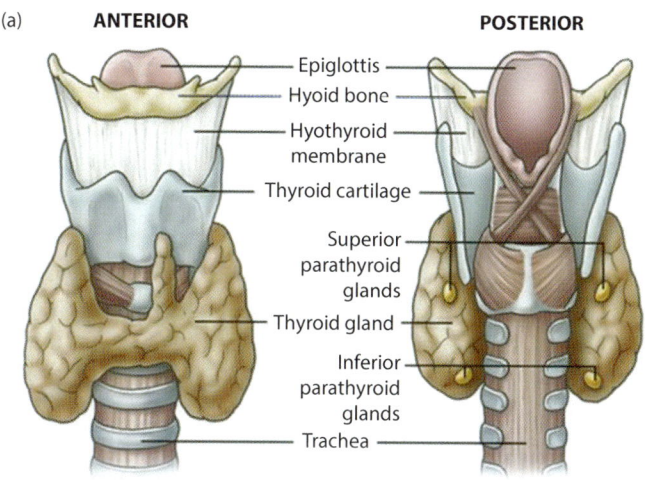

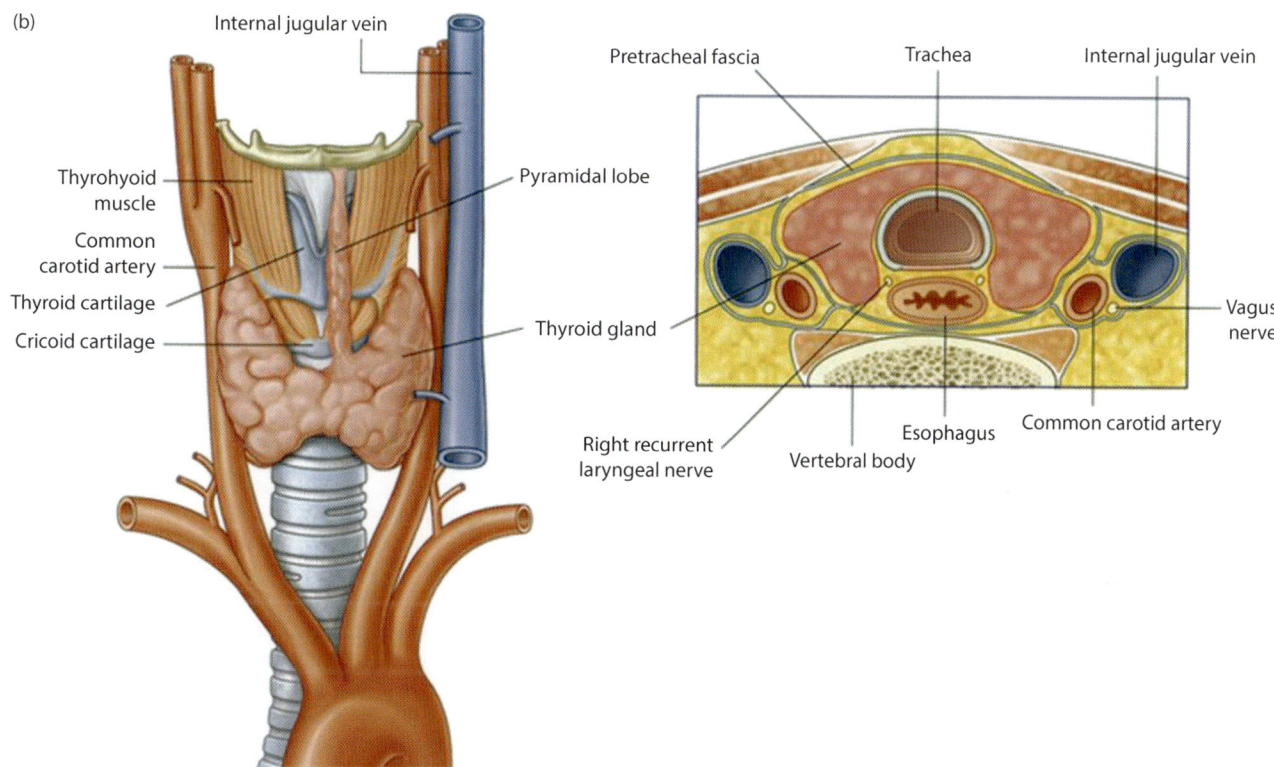

FIGURE 3.1 (a) The thyroid and parathyroid glands. (b) Thyroid in relation to surrounding structures. (Reprinted from (5), with permission from Elsevier, 2018.)

the external laryngeal nerve (ELN). The artery divides into an anterior and posterior branch, with ELN lying posteromedially. *Ligation of the superior pedicle during thyroidectomy poses the risk of injury to the ELN.*

STA can have a variant origin in that it may arise from common carotid artery (CCA) and carotid bifurcation (CB). The artery may also run as common trunks with lingual or facial artery or both and, in rare cases, may arise in common with the occipital artery or ascending pharyngeal artery or from the internal carotid artery (ICA) (13). The variation in origin can be seen in 17% on the left side of the neck and 24% on the right and can differ depending on the demographics (14). Occasionally, there can be a double STA or unilateral STA, which may replace the contralateral STA or the ITA on the same side (15). The STA is wider in Caucasians than in Asians and sometimes may be even absent in Caucasians (16). Congenital anomalies such as hemiagenesis, presence of accessory or ectopic thyroid tissues may have altered vascular anatomy and surgical approaches would likewise have to be altered when dealing with them.

An interesting observation is that thyroid functions may be affected in conditions affecting the cervical sympathetic chain due to variations in thyroid arterial system (16). *Surgeons should be aware of the variations of the STA, for instance in a patient with uncontrollable bleeding from the upper pole, ligation of the*

ECA alone may not be sufficient to stop the hemorrhage if there is presence of a double STA (17). A branch of STA that is commonly encountered and known to cause bleeding is the cricothyroid artery, seen during thyroglossal cyst surgery or excision of pyramidal lobe or isthmusectomy.

The ITA originates most frequently from the thyrocervical trunk and less frequently from the subclavian artery. The artery loops upward behind the carotid sheath, anterior to the vertebral artery, descends on the longus colli and divides into two or more branches crossing the RLN. The nerve may pass anterior or posterior to the artery, or between its branches. The ITA also supplies the parathyroids. *Hence, ligation of the ITA during thyroidectomy should be performed closer to the gland to preserve the vascularity to the parathyroid glands.*

Variants of ITA have also been described in the literature. ITAs have been shown to arise from CCA in about 1% but can also arise from a common stem with the vertebral artery, internal thoracic artery, suprascapular artery and ascending cervical arteries (18). Absent ITA is observed in about 6.1% of cases on the right and 15.2% on the left (19) and appears to be more common in East Asians than Caucasians (20). Double ITA has been reported in 9% of cases on the right and in 4.6% on the left side (21). As the artery comes into the thyroid gland, it has a variable branching pattern and is closely related to the RLN. Observations in cadavers have shown that the RLN on the right is located predominantly posterior to the ITA (60–70%) or anterior to the ITA (18–20%) and in between the branches of ITA (14–18%) (22). Other variations have also been reported such as ITA being placed between the branches of RLN (1–2%) and interpenetration of the nerve in about 2–3% (23). *Therefore, surgeons operating on the thyroid gland should be aware of the variations of the ITA and its relationship to the RLN, so as to avoid any potential injury to the RLN.*

Venous drainage

There are three paired veins draining the thyroid gland, namely the *superior, middle* and *inferior thyroid veins*. These veins form a plexus on the surface of the thyroid gland. The superficial and deep venous tributaries of the upper part of the thyroid gland join to form the superior thyroid vein. It accompanies the STA and empties into the internal jugular vein (IJV) or the facial vein. Superior thyroid veins tend to be single and constant in position on both sides (24).

The lower half of the thyroid gland is drained by the middle thyroid vein, which usually crosses the CCA and the RLN anteriorly to empty into the IJV posterior to the omohyoid belly. The vein may also cross posterior to the RLN and the surgeon should be aware of these variations. The middle thyroid veins, which normally drain into the IJV, occasionally drain into the brachiocephalic vein or may be absent (18). It has been observed that the size of the middle thyroid veins varies directly with the size of the goiters and hyperthyroid state (25). Large goiters extending into the mediastinum can increase the pressure in IJV, causing significant engorgement of the middle thyroid veins. *Therefore, it is important that these veins be identified early and ligated to decrease the risk of significant bleeding.*

The inferior thyroid vein is the largest and also the most variable of the three veins. The veins on both sides may join to form a transverse venous arch across the trachea and receive the veins of the thymus. The veins tend to be constant in their position but the number of branches tends to vary between 1 and 5 (24). The presence of an additional fourth vein may be seen between the middle and inferior thyroid vein. Another vein that has been described is the posterior thyroid vein which is present only on rare occasions.

Lymphatic drainage

Lymphatics of the thyroid gland run parallel to the venous drainage. The upper deep cervical lymph nodes drain the lymphatics accompanying the superior and the middle thyroid veins. The lymphatics that accompany the inferior thyroid veins drain into the lower cervical lymph nodes, namely the supraclavicular, paratracheal and parapharyngeal nodes (26). The posterior part of the thyroid lobe drains into the parapharyngeal and retropharyngeal nodes (27). Lymphatics of the parathyroid glands drain into the deep cervical lymph nodes and paratracheal lymph nodes and are the reason why central compartment nodal clearance is required in the treatment of parathyroid cancer. Understanding the lymphatic drainage is important in managing patients with thyroid cancer, especially in determining the extent and level of nodal surgery (28).

Nerve supply

The innervation of the thyroid gland is by the sympathetic nerves from the sympathetic trunk, which play no role in the regulation of thyroid hormone secretion. The nerves that run close to the thyroid gland are the SLN and the RLN which branch from the vagus nerve. The RLN hooks under the right subclavian artery (embryological derivative of the fourth pharyngeal arch artery) and on the left side curls upward under the ligamentum arteriosum (embryological derivative of the sixth pharyngeal arch artery) (29). The ELN is a branch of the SLN, which is the motor nerve to the cricothyroid muscle that serves as the main tensor of the vocal cords. The internal laryngeal nerve (ILN), another branch of the SLN, acts as a sensory nerve to the mucosal lining of the supraglottic larynx. The SLN is closely related to the STA but the position can be variable. Cernea et al. proposed a system of classification based on the relationship of the SLN to the STA as: type 1 anatomy, where the nerve crosses the superior thyroid vessels by more than 1 cm above the superior pole; type 2 anatomy, the nerve crosses the vessels less than 1 cm above (type 2a) or even below (type 2b) the superior *vascular pedicle* (30).

During thyroid surgery, the RLN is commonly injured (31), and therefore, it is important for surgeons to recognize and identify the nerve using reliable landmarks. The nerve can be typically identified in the Simon triangle bordered by the esophagus medially, CCA laterally and ITA superiorly (32) or by finding the Zuckerkandl tubercle (described later in the chapter). The RLN is a motor nerve to the intrinsic muscles of the larynx and ascends into the larynx in the trachea-esophageal groove. The right RLN runs more obliquely than the left RLN in the neck; however, many variations of the nerves have been reported. The RLN typically runs deep to the ITA (18, 33). *The two landmarks that help identify the RLN close to the insertion of the cricothyroid muscle are the ligament of Berry* (34) *and the tubercle of Zuckerkandl* (35).

Nonrecurrent laryngeal nerve

The non-RLN (NRLN) is a rare anatomical variation of RLN and takes an aberrant course, whereby the nerve does not descend into the thorax and enters directly into the larynx from the vagus nerve. It was first described by Stedman and is usually seen on the right side (36). The incidence of NRLN is about 0.5–1% and associated with an aberrant right subclavian artery (37). However, with intraoperative neuromonitoring (IONM), the incidence of NRLN has been reported to be closer to around 6% (38).

Embryology and Surgical Anatomy

Disappearance of the fourth pharyngeal arch leads to the subclavian artery arising directly from the aorta, resulting in the nerve migrating cranially and originating from the vagus. NRLN on the left side is associated with significant pathology such as situs inversus (39, 40). Three types of NRLN are described: type 1, the nerve runs along with the superior thyroid pedicle, type 2a, where it runs below the ITA and type 2b where it lies between the ITA (39). *The surgical relevance of NRLN is that the nerve is at sixfold higher risk of injury during thyroid and parathyroid surgery.* A meticulous dissection and use of IONM helps identify the NRLN and prevent injury. *It is very important that the surgeon must not divide any transverse band until the RLN is first identified and if the nerve is not found in conventional position, it should raise the possibility of a NRLN being present.*

Histology of the thyroid and parathyroid glands

The main structural and functional unit of the thyroid gland is the follicle, which is lined by a single layer of epithelial cells, surrounded by a basement membrane. The gland has millions of epithelial thyroid follicles. Each follicle has simple cuboidal epithelium and a central lumen filled with gelatinous acidophilic colloid (Figure 3.2(a)) (41). The colloid has a large glycoprotein, thyroglobulin (600 kDa), a precursor for the active forms of T3 and T4. The follicles vary in size significantly but usually each follicle measures about 200 µm and separated by septa. These septa carry blood vessels, nerves and lymphatics. Fenestrated capillaries in the highly vascularized stroma mediate the release of hormones from the follicles to the bloodstream. Lying in between the follicles are the supporting connective tissue and parafollicular cells that produce calcitonin. Parafollicular cells, derived from the neural crest, are seen inside the basal lamina of the follicular epithelium or separate clusters between follicles. These cells are somewhat large and have less staining. They contain rough endoplasmic reticulum, Golgi complexes and small granules containing calcitonin. The parafollicular C-cells are predominantly located in the upper third of the thyroid gland, which explains why medullary thyroid cancers are seen in the upper half of the thyroid gland. The histological features of thyroid follicular cells are summarized in Table 3.1.

TABLE 3.1: The Histological Features of Thyroid Follicular Cell

Apical junctional complexes
Basal lamina
Round and central nucleus
Basally cells are rich in rough endoplasmic reticulum
Apically facing the lumen cells have Golgi complexes, secretory granules, phagosomes, lysosomes and microvilli

The parathyroid glands are normally the size of a grain and have a thin connective tissue capsule. The chief cell is the most important component of the parathyroid gland, is usually small and has a centrally located nucleus and pale granular cytoplasm (Figure 3.2(b)). The cells are usually arranged in a solid pattern surrounded by capillary network, with the presence of stromal fat. Chief cells contain numerous secretory granules within their cytoplasm that synthesize and secrete parathyroid hormone (PTH) (42). Oxyphil cells, which are the second type of cells, have polygonal shapes with abundant eosinophilic granular cytoplasm, higher amounts of mitochondria but fewer organelles and granules than chief cells (43, 44). The exact role of oxyphil cells is unclear but they may secrete PTH in the presence of secondary parathyroid hyperplasia. Ageing and chronic diseases lead to the chief cells being replaced by adipocytes (45). Besides PTH, the parathyroid glands also synthesize chromogranin A (46, 47), cytokeratins and PTH-related protein (PTHrP) (47, 48).

Embryology of the thyroid and parathyroid glands

The thyroid gland is the first endocrine gland to develop in the human body. It develops from an endodermal diverticulum in the third week of intrauterine life, located in the midline of the

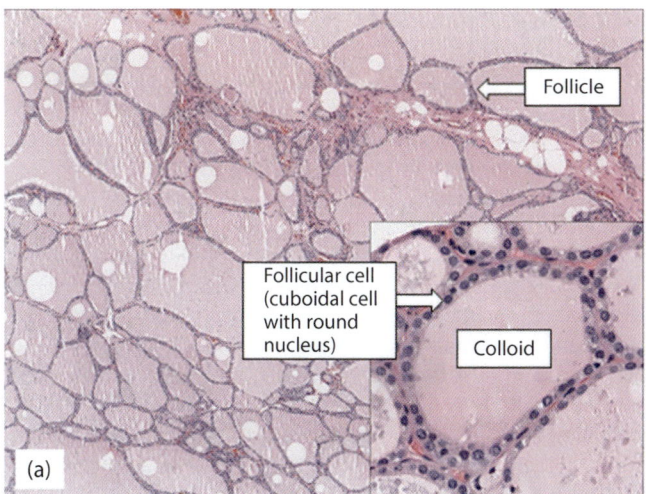
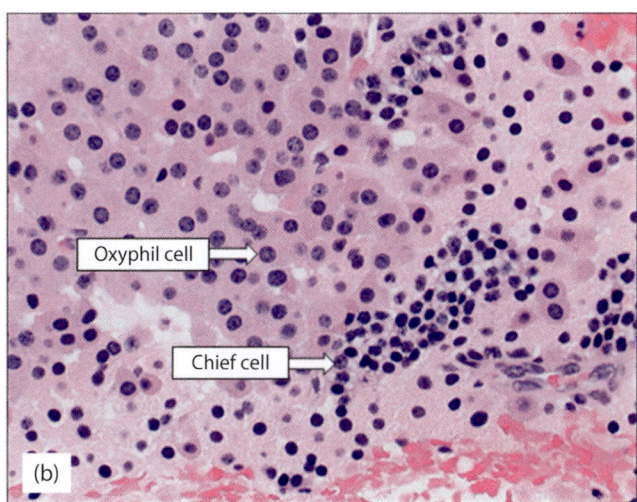

FIGURE 3.2 (a) Microscopic image of thyroid gland with the follicles. The inset shows higher magnification image of a thyroid follicle showing the lining of cuboidal cells with the colloid. (b) Microscopic image of parathyroid gland with the oxyphil and chief cells. (Reprinted from (41), with permission from National University of Singapore, Singapore. https://medicine.nus.edu.sg/pathweb/ (accessed 01 May 2020).)

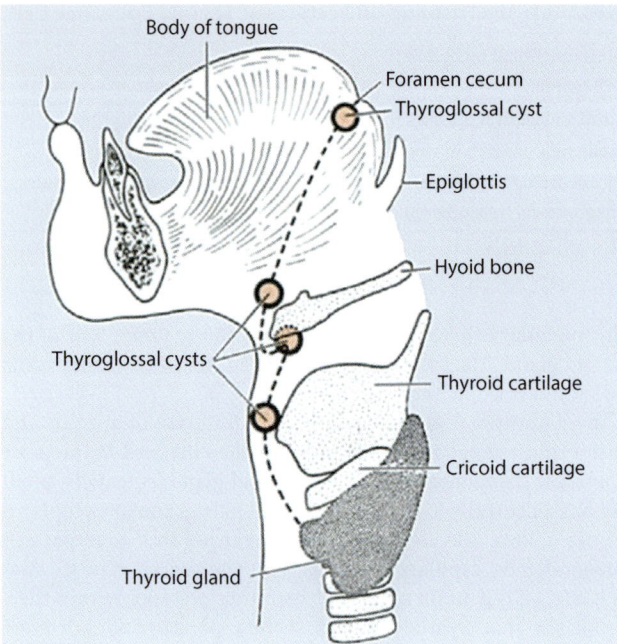

FIGURE 3.3 Thyroglossal cysts. These cysts, most frequently found in the hyoid region, are always close to the midline. (Reprinted from (29), with permission from Lippincott Williams & Wilkins, 2010.)

floor of primitive pharynx between the tuberculum impar and copula (foramen caecum) (Figure 3.3). The thyroid descends in front of the pharyngeal gut as a bilobed diverticulum through the thyroglossal duct (29). The proximal opening of the thyroglossal duct persists as the foramen caecum on the dorsum of the tongue. The distal part of the duct normally disappears once the thyroid reaches its final position in the neck. The thyroid descends in front of larynx and reaches in front of trachea by the seventh week of gestation. The thyroid gland attains its bilobed pattern with a central isthmus at this juncture. The cells of the thyroid follicles start functioning at the end of the third month and the parafollicular cells from the ultimobranchial body are incorporated into them. In about half of the population, the pyramidal lobe is attached to the hyoid bone by a fibrous band called the ***levator glandulae thyroideae***, after it differentiates from the distal end of the thyroglossal duct.

Aberrations in the embryological descent of the thyroid gland can occur and can lead to anomalies of position, ectopic thyroids, anomalous lobes, thyroglossal cyst and fistula and development of accessory thyroid glands. Anomalous positions of the thyroid gland include the *lingual thyroid* (due to its formation on the tongue at the foramen caecum or within the muscles) (49), *sublingual thyroid* – present high in the neck or below the hyoid bone (50) and *intrathoracic thyroid* (situated in the thoracic cavity) (51). Ectopic thyroids have reported to present at sites other than in the neck such as the larynx, trachea, pericardium or the ovaries. Absence of a lobe (hemiagenesis) and the isthmus of the thyroid have also been reported (52).

The presence of a pyramidal lobe, usually arising from the left lobe is very well described. The thyroglossal cyst may develop anywhere along the course of the thyroglossal duct and is usually formed in the midline of the front of the neck. Following the rupture of a thyroglossal cyst, a fistula develops with communication to the exterior via the surface of the neck. Occasionally, small nodules of thyroid tissues are seen in proximity to the main thyroid gland known as *accessory* thyroid.

The parathyroid glands arise from the third and fourth pharyngeal pouches and differentiate in the fifth week of embryonic life. The dorsal portion of the third pharyngeal pouch forms the inferior parathyroid glands, whereas the ventral portion develops forms the thymus gland. The dorsal portion of the fourth pharyngeal pouch forms the superior parathyroid glands whereas the ventral portion forms the ultimobranchial body. Both these glands lose their attachment from the pharyngeal wall and migrate with the thyroid gland. Because of the common embryological origin with the thyroid gland, the superior parathyroids are usually located at the posterior part of the cricothyroid junction (77%), less commonly behind the upper pole (22%) and rarely (less than 1%) behind the lower pharyngeal and upper esophageal junction in the midline (16).

The position of the superior glands can be aberrant such as above the superior pole of the thyroid (53) in a retrolaryngeal or retropharyngeal position (54). Majority of the glands are located on the posterior aspect of the thyroid gland within a circumscribed area of 2 cm in diameter, about 1 cm above the crossing point of the RLN and ITA (55). The inferior parathyroids are usually located at an anterior or a latero-posterior surface of the lower thyroid pole (42%) and in the thymic tongue (39%) (56). Bilateral symmetry is seen in 80% of the superior parathyroid glands and in 70% of the inferior parathyroid glands (55).

Ectopic positions of the parathyroid glands are not uncommon and have an incidence of about 28–42.8% in autopsy findings (57, 58). It is a common cause of failed parathyroid surgery in both primary and secondary hyperparathyroidism. Similarly, multiple glands or supernumerary glands (more than four) have been reported with an incidence ranging between 3 and 13%, even though typically there are only four parathyroid glands (59, 60). Most supernumerary glands are located in close proximity to normal glands but can also be seen in the thymus or the mediastinum (58). Supernumerary glands are also a major cause for both persistent and recurrent hyperparathyroidism (60, 61).

Zuckerkandl tubercle and its relevance

The tubercle of Zuckerkandl was described by Emil Zuckerkandl in 1902, as a projection from the posterior surface of the thyroid, which he termed the "tuberculum" or "processus posterior glandulae thyroideae" (62). It is an important landmark for identification of the RLN and superior parathyroid during thyroidectomy (63–65). The tubercle is the point of embryological fusion of the ultimobranchial body and principal median thyroid process. It is found in over two-thirds of patients undergoing thyroid surgery and is usually found between the upper and lower thyroid poles pointing toward the tracheoesophageal groove. Pelizzo et al classified the tubercle into various grades: grade 0 (unrecognizable), grade 1 (only a thickening of the lateral edge of the thyroid lobe), grade 2 (smaller than 1 cm) or grade 3 (larger than 1 cm) (65). *The majority of the patients with a Zuckerkandl tubercle have the RLN medial to it, although the nerve has been shown to be placed laterally in 7% of patients (63). The superior parathyroid glands are usually found superior to the tubercle and posterior to the RLN.*

Physiology of the thyroid and parathyroid glands

The physiology of the thyroid gland was discussed in detail in Chapter 2. In brief, the thyroid gland synthesizes the hormones triiodothyronine (T3) and thyroxine (T4) and is responsible for regulation of metabolism. Synthesis of the hormones is tightly regulated by a negative feedback mechanism involving the pituitary and hypothalamus glands. *The biosynthesis of thyroid hormones has clinical relevance as they may be altered or aberrant in the various pathologies of the thyroid gland, including thyroid cancer.*

The synthesis of thyroid hormones is unique in many ways:

a. *Thyroid hormones have large amounts of iodine obtained via an efficient energy-dependent mechanism (sodium iodine symporter – NIS) which enables the thyroid follicular cells to take up and concentrate iodine (66).*
b. *Partial synthesis of the hormones takes place at the extracellular luminal surface, which are then stored in the extracellular lumen of the follicle.*
c. *Thyroid hormones are secreted, reabsorbed and re-secreted in that thyroglobulin, which is the precursor molecule, is first released into the follicular lumen from the apical surface. This is then taken up again by the follicular cells and broken down to release the thyroid hormones, from where it is then secreted into the bloodstream.*
d. *The major hormone secreted is the biologically inactive hormone which is converted to the active form T3 in the peripheral tissues.*

Parathyroid glands synthesize PTH. The major regulator of PTH secretion is ionized calcium and vitamin D, which plays a minor role. The three primary target organs for PTH activity are the kidneys, intestines and bones. PTH causes increased renal excretion of phosphate and increased reabsorption of calcium from the renal tubules. It also increases the formation of 1,25-dihydroxycholecalciferol that leads to increased intestinal absorption of calcium. In the bone, the number of osteoblasts, osteoclasts and their phagocytic activities are increased, resulting in increased resorption of bone tissue. *Increased secretion of PTH from an intrinsic tumor or cancer or hyperplasia of the parathyroid glands can cause hypercalcemia resulting in primary hyperparathyroidism.*

Conclusion

The thyroid and parathyroid glands are endocrine glands situated in the neck. These glands release the hormones that play an important role for metabolism and calcium regulation. Many key structures, which are related to the thyroid gland namely the parathyroid glands, SLNs and RLNs, have to be preserved during thyroid surgery. The size of the thyroid gland varies with pathologies such as endemic goiter, tumors and hyperthyroid states. Aberrations in development and disease give rise to problems such as thyroglossal cyst and ducts, agenesis, ectopic glands and tubercle of Zuckerkandl. Parathyroid glands are derivatives of the third and fourth pharyngeal pouches and can have aberrations in number and position. Both the SLN and RLN are prone to variations and a thorough understanding is essential to preserve their integrity during surgery. A comprehensive knowledge of thyroid and parathyroid surgical anatomy and physiology, good and meticulous surgical techniques and vigilant postoperative care will reduce the complications of surgery.

References

1. Lydiatt, Daniel D., and Gregory S. Bucher. 2011. "Historical vignettes of the thyroid gland." Clinical Anatomy 24 (1):1–9.
2. Martensen, Robert L. 1998. "Thomas Wharton's Adenographia (review)." Bulletin of the History of Medicine 72 (4):762–763.
3. Gray, Stephen Wood, and John Elias Skandalakis. 1972. Embryology for surgeons: the embryological basis for the treatment of congenital defects. Philadelphia, PA: Saunders.
4. Hannan, S. Alam. 2006. "The magnificent seven: a history of modern thyroid surgery." International Journal of Surgery 4 (3):187–191.
5. Duffy, C. 2018. "Thyroid and parathyroid surgery." In: Alexander's care of the patient in surgery, 16th ed., ed. Rothrock J. C. Missouri: Elsevier, 1639–1646.
6. Crumley, Roger L. 1991. "Update: ansa cervicalis to recurrent laryngeal nerve anastomosis for unilateral laryngeal paralysis." The Laryngoscope 101 (4):384–388.
7. Braun, Eva Maria, Eva Maria Braun, Gunther Windisch, Gunther Windisch, Gerhard Wolf, Gerhard Wolf, Lisa Hausleitner, Lisa Hausleitner, Friedrich Anderhuber, and Friedrich Anderhuber. 2007. "The pyramidal lobe: clinical anatomy and its importance in thyroid surgery." Surgical and Radiologic Anatomy 29 (1):21–27.
8. Gurleyik, Emin, Gunay Gurleyik, Sami Dogan, Utku Cobek, Fuat Cetin, and Ufuk Onsal. 2015. "Pyramidal lobe of the thyroid gland: surgical anatomy in patients undergoing total thyroidectomy." Anatomy Research International 2015:384148.
9. Dos Reis, L. L., S. Mehra, S. Scherl, J. Clain, J. Machac, and M. L. Urken. 2014. "The differential diagnosis of central compartment radioactive iodine uptake after thyroidectomy: anatomic and surgical considerations." Endocrine Practice 20 (8):832–838.
10. Sawicka-Gutaj, N., A. Klimowicz, J. Sowinski, R. Oleksa, M. Gryczynska, A. Wyszomirska, A. Czarnywojtek, and M. Ruchala. 2014. "Pyramidal lobe decreases endogenous TSH stimulation without impact on radio-iodine therapy outcome in patients with differentiated thyroid cancer." Annales D'endocrinologie (Paris) 75 (3):141–147.
11. Ghossein, Ronald. 2009. "Update to the College of American Pathologists reporting on thyroid carcinomas." Head and Neck Pathology 3 (1):86–93.
12. Gillanders, S. L., and J. P. O'Neill. 2018. "Prognostic markers in well differentiated papillary and follicular thyroid cancer (WDTC)." European Journal of Surgical Oncology 44 (3):286–296.
13. Aggarwal, Nilesh R., Thamburaj Krishnamoorthy, Bobby Devasia, Girish Menon, and Kesavadas Chandrasekhar. 2006. "Variant origin of superior thyroid artery, occipital artery and ascending pharyngeal artery from a common trunk from the cervical segment of internal carotid artery." Surgical and Radiologic Anatomy 28 (6):650–653.
14. Ongeti, Kevin W., and Julius A. Ogeng'o. 2012. "Variant origin of the superior thyroid artery in a Kenyan population." Clinical Anatomy 25 (2):198–202.
15. Skandalakis, Lee John, and John Elias Skandalakis. 2014. Surgical anatomy and technique: a pocket manual. 4th ed. New York, NY: Springer.
16. Toni, Roberto, Claudia Della Casa, Sergio Castorina, Anna Malaguti, Salvatore Mosca, Elio Roti, and Giorgio Valenti. 2004. "A meta-analysis of superior thyroid artery variations in different human groups and their clinical implications." Annals of Anatomy 186 (3):255–262.
17. Ozgur, Zuhal, Govsa, Figen, Celik, Servet, and Ozgur, Tomris. 2009. "Clinically relevant variations of the superior thyroid artery: an anatomic guide for surgical neck dissection." Surgical and Radiologic Anatomy 31 (3):151–159.
18. Yalcin, Bulent. 2016. "Thyroid gland." In Bergman's comprehensive encyclopedia of human anatomic variation, 1189–1204.
19. Kitagawa, W. 1993. "Arterial supply of the thyroid gland in the human fetuses." Nihon Ika Daigaku zasshi 60 (3):140–155.
20. Toni, Roberto, Claudia Della Casa, Sergio Castorina, Elio Roti, Gianpaolo Ceda, and Giorgio Valenti. 2005. "A meta-analysis of inferior thyroid artery variations in different human ethnic groups and their clinical implications." Annals of Anatomy 187 (4):371–385.
21. Yalcin, Bülent. 2006. "Anatomic configurations of the recurrent laryngeal nerve and inferior thyroid artery." Surgery 139 (2):181–187.
22. Özgüner, G., and O. Sulak. 2014. "Arterial supply to the thyroid gland and the relationship between the recurrent laryngeal nerve and the inferior thyroid artery in human fetal cadavers." Clinical Anatomy 27 (8):1185–1192.
23. Tang, W. J., S. Q. Sun, X. L. Wang, Y. X. Sun, and H. X. Huang. 2012. "An applied anatomical study on the recurrent laryngeal nerve and inferior thyroid artery." Surgical and Radiologic Anatomy 34 (4):325–332.
24. Wafae, N., K. Hirose, C. Franco, G. C. Wafae, C. R. Ruiz, L. Daher, and O. C. Person. 2008. "The anatomy of the human thyroid veins and its surgical application." Folia Morphologica 67 (4):221.
25. Dionigi, Gianlorenzo, Gianlorenzo Dionigi, Terenzio Congiu, Terenzio Congiu, Francesca Rovera, Francesca Rovera, Luigi Boni, and Luigi Boni. 2010. "The middle thyroid vein: anatomical and surgical aspects." World Journal of Surgery 34 (3):514–520.
26. Hoyes, A. D., and D. R. Kershaw. 1985. "Anatomy and development of the thyroid gland." Ear, Nose & Throat Journal 64 (7):318–333.
27. Nixon, Iain J., and Ashok R. Shaha. 2013. "Management of regional nodes in thyroid cancer." Oral Oncology 49 (7):671–675.
28. Gimm, O., F. W. Rath, and H. Dralle. 1998. "Pattern of lymph node metastases in papillary thyroid carcinoma." British Journal of Surgery 85 (2):252–254.

29. Sadler, T. W. 2010. Langman's medical embryology. 12th ed. Philadelphia, PA: Lippincott Williams & Wilkins, a Wolters Kluwer business.
30. Cernea, Claudio R., Sunao Nishio, and Flávio C. Hojaij. 1995. "Identification of the external branch of the superior laryngeal nerve (EBSLN) in large goiters." American Journal of Otolaryngology – Head and Neck Medicine and Surgery 16 (5):307–311.
31. Lynch, Jeremy, and Rajeev Parameswaran. 2017. "Management of unilateral recurrent laryngeal nerve injury after thyroid surgery: a review." Head & Neck 39 (7):1470–1478.
32. Simon, Max Michael. 1943. "Recurrent laryngeal nerve in thyroid surgery: triangle for its recognition and protection." The American Journal of Surgery 60 (2):212–220.
33. John, Alana, Denzil Etienne, Zachary Klaassen, Mohammadali M. Shoja, R. Shane Tubbs, and Marios Loukas. 2012. "Variations in the locations of the recurrent laryngeal nerve in relation to the ligament of Berry." The American Surgeon 78 (9):947.
34. Leow, C. K., and A. J. Webb. 1998. "The lateral thyroid ligament of Berry." International Surgery 83 (1):75–78.
35. Pelizzo, M. R., A. Toniato, and G. Gemo. 1998a. "Zuckerkandl's tuberculum: an arrow pointing to the recurrent laryngeal nerve (constant anatomical landmark)." Journal of the American College of Surgeons 187 (3):333–336.
36. Stedman, George William. 1823. "A singular distribution of some of the nerves and arteries in the neck, and the top of the thorax." Edinburgh Medical and Surgical Journal 19 (77):564–565.
37. Henry, J. F., J. Audiffret, A. Denizot, and M. Plan. 1988. "The nonrecurrent inferior laryngeal nerve: review of 33 cases, including two on the left side." Surgery 104 (6):977–984.
38. Donatini, G., B. Carnaille, and G. Dionigi. 2013. "Increased detection of non-recurrent inferior laryngeal nerve (NRLN) during thyroid surgery using systematic intraoperative neuromonitoring (IONM)." World Journal of Surgery 37 (1):91–93.
39. Toniato, Antonio, Renzo Mazzarotto, Andrea Piotto, Paolo Bernante, Costantino Pagetta, and Maria Rosa Pelizzo. 2004. "Identification of the nonrecurrent laryngeal nerve during thyroid surgery: 20-year experience." World Journal of Surgery 28 (7):659–661.
40. Hong, K. H., H. T. Park, and Y. S. Yang. 2014. "Characteristic travelling patterns of non-recurrent laryngeal nerves." The Journal of Laryngology and Otology 128 (6):534–539.
41. Virtual Pathology Museum. 2015. Pathweb online resource. Singapore: Department of Pathology, Yong Loo Lin School of Medicine, National University of Singapore, Singapore.
42. Rubén Harach, H. 2010. The parathyroid. New York, NY: Springer New York, 131–156
43. Cinti, Saverio, Andrea Sbarbati, Manrico Morroni, Vittorio Carboni, Carlo Zancanaro, Vincenzo Lo Cascio, and G. Richard Dickersin. 1992. "Parathyroid glands in primary hyperparathyroidism: an ultrastructural morphometric study of 25 cases." The Journal of Pathology 167 (3):283–290.
44. Roth, S. I., and C. C. Capen. 1974. "Ultrastructural and functional correlations of the parathyroid gland." International Review of Experimental Pathology 13:161.
45. Dufour, D. Robert, and Stephen Y. Wilkerson. 1982. "The normal parathyroid revisited: percentage of stromal fat." Human Pathology 13 (8):717–721.
46. Khan, Ashraf, Arthur S. Tischler, Nilima A. Patwardhan, and Ronald A. Delellis. 2003. "Calcitonin immunoreactivity in neoplastic and hyperplastic parathyroid glands: an immunohistochemical study." Endocrine Pathology 14 (3):249–255.
47. Kitazawa, Riko, Sohei Kitazawa, Masaaki Fukase, Takuo Fujita, Akira Kobayashi, Kazuo Chihara, and Sakan Maeda. 1992. "The expression of parathyroid hormone-related protein (PTHrP) in normal parathyroid: histochemistry and in situ hybridization." Histochemistry 98 (4):211–215.
48. Miettinen, M., R. Clark, V. P. Lehto, I. Virtanen, and I. Damjanov. 1985. "Intermediate-filament proteins in parathyroid glands and parathyroid adenomas." Archives of Pathology & Laboratory Medicine 109 (11):986–989.
49. Guerra, G., M. Cinelli, M. Mesolella, D. Tafuri, A. Rocca, B. Amato, S. Rengo, and D. Testa. 2014. "Morphological, diagnostic and surgical features of ectopic thyroid gland: a review of literature." International Journal of Surgery 12 (Suppl 1):S3–S11.
50. Topaloglu, A. K. 2006. "Athyreosis, dysgenesis, and dyshormonogenesis in congenital hypothyroidism." Pediatric Endocrinology Reviews 3 (Suppl 3):498–502.
51. Sohail, A. A., S. Shahabuddin, and M. I. Siddiqui. 2019. "Ectopic thyroid mass separately present in mediastinum and not a retrosternal extension: a report of two cases." Surgical Case Reports 2019:3821767.
52. Greening, W. P., S. K. Sarker, and M. P. Osborne. 1980. "Hemiagenesis of the thyroid gland." British Journal of Surgery 67 (6):446–448.
53. Randolph, Gregory. 2013. Surgery of the thyroid and parathyroid glands. 2nd ed. Philadelphia, PA: Saunders/Elsevier.
54. Scharpf, Joseph M. D. Facs, Natalia B. S. M. S. Kyriazidis, Dipti M. D. Kamani, and Gregory M. D. Facs Face Randolph. 2016. "Anatomy and embryology of the parathyroid gland." Operative Techniques in Otolaryngology – Head and Neck Surgery 27 (3):117–121.
55. Akerstrom, G., J. Malmaeus, and R. Bergstrom. 1984. "Surgical anatomy of human parathyroid glands." Surgery 95 (1):14–21.
56. Wang, C. 1976. "The anatomic basis of parathyroid surgery." Annals of Surgery 183 (3):271–275.
57. Nanka, O., P. Libánský, and J. Sedý. 2006. "Surgical-anatomical study as a part of operative treatment of primary hyperparathyroidism." Rozhl Chir 85:618–623.
58. Hojaij, F., F. Vanderlei, and C. Plopper. 2011. "Parathyroid gland anatomical distribution and relation to anthropometric and demographic parameters: a cadaveric study." Anatomical Science International 86:204–212.
59. Gomes, E. M., R. C. Nunes, and P. G. Lacativa. 2007. "Ectopic and extranumerary parathyroid glands location in patients with hyperparathyroidism secondary to end stage renal disease." Acta Cirúrgica Brasileira 22:105–109.
60. Uludag, M., A. Isgor, and G. Yetkin. 2009. "Supernumerary ectopic parathyroid glands. Persistent hyperparathyroidism due to mediastinal parathyroid adenoma localized by preoperative single photon emission computed tomography and intraoperative gamma probe application." Hormones (Athens) 8:144–149.
61. Pattou, F. N., L. C. Pellissier, and C. Noël. 2000. "Supernumerary parathyroid glands: frequency and surgical significance in treatment of renal hyperparathyroidism." World Journal of Surgery 24:1330–1334.
62. Zuckerkandl, E. 1902. "Nebst Bermerkungen uber die Epithelkorperchen des Menschen." Anatomische Hefte 61.
63. Gauger, Paul G., Leigh W. Delbridge, Norman W. Thompson, Patricia Crummer, and Thomas S. Reeve. 2001. "Incidence and importance of the tubercle of Zuckerkandl in thyroid surgery." European Journal of Surgery 167 (4):249–254.
64. Hisham, Abdullah N, and Mohd R. Lukman. 2002. "Recurrent laryngeal nerve in thyroid surgery: a critical appraisal." ANZ Journal of Surgery 72 (12):887–889.
65. Pelizzo, Maria Rosa, Antonio Toniato, and Giancarlo Gemo. 1998b. "Zuckerkandl's tuberculum: an arrow pointing to the recurrent laryngeal nerve (constant anatomical landmark)." Journal of the American College of Surgeons 187 (3):333–336.
66. Dohán, Orsolya, Antonio De la Vieja, Viktoriya Paroder, Claudia Riedel, Mona Artani, Mia Reed, Christopher S. Ginter, and Nancy Carrasco. 2003. "The sodium/iodide symporter (NIS): characterization, regulation, and medical significance." Endocrine Reviews 24 (1):48–77.

4

INVESTIGATIONS IN THYROID DISEASES
Imaging

Alka Ashmita Singhal

Introduction

Imaging forms the mainstay of management of thyroid disorders for both diffuse and focal thyroid pathologies. It is utilized in initial diagnosis, to monitor response to treatment and for follow-up. Commonest diagnostic modality utilized for thyroid imaging is ultrasound neck, with added color Doppler for the evaluation of vascularity. Ultrasound elastography is being used as an adjunct in diagnosis by providing the information regarding the stiffness of the tissue. Technetium-99m pertechnetate (99mTcO4−) scan and radioactive iodine are used to assess activity of the thyroid gland and to localize ectopic thyroid tissue. Contrast-enhanced computed tomography (CT) (CECT) or contrast-enhanced magnetic resonance imaging (MRI) (CEMRI) is valuable in cases of lesions extending beyond the thyroid or with the possibility of being extending beyond the thyroid. Positron emission tomography (PET) CT is advised in cases of suspected distant metastasis. Ultrasound-guided fine needle aspiration (FNA) and Bethesda cytopathology provides definitive diagnosis. The chapter aims to provide this information in a simple illustrative manner well understood by both novice and advanced professionals.

Ultrasound thyroid

Thyroid gland has been among the first organs to have been evaluated by ultrasound as early as in late 1960 [1]. Since then, with the further development of B mode imaging and with the advent of high-resolution transducers, there is been a phenomenal change in the quality of imaging and ability to detect tiny micronodular lesions. Using color Doppler the vascularity of gland can be assessed and is helpful in both diagnosis and monitoring response to treatment of thyroid disorders. Ultrasound elastography is used as an adjunct in diagnosis. Ultrasound-guided FNA biopsy improves diagnostic yield and accuracy.

Basic principles of ultrasound and common artifacts

Typical ultrasound equipment consists of a transducer containing a sensitive crystal, appropriate software, hardware, keyboard and a display screen. Medical ultrasound waves are sound waves in the frequency range of 2–20 MHz The basic principle guiding transducer selection is that higher the transducer frequency, better is the image resolution; however, depth penetration is limited with increasing transducer frequency [2, 3]. We use 9–12 MHz linear for most thyroid and neck scans, however, higher frequencies up to 16–18 MHz are used to evaluate further finer details of any pathology as required (Figure 4.1(a) and (d)). A lower frequency transducer such as 5–7 MHz or lower may be required to penetrate the depth of a large multinodular goiter. The ultrasound beam focus is adjusted to the area of interest for better image resolution.

Most modern transducers use piezoelectric crystals. Sound waves are emitted from the transducer due to vibration of the crystals with electric current, whereby electrical energy is converted into mechanical energy and sound energy. A coupling medium such as an ultrasound gel is used to make contact with the skin or mucosal surface and acts by overcoming the air barrier allowing the waves to enter the body and propagate through the different tissues. Part of these waves return to the transducer as reflected echoes. The way the sound waves are reflected between the various tissues is proportional to the difference in their impedance and forms the basis of image formation of the scanned area. The greater the difference in density or impedance between the tissues, more of the sound is reflected back and less is transmitted. If the difference in impedance between the two tissue surfaces is extremely high, example as in the case of a fluid-filled structure or soft tissue versus calcification, it leads to an almost complete reflection of the sound waves, with near negligible sound waves passing posterior to this area. This results in the area behind the calcifications appearing completely black due to acoustic shadowing or lack of insonation (Figure 4.2(a) and (b)).

If the area through which the sound waves travel is completely homogenous as in a fluid-filled structure such as a clear cyst or a blood vessel, the area appears uniformly black or anechoic. Often posterior acoustic enhancement is noted beyond the fluid-filled structures such as a simple cyst as compared to the adjacent parenchymatous tissue. This is due to less absorption of sound energy into the cystic area and more being transmitted as compared to adjacent parenchyma. Reverberating artifacts (Figure 4.3) are noted behind the sharp tracheal reflecting surface and behind the colloid particles. When identified, the tiny triangular comet-tail artifacts (Figure 4.4) behind the colloid particles are an important distinguishing feature between punctate echogenic foci seen in papillary thyroid cancer (Figure 4.5).

To assess vascularity of the tissue color, power and spectral Doppler are used. Color Doppler provides the information regarding the vascularity of the thyroid gland and other vascular structures. Appropriate machine settings are important for correct interpretation; the Doppler gain can be set using the common carotid vessels as a benchmark. Power Doppler has improved sensitivity to low flow; however, it is very prone to motion and flash artifacts [4]. Spectral Doppler allows for sampling of selected site and quantification of flow with various parameters such as peak systolic velocity, resistive index and pulsatility index. Peak systolic velocities in inferior thyroid arteries are higher (>40 cm/s) in patients with Graves' disease than in patients with thyroiditis [5]. This is especially valuable in Grave's disease when thyroid scintigraphy by technetium-99m (Tcm99) pertechnetate or iodine 123 radioisotopes is contraindicated, and the clinical disease is mild or subclinical.

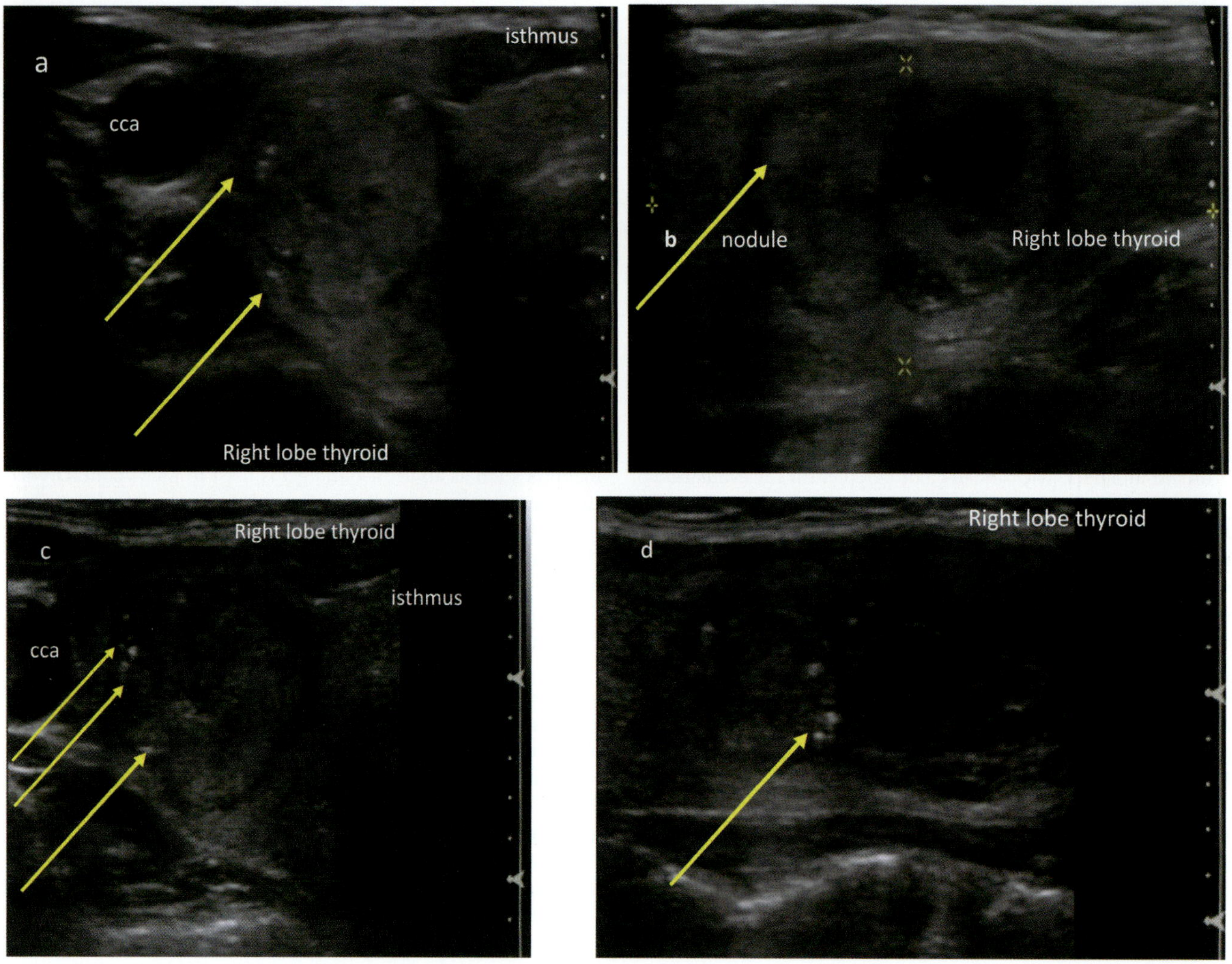

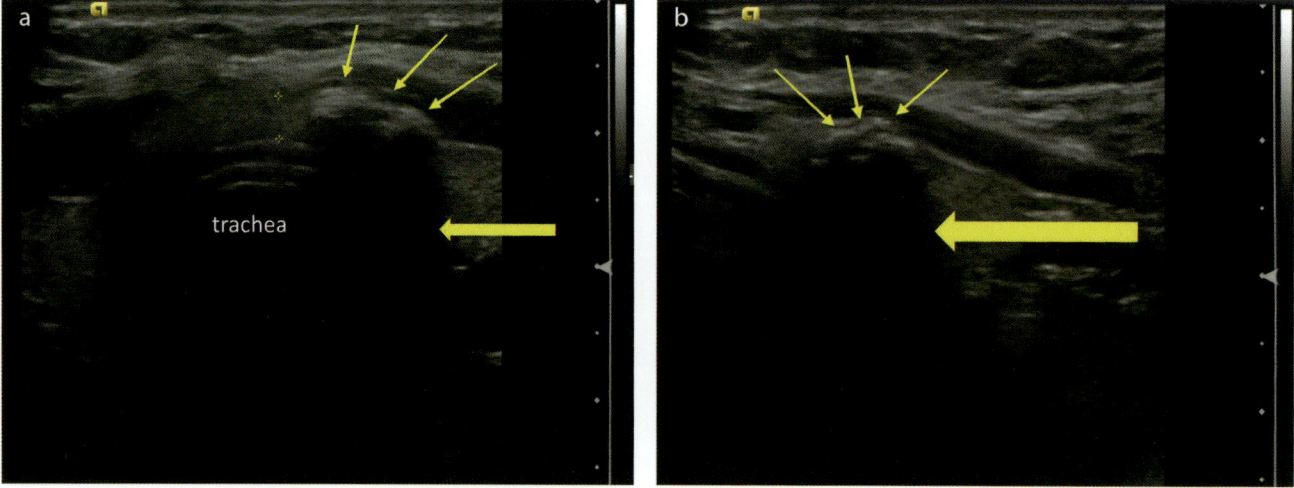

FIGURE 4.1 (a)–(d) Transverse and longitudinal scan of same heterogenous thyroid nodule with 9 MHz transducer in (a) and (b) and with 14 MHz transducer in image (c) and (d). There is increased contrast resolution of the image with higher frequency transducer and better delineation of the tiny punctate echogenic foci (arrows), and the lobulated nodule margins in this case of biopsy-proven papillary thyroid cancer.

FIGURE 4.2 (a) and (b) Transverse and longitudinal scan of isthmus showing posterior acoustic shadowing (long thick arrow) distal to a calcification in the isthmus (short thin arrow). As most of the sound is reflected back from dense calcifications, very less penetrates through, the area posterior to them is not insonated and appears dark or shadows.

Investigations in Thyroid Diseases

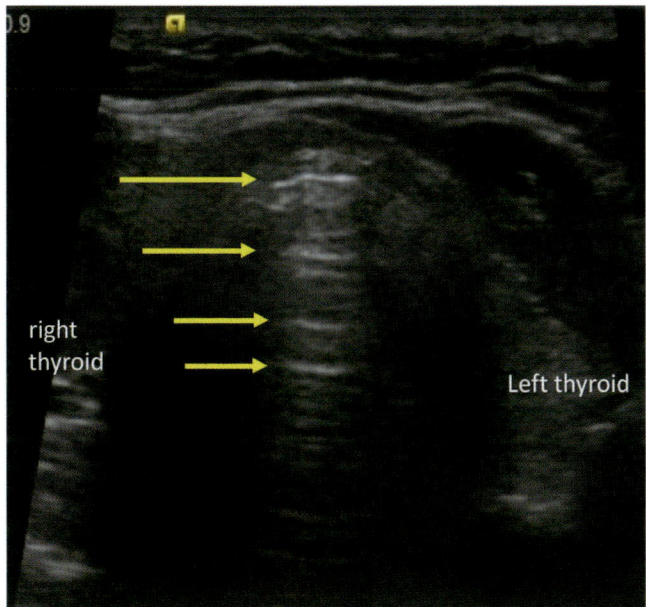

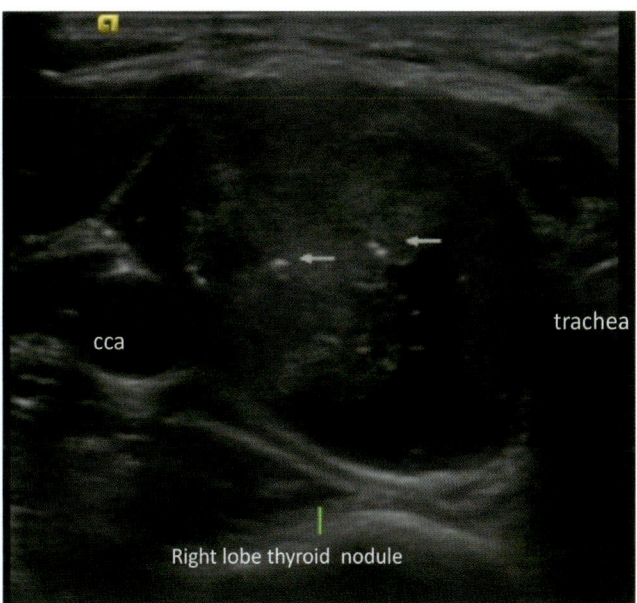

FIGURE 4.3 Reverberation artifacts (lower arrows) from the anterior wall of trachea (top arrow). These occur due to sound waves reflecting many times from a sharp acoustic interface (tracheal wall in this case) into the deeper tissues with diminishing intensity.

FIGURE 4.5 Tiny punctate echogenic foci (arrows) or microcalcifications that are seen in papillary thyroid carcinoma are due to the psammoma bodies. These do not show the comet-tail artifact or any posterior shadowing.

Ultrasound scanning technique and patient positioning

The patient is usually positioned in a supine position with a pillow placed under the neck to allow for slight extension of the neck. If that is not possible as sometimes in elderly patients or in children, the examination may be performed in supine position without the pillow or in sitting position. Patient is advised to refrain from swallowing or talking during the scan, unless required.

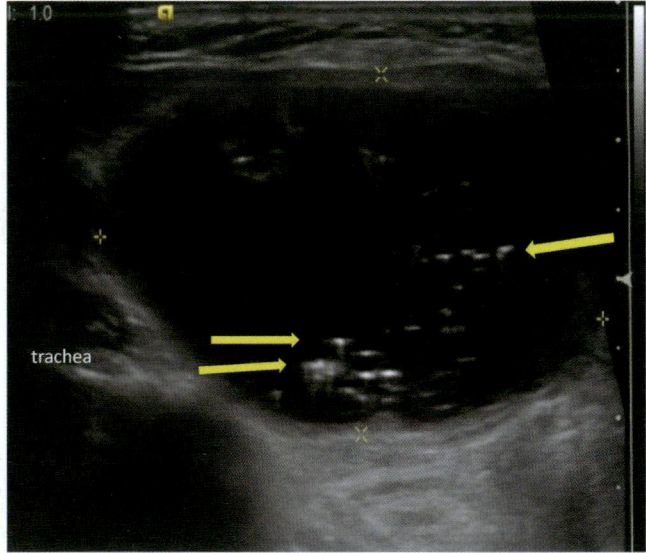

FIGURE 4.4 Comet-tail artifact – a type of reverberation artifact seen due to crystallization of the colloid which gives a tiny sharp interface and leads to a triangular tapering echo (arrows) as in this case of biopsy-proven colloid cyst.

Ultrasound anatomy of normal thyroid glands

Normal thyroid is an H-shaped bilobed gland located in anterior neck and connected by a narrow isthmus across the trachea. On gray-scale imaging, the normal thyroid parenchyma shows diffuse smooth homogenous hyperechoic echoes (Figure 4.6(a) and (b)). A thin rim of echogenic thyroid capsule can be appreciated in the peripheral part of the gland. The size, shape and volume of thyroid gland vary with the age and sex of the patient [6]. Normal adult thyroid gland measures 40–60 mm in longitudinal and 13–18 mm in anteroposterior (AP) dimensions.

The anterior strap muscles sternohyoid and sternothyroid along with sternocleidomastoid are seen anterolaterally and appear as hypoechoic structures. The carotid vessels along with internal jugular vein, vagus nerve and scalenus anterior muscles are seen poster laterally. Esophagus is seen posteriorly and is well identified with fluid and gas within and peristaltic activity. Arterial supply to thyroid is from the superior thyroid artery, a branch of external carotid artery and inferior thyroid artery, a branch of subclavian artery. Venous drainage is mainly to internal jugular vein. Thyroid has rich subcapsular and intrathyroidal lymphatic network. Metastasis from thyroid is commonly seen to level 6 and levels 2–4 cervical lymph nodes. The recurrent laryngeal nerve lies in the posterior relation to mid-part of the thyroid along with the inferior thyroid artery, and this is an important point in evaluation of pathologies in this area. Tubercle of Zuckerkandl may be seen as a pseudo mass in the posterior part of mid thyroid [7]. The superior parathyroid glands are usually located behind the mid thyroid around the crossing of the recurrent laryngeal nerve and inferior thyroid artery. The inferior parathyroid glands are located close to the lower pole of thyroid glands. The parathyroid glands are ectopic in location in approximately 15% cases [8].

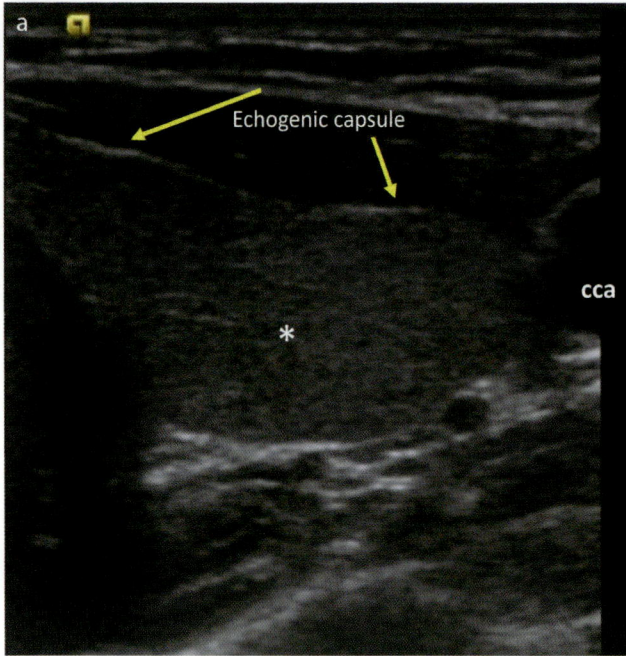
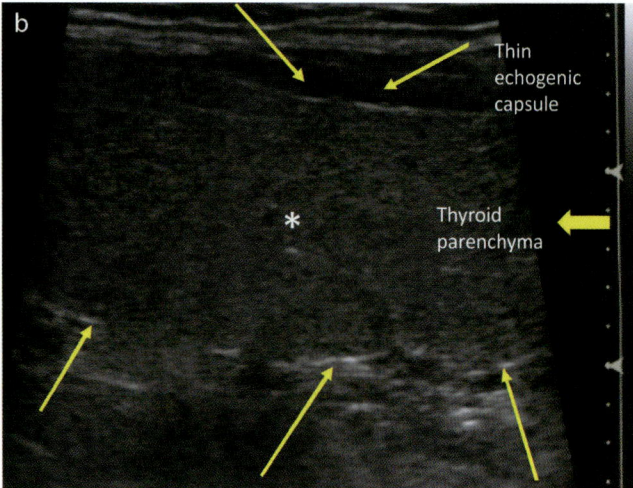

FIGURE 4.6 (a) and (b) Transverse and longitudinal sonogram of a normal thyroid gland showing diffuse smooth homogenous hyperechoic echoes in the parenchyma. Thin echogenic capsule is well seen at the periphery (denoted by thin arrows).

Ultrasound imaging in diffuse thyroid disorders

Evaluation of the background thyroid parenchyma is important and precedes detailed evaluation of any focal pathology [9]. Most common diffuse disorders are the chronic lymphocytic thyroiditis and Grave's disease. Chronic lymphocytic thyroiditis could be atrophic thyroiditis or Goitrous Hashimoto's thyroiditis. A diffuse or patchy decrease in echogenicity or hypoechoic echotexture of the gland (Figure 4.7(a)–(e)) demonstrated on ultrasound is highly suggestive of thyroiditis [10]. The decrease in echogenicity is due to an increase in the intrathyroidal blood flow, increased cellularity of the thyroid follicles with decreased colloid production and or due to lymphocytic infiltration. The decrease in echogenicity occurs even before the bio-clinical abnormality and correlates with the circulating level of thyroid antibodies [11], and, hence, stresses the importance of adequate evaluation of background thyroid parenchyma on gray-scale ultrasound. Associated reactive sub-centimeter hypoechoic level 6 lymph nodes are a common finding (Figure 4.8(a)–(c)).

Color Doppler and power Doppler show increased vascularity of the thyroid gland, often corresponding with the activity of the disease. The hypoechogenicity and the increased vascularity often return to normal with the resolution of the thyroiditis.

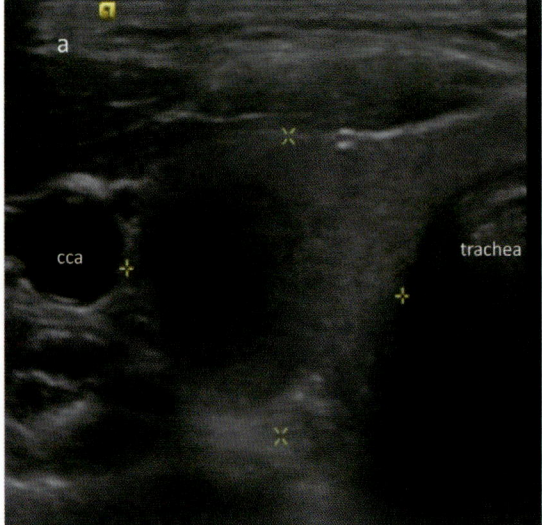
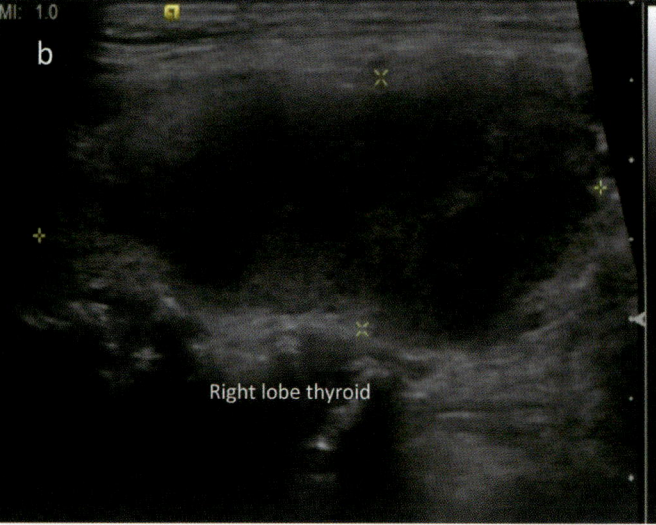

FIGURE 4.7 (a)–(e) Subacute thyroiditis: (a)–(d): Transverse and longitudinal scan of both right and left lobes of thyroid showing a diffuse patchy decrease in echogenicity of the thyroid gland. The echogenicity is almost as hypoechoic as the overlying anterior strap muscles. Image (e): color Doppler scan showing mild vascularity at the time of scan.

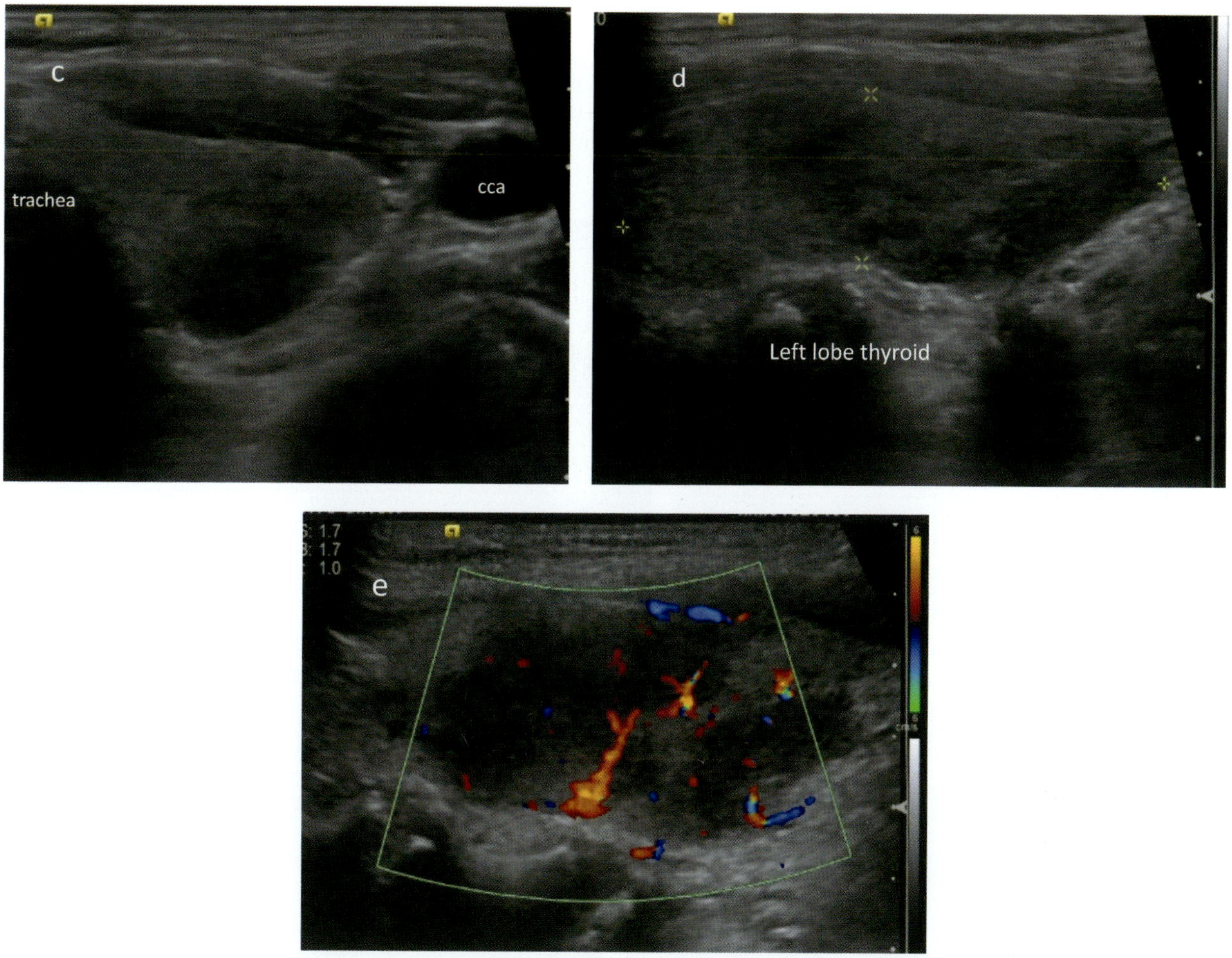

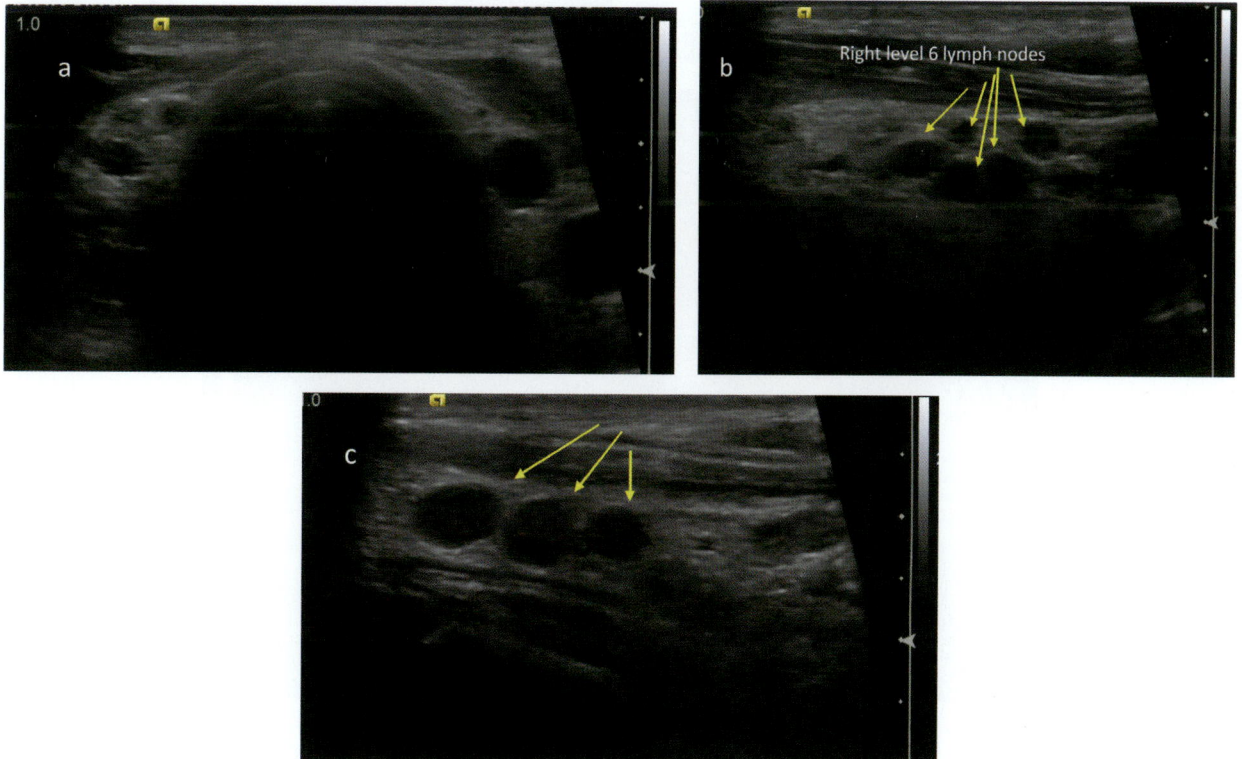

FIGURE 4.7 *(Continued)*

FIGURE 4.8 (a)–(c) Transverse and longitudinal scan at the region of right and left central compartment shows well-defined hypoechoic bilateral reactive level 6 lymph nodes (arrows).

If chronic thyroiditis ensues, the gland may show coarsened echotexture and thin echogenic strands due to fibrosis.

Graves' disease is an autoimmune disease of overactive thyroid gland due to autoantibodies to the TSH receptor that activates it and results also in overgrowth, i.e. diffusely enlarged goiter. It is the most common cause of thyrotoxicosis [12]. On ultrasound thyroid, gland is mildly enlarged with hypoechoic and slightly heterogeneous echotexture (Figure 4.9(a)–(e)).

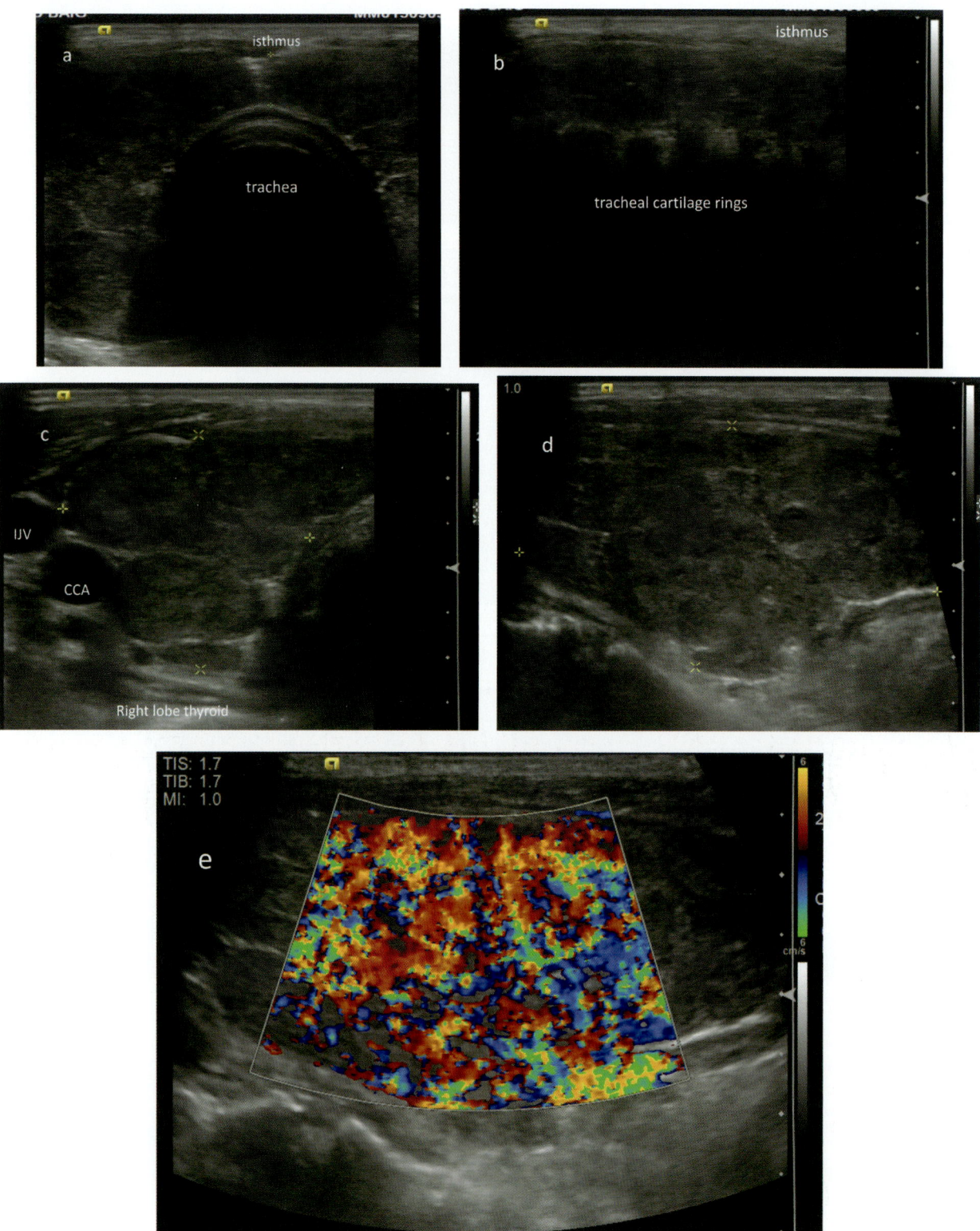

FIGURE 4.9 (a)–(e) A 35-year female with thyrotoxicosis. (a)–(d) Gray-scale ultrasound showing diffuse enlargement of both the lobe of thyroid and isthmus with decreased echogenicity with slightly heterogenous echotexture. The hypoechogenicity is similar to the overlying strap muscles. Image (e): Color Doppler ultrasound showing profound increase in vascularity of the thyroid, giving the appearance of "thyroid inferno".

Investigations in Thyroid Diseases

Ultrasound is required to evaluate size, echotexture, vascularity and nodules. A characteristic hypervascular; "thyroid inferno" pattern is noted on color Doppler in Graves thyrotoxicosis. Ultrasound is also used in evaluating response to treatment as the degree of hypoechogenicity and vascularity corresponds to the level of circulating antithyroid antibodies. Radionuclide scan with iodine-123 and 99mTcO4− classically demonstrates homogeneously increased activity in an enlarged thyroid gland in Grave's disease [13]. Autonomously functioning toxic nodule (AFTN) is an important differential diagnosis for the cause of thyrotoxicosis and is seen as a "hot nodule" on radionuclide imaging with suppression of the remaining thyroid parenchyma.

Hashimoto's thyroiditis

Hashimoto thyroiditis [14] also known as chronic lymphocytic thyroiditis or chronic autoimmune thyroiditis is a subtype of autoimmune thyroiditis. Patients are usually hypothyroid, although there may be a brief hyperthyroid early phase. Ultrasound features depend on the severity and phase of disease (Figure 4.10(a)–(c)).

Usually, the gland is diffusely enlarged with a heterogeneous echotexture. The presence of hypoechoic micronodules (1–6 mm) with surrounding echogenic septation is also considered to have a relatively high positive predictive value. Color Doppler usually shows normal or decreased flow, but rarely hypervascular flow may be seen. Associated enlarged reactive cervical nodes are often seen, especially in level VI. Larger thyroid nodules may be present in nodular Hashimoto thyroiditis. In long-standing cases, a typical nodular "Swiss-cheese" appearance is seen. There is a higher predisposition for papillary thyroid cancer in cases of Hashimoto's thyroiditis, and hence, thyroid nodules need to be carefully evaluated and suspicious nodules biopsied [15, 16]. Riedel thyroiditis typically presents as a hard goiter with compression symptoms on trachea and the inflammation extends beyond the thyroid gland to the adjacent tissues.

Ultrasound evaluation of focal thyroid nodules

A focal thyroid nodule is defined as an area of sonographic abnormality which is distinct from the remainder of thyroid parenchyma, irrespective of its size, shape and character. With the advent high-resolution ultrasound and large number of incidentalomas reported on CT and PET CT, there has been an increase in the reported incidence of thyroid nodules and thyroid cancer. Most thyroid nodules are benign. To screen out and select suspicious nodules for FNAC (FNA cytology) is still a challenge.

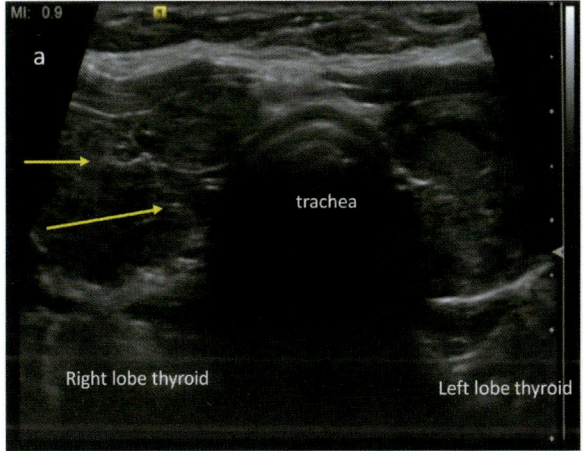
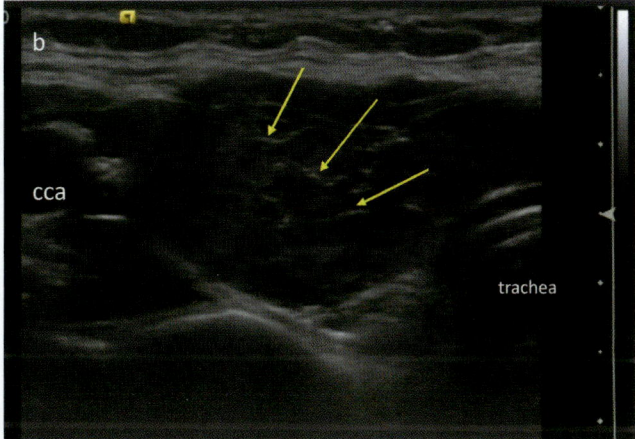
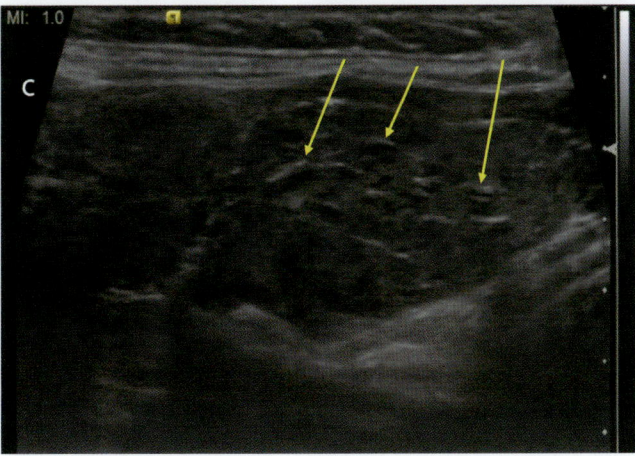

FIGURE 4.10 (a)–(c) Transverse and longitudinal sonogram with color Doppler in patient with long-standing hypothyroidism due to Hashimoto's disease showing the marked hypoechogenicity with echogenic fibrous septa (arrows) giving the gland a characteristic "Swiss-cheese" appearance.

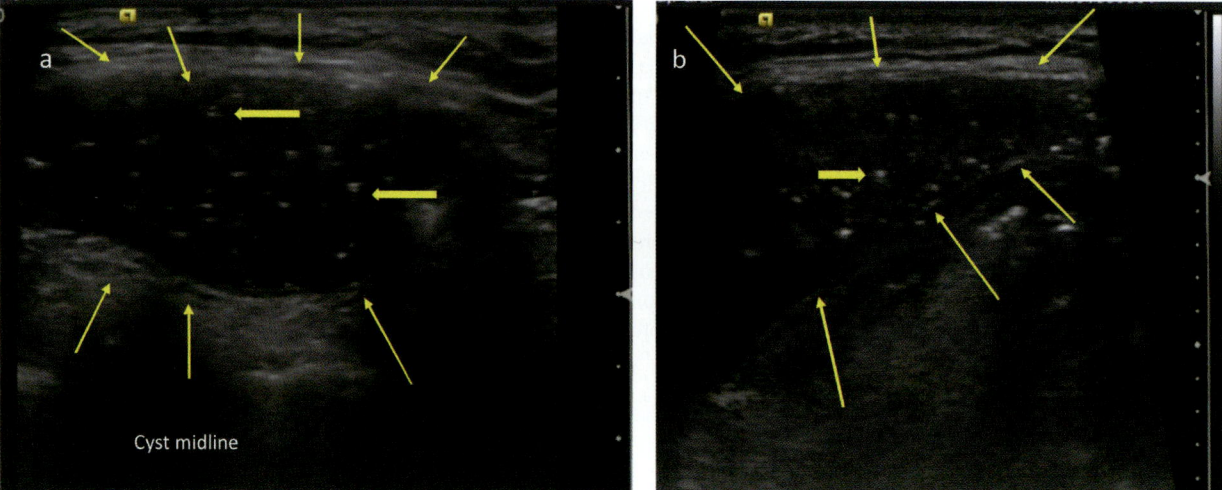

FIGURE 4.11 (a) and (b) Transverse and longitudinal sonogram of neck in a 22-year female who presented with a midline lump just at the level of hyoid bone. The swelling moved with deglutition. Corresponding area shows a well-defined hypoechoic cyst containing numerous echogenic foci with comet-tail artifacts, findings consistent with thyroglossal cyst.

Various criteria have been proposed in literature for evaluation of thyroid nodules and their subsequent management. The authors follow the ATA (American thyroid association) [17] guidelines along with ACR-TIRADS (American College of Radiology-Thyroid Imaging, Reporting and Data System) [18] for scoring and selecting thyroid nodules for FNA and management planning.

Thyroglossal cyst

A thyroglossal cyst [19] forms from the persistent thyroglossal duct and is one of the most frequent congenital cervical anomalies with a population prevalence of 7%. They are usually asymptomatic cystic mobile midline swellings (Figure 4.11(a) and (b). Associated malignancy risk in thyroglossal cyst is 1% and most commonly is papillary thyroid carcinoma. It is often reported on a postsurgery histopathology as an unexpected outcome. Adequate preoperative investigations must be done prior to surgery for thyroglossal cysts. Total thyroidectomy is advised in selected cases.

Colloid nodules and cysts

Colloid nodules, also known as adenomatous colloid goiter, include small colloid cysts to large nodules as seen in multinodular colloid goiter. These are composed of enlarged follicles containing abundant colloid and are seen as cystic or mixed cystic nodules. A typical comet-tail artifact is noted posterior to the colloid crystal aggregate (Figure 4.12(a) and (b)). The nodules may show areas of hemorrhage necrosis and calcification.

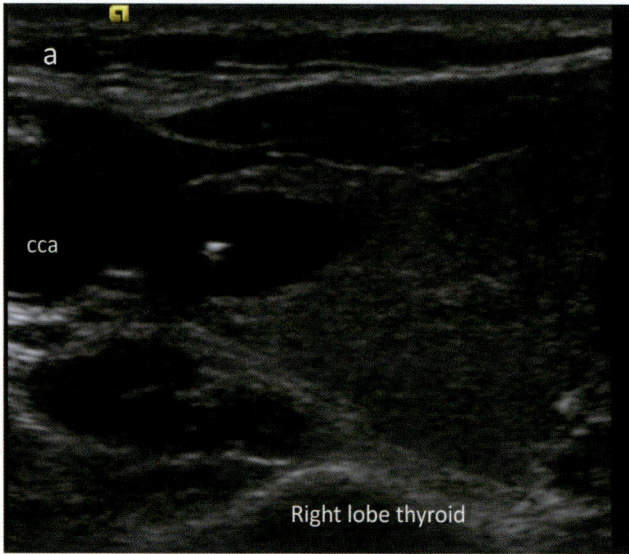
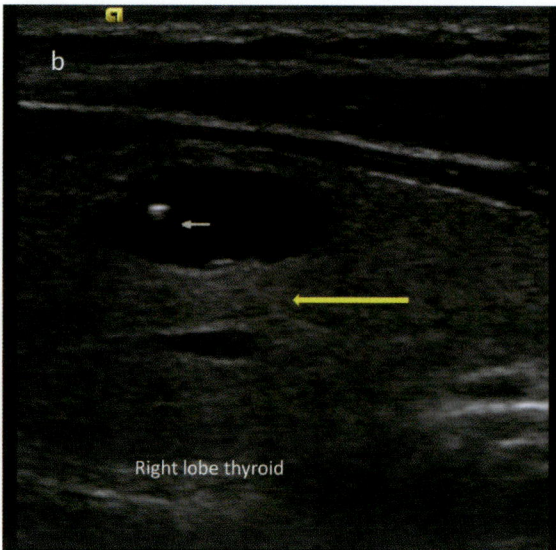

FIGURE 4.12 (a) and (b) Transverse and longitudinal sonogram of right lobe thyroid showing a well-defined anechoic cystic area with echogenic foci with a comet-tail artifact (short arrow). Posterior acoustic enhancement is noted distal to the cyst (long arrow).

Spongiform nodules

Spongiform nodules are defined as being composed of microcystic aggregates or clusters of more than 50% in an isoechoic nodule (Figure 4.13). They are also known as "honey comb" or "puff pastry" nodules. These are generally regarded as benign nodules and larger ones (>2 cm) may be followed up with ultrasound [20].

TIRADS scoring

TIRADS scoring (Table 4.1) is done by choosing the correct lexicon and then risk stratification is done to select the nodules for FNA or follow up depending on the size criteria and features. With multiple nodules, each nodule should be scrutinized for suspicious features and selected for FNA on the basis of sonographic features. Scoring is determined from five categories of ultrasound findings. The higher the cumulative score, the higher the TIRADS level and the likelihood of malignancy (Figures 4.14–4.18).

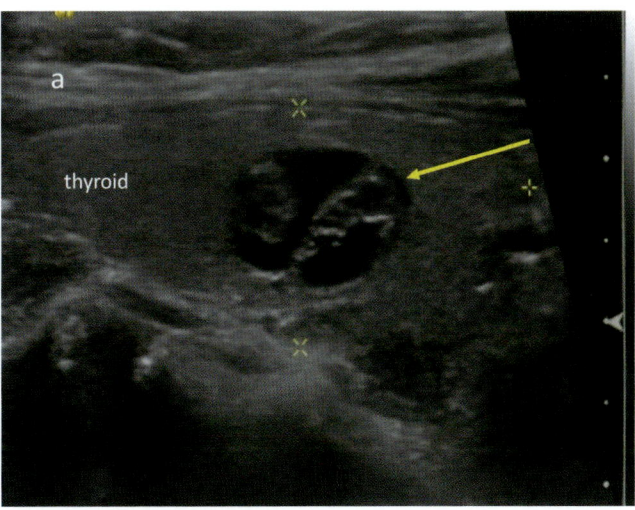

FIGURE 4.13 Longitudinal gray-scale sonogram showing a typical spongiform thyroid nodule consisting of aggregates of microcystic components of at least 50% of nodule volume. These nodules are benign and do not need any further investigations.

TABLE 4.1: (TIRADS Scoring)

Composition		Echogenicity		Shape		Margin		Echogenic Foci	
Cystic/almost completely cystic	0	Anechoic	0	Not taller than wide	0	Smooth	0	None	0
Spongiform	0	Hyperechoic	1	Taller than wide	3	Ill defined	0	Comet-tail artifact	1
Mixed cystic and solid	1	Isoechoic	1			Lobulated/irregular	2	Macrocalcification	1
Solid/almost completely solid	2	Hypoechoic	2			Extra thyroidal extension	3	Peripheral calcification	2
Cannot determine	2	Very hypoechoic	3			Not determined	0	Punctate echogenic foci	3

Cervical lymph node assessment, color Doppler evaluation and assessment are also to be done

TIRADS risk category

TR 1	0
TR 2	2
TR 3	3
TR 4	4–6
TR 5	>7

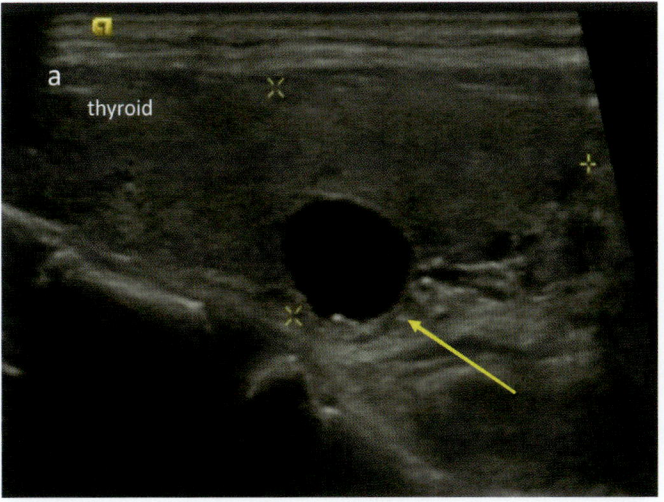
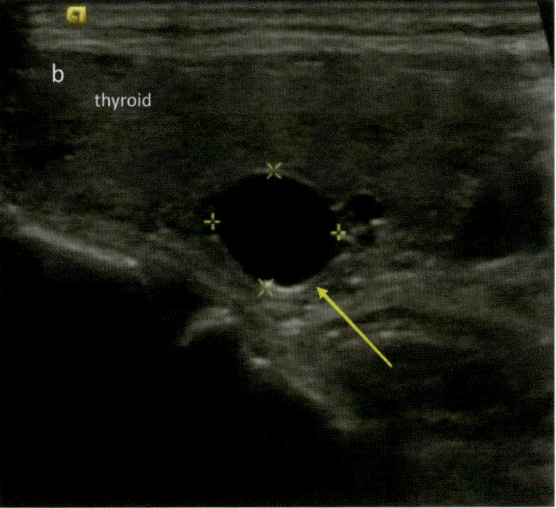

FIGURE 4.14 (a) and (b) Transverse and longitudinal scan gray-scale sonogram showing a well-defined clear anechoic thyroid cyst (arrow) TIRADS 1. No calcification or soft tissue component is seen within the cyst.

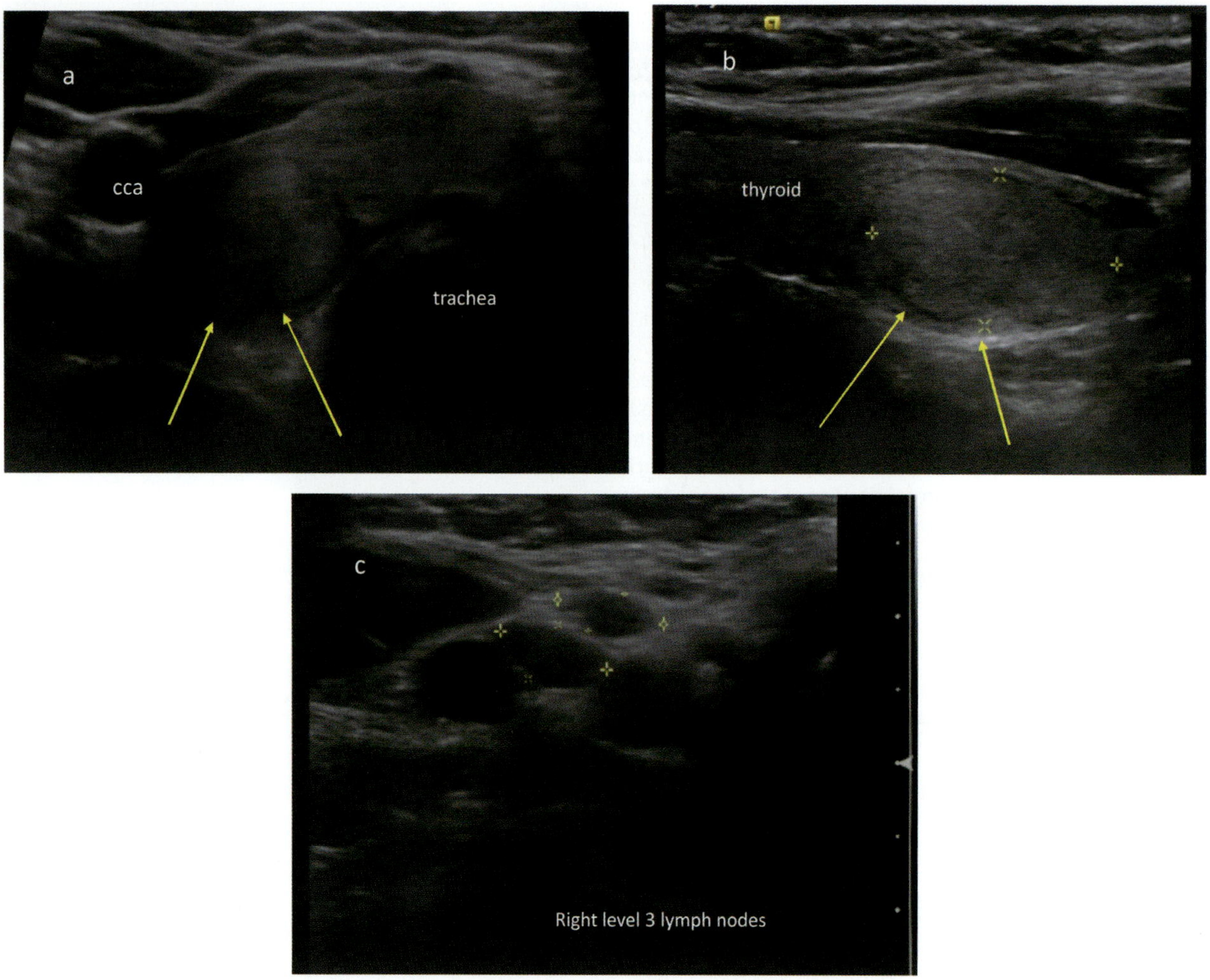

FIGURE 4.15 (a) and (b) Transverse and longitudinal sonogram of right thyroid gland showing a well-defined solid 17 mm × 10 mm iso to hypoechoic nodule with slightly indistinct and lobulated margins (arrows) TIRADS 3. FNAC showed Bethesda II – suggestive of benign follicular nodule. Patient underwent hemithyroidectomy, and the final histopathology reported was noninvasive follicular thyroid neoplasm with papillary like nuclear features (NIFTP). (c) The three lymph 3 nodes removed were free of tumor (0/3).

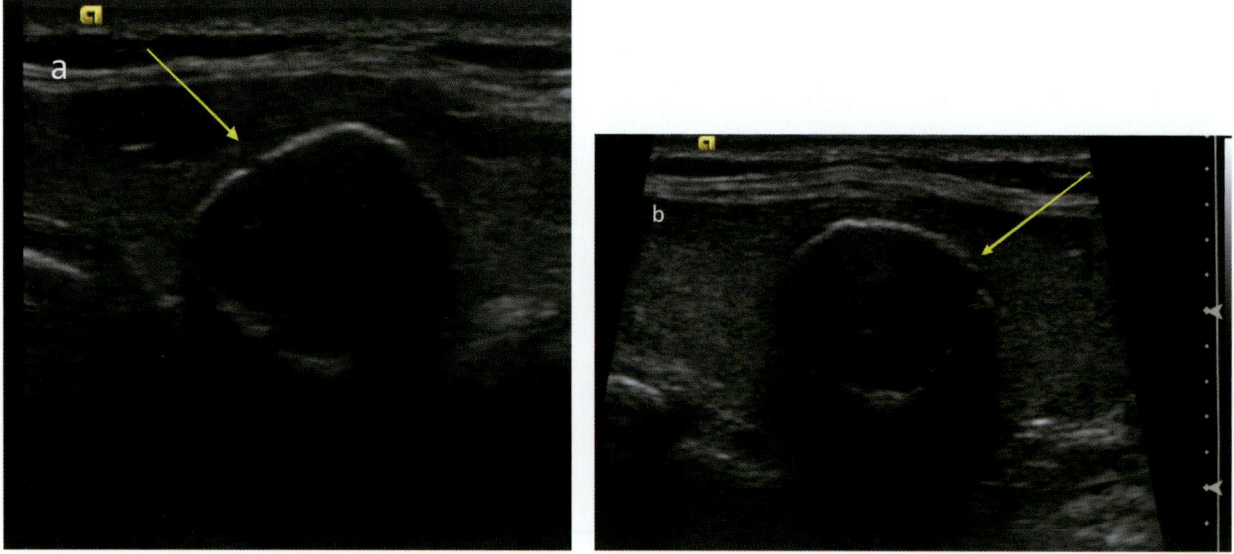

FIGURE 4.16 (a) and (b) Ultrasound neck showing a hypoechoic nodule with broken peripheral calcific rim (arrow) in the mid-part of the thyroid. Patient underwent hemithyroidectomy and the histopathology revealed follicular carcinoma.

Investigations in Thyroid Diseases

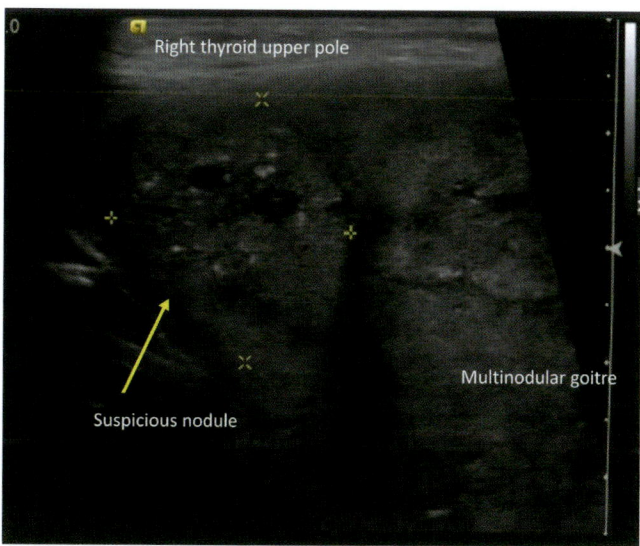

FIGURE 4.17 Longitudinal sonogram of a 45-year female with multinodular goiter showing a suspicious 22 mm × 23 mm heterogenous hypoechoic nodule at the upper pole of right thyroid containing multiple tiny punctate echogenic foci (arrows) TIRADS 5. Biopsy showed papillary thyroid cancer.

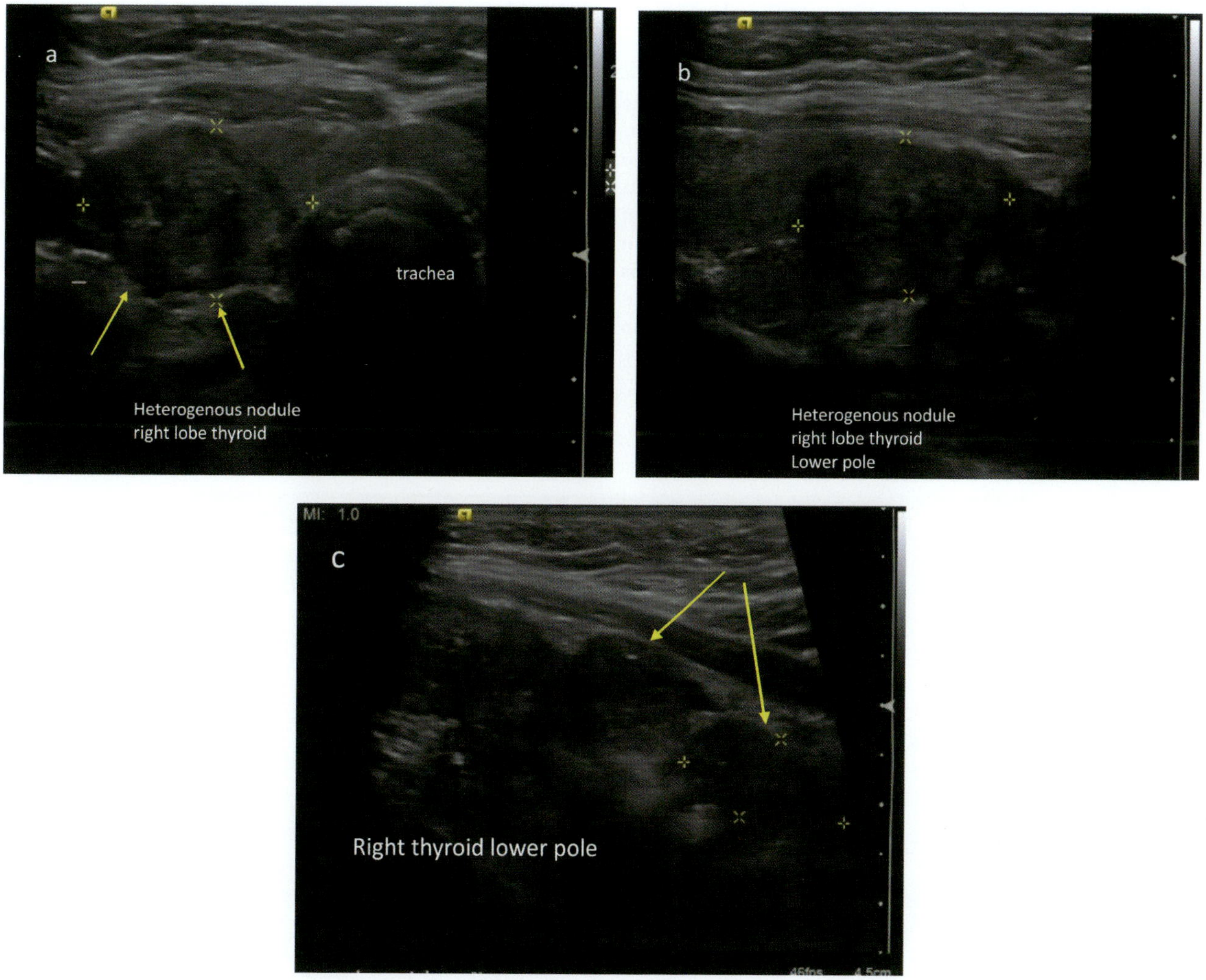

FIGURE 4.18 (a)–(c) Ultrasound thyroid transverse and longitudinal scan showing a heterogeneous hypoechoic solid right thyroid nodule (small arrows) with ill-defined/irregular margins and multiple tiny punctate echogenic foci TIRADS 5. Biopsy showed papillary carcinoma. Image c showing associated metastatic level 6 lymph nodes.

Each nodule is evaluated for its size; composition: [cystic/almost completely cystic (0), spongiform (0), mixed cystic and solid (1), solid/almost completely solid (2), cannot determine (2)]; echogenicity: [anechoic (0), hyperechoic (1), isoechoic (1), hypoechoic (2), very hypoechoic (3), cannot determine (1)]; shape: [not taller than wide (0), taller than-wide (3)]; margins: [smooth (0), ill-defined (0), lobulated/irregular (2), extrathyroidal extension (3), cannot determine (0)]; echogenic foci: [none (0), large comet-tail artifacts (0), macrocalcifications (1), peripheral calcifications (2), punctate echogenic foci (3)]. Thorough cervical lymph node assessment is done. Color Doppler to assess vascularity and elastography to assess the stiffness of the nodules is done. Correlation with cytopathology and Bethesda scoring is done. TIRADS risk category: [TR1 (0 points), TR2 (2 points), TR3 (3 points), TR4 (4–6 points), TR5 (≥7 points)] The recommendations for FNA/follow-up as per size and TIRADS [24] category are then followed.

TIRADS 1 nodules include the clear cystic nodules (Figure 4.14(a) and (b)) with or without comet-tail artifacts and the spongiform nodules. No further investigation is advised for these nodules.

Role of elastography

Ultrasound elastography [21, 22] measures tissue elasticity or stiffness, which is in turn used as an adjunct to characterize the lesions. The technique involves application of a small mechanical force during scanning and the degree of distortion is used to estimate the stiffness of the tissue of interest (Figure 4.19) and is accordingly color coded as per manufacturer. Soft tissues deform more than hard tissues. There are various studies on its role in predicting malignancy; however, currently it is being used as an adjunct in both thyroid nodule and lymph node assessment. The main role is to indicate which nodules may be followed up without resorting to FNA or surgery because of its high negative predictive value (NPV) especially in patients who have nondiagnostic or indeterminate FNA cytology results.

Follicular neoplasm

Follicular neoplasms account for 15% of thyroid cancer are the second most common type after papillary thyroid cancer. Follicular neoplasms include benign follicular hyperplasia, follicular adenoma, follicular thyroid carcinoma (FTC), follicular variant of papillary thyroid cancer (PTC) and Hurthle cell neoplasms. Peak age of onset is 40–60 years and has a female preponderance in the ratio of 3:1. Prognosis depends on the tumor size and is better for <1 cm lesion. Vascular invasion is common leading to distant metastasis, commonly to lung and bone. On ultrasound, most follicular neoplasms are usually well-defined predominantly solid iso to hypoechoic homogenous nodules with often a complete halo or slightly indistinct margins (Figure 4.20(a)–(c)). Hurthle cell neoplasms may show slightly heterogenous echotexture with both hyperechoic and hypoechoic components. They have ill-defined margins and an indistinct halo [23]. Ultrasound-guided FNA and Bethesda cytopathology is advised; however, it is not reliable in distinguishing between follicular adenoma versus carcinoma (which is based on the presence of capsular or vascular invasion). The current recommendation is resection of biopsy-proven follicular neoplasms to exclude malignancy. Postoperative radioactive iodine treatment is often advised and follow-up is done with thyroglobulin levels.

Papillary thyroid carcinoma (PTC)

Papillary thyroid carcinoma is the most common differentiated thyroid cancer (DTC) and accounts for 60–70% of thyroid cancers. Peak age of onset is 30–50 years and has a female preponderance of 3:1. Ultrasound appearances range from solid to mixed solid cystic or cystic mass lesions, usually hypoechoic and with irregular or indistinct margins. Often characteristic tiny punctate echogenic foci (Figure 4.21(a) and (b) are seen and these are due to psammoma bodies and these have a very high sensitivity and specificity for papillary thyroid cancer [24].

Lymphatic spread is common, usually to level 3, level 4 and central compartment lymph nodes. Cervical metastasis is seen at

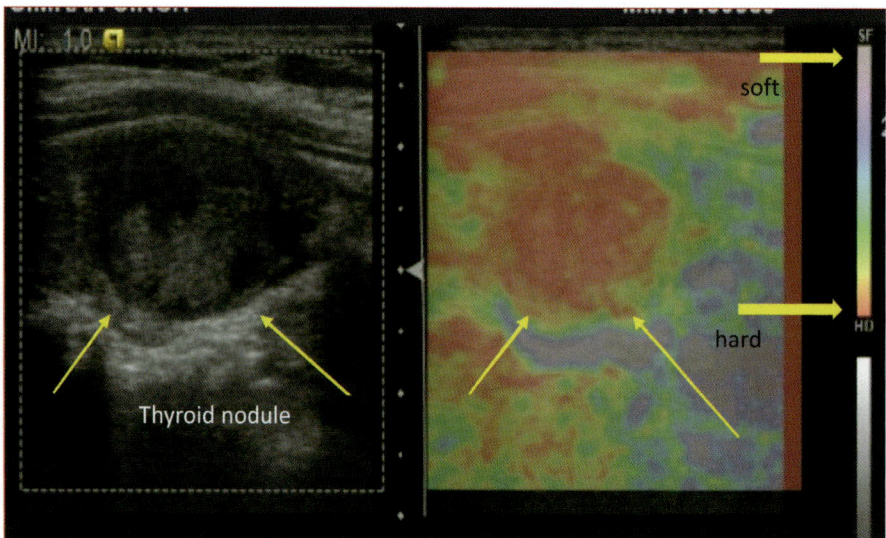

FIGURE 4.19 Longitudinal scan showing a heterogeneous hypoechoic nodule with lobulated margins (thin arrows). Corresponding real-time qualitative elastogram showing the lesion in the red zone, suggesting a moderately stiff to hard nodule (thick arrows), suggesting malignancy on elastography. FNA showed Bethesda V, papillary thyroid carcinoma.

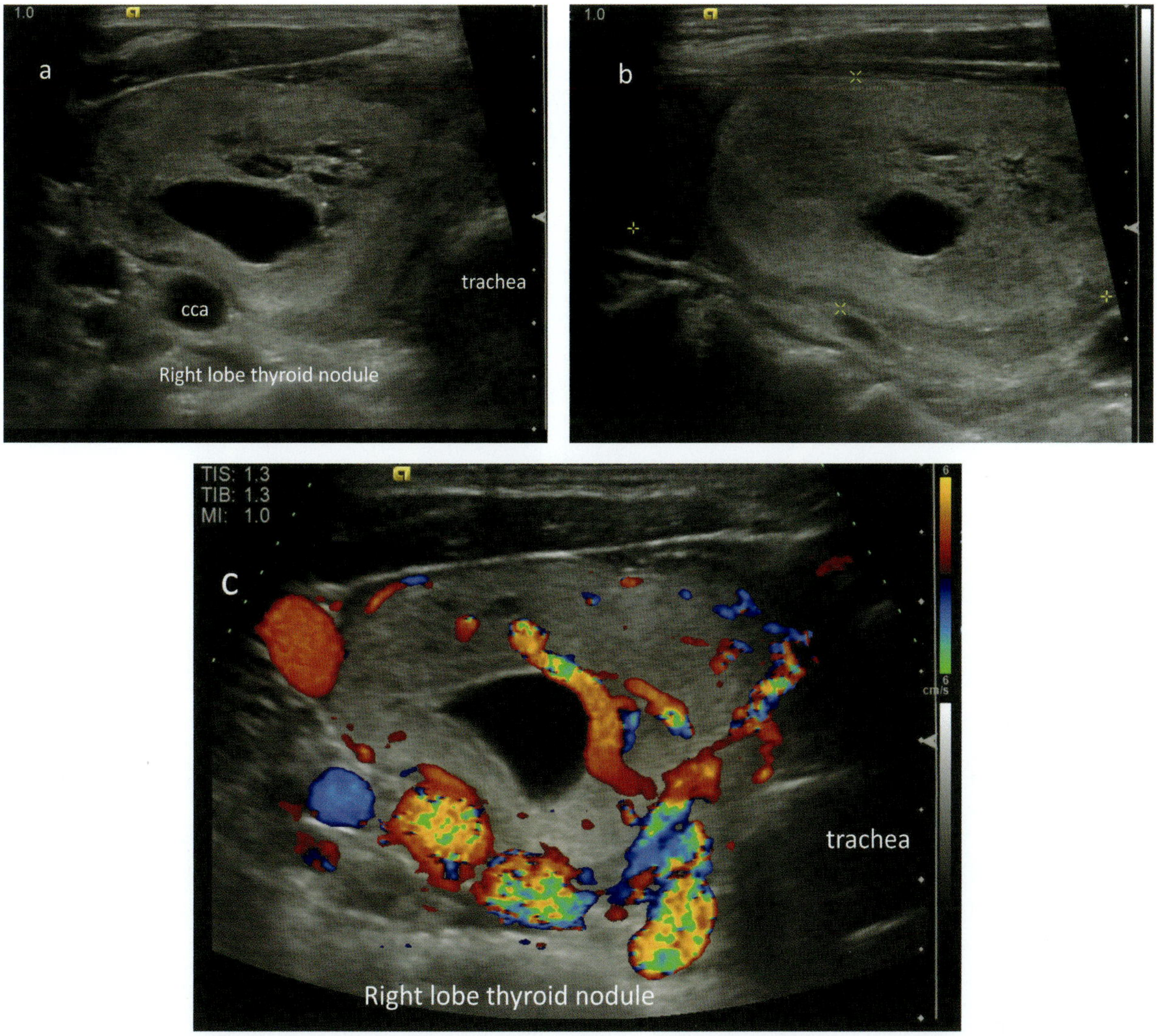

Investigations in Thyroid Diseases

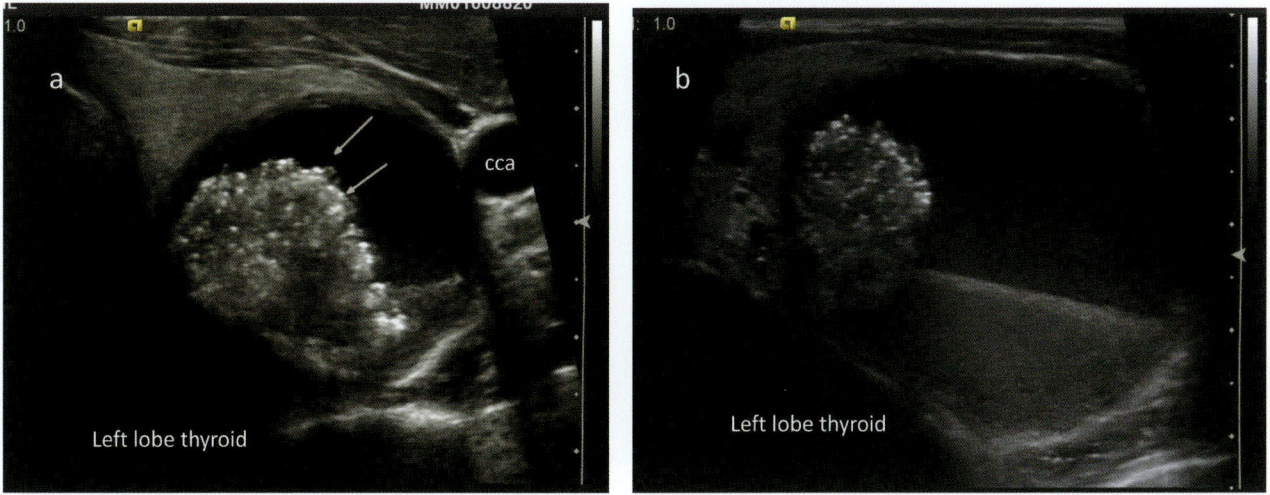

FIGURE 4.20 (a)–(c) Transverse and longitudinal sonogram with color Doppler showing a well-defined predominantly solid iso to hypoechoic nodule in right lobe thyroid. TIRADS 3. On color Doppler peripheral and mild central vascularity is seen. Biopsy showed follicular adenoma.

FIGURE 4.21 (a) and (b) Transverse and gray-scale sonogram of left lobe thyroid showing a large heterogenous hypoechoic mixed solid cystic nodule with eccentric soft tissue containing numerous punctate echogenic foci. Layering of fluid contents is noted within the lesion. Biopsy Bethesda V – Papillary thyroid cancer.

presentation in about 50–75% cases. The metastatic lymph nodes often show cystic change and punctate echogenic foci. PTC has the ability to invade the adjacent structures and extrathyroidal extension can be seen in lesions located close to the thyroid capsule. The authors report here a case 33-year female with a lump in right upper neck at the level of hyoid cartilage, on ultrasound this showed as a heterogenous calcific mass within the strap muscles of anterior neck (Figure 4.22(a)–(e)). FNA confirmed PTC. Distant metastasis is mainly to lung and bone. Mainstay of management is surgery followed by radioactive iodine in select cases.

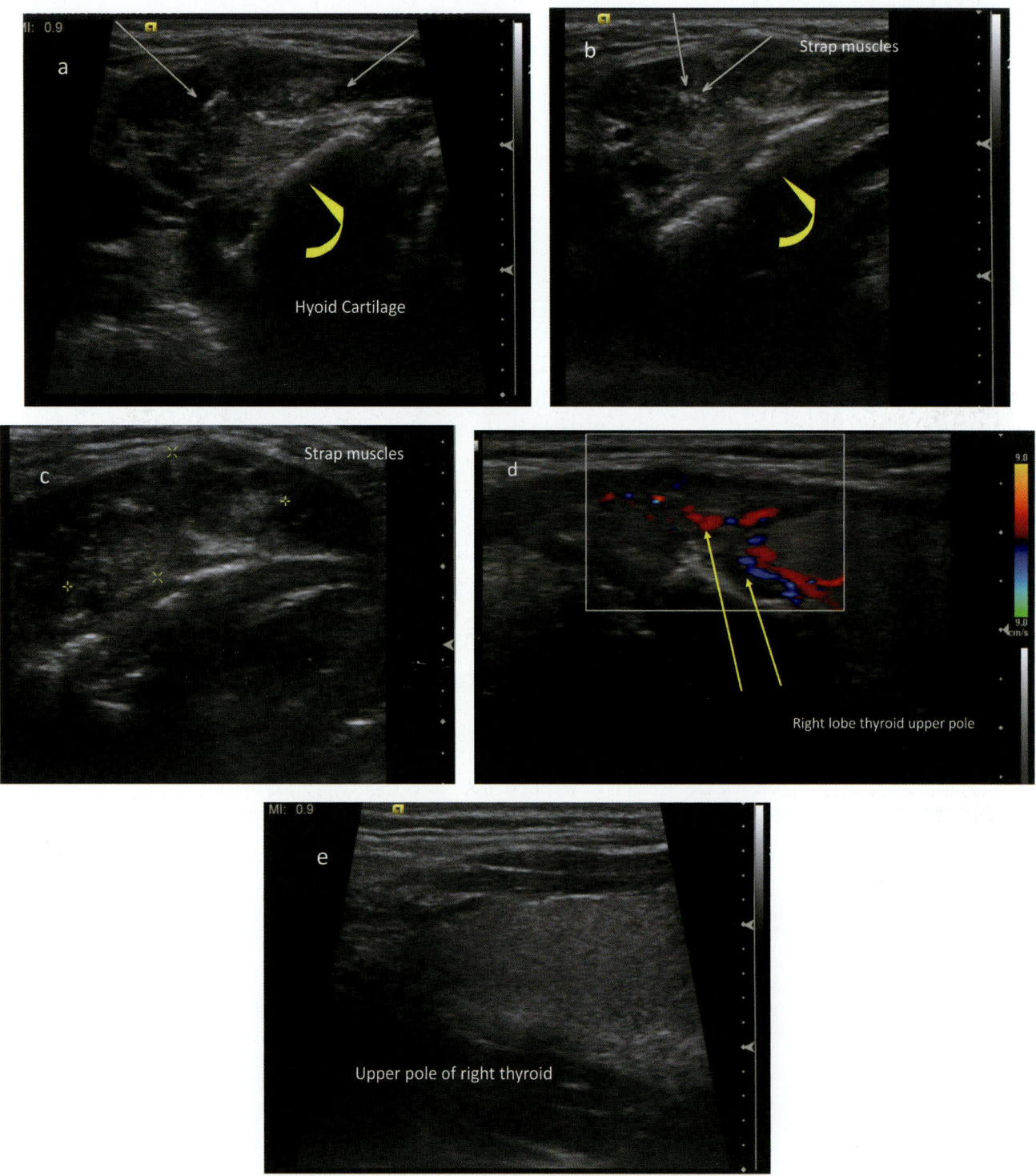

FIGURE 4.22 (a)–(e) A 39-year female presented with a palpable lump in right upper anterior neck, corresponding to a heterogenous hypoechoic lesion of size 15 mm × 8 mm in the right strap muscle at the level of hyoid, just above the upper lobe of right thyroid. Tiny punctate echogenic foci are seen within the lesion (arrows). Biopsy showed papillary thyroid cancer. No lesion was demonstrated in either thyroid glands on ultrasound; however, prominent vessels were noted leading to the lesion from the upper pole of thyroid.

Investigations in Thyroid Diseases

Papillary thyroid microcarcinoma (PTMC)

Papillary thyroid microcarcinoma (PTMC) is a subtype of PTC where the tumor size is less than 10 mm diameter [25, 26]. It is one of the most common thyroid malignancies with an increasing prevalence. The prognosis is generally good. Multicentric and bilateral PTMC with size >5 mm are treated aggressively with lymph node dissection along with thyroidectomy. Clinical presentation of PTMC is usually silent and is often noted incidentally on thyroidectomy specimens done for other purposes or may present with palpable metastatic cervical lymph nodes. These are often called occult PTMCs (Figure 4.23(a)–(e)).

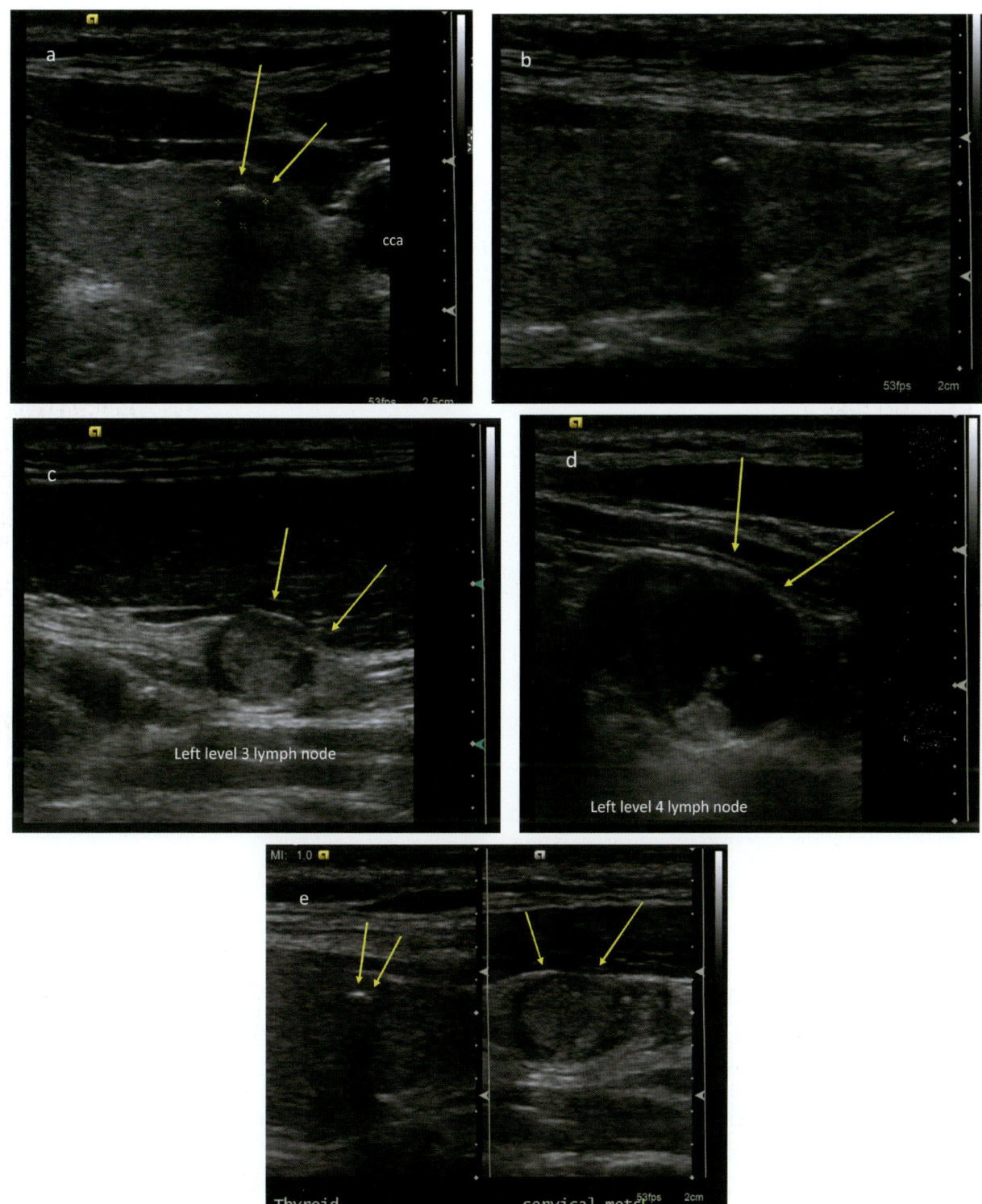

FIGURE 4.23 (a)–(e) Papillary thyroid microcarcinoma (PTMC): Transverse and longitudinal gray-scale sonogram of thyroid and neck in a 45 years male who presented with palpable neck lump and biopsy-proven metastatic papillary thyroid cancer (level 3 and level 4 heterogenous hypoechoic cervical lymph nodes with cystic changes and calcification). The primary calcific lesion in left lobe measured 3.2 mm × 2.6 mm on ultrasound and on postoperative histopathology a corresponding 2 mm focus of microcarcinoma was confirmed.

Medullary carcinoma thyroid (MTC)

Medullary thyroid cancer originates from the parafollicular C cells which secrete calcitonin. MTC is the rarest of all thyroid cancers amounting to 3–4% of all thyroid cancers [27]. MTC is sporadic in 75% case. Inherited MTC is associated with MEN type 2A and 2B syndromes and is carried by a change in the RET gene. MEN2A is also called Sipple syndrome and has 90% risk of having MTC and 50% risk of having pheochromocytoma. Associated hyperparathyroidism may be seen. MEN2B is also called Wagenmann-Froboese syndrome or MEN3 and has a 100% risk of having MTC and 50% risk of having pheochromocytoma. Associated mucosal ganglioneuromas may be seen. Non-MEN familial MTC is also seen [28]. Regional metastasis to cervical lymph nodes is early and patients usually present with a lump in the neck. Symptoms of chemical diarrhea (due to excess calcitonin and prostaglandins) may be noted. Ultrasound features of MTC are similar to any malignant thyroid nodule, appearing as hypoechoic nodules with increased vascularity and calcifications. Metastatic cervical lymph nodes often show similar calcifications and increased vascularity. Distant metastasis is to lungs, bone, liver and rarely to brain. PET CT is required in select cases to evaluate complete extent of the disease. Management is a combination of surgery followed by radiation therapy, chemotherapy and targeted therapy. Follow-up is done by serum calcitonin and carcinoembryonic antigen (CEA) levels.

Anaplastic thyroid carcinoma (ATC)

Anaplastic thyroid carcinoma (ATC) [29] is an undifferentiated high-grade carcinoma and most aggressive thyroid malignancy accounting for less than 2% of all thyroid cancers. Patients are usually elderly with mean age at presentation of 70 years with female preponderance in the ratio of 2:1. It presents as a rapidly enlarging large firm neck mass with symptoms of dyspnea, dysphagia and hoarseness of voice due to involvement of adjacent structures. Local and distant metastasis (lung, bone and brain) are seen at presentation. On ultrasound, a large ill-defined heterogenous hypoechoic firm mass lesion is seen with extra thyroidal extension. Differential diagnosis is from primary thyroid lymphoma (PTL). The prognosis of anaplastic carcinoma is poor and the disease is fatal if unresectable. Management is with multimodality therapy along with surgery.

Thyroid lymphoma

Thyroid lymphoma [30] represents 5% of thyroid malignancies. Non-Hodgkin's lymphoma is the commonest and may be primary as with preexisting Hashimoto's thyroiditis or secondary to generalized lymphoma. On ultrasound, they may be seen as focal or multiple hypoechoic nodules with or without associated cervical lymphadenopathy. Extrathyroidal extension may be seen.

Metastasis to thyroid

Non-thyroid metastasis [31] to thyroid is rare and represents 1.4–3% of all malignancies, the commonest primary being renal cell carcinoma. In autopsy series, most common primary reported has been lung cancer.

Role of computed tomography (CT) and magnetic resonance imaging (MRI)

Normal thyroid parenchyma has homogenous high attenuation CT values as compared to strap muscles and shows homogenous contrast enhancement owing to its hypervascularity. Focal and diffuse thyroid abnormalities are commonly encountered on CT and MRI scans done for various clinical purposes. These incidental thyroid abnormalities pose a diagnostic dilemma as the appearances on CT are nonspecific. Incidentalomas of thyroid have varied appearances such as calcific foci or subtle hypoechoic nodules or gland enlargement (Figure 4.24(a)–(c)). Ultrasound correlation is advised for its better spatial resolution and detailed evaluation and appropriate management. Primary indications of CT and MRI are large masses in neck such as multinodular goiter or large malignant thyroid or lymph nodal mass, where CT or MRI is advised to assess the extent of pathology, its mass effect, invasion and recurrence.

Positron emission tomography (PET) scan

PET [32, 33] is a highly sensitive, low invasive technology for cancer biology imaging. Cancer cells being metabolically more active than normal cells, preferentially take up glucose to a higher degree than normal cells. PET/CT with the use of radiolabelled glucose (18F-2-fluoro-2-deoxy-d-glucose, FDG) is well established in cases of DTC particularly in patients presenting with elevated thyroglobulin levels.

Ultrasound surveillance in a postthyroidectomy patient

Apart from bioclinical follow-up in postoperative cases (example with thyroglobulin in cases of PTC), imaging has a definite role in postoperative surveillance. The common modalities utilized are ultrasound, CT and FDG PET.

In a postthyroidectomy patient, the normal thyroid fossa appears devoid of any heterogenous hypoechoic echoes, and any suggestion of the same should be evaluated further with color Doppler and ultrasound-guided FNA to exclude recurrence (Figure 4.25(a)–(d)).

Southeast Asian perspective in thyroid disorders

The prevalence of large multinodular goiters around the globe is largely related to endemicity of iodine deficiency and can be as high as up to 80% in areas of iodine deficiency in Southeast Asia, South America and Africa [34]. While the iodine deficiency and large multinodular goiters commonly coexist with areas of poor socioeconomic development and mountainous terrain, their prevalence is not restricted to areas with such conditions. Southeast Asian countries primarily affected are India, Pakistan, Bangladesh, Tibet, Myanmar, Thailand, Indonesia and parts of southwestern China and pacific island countries. Large multinodular goiters are seen to be endemic in

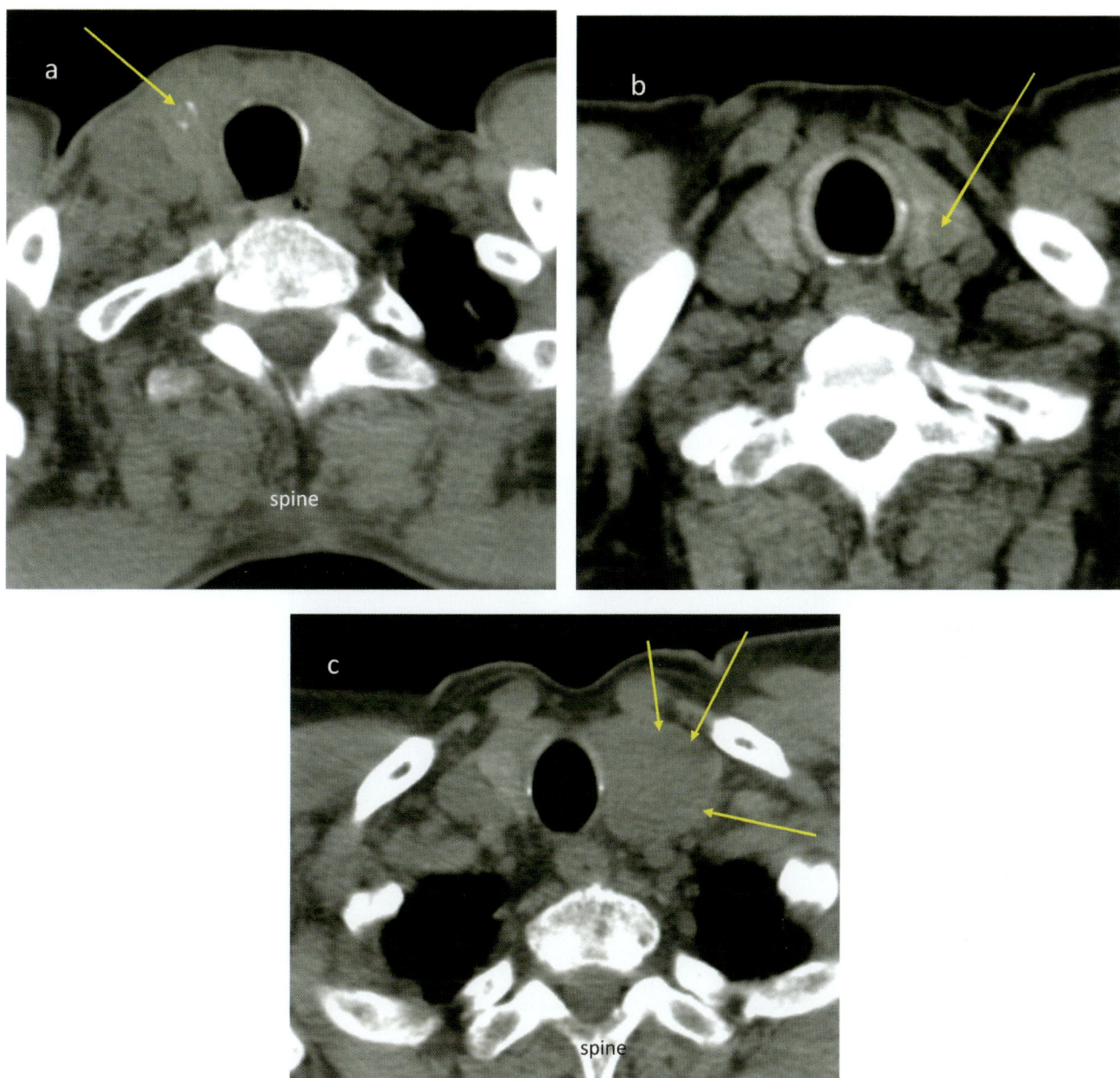

FIGURE 4.24 (a)–(c) Various incidental thyroid nodules (arrows) noted on computed tomography. Image (a) showing a calcific nodule in right lobe, image (b) showing a hypoechoic nodule in left lobe and image (c) showing an enlarged left lobe thyroid.

the hilly parts of the Himalayan region and in parts of central and southern India.

Management of large multinodular goiters is a challenge both for the anesthetist and the operating surgeon and is associated with increased risk of complications and patient morbidity [35]. Ultrasound evaluation of each and every nodule in the thyroid for any suspicious features of malignancy needs to be done very meticulously. Application of appropriate ultrasound techniques and use of transducers with variable frequency and depth penetration is often required to achieve a good image resolution, and appropriate modifications in the technique must be adopted to improve diagnostic outcomes. Comprehensive preoperative imaging by CT is recommended to evaluate the complete extent of the goiter into the neck and mediastinum and identify its anatomical relations with the surrounding structures to aid in surgical planning and preoperative patient counseling.

Conclusion

Imaging forms the fundamental basis of diagnosis and management of various thyroid pathologies. Choice of modality depends on the indication, clinical scenario, age of the patient and various other factors. Authors have aimed to give a comprehensive review with special emphasis on ultrasound imaging, as it is the modality of choice for thyroid gland evaluation. When indicated further additional imaging and appropriate investigations must be advised to improve patient outcomes.

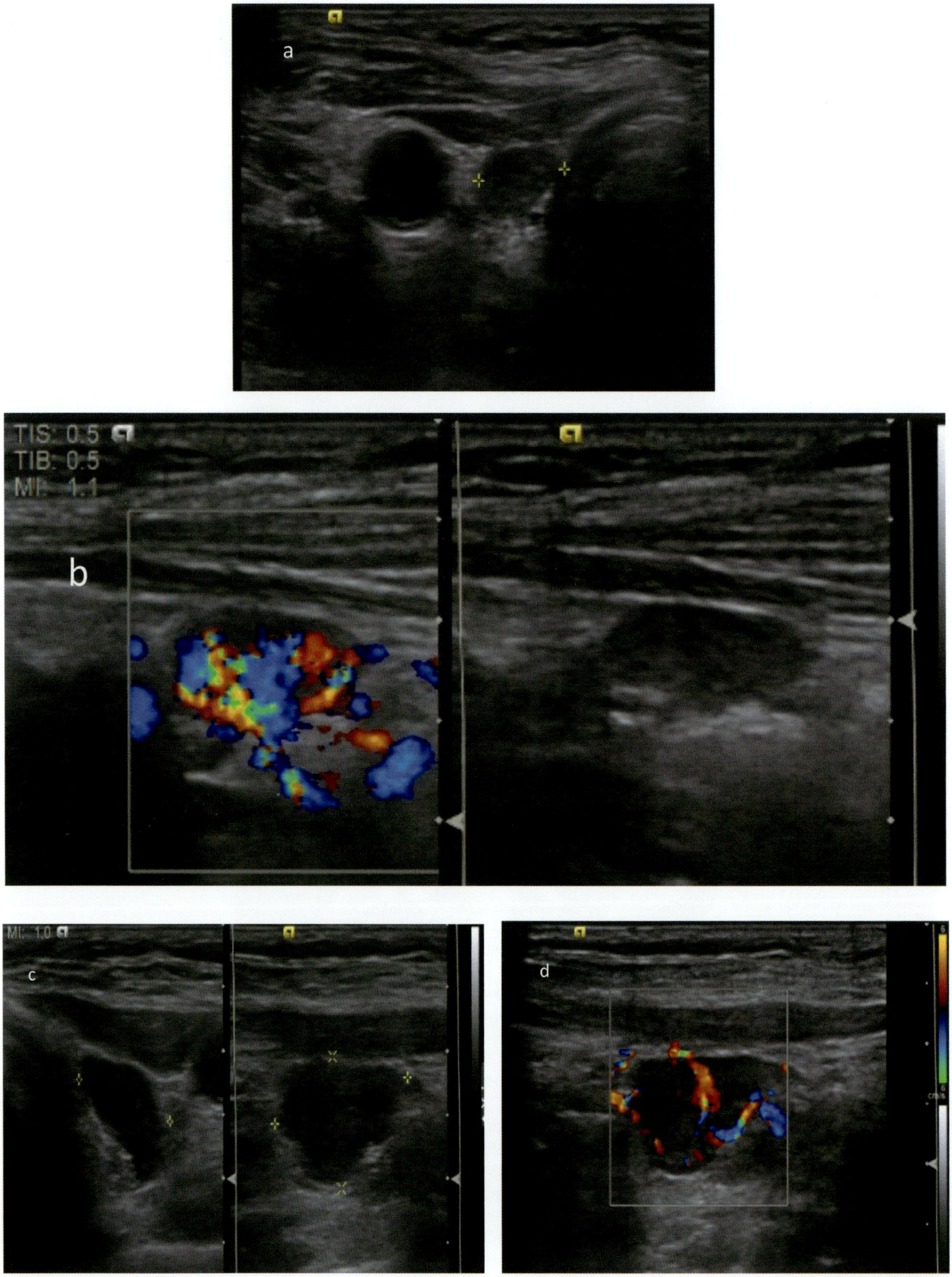

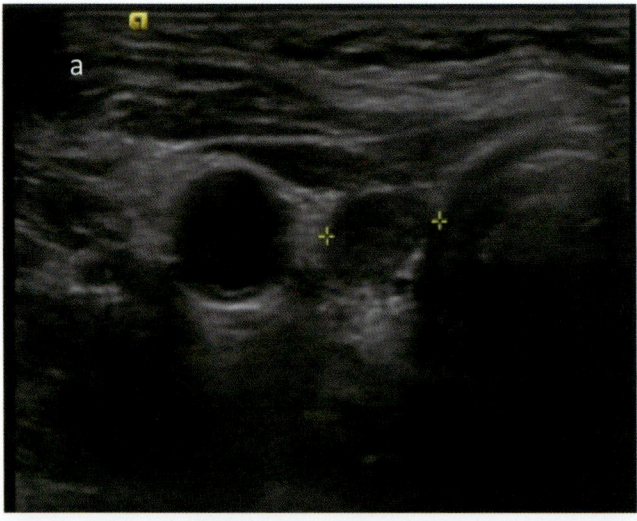

FIGURE 4.25 (a)–(d) Transverse and longitudinal sonogram of right and left thyroid fossa showing heterogenous hypoechoic lymph nodes in bilateral paratracheal region. Thyroglobulin levels were mildly elevated. FNA showed papillary thyroid carcinoma on both sides.

References

1. Levine RA. History of thyroid ultrasound. In: H.J. Baskin, D.S. Duick and R.A. Levine, (ed.), Thyroid Ultrasound and Ultrasound-Guided FNA. Boston, MA: Springer; 2008.
2. Robinson TM. Basic principles of ultrasound. In: Y. Lemoigne, A. Caner and G. Rahal, (ed.), Physics for Medical Imaging Applications. NATO Science Series, vol 240. Dordrecht: Springer; 2007.
3. Kremkau FW. Physics and principles of ultrasound. In: Diagnostic Ultrasound. 6th ed. Philadelphia, PA: WB Saunders; 2002. pp.10, 18–37, 62–64, 71–76, 86–92, 167–194, 273–318.
4. Terslev L, Diamantopoulos AP, Døhn UM, Schmidt WA, Torp-Pedersen S. Settings and artefacts relevant for Doppler ultrasound in large vessel vasculitis. Arthritis Res Ther. 2017;19(1):167.
5. Donkol RH, Nada AM, Boughattas S. Role of color Doppler in differentiation of Graves' disease and thyroiditis in thyrotoxicosis. World J Radiol. 2013;5(4):178–183.
6. Chaudhary V, Bano S. Thyroid ultrasound. Indian J Endocrinol Metab. 2013;17(2):219–227.
7. Lee TC, Selvarajan SK, Curtin H, Mukundan S. Zuckerkandl tubercle of the thyroid: A common imaging finding that may mimic pathology. AJNR Am J Neuroradiol. 2012 Jun;33(6):1134–1138.
8. Roy M, Mazeh H, Chen H, et al. Incidence and localization of ectopic parathyroid adenomas in previously unexplored patients. World J Surg. 2013;37:102.
9. Park M, Park SH, Kim EK, et al. Heterogeneous echogenicity of the underlying thyroid parenchyma: How does this affect the analysis of a thyroid nodule?. BMC Cancer. 2013;13:550.
10. Pishdad P, Pishdad GR, Tavanaa S, Pishdad R, Jalli R. Thyroid ultrasonography in differentiation between Graves' Disease and Hashimoto's thyroiditis. J Biomed Phys Eng. 2017;7(1):21–26.
11. Tam AA, Kaya C, Üçler R, Dirikoç A, Ersoy R, Çakır B. Correlation of normal thyroid ultrasonography with thyroid tests. Quant Imaging Med Surg. 2015;5(4):569–574.
12. Pearce EN. Diagnosis and management of thyrotoxicosis. BMJ. 2006;332(7554):1369–1373.
13. Avs AK, Mohan A, Kumar PG, Puri P. Scintigraphic profile of thyrotoxicosis patients and correlation with biochemical and sonological findings. J Clin Diagn Res. 2017;11(5):OC01–OC03.
14. Anderson L, et al. Hashimoto thyroiditis: Part 1, Sonographic analysis of the nodular form of Hashimoto thyroiditis. Am J Roentgenol. 2010;195(1):208–215.
15. Chen YK, Lin CL, Cheng FT, Sung FC, Kao CH. Cancer risk in patients with Hashimoto's thyroiditis: A nationwide cohort study. Br J Cancer. 2013;109(9):2496–2501.
16. Lai X, Xia Y, Zhang B, Li J, Jiang Y. A meta-analysis of Hashimoto's thyroiditis and papillary thyroid carcinoma risk. Oncotarget. 2017;8(37):62414–62424.
17. Cooper DS, Doherty GM, Haugen BR, et al.; American Thyroid Association (ATA) Guidelines Taskforce on Thyroid Nodules and Differentiated Thyroid Cancer. Revised American Thyroid Association management guidelines for patients with thyroid nodules and differentiated thyroid cancer. Thyroid. 2009;19:1167–1214.
18. Tessler FN, Middleton WD, Grant EG. Thyroid imaging reporting and data system (TI-RADS): A user's guide. Radiology. 2018;287(1):29–36.
19. Soni S, Poorey VK, Chouksey S. Thyroglossal duct cyst, variation in presentation, our experience. Indian J Otolaryngol Head Neck Surg. 2014;66(4):398–400.
20. Kim JY, Jung SL, Kim MK, Kim TJ, Byun JY. Differentiation of benign and malignant thyroid nodules based on the proportion of sponge-like areas on ultrasonography: Imaging-pathologic correlation. Ultrasonography. 2015;34(4):304–311.
21. Zhao CK, Xu HX. Ultrasound elastography of the thyroid: Principles and current status. Ultrasonography. 2019;38(2):106–124.
22. Ghajarzadeh M, Sodagari F, Shakiba M. Diagnostic accuracy of sonoelastography in detecting malignant thyroid nodules: A systematic review and meta-analysis. Am J Roentgenol. 2014;202(4):W379–W389.
23. Sillery JC, Reading CC, Charboneau JW, Henrichsen TL, Hay ID, Mandrekar JN. Thyroid follicular carcinoma: Sonographic features of 50 cases. Am J Roentgenol. 2010;194:44–54.
24. Stulak JM, Grant CS, Farley DR, et al. Value of preoperative ultrasonography in the surgical management of initial and reoperative papillary thyroid cancer. Arch Surg. 2006;141(5):489–496.
25. Hughes DT, Hymart MR, Miller BS, Gauger PG, Doherty GM. The most commonly occurring papillary thyroid cancer in the United States is now a microcarcinoma in a patient older than 45 years. Thyroid. 2011;21:231–236.
26. Hay, Ian D, et al. Papillary thyroid microcarcinoma: A study of 900 cases observed in a 60-year period. Surgery. 2008;144(6):980–988.
27. Liu MJ, Liu ZF, Hou YY, et al. Ultrasonographic characteristics of medullary thyroid carcinoma: A comparison with papillary thyroid carcinoma. Oncotarget. 2017;8(16):27520–27528.
28. Ganeshan D, Paulson E, Duran C, Cabanillas ME, Busaidy NL, Charnsangavej C. Current update on medullary thyroid carcinoma. Am J Roentgenol. 2013;201(6):W867–W876.
29. Ahmed S, Ghazarian MP, Cabanillas ME, Zafereo ME, Williams MD, Vu T, Schomer DF, Debnam JM. Imaging of anaplastic thyroid carcinoma. Am J Neuroradiol. 2018 Mar;39(3):547–551.
30. Stein SA, Wartofsky L. Primary thyroid lymphoma: A clinical review. J Clin Endocrinol Metab. 2013 Aug;98(8): 3131–3138.
31. Nixon IJ, et al. Metastasis to the thyroid gland: A critical review. Ann Surg Oncol. 2017;24(6):1533–1539.
32. Makis W, Ciarallo A. Thyroid incidentalomas on 18F-FDG PET/CT: Clinical significance and controversies. 18F-FDG PET/BT'de Tiroid İnsidentalomalar: Klinik Önem ve Tartışmalar. Mol Imaging Radionucl Ther. 2017;26(3):93–100.
33. Marcus C, Whitworth PW, Surasi DS, Pai SI, Subramaniam RM. PET/CT in the management of thyroid cancers. Am J Roentgenol. 2014;202(6):1316–1329.
34. Kaur H, Kataria AP, Muthuramalingapandian M, Kaur H. Airway considerations in case of a large multinodular goiter. Anesth Essays Res. 2017;11(4):1097–1100.
35. Berri T, Houari R. Complications of thyroidectomy for large goiter. Pan Afr Med J. 2013;16:138.

5

INVESTIGATION IN THYROID DISEASES
Pathology

Chanchal Rana

Introduction

Thyroid disorders are one of the commonest endocrine disorders worldwide. In South East Asia too, there is a significant burden of this disease. Thyroid nodule has a prevalence of 3–7% by palpation but with the use of high-resolution ultrasonography, this incidence has increased to 19–67% with an increasing trend worldwide (1, 2).

The main concern in the patients with thyroid nodules is related to the potential of malignancy in them. Cosmetic, compressive symptoms, hypothyroidism and hyperthyroidism are other reasons for which the patients seek medical attention. In such scenario, it becomes extremely important to identify the cause followed by appropriate management. This chapter deals with role of cytology, histology and other ancillary techniques in the diagnosis of thyroid lesions.

Fine needle aspiration cytology in thyroid

A thyroid fine needle aspiration (FNA) biopsy is a procedure that removes a small sample of tissue from your thyroid gland. Cells are removed through a small, hollow needle. The sample is sent to the lab for analysis. The role of FNA in diagnosis of thyroid lesions dates back to 1930, when Martin and Ellis documented the use of aspiration technique at several sites, including few cases from thyroid (3). Many Studies were conducted in following years; however, the method became widely used only after 1952 (4). Since then FNA has emerged as the most important initial step in diagnostic evaluation of thyroid nodules as well as has assumed a dominant role in deciding the management of patients with these nodules. Numerous studies till date have documented FNA thyroid as a safe, reliable and cost-effective method for pre-diagnostic evaluation of thyroid nodules. The reported sensitivity of thyroid FNA ranges from 65 to 99% and its specificity from 72 to 100% (5). It helps the surgeon to triage the patients thereby avoiding unnecessary surgery and psychological trauma to the patients with benign thyroid nodules.

Indications of FNA in thyroid nodules

Traditionally, the main indication for FNA of the thyroid has been the presence of a solitary nodule. According to the *2015 American Thyroid Association Management Guidelines for Adult Patients with Thyroid Nodules and Differentiated Thyroid Cancer* (6), diagnostic FNA is strongly recommended for nodules ≥1 cm in greatest dimension with high-to-intermediate suspicion sonography pattern and nodules ≥1.5 cm in greatest dimension for low suspicion ultrasonography pattern. FNA may be considered for nodules ≥2 cm in greatest dimension with very low suspicion sonographic pattern. However, in this scenario, observation without FNA is also a reasonable option. FNA thyroid is not required if a nodule does not meet any of the above mentioned criteria or is purely cystic.

There are certain other indications as well, which include (7):

- For confirmation and characterization of clinically obvious thyroid malignancy.
- Evaluation of diffuse swelling (to differentiate between autoimmune/inflammatory pathology and goiter).
- To obtain material for ancillary tests.

Procedure and processing of thyroid FNA

FNA procedure can be performed directly for obvious lesions or under ultrasound guidance for smaller or nonpalpable nodules. After cleaning the area, a thin needle is inserted into the gland with back and forth action (for cell detachment) for few seconds. This is followed by suction through the syringe which is attached to the needle.

The sample obtained is immediately placed on glass slides followed by smear preparation. Thyroid being vascular gland, the smears should be prepared as soon as possible to prevent the cells to get entrapped in the clot. Both air-dried and wet smears should be prepared for each case. The air-dried smears are followed by Romanowsky stains (Giemsa, May graunwald giemsa, Leishman) which provide better cytoplasmic and background details whereas the alcohol-fixed smears are stained with hematoxylin and eosin or Papanicolaou stain for better nuclear details.

Local hemorrhage may be caused due to needling; however, complications like carotid hematoma, transient vocal cord paralysis; acute suppurative thyroiditis, chemical neuritis and puncture of trachea are uncommon and rare (7–10).

Cytopathology reporting of thyroid lesions

It is critical for the cytopathologist to communicate thyroid FNA interpretations to the referring physician/surgeon in clear and unambiguous manner which is clinically helpful. Historically, terminology for thyroid FNA has varied significantly from one laboratory to another, creating confusion in some instances and hindering the sharing of clinically meaningful data among multiple institutions. In 2007, National Cancer Institute (NCI) hosted a conference in Bethesda and developed uniform terminologies for reporting thyroid cytology known as *The Bethesda System for Reporting Thyroid Cytopathology (TBSRTC)* (Table 5.1) (11). It is now most favored and robust guidelines for reporting of thyroid lesions, internationally. These guidelines have recently been revised in the year 2017 with the introduction of molecular testing as an adjunct to cytopathologic examination (12). TBSRTC is a six-tier system that includes six different diagnostic categories each having its own implied risk of malignancy (ROM) and recommended management.

With a recent introduction of a new entity, *Noninvasive follicular thyroid neoplasm with papillary-like nuclear features*

Investigation in Thyroid Diseases

TABLE 5.1: The Various Diagnostic Categories in TBSRTC

I	Nondiagnostic or unsatisfactory (ND/UNS)	• Cyst fluid only (CFO) • Virtually acellular specimen (need at least 6 groups of benign follicular cells, composed of at least 10 cells each for benign) • Other (obscuring blood, clotting artifact, overly thick smear, etc.)
II	Benign	• Consistent with a benign follicular nodule (includes adenomatoid nodule, colloid nodule, etc.) • Consistent with lymphocytic (Hashimoto) thyroiditis in the proper clinical context • Consistent with granulomatous (subacute) thyroiditis • Other (abundant colloid, black thyroid, reactive changes, radiation changes, cyst lining cells, etc.)
III	Atypia of undetermined significance/follicular lesion of undetermined significance (AUS/FLUS)	• Broad category of not easily classified FNAs
IV	Follicular neoplasm (or suspicious for a follicular neoplasm)	• Specify if exclusively Hürthle cell (oncocytic) type
V	Suspicious for malignancy	• Suspicious for papillary carcinoma (only 1–2 features of PTC present, focal changes or sparsely cellular) • Suspicious for medullary carcinoma • Suspicious for metastatic carcinoma • Suspicious for lymphoma • Other
VI	Malignant	• Papillary thyroid carcinoma • Poorly differentiated carcinoma • Medullary thyroid carcinoma • Undifferentiated (anaplastic) carcinoma • Squamous cell carcinoma • Carcinoma with mixed features (specify) • Metastatic carcinoma • Non-Hodgkin lymphoma • Other

(NIFTP), the revised system has documented the ROM in two different ways, by including as well as excluding NIFTP from malignancy tally (Table 5.2). However, it is recommended that ROM in each of the six diagnostic categories should be independently defined at each cytology center or institution to guide clinicians on risk estimates and help choose appropriate molecular testing for patients with indeterminate cytology (11, 12).

Limitations and pitfalls in thyroid cytology

FNA cytology (FNAC) thyroid has now been widely used and established technique worldwide, to determine the presence or absence of a neoplasm, to determine its benign or malignant nature and finally to typing of the tumor present. However, it has its fair share of false positives and negatives, and hence, misdiagnosis of cancer by cytopathology examination has remained one of the most problematic issues in thyroid pathology.

The positive predictive value of FNAC for malignancy according to TBSRTC is 97–99%, and this figure includes noninvasive follicular thyroid neoplasm with papillary-like nuclear features (NIFTP) tumors; the sensitivity and specificity of thyroid FNAC have been reported as 65–99% and 72–100%, respectively (12–14).

The common causes of false-negative results are follicular adenoma mistaken for adenomatous goiter, cystic lesions harboring malignancy, low- and intermediate-grade lymphomas

TABLE 5.2: The 2017 Bethesda System for Reporting Thyroid Cytopathology: Implied Risk of Malignancy and Recommended Clinical Management

Diagnostic Categories	Risk of Malignancy Excluding NIFT from Malignant Tally (%)	Risk of Malignancy, Including NIFT in Malignant Tally (%)	Management
Unsatisfactory/Nondiagnostic	5–10	5–10	Ultrasound guided repeat FNA
Benign	0–3	0–3	Clinical and radiological follow up
Atypia of undetermined significance/follicular lesion of undetermined significance	6–18	~10–30	Repeat FNA, molecular testing or lobectomy
Follicular neoplasm/suspicious for follicular neoplasm	10–40	25–40	Molecular testing, lobectomy
Suspicious for malignancy	45–60	50–75	Near total thyroidectomy or lobectomy
Malignant	94–96	97–99	Near total thyroidectomy or lobectomy

in background of lymphocytic thyroiditis, malignancies with marked necrosis and focal involvement of glands or inadequate smears. Performing FNA under ultrasound guidance can minimize the false-negative rate (15–17).

A false-positive diagnosis can be also be given in situations like cellular colloid goiter mistaken for follicular neoplasm or chronic lymphocytic thyroiditis misdiagnosed for malignant lymphoma (14, 17).

Histopathological evaluation of thyroid

Depending on the preliminary diagnosis established on FNAC of thyroid swelling, various types of specimens can be received for histopathological evaluation. They include core-needle biopsy (CNB), lobectomy, hemithyroidectomy, total thyroidectomy with or without modified radical neck dissection. With the advent of thinner needle, automated devices and high-resolution ultrasound, CNB is now been increasingly used, especially in cases where the previous FNA results had been atypia of undetermined significance or nondiagnostic (18, 19). CNB is a useful technique as it provides more samples as well as can be used for ancillary techniques like immunohistochemical as well as molecular analysis. Unfortunately, it is less useful, like FNA, to distinguish between follicular adenoma vs. follicular carcinoma, noninvasive follicular neoplasm with papillary-like nuclear features vs. invasive follicular variant of papillary thyroid carcinoma (20, 21). In these scenarios, resection specimen still forms the basis for final histopathological diagnosis in thyroid (Figures 5.1–5.4).

Reporting of thyroid surgical pathology

The surgical pathology reports are very important and critical to not only provide histopathological diagnosis but also supply information related to surgical adequacy, prognostic factors, staging as well as guidance for postoperative management. Traditionally, the surgical pathology reports were presented in a narrative manner and were prone to errors and omissions with variability in content and completeness (22, 23). These inconsistencies were the

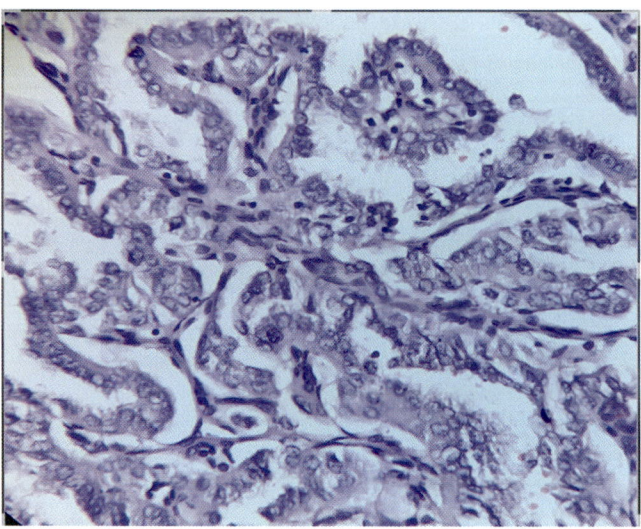

FIGURE 5.2 Conventional papillary thyroid carcinoma: A neoplasm with papillary architecture with well-developed fibrovascular core lined by atypical cells displaying optically clear oval overlapping nuclei with nuclear grooving and inclusion (hematoxylin and eosin, 400× magnification).

primary cause of delay in treatment, incomplete adjuvant therapies and inappropriate postoperative cancer surveillance (24).

Synoptic pathologic reporting has now been developed to improve the quality of pathology reporting and to facilitate standardization and efficiency. Synoptic reporting refers to the presentation of information in tabular rather than narrative format and is based upon predetermined checklists of reportable

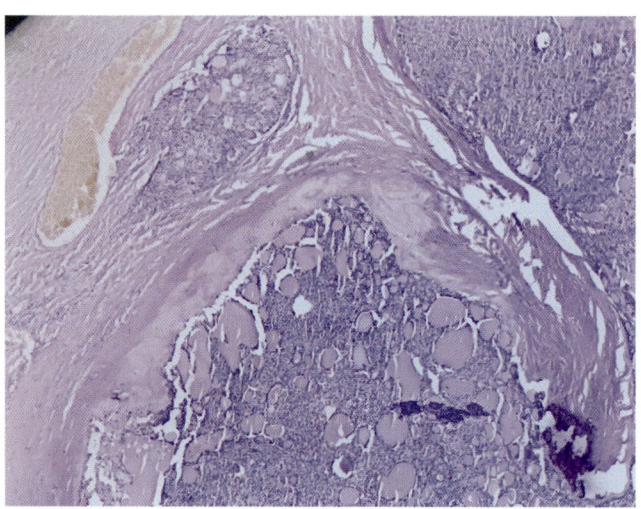

FIGURE 5.1 Follicular carcinoma thyroid: Microphotographs shows a neoplasm with microfollicular pattern with capsular infiltration. A pseudocapsule formation at infiltrating end and focus of calcification is also seen (hematoxylin and eosin, 100× magnification).

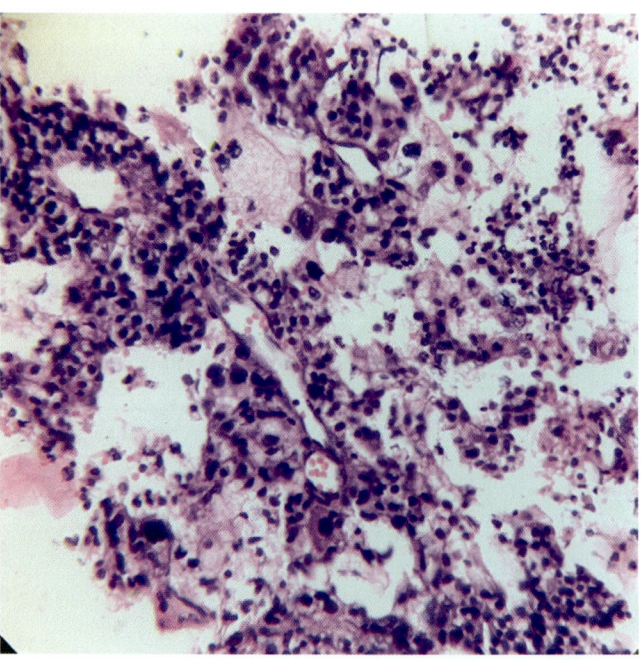

FIGURE 5.3 Anaplastic carcinoma thyroid: A neoplasm with atypical cells arranged in sheets with marked nuclear hyperchromasia and pleomorphism (hematoxylin and eosin, 400× magnifications).

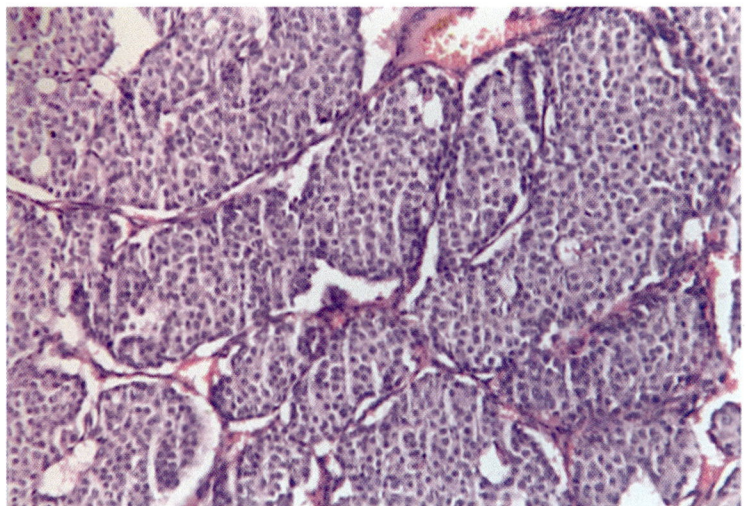 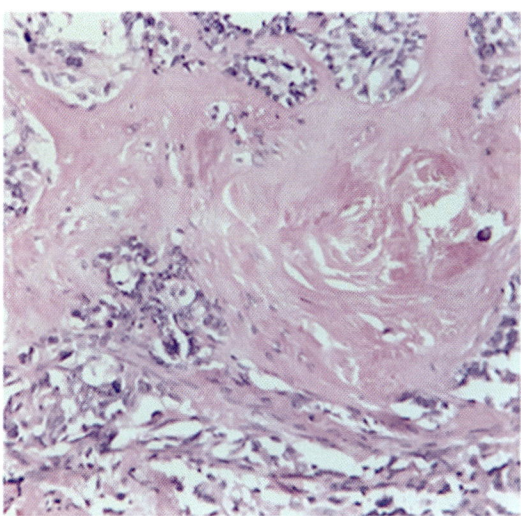

FIGURE 5.4 Medullary thyroid carcinoma: (a) Microphotograph displays a neoplasm with atypical cells arranged in acinar pattern surrounded by thin fibrovascular septa. Cells show minimal nuclear anisomorphism and presence of salt pepper chromatin; (b) presence of extracellular eosinophilic homogeneous material called amyloid.

data elements (25). The College of American Pathologists has developed templates for surgical pathology reporting for 60 site-specific cancers, including thyroid. These templates can be easily accessed through their official website www.cap.org.

WHO classification system in thyroid

The World Health Organization (WHO) classification of tumors serves as an international standard of histopathological diagnosis and the essential basis of clinical practice for neoplastic diseases for all organ systems. The 4th edition (latest) *WHO Classification of Tumors of Endocrine Organs* was published in 2017 (Table 5.3) (26).

This latest classification has incorporated several important modifications to follicular cell tumors listed as follows:

- Introduction of borderline tumors (UMP [uncertain malignant potential], NIFTP [noninvasive follicular thyroid neoplasm with papillary-like nuclear features] and HTT [hyalinizing trabecular tumor]) in the thyroid tumor classification.
- Histological variants of papillary thyroid carcinoma (PTC) were emphasized that may have more aggressive biological behavior or may related to hereditary tumor syndrome.
- Follicular thyroid carcinoma (FTC) was divided into three prognostic categories,
  - minimally invasive (capsular invasion only),
  - encapsulated angioinvasive and
  - widely invasive.
- Poorly differentiated carcinoma (PDC) was defined with Turin consensus criteria more precisely for its histopathological diagnosis, and PTC with solid growth without increased mitosis and/or tumor necrosis was removed from PDC and was placed in PTC as an aggressive variant (solid variant of PTC).
- A new chapter of Hurthle cell (oncocytic) tumors was established acknowledging the peculiar biological and clinical features.
- Prognostic values of genetic markers such as BRAFV600E and TERT promoter mutation in thyroid carcinoma of follicular cell derivation were emphasized and detailed.

- Entire tissue sampling and analysis of the interface between the tumor and its surrounding thyroid parenchyma was emphasized.

Application of immunohistochemistry in thyroid pathology

Diagnosis of thyroid malignancy is quite straightforward most of the times; however, still pathologist may be confronted with situations where due to equivocal findings differentiation between benign and malignant lesions become difficult. In recent years, tremendous efforts had been made to identify various immunohistochemical as well as molecular markers which could help in solving this important issue. Another important use of immunohistochemistry is to identify the follicular origin in tumors that are poorly differentiated or undifferentiated, not follicular derived, and exhibit equivocal histomorphologic features. The application of immunohistochemical biomarkers may play an active or complementary role in their accurate classification.

Hence, based on the abovementioned indications, the immunomarkers can be grouped in two categories: (a) organ-specific markers and (b) marker for differential diagnosis. The important markers used in thyroid pathology as well as their propertied are discussed next (27, 28):

1. *Thyroglobulin*: It is a thyroid hormone precursor and thyroid organ specific. However, it cannot be used to differentiate benign and malignant lesions, also it may not be expressed in poorly or undifferentiated thyroid carcinoma.
2. *TTF-1*: It is a thyroid transcription factor 1 that plays a crucial role in the organogenesis and differentiation of thyroid and lung. Apart from the limitation like for thyroglobulin, it is also expressed in lung, colorectal, ovarian, breast and endocervical adenocarcinomas.
3. *Hector Battifora mesothelial-1 (HBME-1)*: It is a membrane antigen found in the microvilli of mesothelial cells, normal tracheal epithelium and adenocarcinoma of the lung, pancreas and breast. It is known to have an overexpression or diffuse expression in malignant thyroid neoplasm especially PTC. It is virtually not expressed in normal thyroid

TABLE 5.3: 2017 WHO Classifications of Tumors of Thyroid Gland

- Follicular adenoma 8330/0
- Hyalinizing trabecular tumor 8336/1
- Other encapsulated follicular patterned thyroid tumors
- Follicular tumors of uncertain malignant potential 8335/1
- Well-differentiated tumor of uncertain malignant potential 8348/1
- Noninvasive follicular thyroid neoplasm with papillary-like nuclear features 8349/1
- Papillary thyroid carcinoma
- Papillary carcinoma 8260/3
- Follicular variant of PTC 8340/3
- Encapsulated variant of PTC 8343/3
- Papillary microcarcinoma 8341/3
- Columnar cell variant of PTC 8344/3
- Oncocytic variant of PTC 8342/3
- Follicular thyroid carcinoma (FTC), NOS 8330/3
- FTC, minimally invasive 8335/3
- FTC, encapsulated angioinvasive 8339/3
- FTC, widely invasive 8330/3
- Hürthle (oncocytic) cell tumors
- Hürthle cell adenoma 8290/0
- Hürthle cell carcinoma 8290/3
- Poorly differentiated thyroid carcinoma 8337/3
- Anaplastic thyroid carcinoma 8020/3
- Squamous cell carcinoma 8070/3
- Medullary thyroid carcinoma 8345/3
- Mixed medullary and follicular thyroid carcinoma 8346/3
- Mucoepidermoid carcinoma 8430/3
- Sclerosing mucoepidermoid carcinoma with eosinophilia 8430/3
- Mucinous carcinoma 8480/3
- Ectopic thymoma 8580/3
- Spindle epithelial tumor with thymus-like differentiation 8588/3
- Intrathyroid thymic carcinoma 8589/3
- Paraganglioma and mesenchymal/stromal tumors
- Paraganglioma 8693/3
- Peripheral nerve sheath tumors (PNSTs)
- Schwannoma 9560/0
- Malignant PNST 9540/3
- Benign vascular tumors
- Hemangioma 9120/0
- Cavernous hemangioma 9121/0
- Lymphangioma 9170/0
- Angiosarcoma 9120/3
- Smooth muscle tumors
- Leiomyoma 8890/0
- Leiomyosarcoma 8890/3
- Solitary fibrous tumor 8815/1
- Hematolymphoid tumors
- Langerhans cell histiocytosis 9751/3
- Rosai-Dorfman disease
- Follicular dendritic cell sarcoma 9758/3
- Primary thyroid lymphoma
- Germ cell tumors
- Benign teratoma 9080/0
- 9080/1 Immature teratoma 9080/1
- 9080/3 Malignant teratoma 9080/3
- Secondary tumors

tissue making it an important marker which can differentiate between benign vs. malignant lesions in thyroid. However, it is either negative or weakly expressed in HTT and Hurthle cell neoplasms.

4. *Cytokeratin 19*: Low-molecular-weight cytokeratin found in a variety of simple or glandular epithelia, both normal and their neoplastic counterpart. It has no or weak focal positivity in normal follicular epithelium. Overexpression of CK19 is a good indicator for papillary thyroid carcinoma; however, its sensitivity for follicular carcinoma is low.
5. *Galectin-3 (GAL-3)*: It is a member of a family of beta-galactoside-binding animal lectins shown to be involved in tumor progression and metastasis. It is diffusely overexpressed of in well-differentiated follicular-derived thyroid carcinomas. The positivity in benign lesion is only focal. It has a high sensitivity and specificity for thyroid malignancy expecially papillary thyroid carcinoma. Importantly, the sensitivity for follicular marker is also higher as compared to cytokeratin 19.
6. *Thyroid peroxidase (TPO)*: It is thyroid-specific enzyme reflecting normal thyroid function. It is diffusely expressed in normal follicular epithelial cells; hence, its lack of expression signifies malignancy.

As described, no single marker is completely sensitive or specific for thyroid lesions. Depending on the situation, a panel should be used. Thyroglobulin and TTF-1 are suitable markers to identify thyroidal origin at metastatic sites, while CK19, GAL-3, HBME-1 are better suited in circumstances where the primary aim is to differentiate between benign and malignant thyroid conditions.

Genetic alterations in thyroid neoplasms

FNAC is the mainstay on preoperative diagnosis of thyroid pathologies. However, there are approximately 15–30% cases where it may not be useful, especially in indeterminate categories *(Atypia of undetermined significance, Bethesda category III and Suspicious of follicular neoplasm, Bethesda category IV)* (11, 12). This is where the role of analysis of various genetic alterations comes into play. The primary role of molecular testing in thyroid is not only to reduce overtreatment in indeterminate thyroid nodules but also provide prognostic information thereby leading to proper surgical and therapeutic decisions.

Molecular testing for thyroid nodules has evolved rapidly over the past decade both to help improve the diagnostic accuracy of thyroid cytology for indeterminate cases and potentially to guide the extent of surgery as initial therapy for suspected thyroid malignancies. Table 5.4 briefly describes the common abnormalities encountered in various thyroid malignancies and their significance (29–31).

South Asia perspective

Asia is the largest and most populous continent with geographic, religious, ethnic as well as cultural diversity. It is also the largest contributor of thyroid cancer worldwide with approximately 48% of all new thyroid cancer cases as per the GLOBOCON (32).

TABLE 5.4: Common Molecular Abnormalities Encountered in Various Thyroid Malignancies and Their Significance

Genetic Alteration	Significance
RET/PTC rearrangement	• Involves mutagen-activated protein kinase (MAPK) pathway • 11 RET/PTC rearrangements have been reported • Three forms: RET/PTC 1, RET/PTC 2 and RET/PTC 3 are more common • Clonal RET/PTC is of significance in papillary carcinoma thyroid • More frequently seen in children and young adults as well as those with history of radiation exposure. • RET/PTC 1 most common and seen in 60–70% of positive cases
BRAF mutation	• Also involves mitogen-activated protein kinase (MAPK) pathway • Point mutation is most common genetic alteration which involves nucleotide 1799 and results in a valine-to-glutamate substitution at residue 600 (V600E) • Typically present in classical PTC or tall cell variant • Rare in follicular variant • Absent in benign thyroid nodule, hence a very specific molecular marker • Associated with poor prognosis and less responsiveness to radioiodine therapy
RAS mutation	• Human RAS gene includes KRAS, HRAS and NRAS genes • NRAS codon 61 and HRAS codon 61 are most commonly associated with thyroid tumors • 40–50% of conventional follicular carcinoma • 20–40% of follicular adenomas • Also expressed in 10–20% of FV-PTC • Provide strong evidence of neoplasia but does not establish the diagnosis of malignancy • May be associated with less favorable prognosis, increased chances of metastasis and dedifferentiation
PAX8/PPARγ rearrangement	• t(2;3)(q13;p25) • 30–40% of conventional follicular carcinoma • Associated with younger age, smaller size and more frequent vascular invasion • Detection of PAX8/PPARγ rearrangement in a follicular lesion is not fully diagnostic for malignancy by itself, but it should prompt the pathologist to perform an exhaustive search for vascular or capsular invasion
CTNNB1 mutation	• CTNNB1 proto-oncogene that encodes, a member of Wnt signaling pathway • Seen in ~25% of PDTC and ~60% of ATC • Thyroid neoplasm is associated with somatic CTNBB1 mutation • Very rare in well-differentiated thyroid cancer, mainly associated with cribriform-morular variant PTC
TP53	• TP53/P53 is a tumor suppressor gene that plays part in cell cycle regulation and DNA repair • Seen in 10–40% of PDTC and 50–80% of ATC • Inactivating mutation in TP53 is a late event in thyroid cancer progression, which determines tumor dedifferentiation

FNA has been accepted globally as the first-line intervention in the workup of thyroid nodules and the modern systems for reporting thyroid cytopathology provides important statistical outputs like distribution of thyroid FNA samples by diagnostic category, resection rate, ROM, etc. Most meta-analyses on thyroid FNA and TBSRTC have not included Asian publications (33–35). Comparative studies between Asian and Western series have suggested that the Asian experience varies in several aspects like ROM, resection rate, incidence of various entities, etc. These differences are not acknowledged worldwide, which continues to create confusion among experts due to this lack of communication. It should be reiterated that the Asian continent is a major contributor to the global prevalence of thyroid cancer, and that local experience cannot be ignored (36).

- The Bethesda system of reporting thyroid cytopathology is the most robust and internationally accepted classification system. The surgical pathology reports are very important and critical to not only provide histopathological diagnosis but to also supply information related to surgical adequacy, prognostic factors, staging as well as guidance for postoperative management.
- Situations where due to equivocal findings differentiation between benign and malignant lesions become difficult especially in indeterminate categories *(Atypia of undetermined significance, Bethesda category III and Suspicious of follicular neoplasm, Bethesda category IV)*, immunohistochemical as well as genetic analysis becomes very important. They may play an active or complementary role in such scenario.

Conclusions

- Despite all of advancement in radiological and molecular techniques, FNAC of thyroid lesions is still the mainstay in diagnostic approach.
- FNAC is a rapid and cost-effective technique for diagnosis that avoids unnecessary surgeries, relieves the patient of psychological and financial burden and also helps the surgeons to appropriately triage the patients with thyroid nodules.

References

1. Hegedüs L. Clinical practice. The thyroid nodule. N Engl J Med. 2004 Oct; 351(17):1764–1771
2. Jiang H, Tian Y, Yan W, Kong Y, Wang H, Wang A, Dou J, Liang P, Mu Y. The prevalence of thyroid nodules and an analysis of related lifestyle factors in Beijing communities. Int J Environ Res Public Health. 2016 Apr;13(4):442.
3. Martin HE, Ellis EB. Biopsy by needle puncture and aspiration. Ann Surg. 1930 Aug;92(2):169–181.
4. Soderstrom N. Puncture of goiters for aspiration biopsy. Acta Med Scand. 1952;144(3): 237–244.

5. Sharma C. Diagnostic accuracy of fine needle aspiration cytology of thyroid and evaluation of discordant cases. J Egypt Natl Cancer Inst. 2015 Sep;27(3):147–153.
6. Haugen BR, Alexander EK, Bible KC, Doherty GM, Mandel SJ, Nikiforov YE, et al. 2015 American Thyroid Association management guidelines for adult patients with thyroid nodules and differentiated thyroid cancer: The American Thyroid Association guidelines task force on thyroid nodules and differentiated thyroid cancer. Thyroid. 2016 Jan;26(1):1–133.
7. Orell and Sterrett's Fine Needle Aspiration Cytology – 5th Edition [Internet]. [cited 2019 Mar 14]. Available from: https://www.elsevier.com/books/orell-and-sterretts-fine-needle-aspiration-cytology/9780702031519.
8. Park MH, Yoon JH. Anterior neck hematoma causing airway compression following fine needle aspiration cytology of the thyroid nodule: A case report. Acta Cytol. 2009 Feb;53(1):86–88.
9. Alkan S, Košar AT, Erdurak SC, Dadaš B. Transient vocal cord paralysis following ultrasound-guided fine-needle aspiration biopsy for a thyroid nodule. J Otolaryngol Head Neck Surg. 2009 Feb;38(1):E14–E15.
10. Nishihara E, Miyauchi A, Matsuzuka F, Sasaki I, Ohye H, Kubota S, et al. Acute suppurative thyroiditis after fine-needle aspiration causing thyrotoxicosis. Thyroid. 2005 Oct;15(10):1183–1187.
11. Cibas ES, Ali SZ. The Bethesda system for reporting thyroid cytopathology. Thyroid. 2009 Nov;19(11):1159–1165.
12. Cibas ES, Ali SZ. The 2017 Bethesda system for reporting thyroid cytopathology. Thyroid. 2017;27(11):1341–1346.
13. Canberk S, Gunes P, Onenerk M, Erkan M, Kilinc E, Kocak Gursan N, et al. New concept of the encapsulated follicular variant of papillary thyroid carcinoma and its impact on the Bethesda system for reporting thyroid cytopathology: A single-institute experience. Acta Cytol. 2016;60(3):198–204.
14. Malheiros DC, Canberk S, Poller DN, Schmitt F. Thyroid FNAC: Causes of false-positive results. Cytopathology. 2018;29(5):407–417.
15. La Rosa GL, Belfiore A, Giuffrida D, Sicurella C, Ippolito O, Russo G, et al. Evaluation of the fine needle aspiration biopsy in the preoperative selection of cold thyroid nodules. Cancer. 1991 Apr;67(8):2137–2141.
16. Hsu C, Boey J. Diagnostic pitfalls in the fine needle aspiration of thyroid nodules. A study of 555 cases in Chinese patients. Acta Cytol. 1987 Dec;31(6):699–704.
17. Canberk S, Firat P, Schmitt F. Pitfalls in the cytological assessment of thyroid nodules. Turk J Pathol [Internet]. 2015 [cited 2019 Sep 16]; Available from: http://www.turkjpath.org/doi.php?doi=10.5146/tjpath.2015.01312.
18. Paja M, Del Cura JL, Zabala R, Korta I, Ugalde A, Lopez JI. Core-needle biopsy in thyroid nodules: performance, accuracy, and complications. Eur Radiol. 2019 Sep;29(9):4889–4896.
19. Na DG, Kim J, Sung JY, Baek JH, Jung KC, Lee H, et al. Core-needle biopsy is more useful than repeat fine-needle aspiration in thyroid nodules read as nondiagnostic or atypia of undetermined significance by the Bethesda system for reporting thyroid cytopathology. Thyroid. 2012 May;22(5):468–475.
20. Suh CH, Baek JH, Lee JH, Choi YJ, Kim KW, Lee J, et al. The role of core-needle biopsy in the diagnosis of thyroid malignancy in 4580 patients with 4746 thyroid nodules: A systematic review and meta-analysis. Endocrine. 2016 Nov;54(2):315–328.
21. Jung CK, Baek JH. Recent advances in core needle biopsy for thyroid nodules. Endocrinol Metab. 2017 Dec;32(4):407–412.
22. Lam E, Vy N, Bajdik C, Strugnell SS, Walker B, Wiseman SM. Synoptic pathology reporting for thyroid cancer: A review and institutional experience. Expert Rev Anticancer Ther. 2013 Sep;13(9):1073–1079.
23. Leslie KO, Rosai J. Standardization of the surgical pathology report: Formats, templates, and synoptic reports. Semin Diagn Pathol. 1994 Nov;11(4):253–257.
24. Yunker WK, Matthews TW, Dort JC. Making the most of your pathology: Standardized histopathology reporting in head and neck cancer. J Otolaryngol Head Neck Surg. 2008 Feb;37(1):48–55.
25. Kang HP, Devine LJ, Piccoli AL, Seethala RR, Amin W, Parwani AV. Usefulness of a synoptic data tool for reporting of head and neck neoplasms based on the College of American Pathologists cancer checklists. Am J Clin Pathol. 2009 Oct;132(4):521–530.
26. Lloyd RV, Osamura RY, Kloppel G, Rosai J, ed. Cancer IA for R on. WHO Classification of Tumours of Endocrine Organs. 4th ed. Lyon: World Health Organization; 2017. 355 p.
27. Liu H, Lin F. Application of immunohistochemistry in thyroid pathology. Arch Pathol Lab Med. 2014 Dec;139(1):67–82.
28. Baloch Z, Mete O, Asa SL. Immunohistochemical biomarkers in thyroid pathology. Endocr Pathol. 2018 Jun;29(2):91–112.
29. Ferrari SM, Fallahi P, Ruffilli I, Elia G, Ragusa F, Paparo SR, et al. Molecular testing in the diagnosis of differentiated thyroid carcinomas. Gland Surg. 2018 Aug;7(Suppl 1):S19–S29.
30. Goldblum JR, Lamps LW, McKenney JK, Myers JL, Ackerman LV, Rosai J, ed. Rosai and Ackerman's Surgical Pathology [Internet]. 11th ed. Philadelphia, PA: Elsevier; 2018 [cited 2019 Mar 14]. 2 p.
31. Roth MY, Witt RL, Steward DL. Molecular testing for thyroid nodules: Review and current State. Cancer. 2018;124(5):888–898.
32. Ferlay J, Soerjomataram I, Ervik M, et al. GLOBOCAN 2012 v1.0, Cancer Incidence and Mortality Worldwide: IARC Cancer Base No. 11. Lyon: International Agency for Research on Cancer; 2013.
33. Bongiovanni M, Spitale A, Faquin WC, Mazzucchelli L, Baloch ZW. The Bethesda system for reporting thyroid cytopathology: A meta-analysis. Acta Cytol. 2012;56:333–339.
34. Krauss EA, Mahon M, Fede JM, Zhang L. Application of the Bethesda classification for thyroid fine-needle aspiration: Institutional experience and meta-analysis. Arch Pathol Lab Med. 2016;140:1121–1131.
35. Sheffield BS, Masoudi H, Walker B, Wiseman SM. Preoperative diagnosis of thyroid nodules using the Bethesda system for reporting thyroid cytopathology: A comprehensive review and meta-analysis. Expert Rev Endocrinol Metab. 2014;9:97–110.
36. Bychkov A, Kakudo K, Hong SW. Current practices of thyroid fine-needle aspiration in Asia: A missing voice. J Pathol Transl Med. 2017 Nov;51(6):517–520.

6

INFLAMMATORY DISEASES OF THYROID

Shivendra Verma and Manisha Gupta

Introduction

Thyroid gland is considered as one of the largest endocrine glands in human body and is also associated with most common anatomical and dysfunctional endocrine disorder. Inflammatory diseases of thyroid are a nonspecific term as it includes disorders with various etiologies and presentations. The most common disorder in this category is autoimmune thyroiditis (AIT) that includes classical Hashimoto's thyroiditis, euthyroid goiter as well as Graves' disease, since the common denominator in all these presentations is prominent lymphocytic infiltration on histopathological examination.

While Grave's disease (GD) has entirely different presentation and the pathogenesis involves stimulation of TSH receptors by autoantibodies leading to overproduction of thyroid hormones. On the other end of the spectrum, Hashimoto's thyroiditis is characterized by prominent inflammation of the gland and consequent impaired production of thyroid hormones. The clinical picture may range from euthyroid state with or without goiter to subclinical or overt hypothyroidism. Graves' disease has already been covered elsewhere and will not be discussed further in this chapter.

Apart from autoimmune disorders, thyroiditis may also have other etiologies (Table 6.1) and may present with classic temporal pattern. On the other hand, some of the diseases like Riedel's thyroiditis may present only with slowly progressive goiter while sarcoidosis may be associated with granulomatous inflammation. Thus, it is necessary to understand the pathophysiology of thyroiditis in different scenarios and correctly classify it so that appropriate action can be taken.

Autoimmune thyroiditis (AIT)

AIT is now the most common cause of hypothyroidism. Chronic AIT was first described as '*strumalymphomatosa*' by the surgeon Hakaru Hashimoto in 1912. This entity also known as lymphocytic thyroiditis usually presents in two forms: (1) Goitrous form widely known as Hashimoto's thyroiditis and (2) atrophic form known as atrophic thyroiditis or primary myxedema (no goiter). When it presents in childhood or in adolescents, it is known as juvenile AIT. Worldwide the incidence of AIT is variable and is around 350/100,000/year in women and 80/100,000/year in men but the data is not inclusive of south Asian population (1). A population survey in state of Kerala, India, found about 16.7% of adult subjects had anti-thyroid peroxidase antibodies and about 12.1% had anti-thyroglobulin (Tg) antibodies. In this same study of 971 subjects, subclinical hypothyroidism was seen in greater than 9% of adults. In post iodization phase, a countywide screening of schoolgirls from India found that the prevalence of fine needle aspiration cytology (FNAC) confirmed juvenile AIT was 7.5% (2).

Pathophysiology

T cells are the key players in thyroid follicular cell destruction in autoimmune thyroid disease. Cytotoxic CD8+ T cells are abundant in the lymphocytic infiltrate in Hashimoto thyroiditis (3). The T cells recognize both Tg and TPO. The other mode of follicular destruction is apoptosis using death ligands (Fas–FasL). The follicular injury is further enhanced by cytokines released from T cells that induce expression of chemokines and adhesion molecules on follicular cells (Figure 6.1). The role of various antibodies in pathogenesis of Hashimoto's thyroiditis is uncertain. Their role might be secondary after initial tissue injury mediated by natural killer cells (NK cells) and they may bring further tissue injury by either antibody-dependent cell cytotoxicity (ADCC) or complement-dependent cytotoxicity (CDC) (4). In GD, however, these pathways are not prominent and CD4+ cells predominate leading to the production of TSH-R antibodies (Figure 6.1).

Risk factors for autoimmune thyroid disease (Figure 6.2):

1. *Genetic factors:*(5)
    a. HLA-DR3, HLA-DR5 (goitrous),
    b. HLA-B8 (atrophic),
    c. HLA-DR9,HLA- Bw46,87, CD25, FOXP3 etc. and
    d. Thyroid-specific genes like Tg are involved in autoimmune process.
2. *Gender and pregnancy*: Like other autoimmune disorders, females are more prone to AIT as compared to males and hormones as well as skewed X chromosome inactivation are suggested as possible reasons. Moreover, pregnancy is a state of immunosuppression with recovery in postpartum period; thus, many women especially those with positive anti-TPO have a clinical presentation of thyroiditis (6).
3. *Iodine excess*: Excess iodine may cause either free radical-mediated injury or enhanced immune-reactivity of thyroid gland, and thus, iodine exposure may precipitate AIT (7).
4. *Drugs*: Interleukins drugs like Ilα, Ilβ, IL-2; anticancer agents (8) like tyrosine kinase inhibitors (TKI), e.g. Sunitinib; monoclonal antibodies, e.g. anti-CTLA-4 agent Ipilimumab; antipsychotic drug most notably lithium. On the other hand, smoking (9) and moderate alcohol consumption (10) are protective against AIT.
5. *Irradiation*: Atomic bomb survivors in Japan and Chernobyl disaster survivors had increased incidence of AIT.

TABLE 6.1: Types of Thyroiditis

Types of Thyroiditis

1. Autoimmune thyroiditis
2. Painless subacute thyroiditis
3. Painful subacute thyroiditis
4. Acute infectious thyroiditis
5. Riedel thyroiditis
6. Postirradiation (^{131}I or external beam therapy)
7. Drug induced

DOI: 10.1201/9780429197338-6

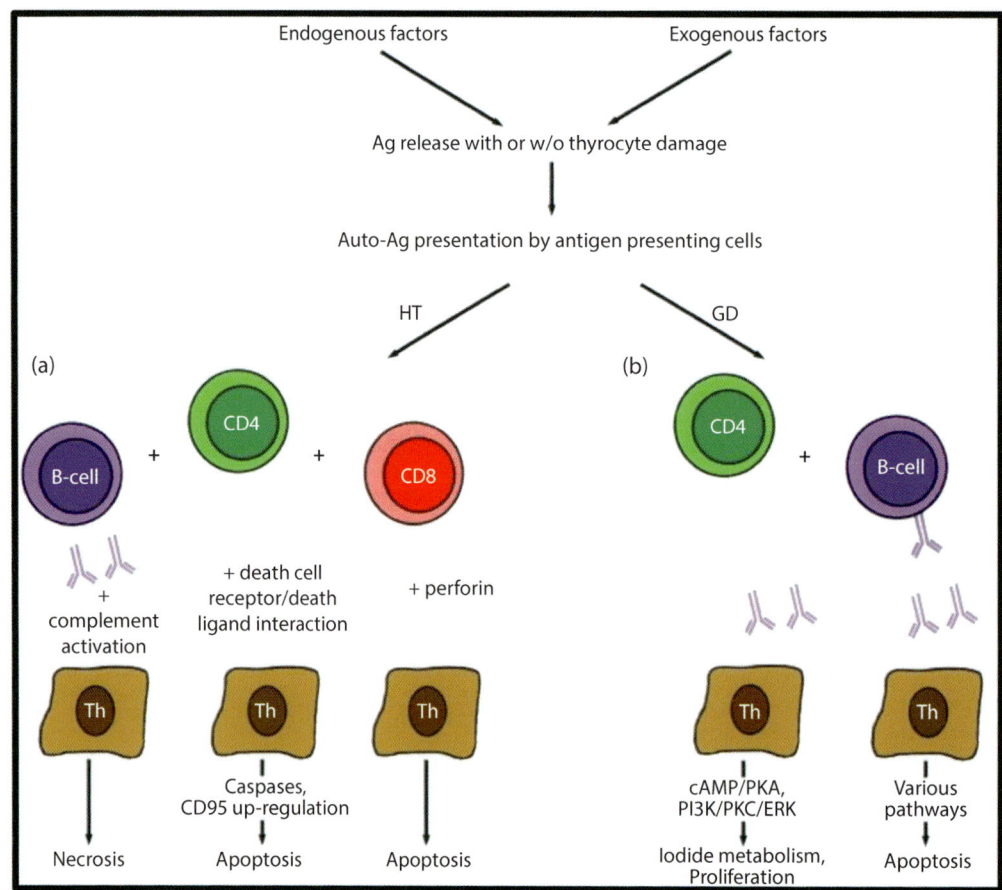

FIGURE 6.1 Pathogenesis of Hashimoto's disease (a) and Graves' disease (b). *Abbreviations:* ERK, extracellular signal-regulated kinase; GD, Graves' disease; HT, Hashimoto's thyroiditis; MAPK, mitogen-activated protein kinase; mTOR, mammalian target of rapamycin; p70S6K, ribosomal protein S6 kinase beta-1; PI3K, phosphatidylinositol-3,4,5-triphosphate kinase; PKA, protein kinase; PKC, protein kinase C. (Reprinted with permission from: Fröhlich E, et al. Thyroid Autoimmunity: Role of anti-thyroid antibodies in thyroid and extrathyroidal diseases. *Front Immunol.* 2017;8:521.)

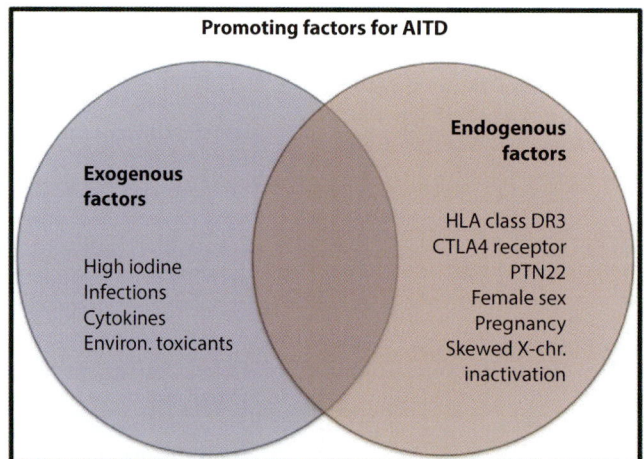

FIGURE 6.2 Promoting factors in Hashimoto's and Graves' disease. *Abbreviations:* chr., chromosome; CTLA4, cytotoxic T-lymphocyte-associated protein 4; Environ., environmental; PTN22, protein tyrosine phosphatase, non-receptor type 22. (Reprinted with permission from: Fröhlich E, et al. Thyroid Autoimmunity: Role of anti-thyroid antibodies in thyroid and extrathyroidal diseases. *Front Immunol.* 2017;8:521.)

Inflammatory Diseases of Thyroid

Pathological features include lymphocytic infiltration with plasma cells and germinal centers, follicular destruction, colloid depletion and fibrosis in goitrous Hashimoto's thyroiditis, whereas in atrophic thyroiditis, the gland is reduced in size with lymphocytic infiltration and fibrosis replacing the thyroid parenchyma (11). The follicular epithelial cells are frequently enlarged and contain an eosinophilic cytoplasm laden with mitochondria (Hürthle cells). Destruction of the gland results in a fall in serum T3 and FT4 and a rise in TSH.

Clinical presentation

Many patients are incidentally diagnosed. Patients with overt hypothyroidism have multisystem involvement (Table 6.2). Symptoms and signs of overt hypothyroidism vary in their prevalence for, e.g., most common symptoms reported in a study were dry skin (76%), cold intolerance (64%), coarse skin (60%), puffy eyelids (60%), decreased sweating (54%) and weight gain (54%), while most common signs were paresthesias (52%), cold skin (50%) and constipation (48%). The same study also found lower negative and positive predictive values for cold intolerance and bradycardia; thus, these symptoms that are presumed to be specific must in fact not lead to the clinical diagnosis of hypothyroidism (12). An often-overlooked sign is poor concentration and rarely patients may present with gait abnormalities as well. However, the data from Indian registry (13) comprising 1500 patients over 33 centers found a very low prevalence of signs and symptoms compared to Caucasian counterparts. In this survey, fatigue (60%) and weight gain (36.22%) were more common symptoms and hair loss was most common sign (30.9%), rest of classic symptoms and signs were present in less than 20% of patients; thus, classical symptoms and signs in Indian patients may not be present and a low threshold for biochemical testing is required.

Among children as well, AIT is the most common cause of goiter and hypothyroidism. One survey from India reported that 80% of children with onset of disease after 5 years had autoimmune cause, but more surprisingly, those with onset less than 5 years also had positive antibodies in greater than 50% children. Moreover, this study also found that those who present with short

TABLE 6.2: Clinical Features and Their Mechanisms in Hypothyroidism

Organ System	Finding	Explanation
Skin	• Non-pitting edema around eyes, hands and feet (*myxedema*) • Dry skin • Poor wound healing • Hair fall	• Accumulation of hygroscopic hyaluronic acid • Reduced sweat and sebaceous gland secretions • Reduced T3 • Reduced T3
Cardiovascular system	• Increased diastolic pressure with reduced pulse pressure • Decreased cardiac output • Pericardial effusion • Decreased amplitude of QRS complex on ECG • Increased PR interval, bradycardia	• Impaired T3-mediated vasodilation secondary to decreased NO synthesis • Decreased expression of SERCA2A, Na^+k^+ATPase, voltage-gated potassium channels and β adrenergic receptors • Increased expression of GAGs • Secondary to pericardial effusion • Decreased chronotropic action
Neurological	• Cerebellar ataxia • Impaired memory • Poor concentration • Entrapment neuropathies	• Altered neurotransmission and growth factors • Decreased cerebral metabolism • Poor blood flow
Psychiatric	• Depression • Schizophrenia • paranoia	• Impaired modulation of serotonin in brain • Altered neurotransmission
Alimentary tract and liver	• Decreased intestinal motility that may lead to constipation and pseudo-obstruction • Elevated liver enzymes • Gall stones • Malabsorption	• Decreased GI motility • Decreased clearance • Decreased gall bladder motility • Intestinal edema
Skeletal system	• Poor growth (if prepubertal onset) (Figure 6.3) • Delayed ossification	• Decreased growth hormone and IGF-1 • Direct action of thyroid hormones at epiphyses
Pituitary	• Increased gland size • Galactorrhea	• Hypertrophy of thyrocytes secondary to increased TRH • Increased TRH stimulates lactotrophs in pituitary
Reproductive	• Delayed puberty • precocious puberty (rare) • Infertility • Decreased libido and erectile dysfunction in men	• Secondary pituitary suppression • Spillover effect of TRH on GnRH receptors and TSH on FSH receptors • Anovulatory cycles, decreased progesterone • Altered androgen metabolism

Abbreviations: FSH, follicle-stimulating hormone; GAGs, glycosaminoglycans; GnRH, gonadotropin-releasing hormone; IGF-1, insulin like growth factor-1; LH, luteinizing hormone; NO, nitric oxide; SERCA2A, sarco/endoplasmic reticulum Ca^{2+}-ATPase; TRH, thyrotropin-releasing hormone; TSH, thyroid-stimulating hormone.

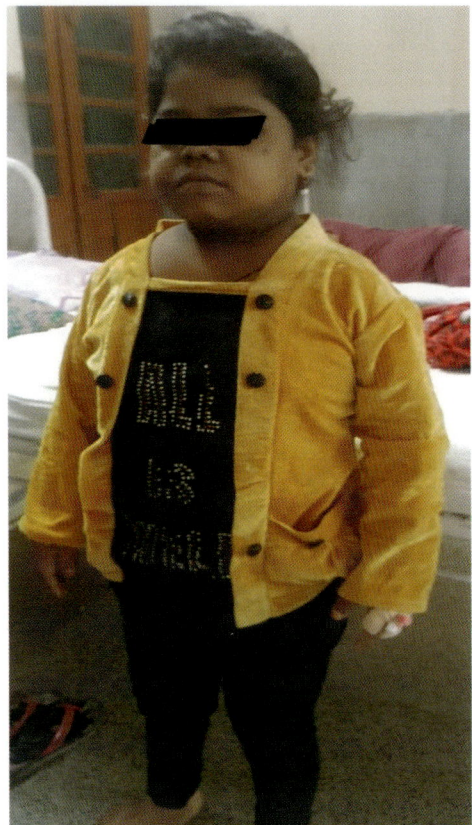

FIGURE 6.3 A late-diagnosed case of Juvenile hypothyroidism presented with decreased final height despite adequate thyroxine replacement.

stature and overt hypothyroid symptoms had lesser prevalence of goiter (see Figure 6.3) (14).

The goiter associated with Hashimoto's thyroiditis has diffuse enlargement, nontender, firm or rubbery in consistency with smooth bosselated surface. Rarely obstruction to nearby structures like trachea, esophagus and recurrent laryngeal nerve may be compressed. Older patients may present with severe hypothyroidism with only a small, firm atrophic thyroid gland (idiopathic myxedema). Laboratory investigation is thus, mandatory to rule out Hashimoto's thyroiditis.

Diagnosis

The diagnostic lab test includes tests for thyroid autoimmunity and assays for TSH and freeT4 (fT4). In 95%, serum TPO antibodies (TPOAb) are detectable with Hashimoto's thyroiditis and 90% of those with atrophic thyroiditis. Tg antibodies (TgAb) are less frequently positive in patients with both types of AIT. Low or undetectable titers of both TPOAb and TgAb are encountered in a few patients with chronic AIT. It is to be noted, however, that 3–8% of the general population has positive antibodies, and thus, the diagnostic significance is not great. One must not rely on autoantibodies to start treatment in euthyroid individual but a higher titer may alarm for future conversion of euthyroid state into subclinical or overt hypothyroidism and periodic monitoring in such a scenario is warranted. Another diagnostic test that may be helpful is fine needle aspiration biopsy (FNAB), which reveals lymphocytic infiltration as well as the presence of Hürthle cells but often is unnecessary and should not be done unless there is suspicion of thyroid nodule suspicious of malignancy on ultrasound. The role of nuclear imaging is also minimal in AIT in contrast to GD as it can be variable and heterogenous.

Treatment

Levothyroxine replacement is the most convenient method of treatment as the drug is orally taken with half-life of 7 days, thus practically can be given once a week. However, the best approach is to take the dose early morning empty stomach with a space of one hour with any subsequent food intake.

Indications of levothyroxine replacement

1. Overt hypothyroidism needs treatment with levothyroxine (LT4) with average daily replacement dose in adult is 1.6 µg/kg body weight. Elderly hypothyroid patients require a dose 20–30% lower dose.
2. *Euthyroid Hashimoto's thyroiditis*: Unsightly goiter or goiter with compressive symptoms (target TSH to lower half of reference range).
3. *Subclinical hypothyroidism*: The elevated TSH must be persistent, i.e. the repeat TSH should be elevated at last after 12 weeks.
   a. *TSH ≥ 10 mU/L*: Consider treatment
   b. women planning pregnancy or having infertility
   c. *TSH between upper limit of reference and 9.9 mU/L*: Consider treatment in <65 years old and in older population if convincing symptoms are present, if >80 years old, treat only if symptoms are present and TSH >7 mU/L.

Other forms of autoimmune thyroiditis

1. Thyrotoxic forms of AIT
   a. silent form
      I. postpartum thyroiditis (PPT)
      II. silent (painless) thyroiditis
   b. *Painful form*: Very rarely seen in patients with rapid onset of symptoms.

Silent (painless) thyroiditis

It is characterized by transient thyrotoxicosis with low radioactive iodine uptake (RAIU) and a small, painless, nontender goiter (15). Silent thyroiditis occurs either sporadically or in the postpartum period where it is called PPT. It is abrupt in onset with mild thyrotoxicosis like symptoms such as tachycardia, heat intolerance, sweating, nervousness and weight loss. Its prevalence has seasonal and geographic variation and a recent exposure to sufficient iodine may precipitate thyroiditis (15). Euthyroid state is ultimately restored in most cases, but persistent hypothyroidism may also develop in 5% of cases. Recurrences may develop in up to 11% of cases. Impaired thyroid reserve or goiter may occur after silent thyroiditis.

Postpartum thyroiditis

PPT is defined as the occurrence of a sporadic destructive thyroiditis in the first year postpartum, in women with no history of overt thyroid disease before pregnancy (16). The reported prevalence of PPT from systematic reviews of prospective studies of women during the first year after delivery is around 4–8% (17, 18). The classical clinical course is observed in about 26% of patients (19). It may have a triphasic clinical course. Most studies reported the onset of thyrotoxic symptoms at a median time of 12–13 weeks postpartum (20). The first phase, within 2–3 months after delivery, is characterized by mild symptoms of thyrotoxicosis and lasts for 1–6 weeks. Mild hypothyroidism of 2–6 weeks' duration may then occur between 3 and 8 months after delivery in 10–50% of cases especially those with positive anti-TPOAb (21). Lack of energy, poor memory, dry skin, palpitation, irritability, excessive fatigue and cold intolerance predominate. Postpartum depression is more common in women with positive thyroid antibodies irrespective of their thyroid status. A small, diffuse, firm, nontender, usually painless goiter is palpable. In women found to be TPOAb positive prenatally, postpartum assessment of thyroid function is recommended at 3, 6 and 12 months (16).

There is often a dilemma between PPT and GD as both are possibilities in postpartum period. While PPT is usually common in early postpartum period (with 3 months) compared to GD which is common 6 months postpartum (20), persistence of symptoms, large goiter, concomitant eye signs and a high TSH-R antibody titer with increased uptake on nuclear imaging favors GD. Figure 6.4 describes the various possibilities associated with AIT in postpartum period (the same principle also follow in differentiating destructive thyroiditis and GD). The most useful test to differentiate the two is nuclear imaging (radioiodine or technetium^{99m} pertechnetate scan) but is contraindicated in lactating women. The management of PPT is largely empirical and directed toward symptom control (19). Administration of β-adrenergic blocking drugs ameliorates symptoms of thyrotoxicosis. Thionamides are not useful in this entity. In patients with marked hypothyroid symptoms, LT4 treatment at medium-low dose (50–75 μg/day) is required, and it should be maintained for the first year after parturition (22).

Viral thyroiditis (subacute thyroiditis)

This entity is also known as subacute thyroiditis or de Quervain's or granulomatous thyroiditis. A tendency to appear in the spring in the northern latitudes has been noted and again it predominates in the female gender. The mumps virus has been implicated in some cases; coxsackievirus, influenza virus, echovirus and adenoviruses may also be etiologic agents. On examination, thyroid is moderately enlarged, firm, nodular and tender. Pathologic examination reveals moderate thyroid enlargement and a mild inflammatory reaction involving the capsule. Histologic features include destruction of thyroid parenchyma and the presence of many large phagocytic cells, including giant cells (23). Patients usually present with pain in thyroid gland (post-viral infection), sore throat, history of fever, pain during swallowing radiates to the ear, jaw and occiput. Hoarseness and dysphagia may be present; along with palpitation, nervousness and lassitude.

Laboratory findings give a thyrotoxicosis-like picture with raised ESR (usually >100 mm/hour). White blood cell count is typically normal whereas Tg level is elevated. On nuclear thyroid scan, gland doesn't take any uptake which confirms the diagnosis however; free T4 and free T3 levels are elevated with normal or slightly low TSH. It is self-limiting disease, resolves completely but might need nonsteroidal anti-inflammatory drugs and beta blockers for palpitation. Severe cases need steroid for short duration such as Prednisolone 20 mg three times a day for 7–10 days.

Acute thyroiditis

It is also known as acute suppurative thyroiditis, rare inflammatory disorder caused by bacteria and fungal infection, rarely accompanied by thyrotoxicosis (24, 25). The causative bacterium includes Staphylococcus, Pneumococcus, Salmonella or Mycobacterium tuberculosis. In addition, infections with certain fungi such as Coccidioides immitis, Candida, Aspergillus and Histoplasma have been reported.

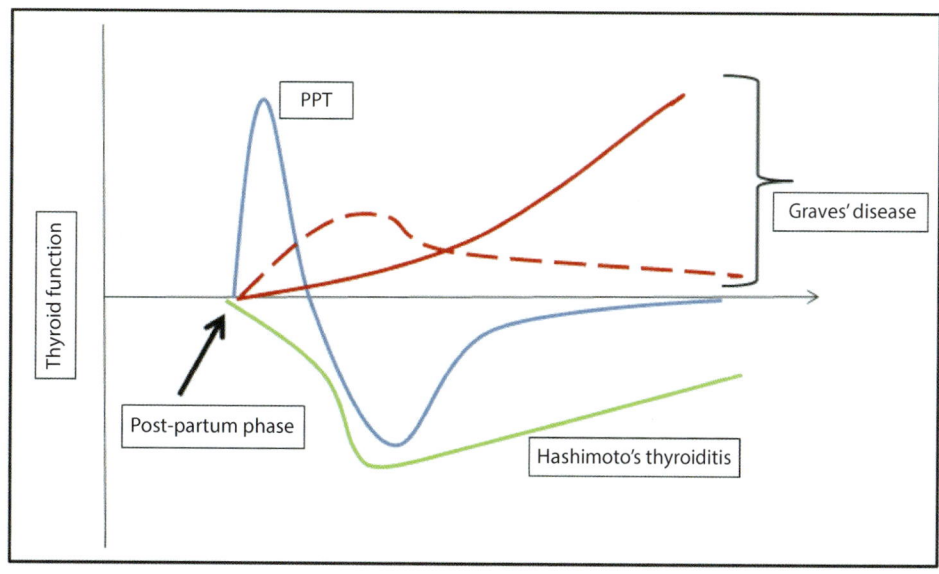

FIGURE 6.4 Outcomes of autoimmune thyroiditis after pregnancy. *Abbreviation:* PPT, postpartum thyroiditis.

Clinically patient presents as abrupt onset of painful thyroid swelling associated with fever. Some adult patients might complaint of firm painful thyroid swelling without any signs of inflammation. Infants with a large cystic fistula may develop acute respiratory distress due to tracheal compression following feeding or crying, and this risk increases markedly with inflammation (26). Laboratory investigations typically show leukocytosis and a positive C-reactive protein reflecting acute inflammation. Notably, serum levels of thyroid hormones, thyrotropin and Tg are normal in most patients, while some patients with severe destruction of thyroid follicles show transient thyrotoxicosis with elevations of serum thyroxine and Tg (27). Thyroid scintigraphy with radioactive iodine or sodium pertechnetate 99mTc demonstrates a decreased uptake in the affected lobe (25). A congenital fistula, pyriform sinus fistula, is the most common route of infection in these patients. Recurrence of inflammation is very common in these patients, and successful surgical removal of fistula is the main line of treatment (28). Successful rate of surgery that has been observed is 85%. Initially abscess can be removed through small incision in the skin but fistulectomy is definite treatment to prevent the recurrence (26). Specific organism should be identified by culture and appropriate antibiotics selection should be done.

Riedel's thyroiditis

Riedel chronic sclerosing thyroiditis is rare and occurs primarily in middle-aged women. It is believed to be a part of IgG4-related disease and may have multisystem involvement in the form of interstitial pneumonia, autoimmune pancreatitis, orbital, sinus or intracranial mass. It is insidious in onset and associated with compression of adjacent structure like trachea, esophagus and recurrent laryngeal nerve due to enlarged thyroid giving the impression of underlying malignancy but there is no associated weight loss. Thyroid gland is moderately enlarged, stony hard and asymmetrical without any lymphadenopathy. Thyroid functions are usually normal but may be associated with hypothyroidism. On histopathology, there is diffuse fibrosis (storiform and keloid type) and inflammatory cells replacing thyroid parenchyma. There is abundance of IgG4 positive cells and the ratio: $IgG4^+/IgG^+$ cells >0.5 in biopsy specimen is suggestive. The RAIU may be normal or low. Elevated circulating thyroid autoantibodies are much less common and are found in lower titers than in Hashimoto's disease. Tamoxifen, 10–20 mg/day (with or without corticosteroids), has been successful in many of these patients and is thought to suppress transforming growth factor-beta (TGFβ).

Drug-induced thyroiditis

Drugs like Amiodarone and lithium cause thyroiditis-like symptoms. Other drugs include IL2, interferon alpha, granulocyte/macrophage colony-stimulating factor (GM-CSF) and the newer immune therapy modulators, all of which can precipitate silent thyroiditis. Thyroiditis has also been associated with multitargeting kinase inhibitors such as sunitinib and sorafenib given for a variety of tumors, including gastrointestinal stromal tumors, hepatocellular carcinoma and renal cell carcinoma. Blood investigations give picture of thyrotoxicosis, but slowly it further progresses to destruction of thyroid gland.

One of the common drugs causing thyroid dysfunction is amiodarone which is a potent class 3 antiarrhythmic drug that resembles thyroid hormone. Amiodarone contains 37.5% iodine by weight and generates iodine excess; one 200-mg tablet/day releases 6 mg of iodide daily that has obligatory and facultative effects on thyroid (29). Due to its high-fat solubility, the drug has a slow turnover, which explains the long elimination half-life of around 40 days for amiodarone and 57 days for its metabolite – desethylamiodarone (DEA) (30). Amiodarone can cause both hypo- and hyperthyroidism. Amiodarone-induced hypothyroidism (AIH) is caused by a failure to escape from the Wolff-Chaikoff effect especially found in TPOAb positive and is more prevalent in iodine sufficient region (31) whereas Amiodarone-induced thyrotoxicosis (AmIT), in contrast, is more prevalent in iodine-deficient regions (32). Table 6.3 describes various drugs implicated in thyroid dysfunction.

TABLE 6.3: Drugs Causing Thyroiditis

Drugs	Manifestation	Therapy
Amiodarone	Hypothyroidism	Thyroxine replacement
	Iodine induced (type 1) (overproduction of hormones)	Supportive care, Antithyroid drugs perchlorate, Surgery
	Thyroiditis (type 2) (destructive thyroiditis)	Supportive care, corticosteroids, surgery
Lithium	Hypothyroidism	Thyroxine replacement
	Painless thyroiditis	Supportive care,
	GD	Antithyroid drugs
Interferon α	Painless thyroiditis	Supportive care
	GD	Antithyroid drugs, Radioactive iodine
Interleukin 2	Painless thyroiditis	Supportive care
	Graves' disease (GD)	Antithyroid drugs, Radioactive iodine
Iodinated contrast	Underlying thyroid autonomy	Antithyroid drugs
Radioactive iodine (early)	Destruction	Observation, if severe administer corticosteroids
Radioactive iodine for TMNG (late)	GD	Antithyroid drugs, repeat radioactive iodine, surgery

Abbreviations: GD, Grave's disease; TMNG, toxic multinodular goiter.
Source: Adapted from Ross DS. Burch, Cooper DS, et al. 2016 American Thyroid Association guidelines for diagnosis and management of hyperthyroidism and other causes of thyrotoxicosis. *Thyroid*. 2016;26(10):1343–1421.

Miscellaneous forms of thyroiditis

Sarcoidosis and radiation are other rare forms of thyroid inflammation. Sarcoidosis is characterized by granulomatous inflammation of the gland resulting in goiter and less commonly hypothyroidism. Postradiation thyroiditis may range from acute classical presentation of destructive thyroiditis to insidious onset hypothyroidism. As discussed previously, radiation is a risk factor for hypothyroidism, and thus, people with underlying thyroid antibodies are more susceptible. One of the very common causes of postradiation thyroiditis is after ^{131}I radioiodine ablation for hyperthyroidism and the risk of hypothyroidism increases with increasing dose of radioiodine and postradiation duration. Therefore, it is of utmost importance to check the TSH levels at regular intervals post thyroid ablation.

South Asian perspective

The presentation of thyroiditis of various forms more or less is similar compared to Western counterparts; however, the prevalence of various signs and symptoms are less common in Indian patients and atypical presentations are far more common for, e.g. there are cases of short stature and delayed puberty among Indian children due to lack of universal screening for congenital hypothyroidism as well as lack of awareness about juvenile AIT (see Figure 6.3). Further, the awareness regarding correct dose and precautions with levothyroxine is scarce. The goiter associated with Hashimoto's thyroiditis not uncommonly leads to unnecessary FNAC when a simple ultrasound should be enough.

The subacute viral thyroiditis has a usual presentation and often patients can pinpoint the onset of symptoms. However, the acute thyrotoxic phase more often than not is being mistreated as Graves' disease that leads to risk of adverse effects due to unnecessary treatment with antithyroid agents. There is also lack of facilities regarding the use of nuclear imaging in thyroid disorders specially in diagnosis of thyroiditis. Clinicians dealing with thyroid disorders should be taught about the differentiating feature between destructive thyroiditis and hyperthyroidism (see Figure 6.4).

The other forms of thyroiditis are quite rare and may require FNAC and other tests to arrive at a diagnosis for, e.g., sarcoidosis and Riedel's thyroiditis. These disorders more commonly present with goiter rather than biochemical abnormalities in thyroid function tests.

Conclusion

Thyroiditis is a disorder of multiple etiologies and with wide spectrum of presentations ranging from local symptoms in acute phase that may be followed by symptoms of thyrotoxicosis to overt hypothyroid symptoms in some patients. Clinicians must be aware of this possibility to avoid unnecessary use of antithyroid drugs or even prolonged use of thyroxine replacements. A careful history of offending medications, temporal pattern of symptoms and concomitant systemic disorder may help in detecting the etiology and planning appropriate treatment.

References

1. McGrogan A, Seaman HE, Wright JW, de Vries CS. The incidence of autoimmune thyroid disease: A systematic review of the literature. Clin Endocrinol (Oxf). 2008 Nov;69(5):687–696.
2. Marwaha RK, Tandon N, Karak AK, Gupta N, Verma K, Kochupillai N. Hashimoto's thyroiditis: Countrywide screening of goitrous healthy young girls in postiodization phase in India. J Clin Endocrinol Metab. 2000 Oct;85(10):3798–3802.
3. Ehlers M, Thiel A, Bernecker C, Porwol D, Papewalis C, Willenberg HS, et al. Evidence of a combined cytotoxic thyroglobulin and thyroperoxidase epitope-specific cellular immunity in Hashimoto's thyroiditis. J Clin Endocrinol Metab. 2012 Apr;97(4):1347–1354.
4. Rebuffat SA, Nguyen B, Robert B, Castex F, Peraldi-Roux S. Antithyroperoxidase antibody-dependent cytotoxicity in autoimmune thyroid disease. J Clin Endocrinol Metab. 2008 Mar;93(3):929–934.
5. Renné C, Ramos Lopez E, Steimle-Grauer SA, Ziolkowski P, Pani MA, Luther C, et al. Thyroid fetal male microchimerisms in mothers with thyroid disorders: Presence of Y-chromosomal immunofluorescence in thyroid-infiltrating lymphocytes is more prevalent in Hashimoto's thyroiditis and Graves' disease than in follicular adenomas. J Clin Endocrinol Metab. 2004 Nov;89(11):5810–5814.
6. Weetman AP. Immunity, thyroid function and pregnancy: Molecular mechanisms. Nat Rev Endocrinol. 2010 Jun;6(6):311–318.
7. Usha Menon V, Sundaram KR, Unnikrishnan AG, Jayakumar RV, Nair V, Kumar H. High prevalence of undetected thyroid disorders in an iodine sufficient adult south Indian population. J Indian Med Assoc. 2009 Feb;107(2):72–77.
8. Torino F, Barnabei A, Paragliola R, Baldelli R, Appetecchia M, Corsello SM. Thyroid dysfunction as an unintended side effect of anticancer drugs. Thyroid. 2013 Nov;23(11):1345–1366.
9. Wiersinga WM. Smoking and thyroid. Clin Endocrinol (Oxf). 2013 Aug;79(2):145–151.
10. Carlé A, Pedersen IB, Knudsen N, Perrild H, Ovesen L, Rasmussen LB, et al. Moderate alcohol consumption may protect against overt autoimmune hypothyroidism: A population-based case-control study. Eur J Endocrinol. 2012 Oct;167(4):483–490.
11. Tomer Y. Mechanisms of autoimmune thyroid diseases: From genetics to epigenetics. Annu Rev Pathol. 2014;9:147–156.
12. Zulewski H, Müller B, Exer P, Miserez AR, Staub JJ. Estimation of tissue hypothyroidism by a new clinical score: Evaluation of patients with various grades of hypothyroidism and controls. J Clin Endocrinol Metab. 1997 Mar;82(3):771–776.
13. Sethi B, Barua S, Raghavendra MS, Gotur J, Khandelwal D, Vyas U. The thyroid registry: Clinical and hormonal characteristics of adult Indian patients with hypothyroidism. Indian J Endocrinol Metab. 2017 Apr;21(2):302–307.
14. Indian Pediatrics – Editorial [Internet]. [cited 2020 Apr 30]. Available from: https://indianpediatrics.net/july1999/july-659-668.htm.
15. Samuels MH. Subacute, silent, and postpartum thyroiditis. Med Clin North Am. 2012 Mar;96(2):223–233.
16. De Groot L, Abalovich M, Alexander EK, Amino N, Barbour L, Cobin RH, et al. Management of thyroid dysfunction during pregnancy and postpartum: An Endocrine Society clinical practice guideline. J Clin Endocrinol Metab. 2012 Aug;97(8):2543–2565.
17. Nicholson WK, Robinson KA, Smallridge RC, Ladenson PW, Powe NR. Prevalence of postpartum thyroid dysfunction: A quantitative review. Thyroid. 2006 Jun;16(6):573–582.
18. Premawardhana LD, Parkes AB, Ammari F, John R, Darke C, Adams H, et al. Postpartum thyroiditis and long-term thyroid status: Prognostic influence of thyroid peroxidase antibodies and ultrasound echogenicity. J Clin Endocrinol Metab. 2000 Jan;85(1):71–75.
19. Approach to the patient with postpartum thyroiditis. – PubMed – NCBI [Internet]. [cited 2020 Apr 17]. Available from: https://www.ncbi.nlm.nih.gov/pubmed/22312089.
20. Ide A, Amino N, Kang S, Yoshioka W, Kudo T, Nishihara E, et al. Differentiation of postpartum Graves' thyrotoxicosis from postpartum destructive thyrotoxicosis using antithyrotropin receptor antibodies and thyroid blood flow. Thyroid. 2014 Jun;24(6):1027–1031.
21. Alexander EK, Pearce EN, Brent GA, Brown RS, Chen H, Dosiou C, et al. 2017 Guidelines of the American Thyroid Association for the diagnosis and management of thyroid disease during pregnancy and the postpartum. Thyroid. 2017;27(3):315–389.
22. Pearce EN. Thyroid disorders during pregnancy and postpartum. Best Pract Res Clin Obstet Gynaecol. 2015 Jul;29(5):700–706.
23. Fatourechi V, Aniszewski JP, Fatourechi GZE, Atkinson EJ, Jacobsen SJ. Clinical features and outcome of subacute thyroiditis in an incidence cohort: Olmsted County, Minnesota, study. J Clin Endocrinol Metab. 2003 May;88(5):2100–2105.
24. Paes JE, Burman KD, Cohen J, Franklyn J, McHenry CR, Shoham S, et al. Acute bacterial suppurative thyroiditis: A clinical review and expert opinion. Thyroid. 2010 Mar;20(3):247–255.
25. Yolmo D, Madana J, Kalaiarasi R, Gopalakrishnan S, Kiruba Shankar M, Krishnapriya S. Retrospective case review of pyriform sinus fistulae of third branchial arch origin commonly presenting as acute suppurative thyroiditis in children. J Laryngol Otol. 2012 Jul;126(7):737–742.
26. Miyauchi A, Matsuzuka F, Kuma K, Takai S. Piriform sinus fistula: An underlying abnormality common in patients with acute suppurative thyroiditis. World J Surg. 1990 Jun;14(3):400–405.
27. Fukata S, Miyauchi A, Kuma K, Sugawara M. Acute suppurative thyroiditis caused by an infected piriform sinus fistula with thyrotoxicosis. Thyroid. 2002 Feb;12(2):175–178.
28. Kim KH, Sung MW, Koh TY, Oh SH, Kim IS. Pyriform sinus fistula: Management with chemocauterization of the internal opening. Ann Otol Rhinol Laryngol. 2000 May;109(5):452–456.
29. Amiodarone-induced thyroid dysfunction. – PubMed – NCBI [Internet]. [cited 2020 Apr 17]. Available from: https://www.ncbi.nlm.nih.gov/pubmed/24067547.
30. Eskes SA, Wiersinga WM. Amiodarone and thyroid. Best Pract Res Clin Endocrinol Metab. 2009 Dec;23(6):735–751.
31. Martino E, Bartalena L, Bogazzi F, Braverman LE. The effects of amiodarone on the thyroid. Endocr Rev. 2001 Apr;22(2):240–254.
32. Cohen-Lehman J, Dahl P, Danzi S, Klein I. Effects of amiodarone therapy on thyroid function. Nat Rev Endocrinol. 2010 Jan;6(1):34–41.

7

HYPOTHYROIDISM

Madhukar Mittal, Parul Gupta and M K Garg

Introduction

Hypothyroidism, a state of thyroid hormone deficiency, is the most common clinical disorder of thyroid function (1). Primary hypothyroidism accounts for most (~99%) of the cases of hypothyroidism and is defined by a decrease in production and secretion of thyroxine (T4) and triidothyronine (T3) from the thyroid gland. Primary hypothyroidism is, thus, biochemically characterized by a high thyrotropin (TSH) with or without a low T4. In less than 1% cases, hypothyroidism is caused by decreased stimulation of thyroid by the TSH/TRH and is referred as central/secondary/hypothyrotropic hypothyroidism. Central hypothyroidism is characterized by low/low normal thyroxine and low or inappropriately normal or even high (but not more than 10–15 mIU/L) serum TSH (1).

Subclinical hypothyroidism is regarded as a sign of early thyroid failure and is defined biochemically by TSH above the reference range (but not more than 10 mIU/L) and free thyroxine concentration within the normal range. The term is a misnomer as the nomenclature does not depend on whether the patient has symptoms or not.

Causes

The causes are enumerated in Table 7.1.

Primary hypothyroidism

Iodine deficiency: Approximately one-third of the world's population lives in iodine-deficient areas. When the intake of iodine is inadequate, the thyroid gland enlarges (goiter) and when it is no longer able to synthesize sufficient amount of thyroid hormones, decompensation occurs and hypothyroidism ensues. Iodine deficiency is presumed to be the most common cause of hypothyroidism in South Asian region (2) although autoimmune hypothyroidism is being commonly seen in the areas of adequate consumption of iodized salt. Recommended daily intake (RDA) of iodine is 90 μg/day for children <6 years, 120 μg/day for 6–12 years, 150 μg/day for adults and 250 μg for pregnant and lactating females. A 24-hour urinary iodine concentration (UIC) ≥100 μg/L indicates sufficient iodine intake. Salt iodization is now mandated in over 120 countries to ensure adequate iodine intake. However, universal fortification has now raised concerns regarding hypothyroidism induced by excess iodine intake (3).

Autoimmune: Chronic autoimmune thyroiditis is the most common cause of hypothyroidism in iodine sufficient areas (2). The average age of onset is between 30 and 60 years. It can be subclassified as atrophic or goitrous variant. The goitrous form can present as either focal or diffuse lymphocytic thyroiditis. The latter when associated with follicular destruction and eosinophilic infiltrate is commonly called as Hashimoto thyroiditis (4). Antibody to thyroid peroxidase (TPO) is found in 90–100% patients with autoimmune thyroiditis but it can also be positive in 8–27% of general population. Antibody to thyroglobulin (Tg) can also be found in 80–90% patients with autoimmunity but has lower affinity and is found in lower concentration, so is less commonly measured (5).

Iatrogenic: Hypothyroidism is common after surgery or radioactive iodine ablation for treatment of hyperthyroidism. It has been estimated that one in five patients who undergoes hemithyroidectomy may develop hypothyroidism. A systematic review of 32 studies estimated the overall risk of hypothyroidism after hemithyroidectomy to be 22% and estimated risk of clinical hypothyroidism as 4% (6). In a study of 130 patients treated with I^{131} for multinodular goiter and followed up for a median of 42 months, hypothyroidism developed in 20% patients who had received prior antithyroid drugs and in 6% of those who did not (7). Similarly, in 265 patients of toxic nodular goiter treated with 150 Gy I^{131}, the incidence of hypothyroidism at 3 months, 1 year and at end of follow-up (max 8 years) was 32%, 55% and 73%, respectively (8).

Drugs: Iodine-containing drugs (amiodarone, contrast agents), lithium, tetracycline, aminoglutethimide, ethionamide cause inhibition of synthesis and/release of thyroid hormones while interferon alpha acts via immune mechanism. Tyrosine kinase inhibitors cause drug-induced thyroiditis leading to hypothyroidism (9).

Central hypothyroidism

It is an uncommon cause of hypothyroidism with an estimated incidence of 1:16,000–1:100,000 (10). It is due to insufficient stimulation of an otherwise normal thyroid gland by TSH/TRH due to either functional or anatomical disorder of pituitary and or hypothalamus. Biochemically, it is characterized by low or low-normal free T4 with inappropriately low/normal TSH. Occasionally, the TSH can even be mildly elevated probably because of the presence of decreased bioactivity of TSH (11).

The common causes of central hypothyroidism are enumerated in Table 7.1 (10). Congenital central hypothyroidism can be isolated or associated with multiple pituitary hormone deficiency (MPHD). Craniopharyngioma is the most common expansile lesion associated with central hypothyroidism in pediatric patients. In adults, macroadenoma of the pituitary or its treatment accounts for most of the cases (10).

Transient hypothyroidism

It is defined as periods of decreased thyroid hormone production that is eventually followed by euthyroid state, e.g. subacute thyroiditis that is usually preceded by features of mild-to-moderate thyrotoxicosis (5). This may also commonly occur post hemithyroidectomy where the rest of the gland is able to compensate over time for the lost thyroid tissue. Thyroxine replacement may be needed in the phase of transient hypothyroidism with gradual reduction of doses and eventual discontinuation. Thyroxine withdrawal may also lead to a transient rise of TSH for a short period of time.

Hypothyroidism

TABLE 7.1: Causes of Hypothyroidism

Primary Hypothyroidism	
Iodine deficiency	Moderate-to-severe iodine deficiency
Autoimmune	Chronic thyroiditis (Hashimoto's thyroiditis)
Iatrogenic	Postsurgical (thyroidectomy)
	Post radioiodine ablation (e.g., for Grave's disease)
	Postradiation (therapeutic radiation for non-thyroidal malignancy)
Drugs	Thionamides, amiodarone, contrast agents, lithium, tetracyclines, interferon alpha, tyrosine kinase inhibitors, others
Infiltration	Amyloidosis, hemochromatosis, sarcoidosis, scleroderma, cystinosis, Riedel struma, lymphoma
Central Hypothyroidism	
Congenital isolated central hypothyroidism	Mutation in TSHβ, TSHR, TBL1X, IRS4
Congenital multiple pituitary hormone deficiency	Mutation in IGSF1, PUO1F1, PROP1, HESX1, SOX3, OTX2, LHX3, LHX4, LEPR
Invasive/compressive lesions of sella turcica	Pituitary macroadenomas
	Craniopharyngioma, meningioma
	Rathke cleft cysts
Iatrogenic	Cranial surgery/irradiation
Injury	Head trauma/traumatic delivery
Infiltrative	Iron overload, TB, syphilis
	Sarcoidosis, histiocytosis X
Autoimmune	Lymphocytic hypophysitis
Vascular	Pituitary infarction
	Sheehan syndrome
	Subarachnoid hemorrhage
Drugs	Bexarotene, CTLA4 inhibitors
Transient Hypothyroidism	
Post thyroiditis	Subacute viral/de Quervain thyroiditis
	Postpartum
	Painless (Silent) thyroiditis
Peripheral Hypothyroidism	
Consumptive	Hemangioma/hemangioendothelioma

Peripheral hypothyroidism

It is described in infants with visceral hemangiomas that show deiodinase 3 enzyme activity and, thus, increased conversion of T4 to rT3 (5). This is a form of consumptive hypothyroidism.

Clinical features

There is a large variation in clinical presentation of hypothyroidism. The underlying pathophysiology is slowing of the physiological processes and deposition of glycosaminoglycans and clinical manifestations reflect this (detailed in Table 7.2) (5). The symptoms are largely nonspecific especially in adults and elderly. Traditionally, it was believed that the number of hypothyroid symptoms was related directly to the level of TSH and more the number of symptoms, stronger was the association with diagnosis of hypothyroidism and patients reporting seven or more changed symptoms were more likely to be hypothyroid (Likelihood ratio 8.7) (12). However, as per a case control study by Carle et al. (13), none of the 34 hypothyroidism-related symptoms had high likelihood ratio/diagnostic odds ratio and neither the presence nor the absence of any individual hypothyroidism symptoms was reliable to decide who should get the thyroid function tested. The highest diagnostic odds ratio was reported for tiredness, dry skin, hair loss (13).

In addition to the biochemical markers of thyroid function, various physiological and tissue biomarkers are available. The physiological parameters are heart rate, basal metabolic rate, pulse wave arrival time, achilles reflex time, voice fundamental frequency and left ventricular function assessed by echocardiography. Various tissue biomarkers of action of thyroid function include SHBG, LDL, creatine kinase, urinary telopeptides, osteocalcin, ferritin, myoglobin, etc. But these are for research settings and not recommended for routine clinical use (14).

Myxedema coma: It occurs as a consequence of long-standing and untreated decompensated hypothyroidism. It is a life-threatening emergency characterized by altered mental status and defective thermoregulation. Precipitating factors include infections, sedative use and discontinuation of thyroid supplementation. Cardiogenic shock, severe respiratory depression, arrhythmia and coma occur due to low intracellular T3. It needs to be recognized and treated early as the prognosis is poor with a mortality of about 25–60% despite treatment (15).

Cretinism: It is a consequence of severe long-standing untreated iodine deficiency and is characterized by intellectual impairment, deaf-mutism and spasticity (16). This severe form of hypothyroidism is less seen clinically nowadays.

Diagnosis

The diagnosis of hypothyroidism relies mainly on TSH and free T4 values (Figure 7.1). As discussed earlier, primary hypothyroidism is defined by TSH concentration above the population-specific reference range (most commonly used 0.4 to 4–5 mIU/L) and free thyroxine concentration in normal or below the reference range.

TABLE 7.2: Clinical Features

System	Symptoms	Signs/Manifestations	Lab Parameter
General metabolism	Weight gain, decreased appetite, fatigue, cold intolerance	low basal body temperature	↓SHBG, ↑Albumin ↑LDL ↓Leptin, ↑Resistin
Cardiovascular	shortness of breath easy fatiguability angina	bradycardia, hypertension, pericardial effusions	↓Cardiac output, ↑peripheral resistance ECG: sinus bradycardia, prolonged PR interval, low amplitude QRS
Respiratory	Dyspnea Sleep apnea	Pleural effusion	CO_2 retention, ↓diffusion capacity
Gastrointestinal	Constipation,	Achlorhydria	Fatty liver
CNS	Hoarseness of voice, decreased taste, vision, hearing paresthesia, intellectual slowing, lethargy, somnolence, headache, myxedema madness, seizures	hung up reflexes, dementia, ataxia, carpal tunnel syndrome	EEG: slow α wave and loss of amplitude
Skin and hair	Dry skin, hair loss, puffy face, delayed wound healing, vitiligo	Non-pitting edema, loss of lateral eyebrows, alopecia, pale cool skin	Skin histopathology: hyperkeratosis with plugging of hair follicles, PAS+ mucinous material
Musculoskeletal	Muscle cramps, arthralgia, growth failure	Calf hypertrophy, short limb dwarfism, myoclonus	Epiphyseal dysgenesis: stippled epiphysis, ↑PTH
Hematopoietic	Anemia, bleeding tendency		Normocytic/macrocytic anemia, ↓factors VIII and IX, ↑capillary fragility, ↓ platelet adhesiveness
Endocrine	Decreased libido, menorrhagia, infertility/subfertility, short stature, delayed puberty, rarely precocious puberty	Galactorrhea	Failure of ovulation, oligospermia, ↓SHBG, ↓response to GH stimulation tests, including insulin Rarely, pituitary enlargement on MRI
Renal and electrolyte	Deterioration of renal function	Hypertension, edema	↓Plasma rennin activity ↓GFR, hyponatremia

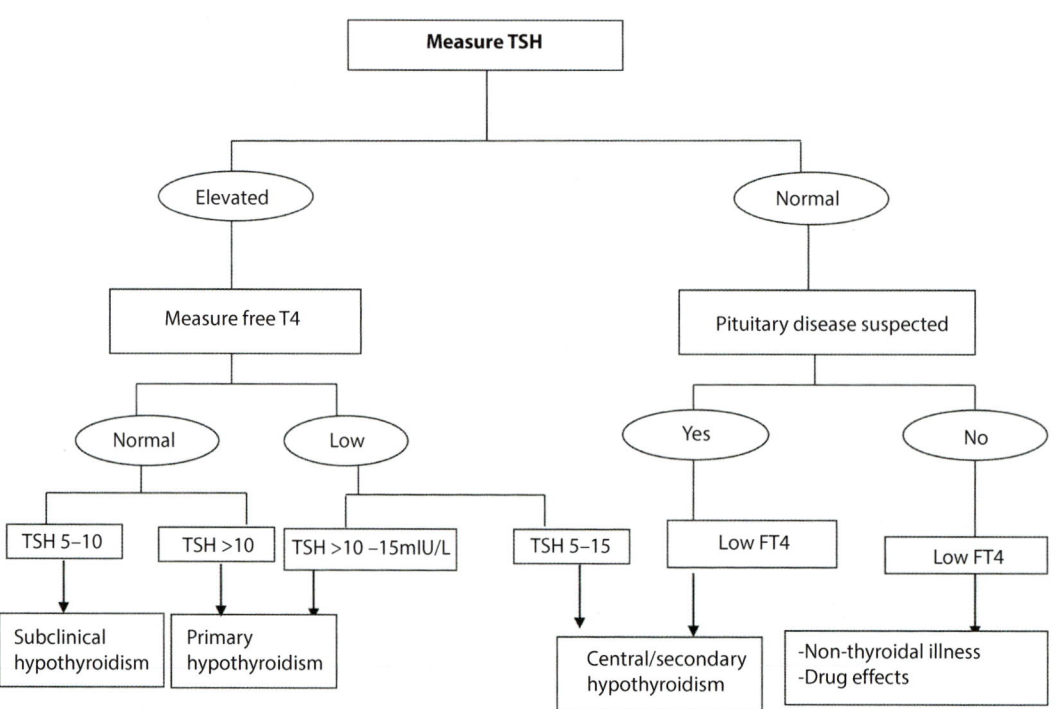

FIGURE 7.1 Evaluation of suspected hypothyroidism.

Hypothyroidism

The reference range differs with age, sex, ethnic origin and appropriate reference limits should be used for interpreting thyroid function tests (TFTs). Reference ranges for thyroid function (FT3, FT4 and TSH) for Indian population generated through cross-sectional studies are available for school-aged children, adults and pregnant females (17–19).

Both TSH and FT4 are higher in infants, especially in first week of life. Similarly, with each decade, there is a rise in TSH value and there is increased variability around mean. There is circadian and seasonal variation in TSH values with higher concentrations toward evening and in winter and spring. Also patients with severe hypothyroidism show even more irregularity in TSH secretion. Thus, the TSH and FT4 values should be interpreted keeping these variations in mind (20).

Serum TSH may be anomalously low for several months after either surgical or I^{131} ablation especially if TSH synthesis was suppressed for a long period prior to ablation. Thus, in such cases, diagnosis of hypothyroidism should rely on FT4 rather on TSH (5).

The diagnosis of central hypothyroidism may be missed if clinicians are not aware of interpreting TFTs. This is because especially in developing regions like South Asia, where clinicians may rely only on TSH values for diagnosis of hypothyroidism. This "reflex TSH strategy" of screening for hypothyroidism will miss central hypothyroidism cases (21), and thus, both TSH and free thyroxine should be checked especially in patients with suspected pituitary/hypothalamic cause.

It is important to differentiate certain conditions where abnormalities in TSH/T4/T3 may be there but not within the parameters of a classic primary hypothyroidism. In such cases, instead of starting blanket levothyroxine therapy, it may be appropriate to take opinion of an endocrinologist for reaching a conclusive diagnosis. These include:

- *Resistance to thyroid hormone (RTH)*: Autosomal dominant mutations in the thyroid hormone receptor genes α and β can lead to resistance to thyroid hormone. RTH α is characterized by high or high normal TSH and T3 and a low normal T4. Clinically, patients may be asymptomatic or present with features of hypothyroidism, including bradycardia, constipation, macroglossia and growth retardation. It can be differentiated by childhood presentation, dysmorphism and presence of family history (TFTs may need to be done in first degree relatives) and low T4/T3 ratio. The confirmation is done with genetic analysis (22). RTH β presents with thyroid enlargement and a mixture of symptoms of hyperthyroidism and hypothyroidism (palpitations, tachycardia and growth retardation) with raised FT4 and normal or slightly raised TSH levels (5).
- *TSH-secreting pituitary adenoma*: Although difficult, it is important to differentiate RTH β from a TSHoma. Discriminatory tests include peripheral tissue markers (viz., SHBG), dynamic testing (diminished TSH response to intravenous TRH 200 μg before and after administration of liothyronine – the "T3 suppression test"), elevated serum concentrations of pituitary glycoprotein hormone α-subunit (ASU) or a raised ASU/TSH molar ratio (>1.0) and the presence of an obvious lesion on pituitary imaging all favor a TSHoma. Microadenomas (microTSHomas) may complicate this picture further and may not be easy to differentiate especially in the light of more pituitary incidentalomas being detected with higher resolution MRIs (5).
- *Disorders of thyroid hormone transport or metabolism*: Altered TBG concentrations and thyroid hormone-binding proteins, MCT8 mutations
- *Drugs inhibiting TSH secretion*: Glucocorticoids, dopamine, metformin, cocaine, antiepileptics and antipsychotics.
- Levothyroxine withdrawal/prolonged suppression of TSH after recovery from thyrotoxicosis.

Severe non-thyroidal illness can cause low FT4, but TSH is usually in normal range (except during recovery). Thus, thyroid function testing should be interpreted with caution in these patients who are clinically in a sick state (sick euthyroid syndrome) (23).

Assay interference – several conditions can interfere with laboratory measurements of thyroid analytes and interference should be suspected if TFTs do not match the clinical presentation. In cases of suspected FT4 assay interference, equilibrium dialysis method for FT4 estimation should be used. If it not available, two-step immunoassay method or mass spectrometry should be used (24). Heterophile antibodies such as anti-mouse antibody can cause errors in TSH values with immunometric assays. Macro-TSH can also cause erroneously high TSH values and can be excluded by PEG precipitation test. Heparin and biotin can also interfere with the results (24). Interference in TSH assay occurs with biotin use in certain chemiluminescence assay systems. If interference is suspected, it is advisable to repeat TFTs from a different laboratory along with means to avoid suspected cause of interference.

Screening

American Thyroid Association (ATA) (25) recommends screening for hypothyroidism every 5 years for individuals aged >35 years while the American Association of Clinical Endocrinologists (AACE) (26) and American Academy of family physicians (AAFP) (27) recommend screening for older patients >60 years especially women. As per London Royal College of physicians (28) and US preventive task force (29), screening of general population is not justified.

Regarding screening of pregnant women, ATA (24) and Indian Thyroid Society (30) recommend screening TSH for all pregnant women at their first visit. However, national guidelines by Government of India (31) recommend screening only in high-risk cases.

Treatment

Levothyroxine (LT4) monotherapy is the treatment of choice (14). It should be taken either 60 minutes before breakfast and there should be at least 4-hour separation with other supplements, e.g. calcium and iron. Alternatively, dosing may be given at bedtime (≥3 hours after the evening meal) in certain circumstances. The other medications that potentially affect levothyroxine absorption include proton pump inhibitors, H2 blockers, raloxifene, cholestyramine, colesevelam, sevelamer and sucralfate. Switching between different brands of levothyroxine should normally be avoided as it can potentially result in variation in the dose administered. It is recommended that after any change in the formulation or after initiation or discontinuation of drugs affecting thyroxine metabolism (phenobarbital, rifampicin, phenytoin, carbamazepine, sertraline and tyrosine kinase inhibitors) or protein binding (estrogen and androgens), serum TSH should be measured after steady state, i.e. at 4–6 weeks (14).

The following should be considered before deciding the initial dose of levothyroxine:

- Patient's weight
- Lean body mass
- Pregnancy status
- Etiology of hypothyroidism
- Degree of thyrotropin elevation
- Age
- General clinical context especially the cardiac status

The recommended dose is 1.6–1.8 µg/kg of actual body weight in patients with minimal endogenous thyroid function. Post-thyroidectomy patients require higher dose as compared to patients with Hashimoto thyroiditis. The doses to be used in children are as follows (14):

- *Newborn*: 10–15 µg/kg/day
- *1–3 years*: 4–6 µg/kg/day
- *3–10 years*: 3–5 µg/kg/day
- *10–16 years*: 2–4 µg/kg/day

The dose of thyroxine in children can also be calculated as per body surface area as 100 µg/m^2/day (14). Children and young adults can be started on full calculated LT4 dose but in elderly and patients with cardiac disease, the recommendation is to "start low and go slow". In patients with coronary artery disease, LT4 should be started at 12.5–25 µg per day and should be gradually increased to target TSH levels over time.

In cases of primary hypothyroidism, TSH levels should be used to adjust LT4 dose with target TSH being 0.5–4 mIU/L (4–6 mIU/L in patients >70 years). Serum TSH should be repeated after 4–6 weeks of treatment initiation and dose adjustments of 12.5–25 µg/day should be made till a target TSH is reached. Thereafter, TSH should be measured in 4–6 months and then yearly. TSH below 0.1 mIU/L (iatrogenic thyrotoxicosis) should be avoided as it can lead to atrial fibrillation and osteoporosis especially in elderly and postmenopausal females. In secondary hypothyroidism, the treatment goal should be to maintain serum-free T4 in upper half of reference range. Although advocated by certain groups, currently there is insufficient evidence to support use of liothyronine (LT3) and LT4 combination for any indication.

Myxedema coma treatment involves early administrative of thyroid hormones along with supportive treatment. ATA guidelines recommend that 200–400 µg of levothyroxine to be given as loading dose followed by 1.6 µg/kg daily (reduced to 75% intravenous) along with intravenous glucocorticoid administration. Intravenous liothyronine (5–20 µg loading dose followed by 2.5 to 10 mcg 8 hourly maintenance dose) may also be added where available. Intravenous thyroxine is preferred over oral drug delivery due to altered gut absorption in myxedema coma, but due to unavailability of intravenous thyroxine, usually oral thyroxine is given via nasogastric tube. Therapeutic end points include improved mental status, cardiac and pulmonary function (14).

Monitoring response

Most of the hypothyroid patients are well controlled with levothyroxine in doses of 1.3–1.6–1.8 µg/kg/day. Persistent elevation of TSH warrants further increase of dose but more importantly needs checking for nonadherence/noncompliance. Once good compliance is confirmed, one needs to look into other important causes like concomitant medications (e.g., ferrous sulfate, calcium carbonate, antacids), pharmacokinetics/pharmacodynamics modifying drugs (e.g. rifampicin, carbamazepine, phenytoin, amiodarone) and anti-T4 antibodies. This is termed as pseudomalabsorption of levothyroxine. Malabsorption due to gastrointestinal disorders (e.g. celiac disease, tropical sprue, resection of small intestine, atrophic gastritis and others) or altered gut microbiota needs to be evaluated. Assessment for levothyroxine absorption may help in deciding whether an extensive evaluation for malabsorption syndromes is needed or not. Subjects with persistent elevations of TSH on higher dose of levothyroxine can be reliably diagnosed to be nonadherent to treatment with levothyroxine absorption test [10 mcg/kg or 600 mcg maximum levothyroxine is given and free T4 measured hourly for 5 hours; value >0.40 ng/dL at 3 h suggests that workup for malabsorption is unwarranted] (32). For increasing compliance, weekly supervised dose of levothyroxine may be an option.

Special consideration

Subclinical hypothyroidism: It is defined biochemically by TSH above the reference range up to 10 mIU/L and free thyroxine concentration within the normal range. It has been associated with altered metabolic profile, increased cardiovascular risk, increased pregnancy loss and infertility. The risk of progression to overt hypothyroidism annually is 4% in women with raised TSH and positive antithyroid antibody and 2–4% in those who are negative for antibodies. Treatment of subclinical hypothyroidism with levothyroxine is recommended in those who have positive TPO antibodies, goiter, and in pregnant females with serum TSH above the reference range for pregnancy. Treatment can also be considered in patients who have symptoms suggestive of hypothyroidism and patients who wish to conceive and have history of pregnancy loss or infertility (33). The dose of levothyroxine to treat subclinical hypothyroidism is much lower, usually 12.5–25 µg/day.

Hypothyroidism in pregnancy: Hypothyroidism in pregnancy is defined as increased TSH with/without decreased FT4 as per trimester-specific range. Trimester-specific ranges for Indian population are available and should be used to interpret TFT in South Asian population (19). Early recognition of maternal hypothyroidism is important since if untreated, it can lead to pregnancy loss, preterm birth, low birth weight and low IQ in offspring. As per ATA guidelines (34), anti-TPO antibody should be done if TSH is >2.5 mIU/L. Levothyroxine should be started in all cases of TSH >10 mIU/L irrespective of TPO positivity and in TPOAb positive women with TSH greater than pregnancy-specific range. The upper reference limit for TSH as 4 mIU/L as suggested by ATA is different from the normative data in Indian pregnant females (35) and one may consider 3 mIU/L in first trimester and 3.5 mIU/L in second and third trimesters for South Asian population based on this data. The target should be to maintain TSH <2.5 mIU/L or in lower half of trimester-specific range. Thyroid functions should be monitored 4 weekly till mid-gestation and at least once near 30 weeks. In a known hypothyroid female, LT4 dose should be increased to 20–30% of the prepregnancy dose and should be reduced to preconceptional dose in postpartum period. In those women where LT4 was started during pregnancy, it can be stopped postpartum especially if the dose was <50 µg/day (34).

Congenital hypothyroidism: It is the most common cause of preventable mental retardation worldwide. As per Indian Society for Pediatric and Adolescent Endocrinology (ISPAE) guidelines

Hypothyroidism

TABLE 7.3: Prevalence of Hypothyroidism in South Asia

	India (38)	Nepal (41)	Bangladesh (42)
No. of participants	5376	671	925
Overall prevalence of thyroid disorder (%)	–	4.32	20.43
Subclinical hypothyroidism (%)	8.02	3.12	6.59
Overt hypothyroidism (%)	10.59	0.59	4.97
Age-group with max prevalence	46–54 years	–	11–45
TPO positivity	21.85%	–	15.09%
Overt hypothyroid male:female	1:3	1:2	1:2.5
Goiter	18.68%	NA	10.49%

for diagnosis and management of congenital hypothyroidism, screening TSH should be done for all newborns at 48–72 hours of life. If the TSH is >20 mIU/L, a confirmatory venous sampling should be done and labeled as congenital hypothyroidism if venous TSH is >20 mIU/L in <2 weeks or >10 mIU/L in >2 weeks of age with a low T4. Levothyroxine should be started at 10–15 µg/kg/day and neck imaging with ultrasound and radionuclide scan should be performed. If the thyroid gland is not visualized on ultrasound or nuclear scan, it suggests thyroid agenesis. A normal-sized or enlarged gland with increased uptake suggests iodine deficiency while reduced uptake could be due to thyroid dysgenesis, iodide symporter gene mutation or maternal antithyroid drug intake (36, 37). Thyroid dysgenesis is the most common cause of congenital hypothyroidism.

South Asian perspective

Epidemiology: The prevalence of hypothyroidism in South Asian region is much higher as compared to Europe (0.2–5.3%) and the United States (0.3–3.7%) (2) as shown in Table 7.3. A survey conducted pan India over 2014–2016 screened a population of 33 lakh for thyroid disorders and found that 32% of population had thyroid dysfunction (38). A cross-sectional study in India showed that the prevalence is higher in inland cities as compared to coastal cities (11.73 vs. 9.45%) (39). The prevalence of hypothyroidism in pregnancy in Indian population was reported as 6.47% with 4.58% as overt hypothyroidism (40). Nomogram of thyroid gland size in normal population in Bangladesh found some thyroid pathology in 9.08% (41).

Clinical features: The percentage frequency of symptoms, signs and associated comorbidity in decreasing order as per reports of a multicenter registry that included 1500 newly diagnosed, treatment naïve adult hypothyroid patients from 33 centers across India is enumerated in Table 7.4 (44). Comorbidities were associated with hypothyroidism in 36.36% of patients. Most common presenting symptom overall was fatigue and menstrual abnormalities were reported in all premenopausal females included in the study. In a cross-sectional study in Bangladesh, 11.5% dyslipidemic patients had hypothyroidism (9.5% subclinical and 2% overt hypothyroidism) and there was a positive association of BMI and diastolic blood pressure with FT4 and TSH (45). A study of 1056 diabetic patients with unknown thyroid status reported subclinical hypothyroidism in 14.1%, overt primary hypothyroidism in 4%, central hypothyroidism in 0.9% and TPO positivity in 32.9% patients (46). Metabolic syndrome was associated with thyroid dysfunction in 28% (47).

Etiology: Iodine deficiency remains the most common cause of hypothyroidism in South Asia unlike the Western world where autoimmune thyroiditis is the most common cause. In a study of 764 goitrous girls in India, juvenile autoimmune thyroiditis was found in only 7.5% (Hashimoto in 5.6% and focal lymphocytic in 1.9%) (48). But, there seems to be a rise in TPO positivity over the years in last two decades probably due to complex genetic and environmental factors (49).

Legislation for universal salt iodization was passed in various countries in South Asia starting from Bangladesh in the late 1980s. Since then the iodine status has improved and prevalence of goiter has declined considerably. Iodine nutrition status was assessed by WHO as per urine iodine concentration data collected over 1993–2004 (50). In South Asian region, India, Bangladesh, Maldives, Nepal, Sri Lanka had adequate iodine status, while Pakistan had mild iodine deficiency and Afghanistan had moderate iodine deficiency while Bhutan had more than adequate iodine intake. But as per the latest report by Iodine Global Network, all the countries included in South Asia currently have optimal iodine intake as per their median urine iodine concentration apart from Nepal that has excess iodine intake (51).

But despite improvement in iodine status, prevalence of goiter is 20 and 50%, respectively, in school-aged children and women in Afghanistan (52). In Pakistan, 79.5% pregnant females were iodine deficient, 24.7% had moderate iodine deficiency, 34.5% had goiter and only 34.2% were consuming iodized salt (53, 54). Thus, it is very important to ensure iodination and screen pregnant females for hypothyroidism to prevent adverse fetal outcomes. However, in a case control study in India, increased prevalence of hypothyroidism was found in patients with higher median UIC but further studies are needed to confirm this trend (55).

High consumption of cyanogenic foods in South Asian region could also be implicated for the high prevalence of

TABLE 7.4: Clinical Features of Hypothyroidism: A Study from India (43)

Symptoms	%	Signs	%	Comorbidity	%
Fatigue	60.1	Hair loss	30.89	Type 2 diabetes	13.54
Weight gain and poor appetite	36.22	Limb swelling	18.08	Hypertension	11.34
Poor memory	19.81	Dry, coarse skin	17.01	Dyslipidemia	4.27
Constipation	18.1	Others	10.41	Hypocalcemia	2.87
Shortness of breath	16.7	Delayed relaxation of tendon reflex	7.47	Vitamin D deficiency	1.73
Feeling cold	15.2	Cool extremity	4.4	Anemia	1.27
Periorbital puffiness	11.4	Slow pulse rate	3.20	Obesity	1.27
Hoarseness of voice	8.74	Carpal tunnel	1.27	Vitamin B12 deficiency	0.53

hypothyroidism in this part of world but the exact role is unclear (56). Goiter was reportedly more common in people using subterranean water and less common in those using turmeric, spices, chilis and dairy products, including milk and ghee (57). The use of pesticides, unclean drinking water, exposure to industrial pollutants, e.g. resorcinol and phthalic acid and other endocrine disruptors could also be amongst the causes and needs further research (58).

Diagnosis and treatment: Despite the guidelines recommending both TSH and T4 for diagnosis of hypothyroidism, 81% percent patients in India were diagnosed and treated solely on the basis of TSH alone (44). Thus, if TSH only approach is followed, it misses out central hypothyroidism. In another cross-sectional study from India, 379 patients who self-reported themselves as hypothyroid, 28% still had high TSH values (39). This highlights the need for awareness and scientific education amongst the clinicians in South Asia regarding appropriate diagnosis and management of hypothyroidism.

Also, the importance of screening and regular monitoring of thyroid functions cannot be underscored. The reference range for TSH and T4 for newborns, school children, pregnant females and adults are available for Indian population and should be used for interpreting TFTs in the South Asian region (17, 18, 35, 37). Since pregnant females are the most vulnerable population and untreated hypothyroidism has grave consequences on maternal and fetal health, all efforts should be made to screen all pregnant females for hypothyroidism (30). If due to resource constraints, universal screening is not possible, all high-risk cases enumerated next should be screened for hypothyroidism (31) as follows:

- Residing in moderate-to-severe iodine-deficient areas
- Symptom of thyroid dysfunction or presence of goiter
- Obesity (BMI > 30 kg/m^2)
- History of prior thyroid dysfunction in self or first-degree relative
- History of preterm delivery, miscarriage, abruption, mental retardation in previous births
- History of infertility or other autoimmune conditions
- Use of amiodarone or lithium or recent use of iodinated contrast

Conclusion

Hypothyroidism is one of the most commonly prevalent endocrine disorders and is the commonest thyroid disorder. Factors both genetic and environmental, pertaining specifically to people residing in South Asia, play an important role. Iodine deficiency followed by autoimmune thyroiditis remains the common etiologies. The spectrum of hypothyroidism covers all ages from newborn to elderly with characteristic clinical features. Clinical manifestations may be nonspecific and, hence, screening may be required. The diagnosis of hypothyroidism is made by thyroid function hormonal testing. Although primary hypothyroidism is the commonest form, it is important to differentiate between the different forms of hypothyroidism. Laboratory assessments with third-generation electrochemiluminescence assays are the current gold standard. The treatment remains levothyroxine (T4) replacement which is simple, effective and cheap. Care needs to be taken while treating specific populations like newborn and infants, growing children, pregnant females and elderly with cardiac comorbidities. Long-term public health measures in South Asia with regards to iodination of salt need to be looked into while balancing concerns of persisting iodine deficiency and increased autoimmunity.

References

1. Braverman LE, Cooper DS, Kopp P. Werner & Ingbar's The Thyroid, 11th ed, Wolters Kluwer, 2021.
2. Taylor PN, Albrecht D, Scholz A, Gutierrez-Buey G, Lazarus JH, Dayan CM, et al. Global epidemiology of hyperthyroidism and hypothyroidism. Nat Rev Endocrinol. 2018 May;14(5):301–316.
3. WHO | Fortification of food-grade salt with iodine for the prevention and control of iodine deficiency disorders [Internet]. WHO. World Health Organization; [cited 2020 Apr 6]. Available from: http://www.who.int/nutrition/publications/guidelines/fortification_foodgrade_saltwithiodine/en/
4. Dayan CM, Daniels GH. Chronic autoimmune thyroiditis. N Engl J Med. 1996 Jul;335(2):99–107.
5. Melmed S, Auchus R, Goldfine A, Koenig R, Rosen C. Williams Textbook of Endocrinology,14th ed., Philadelphia, PA: Elsevier; 2016. pp. 361, 405, 422.
6. Verloop H, Louwerens M, Schoones JW, Kievit J, Smit JWA, Dekkers OM. Risk of hypothyroidism following hemithyroidectomy: systematic review and meta-analysis of prognostic studies. J Clin Endocrinol Metab. 2012 Jul;97(7):2243–2255.
7. Nygaard B, Hegedüs L, Ulriksen P, Nielsen KG, Hansen JM. Radioiodine therapy for multinodular toxic goiter. Arch Intern Med. 1999 Jun;159(12):1364.
8. Kahraman D, Keller C, Schneider C, Eschner W, Sudbrock F, Schmidt M, et al. Development of hypothyroidism during long-term follow-up of patients with toxic nodular goitre after radioiodine therapy: long-term follow-up of patients with toxic nodular goitre treated with radioiodine. Clin Endocrinol (Oxf). 2012 Feb;76(2):297–303.
9. Rizzo LFL, Mana DL, Serra HA. Drug-induced hypothyroidism. Medicina (B Aires). 2017;77(5):394–404.
10. Persani L, Cangiano B, Bonomi M. The diagnosis and management of central hypothyroidism in 2018. Endocr Connect. 2019 Feb;8(2):R44–R54.
11. Persani L, Ferretti E, Borgato S, Faglia G, Beck-Peccoz P. Circul Thyrotropin Bioactiv Sporadic Central Hypothyroidism. 2000;85(10):5.
12. Canaris GJ, Steiner JF, Ridgway EC. Do traditional symptoms of hypothyroidism correlate with biochemical disease? J Gen Intern Med. 1997 Sep;12(9):544–550.
13. Carlé A, Pedersen IB, Knudsen N, Perrild H, Ovesen L, Laurberg P. Hypothyroid symptoms and the likelihood of overt thyroid failure: a population-based case–control study. Eur J Endocrinol. 2014 Nov;171(5):593–602.
14. Jonklaas J, Bianco AC, Bauer AJ, Burman KD, Cappola AR, Celi FS, et al. Guidelines for the treatment of hypothyroidism: prepared by the American Thyroid Association Task Force on Thyroid Hormone Replacement. Thyroid. 2014 Dec;24(12):1670–1751.
15. Mathew V, Misgar RA, Ghosh S, Mukhopadhyay P, Roychowdhury P, Pandit K, et al. Myxedema coma: a new look into an old crisis. J Thyroid Res. 2011;2011:1–7.
16. Srivastav A, Maisnam I, Dutta D, Ghosh S, Mukhopadhyay S, Chowdhury S. Cretinism revisited. Indian J Endocrinol Metab. 2012 Dec;16(Suppl 2):S336–S337.
17. Marwaha RK, Tandon N, Desai A, Kanwar R, Grewal K, Aggarwal R, et al. Reference range of thyroid hormones in normal Indian school-age children. Clin Endocrinol (Oxf). 2007 Sep;0(0):070926054724001.
18. Marwaha RK, Tandon N, Ganie MA, Mehan N, Sastry A, Garg MK, et al. Reference range of thyroid function (FT3, FT4 and TSH) among Indian adults. Clin Biochem. 2013 Mar;46(4–5):341–345.
19. Rajput R, Singh B, Goel V, Verma A, Seth S, Nanda S. Trimester-specific reference interval for thyroid hormones during pregnancy at a Tertiary Care Hospital in Haryana, India. Indian J Endocrinol Metab. 2016;20(6):810.
20. Chaker L, Bianco AC, Jonklaas J, Peeters RP. Hypothyroidism. Lancet. 2017 Sep;390(10101):1550–1562.
21. Persani L. Central hypothyroidism: pathogenic, diagnostic, and therapeutic challenges. J Clin Endocrinol Metab. 2012 Sep 1;97(9):3068–3078.
22. Moran C, Chatterjee K. Resistance to thyroid hormone due to defective thyroid receptor alpha. Best Pract Res Clin Endocrinol Metab. 2015 Aug;29(4):647–657.
23. Fliers E, Bianco AC, Langouche L, Boelen A. Thyroid function in critically ill patients. Lancet Diabetes Endocrinol. 2015 Oct;3(10):816–825.
24. Gurnell M, Halsall DJ, Chatterjee VK. What should be done when thyroid function tests do not make sense? Clin Endocrinol (Oxf). 2011 Jun;74(6):673–678.
25. Ladenson PW, Singer PA, Ain KB, Bagchi N, Bigos ST, Levy EG, et al. American Thyroid Association guidelines for detection of thyroid dysfunction. Arch Intern Med. 2000 Jun;160(11):1573–1575.
26. Garber J, Cobin R, Gharib H, Hennessey J, Klein I, Mechanick J, et al. Clinical Practice Guidelines for Hypothyroidism in Adults: Cosponsored by the American Association of Clinical Endocrinologists and the American Thyroid Association. 41.
27. Ressel G. Introduction to AAFP Summary of Recommendations for Periodic Health Examinations. Am Fam Physician. 2002 Apr;65(7):1467.
28. Vanderpump MP, Ahlquist JA, Franklyn JA, Clayton RN. Consensus statement for good practice and audit measures in the management of hypothyroidism and hyperthyroidism. The Research Unit of the Royal College of Physicians of London, the Endocrinology and Diabetes Committee of the Royal College of Physicians of London, and the Society for Endocrinology. BMJ. 1996 Aug;313(7056):539–544.
29. Helfand M, U.S. Preventive Services Task Force. Screening for subclinical thyroid dysfunction in nonpregnant adults: a summary of the evidence for the U.S. Preventive Services Task Force. Ann Intern Med. 2004 Jan;140(2):128–141.
30. Indian Thyroid Society guidelines for management of thyroid dysfunction during pregnancy. Clinical practice guidelines. New Delhi: Elsevier; 2012.

31. Ray Arunabh (2014). National Guidelines for Screening of Hypothyroidism during Pregnancy. MoHFW, Government of India.
32. Ghosh S, Pramanik S, Biswas K, Bhattacharjee K, Sarkar R, Chowdhury S, et al. Levothyroxine absorption test to differentiate pseudomalabsorption from true malabsorption. Eur Thyroid J. 2020;9(1):19–24.
33. Cooper DS, Biondi B. Subclinical thyroid disease. Lancet. 2012 Mar;379(9821):1142–1154.
34. Alexander EK, Pearce EN, Brent GA, Brown RS, Chen H, Dosiou C, et al. 2017 Guidelines of the American Thyroid Association for the diagnosis and management of thyroid disease during pregnancy and the postpartum. Thyroid. 2017 Mar;27(3):315–389.
35. Kalra S, Agarwal S, Aggarwal R, Ranabir S. Trimester-specific thyroid-stimulating hormone: an Indian perspective. Indian J Endocrinol Metab. 2018;22(1):1.
36. Desai MP, Sharma R, Riaz I, Sudhanshu S, Parikh R, Bhatia V. Newborn Screening Guidelines for Congenital Hypothyroidism in India: Recommendations of the Indian Society for Pediatric and Adolescent Endocrinology (ISPAE) – Part I: Screening and Confirmation of Diagnosis. Indian J Pediatr. 2018;85(6):440–447.
37. Sudhanshu S, Riaz I, Sharma R, Desai MP, Parikh R, Bhatia V. Newborn Screening Guidelines for Congenital Hypothyroidism in India: Recommendations of the Indian Society for Pediatric and Adolescent Endocrinology (ISPAE) – Part II: Imaging, Treatment and Follow-up. Indian J Pediatr. 2018;85(6):448–453.
38. Over 30% Indians suffering from thyroid disorder: survey [Internet]. https://www.outlookindia.com/. [cited 2020 Apr 5]. Available from: https://www.outlookindia.com/newsscroll/over-30-indians-suffering-from-thyroid-disorder-survey/1059092
39. Unnikrishnan AG, Kalra S, Sahay RK, Bantwal G, John M, Tewari N. Prevalence of hypothyroidism in adults: an epidemiological study in eight cities of India. Indian J Endocrinol Metab. 2013;17(4):647–652.
40. Sahu MT, Das V, Mittal S, Agarwal A, Sahu M. Overt and subclinical thyroid dysfunction among Indian pregnant women and its effect on maternal and fetal outcome. Arch Gynecol Obstet. 2009 May;281(2):215.
41. Rashid SQ. Thyroid Gland Standard for Bangladeshi Population and Prevalence of Unknown Pathologies in the Normal Population. J Med Ultrasound. 2016 Sep;24(3):101–106.
42. Joshi A, Yonzon P. Community based study of thyroid disorder prevalence in Nepal. In BioScientifica; 2019 [cited 2020 Mar 27]. Available from: https://www.endocrine-abstracts.org/ea/0063/ea0063p776
43. Paul AK, Miah SR, Mamun AA, Islam S. Thyroid disorders in Khulna district: a community based study. Bangladesh Med Res Counc Bull. 2006 Dec;32(3):66–71.
44. Sethi B, Barua S, Raghavendra M, Gotur J, Khandelwal D, Vyas U. The thyroid registry: Clinical and hormonal characteristics of adult indian patients with hypothyroidism. Indian J Endocrinol Metab. 2017;21(2):302.
45. Rabeya R, Zaman S, Chowdhury AB, Nabi MH, Hawlader MDH. Magnitude and determinants of hypothyroidism among dyslipidemic patients in Bangladesh: a hospital-based cross-sectional study. Int J Diabetes Metab. 2019;25(1–2):19–25.
46. Kamrul-Hasan ABM, Akter F, Selim S, Asaduzzaman M, Rahman MH, Chanda PK, et al. Thyroid function and autoantibody status in Bangladeshi patients with type 2 diabetes mellitus. Thyroid Res Pract. 2018 Sep;15(3):132.
47. Deshmukh V, Farishta F, Bhole M. Thyroid dysfunction in patients with metabolic syndrome: a cross-sectional, epidemiological, pan-India Study. Int J Endocrinol. 2018 Dec;2018:1–6.
48. Marwaha RK, Tandon N, Karak AK, Gupta N, Verma K, Kochupillai N. Hashimoto's thyroiditis: countrywide screening of goitrous healthy young girls in postiodization phase in India. J Clin Endocrinol Metab. 2000;85(10):5.
49. Marwaha RK, Tandon N, Ganie MA, Kanwar R, Sastry A, Garg M, et al. Status of thyroid function in Indian adults: two decades after universal salt iodization. J Assoc Physicians India. 2012;60:32–36.
50. WHO | Summary tables and maps on iodine status worldwide [Internet]. WHO. World Health Organization; [cited 2020 Mar 27]. Available from: https://www.who.int/vmnis/database/iodine/iodine_data_status_summary/en/
51. Iodine Global Network (IGN) - Home [Internet]. [cited 2020 Mar 27]. Available from: https://www.ign.org/
52. Oberlin O, Plantin-Carrenard E, Rigal O, Wilkinson C. Goitre and iodine deficiency in Afghanistan: a case—control study. Br J Nutr. 2006 Jan;95(1):196–203.
53. Elahi S, Rizvi NB, Nagra SA. Iodine deficiency in pregnant women of Lahore. J Pak Med Assoc. 2009 Nov;59(11):741–3.
54. Afzal R. Thyroid disorders in pregnancy: an overview of literature from Pakistan. Indian J Endocrinol Metab. 2013 Sep;17(5):943.
55. Shrestha U, Gautam N, Agrawal K, Jha A, Jayan A. Iodine status among subclinical and overt hypothyroid patients by urinary iodine assay: a case–control study. Indian J Endocrinol Metab. 2017;21(5):719.
56. Chandra AK, Mukhopadhyay S, Lahari D, Tripathy S. Goitrogenic content of Indian cyanogenic plant foods & their in vitro anti-thyroidal activity. Indian J Med Res. 2004 May;119(5):180–185.
57. Jawa A, Jawad A, Riaz S, Assir MZ, Chaudhary A, Zakria M, et al. Turmeric use is associated with reduced goitrogenesis: Thyroid disorder prevalence in Pakistan (THYPAK) study. Indian J Endocrinol Metab. 2015;19(3):347.
58. Bagcchi S. Hypothyroidism in India: more to be done. Lancet Diabetes Endocrinol. 2014 Oct;2(10):778.

8

HYPERTHYROIDISM
Surgeon's Perspective

Sasi Mouli, PV Pradeep and Anand Kumar Mishra

Introduction

Thyrotoxicosis is a clinical syndrome of increased circulating thyroid hormone due to any etiology irrespective of the source. On the contrary, hyperthyroidism is a condition of excess in both synthesis and secretion of thyroid hormone (Figure 8.1). Hyperthyroidism is the most common cause of thyrotoxicosis. Graves' disease (GD) is the commonest cause of hyperthyroidism in iodine sufficient area (1). In iodine-deficient areas, toxic multinodular goiter (TMNG), toxic adenoma (TA) constitutes nearly 50% of hyperthyroidism (1, 2). Hence thyrotoxicosis can be present with or without hyperthyroidism. This chapter deals with hyperthyroidism and surgical treatment of hyperthyroidism

Epidemiology

Prevalence of hyperthyroidism varies across world as it depends on the population selection and its dynamics, threshold levels, assay sensitivity and iodine intake. It ranges from 0.2 to 1.6% (3). Australia has a prevalence of 0.3% for both overt and subclinical hyperthyroidism (4). Prevalence of overt hyperthyroidism in the United States and Europe is 0.5%, 0.7% respectively (3). Unnikrishnan et al. from India quoted a prevalence of overt hyperthyroidism in 1.6% and subclinical hyperthyroidism in 1.3% (5). Any age-group may be involved, but more commonly, GD involves relatively younger age-group, whereas TMNG is more common in elderly. Females are more commonly affected than males (6, 7). Iodine-replete areas have a higher incidence of autoimmune thyrotoxicosis whereas iodine-deficient areas have a predominance of toxic goiters (3). One cross-sectional study from China found that the prevalence of hyperthyroidism in iodine-repleted areas is higher than iodine-depleted areas (8).

GD occurs with an incidence of 20–50 cases per 100,000 persons per annum. It is more common to occur in third to fifth decades (3, 9). Females are more commonly affected than males with almost 8:1 ratio (10). On the contrary, TMNG occurs in elderly, with a female preponderance (5:1) and are commoner in iodine-depleted areas of the world (18 per 100,000 per annum) vs. iodine-repleted areas (1.5 per 100,000 per annum). The incidence of TA has a similar distribution with iodine-depleted areas (3.6 per 100,000 per annum) vs. iodine sufficient areas (1.6 per 100,000 per annum) (3, 11). Thyroiditis is another cause of thyrotoxicosis, with a slight female preponderance (1.5:1). Though thyroiditis has a triphasic clinical course, having thyrotoxic, hypo-thyroid and a euthyroid phase, reported incidence of thyrotoxicosis in thyroiditis varies from 10% in Japan to 2.4% in New York (3). Drug-induced hyperthyroidism (discussed below in a separate section) with a prevalence of 1–38% occurs more commonly with amiodarone, in iodine-depleted areas with a higher male preponderance (3:1) (12).

Etiology and classification

Hyperthyroidism as explained above is both as a result of excess synthesis and secretion of thyroxine. Hyperthyroidism can be either overt or subclinical. In overt hyperthyroidism, serum thyroid-stimulating hormone (TSH) is reduced, with increase in free thyroxine (FT4). In the case of subclinical hyperthyroidism, serum TSH is lower than the normal range but thyroxine (T4) and/or triiodothyronine (T3) levels remain within normal range. Thyrotoxicosis can occur with or without hyperthyroidism. The most common cause in iodine sufficient areas is GD (70–80%). In iodine-deficient areas, nearly half the cases are attributable to TMNG and TA (1, 10). Table 8.1 shows classification and various mechanisms of thyrotoxicosis.

Pathogenesis

Graves' disease: It is the commonest cause of hyperthyroidism that has autoimmune origin. GD is an autoimmune disease which is organ specific. This is due to the circulating autoantibodies (Ab) that stimulate the TSHR (TSH receptor). The TSHR-stimulating antibody (TSI) binds to the leucine-rich extracellular domain of the TSHR. TSHR Ab also interacts with the IGF1 receptors on the surface of thyrocytes and on orbital fibroblasts. The TSHR Ab after binding to the TSHR increases the production of intracellular cyclic AMP which leads to thyrocyte growth and thyroid hormone production. Studies in twins have shown 80% susceptibility to GD, and it's also seen that about 30% of GD patients have family members affected with autoimmune thyroid disease (13). Thyroid gland has patchy infiltrates of T-helper cells (both types 1,2). The development of autoimmunity in GD can occur as a result of various processes undergoing in human body (13).

1. Reduction in self-elimination of auto-activated T cells results in stimulating TSH receptor.
2. Inflammatory markers of non-thyroidal origin (such as interferon-γ) may infiltrate thyroid gland resulting in stimulation of T cells.
3. Segmentation in presentation of thyroid antigen causing stimulation in autoimmune conditions as a result of overexpression of major histocompatibility complex (MHC) class-II.
4. Though not proven, cross-reactivity between some bacterial antigens (like Yersinia enterocolitica and Borrelia) and autoantigens may also result in autoimmunity (13).

Hyperthyroidism

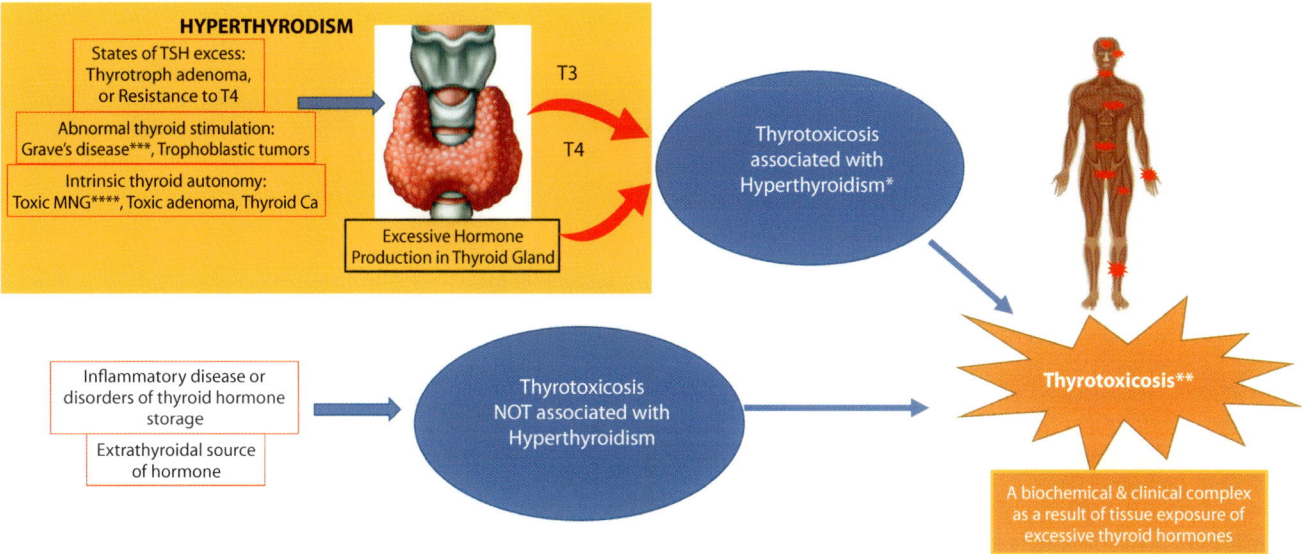

FIGURE 8.1 Causes of thyrotoxicosis. *****Hyperthyroidism** refers to disorders in which thyrotoxicosis results from overproduction of hormone by the thyroid itself, the most common being Graves' disease (yellow block). ******Thyrotoxicosis** is the biochemical and clinical complex that results when the tissues are presented with excessive quantities of the thyroid hormones. *******Primary thyrotoxicosis** is defined as goiter appearing at the same time as the hyperthyroidism, e.g. Grave's disease. ********Secondary thyrotoxicosis** is defined as nodular goiter is present for a long time before the hyperthyroidism, e.g. toxic multinodular goiter.

GD has a polygenic inheritance; the human leukocyte antigen (HLA) association is well established with GD. Most important involved are HLA-b8 (in Caucasians) (14), HLA-B25, HLA-DPB1*0501 (Japanese), HLA-DR3, HLA-DRB1*03, and HLA-DRB1*08. Other genetic factors involve increase in expression of CD40 resulting in enhanced autoimmunity, FOXP3 gene (located on chromosome Xp11) and CTLA-4 (10). Environmental factors that are quoted in the context of GD are female gender, tobacco smoking, dietary iodine, stress, infections as mentioned above (Yersinia and Borrelia), pregnancy/postpartum and neck irradiation (9, 13). Overall, the immunoglobulins (Ig) belonging to IgG1 subclass produce the stimulating antibodies against TSH receptor which are responsible for GD (9).

Graves' ophthalmopathy (GO) is infiltrative disease with lymphocyte infiltrating the orbital tissue with a target effect on

TABLE 8.1: Classification and Mechanism of Thyrotoxicosis

Radioactive Iodine Uptake (RAIU)	Underlying Cause	Diseases	Molecular Mechanism
Increased	Increased TSHR stimulation	• Graves' disease • hCG related: pregnancy associated/trophoblastic disease • TSH-producing pituitary tumors	TSHR-stimulating antibody hCG mediated Elevated TSH
	Autonomous secretion of thyroid hormone	• Toxic adenoma • Toxic multinodular goiter • TSH receptor activating mutations	TSHR mutation and GSα point mutation
Low or near absent	Release of preformed hormones due to destruction of follicles	• Acute thyroiditis • Autoimmune thyroiditis (hashitoxicosis) • Drug-induced (amiodarone) • Palpation thyroiditis • Postpartum thyroiditis • Subacute thyroiditis (Granulomatous thyroiditis/ de Quervain's thyroiditis, painless thyroiditis)	Preformed thyroxine release Destruction of follicles Preformed thyroid hormone release Post-viral infection
	Extrathyroidal sources	• Excessive supplementation of thyroid hormone (Iatrogenic/self-administration) • Food supplements/iodine • Functional metastases from follicular thyroid cancer • Struma ovarii	Exogenous Jod-Basedow phenomenon Extrathyroidal hormone production in metastases; ovarian tumor

fibroblasts and adipocytes. Orbital tissues are infiltrated with lymphocytes. The interaction between the T cells and fibroblasts result in tissue activation and induction of genes involved in inflammation. The T cell produces cytokines like interleukin-1β, 6, 12, 16, TNF-α, interferon-γ (IFN-γ) and CD-40 ligand. There is a resultant tissue inflammation and remodeling with accumulation of glycosaminoglycans (GAGs) in adipocytes and extraocular muscles (EOMs) causing tissue and volume expansion of orbit with optic nerve compression (13). Accumulation of hyaluronidase digestible material and adipogenesis results in expansion of EOMs. Initially, the EOM fibers become widely separated and later fibrotic (1). A shared antigen in the orbit and thyroid gland like thyrotropin receptor may be the one initiating lymphocytic infiltration (5). It's also now proven that fibroblasts express proteins like thyrotropin receptor, thyroglobulin, thyroperoxidase and sodium iodide symporter. Insulin-like growth factor-1 is also involved in pathogenesis as evidenced by its overexpression on the orbital fibroblasts (1).

Toxic multinodular goiter and toxic adenoma: Iodine deficiency is one of the most important risk factors in the formation of goiter. In long-standing goiters the TSHR and GSα (type α1b) protein genes are activated due to somatic point mutations which cause benign clonal expansion of thyroid follicles responsible for autonomous functioning. Single hyperfunctioning nodule results in TA, whereas multiple nodule formation with one or more hyperfunctioning nodules results in TMNG. Few other growth factors that may also result in add on effect in causing clonal expansion, such as insulin-like growth factor-1 (IGF-1), transforming growth factor (TGF), fibroblast growth factor, epidermal growth factor. There is a resultant activation of cyclic adenosine monophosphate (cAMP) leading to hyperplasia of follicular cells (13).

Other causes of hyperthyroidism with their possible mechanism are explained in Table 8.1.

Clinical features and complications

Wide variety of symptom occurs in hyperthyroidism. Most significant symptoms are loss of weight despite a good appetite, a recent preference for cold, sweating and palpitations. The onset is abrupt. Primary hyperthyroidism is often more severe than secondary. Orbital proptosis, ophthalmoplegia and pretibial myxedema may be associated with primary type. Goiter in secondary hyperthyroidism is usually nodular, with an insidious onset. Usually only eye signs secondary to sympathetic overdrive are observed. Patient may present with cardiac failure or atrial fibrillation. Neuromuscular symptoms include tremors, nervousness, anxiety, restlessness, insomnia, fatigue, weakness. The main cardiovascular symptom is palpitations, whereas signs include tachycardia, hypertension (with increased systolic pressure and wide pulse pressure), irregular heartbeat (atrial fibrillation). Respiratory ones include breathlessness, tachypnea. Gastrointestinal symptoms include increased frequency of bowel movements, intestinal motility and malabsorption. Severe thyrotoxicosis may result in hepatic dysfunction. The possible mechanisms are mentioned in Table 8.2. Severe GD patients may have rare (0.5–4.3%) features such as dermopathy and acropachy (13).

The most significant signs are the excitability of the patient, the presence of a goiter, exophthalmos and tachycardia or cardiac arrhythmia. In primary thyrotoxicosis, goiter is diffuse and vascular; it may be large or small, firm or soft, and a thrill and a bruit may be present. Uniform diffuse soft goiter is characteristic of GD. There may be palpable thrill or audible bruit over the superior pole of thyroid in the case of severe GD. Single nodule is present in TA. If multiple nodules are palpable, it is labeled as TMNG. Toxic MNG presents in relatively elderly patients and hence the risk of cardiovascular complications is relatively high. Other signs include fine tremors appreciated in palms, outstretched fingers and tongue. Thyroiditis patients usually give history of throat infection with a painful or painless uniform goiter. Table 8.2 has details of clinical features with possible causative mechanism.

In children, thyrotoxicosis should always be considered in situations of a growth spurt, behavior problems or myopathy. In adults, if there is new onset tachycardia or arrhythmia develops or there is unexplained diarrhea or weight loss, it should be considered.

The major symptoms of hyperthyroidism can be remembered by mnemonics: "**D**on't **E**vade **F**eeling **H**ot **A**nd **S**weaty **P**atients" (**D**iarrhea, **E**motional liability, **F**atigued, **H**eat intolerance, increased **A**ppetite, **S**weating, and **P**alpitations or "**FANTOM PWD**" for both symptom and signs (Table 8.3).

Clinical examination

A complete systemic examination along with local examination of neck is required in these patients. The patient appears anxious, restless and palm is moist with warm skin. About 10% of patients may have palmar erythema. Fine tremor in the out-stretched fingers and tongue is characteristic. In general examination, patient may have hypertension with wide pulse pressure, tachycardia or arrhythmias. There may be separation of the fingernail from the nail bed (Plummer's nail), especially observed in the ring finger. There may be audible systolic murmur with signs of heart failure. Abdominal examination may reveal splenomegaly. A weighted scoring index proposed by Wayne to make a clinical diagnosis of hyperthyroidism remains a useful bedside tool. However, it is now of more a historical importance. A diffusely enlarged thyroid gland is seen. A bruit is generally present over the gland signifying that the patient is thyrotoxic.

Wayne's index
In 1960, Sir Edward Wayne described a scale for clinical diagnosis of hyperthyroidism (Table 8.4). It is a clinical scoring tool in which nine symptoms and ten signs are evaluated (range: +45 to −25). Signs are scored both positively and negatively (absence means negative marking). Only two symptoms (decreased appetite and preference for heat) have negative scores. A score less than 11 defines "euthyroidism" while scoring above 19 suggests "toxic hyperthyroidism" (15). In today's era, this has no relevance with availability of thyroid function test at every place. It had shown a diagnostic accuracy of 85%.

Eyes: The eye signs include lid lag or stare (sympathetic overactivity), infrequent blinking, failure to wrinkle the brow on upward gaze, proptosis and congestive oculopathy (chemosis, conjunctivitis, periorbital swelling, corneal ulceration in severe cases). Exophthalmic ophthalmoplegia occurs with ocular muscle weakness and impaired upward gaze and convergence. Clinicians in last two centuries have described a number of clinical signs for

Hyperthyroidism

TABLE 8.2: Clinical Features with Possible Mechanisms

System Involved	Clinical Features	Possible Mechanisms
Cardiovascular system	Palpitations	Increased sympathetic activity and decreased vagal tone, upregulation of β-adrenergic receptors
	Tachycardia	
	Hypertension (high systolic low diastolic, high pulse pressure)	Increased sensitivity to catecholamines, reduced peripheral vascular resistance
	Increased contractility	Increased ratio of α- to β-myosin heavy-chain expression, reduction in phospholamban, increased calcium ion movement across the sarcoplasmic reticulum
	Cardiac arrhythmias (atrial fibrillation, supraventricular arrhythmias)	
	Increased stroke volume	Direct action of T3 hormone excess levels
	High output cardiac failure	Stimulating autoantibodies to β-adrenergic receptors
	Pleuropericardial rub (Means-Lerman scratch)	Overexpression of type 2 deiodinase in myocardium
Neuromuscular system and nervous system	Nervousness	Direct effect of thyroxine excess
	Proximal muscle weakness	Increased type II muscle fibers breakdown and atrophy more than type I muscle fibers
	Easy fatigability	
	Restlessness	
	Tremors	
	Jerky movements	
	Anxiety	
	Insomnia	
	Poor memory	
Bone and skeletal system	Reduced bone mineral density	T3-induced osteoclastic activity >osteoblastic activity
	Osteoporosis	Increased bone turnover
	Pathological bone fracture	Loss of calcium and phosphorous through urine and stool
		Net demineralization
Alimentary system	Higher frequency of bowel movements	Altered adrenergic activity in bowel
	Malabsorption	Direct thyroid hormone excess effects
	Hepatic dysfunction	
Respiratory system	Dyspnea	Vital capacity reduced
	Tachypnea	Respiratory muscle fatigue (specially during exercise)
Skin and hair	Warm	Increased metabolism
	Moist	Increased Na+/K+ ATPase activity leading to increased thermogenesis
	Soft friable nails	
	Hair loss	
Metabolism	Increased appetite but weight loss	Increased metabolism in general is insufficient to meet the caloric requirements
	Fats	Increased lipolysis >> lipogenesis
	Proteins	Increased proteolysis >> protein synthesis
Eyes	Retraction of upper eyelids	Increased adrenergic tone causing persistent Muller's muscle contraction
	Exophthalmos and Grave's ophthalmopathy	Infiltrative ophthalmopathy, fibroblasts overgrowth, cytokine and IGF-1-mediated inflammation
		Accumulation of glycosaminoglycans

TABLE 8.3: Symptoms and Signs of Thyrotoxicosis Mnemonic "FANTOM PWD"

F	Fatigue
A	Increased Appetite
N	Nervousness and Anxiety
T	Tremors
O	Ophthalmopathy
M	Menstrual irregularities, Myopathy esp proximal muscle weakness
P	Palpitations, High Pulse rate, Perspiration
W	Weather liking (Heat intolerance), Weight loss, Water hammer pulse
D	Dyspnea, Dysphagia, Dysarthria, Diarrhea

TABLE 8.4: Wayne's Index for Evaluation of Hyperthyroidism

Symptoms of Recent Onset and/or Increased Severity	Score	Signs	Present	Absent
Dyspnea on effect	+1	Palpable thyroid	+3	−3
Palpitations	+2	Bruit over thyroid	+2	−2
Tiredness	+2	Exophthalmoses	+2	−
Preference for heat	−5	Lid retraction	+2	−
Preference for cold	+5	Lid lag	+1	−
Excessive sweating	+3	Hyperkinesis	+4	−2
Nervousness	+2	Hands – hot	+2	−2
		– Moist	+1	−1
Appetite: increased Decreased	−3	Casual pulse rate: >80/min >90/min	+3	−3 −
Weight increased Decreased	+3	Atrial fibrillation	+4	−

TABLE 8.5: List of the Signs Described in Graves' Ophthalmopathy

Name of the Sign	Clinician After Whom It Was Named	Details of the Sign
Abadie's sign	Jean Marie Charles Abadie (1842–1932)	Spasticity of upper eyelid elevators
Ballet's sign	Louis Gilbert Simeon Ballet (1853–1916)	Paresis/Paralysis of ≥1 extraocular muscles
Becker's sign	Otto Heinrich Enoch Becker (1828–1890)	Exaggerated retinal artery pulsations
Boston's sign	Leonard Napoleon Boston (1871–1931)	Twitching of upper eyelids on lower gaze
Cowen's sign	Jack Posner Cowen, (1906–1989)	Spasmodic contraction of pupil on consensual pupillary reflex
Dalrymple's sign	John Dalrymple (1803–1852)	Retraction of upper eyelids
Enroth's sign	Emil Emanuel Enroth (1879–1953)	Eyelid edema especially upper eyelid
Gifford's sign	Harold Gifford Sr. (1858–1929)	Inability to evert upper eyelid
Goldzeiher's sign	Wilhelm Goldzieher (1849–1916)	Injected temporal conjunctiva
Griffith's sign	Alexander James Hill Griffith (1858–1937)	Lower lid lags on superior gaze
Hertoghe's sign	Eugene Louis Chretien Hertoghe (1860–1928)	Loss of lateral eyebrows
Jellinek's sign	Edward Jellinek (1890–1963)	Hyperpigmentation of upper eyelid folds
Joffroy's sign	Alexis Joffroy (1844–1908)	Forehead creases do not become evident on upward gaze
Jendrassik's sign	Ernő Jendrassik (1858–1921)	Limitation of eyeball abduction and rotation
Knies's sign	Max Knies, (1851–1917)	Un symmetrical pupillary dilatation in low light
Kocher's sign	Emil Theodor Kocher (1841–1917)	Spastic retraction of fixated upper eyelid
Loewi's sign	Otto Loewi (1873–1961)	Dilation of pupil on adrenaline drops (1:1000)
Mann's sign	John Dixon Mann, (1840–1912)	Apparent situation of eyes at different levels
Mean sign		Upper sclera is visible on upward gaze because of globe lag
Möbius's sign	Paul Julius Möbius (1853–1907)	Absence of symmetrical convergence of eyes
Payne–Trousseau's sign	John Howard Payne (1916–1983), Armand Trousseau (1801–1867)	Misplaced globe
Pochin's sign	Sir Edward Eric Pochin (1909–1990)	Reduction in magnitude of blinking
Riesman's sign	David Riesman (1867–1940)	Bruits over eyelids on auscultation
Movement's cap phenomenon		Incomplete, abrupt and difficult eyeball movements
Rosenbach's sign	Ottomar Ernst Felix Rosenbach (1851–1907)	Active fine tremors of upper eyelids
Snellen–Riesman's sign	Herman Snellen (1834–1908), David Riesman, American physician (1867–1940)	Systolic murmur over closed eyelids
Stellwag's sign	Karl Stellwag (1823–1904)	Decreased frequency and amplitude of blinking
Suker's sign	George Francis "Franklin" Suker (1869–1933)	Difficulty in fixation of lateral gaze
Topolanski's sign	Alfred Topolanski (1861–1960)	Appreciation of interconnected vascular band at insertion of four rectus muscles
von Graefe's sign	Friedrich Wilhelm Ernst Albrecht von Gräfe (1828–1870)	Lag of upper eyelids on lower gaze
Wilder's sign	Helenor Campbell Wilder (1895–1998)	Twitching of eyes on change of gaze from abduction to adduction

assessment of eyes that are summarized in Table 8.5. The exophthalmos can be assessed with a Hertel's exophthalmometer that measures the distance between lateral bony orbital margin and the anterior surface of the cornea. Upto 50% of individuals with GD have clinical involvement of the eyes known as GO. GO is a biphasic disease, with an initial "active phase" of inflammation which may last up to 3 years, followed by "inactive phase" with stable proptosis and impaired eye muscle mobility. Most common clinical features of GO are eyelid retraction, 92%; exophthalmos, 62%; EOM dysfunction, 43%; ocular pain, 30%; increased lacrimation, 23%; and optic neuropathy, 6% (16). Cigarette smoking is the strongest modifiable risk factor. The intensity of eye inflammation is assessed by a scoring system first published in 1997, known as "Clinical Activity Score (CAS). CAS includes scoring of four classical signs of inflammation (pain, redness, swelling and impaired function). A CAS ≥ 4 implies an active inflammatory stage of GO (17). The higher the CAS, the greater is the response to immunosuppression (Table 8.6).

The severity of eye changes can be objectively classified by using the "NO SPECS" system. It scores the disease based on soft tissue involvement, corneal involvement and sight loss (18).

Class 0: **N**o Symptoms or signs
Class: **O**nly signs (Limited only signs, no symptoms (signs limited to upper lid retraction and stare, with or without lid lag and proptosis)
Class 2: **S**oft-tissue involvement with symptoms and signs
Class 3: **P**roptosis
Class 4: **E**OMs involvement usually with diplopia
Class 5: **C**orneal involvement, primarily due to lag opthalmos
Class 6: **S**ight loss due to optic nerve involvement

GO should be assessed by CAS to evaluate the activity and, by NO SPECS or VISA score (vision, inflammation, strabismus and appearance) for the severity of the disease (19, 20). EUGOGO classification includes both activity and severity parameters (21).

Hyperthyroidism

TABLE 8.6: Clinical Activity Scoring System for Graves' Ophthalmopathy Evaluation

Pain	1. Painful, oppressive feeling on or behind the globe during the last 2 weeks
	2. Pain on attempted up, side or down gaze during the last 4 weeks
Redness	3. Redness of the eyelids
	4. Diffuse redness of the conjunctiva covering at least one quadrant
Swelling	5. Swelling of eyelids
	6. Chemosis
	7. Swollen caruncle
	8. Increase of proptosis ≥2 mm during a period of 1–3 months
Impaired function	9. Decrease of eye movements in any direction ≥5° during a period of 1–3 months
	10. Decrease of visual acuity of ≥1 line on the Snellen chart (using a pinhole) during a period of 1–3 months

TABLE 8.7: Differential Diagnosis of Thyrotoxicosis

High Uptake of Iodine	Low Uptake of Iodine
Graves' disease (Basedow's disease)	Exogenous thyroid hormone (medicine, or Factitious)
Functioning nodule/toxic adenoma	Dietary (hamburger thyrotoxicosis)
Toxic multinodular goiter	
Pituitary tumor secreting excess TSH	Thyroiditis (subacute, silent, postpartum)
Tumors of placenta secreting large quantities of human chorionic gonadotropin	Excess iodine intake
	Drug; amiodarone
	Uptake at extrathyroidal sites like struma ovarii, functioning thyroid metastases

VISA classification was developed by Dolman and Rootman in 2006 and modified by International Thyroid Eye disease society. Four severity parameters are assessed: V (vision), I (inflammation/congestion), S (strabismus/motility restriction) and A (appearance/exposure). The management of the ophthalmopathy is guided by the severity of disease calculated by a global severity score which includes vision (1 point), inflammation (10 points), strabismus (6 points) and appearance (3 points).

Initial management involves absolute Tobacco abstinence, attaining Euthyroidism, Artificial tears, Referral to specialist center and enrollment in Self-help groups. These measures can be remembered by the mnemonic TEARS.

Skin dermopathy is uncommon (1–4%) and usually observed over the dorsum of the legs or feet and is also called pretibial myxedema. The affected area is raised, thickened and may be hyperpigmented. It is always seen in association with severe opthlmoplegia (22).

Thyroid storm: This manifests with high fever, heart failure, diarrhea, jaundice and impaired consciousness. Patients develop hyperpyrexia, tachycardia, arrhythmia, congestive cardiac failure, agitation, delirium, psychosis, stupor or coma (22). Usually, there may be a precipitant cause. The "Burch-Wartofsky" point scale is used to grade the severity. Score >45 indicates that the patient is in thyroid storm, 25–44 indicates impending storm and <25 that the storm is unlikely. The most common cause of mortality in thyroid storm is multiple organ failure, arrhythmias, DIC, hypoxic brain syndrome. Treatment of thyroid storm includes ATD therapy, glucocorticoids, beta blockers, cooling blankets, volume resuscitation, nutritional support and respiratory care.

Diagnosis

Biochemical diagnosis of thyrotoxicosis is by measuring serum TSH, T3 and free T4. Serum TSH is low or undetectable in hyperthyroidism. The second-generation TSH assays detect up to 0.1 µIU/ml whereas the newer third-generation immune chemiluminescent assays detect <0.01 µIU/ml (23). Subclinical hyperthyroidism is differentiated from overt hyperthyroidism by measuring serum T4 (or fT4) levels that are usually normal in subclinical hyperthyroidism but elevated in overt. If TSH is low with a normal fT4 levels, serum T3 levels are to be measured to diagnose isolated T3 toxicity. A TSH-producing pituitary adenoma is suspected if serum levels of TSH are normal or mildly elevated along with elevated levels of fT4 levels (1). In the case of GD, serum TSH receptor antibodies (TSHR Ab) are elevated with more than 99% sensitivity and specificity (9). However, in iodine-deficient areas, the TSHR Ab can be present in about 17% of the TMNG and nearly 6–9% of thyroiditis. Antithyroid peroxidise (TPO) antibody is commonly elevated in GD, but has limited diagnostic value with 75–80% sensitivity (10).

After biochemical diagnosis of hyperthyroidism, the next step is to define the etiology of hyperthyroidism. Thyroid scan is used to identify the etiology. Technetium (Tc^{99}) is commonly used than iodine (I^{123}) nowadays. Pattern of uptake of the radionuclide scan guides to etiology (Table 8.7). Complete diffuse uptake is present in GD (Figure 8.2), single hyperfunctioning area with suppression of surrounding thyroid tissue is

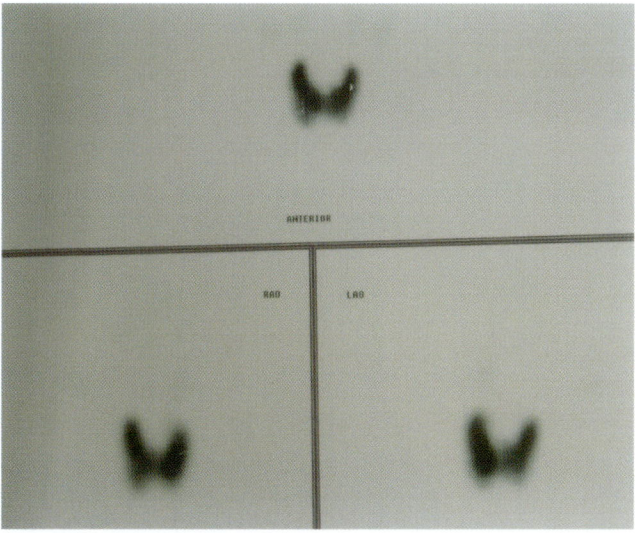

FIGURE 8.2 Technitium-99 scan showing diffuse intense uptake suggestive of Graves' disease.

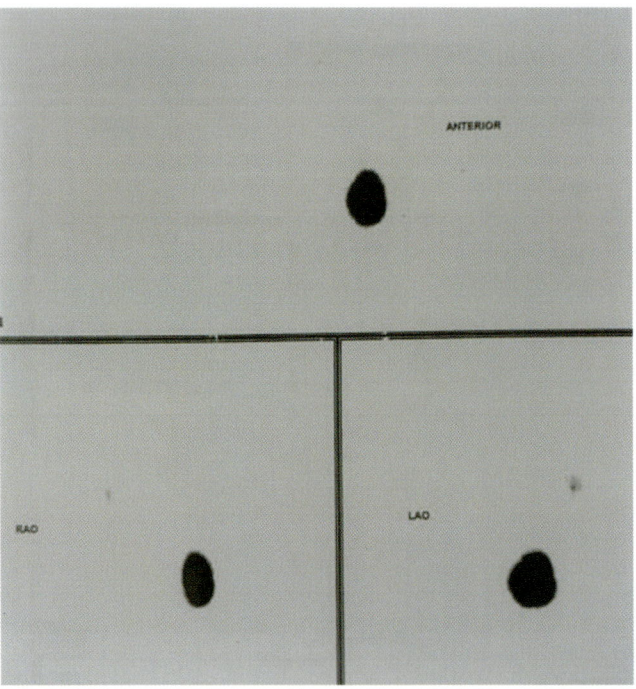

FIGURE 8.3 Tc99 scan showing hot area with surrounding gland suppressed suggestive of toxic adenoma.

diagnostic of TA (Figure 8.3). In TMNG, multiple areas of hot nodules with a suppressed surrounding non-nodular thyroid tissue are present (Figure 8.4). Low or minimal activity that is slightly higher than the background is suggestive of thyroiditis.

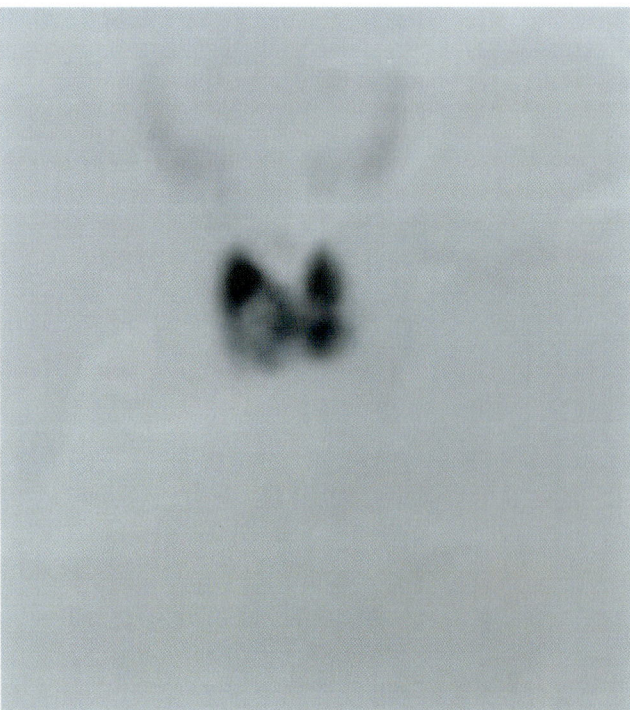

FIGURE 8.4 Tc99 scan showing multiple hot areas with surrounding cold and suppressed areas suggestive of toxic multinodular goiter.

Cold areas on scintigraphy in GD represent nodular GD, previously called "Marine-Lenhart syndrome" (24).

Metastatic functional FTC shows increased uptake at the metastatic site. Headache and diplopia maybe present in those with hyperthyroidism due to a pituitary TSH-secreting adenoma. Though the scintigraphy of neck simulates GD, a computed tomography (CT) or magnetic resonance imaging (MRI) of brain clinches the diagnosis of pituitary adenoma. Ultrasound is the radiological investigation of choice when a nodular goiter is present and a guided fine needle aspiration cytology (FNAC) is warranted in the case of suspicious nodules. Sonography of thyroid is important in the case of TA to visualize the rest of thyroid gland, which guides the surgeon to decide on the extent of thyroidectomy. Recently, color Doppler of thyroid gland has been also used with diagnostic sensitivity of 87% and specificity of 100% for GD diagnosis (10).

Treatment

The treatment of hyperthyroidism is mainly divided into initial phase of controlling symptoms due to thyroid hormone excess and definitive management in the form of radioactive iodine (RAI) ablation or surgery.

Medical management

Antithyroid drugs (ATDs): Thionamide group of drugs include methimazole (MMI), carbimazole (CBZ) and propylthiouracil (PTU). The ATDs have multiple actions. It has intrathyroidal action and extrathyroidal action. It affects iodine oxidation/organification, iodotyrosine coupling, follicular cell growth and inhibition of T4–T3 conversion (PTU). ATDs are considered to have immunosuppressive action. This action has been attributed in remission though not yet completely proven. There is increased apoptosis of intraparenchymal lymphocytes in thyroid. CBZ is decarboxylated to MMZ in liver in which 10 mg of CBZ gets metabolized into 6 mg of MMI. Plasma half-life of MMI is 6–10 hours vs. 1–2 hours of PTU. The compliance with MMI is better than PTU as it can be given in a single daily dose (10–30 mg, up to maximum of 80 mg MMI vs. 100–300 mg; maximum dose 1000 mg) (25, 26). Initial dose of MMZ is 10–30 mg once daily dose, PTU is given 100 mg 8 hourly. The dose of ATD is based on the T4/FT4 levels that is checked after 4 weeks (titration regime). TSH remains suppressed for several months and is not a sensitive index of early treatment response. MMZ in high doses can be combined with levothyroxine (block and replace treatment). Both PTU and MMZ cross placenta and secreted in milk (25).

There has been no advantage of BR regimen as compared to titration regiment for rendering euthyroid or in remission rates (remission is defined as a state of euthyroidism for more than 1 year after halting the ATDs). The possible advantage of BR regimen is to delay the definitive therapy in the case of pediatric GD (27).

Adverse effects of ATDs may be minor like skin reactions such as urticaria, rash, allergy, arthralgia, nausea and altered taste occurring in up to 5% of patients. Major side effects are rare include polyarthritis, agranulocytosis and vasculitis (1%) (ANCA-positive i.e. dose and duration dependant) (Table 8.8). Agranulocytosis

Hyperthyroidism

TABLE 8.8: Comparing the Side Effects of Thionamide Antithyroid Drugs

Adverse Effect	Propylthiouracil (PTU)	Methimazole (MMI)
Minor reactions	5–20%	5–20% (dose related)
Fever, rash, arthralgia (polyarthritis called antithyroid arthritis syndrome)	Nausea	Metallic taste Nausea
Abnormal taste, gastrointestinal upset		
Major reactions		
Agranulocytosis (immune mediated) Mostly within three months of ATD starting More likely in older age	0.2–0.5% (not clearly dose related)	0.2–0.5% (dose related)
Hypatotoxicity (hepatitis) More seen in age >40 years	30% (<1% serve)	Cholestatic (usually reversible, with few death reported)
Vasculitis PTU>MMI	Antineutrophil cytoplasmic antibody positive	Rare
Hematologic abnormalities	Pancytopenia, aplastic anemia, thrombocytopenia	
Insulin autoimmune syndrome	Not seen	In Asian population

occurs abruptly within 3 months of initiating ATD. Carrying HLA-B* 38:02, HLA DR-B1* 08:03 increase the odds ratio to 48.41. PTU-associated hepatotoxicity occurs commonly in children whereas with MMZ it is mild and has cholestatic pattern.

Routine assessment of liver function tests and WBC counts are not recommended for patients on ATD.

Fulminant hepatic failure is the most feared complication occurring more commonly with PTU as it causes hepatocellular damage (cholestatic with MMI). All the drugs cross placenta though MMI has higher propensity than PTU, hence PTU is considered as drug of choice in first trimester of pregnancy (25, 28).

Non-thionamide drugs:

These include organic and inorganic iodides, glucocorticoids, beta blockers, perchlorate, lithium, cholestyramine, the details of which have been discussed in Table 8.9.

Radioactive iodine ablation therapy (RAIT)

RAI therapy (RAIT) is definitive method of choice once the patient is euthyroid with persistent GD, TA or TMNG. The iodine (I131) is taken up by sodium iodine symporter (NIS), following which emission of radiation intra-parenchymally leads to destruction of thyroid tissue. It is indicated in persistent GD post-ATDs, small goiters (40–60 ml volume), preferably without ocular involvement. As RAI worsens GO or induces overt GO in patients with approximately 20% of GD, RAI is not advisable. However, in mild GO, RAI is administered cautiously with steroid cover (0.5 mg/kg of prednisolone for 1–3 months). The dose of RAIT in GD is about 10–15 mCi and for TA or TMNG is up to 20 mCi when fixed doses are administered. Contraindications for RAIT are pregnancy, suspected or proven thyroid malignancy, pediatric age-group and GO (28, 29).

ATDs are withheld for 5–7 days prior to administration of RAIT and restarted 3–5 days post-RAIT. The remission rates are 80–90% with RAIT. Few side effects occur post-RAIT like thyroiditis. Patients with persistent hyperthyroidism are candidates for a second sitting of RAIT (1, 10, 29).

TABLE 8.9: Non-Thionamide Drugs Used in Grave's Disease

Group and Drug	Dose	Mechanism of Action	Indications	Side Effects
Iodine: Lugol's Iodine SSKI	50 mg/day (up to 2000 mg/day)	Inhibits thyroid hormone release (thyroid constipation) Transient reduction in thyroid hormone synthesis (Wolff–Chaikoff effect)	GD Thyroid storm	Rash Fever Sialadenitis Mucositis Conjunctivitis
Lithium	750 mg/day (500–1500 mg/day)	Inhibits action of TSH thereby inhibiting thyroid hormone release and to some extent synthesis	GD AIT-type 1	Narrow therapeutic index drug (0.5–1.5 mEq/L) Mild/moderate/severe toxicity – GI symptoms in mild, neuromuscular in moderate, CNS effects in severe
Perchlorate	1 g/day	Inhibits iodine uptake Decreases thyroid hormone synthesis	AIT-type 1	Rash, fever, agranulocytosis, Lymphadenopathy, nephritic syndrome
Glucocorticoids Hydrocortisone Dexamethasone	100–300 mg/day 2–8 mg/day	Reduced peripheral conversion of T4–T3 (dexamethasone reduces synthesis of thyroxine synthesis)	Thyroid storm GD	Increased blood glucose and blood pressure
Beta blockers	20–80 mg/day	Reduction in peripheral conversion of T4–T3	GD TMNG/TA	Blood pressure Cautious in asthmatics
Cholestyramine	50 mg/day	Reduction in absorption of thyroxine from intestines	GD TMNG	Bloating Flatulence Constipation

Abbreviations: AIT, Amiodarone-induced thyrotoxicosis; GD, Graves' disease; TMNG, toxic multinodular goiter; TA, toxic adenoma.

Surgery

Surgical ablation in the form of near-total thyroidectomy (nTT) or TT is the standard of surgical therapy. Surgery is indicated in patients with persistent hyperthyroidism after ATDs, those with suspicious or proven malignancy, pregnant ladies, pediatric age-group, large goiters (>80 ml), GD with concomitant nodules or hyperparathyroidism, in cases of GO and those who opt for surgery. Preoperatively establishing euthyroidism is mandatory which is done with ATDs. Those patients with GD may also be administered inorganic iodide preparations such as Lugol's or supersaturated potassium iodide (SSKI) solution for 7–10 days prior to surgery which helps reduce the gland vascularity and hormone secretion. Remission in high-volume thyroid surgeon is almost 100%. Side effects of surgical intervention include hypocalcemia (1–3%) and recurrent laryngeal nerve (RLN) palsy (<1%) (1).

Graves' disease treatment

Spontaneous remission occurs in a small proportion of patients. Autoimmune hypothyroidism develops in 10–20% of patients during long-term follow-up. The definitive treatment includes ATDs, RAI and thyroidectomy. Each treatment option has its indications, advantages and disadvantages. In uncomplicated cases, ATDs remain the first line of treatment in Europe and North America. Both RAI ablation and TT result in permanent hypothyroidism and need thyroxine replacement lifelong. In all GD patients, a rapid and static hormone control is desirable as:

1. In a retrospective cohort study of 4189 GD patients regardless of the method of treatment, low TSH at 1 year following GD diagnosis was associated with a 55% increase in cardiovascular mortality (30).
2. Similarly, Lillevang et al. in a cohort study of 235,547 individual investigated the association between hyperthyroidism and mortality in both treated and untreated GD patients and concluded that suppressed TSH increases mortality in both groups and every 6 months' duration of suppressed TSH was associated with a 11–13% increase in total mortality (31).
3. Dale et al. in a study of 162 consecutive hyperthyroid patients found that even transient hypothyroidism during treatment was associated with greater weight gain during medical treatment. (32).
4. Consensus statement of the European Group on Graves' orbitopathy (EUGOGO) on management of GO recommends avoidance of hypothyroidism as it can cause exacerbation of thyroid eye disease (33).

Antithyroid drugs

The optimal duration of ATD for the titration regime is 12–18 months. Maximum remission rate that is expected is 50–55%. Normalization of TSHR antibody indicates greater chance of remission. If TSHR antibody is high after initial 12–18 months of treatment, continue ATD for another 12 months or can go for RAIT/surgery. Relapse occurs after 6 months of stopping ATD or may be years later. Patients with high TSHR Ab, large goiter are more likely to relapse (34). The poor prognostic factors in Grave's disease include male sex, age less than 40 years, smoker, the presence of large goiter, severe biochemical disease, high T3 TSH ratio, repeated episodes of relapse and very high receptor antibodies. Graves' Recurrent Events After Therapy (GREAT) score has been suggested for prediction of recurrent Graves' hyperthyroidism for the outcome with ATDs and it includes age, free T4, thyroid-binding inhibitory immunoglobulin and goiter size. GREAT scores with classes I and III have remission rate of 84% and 32%, respectively. So ATD would be a reasonable option in class I while thyroidectomy or RAI might be preferred option in class III patients (35).

Beta blockers: Propranolol 20–40 mg 6th hourly or longer acting atenolol/bisoprolol is used to control palpitations and tremor. Cardio-selective beta blockers can be used in patients with asthma. Atrial fibrillation may necessitate anticoagulants.

A meta-analysis has confirmed high relapse rate after ATD (52.5%), whereas it was 15% with RAIT and 10% with surgery (36).

Radioactive iodine therapy

Ionizing radiation has multiple effects at cellular level. The DNA damage is due to combination of direct effect, through breakage of molecular bonds, or indirectly through free radical formation. The common indications for RAIT in GD are side effects to/relapse after ATD therapy, thyrotoxic periodic paralysis and cardiac arrhythmias. RAIT is contraindicated in pregnancy, breastfeeding mothers and conception should be postponed to >6 months after RAI treatment. The thyroid function becomes normal within 3–12 months after RAIT in about 90% of patients. Few patients may need repeat RAIT. ATD needs to be stopped for 5–7 days prior to RAIT (6). Adverse effects described are pain in the region of thyroid gland, sialadenitis. Transient hyperthyroidism occurs in a few and managed with beta blockers. If hyperthyroidism does not improve after 3 months of RAIT, it is due to treatment failure. Flare-up of GO is seen in 15–33% of the cases (6).

Surgical ablation

Thyroidectomy is not the first line of management in a newly diagnosed case of GD. However, in large goiters, suspicion of malignancy, presence of ophthalmopathy and if patient does not opt for ATD and RAIT, thyroidectomy is advocated. There are advantages with thyroidectomy since it provides rapid control of hyperthyroidism, the absence of radiation risk and the absence of side effects of ATD (11). Thyroiditis should be ruled out in hyperthyroid diffuse goiters before subjecting them to surgery (12). Disadvantage of surgery include complications like hypocalcemia, voice change if not operated by experienced surgeons. Total thyroidectomy is the procedure of choice since there will not be any recurrence. Prior to surgery hyperthyroidism has to be controlled with ATD. Normal T4/FT4 indicates control of hyperthyroidism. The use of saturated solution of potassium iodide (SSKI) is used by 40% of thyroidologists for 10 days prior to surgery as it is said to decrease vascularity. Absolute indication of surgery are suspicious or biopsy-proven malignant nodules in the parenchyma of gland, associated hyperparathyroidism which require surgery, inability to use RAI ablation as definitive treatment in situations of pregnancy, lactation or children with <16 years of age, severe intolerance to ATD and large goiter with compressive or obstructive symptoms. Relative indication of surgery are associated severe GO, poorly controlled GD, patients desiring pregnancy within 6–12 months of treatment or patients with poor follow-up and patients having incomplete cure by initial attempt at RAIT.

Pregnancy and Graves' disease

Pregnancy should be postponed if hyperthyroidism is inadequately controlled until euthyroid state is achieved as confirmed by normal thyroid function at least twice over a 2-month period. Pregnancy also should be delayed 6 months post-RAIT. If thyroidectomy was performed for GD, euthyroidism should be ensured prior to conception. Patients planning pregnancy/who are pregnant should be informed about the risk of ATD-associated birth defects, possibility of stopping the ATD/changing it to PTU.

The initial ATD dose in pregnancy depends on severity of hyperthyroidism: MMI 5–15 mg or PTU 50–200 mg. The lowest possible dose of ATD is used. Block and replace therapy is not indicated in pregnancy (9). 2–4% of children can have embryopathy, including dysmorphic facies, aplasia cutis, choanal atresia, abdominal wall defects and ventricular septal defects. PTU is also associated with birth defects but with less severity. The use of propranolol may cause intrauterine growth retardation, fetal bradycardia and neonatal hypoglycemia. The thyroid function is monitored every 4 weeks. Maternal FT4 is maintained at upper limit of normal. Neonatal dysthyroidism should be suspected in those with a high titre of TSHR Ab in early first trimester and late second trimester (9). If ATD are required after 16th week of gestation, change from PTU to MMI is indicated. Both PTU and MMI enter breast milk, doses of <250 mg PTU and <20 mg MMI are safe for mother in postpartum phase (37).

Graves' disease in children

Of all the GD occurring, this age-group contributes around 1–5% with a female preponderance in children as well. Pathogenesis remains the same as explained earlier with genetic factors involving HLA type 2 and CTLA-4. The involvement of first-degree relative is nearly 80% (38). Initial management is with ATDs to render euthyroid. As the relapse rates in children in more than 75–80%, with only ATDs, definitive therapy is must. Definitive therapy in children is surgery as they may be noncompliant to ATDs. Administration of RAIT in children is considered only when the child and/or the guardian does not want the child to undergo surgery. In high-volume thyroid surgeon, surgical complications like hypocalcemia and RLN palsy are similar to adult rates (38, 39). Other complications include bleeding and scarring.

Toxic adenoma and toxic multinodular goiter

Iodine deficiency is one of the most common predisposing factors to goiter and in long-standing goiters, the somatic point mutations of TSHR and GSα (in TA) lead to benign clonal expansion of thyroid follicular cells, which result in TA (when unifocal) and TMNG (when multifocal). Toxic MNG is more common, representing 40–50% of total cases of hyperthyroidism in iodine-deficient areas. It has female preponderance 5:1 and occurs at a later age than GD (3, 11). The presenting features are goiter, single nodule in TA and multiple nodules in TMNG, with features of hyperthyroidism. As this occurs at a later age, cardiovascular symptoms and complications are more common up to 15% (10).

Thyroid profile shows reduced levels of TSH and elevated fT4 levels. In contrast to GD, TSHR Abs are rarely (less than 10%) elevated in TA or TMNG. Thyroid scan in TA shows single hyperfunctioning nodule with surrounding suppressed thyroid. In TMNG, there are multiple hot nodules with interspersed normal or suppressed thyroid tissue. Ultrasound of thyroid gland shows single nodule in TA and multiple nodules in TMNG. Ultrasound can also guide in case of suspicious lesion for FNAC (10, 11).

Definitive treatment for both TA and TMNG is by RAIT or surgery as medical management alone using ATDs is not curative with a relapse of almost 95% at 2 years (40). Initial ATDs may be required to control hyperthyroidism. Beta blockers are frequently required due to cardiovascular effects of hyperthyroidism. Iodides are contraindicated in preoperative preparation of TMNG and TA (28).

RAIT for TA and TMNG: RAIT is indicated in both TA and TMNG. Those patients with TMNG have shown a response rate of 80% by 6 months. Recent study by Saki et al observed 93.8% cure rates in TMNG (41). The goiter may reduce in up to 21%, with hypothyroidism occurring in 4–30% of the patients (28, 41, 42). In patients with TA, the response rates were similar to TMNG. Saki et al observed 94.7% of cure rates in TA. Hyperthyroidism may remain in 6–25% at 6 months of the patients treated with RAI (28, 41). Recurrence or need of retreatment may occur in nearly 5% of patients with TA and up to 20% of the patients in TMNG. Goiter does not disappear in majority of the patients undergoing RAIT. RAI is an absolute contraindication in pregnancy, lactation and malignancy. A relative contraindication is in patients who do not comply with radiation safety guidelines (28, 40, 41).

Surgery for TA and TMNG: Surgical treatment of TA depends on the involvement of the lobe, the presence of nodules in opposite lobe and suspicion of malignancy. Surgical options for TA include lobectomy, isthmectomy, nTT or TT. For those with TMNG, the surgical treatment is nTT or TT. Patients should be euthyroid prior to surgery. The use of Lugol's iodine is contraindicated in preoperative preparation of TA or TMNG as compared to GD. Recurrence after nTT or TT in TA and TMNG is <1% when performed by high-volume thyroid surgeon (27). Recurrence after subtotal thyroidectomy across various studies ranges up to 30% (43). Pregnancy may be considered as a relative contraindication (28).

Newer modalities: Ethanol ablation (EA), radiofrequency ablation (RFA) and laser thermal ablation (LTA), microwave ablation (MWA), high-frequency ultrasound (HIFU) are available nonsurgical ablation modalities to benign thyroid nodules. RFA, LTA and EA are amongst the more commonly used modalities for TA and TMNG. These modalities are used as an alternative for definitive therapy or in those patients who opt out of RAI and surgery. These modalities are indicated in nodules up to 30 mm size, after excluding malignancy (44–46). Multiple sittings are necessary for ethanol injection. Tarantino et al followed 125 patients over 5 years and found nearly 92% having greater than 50% reduction in size with EA (28). RFA and LTA have been effective in reducing nodule size up to 80% in half of the patients at 12 months. The best candidates were those with nodule volume less than 10ml, whereas those with higher volume had lower reduction in nodule size. HIFU was found to be less effective with volume reduction of about 53% at 12 months (45). Combination of LTA with RAI has found to be more effective in volume reduction than RAI alone in larger nodules (46, 47).

Thyroiditis

Most common cause of thyrotoxicosis without hyperthyroidism is thyroiditis. Preformed thyroid hormone is released rather than excess synthesis as compared to hyperthyroidism. Among various thyroiditis, transient thyrotoxic phase is usually present in painless sporadic thyroiditis, painful subacute thyroiditis, and postpartum thyroiditis. Painless thyroiditis presents between 30 and 40 years, with female preponderance (2:1). It is considered to have autoimmune etiology and presents as thyromegaly without neck pain. Painful subacute thyroiditis presents between 20 and 60 years, also with a female preponderance (5:1). There is usually history of viral throat infection and presents with painful thyromegaly. Postpartum thyroiditis presents immediately up to 1-year post-termination of pregnancy. There is no neck pain associated. On histology, there is lymphocytic infiltration seen in all three types of thyroiditis, also granulomas may be present in painful subacute thyroiditis (10, 48, 49).

In thyroiditis, thyroid hormone profile shows reduced TSH and elevated fT4 levels. One of the first markers to be elevated in thyroiditis is thyroglobulin (Tg). Antithyroid peroxidise (Anti-TPO) is elevated in painless and postpartum thyroiditis, whereas in subacute thyroiditis, it may be raised or normal. Additionally, erythrocyte sedimentation rate is raised in subacute thyroiditis but remains normal in the former two. RAI uptake scan shows reduced tracer uptake in all three conditions. As mostly they are self-limiting and also have a thyrotoxic phase followed by hypothyroid phase, treatment during thyrotoxic phase includes medication for pain with nonsteroidal anti-inflammatory drugs (NSAIDs). Few may require steroids for pain. Beta blockers are administered for effects of thyrotoxicosis (10, 48, 49).

Drug-induced thyroiditis

Drug-induced thyroiditis is caused by amiodarone, iodine, lithium, interferon- α and other drugs. Of these, amiodarone is the most important drug. Amiodarone-induced thyrotoxicosis (AIT) occurs approximately with an average incidence of 20–25%. Amiodarone contains 37% of iodine by weight, of which 10% is deiodinated every day that results in release of 7–21 mg of iodine for uptake per day. Two types of AIT are known, type 1 is increased synthesis and type 2 is destructive type (12, 48). Table 8.10 describes differences between two types of AIT.

TABLE 8.10: Types of Amiodarone-Induced Thyrotoxicosis (AIT)

	AIT-Type 1	AIT-Type 2
History	Sudden, explosive Early or late during the course of treatment	Gradual Usually after prolonged administration
Predisposing factors	Preexisting thyroid disease Iodine-deficient areas 29% with diffuse goiter 38% with nodular goiter	No preexisting thyroid disorder
Pathology	Increased hormone synthesis	Destruction of follicles Release of preformed hormone
Antibodies	TSHR Abs may be present in preexisting thyroid disease	Absent
RAI uptake	Normal or low or increased	Low
Cytokines	Normal or mildly elevated IL-6	Highly elevated levels of IL-6
Sonography – color Doppler	Increased vascularity	Normal
Treatment	ATDs (thionamides) Perchlorates Organic iodide (iopanoic acid)	Steroids
Sequel hypothyroidism	Absent	Possible

Other causes of thyrotoxicosis

Other causes include excess thyroxine supplementation (factitious thyrotoxicosis) which can be diagnosed on history of thyroxine supplementation. Pituitary tumors with TSH secretion are diagnosed biochemically with a suspicion when serum TSH and fT4 are raised and confirmed with CT or MRI of brain. Treatment is removal of pituitary tumor. Metastatic FTC rarely presents with thyrotoxicosis, and its treatment is multimodal. Struma ovarii presents in females as pelvic mass with features of thyrotoxicosis more commonly when greater than 50% of tumor contains thyroid tissue. Treatment is essentially surgical after rendering patient euthyroid. Metastatic lesions may need adjuvant RAIT (10).

Hyperthyroidism with Thyroid carcinoma

Reduced TSH levels are believed to be a protective factor for thyroid carcinoma due to increased iodine uptake and hormone synthesis, nevertheless hyperthyroidism and thyroid carcinoma coexist. The exact incidence of hyperthyroidism with thyroid carcinoma is not well known, the prevalence of nodule is approximately 10–15% with GD with malignancy rates between 2.3 and 45.8% vs. 5% malignancy in euthyroid nodular goiter (50). All pathological variants of differentiated thyroid cancer (DTC) may occur with hyperthyroidism but the most common is papillary variant. Main mechanism in GD includes stimulation of DTC cells by the TSHR Ab and increase in vascular endothelial growth factor (VEGF) resulting in neo-angiogenesis. The mechanisms attributed to TMNG and TA are due to cytokines like TGF-β (50–51).

Diagnosis of hyperthyroidism is established biochemically with low TSH and elevated fT4 levels. Concomitant DTC with hyperthyroidism is diagnosed by FNAC preferably ultrasound guided. The use of ultrasound increases nodule detection up to 33.6% in GD (52). Diffuse goiter is present in GD, nodules in TA and TMNG. Clinical features of hyperthyroidism coexist. Surgical removal is the only curative therapy, but patients to be made euthyroid preoperatively. TT or nTT is the surgical treatment of choice.

Retrospective study by Medas et al. operated on 2820 thyroid nodules, of which 909 had thyroid cancer and 87 were associated with hyperthyroidism. They found higher lymph node metastases (12.6%) associated in patients of thyroid carcinoma with hyperthyroidism vs. euthyroid nodules (6.1%) which was statistically significant ($p = 0.03$). In postoperative outcomes, rate of hypoparathyroidism is more in hyperthyroidism group (28.1 vs. 13.2%; $p < 0.01$) and 5-year disease-free survival was less in hyperthyroidism group (89.1 vs. 96.6%; $p = 0.03$) (53). Similarly, Menon et al found PTC in 29 (18%) associated with hyperthyroidism in a cohort of 308 patients. In this study, they also found that patients of PTC with GD as compared to carcinoma in euthyroid patients were found to have higher locoregional recurrence (3.4 vs. 1.7% $p = 0.246$), distant metastases (10.3 vs. 2.5% $p = 0.027$) and mortality (3.4 vs. 1.3%; $p = 0.358$) (51). Overall, thyroid carcinoma associated with hyperthyroidism is aggressive than euthyroid nodules with carcinoma.

South-Asian perspective

In India, the exact prevalence of hyperthyroidism is not documented, but studies show that prevalence of hyperthyroidism range from 1.79 to 2.5% in various series reported by Arindam

Bose et al. (54), Rebecca et al. (55), Deokar et al. (56). Unnikrishnan et al have found prevalence rate in hyperthyroidism of 1.8% with 0.6% constituting subclinical and 1.2% overt hyperthyroidism (5). One cross-sectional study from China found that the prevalence of hyperthyroidism in iodine-repleted areas is higher than iodine-depleted areas (8). In iodine-deficient areas, nearly 40–50% of hyperthyroidism occurs due to toxic nodular goiters (TA or TMNG) (3, 11).

Thyroiditis is more common in iodine sufficient areas of India than nodular goiters. TMNG presents in elderly females with more prominent cardiovascular complications. Drug-induced thyrotoxicosis (AIT) in iodine-deficient areas predominantly is of type 1 with preexisting or underlying thyroid nodular disease. Management for hyperthyroidism is by initial medical management, followed by RAIT or surgery.

Conclusion

Etiology of hyperthyroidism has to be diagnosed meticulously in order to determine the line of management. Thyrotoxicosis presentation varies according to the underlying causative factor. Diagnosis is essentially made by elevated thyroid hormones and the etiology can be ascertained by clinical history and thyroid scan. RAI ablation or surgery is the mainstay of treatment in GD. ATD is essential to make the patient euthyroid prior to definitive therapy. Prompt discussion with patients regarding delayed outcome and retreatment in those who opt for RAI is mandatory. Surgical treatment of choice in the form of nTTx or TTx ought to be performed in a high-volume center to reduce complication and recurrence. TA and TMNG are managed similarly to GD i.e. rendering euthyroid with ATDs, followed by definitive therapy. Extent of surgery in toxic solitary adenoma depends on radiology, nuclear imaging after malignancy is ruled out. Newer ablative therapies like RFA, EA and LTA are considered as a substitute for definitive therapy in selective patients. Nonetheless, malignancy should always be treated by surgery. Other causes of thyrotoxicosis are to be treated accordingly. Thyroid malignancy coexists with hyperthyroidism. This subset is more aggressive in nature than the euthyroid counterpart.

References

1. De Leo S, Lee SY, Braverman LE. Hyperthyroidism. Lancet. 2016 Aug;388(10047):906–918.
2. Laurberg P, Cerqueira C, Ovesen L, Rasmussen LB, Perrild H, Andersen S, et al. Iodine intake as a determinant of thyroid disorders in populations. Best Pract Res Clin Endocrinol Metab. 2010 Feb;24(1):13–27.
3. Taylor PN, Albrecht D, Scholz A, Gutierrez-Buey G, Lazarus JH, Dayan CM, et al. Global epidemiology of hyperthyroidism and hypothyroidism. Nat Rev Endocrinol. 2018;14(5):301–316.
4. Walsh JP. Managing thyroid disease in general practice. Med J Austr. 2016 Aug;205(4):179–184.
5. Unnikrishnan AG, Menon UV. Thyroid disorders in India: an epidemiological perspective. Indian J Endocrinol Metab. 2011 Jul;15(Suppl2):S78–S81.
6. Gopinath B, Wang JJ, Kifley A, Wall JR, Eastman CJ, Leeder SR, et al. Five-year incidence and progression of thyroid dysfunction in an older population. Inter Med J. 2010;40(9):642–649.
7. Tunbridge WM, Evered DC, Hall R, Appleton D, Brewis M, Clark F, et al. The spectrum of thyroid disease in a community: the Whickham survey. Clin Endocrinol (Oxf). 1977 Dec;7(6):481–493.
8. Du Y, Gao Y, Meng F, Liu S, Fan Z, Wu J, et al. Iodine deficiency and excess coexist in China and induce thyroid dysfunction and disease: a cross-sectional study. PLOS ONE [Internet]. 2014 Nov 6 [cited 2020 Nov 12];9(11). Available from: https://www.ncbi.nlm.nih.gov/pmc/articles/PMC4223066/
9. Smith TJ, Hegedüs L. Graves' disease. N Engl J Med. 2017;376(2):185.
10. Sharma A, Stan MN. Thyrotoxicosis: diagnosis and management. Mayo Clin Proc. 2019 Jun;94(6):1048–1064.
11. Laurberg P, Pedersen KM, Vestergaard H, Sigurdsson G. High incidence of multinodular toxic goitre in the elderly population in a low iodine intake area vs. high incidence of Graves' disease in the young in a high iodine intake area: comparative surveys of thyrotoxicosis epidemiology in East-Jutland Denmark and Iceland. J Intern Med. 1991 May;229(5):415–420.
12. Martino E, Bartalena L, Bogazzi F, Braverman LE. The effects of amiodarone on the thyroid. Endocr Rev. 2001 Apr;22(2):240–254.
13. Singh I, Hershman JM. Pathogenesis of hyperthyroidism. Compr Physiol. 2016 06;7(1):67–79.
14. Jacobson EM, Huber A, Tomer Y. The HLA gene complex in thyroid autoimmunity: from epidemiology to etiology. J Autoimmun. 2008 Mar;30(1–2):58–62.
15. Crooks J, Murray IPC, Wayne EJ. Statistical methods applied to the clinical diagnosis of thyrotoxicosis. Q J Med. 1959;28:211–234.
16. Bartley GB, Fatourechi V, Kadrmas EF, et al. Clinical features of Graves' ophthalmopathy in an incidence cohort. Am J Ophthalmol. 1996;121:284–290.
17. Mourits MP, Koornneef L, Wiersinga WM, Prummel MF, Berghout A, van der Gaag R. Clinical criteria for the assessment of disease activity in Graves' Opthalmopathy: a novel approach. Br J Ophthalmol. 1989;73:639–644.
18. Werner SC. Classification of the eye changes of Graves' disease. Am J Ophthalmol. 1969;68:646–648.
19. Jesús Barrio-Barrio, Alfonso L. Sabater, Elvira Bonet-Farriol, Álvaro Velázquez-Villoria, Juan C. Galofré Graves' Ophthalmopathy: VISA versus EUGOGO classification, assessment, and management. J Ophthalmol. 2015;2015:249125.
20. Dolman P. J., Rootman J. VISA classification for Graves orbitopathy. Ophthalm Plastic Reconstr Surg. 2006;22(5):319–324.
21. European Group on Graves' Orbitopathy, Clin Eval Eugogo Atlas. 2009, http://www.eugogo.eu/_downloads/clincial_evaluation/Clinical_Evaluation_GO.pdf
22. Fatourechi V, Debra DFA, Schwartz KM. Thyroid acropachy: report of 40 patienst treated at a single institution in a 26-year period. J Clin Endocrinol Metab. 2002;87:5435–5441
23. Hollenberg, A. and M Weirsinga, W., 2020. Hyperthyroid disorders. In: S. Melmed, R. Auchus, A. Goldfine, R. Koenig and C. Rosen, eds., Hyperthyroid Disorders Williams Textbook of Endocrinology, 14th ed. Philadelphia: Elsevier, pp. 364–403.
24. Intenzo CM, dePapp AE, Jabbour S, Miller JL, Kim SM, Capuzzi DM. Scintigraphic manifestations of thyrotoxicosis. RadioGraphics. 2003 Jul;23(4):857–869.
25. Cooper DS. Antithyroid drugs. N Engl J Med. 2005 Mar;352(9):905–917.
26. Cooper DS. Antithyroid drugs in the management of patients with Graves' disease: an evidence-based approach to therapeutic controversies. J Clin Endocrinol Metab. 2003 Aug;88(8):3474–3481.
27. Vigone MC, Peroni E, Di Frenna M, Mora S, Barera G, Weber G. "Block-and-replace" treatment in Graves' disease: experience in a cohort of pediatric patients. J Endocrinol Invest. 2020 May;43(5):595–600.
28. Ross DS, Burch HB, Cooper DS, Greenlee MC, Laurberg P, Maia AL, et al. 2016 American Thyroid Association Guidelines for diagnosis and management of hyperthyroidism and other causes of thyrotoxicosis. Thyroid. 2016;26(10):1343–1421.
29. Kahaly GJ. Management of Graves thyroidal and extrathyroidal disease: an update. J Clin Endocr Metab. 2020;105(12):1–17.
30. Okosieme OE, Taylor PN, Evans C, Thayer D, Chai A, Khan I, Draman MS, Tennant B, Geen J, Sayers A, French R, Lazarus JH, Premawardhana LD, Dayan CM. Primary therapy of Graves' disease and cardiovascular morbidity and mortality: a linked-record cohort study. Lancet Diabetes Endocrinol. 2019 Apr;7(4):278–287.
31. Lillevang-Johansen M, Abrahamsen B, Jørgensen HL, Brix TH, Hegedüs L. Excess mortality in treated and untreated hyperthyroidism is related to cumulative periods of low serum TSH. J Clin Endocrinol Metab. 2017 Jul; 102(7):2301–2309.
32. Dale J, Daykin J, Holder R, Sheppard MC, Franklyn JA. Weight gain following treatment of hyperthyroidism. Clin Endocrinol (Oxf). 2001 Aug; 55(2):233–239.
33. Bartalena L, Baldeschi L, Dickinson A, Eckstein A, Kendall-Taylor P, Marcocci C, et al, Consensus statement of the European Group on Graves' orbitopathy (EUGOGO) on management of GO. Eur J Endocrinol. 2008 Mar;158(3):273–285.
34. Goichot B, Bouee S, Castello-Bridoux C, Caron P. Survey of clinical practice patterns in management of 992 hyperthyroid patients in France. Eur Thyroid J. 2017;6:152–159.
35. Vos XG, Endert E, Zwinderman AH, Tijssen JG, Wiersinga WM. Predicting the risk of recurrence before the start of antithyroid drug therapy in patients with Graves' hyperthyroidism. J Clin Endocrinol Metab. 2016;101:1381–1389.
36. Sundaresh V, Brito JP, Wang Z, Prokop LJ, Stan MN, Murad MH, Bahn RS. Comapritive effectiveness of therapies for Graves hyperthyroidism: a systematic review and network meta-analysis. J Clin Endocrinol Metab. 2013;98:3671–3677.
37. Mandel SJ, Cooper DS. The use of antithyroid drugs in pregnancy and lactation. J Clin Endocrinol Metab. 2001;86:2354–2359.
38. Léger J, Carel JC. Hyperthyroidism in childhood: causes, when and how to treat. J Clin Res Pediatr Endocrinol. 2013 Mar;5(Suppl 1):50–56.
39. Minamitani K, Sato H, Ohye H, Harada S, Arisaka O. Guidelines for the treatment of childhood-onset Graves' disease in Japan, 2016. Clin Pediatr Endocrinol. 2017;26(2):29–62.
40. Kang AS, Grant CS, Thompson GB, van Heerden JA. Current treatment of nodular goiter with hyperthyroidism (Plummer's disease): surgery versus radioiodine. Surgery. 2002 Dec;132(6):916–923; discussion 923.
41. Şakı H, Cengiz A, Yürekli Y. Effectiveness of radioiodine treatment for toxic nodular goiter. Mol Imaging Radionucl Ther. 2015 Oct;24(3):100–104.
42. Ahmad T, Khoja A, Rashid NH, Ashfaq MA. Outcome of radioactive iodine therapy in Toxic Nodular Goiter in Pakistan. Pak J Med Sci. 2018;34(5):1146–1151.
43. Hedley AJ, Ross IP, Beck JS, Donald D, Albert-Recht F, Michie W, et al. Recurrent thyrotoxicosis after subtotal thyroidectomy. Br Med J. 1971 Oct;4(5782):258–261.
44. Tarantino L, Francica G, Sordelli I, Sperlongano P, Parmeggiani D, Ripa C, et al. Percutaneous ethanol injection of hyperfunctioning thyroid nodules: long-term follow-up in 125 patients. Am J Roentgenol. 2008 Mar;190(3):800–808.
45. Papini E, Monpeyssen H, Frasoldati A, Hegedüs L. 2020 European Thyroid Association Clinical Practice Guideline for the use of image-guided ablation in benign thyroid nodules. ETJ. 2020;9(4):172–185.

46. Hahn SY, Shin JH, Na DG, Ha EJ, Ahn HS, Lim HK, et al. Ethanol ablation of the thyroid nodules: 2018 consensus statement by the korean society of thyroid radiology. Korean J Radiol. 2019 Apr;20(4):609–620.
47. Chianelli M, Bizzarri G, Todino V, Misischi I, Bianchini A, Graziano F, et al. Laser ablation and 131-Iodine: a 24-month pilot study of combined treatment for large toxic nodular goiter. J Clin Endocrinol Metab. 2014 Jul;99(7):E1283–E1286.
48. Pearce EN, Farwell AP, Braverman LE. Thyroiditis. N Engl J Med. 2003 Jun;348(26):2646–2655.
49. Begum A, Bari M, Ayaz K, Yasmin R, Rajib N, Rashid M, et al. Thyroiditis – a review. J Med. 2006 Jan 1;7:58–63.
50. Fu H, Cheng L, Jin Y, Chen L. Thyrotoxicosis with concomitant thyroid cancer. Endocr Relat Cancer. 2019;26(7):R395–R413.
51. Menon R, Nair CG, Babu M, Jacob P, Krishna GP. The outcome of papillary thyroid cancer associated with Graves' disease: a case control study [Internet]. J Thyroid Res Hindawi. 2018;2018 [cited 2020 Nov 21]. p. e8253094. Available from: https://www.hindawi.com/journals/jtr/2018/8253094/
52. Cantalamessa L, Baldini M, Orsatti A, Meroni L, Amodei V, Castagnone D. Thyroid nodules in Graves disease and the risk of thyroid carcinoma. Arch Intern Med. 1999 Aug;159(15):1705–1708.
53. Medas F, Erdas E, Canu GL, Longheu A, Pisano G, Tuveri M, et al. Does hyperthyroidism worsen prognosis of thyroid carcinoma? A retrospective analysis on 2820 consecutive thyroidectomies. J Otolaryngol - Head Neck Surg. 2018 Jan;47(1):6.
54. Bose A, Sharma N, Hemvani N, Chitnis DS. A hospital based prevalence study on thyroid disorders in Malwa region of Central India. Int J Curr Microbiol App Sci. 2015;8.
55. Abraham R, Srinivasa Murugan V, Pukazhvanthen P, Sen SK. Thyroid disorders in women of Puducherry. Indian J Clin Biochem. 2009 Jan;24(1):52–59.
56. Deokar PG, Nagdeote AN, Lanje MJ, Basutkar DG. Prevalence of thyroid disorders in a tertiary care center. Int J Cur Res Rev 2016; 8(9):26–30.

9

APPROACH TO THYROID NODULES

Chiaw-Ling Chng

Introduction

Thyroid nodules are a prevalent clinical problem, with palpable thyroid nodules detected in about 5% of women and 1% of men living in iodine-sufficient countries (1, 2). The use of high-resolution ultrasound (US) further inflates this figure, detecting thyroid nodules in 19%–68% of randomly selected individuals (3, 4). Approximately 10% of patients who present with thyroid nodules are malignant (5). The incidence of thyroid cancer has increased about fivefold in the last 50 years, mostly due to small papillary thyroid cancers, a mostly indolent form of thyroid cancer (6). The main goal in evaluating the thyroid nodule is the identification of thyroid cancers, although some may be clinically relevant due to compressive symptoms or thyroid dysfunction. The aim of this chapter is to provide guidance to aid clinical decisions in the selection of thyroid nodules for further evaluation and interpretation of results of evaluation.

History and physical examination

Most patients with thyroid nodules are asymptomatic as many are incidentally diagnosed due to imaging for unrelated causes, e.g. carotid duplex US after cerebrovascular accident. However, focal uptake on the PET scan and an increased maximum standardized uptake value (SUV) is associated increased risk of malignancy (ROM) (55%) (7) in a thyroid nodule and warrants further investigations such as fine-needle aspiration biopsy. Careful history taking should include information of previous childhood radiation exposure to the head and neck, growth of the thyroid nodule, any associated local symptoms such as pain, hoarseness of voice, dysphagia and symptoms of hyper or hypothyroidism. Familial history of thyroid cancer or hereditary syndromes that include thyroid cancer (e.g. multiple endocrine neoplasia syndrome type 2, familial adenomatous polyposis, Cowden disease) are risk factors for thyroid malignancy. Physical examination should concentrate on inspection for visible lumps and palpation of the thyroid and cervical lymph nodes. The presence of a firm thyroid nodule fixed to adjacent structures and cervical lymphadenopathy with thyroid nodule requires early evaluation. Potential "red flags" the initial evaluation of thyroid nodule is summarized in Table 9.1.

Laboratory evaluation and imaging

The initial evaluation of the thyroid nodule should include a measurement of serum thyrotropin (TSH). The finding of a suppressed TSH suggests the presence of hyperfunctional thyroid nodule which should be followed by a radionuclide scan, i.e. I-123 or technetium pertechnetate scintigraphy. A radioiodine uptake scintigraphy measures the percentage of administered radioiodine (I-123) that is concentrated into the thyroid gland after a fixed interval, usually 24 hours. Unlike I-123, which is both concentrated and organified within the thyroid, technetium pertechnetate is only concentrated in the thyroid. A technetium uptake scintigraphy measures the percentage of administered technetium that is trapped in the thyroid after a fixed interval, usually 20 minutes. Technetium pertechnetate is readily available and associated with less total body radiation, thus more widely used than I-123 (8). The purpose of the radionuclide scan would be to investigate the presence of autonomously functional thyroid nodule (≤5% of all thyroid nodules) (9). Hyperfunctional thyroid nodules ("hot" nodules) are almost always benign, thus do not require cytologic evaluation (Figure 9.1). In the case of multinodular goiter, a mixture of "hot" and "cold" (nonfunctioning) nodules may be present. These "cold" nodules should be evaluated with a US thyroid. Routine measurement of serum thyroglobulin to detect thyroid malignancy is not recommended, since the marker can be elevated in benign thyroid diseases, e.g. thyroiditis. Serum calcitonin is a marker for medullary thyroid cancer. Currently, there is insufficient evidence to recommend routine measurement of serum calcitonin (10). Although routine use of serum calcitonin may detect medullary thyroid cancer at an earlier stage, consequent reduction of cancer-specific mortality cannot be ascertained. In addition, assay performance, specificity and cost-effectiveness are suboptimal (11).

Ultrasound thyroid

US is the primary tool used for the initial risk stratification of thyroid nodules and aids the clinician to subsequently decide that nodules require further evaluation by fine-needle aspiration biopsy. Diagnostic US should be performed in all patients with suspected thyroid nodule or incidentally thyroid nodules detected on another imaging study such as CT, MRI or ^{18}FDG-PET scans. A diagnostic US thyroid report should include the nodule size in three dimensions, location and description of the nodule's sonographic features, including composition (solid,

TABLE 9.1: Potential "Red Flags" in the Initial Evaluation of Thyroid Nodule

---

Family history of thyroid cancer or hereditary syndromes, e.g. multiple endocrine neoplasia 2A (primary hyperparathyroidism, pheochromocytoma and medullary thyroid cancer), MEN 2B (pheochromocytoma, medullary thyroid cancer, marfanoid habitus, mucosal and digestive neurofibromatosis), Cowden disease, familial adenomatous polyposis

Personal history of head and neck irradiation, particularly as a child

Enlarging thyroid mass

Symptoms of compression such as hoarseness of voice, dysphagia, dyspnea

Firm nodule fixed to adjacent structures

Associated cervical lymphadenopathy

PET-positive thyroid nodule

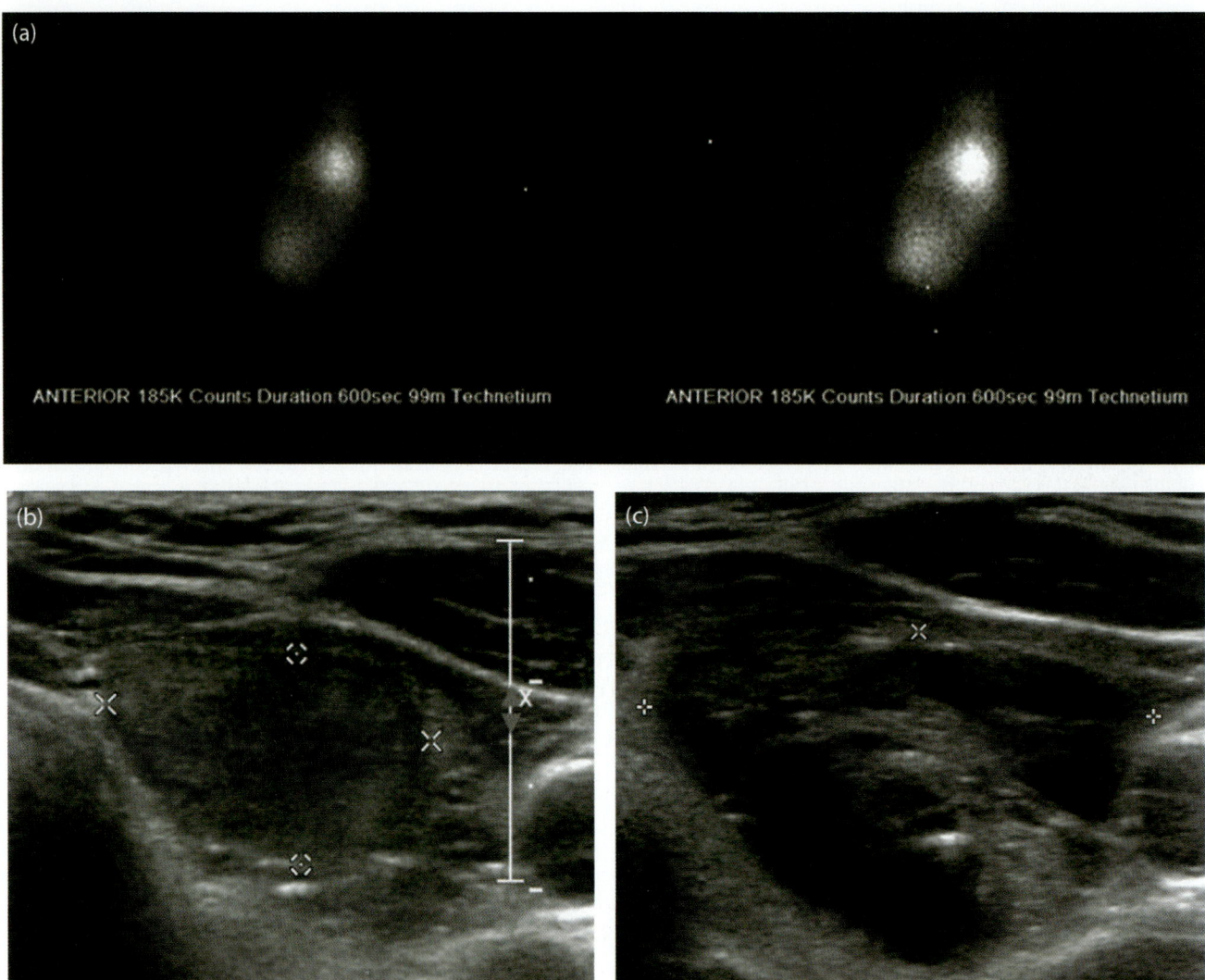

FIGURE 9.1 (a) Technetium pertechnetate thyroid uptake scan showing enlarged left thyroid lobe with two foci of increased tracer uptake of the left thyroid gland suggestive of "hot" nodules. There is suppression of tracer uptake in the right thyroid. (b) and (c) Correlative ultrasound showing the left upper pole and left lower pole nodules respectively.

cystic, mixed solid-cystic or spongiform), echogenicity, margins, presence and type of calcifications, and shape if taller than wide, and vascularity. Routine US examination of the internal jugular chain of cervical lymph nodes, particularly on the ipsilateral side of a suspicious thyroid lesion, should be performed. The pattern of sonographic features of the nodule confers a ROM and guides fine needle aspiration cytology (FNAC) decision-making (10).

Certain features of thyroid nodules on US are associated with higher ROM (Figure 9.2). The most commonly highlighted malignant US features are (12):

1. Microcalcification, which represent psammoma bodies, which are 10–100 μm round laminar crystalline calcific deposits. On US, microcalcifications appear as punctuate hyperechoic foci without acoustic shadowing
2. Interrupted rim calcifications: suggest tumor invasion in the area of disrupted calcification
3. Marked hypoechogenicity: thyroid nodule with a darker appearance than that of infrahyoid or strap muscles of the neck
4. Ill-defined or irregular margins: suggest malignant infiltration of adjacent parenchyma
5. Taller-than-wide shape: this appearance is thought to be due to centrifugal tendency in tumor growth, which does not occur at a uniform rate in all dimensions
6. Associated suspicious cervical lymphadenopathy: suspicious features are a round shape, increased size, absence of fatty hilum, heterogeneous echotexture, calcifications, cystic areas and vascularity throughout the lymph node on Doppler imaging

In our study of 167 histologically proven thyroid nodules in the author's institution, we found significantly higher percentages of malignant nodules were solid, hypoechoic, had irregular margins, taller-than-wide morphology, microcalcifications, disrupted rim calcifications or associated abnormal cervical lymphadenopathy (13).

Three meta-analyses have been conducted to date to evaluate the diagnostic performance of these US features found largely

Approach to Thyroid Nodules

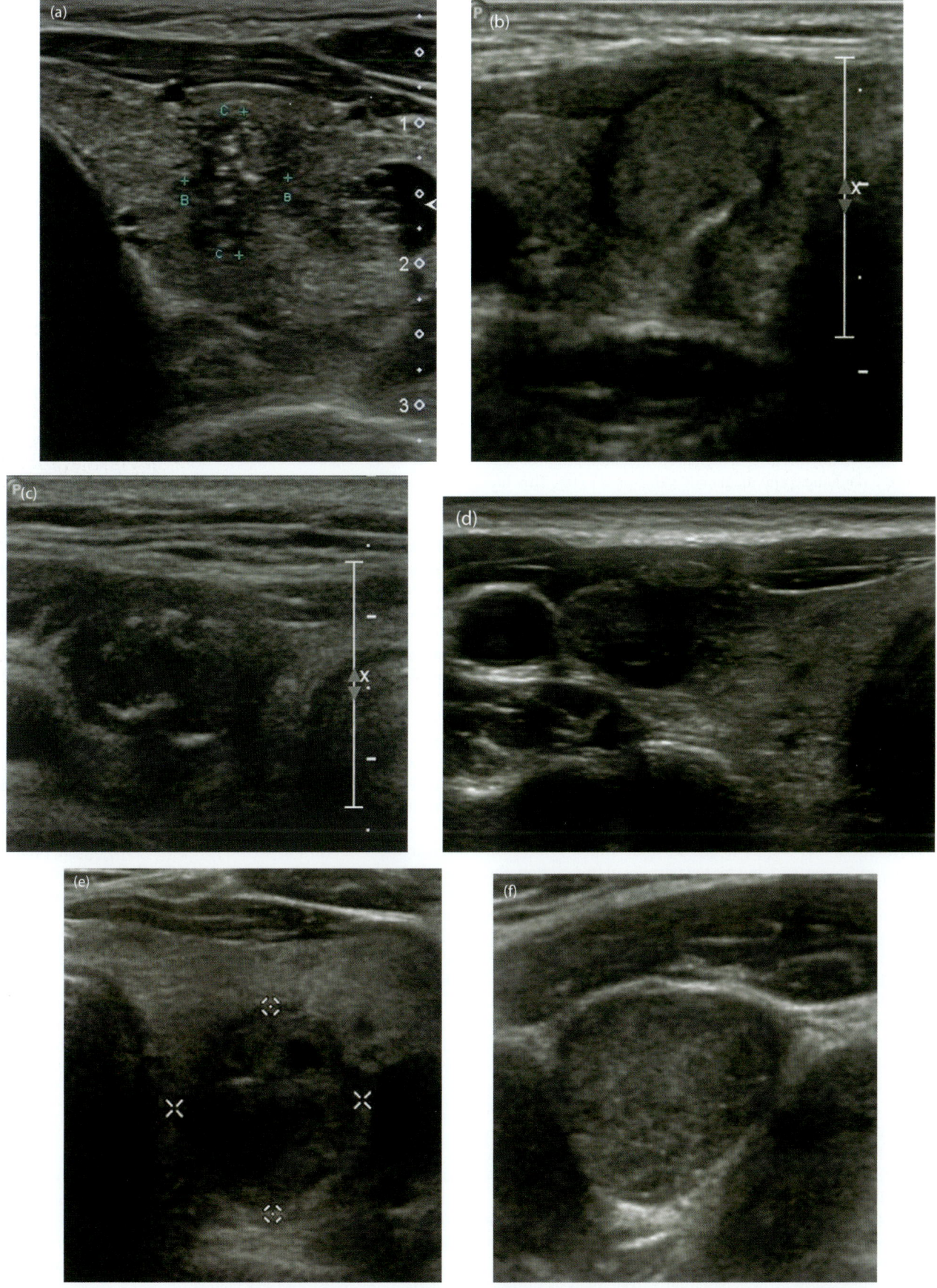

FIGURE 9.2 Ultrasound features of suspicious thyroid nodules. (a) Microcalcifications (b) interrupted rim calcification (c) marked hypoechogenicity (d) ill-defined margins (e) taller-than-wide morphology (f) suspicious cervical lymphadenopathy (left level II cervical lymph node).

TABLE 9.2: The Three Meta-Analyses That Have Been Conducted to Date to Evaluate the Diagnostic Performance of Thyroid Nodule Ultrasound Features in Predicting Malignancy

Study	Study Inclusion	Results
Brito et al. (14)	31 Studies with 18,288 nodules	The US features with the highest diagnostic odds ratio (DOR) correctly indicating malignancy were taller than wide shape (11.14; 95% CI 6.6–18.9) and internal calcifications (6.78; 95% CI 4.48–10.24). A spongiform (12; 95% CI: 0.6–234.3) and a cystic appearance (6.8; 95% CI: 2.3–20.3) most reliably predicted benignity
Campanella et al. (15)	41 Studies with 29,678 nodules	Highest risk of malignancy was associated with a taller-than-wide shape (DOR of 10.2; 95% CI: 6.7–15.3), an absent halo sign (7.1; 95% CI: 3.7–13.7), microcalcifications (6.8; 95% CI: 4.7–9.7) and irregular margins (6.1; 95% CI: 3.1–12.0)
Remonti et al. (16)	52 Studies with 12,786 nodules	Highest specificities for malignancy were the absence of elasticity (86.2%), microcalcifications (87.8%), irregular margins (83.1%) and a taller-than-wide shape (96.6%), respectively

similar results, as summarized in Table 9.2 (14–16). However, all the authors concluded that none of the US characteristics alone is reliable to predict malignancy. This deficiency is further crippled by substantial interobserver variation in the assessment and reporting of some of the US patterns (17). Although no single US feature can reliably predict malignancy, a combination of several features enhances the diagnostic value of US (18). This has prompted the development of standardized systems for reporting US features using "pattern recognition" technique, in an attempt to delineate sets of characteristics associated with specific risk levels for malignancy.

Horvath et al. in 2009 developed a US risk classification system known as the Thyroid Imaging Reporting and Data System (TIRADS) (19). This is a system similar to the one used for breast imaging. It consists of a 6-point scale for risk stratification with increasing risks of malignancy. This was subsequently modified and validated in a large prospective study (20). Following this, US risk stratification systems recommendations have been issued by the Korean Society of Radiology, American College of Radiology (ACR), the American Thyroid Association (ATA), European Thyroid Association, the American Association of Clinical Endocrinologists, the American College of Endocrinology and the Italian Associazione Medici Endocrinologi (10, 21–24). It is not the intent of this chapter to discuss in detail the various US risk stratification systems, but for the purpose of this section, the two most widely adopted systems, which are the ATA, a more pattern based system and ACR TI-RADS, a point-based system will be highlighted (Figure 9.3).

According to the 2015 ATA US risk stratification, thyroid nodules are classified into five categories according to the combination of US features: benign, very low suspicion, low suspicion, intermediate suspicion and high suspicion with increasing estimated ROM, i.e. <1%, <3%, 5%–10%, 10%–20% and >70%–90%, respectively. FNAC is recommended in high- and intermediate-suspicion categories for nodules larger than 1 cm and in low-suspicion categories for nodules >1.5 cm. In very low–suspicion categories, FNAC should be considered for nodules larger than 2.0 cm, whereas it is not recommended for benign nodules. The ACR TI-RADS guidelines were published in 2017. This system assigns points for five US features, including composition, echogenicity, shape, margins, echogenic foci and more suspicious features were awarded additional points. Finally, total points determined the nodule's ACR TI-RADS level (TI-RADS level, TR 1-5). The projected ROM was based on partial analysis of 3433 nodules with cytological results which showed cancer risk levels of no more than 2% for TR1 and TR2 nodules, 5% for TR3 nodules, 5%–20% for TR4 nodules, and at least 20% for TR5 nodules. The ACR TI-RADS is consistent with most other guidelines in recommending FNAC for highly suspicious nodules 1 cm or larger. However, the thresholds for mildly suspicious and moderately suspicious nodules (2.5 and 1.5 cm, respectively) are higher than the cutoffs advocated by the ATA. In addition, the ACR TI-RADS made recommendations to the interval US follow-up for the various TI-RADS categories. The main drawback of ATA system is the existence of a "not specified" pattern with an 18.2%–19.0% malignancy risk (25, 26). Direct comparison between these two guidelines yielded variable results. However, the rate of unnecessary FNAC was lowest with the ACR guidelines (27, 28).

Notably, both central vascularity and elasticity of nodule were not included in both guidelines as suspicious US features. Vascular flow within a thyroid nodule can be detected with color or power Doppler US. The most common pattern of vascularity in thyroid malignancy is marked intranodular hypervascularity, which is defined as flow in the central part of the nodule that is greater than that in the surrounding thyroid tissue. The utility of this feature in identifying thyroid cancer remains controversial (29). The ATA guidelines suggest intranodular vascularity may correlate better with follicular thyroid cancers rather than the more common papillary thyroid cancers (10). Elastography is the measurement of stiffness of the thyroid nodule, on the premise that malignant thyroid nodules are stiffer than benign nodules. The two frequently used elastography techniques are (1) strain elastography that measures the amount of distortion that occurs when the nodule responds to an external pressure (2) shear-wave elastography, uses an acoustic radiation force impulse created by a focused US beam, which allows measurement of the propagation speed of shear waves within the tissue to locally quantify its stiffness in kilopascals or meters per second. Several limitations exist in the employment of this technique, coupled with interobserver variability precludes its widespread adoption (30).

Cytological evaluation

In practice, ATA benign and TIRADS 1 and 2 nodules may be observed; ATA very low to high suspicion and TIRADS 3–5 nodules should undergo FNAC depending on nodule size, with biopsy cutoff points different between the two systems. Thyroid nodules in these categories that do not meet the size criteria for FNAC may be observed with close monitoring or biopsied based on patient preference and risk factors.

US-guided FNAC (US-FNAC) is a valuable and simple approach for the diagnosis of thyroid nodules and has a much higher

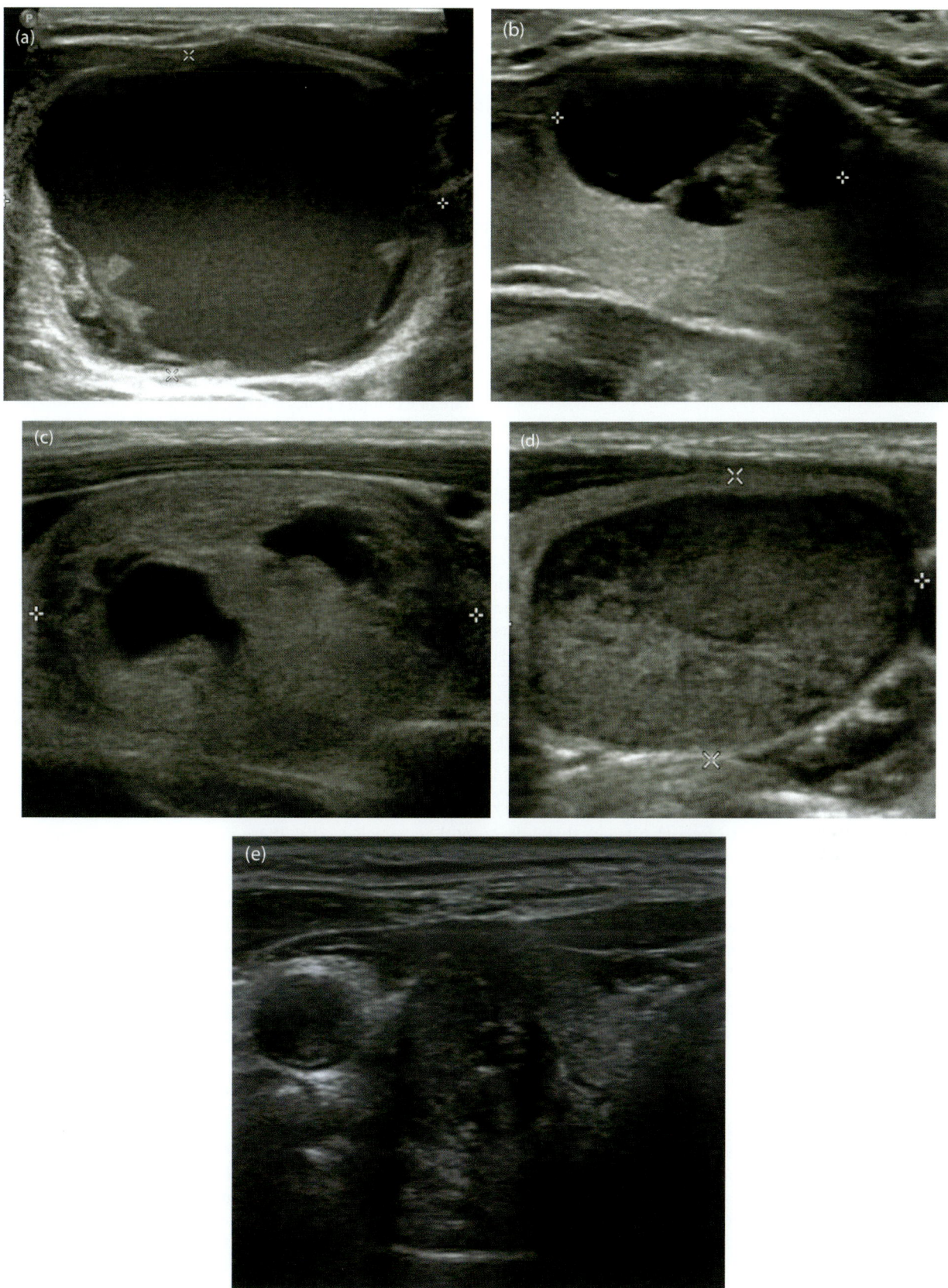

FIGURE 9.3 Sonographic appearance of thyroid nodules. (a) Pure cyst, TIRADS 1 or ATA benign category (b) partially cystic nodule, TIRADS 2 or ATA very low suspicion category (c) solid-cystic nodule, TIRADS 3 or ATA low suspicion nodule (d) solid hypoechoic nodule, TIRADS 4 or ATA intermediate suspicion nodule (histology: follicular thyroid cancer, encapsulated, angioinvasive) (e) solid hypoechoic nodule with microcalcifications, TIRADS 5 or ATA high-suspicion nodule (histology: papillary thyroid cancer).

accuracy compared to conventional palpation-directed biopsy techniques (31). The performance of FNAC under US guidance is essential for non-palpable incidental nodules or have predominantly cystic component. In the author's institution, US-FNAC is performed freehand using a 27-gauge needle with non-aspiration technique. The smears are immediately examined for adequacy and prepared by an on-site cytotechnologist. These are then sent to the pathology laboratory on the same day and interpreted by cytopathologists with experience in thyroid cytology. In the author's experience, the presence of a cytotechnologist on-site examining the specimen has been shown to improve diagnostic adequacy through improved sampling and has largely contributed to a consistent nondiagnostic rate of below 5%. One of the main advantages of on-site assessment is that it allows additional material to be aspirated if the sample is insufficient or if material is needed for ancillary tests. Furthermore, the presence of a trained biomedical scientist enables good-quality preparations to be made.

Currently, several thyroid cytology classification systems exist – e.g. The Bethesda System for Reporting Thyroid Cytopathology (TBSRTC categories) (32), UK Royal College of Pathologists (RCPATH) Guidance on the Reporting of Thyroid Cytology Specimens (Thy 1–5) (33), The Italian reporting system (TIR 1-5) (34), The Australian System for reporting thyroid cytology (RCPA/ASC categories 1–6) (35). By far, TBSRTC has been used in the majority of pathology practices in North America and has been widely accepted in many European and Asian countries. The Bethesda classification system consists of six categories: Bethesda I: nondiagnostic or unsatisfactory; Bethesda II: benign; Bethesda III: atypia of undetermined significance (AUS) or follicular lesion of undetermined significance (FLUS); Bethesda IV: follicular neoplasm (FN) or suspicious of FN (SFN); Bethesda V: suspicious for malignancy; Bethesda VI: malignant. Each category has an implied cancer risk that ranges from 0% to 3% for Bethesda II to virtually 100% for Bethesda VI, as well as recommendations for clinical management. The 2017 revision provides an updated ROM for each category that differs from that in the first edition, due to greater consistency in using TBSRTC, robust published data based on large prospective studies and the recent recategorization of encapsulated follicular variant of papillary carcinoma as noninvasive follicular thyroid neoplasm with papillary-like nuclear features (NIFTP) (36). Most NIFTPs were interpreted cytologically as Bethesda III–V. These tend to follow an indolent course and can be treated conservatively, but accurate diagnosis requires a surgical excision. The 2017 revision considers the impact of NIFTP on the ROM for the various diagnostic categories, and two separate ROM calculations are made, depending on whether or not NIFTP is considered as a "malignancy." Excluding NIFTP from the tally of malignancies in the Bethesda III-V substantially reduces the ROM across these categories – ROM if NIFTP not considered malignant vs ROM if NIFTP considered malignant: Bethesda III: 6%–18% vs 10%–30%; Bethesda IV: 10%–40% vs 25%–40% and Bethesda V: 45%–60% vs 50%–75%.

A satisfactory thyroid FNAC specimen requires at least six groups of 10 benign follicular cells. Reaspiration is generally recommended for Bethesda I (nondiagnostic or unsatisfactory) specimens although several exceptions to this numerical requirement exist. These include specimens with abundant colloid even in the absence of sufficient benign follicular cells, the presence of specific diagnosis such as lymphocytic thyroiditis or specimens with significant atypia, which by definition, the specimen is adequate for evaluation. Correlation with US findings is recommended in specimens which show cyst contents, since the same cytological diagnosis will be interpreted differently in the case of a pure cyst (benign) vs a case where worrisome US features are present. Repeat aspiration will yield diagnostic specimen in 60%–80% of nodules, especially if the cystic component is <50% (37–39). Core needle biopsy has been suggested as an alternative to repeat FNAC for thyroid nodules with previous nondiagnostic results and could reduce the rate of nondiagnostic results or diagnostic surgery in calcified thyroid nodules (40). Surgical excision should be considered in repeatedly nondiagnostic or unsatisfactory specimens, especially if suspicious sonographic features or risk factors for malignancy are present (10).

The Bethesda II (benign) category has a very low ROM and is the most common cytological diagnosis. The false-negative rate of a benign cytological diagnosis is 3.2% based on the largest pooled analysis of 12 studies (41). Current evidence does not suggest larger size is associated with higher false-negative rate (42, 43). Optimal follow-up strategy with thyroid nodules with benign cytology remains debatable. In a prospective, observational study involving 992 consecutive patients with 1–4 asymptomatic, sonographically or cytologically benign thyroid nodules in an attempt to delineate the natural history of such nodules, the authors noted significant nodule growth (defined as increase involving at least 2 nodule dimensions, each amounting to at least 2 mm and representing at least 20% of the baseline diameter) occurred in 15% of cases, new nodules developed in 9.3% of patients, and thyroid cancer was diagnosed in 0.3% of nodules. The indolent and limited growth in majority of these thyroid nodules suggests longer interval reassessment can be considered (44). Similarly, in a retrospective study of 2010 cytologically benign thyroid nodules with average follow-up of 8.5 years, only 18 false-negative malignancies were identified, and no deaths were attributable to thyroid cancer. Hence, the authors conclude that these data support a recommendation for repeat thyroid nodule evaluation 2–4 years after the initial benign FNAC (45). The need for repeat FNAC of thyroid nodules with benign cytology should be guided by suspicious US characteristics rather than nodule growth (46). In asymptomatic patients with thyroid nodules with a repeated benign cytology and no suspicious clinical or US features, routine follow-up may not be necessary (24). However, large thyroid nodules may require monitoring for potential development of compressive symptoms.

Molecular testing

The indeterminate category based on TBSRTC criteria includes AUS/FLUS, SFN/FN and suspicious for malignancy cytological diagnoses (Bethesda III–V). Before the advent of molecular diagnostics, repeat FNAC was recommended for Bethesda III and diagnostic lobectomy was recommended for Bethesda IV nodules. Molecular testing is increasingly utilized in these cytology results to guide recommendations for initial surgery. The ATA guidelines has described an ideal "rule-in" test would have a positive predictive value (PPV) for histopathologically proven malignancy similar to a malignant cytologic diagnosis (98.6%), and an ideal "rule-out" test would have a negative predictive value (NPV) similar to a benign cytologic diagnosis (96.3%) (10).

However, it should be noted that application and interpretation of molecular testing result is dependent on the prevalence of malignancy in the cytology category in the institution, since the prevalence will impact on the positive and negative predictive value of the molecular test. In addition, molecular testing is likely not required if the pretest probability of thyroid cancer is high, such as presence of strong risk factors for thyroid cancer (e.g. previous head and neck radiation), highly suspicious US features or Bethesda V cytology (47).

The Afirma gene expression classifier (GEC) examines the expression of 167 genes associated with thyroid cancer, and the results are reported as GEC-suspicious or GEC-benign. The initial multicenter clinical validation study investigated 4812 cytological specimens, including 12% with indeterminate cytology results. Subsequent analysis of 265 specimens showed that Bethesda III and IV nodules reported as GEC-benign result have an NPV of 95%, which essentially supports the GEC as a rule-out test (48). Hence, Bethesda III/IV nodules with GEC-benign results can be monitored without surgical intervention. Several studies have demonstrated site-to-site variability in PPV in the GEC-suspicious nodules (16%–57%), corresponding to differences in prevalence of malignancy (48–51). The low specificity of GEC-suspicious results suggests diagnostic lobectomy will still be necessary for this result (52). Recently, the GEC test was migrated from a microarray mRNA expression platform to next-generation RNA sequencing (NGS) platform that utilizes NGS and machine learning algorithms. The test incorporates measurement of RNA transcriptome expression and sequencing of nuclear and mitochondrial RNAs and genomic copy number analysis, including loss of heterozygosity (53). The purpose of the gene sequencing classifier (GSC) is to maintain high original sensitivity while increasing its specificity. A blinded clinical validation study that examines the same cohort as the GEC validation study assessed GSC performance in 191 Bethesda III/IV thyroid nodules from 49 sites. The test performance was as follows: sensitivity 93%, specificity 71%, PPV 51% and NPV 97% for Bethesda III nodules; sensitivity 88%, specificity 64%, PPV 42% and NPV 95% for Bethesda IV nodules. The overall cancer prevalence in this study for Bethesda III/IV nodules was 24%. Subsequent studies demonstrated significantly higher specificity and PPV, with maintenance of high NPV and sensitivity, and reduction in surgical intervention (up to 68%) when comparing GSC with GEC (54, 55). Another major change from GEC to GSC was the incorporation of an algorithm for nodules with Hürthle cell changes, with recent studies showing improvement in specificity among Hürthle cell neoplasms with the use of GSC compared to GEC, translating to fewer unnecessary diagnostic lobectomy (55–57).

The Thyroid Sequencing test (ThyroSeq) is based on the detection of thyroid cancer–associated molecular alterations in cell DNA and RNA. The earliest version was introduced into routine clinical practice in 2007 as a seven-gene panel composed of a panel of mutations (BRAF, N-/H-/K-RAS) as well as the translocations RET/PTC and PAX8/PPAR (ThyroSeq v0). The next versions of the test migrated to the NGS platforms and included a 13-gene panel that was launched in 2013 (ThyroSeq v1) and a 56-gene panel to include several point mutations and gene fusions was launched in 2014 (ThyroSeq v2). In the largest independent postvalidation study consisted of 190 Bethesda III/IV thyroid nodules, including 102 nodules with surgical histology, the ThyroSeq v2 test performance was as follows: sensitivity 70%, specificity 77%, PPV 42% and NPV 91%, with cancer/NIFTP prevalence of 20% in this study. Notably, the authors found that the test performs better for Bethesda IV than III nodules, achieving NPV of 94% in this subset of indeterminate cytology, which may be high enough to consider observation instead of surgery (58). The ThyroSeq v3 Genomic Classifier was released for clinical use in 2017 and includes more than 12,000 mutation hotspots and more than 120 gene fusion types, which aims to achieving both high sensitivity and specificity in detecting all types of thyroid cancers and providing detailed genomic information of the nodule sampled by FNAC. In a prospective blinded multicenter study by Steward et al., ThyroSeq v3 demonstrated sensitivity 91%, specificity 85%, PPV 64% and NPV 97% in Bethesda III nodules (cancer/NIFTP prevalence 23%) and sensitivity 97%, specificity 75%, PPV 68% and NPV 98% in Bethesda IV nodules (cancer/NIFTP prevalence 35%). These findings indicate the test is more sensitive but less specific than earlier versions. The authors conclude the high sensitivity/NPV and reasonably high specificity/PPV may obviate surgery in up to 61% of patients with Bethesda III/IV nodules (59).

ThyGenX is a targeted NGS test that assays for a small number of mutations in five genes (BRAF, KRAS, HRAS, NRAS and PIK3CA) and three gene fusions (RET-PTC1, RET-PTC3 and PAX8-PPARG) associated with thyroid cancers. ThyraMIR measures the expression levels of 10 microRNAs (miRNAs) by quantitative real-time polymerase chain reaction and uses a proprietary algorithm to classify each nodule as having either a high- or low-risk miRNA profile. ThyraMIR is an additional reflex test for cases where ThyGenX is negative for genetic alterations or if a mutation with a lower specificity for malignancy is detected. The clinical validation study included 109 Bethesda III/IV nodules from 12 endocrinology centers and compared qualitative molecular results with surgical histopathology. The combined algorithm showed sensitivity 89%, specificity 85%, PPV 74% and NPV 94% (cancer prevalence 32%). The authors conclude that independent of cancer prevalence, the test decreased the rate of avoidable surgeries by 69% (60).

The introduction of the term NIFTP made a significant impact on thyroid cytology on the ROM of the different diagnostic categories in TBSRTC, particularly in the indeterminate subsets. NIFTP is considered a premalignant tumor and its diagnosis primarily relies on histologic examination of the capsule. In general, molecular tests in these cases will likely prompt diagnostic lobectomy (61).

Conclusion

Thorough history and physical examination with identification of potential clinical "red flags" remains an integral part of the approach to thyroid nodules. Subsequent thyroid function evaluation and US risk stratification are pivotal in the evaluation of thyroid nodules as they provide essential information on autonomous nodules and presence of suspicious US features. Fine-needle aspiration biopsy, especially under US guidance in selected nodules provides a simple, reliable and accurate tool for diagnosing thyroid cancers. The field of molecular testing in thyroid nodules is evolving rapidly with much progress made in the recent years. However, each test has different advantages and limitations in the evaluation of indeterminate thyroid FNAC result. In addition, they may not be available in many countries and in resource-limited settings. In such circumstances, a pragmatic approach to indeterminate cytological results based on clinical risk factors and US pattern risk stratifications is prudent (62, 63).

References

1. Vander JB, Gaston EA, Dawber TR. The significance of nontoxic thyroid nodules. Final report of a 15-year study of the incidence of thyroid malignancy. Ann Intern Med. 1968;69(3):537–40.
2. Tunbridge WM, Evered DC, Hall R, Appleton D, Brewis M, Clark F, et al. The spectrum of thyroid disease in a community: the Whickham survey. Clin Endocrinol (Oxf). 1977;7(6):481–93.
3. Tan GH, Gharib H. Thyroid incidentalomas: management approaches to nonpalpable nodules discovered incidentally on thyroid imaging. Ann Intern Med. 1997;126(3):226–31.
4. Guth S, Theune U, Aberle J, Galach A, Bamberger CM. Very high prevalence of thyroid nodules detected by high frequency (13 MHz) ultrasound examination. Eur J Clin Invest. 2009;39(8):699–706.
5. Brito JP, Yarur AJ, Prokop LJ, McIver B, Murad MH, Montori VM. Prevalence of thyroid cancer in multinodular goiter versus single nodule: a systematic review and meta-analysis. Thyroid. 2013;23(4):449–55.
6. Brito JP, Morris JC, Montori VM. Thyroid cancer: zealous imaging has increased detection and treatment of low risk tumours. BMJ. 2013;347:f4706.
7. Sharma SD, Jacques T, Smith S, Watters G. Diagnosis of incidental thyroid nodules on 18F-fluorodeoxyglucose positron emission tomography imaging: are these significant? J Laryngol Otol. 2015;129(1):53–6.
8. Czepczyński R. Nuclear medicine in the diagnosis of benign thyroid diseases. Nucl Med Rev Cent East Eur. 2012;15(2):113–9.
9. Bomeli SR, LeBeau SO, Ferris RL. Evaluation of a thyroid nodule. Otolaryngol Clin North Am. 2010;43(2):229–38, vii.
10. Haugen BR, Alexander EK, Bible KC, Doherty GM, Mandel SJ, Nikiforov YE, et al. 2015 American Thyroid Association management guidelines for adult patients with thyroid nodules and differentiated thyroid cancer: the American Thyroid Association Guidelines Task Force on thyroid nodules and differentiated thyroid cancer. Thyroid. 2016;26(1):1–133.
11. Costante G, Durante C, Francis Z, Schlumberger M, Filetti S. Determination of calcitonin levels in C-cell disease: clinical interest and potential pitfalls. Nat Clin Pract Endocrinol Metab. 2009;5(1):35–44.
12. Hoang JK, Lee WK, Lee M, Johnson D, Farrell S. US features of thyroid malignancy: pearls and pitfalls. Radiographics. 2007;27(3):847–60; discussion 861–5.
13. Chng CL, Tan HC, Too CW, Lim WY, Chiam PPS, Zhu L, et al. Diagnostic performance of ATA, BTA and TIRADS sonographic patterns in the prediction of malignancy in histologically proven thyroid nodules. Singapore Med J. 2018;59(11):578–83.
14. Brito JP, Gionfriddo MR, Al Nofal A, Boehmer KR, Leppin AL, Reading C, et al. The accuracy of thyroid nodule ultrasound to predict thyroid cancer: systematic review and meta-analysis. J Clin Endocrinol Metab. 2014;99(4):1253–63.
15. Campanella P, Ianni F, Rota CA, Corsello SM, Pontecorvi A. Quantification of cancer risk of each clinical and ultrasonographic suspicious feature of thyroid nodules: a systematic review and meta-analysis. Eur J Endocrinol. 2014;170(5):R203–11.
16. Remonti LR, Kramer CK, Leitão CB, Pinto LCF, Gross JL. Thyroid ultrasound features and risk of carcinoma: a systematic review and meta-analysis of observational studies. Thyroid. 2015;25(5):538–50.
17. Choi SH, Kim E-K, Kwak JY, Kim MJ, Son EJ. Interobserver and intraobserver variations in ultrasound assessment of thyroid nodules. Thyroid. 2010;20(2):167–72.
18. Reading CC, Charboneau JW, Hay ID, Sebo TJ. Sonography of thyroid nodules: a 'classic pattern' diagnostic approach. Ultrasound Q. 2005;21(3):157–65.
19. Horvath E, Majlis S, Rossi R, Franco C, Niedmann JP, Castro A, et al. An ultrasonogram reporting system for thyroid nodules stratifying cancer risk for clinical management. J Clin Endocrinol Metab. 2009;94(5):1748–51.
20. Russ G, Royer B, Bigorgne C, Rouxel A, Bienvenu-Perrard M, Leenhardt L. Prospective evaluation of thyroid imaging reporting and data system on 4550 nodules with and without elastography. Eur J Endocrinol. 2013;168(5):649–55.
21. Na DG, Baek JH, Sung JY, Kim J-H, Kim JK, Choi YJ, et al. Thyroid imaging reporting and data system risk stratification of thyroid nodules: categorization based on solidity and echogenicity. Thyroid. 2016;26(4):562–72.
22. Tessler FN, Middleton WD, Grant EG, Hoang JK, Berland LL, Teefey SA, et al. ACR Thyroid Imaging, Reporting and Data System (TI-RADS): white paper of the ACR TI-RADS Committee. J Am Coll Radiol. 2017;14(5):587–95.
23. Russ G, Bonnema SJ, Erdogan MF, Durante C, Ngu R, Leenhardt L. European Thyroid Association guidelines for ultrasound malignancy risk stratification of thyroid nodules in adults: the EU-TIRADS. Eur Thyroid J. 2017;6(5):225–37.
24. Gharib H, Papini E, Garber JR, Duick DS, Harrell RM, Hegedüs L, et al. American Association of Clinical Endocrinologists, American College of Endocrinology, and Associazione Medici Endocrinologi Medical Guidelines for clinical practice for the diagnosis and management of thyroid nodules – 2016 update. Endocr Pract. 2016;22(5):622–39.
25. Yoon JH, Lee HS, Kim E-K, Moon HJ, Kwak JY. Malignancy risk stratification of thyroid nodules: comparison between the thyroid imaging reporting and data system and the 2014 American Thyroid Association Management Guidelines. Radiology. 2016;278(3):917–24.
26. Ha EJ, Na DG, Baek JH, Sung JY, Kim J-H, Kang SY. US fine-needle aspiration biopsy for thyroid malignancy: diagnostic performance of seven society guidelines applied to 2000 thyroid nodules. Radiology. 2018;287(3):893–900.
27. Grani G, Lamartina L, Ascoli V, Bosco D, Biffoni M, Giacomelli L, et al. Reducing the number of unnecessary thyroid biopsies while improving diagnostic accuracy: toward the 'right' TIRADS. J Clin Endocrinol Metab. 2019;104(1):95–102.
28. Wu X-L, Du J-R, Wang H, Jin C-X, Sui G-Q, Yang D-Y, et al. Comparison and preliminary discussion of the reasons for the differences in diagnostic performance and unnecessary FNA biopsies between the ACR TIRADS and 2015 ATA guidelines. Endocrine. 2019;65(1):121–31.
29. Moon HJ, Kwak JY, Kim MJ, Son EJ, Kim E-K. Can vascularity at power Doppler US help predict thyroid malignancy? Radiology. 2010;255(1):260–9.
30. Azizi G, Malchoff CD. Ultrasound elastography of thyroid nodules. In: Duick DS, Levine RA, Lupo MA, editors. Thyroid and parathyroid ultrasound and utrasound-guided FNA. Cham: Springer International Publishing. [Internet]. 2018. pp. 489–516. Available from: https://doi.org/10.1007/978-3-319-67238-0_16.
31. Koike E, Yamashita H, Noguchi S, Murakami T, Ohshima A, Maruta J, et al. Effect of combining ultrasonography and ultrasound-guided fine-needle aspiration biopsy findings for the diagnosis of thyroid nodules. Eur J Surg. 2001;167(9):656–61.
32. Cibas ES, Ali SZ. The 2017 Bethesda system for reporting thyroid cytopathology. Thyroid. 2017;27(11):1341–6.
33. Cross P, Chandra A, Giles T, Johnson S, Kocjan G, Poller D, et al. Guidance on the reporting of thyroid cytology specimens. 2nd ed. London: Royal College of Pathologists. [Internet]. 2016 [Cited October 23, 2019]. Available from: www.rcpath.org/uploads/assets/7d693ce4-0091-4621-97f79e2a0d1034d6/g089_guidancereportingthyroidcytology_jan16.pdf.
34. Fadda G, Straccia P. The Italian reporting system for thyroid cytology. In: Kakudo K, editor. Thyroid FNA cytology: differential diagnoses and pitfalls. Singapore: Springer Singapore. [Internet]. 2019. pp. 53–7. Available from: https://doi.org/10.1007/978-981-13-1897-9_6.
35. Kumarasinghe P. Australian system for reporting thyroid cytology. In: Kakudo K, editor. Thyroid FNA cytology: differential diagnoses and pitfalls. Singapore: Springer Singapore. [Internet]. 2019. pp. 69–76. Available from: https://doi.org/10.1007/978-981-13-1897-9_8.
36. Nikiforov YE, Seethala RR, Tallini G, Baloch ZW, Basolo F, Thompson LDR, et al. Nomenclature revision for encapsulated follicular variant of papillary thyroid carcinoma: a paradigm shift to reduce overtreatment of indolent tumors. JAMA Oncol. 2016;2(8):1023–9.
37. Alexander EK, Heering JP, Benson CB, Frates MC, Doubilet PM, Cibas ES, et al. Assessment of nondiagnostic ultrasound-guided fine needle aspirations of thyroid nodules. J Clin Endocrinol Metab. 2002;87(11):4924–7.
38. Orija IB, Piñeyro M, Biscotti C, Reddy SSK, Hamrahian AH. Value of repeating a nondiagnostic thyroid fine-needle aspiration biopsy. Endocr Pract. 2007;13(7):735–42.
39. Choi YS, Hong SW, Kwak JY, Moon HJ, Kim E-K. Clinical and ultrasonographic findings affecting nondiagnostic results on the second fine needle aspiration for thyroid nodules. Ann Surg Oncol. 2012;19(7):2304–9.
40. Na DG, Baek JH, Jung SL, Kim J-H, Sung JY, Kim KS, et al. Core needle biopsy of the thyroid: 2016 consensus statement and recommendations from Korean Society of Thyroid Radiology. Korean J Radiol. 2017;18(1):217–37.
41. Tee YY, Lowe AJ, Brand CA, Judson RT. Fine-needle aspiration may miss a third of all malignancy in palpable thyroid nodules: a comprehensive literature review. Ann Surg. 2007;246(5):714–20.
42. Porterfield JR, Grant CS, Dean DS, Thompson GB, Farley DR, Richards ML, et al. Reliability of benign fine needle aspiration cytology of large thyroid nodules. Surgery. 2008;144(6):963–8; discussion 968–9.
43. Yoon JH, Kwak JY, Moon HJ, Kim MJ, Kim E-K. The diagnostic accuracy of ultrasound-guided fine-needle aspiration biopsy and the sonographic differences between benign and malignant thyroid nodules 3 cm or larger. Thyroid. 2011;21(9):993–1000.
44. Durante C, Costante G, Lucisano G, Bruno R, Meringolo D, Paciaroni A, et al. The natural history of benign thyroid nodules. JAMA. 2015;313(9):926–35.
45. Nou E, Kwong N, Alexander LK, Cibas ES, Marqusee E, Alexander EK. Determination of the optimal time interval for repeat evaluation after a benign thyroid nodule aspiration. J Clin Endocrinol Metab. 2014;99(2):510–6.
46. Rosário PW, Calsolari MR. What is the best criterion for repetition of fine-needle aspiration in thyroid nodules with initially benign cytology? Thyroid. 2015;25(10):1115–20.
47. Mayson SE, Haugen BR. Molecular diagnostic evaluation of thyroid nodules. Endocrinol Metab Clin North Am. 2019;48(1):85–97.
48. Alexander EK, Kennedy GC, Baloch ZW, Cibas ES, Chudova D, Diggans J, et al. Preoperative diagnosis of benign thyroid nodules with indeterminate cytology. N Engl J Med. 2012;367(8):705–15.
49. Alexander EK, Schorr M, Klopper J, Kim C, Sipos J, Nabhan F, et al. Multicenter clinical experience with the Afirma gene expression classifier. J Clin Endocrinol Metab. 2014;99(1):119–25.
50. Harrell RM, Bimston DN. Surgical utility of Afirma: effects of high cancer prevalence and oncocytic cell types in patients with indeterminate thyroid cytology. Endocr Pract. 2014;20(4):364–9.
51. McIver B, Castro MR, Morris JC, Bernet V, Smallridge R, Henry M, et al. An independent study of a gene expression classifier (Afirma) in the evaluation of cytologically indeterminate thyroid nodules. J Clin Endocrinol Metab. 2014;99(11):4069–77.
52. Wang TS, Sosa JA. Thyroid surgery for differentiated thyroid cancer – recent advances and future directions. Nat Rev Endocrinol. 2018;14(11):670–83.
53. Patel KN, Angell TE, Babiarz J, Barth NM, Blevins T, Duh Q-Y, et al. Performance of a genomic sequencing classifier for the preoperative diagnosis of cytologically indeterminate thyroid nodules. JAMA Surg. 2018;153(9):817–24.

54. Endo M, Nabhan F, Porter K, Roll K, Shirley LA, Azaryan I, et al. Afirma gene sequencing classifier compared with gene expression classifier in indeterminate thyroid nodules. Thyroid. 2019;29(8):1115–24.
55. San Martin VT, Lawrence L, Bena J, Madhun NZ, Berber E, Elsheikh TM, et al. Real world comparison of Afirma GEC and GSC for the assessment of cytologically indeterminate thyroid nodules. J Clin Endocrinol Metab. 2020;105(3):e428–35.
56. Angell TE, Heller HT, Cibas ES, Barletta JA, Kim MI, Krane JF, et al. Independent comparison of the Afirma genomic sequencing classifier and gene expression classifier for cytologically indeterminate thyroid nodules. Thyroid. 2019;29(5):650–6.
57. Hao Y, Duh Q-Y, Kloos RT, Babiarz J, Harrell RM, Traweek ST, et al. Identification of Hürthle cell cancers: solving a clinical challenge with genomic sequencing and a trio of machine learning algorithms. BMC Syst Biol. 2019;13(Suppl 2):27.
58. Valderrabano P, Khazai L, Leon ME, Thompson ZJ, Ma Z, Chung CH, et al. Evaluation of ThyroSeq v2 performance in thyroid nodules with indeterminate cytology. Endocr Relat Cancer. 2017;24(3):127–36.
59. Steward DL, Carty SE, Sippel RS, Yang SP, Sosa JA, Sipos JA, et al. Performance of a multigene genomic classifier in thyroid nodules with indeterminate cytology: a prospective blinded multicenter study. JAMA Oncol. 2019;5(2):204–12.
60. Labourier E, Shifrin A, Busseniers AE, Lupo MA, Manganelli ML, Andruss B, et al. Molecular testing for miRNA, mRNA, and DNA on fine-needle aspiration improves the preoperative diagnosis of thyroid nodules with indeterminate cytology. J Clin Endocrinol Metab. 2015;100(7):2743–50.
61. Nishino M, Nikiforova M. Update on molecular testing for cytologically indeterminate thyroid nodules. Arch Pathol Lab Med. 2018;142(4):446–57.
62. Barbosa TLM, Junior COM, Graf H, Cavalvanti T, Trippia MA, da Silveira Ugino RT, et al. ACR TI-RADS and ATA US scores are helpful for the management of thyroid nodules with indeterminate cytology. BMC Endocr Disord. 2019;19(1):112.
63. Seshadri KG. A pragmatic approach to the indeterminate thyroid nodule. Indian J Endocrinol Metab. 2017;21(5):751–7.

10

NONSURGICAL MANAGEMENT OF THYROID NODULES

Anand Kumar Mishra

Introduction

Palpable thyroid nodule disease is present in 1% men and 5% women in iodine-sufficient regions and autopsy data suggest 50% prevalence of nodules in clinical normal thyroid gland (1–3). Moderate-to-severe iodine deficiency has contributed to this high prevalence of thyroid nodules in the past. High-resolution ultrasound (US) (HRUS) can detect thyroid nodules in 19–67% of population in a random selection with higher frequencies in elderly people and females (4). Most of these nodules are benign, and thyroid cancer has been detected in 5–15% of nodules depending upon age, sex, radiation exposure, family history and other factors (5, 6). All nodules should undergo fine needle aspiration cytology (FNAC) with sufficient diagnostic value (at least six groups of follicular cells with 10–15 cells each). Autonomously functioning nodules do not require a FNAC. American Thyroid Association recommends FNAC in all nodules more than 1.5-cm size with benign features and 1 cm with suspicious features. Treatment of nodules is dependent upon the result of triple test (thyroid stimulating hormone [TSH], HRUS and FNAC). There is no indication of therapeutic intervention in sonographically detected asymptomatic, biochemically euthyroid nodules without suspicious features and patients who don't have high-risk history (history of radiation to head, neck in childhood) or family history of thyroid cancer. In these patients, only watchful waiting may be sufficient (7). Surgery is the standard treatment for nodules with symptomatic, suspicious or proven malignancy and cosmetic concern. Radioiodine treatment is applied for autonomously functioning nodules. Percutaneous ethanol injection was first used for the treatment of autonomous thyroid nodules by an Italian group in 1990 (7). In the following three decades, other nonsurgical and non-radioiodine ablative methods for thyroid nodules treatment have developed: radiofrequency (RF) ablation (RFA), percutaneous microwave ablation (PMWA), laser thermal ablation (LTA) and high-frequency US ablation (HFUA). Prerequisites for these nonsurgical techniques are that one should confirm the benign nature of the nodule at least twice by separate US-guided FNAC (8).

Clinical and diagnostic evaluation of thyroid nodules

Important components on history that need to be considered when evaluating thyroid nodules are sex of the patient, age, onset and duration of thyroid nodule, rate of nodular growth, any recent symptoms suggestive of dysphagia, dyspnea, cough, hoarseness, dysphonia, history of external neck irradiation during childhood and a family history of benign or malignant thyroid disease. Important signs on physical examination are consistency, motility of thyroid nodules and the presence of palpable neck lymph nodes. All patients with thyroid nodules should be subjected to triple investigation to know the function, morphology and nature of the nodule, viz., TSH, free T4 (first line), HRUS and FNAC, preferably guided. There should be very clear goals when a nodule management is being planned. One is that a nodule that is malignant or at risk of developing cancer should be treated. All symptomatic nodules or at risk of producing symptoms should be treated. Surgery is the standard treatment of all symptomatic nodules, nodules with compressive symptoms, nodules with suspicion or proven malignancy and with cosmetic concern. Benign nodules that have a retrosternal extension or large size also need surgery.

Natural history of benign thyroid nodules

Current knowledge regarding the natural history of benign thyroid nodules is limited as there is very little data available. An untreated thyroid nodule is expected to grow, and new nodules might appear if it is not treated. Data from following clinical studies indicate that most benign nodules grow but very slowly over time.

1. During a follow-up of 15 years, only 14% of benign nodules (n = 140) displayed any growth at all (9).
2. During mean follow-up of 3 years, volume increases of 30% or more in almost 50% benign nodules (n = 139) were seen (10).
3. During mean follow up of 20 months, a 15% volume increase was documented in 39% of benign nodules (11).
4. In women, nodules often stop growing after the onset of menopause (12).

During follow-up, if a nodule is enlarging, it is more likely that it has developed malignant transformation than those that shrink or remain stable in size (12).

Nonsurgical management

Surveillance alone
Benign euthyroid and asymptomatic small thyroid nodule without high-risk history or imaging features do not require any treatment and can be followed up periodically. But this approach can be followed only after discussion with a compliant patient. Triple evaluation should be carried out when there is significant nodule growth (20% increase diameter) or at 6- to 12-months interval or at longer intervals. Rapid growth of nodule is a relative indication for immediate surgery, even if FNAC does not suggest malignancy.

Iodine supplementation
Individual iodine supplementation does not shrink thyroid nodules or prevent further growth (13–14). Iodine supplementation may be used for volume control of endemic goiters. Rarely, it can cause iodine-induced thyrotoxicosis in long-standing goiters especially in elderly patients (15).

Thyroid hormone suppressive therapy
Current knowledge regarding the impact of thyroid hormone suppressive therapy for solitary nodules is conflicting. It is expected that levothyroxine will suppress thyrocyte growth by preventing

TSH growth-promoting effect on thyroid cells shrinks thyroid nodules and prevents the appearance of new nodules. However, there are many questions that need to be considered before deciding the suppressive therapy:

1. There are many other factors like insulin-like growth factors, and growth factors besides TSH that can cause nodule growth (16).
2. TSH interferes with oncogenesis in nodular thyroid tissue (17).
3. What should be the target levels of TSH suppression and treatment duration? The degree of TSH suppression required to produce the therapeutic effect is not defined clearly in the studies and it varies in different studies.
4. Long-term thyroid-hormone-suppressive therapy induces a state of subclinical hyperthyroidism (18–19). Possible adverse effects are unpleasant symptoms and higher morbidity of cardiovascular system (elevated heart rate; supraventricular arrhythmias, particularly atrial fibrillation, increased left ventricular mass; increased cardiac contractility; and impaired diastolic function). It also causes significant bone mineral density loss in postmenopausal women (20, 21). Elderly patient can have higher mortality from cardiovascular events (22) and as nodules in this age are characterized by slow growth, so TSH suppressive therapy should not be used.
5. There is always a question of how to assess dimensions of nodule (palpation versus ultrasonography) and degree of volume reduction to define therapeutic efficacy.
6. Long-term administration of levothyroxine is needed as nodules rapidly return to their pretreatment size or show regrowth after stoppage of therapy.

Literature suggest that a subset of benign thyroid nodules do respond to thyroid-hormone-suppressive therapy (34), but markers for this subset are not yet identified:

1. Levothyroxine therapy is effective in solid nodules, however cystic nodules do not show effect (23–25).
2. In iodine-sufficient regions, 17–25% of patients with a solitary (or dominant) thyroid nodule will have a modest decrease in nodule size (>50%) as a result of TSH suppression therapy.
3. Other nodule characteristics associated with responsiveness are recent diagnosis, relatively small volumes (<10, <2.5 or <1.5 ml), have an abundance of colloid in FNAC, and the absence of hyperplastic or fibrotic changes (12, 26-27).

In selected patients (iodine-deficient, younger patients with growing diffuse or nodular goiter who are concerned about growth of their goiter), a trial of levothyroxine therapy with the aim of TSH suppression or low-normal TSH can be tried but it will be not useful if the TSH is already subnormal. However, routine TSH suppressive therapy is not recommended for benign thyroid nodules (28).

Percutaneous ethanol ablation

The percutaneous US-guided ethanol injection (PEI) of strength 95–99% has been used as an alternative for surgery to treat thyroid nodules. In this technique, ethanol is injected inside the nodule under HRUS guidance. Ethanol causes cellular dehydration, thrombosis of small vessels, protein denaturation, cellular coagulation necrosis and subsequent reactive tissue fibrosis inside nodule (29-32), leading to shrinkage of nodule over time. The best results are obtained in symptomatic recurrent cystic thyroid nodules, predominantly cystic nodules and autonomously functioning nodules. PEI is less effective in nodules that have a solid component > 50%. Adverse effects associated with this procedure are pain, ethanol seepage outside the nodule, transient hyperthyroidism, recurrent nerve damage (transient or permanent), permanent ipsilateral facial dysesthesia and paranodular fibrosis, which may need surgery.

Technique
A 12- to 21-ga needle is inserted through the isthmus of the gland, and the needle tip is placed into the center of the nodule. Initially, all fluid is aspirated, and if it is thick, a larger needle can be used for this purpose. After aspiration, normal saline irrigation is done to remove colloid attached with the cyst wall. Sterile ethanol of 95–99% strength is injected inside the nodule, and the volume injected is more than 50% of the fluid aspirated initially. After 2 minutes, injected ethanol is aspirated completely and needle removed.

Effectiveness
In cystic nodules, mean volume reduction is 85–98.5% (29-37). In predominantly cystic nodules, which have a solid component between 10 and 50%, mean volume reduction is 64–73%, but there is more recurrence (32, 33). Main reason of recurrence after PEI has been the solid component with increased vascularity. Long-term cure in the treatment of toxic nodules could be achieved in only 70% of the cases (34).

Thermal ablation techniques

There are mainly four thermal techniques that are used for the treatment of thyroid nodules:

- Radiofrequency ablation
- Microwave ablation
- Laser ablation
- High-frequency ultrasound ablation

Radiofrequency ablation (RFA)

In this technique, RF current is delivered through a probe inside the nodule, which causes thermal tissue necrosis. RFA uses an alternating electric current with frequencies usually below 900 kHz generated by an RF generator. Just like electric cautery, there are monopolar and bipolar RF electrode. When using monopolar RF electrode, grounding pads are required. Bipolar probes are safer in patients with implanted electrical devices such as pacemakers. There are also cooled probes, which cause less skin burning and destruction of tissue by shaft of the probe. RF current causes generation of microbubbles in the tissue, which produce an additional mechanical damaging effect. Conducted heat leads to slow-growing temperatures in more remote tissue. These mechanisms are responsible for most of the therapeutic effect of RFA.

The adverse effects of RFA are brachial plexus damage, nodule rupture, change in thyroid function (mostly transient), bleeding, subsequent hematoma, cough, vomiting, vago-vagal reaction, skin burns and infection. Patient usually complains of pain at local site, which resolves after some time, and can be treated with analgesics, if necessary.

Procedure

There are two methods of electrode placement – fixed electrode technique and moving shot technique. For thyroid nodules, moving shot technique is safe and effective. For moving shot technique, straight-type internally cooled electrode (monopolar) is best. The procedure is performed under local anesthesia and under HRUS guidance. Electrode is placed through isthmus as it travels through sufficient thyroid parenchyma, which prevents change in the electrode position when patients are swallowing or talking and also prevents the leakage of ablated hot fluid outside the thyroid gland. The tip is initially placed in the deepest and most remote portion of nodule and gradually is pulled back to superficial portion as procedure ablation starts. The ablation produced by the RF current is visible as transient hyperechoic zones on HRUS. RF power and size of active tip depend upon target nodule size and its internal characteristics. Procedure is started with 30–50 W of RF power and a 1-cm active tip. If a transient hyperechoic zone does not appear within 5–10 seconds, power is increased by 10-W increments, to a maximum of 120 W. The procedure is finished when entire nodules have become transient hyperechoic zones (38).

Effectiveness

The volume reduction of nodule depends upon (35–37, 39-40):

- Number of treatment sessions
- Proportion of the solid nodule component
- Size of initial nodule
- Follow-up period duration

Volume reduction ratio of 90–92% in cystic (solid component <10%), 85–89% in predominantly cystic (solid component 10–50%) and 84–87% in solid (solid > 50%) nodules has been reported. In nodules, which are predominantly cystic, a combination of initial percutaneous ethanol ablation (PEA) and RFA can be used for best output. The moving shot technique of thyroid RFA has low complication rate, and is also effective for hypervascular nodules.

Laser thermal ablation (LTA)

LTA has been used for years in palliative care of advanced cancers. In last decade, it has been used in the treatment of thyroid nodules. The procedure is performed under HRUS guidance in which laser light is delivered inside the nodule, which increases temperature up to >60°C in target lesion, causing tissue necrosis visible as hyperechoic zone on HRUS and leads to subsequent fibrosis. Laser light is conducted into the lesion via silical optical fibers. Laser diodes or ND:YAG (neodymium:yttrium aluminum garnet) are the source of energy. Up to four needles are used simultaneously with energy delivered over a time of 5–15 minutes (32). The major disadvantage of LTA technique is that one has to monitor real-time thermal necrosis as echogenic zone on HRUS or Doppler during the procedure and proceed. But hyperechoic zone correlates poorly with area of thermal necrosis on HRUS. So it becomes impossible to identify true boundaries of laser-induced tissue damage during the procedure. Accurate estimate of volume of thermal necrosis can be noticed only a few hours after the procedure. Patients often experience burning cervical pain, which rapidly decreases once energy delivery ceases.

Procedure

A laser fiber is inserted through sheath of a 21-ga needle with 5 mm of bare fiber allowed in direct contact with thyroid tissue and this technique is called as flat-tip technique. One to four such needles with gap of 1 cm between two fibers are placed along cranio-caudal direction of the nodule. Ablation is started at 1.0 cm from the caudal portion of the thyroid nodule. A transient hyperechoic zone appears, gradually increases over time and then coalesces around each fiber. When echogenic zones coalesce, the operator pulls back the fiber in 1.0-cm increments. Additional doses of laser energy are administered at each step until fibers tip is 5 mm away from cranial portion of the nodule. Number of fibers, number of pullbacks and total energy delivered depend upon nodule volume and ellipsoidal shape of nodule (35-37, 41).

Effectiveness

LTA can be used for solid benign nodules that are symptomatic or with cosmetic concern. It is also used for autonomously functioning nodules, not suitable for surgery or radioiodine therapy. RFA seems to be superior to LTA in terms of volume reduction in solid nodules.

High-intensity focused ultrasound (HIFU): High-frequency ultrasound ablation

High-intensity focused US (HIFU) technique is a computer-aided technique of using heat produced by focused US beams for tissue destruction delivered inside body by probes without skin penetration. US beam is focused by means of a curved or phase-array transducer and energy concentration is highly collimated. Multiple impulses are needed to induce an ablation volume of clinical significance. The data received from the imaging device is used to focus the US energy into the target lesion. The temperature reaches up to 85°C in target lesion and produces hyperthermia locally followed by tissue destruction by coagulative necrosis. Heat causes water vaporization and bubbles formation. Development and expansion of multiple bubbles produce mechanical damage to the cell structures. For treatment purposes, nodule is automatically subdivided into multiple ablation units with a size of approximately 5 mm (width) × 7 mm (thickness). After a treatment pulse of 8 seconds, a cooling phase of about 40 seconds is required before the next pulse can be applied. The advantage with this technique is that it is a noninvasive outdoor procedure performed under conscious sedation, and damage to important structures such as trachea, carotid artery and skin can be prevented. The only disadvantage is cost of equipment, availability of expert and requirement of more than one session. The procedure is painful and may require analgesic therapy (42).

Effectiveness

Indication for HIFU may be small symptomatic nodules (<15 ml), benign nodules with cosmetic indication, autonomously functioning nodule not suitable for surgery or patients refuses conventional therapies (surgery, radioiodine therapy and antithyroid drugs).

South Asia perspective

Nonsurgical methods of treatment techniques are not popular in India and only PEA methods have been used at some centers. HIFU is a promising method, and it is popular in other Asian countries. RFA is especially popular in Korea.

Conclusion

In non-palpable benign asymptomatic thyroid nodules, periodic clinical and morphological surveillance seem to be sufficient. Nonsurgical management decisions should always be based on a careful analysis of benefits and risks to the patient. PEA should be used as the first-line option in cystic thyroid nodules, although it has comparable efficacy with RFA and LTA but is preferred being less expensive. In predominantly cystic thyroid nodules, combination therapy of PEA followed by RFA or LTA seems to be more effective and practical. In solid thyroid nodules, PEA is an inappropriate treatment and between RFA and LTA, and RFA seems to have a superior efficacy. HIFU is the latest advance in treatment modality. It has an advantage of being a noninvasive procedure and permits tissue destruction without affecting the surrounding tissue.

References

1. Tunbridge WMG, Evered DC, Hall R, Appleton D, Brewis M, Clark F, Evans JG, Young E, Bird T, Smith PA (1977) The spectrum of thyroid disease in a community: the Whickham Survey. Clin Endocrinol (Oxf) **7**: 481–493.
2. Vander JB, Gaston EA, Dawber TR (1968) The significance of nontoxic thyroid nodules. Ann Intern Med **69**: 537–540.
3. Mortensen JD et al. (1955) Gross and microscopic findings in clinically normal thyroid glands. J Clin Endocrinol Metab **15**: 1270–1280.
4. Tan GH, Gharib H (1997) Thyroid incidentalomas: management approaches to nonpalpable nodules discovered incidentally on thyroid imaging. Ann Intern Med **126**: 226–231.
5. Hegedus L (2004) Clinical practice. The thyroid nodule. N Engl J Med **351**: 1764–1771.
6. Mandel SJ (2004) A 64-year-old woman with a thyroid nodule. JAMA **292**: 2632–2642.
7. Livraghi T, Paracchi A, Ferrari C et al. (1990) Treatment of autonomous thyroid nodules with percutaneous ethanol injection: preliminary results. Work in progress. Radiology **175**: 827–829.
8. Na DG, Lee JH, Jung SL et al. (2012) Radiofrequency ablation of benign thyroid nodules and recurrent thyroid cancers: consensus statement and recommendations. Korean J. Radiol **13**(2), 117–125.
9. Kuma K et al. (1992) Outcome of long standing solitary thyroid nodules. World J Surg **16**: 583–587.
10. Quadbeck B et al. (2002) Long-term follow-up of thyroid nodule growth. Exp Clin Endocrinol Diabetes **110**: 348–354.
11. Alexander EK et al. (2003) Natural history of benign solid and cystic thyroid nodules. Ann Intern Med **138**: 315–318.
12. Costante G et al. (2004) Slow growth of benign thyroid nodules after menopause: no need for long-term thyroxine suppressive therapy in post-menopausal women. J Endocrinol Invest **27**: 31–36.
13. Bennedbæk FN and Hegedüs L (2000) Management of the solitary thyroid nodule: results of a North American survey. J Clin Endocrinol Metab **85**: 2493–2498.
14. Bonnema SJ et al. (2000) Management of the nontoxic multinodular goitre: a European questionnaire study. Clin Endocrinol (Oxf) **53**: 5–12.
15. Azizi F et al. (2005) Reappraisal of the risk of iodineinduced hyperthyroidism: an epidemiological population survey. J Endocrinol Invest **28**: 23–29.
16. Biondi B et al. (2005) Thyroid-hormone therapy and thyroid cancer: a reassessment. Nat Clin Pract Endocrinol Metab **1**: 32–40.
17. Bruno R et al. (2005) Modulation of thyroid-specific gene expression in normal and nodular human thyroid tissues from adults: an in vivo effect of thyrotropin. J Clin Endocrinol Metab **90**: 5692–5697.
18. Surks MI et al. (2004) Subclinical thyroid disease. Scientific review and guidelines for diagnosis and management. JAMA **291**: 228–238.
19. Biondi B et al. (2005) Subclinical hyperthyroidism: clinical features and treatment options. Eur J Endocrinol **152**: 1–9.
20. Uzzan B et al. (1996) Effects on bone mass of longterm treatment with thyroid hormones: a metaanalysis. J Clin Endocrinol Metab **81**: 4278–4289.
21. Faber J and Galloe AM (1994) Changes in bone mass during prolonged subclinical hyperthyroidism due to L-thyroxine treatment: a meta-analysis. Eur J Endocrinol **130**: 350–356.
22. Biondi B et al. (2002) Mortality in elderly patients with subclinical hyperthyroidism. Lancet **359**: 799–800.
23. McCowen K et al. (1980) The role of thyroid therapy in patients with thyroid cysts. Am J Med **68**: 853–855.
24. La Rosa G et al. (1995) Levothyroxine and potassium iodide are both effective in treating benign solitary solid cold nodules of the thyroid. Ann Intern Med **122**: 1–8.
25. Wemeau JL et al. (2002) Effects of thyroid-stimulating hormone suppression with levothyroxine in reducing the volume of solitary thyroid nodules and improving extranodular nonpalpable changes: a randomized, double-blind, placebo-controlled trial by the French Thyroid Research Group. J Clin Endocrinol Metab **87**: 4928–4934.
26. La Rosa G et al. (1996) Cold thyroid nodule reduction with L-thyroxine can be predicted by initial nodule volume and cytological characteristics. J Clin Endocrinol Metab **81**: 4385–4387.
27. Lima N et al. (1997) Levothyroxine suppressive therapy is partially effective in treating patients with benign, solid thyroid nodules and multinodular goiters. Thyroid **7**: 691–697.
28. Haugen BR, Alexander EK, Bible KC, et al. (2016) 2015 American Thyroid Association management guidelines for adult patients with thyroid nodules and differentiated thyroid cancer: the American Thyroid Association guidelines task force on thyroid nodules and differentiated thyroid cancer. Thyroid Jan;**26**(1): 1–133.
29. Monzani F, Lippi F, Goletti O et al. (1994) Percutaneous aspiration and ethanol sclerotherapy for thyroid cysts. J. Clin. Endocrinol. Metabol **78**(3): 800–802.
30. Valcavi R, Frasoldati A (2004) Ultrasound-guided percutaneous ethanol injection therapy in thyroid cystic nodules. Endocr. Pract **10**(3): 269–275.
31. Zieleznik W, Kawczyk-Krupka A, Barlik MP, Cebula W, Sieron A (2005) Modified percutaneous ethanol injection in the treatment of viscous cystic thyroid nodules. Thyroid **15**(7): 683–686.
32. Jang SW, Baek JH, Kim JK et al. (2012) How to manage the patients with unsatisfactory results after ethanol ablation for thyroid nodules: role of radiofrequency ablation. Eur. J. Radiol **81**(5): 905–910.
33. Lee JH, Kim YS, Lee D, Choi H, Yoo H, Baek JH (2010) Radiofrequency ablation (RFA) of benign thyroid nodules in patients with incompletely resolved clinical problems after ethanol ablation (EA). World. J. Surg **34**(7): 1488–1493.
34. Lippi F, Ferrari C, Manetti L et al. (1996) Treatment of solitary autonomous thyroid nodules by percutaneous ethanol injection: results of an Italian multicenter study. The Multicenter Study Group. J Clin Endocrinol Metab **81**: 3261–3264.
35. Ha E J, Baek J H (2014) Advances in nonsurgical treatment of benign thyroid nodules. Future Oncol **10**(8): 1399–1405.
36. Feldkamp J, Grünwald F, Luster M, Lorenz K, Vorländer C, Führer D (2020) Non-Surgical and Non-Radioiodine Techniques for Ablation of Benign Thyroid Nodules: consensus Statement and Recommendation. Exp Clin Endocrinol Diabetes;**128**(101):687–692.
37. Filetti S, Durante C, Torlontano M (2006) Nonsurgical approaches to the management of thyroid nodules. Nat Clin Pract Endocrinol Metab **2**(7): 384–394.
38. Shin JH, Baek JH, Ha EJ, Lee JH (2012) Radiofrequency ablation of thyroid nodules: basic principles and clinical application. Int J Endocrinol **2012**: 919650.
39. Lim HK, Lee JH, Ha EJ, Sung JY, Kim JK, Baek JH (2013) Radiofrequency ablation of benign non-functioning thyroid nodules: 4-year follow-up results for 111 patients. Eur Radiol **23**(4): 1044–1049.
40. Huh JY, Baek JH, Choi H, Kim JK, Lee JH (2012) Symptomatic benign thyroid nodules: efficacy of additional radiofrequency ablation treatment session – prospective randomized study. Radiology **263**(3): 909–916.
41. Baek JH, Lee JH, Valcavi R, Pacella CM, Rhim H, Na DG (2011) Thermal ablation for benign thyroid nodules: radiofrequency and laser. Korean J Radiol **12**(5), 525–540.
42. Lang BHH, Woo YC, Chiu KW (2018) Evaluation of pain during high-intensity focused ultrasound ablation of benign thyroid nodules. Eur Radiol **28**: 2620–2627.

11
MANAGEMENT OF NON-ENDEMIC GOITERS
Anand Kumar Mishra

Introduction

Goiter is chronic enlargement of the thyroid gland caused by various reasons. Morphologically, an enlarged thyroid gland or goiter can be diffuse or nodular. The nodular goiter can be a solitary nodule or multinodular (MNG). Nodules larger than 1 cm may be detected clinically by palpation and clinically found in at least 4% of the general population. Nodules less than 1 cm in diameter cannot be palpated unless they are located on the surface of the gland. All malignant and suspicious nodules on clinical basis, which include history and examination, or investigation should be managed by surgery. Toxic goiters are managed initially medically and later with definitive therapy of surgery or radioiodine therapy. All benign diffuse or multinodular nontoxic goiters that are asymptomatic may be observed and symptomatic patients with compressive symptoms, cosmetic concerns or concern for malignancy should also be managed by surgery. Levothyroxine therapy is controversial and may reduce the volume of goiter up to 50% but regrowth starts rapidly after cessation of therapy. Radioiodine (RAI) therapy alone or in combination of recombinant human thyroid stimulating hormone (TSH) (rhTSH) is another safe and effective option. In all nontoxic diffuse or nodular goiter diagnosis, the treatment goals are:

1. Correction of underlying thyroid dysfunction if present.
2. Exclude cancer in the nodular goiter by investigations.
3. Decide whether benign goiter needs treatment or observation. The benefits and risk of medical or surgical therapy should be discussed with the patient and then individualized treatment should be administered.

Incidence

The incidence of diffuse and nodular goiter depends on many etiological factors and the method of population survey. Routine autopsy surveys (30–50%) and ultrasound (US) screening (16–67%) of population have yielded higher incidence of nodular goiter (1). In iodine-sufficient countries, prevalence of clinical nodularity is approximately 4% (2). Iodine-deficient regions with universal salt iodination program, incidence of nodular goiter and MNG in elderly subjects is approximately 10%, which is attributed to the lack of nutritional iodine in early adult life (3). In iodine-deficient areas, goiter prevalence may be very high.

Etiology

The initial comprehensive theory for development of MNG was proposed by David Marine and Selwyn Taylor (4, 5). Most important etiological factor for goiter formation is iodine. In iodine-deficient areas, TSH causes hyperplasia of follicular cells, so that more iodine can be trapped from circulation. There is a heterogeneous response of chronic and intermittent stimulus by polyclonal follicular cells and ultimately leads to nodule formation. While in iodine-sufficient areas, thyroid follicles are heterogeneous in growth and activity potential in response to genetic, intrinsic and environmental factors, which leads to nodule formation. In summary, chronic low-grade, intermittent environmental and other intrinsic stimulus leads to thyroid hyperplasia initially and later nodular goiter. Some individuals may have genetic predisposition also (Figures 11.1 and 11.2). Goiter can be classified into diffuse and nodular goiter on the basis of morphology. The nodular goiter can be solitary or multinodular. Functionally, goiter can be toxic (hyperthyroid) or nontoxic (hypothyroid or euthyroid).

Natural history

The natural history of thyroid nodules is poorly understood. Minimal diffuse enlargement of thyroid gland in teenage boys and girls is physiological due to the increasing demand of thyroid hormone during this period in response to the complex structural and hormonal changes occurring at this time. It is reversible and usually regresses but may persist more commonly in girls. It may grow further during pregnancy and lead to sporadic nodular goiter. Diffuse or nodular goiter can be asymptomatic or symptomatic for pressure symptoms, such as difficulty in swallowing, choking sensation in neck, dry cough, respiratory distress or just feeling of a lump in the throat. Size, duration or morphology of the goiter does not have any correlation with symptoms or pathology. Most of the patients notice very slow growth of nodules, but rarely a patient may have rapid growth giving suspicion of malignancy. The asymmetrical or retrosternal nodule may impinge upon or stretch the recurrent laryngeal nerve and produce voice symptoms and dry cough. In long-standing goiter, some nodule may become autonomous and patients become thyrotoxic (9–10%). The true rate of progression from normal thyroid function to subclinical and finally overt hyperthyroidism in long-standing nontoxic goiters is poorly understood. Factors influencing this progression are genetic predisposition of individual, somatic mutations of individual nodules, size of nodule (>3 cm and goiter volume 16 ml) and iodine intake (6–8). These elderly patients may present with rhythm irregularities or congestive heart failure. In a goiter, all types of growth patterns are possible depending upon age, iodine status and pathology including stable, slow over many years, spontaneous reduction and even fluctuation in the size (9–12). A growing goiter characteristically presets as a progressive swelling in neck. This growth if it is in the downward direction can produce a substernal goiter. This type of history is sometimes elucidated in an older patient who narrates that the goiter once present in the neck has disappeared. Sudden increase in size of nodule suggests hemorrhage or the appearance of aggressive malignancy but intra-nodular hemorrhage will manifest as a painful and tender nodule. The natural history with respect to growth and function cannot be predicted in a

Management of Non-endemic Goiters

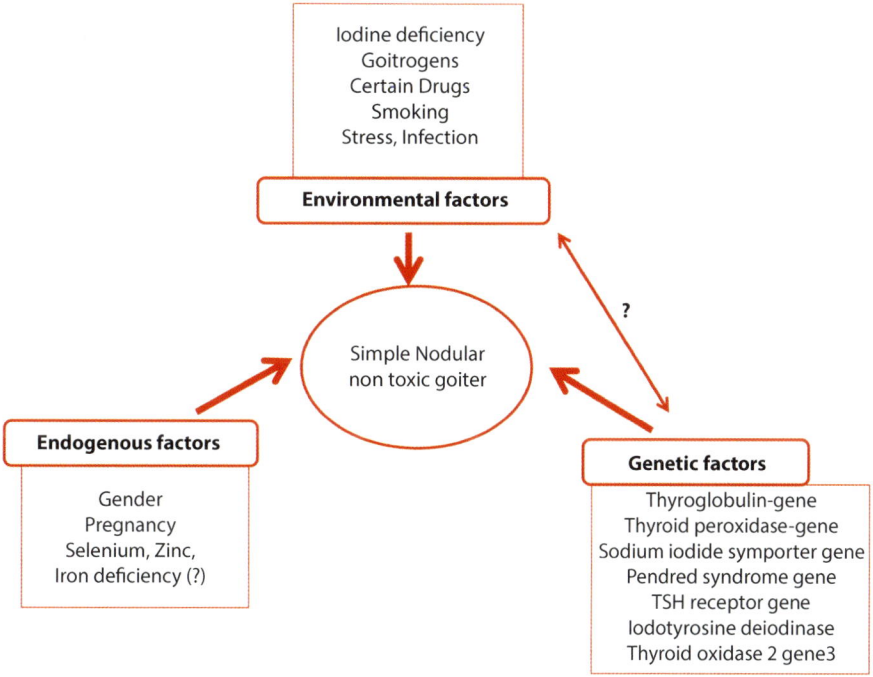

FIGURE 11.1 Multifactorial origin of simple nodular goiter.

given MNG or single nodule because no specific growth parameters exist. Therefore, it is also impossible to decide surveillance vs. treatment before it grows further and possibly affects treatment outcome adversely. Clinicians decide the strategy based on available clinical and investigation results.

Hypothyroidism is seen associated with autoimmune conditions, most common of which is Hashimoto's thyroiditis. In autoimmune diseases, goiter is diffuse. Iodine supplementation programs in iodine-deficient areas have led to an increase of hyperthyroidism (non-autoimmune) possibly by "hot" thyroid nodules. Approximately it is 4–17% of MNG harbor malignancy (13, 14). In MNG, it is impractical to perform US-guided fine needle aspiration (FNA) of all nodules, so only those nodules are subjected that have suspicious features visible on US. In iodine-deficient regions, the most common thyroid cancer (TC) is papillary, and in iodine-deficient areas, follicular lymphoma is seen associated with Hashimoto's thyroiditis and anaplastic cancer are seen in patients with a history of long-standing goiters. Literature suggests a lower prevalence of TC in MNG compared to solitary nodules, particularly in iodine-deficient areas (9, 10).

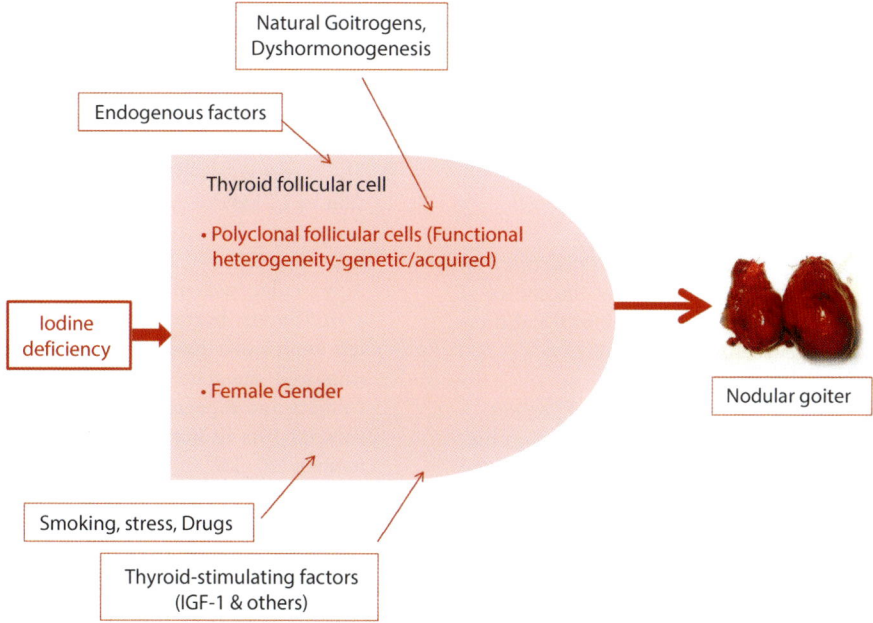

FIGURE 11.2 Multifactorial origin of simple nodular goiter.

With prevalence of 4% clinical nodularity of thyroid gland in general population and approximately 5% of nodular goiter harboring TC, the calculated prevalence of TC in general population would be 2000 per 10 lakhs. It is worth noticing that only about 2 of these 2000 hypothetical TC would become clinically apparent each year (15). Thus, there is a big gap between clinical presentation of TC and its calculated frequency. The reason may be selection bias. Surgically managed MNG selected by their physicians for thyroid surgery probably have clinically significant thyroid disease. Factors controlling the selection process are clinical history examination and results of the investigation. Many MNG patients who are asymptomatic or have inapparent goiter do not seek clinical consultation. To pick all these cancers, one has to do population surveys with proactive screening by US imaging. And higher incidence of nodular disease and TC has been the trend in countries where such surveys have been done (16, 17). Since most of these tumors don't cause any harm to the patients, it is fair not do population surveys. Papillary is the most common TC and also most commonly found tumor in MNG.

Symptoms

Symptoms of goiter can be the presence of a mass in the neck that may be asymptomatic or symptomatic for growth, pressure symptoms like choking sensation in neck, positional symptoms, breathlessness, dysphagia, cough and hoarseness or stridor in late cases. Goiter is painless and associated with pain in infective situations, autoimmune enlargement, intranodular hemorrhage and anaplastic cancer. Long-standing MNG may develop hyperthyroidism, and rarely, patient can develop Horner's syndrome. Size, duration or morphology of the goiter does not have any correlation with symptoms or pathology.

Diagnosis

All patients with nodular disease are investigated for thyroid function assessment (minimal by TSH or combination of Free T4, TSH or total T3, Free T4 and TSH), morphology (high-resolution US) and pathology (FNA cytology) of enlarged thyroid gland. Any patient with suppressed TSH should be subjected to scintigraphy to know the etiology of hyperthyroidism. Further imaging by CT or MRI scan depends upon the nature of the disease and treatment planning. Investigations are discussed in detail in the previous chapters.

Management

In benign nontoxic goiter, size of the goiter and occurrence of symptoms do not have any correlation. Therefore, the choice of treatment in these patients is challenging. In all nontoxic diffuse or nodular goiter diagnosis, the treatment goals are:

1. Correction of underlying thyroid dysfunction if present.
2. All nodular goiters that are suspicious for cancer on history and examination or investigation should be subjected for surgery. All patients with proven cancer on fine needle aspiration cytology (FNAC) should also be managed by surgery.
3. The treatment decision for a benign goiter needs to be individualized. The decision between treatment and observation depends upon benefits and risk of medical or surgical therapy and other factors including patient's wishes, social factors, finances available, availability of experienced thyroid surgeon, belief of clinicians and local practice patterns.

Iodine therapy was used as an initial therapeutic approach of benign goiter. The therapeutic effect of iodine in a nodular goiter has very limited value in reducing the size or nodularity. There is always risk of subclinical/clinical hyperthyroidism (Jod-Basedow) by iodine therapy. Therefore, iodine should not be used to treat nontoxic goiter (13–15). The other nonsurgical modalities are clinical observation only, thyroxine (LT4) suppressive therapy, radioiodine (RAI ^{131}I) alone or with recombinant TSH and nonsurgical ablative therapy. Surgery and ablative nonsurgical treatment modalities have been discussed in other chapters. In the following sections, the benefits and risks of LT4 and RAI ^{131}I will be discussed. The management algorithm is outlined in Figure 11.3.

Clinical observation

Clinical observation is a modality of management in asymptomatic nontoxic goiter where the possibility of malignancy has been excluded by guided FNA cytology. These patients will need clinical assessment at 6 months- to yearly interval and investigations (thyroid function test and ultrasonography) at yearly intervals. Ultrasonography should be used as an extension of clinical examination and may be performed whenever palpation of the thyroid is uncertain. FNAC should be repeated whenever nodule's size is changing. Whenever in the follow-up, the volume of the nodule enlarges more than 20%, a repeat evaluation by FNAC may be performed.

Thyroid hormone suppressive therapy

Current knowledge regarding the therapeutic use of LT4 therapy in reducing nodular growth is still debated. It is expected that exogenous LT4 will suppress thyrocyte growth by preventing TSH-induced growth and shrinks thyroid nodules. However, there are many questions that need to be considered before deciding the suppressive therapy:

1. There are many other factors like insulin-like growth factors, and growth factors besides TSH that can cause nodule growth (18).
2. TSH interferes with oncogenesis in nodular thyroid tissue (19).
3. The target levels of TSH suppression and treatment duration by LT4 is not defined.
4. Long-term LT4 therapy induces a state of subclinical hyperthyroidism (20, 21). There is higher morbidity of cardiovascular system (elevated heart rate; supraventricular arrhythmias, particularly atrial fibrillation and increased left ventricular mass; increased cardiac contractility; and impaired diastolic function) with subclinical hyperthyroidism and especially in elderly people. It also causes significant loss in bone mineral density in postmenopausal women (20–24).
5. There are no defined standards for nodule dimensions assessment (palpation versus ultrasonography) and degree of volume reduction to define therapeutic efficacy.
6. The trials result show that long-term LT4 administration is needed to have any significant benefit, but nodules rapidly return to their pretreatment size or show regrowth once therapy is stopped.

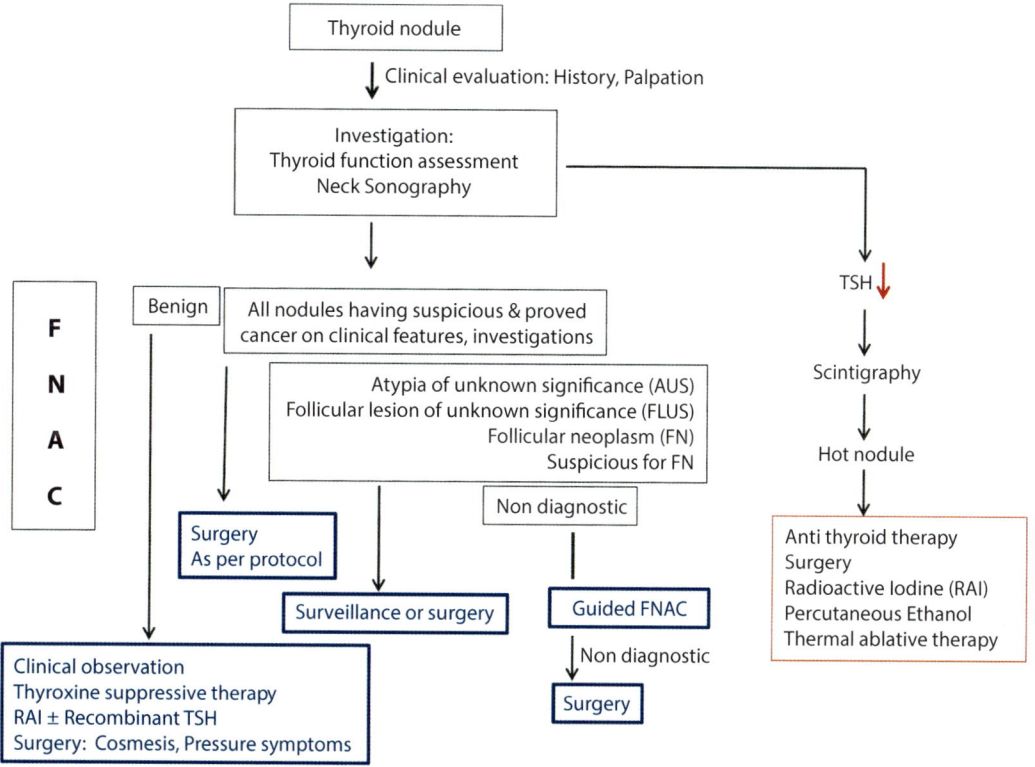

FIGURE 11.3 Algorithm for cost-effective management of nodule.

Literature suggests that a subset of benign thyroid nodules do respond to thyroid-hormone-suppressive therapy but markers for this subset are not yet identified:

1. LT4 therapy is effective only in solid nodules (25–27).
2. In iodine-sufficient regions, 17–25% solitary (or dominant) thyroid nodule will have a modest decrease in nodule size (>50%) by LT4 therapy.
3. Other nodule characteristics that can have benefit of LT4 therapy are recent diagnosis, relatively small volumes (<10, <2.5 or <1.5), contain an abundance of colloid in FNAC and the absence of hyperplastic or fibrotic changes (28–30).

In summary, a trial of LT4 therapy can be tried in patients with low-normal TSH, in younger patients without comorbidity with diffuse goiter, and in patients with benign solitary thyroid nodules who are concerned about subsequent growth; however its use is inappropriate in elderly people (>60 years) and postmenopausal women. But routine LT4 therapy is not recommended for benign thyroid nodules (31).

Therapy with radioiodine

RAI therapy is a treatment option in patients with multiple comorbidities where surgery and anesthesia have very high risk. It can be an option for a patient who refuses surgery. This form of treatment was introduced around three decades ago. It works in reducing the size of the goiter up to 60% but some patients develop temporary mild thyrotoxicosis in the first 2 weeks of treatment. It can be reduced by giving glucocorticoid and beta blockers. The other major disadvantage is the development of unpredictable hypothyroidism in up to 45% of patients. Acute adverse effects of this therapy include painful transient thyroiditis, thyroid swelling, compression of trachea and heart-related symptoms. The lifetime risk of development of cancer in other places than thyroid gland is 1.6% (32, 33). One of the problems with this form of treatment is low isotope accumulation in inactive and partially suppressed areas around nodule. Simultaneous administration of recombinant TSH (rhTSH) increases two- to four-fold more accumulation of RAI. Recombinant TSH reactivates the dormant areas for RAI concentration (34). It not only amplifies the effect of RAI but also causes homogeneous distribution in the goiter. This results in less treatment dose requirement. One to two injection of rhTSH (0.1–0.3 mg) should be administered 24 hour prior to RAI therapy. Recently, a "modified-release rhTSH" has been introduced, which has more delayed peak in comparison to rhTSH. It is being used under trials only (35).

Current literature suggests that RAI therapy results in:

1. RAI can cause volume reduction of 33–66% in 80% of patients.
2. It improves dysphagia or dyspnea in 70–90% of patients.
3. Post RAI hypothyroidism is observed in 60% of patients at 8 years.
4. Post RAI Graves' disease is seen in 10% of patients.
5. Post RAI lifetime cancer risk is 1.6%.

Surgery

In today's era, when surgery and anesthesia have become very safe, the standard treatment for nontoxic goiters that are symptomatic is surgery. Surgery provides immediate relief in compressive symptoms. It allows pathological assessment of the specimen where incidental cancers can be identified in the nodule. Surgery is totally safe in the hands of experienced thyroid surgeons. There remains controversy regarding the ideal surgery in benign thyroid diseases (36). Subtotal thyroidectomy (STT) was considered gold standard operation for MNG with two advantages: less postoperative complications and no need for lifelong LT4 replacement therapy. However, there were high recurrence rates (up to 43%) after this operation, and hypothyroidism was unpredictable. Many clinicians argue that after STT, residual remnant pathology is also left, and there may be malignant transformation in the residual remnant (37). So total thyroidectomy (TT) has the advantages of one-stage removal of incidental TC and a lower risk of recurrence. TT operation is condemned for its high percentage of postsurgical complications. But there is enough evidence to show that TT performed by an experienced thyroid surgeon has same postoperative complications as STT. The transient hypocalcemia rates are high in TT but one should not consider it a complication but as sequelae of this operation. After TT, there is no recurrence and hypothyroidism can be treated by fixed-dose LT4 supplementation that requires, initially, two to three dose adjustments. TT should be considered for safe and effective operation to prevent goiter recurrence. Lobectomy should be the choice for symptomatic unilateral MNG. Current guidelines and evidence favor TT for nontoxic benign MNG (31, 38, 39).

South Asia perspective

India has both iodine sufficient and deficient regions, and same is the pattern seen in many South Asian countries. Sub-Himalayan regions in India and some other parts are iodine deficient while coastal regions are iodine sufficient. In India, there is a universal iodination program from the Government of India. Benign nontoxic goiter is very common in this region, which is reflected in many publications, but people in rural areas do not consider it a disease and seek consultation only when they become symptomatic. Other type of presentation is as thyroid incidentaloma. The evaluation and treatment facilities are available at most of the cities. The preferable surgery of nontoxic bilateral MNG in this region is TT (40, 41). Very few clinicians use suppressive LT4 therapy, and RAI is not used for MNG treatment commonly. RAI with rhTSH therapy is costly, controversial and experimental so not used.

Conclusion

Aims of treatment in patient with nontoxic goiter are correction of thyroid dysfunction if any, reduce the size of the gland and prevent further growth of goiter. Treatment decisions should be individualized and should be evidence-based. Individuals with large benign goiters with pressure symptoms or cosmetic concern require surgery. Asymptomatic patients in whom cancer has been excluded by investigations can be clinically followed. There is controversy regarding the effectiveness of LT4 and RAI therapy in these patients, and it is better to avoid these forms of treatment unless there are compelling reasons. There is no ideal treatment of nontoxic goiter. Treatment decision is influenced by many factors that include beliefs of treating clinician, local availability of experienced thyroid surgeons, patient's age and associated comorbidities, patient's wishes, social factors, finances available and local practice patterns.

References

1. Charib TGH (1997) Thyroid incidentalomas: management approaches to non-palpable nodules discovered incidentally on thyroid imaging. Ann Int Med 126: 226–231.
2. Pinchera A, Aghini-Lombardi F, Antonangeli L, Vitti P (1996) Multinodular goiter. Epidemiology and prevention. Ann Ital Chir 67: 317–325.
3. Jarlob AE, Nygaard B, Hegedus L, Hartling SC, Hansen JM (1998) Observer variation in the clinical and laboratory evaluation of patients with thyroid dysfunction and goiter. Thyroid 8: 393–398.
4. Marine D (1924) Etiology and prevention of simple goiter. Medicine 3: 453.
5. Taylor S (1953) The evolution of nodular goiter. J Clin Endocrinol Metab 13: 1232.
6. Brix TH, Hededus L (2000) Genetic and environmental factors in the aetiology of simple goiter. Ann Med 32: 153–156.
7. Krohn K, Paschke R (2001) Progress in understanding the etiology of thyroid autonomy. J Clin Endocrinol Metab 86: 3336–3345.
8. Laurberg P, Pedersen IB, Knudsen N, Ovesen L, Andersen S (2001) Environmental iodine intake affects the type of non-malignant thyroid disease. Thyroid 11: 457–469.
9. Vanderpump MP, Tunbridge WM, French JM et al. (1995) The incidence of thyroid disorders in the community: a twenty-year follow-up of the Whickham Survey. Clin Endocrinol (Oxf) 43: 55–68.
10. Rallison ML, Dobyns BM, Meikle AW, Bishop M, Lyon JL, Stevens W (1991) Natural history of thyroid abnormalities: prevalence, incidence, and regression of thyroid diseases in adolescents and young adults. Am J Med 91: 363–370.
11. Berghout A, Wiersinga WM, Smits NJ, Touber JL (1990) Interrelationships between age, thyroid volume, thyroid nodularity, and thyroid function in patients with sporadic nontoxic goiter. Am J Med 89: 602–608.
12. Furlanetto TW, Nguyen LQ, Jameson JL (1999) Estradiol increases proliferation and down-regulates the sodium/iodide symporter gene in FRTL-5 cells. Endocrinology 140: 5705–5711.
13. Koh KB, Chang KW (1992) Carcinoma in multinodular goiter. Brit J Surg 79: 266.
14. Bisi H, Fernandes SO, Camargo RYA, Koch L, Abdo AH, Brito T (1989) The prevalence of unsuspected thyroid pathology in 300 sequential autopsies with special reference to the incidental carcinoma. Cancer 64: 1888–1893.
15. Siegel RL, Miller KD, Jemal A (2015) Cancer statistics, 2015. CA Cancer J Clin 65: 5–29.
16. Mao Y, Xing M (2016) Recent incidences and differential trends of thyroid cancer in the USA. Endocr Relat Cancer 23(4): 313–322.
17. Kitahara, C., Sosa, J (2016) The changing incidence of thyroid cancer. Nat Rev Endocrinol 12: 646–653.
18. Biondi B et al. (2005) Thyroid-hormone therapy and thyroid cancer: a reassessment. Nat Clin Pract Endocrinol Metab 1: 32–40.
19. Bruno R et al. (2005) Modulation of thyroid-specific gene expression in normal and nodular human thyroid tissues from adults: an in vivo effect of thyrotropin. J Clin Endocrinol Metab 90: 5692–5697.
20. Surks MI et al. (2004) Subclinical thyroid disease. Scientific review and guidelines for diagnosis and management. JAMA 291: 228–238.
21. Biondi B et al. (2005) Subclinical hyperthyroidism: clinical features and treatment options. Eur J Endocrinol 152: 1–9.
22. Uzzan B et al. (1996) Effects on bone mass of long term treatment with thyroid hormones: a metaanalysis. J Clin Endocrinol Metab 81: 4278–4289.
23. Faber J, Galloe AM (1994) Changes in bone mass during prolonged subclinical hyperthyroidism due to L-thyroxine treatment: a meta-analysis. Eur J Endocrinol 130: 350–356.
24. Biondi B et al. (2002) Mortality in elderly patients with subclinical hyperthyroidism. Lancet 359: 799–800.
25. McCowen K et al. (1980) The role of thyroid therapy in patients with thyroid cysts. Am J Med 68: 853–855.
26. La Rosa G et al. (1995) Levothyroxine and potassium iodide are both effective in treating benign solitary solid cold nodules of the thyroid. Ann Intern Med 122: 1–8.
27. Wemeau JL et al. (2002) Effects of thyroid-stimulating hormone suppression with levo-thyroxine in reducing the volume of solitary thyroid nodules and improving extranodular nonpalpable changes: a randomized, double-blind, placebo-controlled trial by the French Thyroid Research Group. J Clin Endocrinol Metab 87: 4928–4934.
28. La Rosa G et al. (1996) Cold thyroid nodule reduction with L-thyroxine can be predicted by initial nodule volume and cytological characteristics. J Clin Endocrinol Metab 81: 4385–4387.
29. Lima N et al. (1997) Levothyroxine suppressive therapy is partially effective in treating patients with benign, solid thyroid nodules and multinodular goiters. Thyroid 7: 691–697.
30. Costante G et al. (2004) Slow growth of benign thyroid nodules after menopause: no need for long-term thyroxine suppressive therapy in post-menopausal women. J Endocrinol Invest 27: 31–36.
31. Haugen BR, Alexander EK, Bible KC et al. (2016) 2015 American Thyroid Association management guidelines for adult patients with thyroid nodules and differentiated thyroid cancer: the American Thyroid Association guidelines task force on thyroid nodules and differentiated thyroid cancer. Thyroid Jan;26(1): 1–133.
32. Wesche MF, Tiel-V Buul MM, Lips P, Smits NJ, Wiersinga WM (2001) A random-ized trial comparing levothyroxine with radioactive iodine in the treatment of sporadic nontoxic goiter. J Clin Endocrinol Metab 86: 998–1005.
33. Huysmans DA, Buijs WC, van de Ven MT et al. (1996) Dosimetry and risk estimates of radioiodine therapy for large, multinodular goiters. J Nucl Med 37: 2072–2079.
34. Bonnema SJ, Fast S, Hegedüs L (2014) The role of radioiodine therapy in benign nodular goiter. Best Pract Res Clin Endocrinol Metabol 28: 619–631.

35. Graf H, Fast S, Pacini F et al. (2011) Modified- release recombinant human TSH (MRrhTSH) augments the effect of 131I therapy in benign multinodular goiter. Results from a multicenter international, randomized, placebo-controlled study. J Clin Endocrinol Metab 96: 1368–1376.
36. Ozbas S, Kocak S, Aydintug S et al. (2005) Comparison of the complications of subtotal, near total and total thyroidectomy in the surgical management of multinodular goitre. Endocr J 52: 199–205.
37. Röjdmark J, Järhult J (1995) High long term recurrence rate after subtotal thyroidectomy for nodular goitre. Eur J Surg 161: 725–727.
38. Gharib H, Papini E, Garber JR et al. (2016) American Association of Clinical Endocrinologists, American College of Endocrinology, and Associazione Medici Endocrinologi medical guidelines for clinical practice for the diagnosis and management of thyroid nodules-2016 update. Endocr Pract 22: 622–639.
39. Cirocchi R, Trastulli S, Randolph J et al. (2015) Total or near-total thyroidectomy versus subtotal thyroidectomy for multinodular non-toxic goitre in adults. Cochrane Database Syst Rev (8). Art. No.: CD010370. DOI: 10.1002/14651858.CD010370.pub2.
40. Agarwal G, Aggarwal V (2008) Is total thyroidectomy the surgical procedure of choice for benign multinodular goiter? An evidence-based review. World J Surg 32: 1313–1324.
41. Agarwal A, Mishra AK, Gupta SK et al. (2007) High incidence of tracheomalacia in longstanding goiters: experience from an endemic goiter region. World J Surg 31: 832–837.

12

MANAGEMENT OF ENDEMIC GOITER

Ranil Fernando

Introduction

Goiter is a global problem and a common endocrine disorder encountered in medical practice. Certain parts of the world and countries are considered endemic for goiter. The word endemic means frequent in a certain locality. Endemicity was defined as goiter prevalence in the general population of an area exceeding 10% (1). This definition has been debated by some authors (2). There is now a tendency to decrease this figure from 10 to 5%. Therefore, more areas will be classified as having a problem of endemic goiter (2). The endemic goiter map of Asia compiled by Ramalingaswami et al. in 1973 (3) is depicted in Figure 12.1; this depicts only the high-prevalence zones. It must also be remembered that this has changed in the last few decades.

Historical aspects and etiology of endemic goiter

The etiology of endemic goiter remains a topic of debate. It is generally believed that the development of a simple goiter, whether endemic or sporadic, depends on complex interactions between genetic, environmental and endogenous factors (4). The main etiological factor identified worldwide for endemic goiters is the deficiency of iodine. Hence, endemic goiter is classified as part of a spectrum of disorders known as iodine deficiency disorders (IDD). Goiter is considered a determinant of the prevalence and severity of IDD in populations. **Iodine deficiency remains a large global health problem. It is estimated that around 2 billion individuals worldwide do not take adequate iodine in their diet**. This is seen particularly in South Asia and sub-Saharan Africa (5), making endemic goiter still a real problem the health-care system has to deal with particularly in the sub-Saharan Africa and Asia. Some of these patients will need some management including surgical treatment.

In 1979, De Maeyer Lowenstein and Thilly complied with a comprehensive document under the auspices of the WHO to control endemic goiter. The report recommended universal iodization and several other public health measures (6). The WHO launched the universal iodine supplementation of salt in the 1990s. In May 1990, the 43rd World Health Assembly passed a resolution that the "WHO shall aim at eliminating iodine deficiency disorders as a major health problem in all countries by 2000". This resulted in a concerted effort globally to eliminate IDD with some success.

Emergence of the effects of over iodization is now being recognized in several parts of the world. Overiodization may cause hyperthyroidism (iodine-induced hyperthyroidism [IIH] or hypothyroidism [IID]) in vulnerable people and iodization needs close monitoring (7).

The carcinogenic effect of excess iodine needs to be studied further as the evidence for this effect has not yet been demonstrated clearly; on the contrary, chronic iodine deficiency may induce thyroid cancer, especially follicular carcinoma (8). **Hence, the whole question of iodization and endemic goiter needs further study and careful scrutiny**.

Despite elimination of IDD in some countries, goiter remains an endemic problem **in those countries, suggesting that other etiological factors may also be in operation to account for the endemicity**. Other etiological factors may be important in these areas, e.g., cassava consumption and selenium deficiency in sub-Saharan Africa (9). The identification of a main etiological factor will be critical in the management of endemic goiter. Once the correctable etiological factors are rectified, there will be elimination of deficiency goiters in the long term. In many countries, including Asian countries, the enormous goiters seen previously have become a rarity due to the success of iodization and other measures undertaken. These remedial measures must be closely monitored and updated as an important part in the management of endemic goiters. There are a residual number of goiters that will need evaluation and management in iodine sufficient as well as endemic populations.

Clinical presentations of endemic goiters

The endemic goiters present as several clinical entities in various parts of the world. In neonates and children, endemic goiters may be associated with, hypothyroidism, mental retardation deaf-mutism and cretinism in the worst form. These problems should be dealt with by endocrinologists, neonatologists and pediatricians. In **adults**, the endemic goiter may present as one of the variety (Table 12.1).

Majority of patients in endemic areas will present with a diffuse colloid goiter or a euthyroid multinodular goiter (MNG). Some subjects with small goiters may not present at all to clinics and are only detected by goiter studies or community-based surveys. Once goiter is detected, it needs complete evaluation before management decisions are made.

Clinical evaluation

All endemic goiters must be fully evaluated clinically. The size of the goiter must be expressed using the Modified WHO Classification of Goiters (10) given in Table 12.2.

In addition, the other physical characteristics such as symmetry, consistency, position trachea and carotids retrosternal extension need to be assessed and documented.

Traditionally, students are taught that goiters should be palpated from behind, but this is a fallacy. Symmetry, position of trachea consistency can only properly be assessed from the front. In addition, eye sign pulse etc. can only be done from the

Management of Endemic Goiter

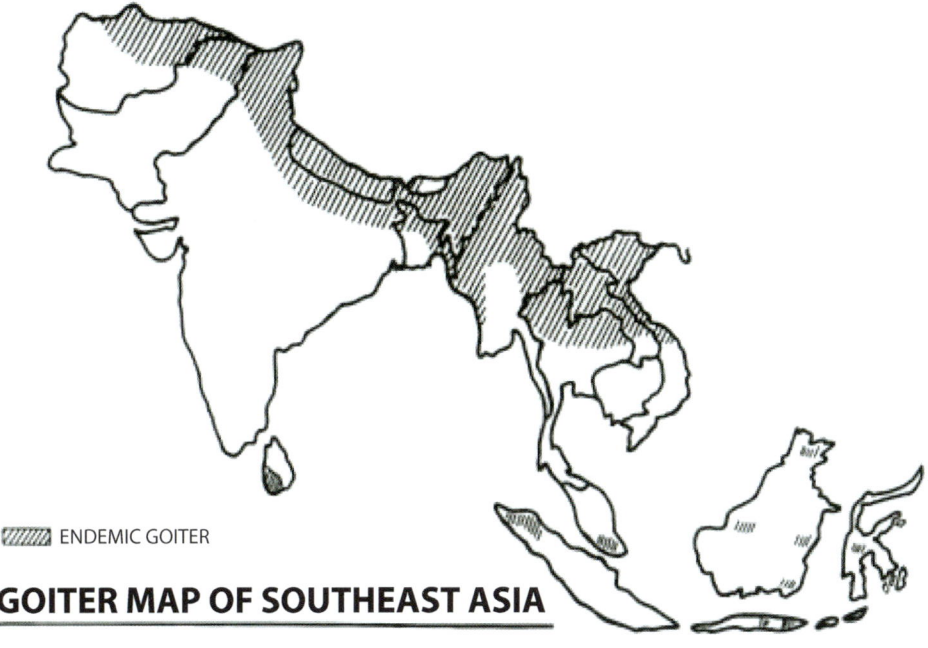

FIGURE 12.1 Endemic regions of the South Asia.

TABLE 12.1: Presentations of Endemic Goiter

1. Simple diffuse goiter with or without dysfunction (colloid goiter)
2. Multinodular goiter (MNG) with or without dysfunction (MNG with or without toxicosis)
3. Multinodular goiter with an occult carcinoma found postoperatively
4. Solitary nodule of the thyroid (STN) with or without dysfunction (STN or AFTN)
5. Diffuse goiter with Hashimoto disease associated with hyper- or hypothyroidism
6. Overt thyroid cancer (long-standing goiter)
7. Recurrent goiter

Imaging

Morphology of goiter is assessed first by clinical examination. **Ultrasonography is the main imaging modality used in the assessment of endemic goiters**. US scan is superior to clinical examination in detecting thyroid nodules. Thyroid nodules as small as 3 mm are detectable on ultrasonography. Clinical methods and ultrasonography are also used in assessing the prevalence of goiter to determine endemicity. There are clear limitations to the use of clinical examination and US scan in assessing the size of a small goiter.

front. The important thing is to get all the signs. Hence, examination from the front as depicted in Figure 12.2, examination from the side Figure 12.3 and from behind – Figure 12.4 must be done to do carry out a proper examination of the thyroid.

On the clinical findings, the goiters can be classified into several types based on morphology and function depicted in Figure 12.5.

Evaluation of an endemic goiter

As in any investigation of goiter, the aims of investigating endemic goiter are to confirm the morphology, assess the function and determine the histopathology of the goiter before making definitive management decisions.

TABLE 12.2: Modified WHO Classification of Goiter

Grade 1: Enlarged thyroid, palpable but not visible when the neck is in the normal position

Grade 2: Thyroid clearly visible when the neck is in the normal position

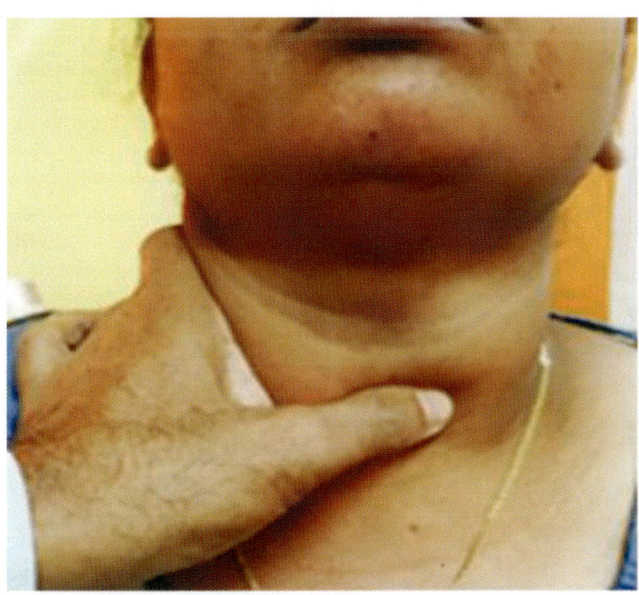

FIGURE 12.2 Examination from the front of the patient.

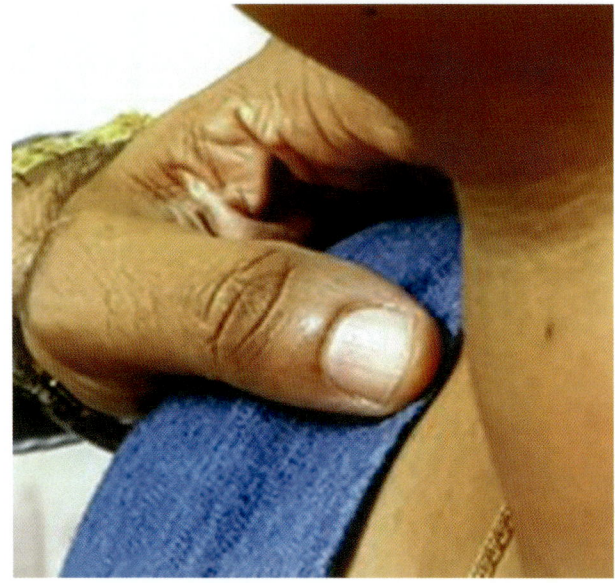

FIGURE 12.3 Inspection of neck from the side.

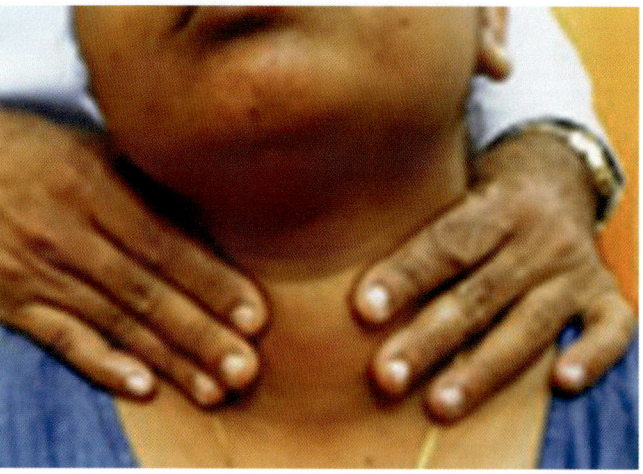

FIGURE 12.4 Examination from the behind.

Several authors, state that "significant inter-observer and intra-observer variation occurs in sonographic measurements of thyroid volume"; proper training and experience is needed before reliance can be placed only on ultrasonography to assess thyroid size (11). In addition, there is evidence to suggest that thyroid size differs in different populations. The size of the thyroid is affected by several factors including the iodine status of a population (12). The best option is for each country and region to develop its own reference values for determining the size and the volume of the thyroid. In spite of limitations, the clinical examination and the US scan will provide sufficient information about the morphology of the thyroid gland to decide on the management plan.

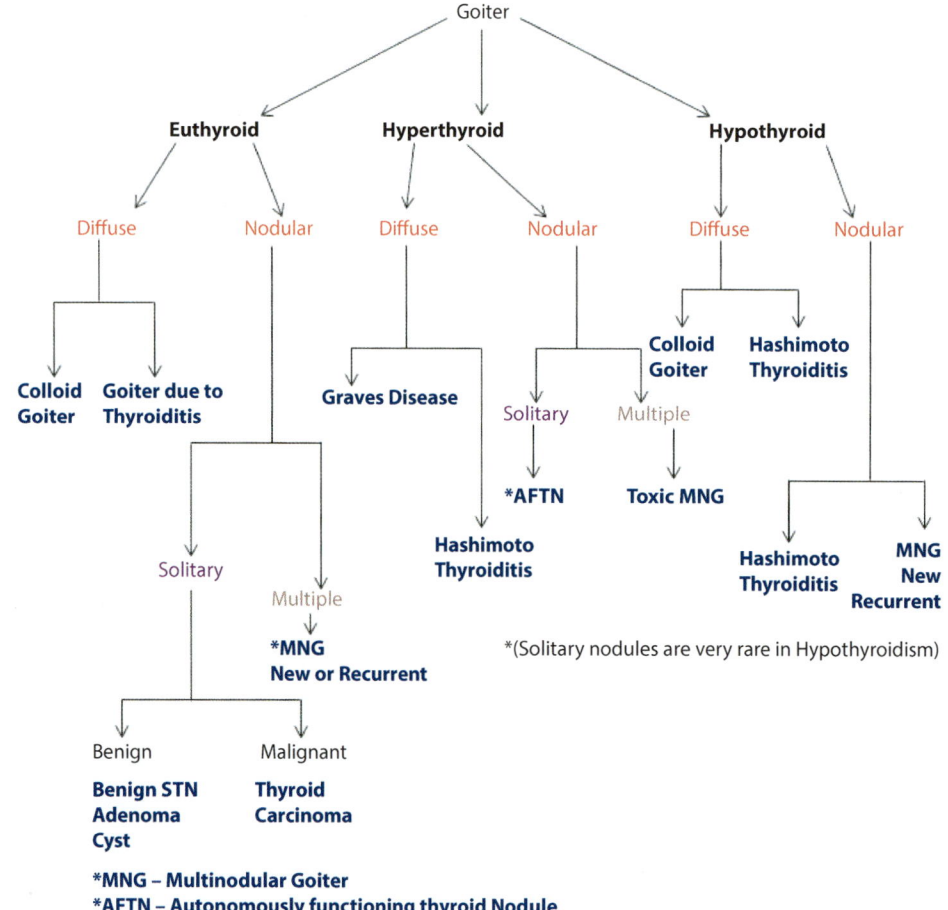

FIGURE 12.5 Clinical classification of endemic goiter.

If retrosternal extension or involvement of surrounding structures such as the carotid artery or the internal jugular vein is detected or suspected clinically, a CT scan has a definitive place in the assessment of an endemic goiter.

X-ray of the cervical area is done to assess the trachea and the cervical vertebrae, especially if there is tracheal deviation or an elderly patient is considered for surgery. Other imaging modalities are rarely needed in the evaluation of an endemic goiter. The cost factor and the cost-effectiveness of investigation must be borne in mind before requesting any imaging modality.

Radioisotope scanning has a very limited role in the evaluation of an endemic goiter. 99mTc, I^{123} and I^{131} are the isotopes commonly used for thyroid isotope scanning. They provide information about the function of the thyroid gland. **Historically cold (hypoactive) nodules were considered to indicate a possible malignancy.** Due to the very low diagnostic accuracy, and the advent of far more sensitive FNC, there is consensus that the role of the isotope is very limited in the initial assessment of thyroid nodules (13). The specific indication for an isotope scan is the suspicion of an autonomously functioning thyroid nodule (AFTN). **It is one indication where a scintiscan is essential when evaluating a nodular thyroid.**

Biochemical evaluation

Functional status is assessed by the thyroid hormone assay – T3, T4 and TSH. These assays are readily available in many countries. If cost constrains do not permit the assay of all three parameters, **initial assay of the TSH, which is a very sensitive assay of thyroid pituitary axis, will provide a useful and reliable guide about the thyroid status** (14). The only exception is the very rare possibility of a TSH-secreting lesion in the pituitary. There are other non-thyroidal illnesses that may change the values of thyroid function (non-thyroidal illness syndrome); these must be borne in mind when interpreting thyroid function tests (15).

Other investigations such as thyroid antibodies will assist in diagnosing Hashimoto thyroiditis and Graves' disease and should be done appropriately. Serum calcitonin is used in screening for medullary carcinoma of thyroid.

There are two types of TSH receptor antibodies (TRAb): thyroid stimulating antibody (TSAb) and TSH-stimulation blocking antibody (TSBAb). These antibodies are most commonly found in Graves' disease and may become adjuncts to diagnosing Graves' disease, especially in pregnant/postpartum women, children and in cases of atypical Graves'. **These antibodies are not required for diagnosis in most patients with Graves' disease, especially if cost is a constraint (16 & 17).**

The thyroid peroxidase (TPO) thyroglobulin (TG) antibodies are immune markers most commonly found in Hashimoto's thyroiditis and will be positive even in a significant percentage of patients with Graves' disease (16 & 17). All antibodies tests are relatively expensive, particularly in the developing world and their measurement must be done judiciously giving careful consideration to the real indication and the cost-effectiveness. Serum TG level has no role in the diagnosis of a thyroid nodular or endemic goiter.

Other biochemical parameters such as serum calcium are not routine assessment of an endemic goiter. They should be considered for specific reasons for individual patients **being cognizant of the cost-effectiveness, especially in the developing economies of South Asia.**

Cyto/histopathology

FNC is the mainstay in the assessment of pathology of the thyroid gland. The British Thyroid Association (BTA)/RCP Thy1–5 system (18) and The Bethesda System for Reporting Thyroid Cytology (TBSRTC) (19) have made the decision-making in thyroid lesions much more uniform. It is the follicular lesions that cause the major issue as there is no way of differentiating between a thyroid adenoma and a thyroid carcinoma on FNC. In addition, in about 10–20% of patients, FNC fails to provide a clear diagnosis to make a decision about a definitive plan of management. These are called indeterminate lesions or AUS/FLUS lesions. AUS stands for atypia of unknown significance and FLUS for follicular lesion of unknown significance. These lesions will require further evaluation and discussion at multidisciplinary meetings. **The cancer risk for this category of lesions is 5–15% and recommended management protocol is repeat FNC after sufficient time gap (20 & 21). Treatment of such goiters must be individualized.**

Once all the evaluations are done, endemic goiter will belong to the categories depicted in Table 12.1 and Figure 12.5. The commonest categories are euthyroid MNG and euthyroid colloid goiter.

Management

Management of euthyroid multinodular and colloid goiter

MNG/colloid goiter will need treatment in certain patients. All patients must have a complete evaluation of the thyroid and the health status. Once all the information is available, an evidence-guided decision must be made in deciding the best form of management. **The first principle of treatment, i.e., "Primum non nocere" – "First do no harm" applies very aptly to the management of endemic goiters.** Some old and infirm patients with small goiters will not require any treatment apart from periodic observation.

There is a tendency to use thyroxine empirically to reduce the size of goiters. This has been debated for many years. While there is some reduction in size initially, it is not sustainable and the gland tends to grow soon after the stoppage of the thyroxine. The dose required is a suppressive dose and the optimal duration is unknown. The cardiovascular, skeletal and other side effects of thyroxine such as iatrogenic hyperthyroidism have prompted **many authors to recommend abandoning the use of thyroxine to reduce the size of thyroids** (22). This will be very relevant in older patients with comorbidities and small goiters. Thyroxine will have very little effect on large goiters. Several guidelines discourage the empirical use of thyroxine. **There is an urgent need to stop the indiscriminate use of thyroxine in general.** Other patients will have large goiters or have symptoms of compression due to the goiter. If these patients require intervention, the only viable option is surgery.

Main indications (**the 5 Cs**) for surgery for MNG/colloid goiter are:

1. Cosmesis
2. Compression (of trachea or superior thoracic aperture)
3. Cancer (fear of it)
4. Comeback (recurrence)
5. Control of toxicity (failed medical therapy in Graves' or toxic MNG)

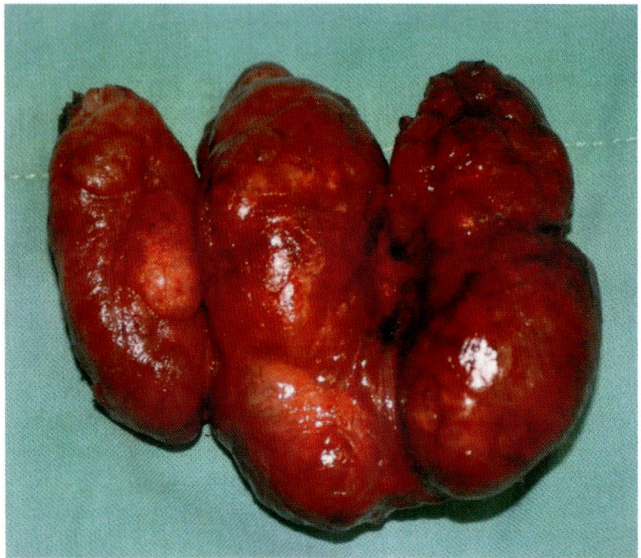

FIGURE 12.6 Total thyroidectomy specimen.

It must be remembered that the disease process affects the whole gland and the treatment must address this. There still debate about surgical options in dealing with euthyroid multinodular/colloid goiter. Though there are a few detractors, most authors agree that the best option for MNG/colloid goiter is total/near-total thyroidectomy (Figure 12.6) (23, 24, 25 & 26). This is more so in very large goiters seen in the Asian subcontinent where other forms of therapy will not be effective (Figure 12.7). It has been the experience of surgeons in the endemic goiter areas that recurrent goiters occur several years after subtotal thyroidectomy, and the surgery is fraught with difficulty (27 & 28). **Most recurrences occur close to vital structures such as the recurrent laryngeal nerve and the parathyroids increasing the risk of complications from surgery significantly.** The first operation must eliminate the need to undertake reoperative surgery. The only drawback is that the patients will need to be on lifelong thyroxine therapy. Most patients tolerate this well. They also need clinic follow-up to ensure that they remain euthyroid.

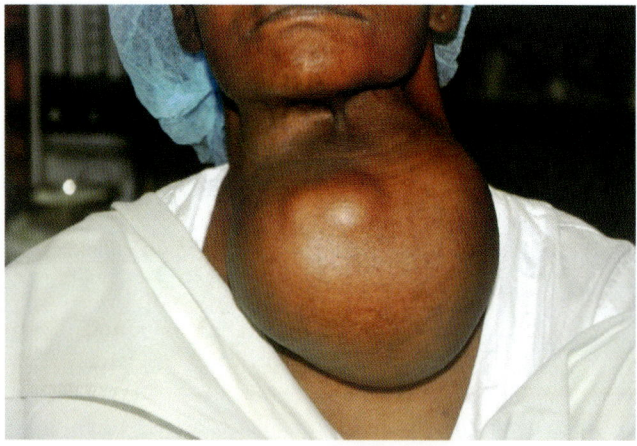

FIGURE 12.7 Endemic goiter.

Occult/incidental carcinoma

Incidental thyroid carcinoma (ITC) or occult carcinoma of the thyroid is a thyroid cancer that is not diagnosed preoperatively and is detected histologically when a thyroidectomy is undertaken for benign disease. **This is seen commonly in patients with long-standing MNG.** The incidence of occult carcinoma (incidental carcinoma) varies in the literature between 3 and 50% (29, 30 & 31). If a subtotal procedure had been undertaken, and the histology report reveals the presence of a carcinoma, the tumor is inappropriately treated. What surgery should to be undertaken to complete the treatment causes several dilemmas.

There is very little doubt that total thyroidectomy is the best option for euthyroid multinodular and colloid goiters.

Toxic goiters

Graves' disease, Hashimoto disease, toxic MNG (Plummer's disease), AFTN constitute the main toxic goiters in an endemic area.

The first priority is to make the patient euthyroid with appropriate drugs. Common drugs used are carbimazole, methimazole and beta-blockers. While azoles block thyroxine production, beta-blockers inhibit the sympathetic overdrive associated with toxicity. Once the patient is euthyroid, a decision has to be made about further management.

Graves' disease is managed mostly medically. Some patients will require surgery for failure of medical therapy. They also can be offered radiotherapy. If surgery is undertaken, best option is to do a total thyroidectomy for the reasons outlined previously.

Hashimoto disease does not require treatment with azoles commonly as there is no increase in thyroxine production. Most will be controlled with beta-blockage. The only very rare exception is the coexistence Graves and Hashimoto Disease (32). Occasionally patients with Hashimoto disease develop compressive symptoms. They will also need a total thyroidectomy.

Significant number of patients with Hashimoto disease will become hypothyroid requiring replacement thyroxine. All these patients will need careful monitoring and follow-up.

Toxic MNG (Plummer's disease) will need control with antithyroid drugs. This group of patients usually belongs to an older age-group and has had long-standing goiters, **unlike Graves' disease; these patients will require surgery once they are euthyroid**. Careful assessment of comorbidities must be done before surgery. They too will require total thyroidectomy for the reasons already outlined under nontoxic MNG.

Autonomously functioning thyroid nodule (AFTN-Goetsch disease)

AFTN constitute about 5% of all thyroid nodules. They are also called autonomous thyroid adenoma. AFTN is characterized by a single-thyroid adenoma, which is functioning autonomously and independently of pituitary stimulation or any other extrathyroidal stimulator. **Many patients with a solitary AFTN are euthyroid**. Progression to persisting hyperthyroidism occurs in only a small number of patients (5–10%). Patients with hyperfunctioning adenomas who are euthyroid initially develop hyperthyroidism at a rate of about 4% per year (33). This depends on the size of the adenoma; iodine intake and the age of the patient toxicity rarely develop in nodules less than 2.5 cm in diameter (33). Spontaneous degeneration of the nodule is also documented. Some AFTNs are left untreated as they are mostly euthyroid.

Treatment consists mainly of surgery or radiotherapy (34) with other less-invasive options such as ethanol injection, RFA, HIFU and laser as alternatives in selected individuals (35). Surgery (hemithyroidectomy) is offered mainly for patients below 50 years, those with compressive features and when malignancy is suspected or is diagnosed during assessment. The other options are offered for other patients especially older patients.

Hypothyroid endemic goiters – These are usually managed by physicians and endocrinologists and will require **lifelong thyroxine therapy**. Rarely may they need surgery due to features of compression.

Thyroid cancer

Some patients with endemic goiter will be shown to have a thyroid cancer on investigations; they will need **evidence-guided stage-appropriate treatment.**

Concluding remarks

Endemic Goiter remains a global health problem. With the institution of the Universal iodization program by the WHO, the prevalence of iodine deficiency goiters has decreased. But in certain parts of the world, endemic goiter remains a problem due to other goitrogens. **A patient with an endemic goiter may or may not require treatment**. If treatment is deemed necessary, a complete clinical, biochemical, sonographic and cytological assessment must be done. **Thyroxine replacement therapy and surgery are the main modes of therapy.**

References

1. McGirr EM, Greig WR. Proceedings of the Royal Society of Medicine Meeting. Thyroid Dis. 1967 Oct. doi: 10.1177/003591576806100428.
2. Koutras DA. Endemic goiter – An update. Hormones. 2002;1(3):157–164.
3. Ramalingaswami V. Endemic goiter in Southeast Asia. New clothes on an old body. Ann Intern Med. 1973;78:277–283.
4. Heiberg TB, Hegedüs L. Genetic and environmental factors in the aetiology of simple goitre. Ann Med. 2000;32(3):153–156.
5. Zimmermann MB, Jooste PL, Pandav CS. Iodine-deficiency disorders. Lancet. 2008;372(9645):1251–1262.
6. De Maeyer EM, Lowenstein FW, Thilly CH. The Control of Endemic Goitre. Geneva: WHO Publications; 1979.
7. Katagiri R, Yuan X, Kobayashi S, Sasaki S. Effect of excess iodine intake on thyroid diseases in different populations: A systematic review and meta-analyses including observational studies. Mar 2017. doi.org/10.1371/journal.pone.0173722.
8. Zimmermann MB, Galetti V. Iodine intake as a risk factor for thyroid cancer: A comprehensive review of animal and human studies. Thyroid Res. 2015 Jun;8:8.
9. Kishosha PA, Galukande M, Gakwaya AM. Selenium deficiency a factor in endemic goiter persistence in sub-Saharan Africa World J Surg. 2011 Jul;35(7):1540–1545.
10. World Health Organization. Indicators for Assessing Iodine Deficiency Disorders and Their Control through Salt Iodization. World Health Organization; 1994. 66 p. WHO/NHD/01.1; WHO/NUT/94.6.
11. Jarlov AE, Nygard B, Hegedüs L, Karstrup S, Hansen JM. Observer variation in ultrasound assessment of the thyroid gland. Br J Radiol. 1993;66:625–627.
12. Zimmermann MB, Hess SY, Molinari L, et al. New reference values for thyroid volume by ultrasound in iodine-sufficient schoolchildren: A World Health Organization/Nutrition for Health and Development Iodine Deficiency Study Group Report 1, 2, 3. Am J Clin Nutr. 2004;79:231–237.
13. Cases JA, Surks MI. The changing role of scintigraphy in the evaluation of thyroid nodules. Semin Nucl Med. 2000 Apr;30(2):81–87.
14. Sheehan MT. Biochemical testing of the thyroid: TSH is the best and, oftentimes, only test needed – A review for primary care. Clin Med Res. 2016 Jun;14(2):83–92.
15. Farwell AP. Non thyroidal illness syndrome Curr Opin Endocrinol Diabetes Obes. 2013 Oct;20(5):478–484.
16. Roti E, Braverman LE, DeGroot LJ. TSH receptor antibody measurement in the diagnosis and management of Graves' disease is rarely necessary. J Clin Endocrinol Metab. 2011 Apr;83(11):3777–3785.
17. Girgis CM, Champion BL, Wall JR. Current concepts in Graves' disease Ther Adv Endocrinol Metab. 2011 Jun;2(3):135–144.
18. British Thyroid Association. Guidelines for the Management of Thyroid Cancer. 3rd ed. Report of the Thyroid Cancer Guidelines Update Group. London: RCP; 2014.
19. Cibas ES, Ali SZ. The Bethesda system for reporting thyroid cytopathology. Am J Clin Pathol. 2009;132:658–665.
20. Renuka IV, Bala GS, Aparna C, Kumari R, Sumalatha K. The Bethesda system for reporting thyroid cytopathology: Interpretation and guidelines in surgical treatment. Indian J Otolaryngol Head Neck Surg. 2012 Dec;64(4):305–311.
21. Ho AS, Sarti EE, Kunal S, et al. Malignancy rate in thyroid nodules classified as Bethesda category III (AUS/FLUS). Thyroid. 2014 May;24(5):832–839.
22. Reeve TS, Delbridge L, Cohen A, Crummer P. Total thyroidectomy. The preferred option for multinodular goiter. Ann Surg. 1987 Dec;206(6):782–786.
23. Papaleontiou M, Haymart MR. Inappropriate use of suppressive doses of thyroid hormone in thyroid nodule management: Results from a nationwide survey. Endocr Pract. 2016 Nov;22(11):1358–1360.
24. Agarwal G, Aggarwal, V. Is total thyroidectomy the surgical procedure of choice for benign multinodular goiter? World J Surg. 2008 Jul;32(7): 1313.
25. Vassiliou I, Tympa A, Arkadopoulos N, Nikolakopoulos F, Petropoulou T, Smyrniotis V. Total thyroidectomy as the single surgical option for benign and malignant thyroid disease: A surgical challenge. Arch Med Sci. 2013 Feb;9(1):74–78.
26. Guidelines for the Surgical Management of Endocrine Disease and Training Requirements for Endocrine Surgery. The British Association of Endocrine Surgeons. https://www.baets.org.uk/wp-content/uploads/2013/02/BAETS-Guidelines-2003.pdf.
27. Müller PE, Jakoby R, Heinert G, Spelsberg F. Surgery for recurrent goitre: Its complications and their risk factors. Eur J Surg. 2001 Nov;167(11):816–821.
28. Cappellani A, Di Vita M, Zanghì A, Lo Menzo E, Cavallaro A, Alfano G, Giuffrida D. The recurrent goiter: Prevention and management. Ann Ital Chir. 2008 Jul-Aug;79(4):247–253.
29. Pinto D, Munasinghe N, Chandrasinghe PC, Fernando R. Incidental thyroid carcinoma in benign thyroid disease: A cohort study World. J Endocr Surg. 2018 Sept-Dec;10(2):154–156.
30. Meyer-Rochow G, Conaglen JV, Elston MS, et al. Rates of unsuspected thyroid cancer in multinodular thyroid disease. NZMJ. 2018 Jan;131(1468):69–74.
31. Nanjappa N, Kumar A, Swain SK, Aroul TT, Smile SR, Kotasthane D. Incidental thyroid carcinoma Indian. J Otolaryngol Head Neck Surg. 2013 Jan;65(1):37–39.
32. Dasari S, Naha K, Hande M, Vivek G. Hot and cold: Coexistent Graves' disease and Hashimoto's thyroiditis in a patient with Schmidt's syndrome. BMJ Case Rep. 2014;2014: bcr2013010432.
33. Corvilain B. The natural history of thyroid autonomy and hot nodules. Ann Endocrinol (Paris). 2003 Feb;64(1):17–22.
34. Burch HB, Shakir F, Fitzsimmons TR, Jaques DP, Shriver CD. Diagnosis and management of the autonomously functioning thyroid nodule: The Walter Reed Army Medical Center experience, 1975-1996. Thyroid. 1998;8(10):872–880.
35. Yukiko Y, Kiminori S, Junko A. Treatment of autonomously functioning thyroid nodules at a single institution: Radioiodine therapy, surgery, and ethanol injection therapy. Ann Nucl Med. 2011;25:749–754.

13

MOLECULAR PATHWAYS OF THYROID CARCINOGENESIS

Chue Koy Min and Rajeev Parameswaran

Introduction

Thyroid cancer is the most common endocrine malignancy, and its incidence has increased over the past three decades (1). In the United States, the incidence of thyroid cancer has gradually increased, from an estimated 5.7–7.2 new cases per 100,000 men and women per year in the 1990s to an estimated 13.8–14.6 new cases per 100,000 men and women per year in the current decade (1), though the survival has remained excellent, accounting for only 0.4–0.5% of all cancer deaths in the last three decades (1). This trend was similarly observed worldwide as well, both in Asia and Europe (2–6).

Broadly speaking, majority of primary thyroid cancers arising from the thyroid follicular cell can be classified into papillary thyroid carcinomas, follicular thyroid carcinomas, Hürthle cell tumors, poorly differentiated thyroid carcinomas and anaplastic thyroid carcinomas (7). In addition to the above, medullary thyroid carcinoma are also considered primary thyroid cancers, being derived from the parafollicular C cells (8).

In 2005, *BRAF* gene mutations were discovered to correlate with poorer clinical prognosis in papillary thyroid cancers (9). Since then over the next ten years, there has been an explosion of knowledge with regards to the molecular pathways in thyroid cancer. Recently, The Cancer Genome Atlas (TCGA) has managed to identify 96.5% of oncogenic drivers in papillary thyroid carcinoma (10). The understanding of the molecular pathways on thyroid tumors will no doubt allow us to better understand the various subtypes of thyroid cancers, identify genetic prognostic factors correlating with poorer prognosis and pave the way for personalized treatment in the future.

Papillary thyroid carcinoma

Papillary thyroid carcinomas are the most prevalent thyroid cancer, accounting for around 70–90% of all differentiated thyroid cancer types (11). They are more common in females, have a peak incidence in the 20–30-year-old age group. Most papillary thyroid carcinomas are indolent, with a predilection for metastases to regional lymph nodes. In around 30% of patients, they can be multifocal as well (12).

Mitogen-activated protein kinase (MAPK) signaling pathway

The Cancer Genome Atlas (TCGA) genetically characterized papillary thyroid carcinomas, leading to a better understanding with regards to the oncogenic drivers for papillary thyroid carcinoma (10, 13). Previously described studies of papillary thyroid carcinoma attributed the main molecular aberrations to BRAF, RET/PTC, RAS and MET (11, 13–15). With a better understanding of molecular interactions between each of these gene products, scientists could map all these molecular aberrations leading to disruptions in the MAPK signaling pathway as a driver in tumorigenesis (8).

The MAPK signaling pathway plays a significant role in incorporating extracellular mitogenic and apoptotic signals and transmitting them intracellularly to result in cell growth and proliferation (8). This pathway is particularly important for tumorigenesis in papillary thyroid carcinomas. The TCGA study reported that a majority of the cohort of papillary thyroid carcinomas studied contain mutations within the MAPK signaling pathway (13).

The MAPK pathway is part of a signal transduction pathway that conveys an extracellular stimulus to a cellular response, utilizing a series of three consecutively activated protein kinases (16). The cellular responses triggered via this signaling pathway are responsible for cell proliferation and growth, apoptosis and differentiation (17). The MAPK pathway consists of three sequential protein kinases, activated in succession: the MAPK kinase kinase (MAPKKK), MAPK kinase (MAPKK) and MAPK (16). Each kinase in turn directly phosphorylates and activates a further downstream kinase until the final MAPK elicits a response at the cellular level (16). Each MAPK pathway can further be grouped into three main groups depending on their receptor family. The extracellular signal–regulated kinases (ERKs) family is an important group in thyroid tumorigenesis (16). The original ERK-MAPK pathway involves transmembrane extracellular receptors that respond to growth factors and mitotic signals, either as receptor tyrosine kinases or G protein–coupled receptors (18). Upon activation, mitotic signals are then transmitted to intracellular proteins, such as *RAS* and subsequently *BRAF*, which serve as the MAPKKK (18). These are then propagated to *MEK1* or *MEK2*, which serve as the MAPKK (8, 18), which then in turn activates *ERK*, which functions as the MAPK (8, 18). *ERK* then eventually crosses the nuclear membrane leading to transcription of gene products responsible for growth and proliferation (8, 18).

BRAF mutations

Papillary thyroid carcinomas are driven by the MAPK pathway, with the two main driver mutations being *BRAF* and *RAS* (8). Indeed, point mutations of the *BRAF* gene were identified in 45% of papillary thyroid carcinomas (14, 15). More than half of these point mutations (61.7%) of the *BRAF* gene involve a missense mutation resulting in an amino acid substitution of valine for glutamate at codon 600, denoted as the *BRAF-V600E* mutation (19). *BRAF-V600E* mutants were associated with classical and tall cell variant papillary thyroid carcinomas (13, 19). Compared to *RAS* mutants, *BRAF-V600E* mutations are associated with an increased MAPK signaling, with varied downstream effects (13). These include having resultant papillary thyroid carcinomas with a reduced sodium iodide symporter expression (20). This may explain why tall cell variants are more resistant to radioiodine treatment and carries a poorer prognosis.

RAS mutations

The second main driver mutation in the MAPK pathway for papillary thyroid carcinoma is *RAS* mutations. *RAS* mutants, in contrast to *BRAF* mutants, are more associated with follicular variant papillary thyroid carcinomas (13, 19). *RAS* is an intracellular GTP-binding protein upstream of *BRAF* and was first reported to be mutated in thyroid carcinomas before the 20th century (21). In the *RAS* gene family, three of them were reported to be mutated in thyroid carcinomas, namely, *HRAS*, *NRAS* and *KRAS* (22). *RAS* mutants can result in increased signaling via the MAPK or the phosphatidylinositol-3-kinase (PI3K)-AKT pathway, with *KRAS* being a preferential activator of MAPK pathway (22, 23). *RAS* mutations were noted to be almost mutually exclusive to *BRAF* mutations in papillary thyroid carcinomas (24). Interestingly, *RAS* mutants in papillary thyroid carcinomas tended to result in a follicular variant phenotype (13), with more benign characteristics such as being encapsulated and with less frequent lymph node metastases (25). This has led the TCGA group to propose the use of a *BRAF-V600E-RAS* score as a genotype-phenotype predictive score, with *RAS*-like mutants generally having more well-differentiated tumors (10).

Rearranged during transfection (RET) gene fusion

The *RET* gene is a receptor tyrosine kinase that is important for the development of neurons and the kidneys (26). The *RET* gene oncogenic gene translocation is another driver for papillary thyroid carcinoma tumorigenesis. The RET proto-oncogene is found on the chromosome 10q11.2 (27), and the RET/PTC gene rearrangement is found in an estimated 20% of papillary thyroid carcinomas (28). The wild-type RET proto-oncogene is expressed in thyroid parafollicular C cells but not in normal thyroid follicular epithelial cells (29).

In 1987, based on tissue from irradiated papillary thyroid carcinoma, a fusion oncogene, subsequently named *RETS/PTC*, was reported (30). The gene product was a chimeric gene containing the *RET* tyrosine-kinase domain (27, 31) with the 5′ terminal region of CCD6 gene (27, 32). The new rearrangement results in a constitutively active receptor tyrosine kinase without the need for ligand binding and subsequent dimerization (8). This results in the activation of downstream signals that eventually feed into the MAPK or PI3K-AKT pathways (33). Interestingly, the RET/PTC gene rearrangement was found to be more prevalent in thyroid cancers following radiation exposure (27), such as in post-Chernobyl (27, 34) or atomic bomb survivors (27, 35) who developed papillary thyroid carcinomas. Such a finding has also been replicated where *RET/PTC* rearrangements have been reported in normal thyroid follicular cells cultured *in vitro* following exposure to radiation (36) and can be attributed to the fact that the *RET* proto-oncogene is susceptible to ionizing radiation (37). At present, the presence of *RET/PTC* rearrangements does not seem to impact on prognosis (27), and studies that have investigated its role in survival and outcomes for papillary thyroid carcinomas have yielded mixed results (27, 38–40).

Other mutations in papillary thyroid carcinoma

Interestingly, while papillary thyroid carcinoma is MAPK driven, it appeared that the tumor microenvironment also plays a part in its aggressiveness. Of note is papillary microcarcinoma, which is defined by the World Health Organization, as being a papillary thyroid carcinoma that is less than 1 cm in diameter (41). Hsu et al. reported through their propensity score-matched analysis between papillary carcinoma and papillary microcarcinoma samples that though they share the similar gene expression classes, being either *BRAF*-like or *RAS*-like, like their carcinoma counterparts, they do display different gene expression patterns, in particular the lack of inactivating mutations in cell cycle regulatory genes and genes involved in extracellular matrix pathways (42).

In addition to the known mutations in the MAPK pathway, the TCGA has also advanced the knowledge and reduced the "dark matter" of the papillary thyroid carcinoma genome to around 4% (10). Through the study, in addition to the main driver mutations of *BRAF* and *RAS* in the MAPK pathway, a novel driver mutation in *EIF1AX* was also reported (10). *EIF1AX* is a protein involved in the ribosomal assembly and gene translation (10). *EIF1AX* mutation was found in the TCGA cohort that was almost mutually exclusive with those harboring the MAPK pathway mutations, hence suggesting its role as a novel driver mutation in papillary thyroid carcinoma (10).

Follicular thyroid carcinoma

Follicular thyroid carcinoma is the second most common thyroid cancer and accounts for approximately 10–15% of all thyroid cancers (43). It is similarly more prevalent in females, tends to occur later in life, at approximately 50–60 years old and with an increased tendency for hematogenous spread (43).

Follicular thyroid carcinoma is primarily driven by the *RAS* mutations (13), which include the PI3K-AKT and the RASSF1-MST1-FOXO3 signaling pathway, as well as the *PAX8/PPARG* gene fusion (44).

Phosphatidylinositol-3-kinase (PI3K)-AKT signaling pathway

The PI3K-AKT pathway was discovered to be instrumental in thyroid tumorigenesis, particularly for follicular thyroid carcinomas, from the study of Cowden's syndrome with its associated germline *PTEN* mutation and its association with follicular thyroid adenoma and follicular thyroid carcinoma (8, 45). Similar to the MAPK pathway for papillary thyroid carcinoma, the PI3K-ATK pathway has a primary role in tumorigenesis for follicular thyroid carcinoma (8).

The PI3K-AKT pathway is also related to *RAS*, which is an upstream signaling protein in the pathway (8). Activation of receptor tyrosine kinases by an extracellular signal leads to eventual dimerization and activation of *RAS*, which in turn activates *PI3K* (8). *PI3K* eventually results in the phosphorylation of *AKT*, which then enters the nuclear membrane to result in the transcription of proto-oncogenes (8).

It is likely that accumulation of mutations in the PI3K-AKT pathway eventually results in the development of follicular thyroid carcinoma is thyroid follicular cells, with point mutations of *RAS* oncogenes possibly being one of the earlier mutations. *RAS* oncogene mutations are seen in almost half of all follicular thyroid carcinomas (46–48). The overactivation of this pathway leads to a more aggressive tumor behavior, eventually resulting in capsular and vascular invasion, which defines follicular thyroid carcinomas from follicular thyroid adenomas. This was shown by the markedly increased number of mutations in the PI3K-AKT pathway for follicular thyroid carcinomas compared to their adenoma counterparts (49). It was also shown using *in vivo* models that the simultaneous activation of *K-ras* with *PI3K* signaling can result in the development of invasive and metastatic thyroid carcinoma (50).

RASSF1-MST1-FOXO3 signaling pathway

RASSF1 belongs to a family of tumor suppressor genes that contain an *RAS*-association domain (51–53), which is frequently associated with loss of function mutations or allelic loss in solid tumors (53, 54). RASSF1 functions in cell cycle regulation, particularly with cell death and apoptosis (53). RASSF1 in turn activates MST1, which activates the transcription factor FOXO3 (8). The translocation of FOXO3 from the cytoplasm into the nucleus allows for the downstream transcription of genes involved in apoptosis, eventually resulting in cell death (8, 55). In thyroid cancers, particularly in follicular carcinoma and also follicular adenoma, promoter silencing secondary to hypermethylation of the RASSF1 gene is frequently encountered (56, 57), and this mutation seems to be mutually exclusive to BRAF mutations (57). Xing et al. also reported in the results that the RASSF1 promoter silencing is more commonly seen in follicular carcinomas (75%), followed by adenomas (44%), and was less common in their papillary counterparts (20%) (57).

PAX8/PPARG gene fusion

The last common driver mutation for follicular thyroid carcinomas is the *PAX8/PPARG* fusion protein. The *PAX8/PPARG* gene fusion with its antecedent gene product is found in up to a third of follicular thyroid carcinomas (44, 58), as well as follicular variants of papillary thyroid carcinomas (44, 59). PAX8 is a transcription factor necessary for the development and function of the thyroid gland (44). PPARG is a nuclear transcription factor responsible for insulin sensitivity and lipid metabolism (44). The gene fusion creates a fusion gene product, driven by the PAX8 promoter, which is highly upregulated in the thyroid follicular cell (44). The fusion protein then works as an oncoprotein (44), resulting in accelerated cell growth and division and limitation of apoptosis (60). It is postulated that the original PPARG functions as a thyroid tumor suppressor gene, which is subsequently negatively inhibited in patients harboring the *PAX8/PPARG* gene fusion, due to the excessive oncoproteins translated due to the PAX8 promoter effect (44). Interestingly, the frequency of *PAX8/PPARG* gene fusions was less commonly seen in the Asian population, reported in only approximately 3% in a Korean (61) and 4% in a Japanese cohort (62).

Hürthle cell carcinoma

Hürthle cell carcinoma is a rare differentiated thyroid carcinoma, accounting for only 5% of all well-differentiated thyroid carcinomas (63). They were previously thought to be a subset of follicular thyroid carcinomas (63), with a more aggressive behavior and poorer prognosis compared to other differentiated thyroid cancers (64). Furthermore, similar to follicular thyroid carcinoma, the distinguishing feature between a Hürthle cell adenoma and that of its carcinoma counterpart is based on the presence pathologically of capsular or vascular invasion (13). However, molecular studies have subsequently identified unique oncogenic features distinct to Hürthle cell carcinomas and, hence, distinguished them as a separate clinical entity (63).

Hürthle cells are oncocytic follicular cells with marked eosinophilic cytoplasm due to the abundance of mitochondria (65), which are abnormal (66). Interestingly, though named after Karl Hürthle in 1894, the cells originally described by Hürthle proved to be the parafollicular C cells (67), distinct from the current oncocytic cells we know about which carry his name (65).

Mitochondrial DNA aberrations

The hallmark of Hürthle cell carcinomas, which differs significantly from other differentiated thyroid cancers, is the presence of mitochondria dysfunction with mitochondrial DNA alterations (66). In Hürthle cell carcinomas, the cytoplasm is filled with an elevated number of mitochondria, which harbors aberrations in their DNA (66). This mitochondrial genomic anomaly showed similarities to those observed in cells of patients with mitochondrial diseases and myopathies (66, 68–72). It has been purported that mitochondria DNA is more susceptible to DNA damage compared to the eukaryotic nuclear DNA, and it lacks mismatch repair machinery unlike the mismatch repair genes encoded for in nuclear DNA (66). It is likely that the mutations in mitochondria DNA may have resulted in cellular hypoxia due to a decline in oxidative phosphorylation with a lack of adenosine triphosphate (ATP) production (66), and this resulted in a compensatory proliferation of cytosolic mitochondria (66). In fact, when contrasting Hürthle cell carcinomas with other non-Hürthle cell subtypes, the presence of mitochondria DNA common deletions were reported to occur in every case (100%) of Hürthle cell adenoma, Hürthle cell follicular carcinoma and Hürthle cell papillary carcinomas as compared to 18.8% in papillary thyroid carcinomas, 0% in follicular thyroid carcinomas and 33.3% in thyroid adenomas (66).

The mechanism for tumorigenesis, and the driver mutations following mitochondrial alterations in Hürthle cells and its development to carcinoma, is uncertain. Habano et al. previously reported a positive correlation between mitochondrial microsatellite instability and nuclear genome microsatellite instability, establishing a possible link between a mitochondrial microsatellite unstable phenotype with carcinogenesis for intestinal gastric-type carcinomas (73). However, this positive correlation was not reported in Hürthle cell carcinomas. In fact, Lazzereschi et al. reported in their analysis of 51 thyroid tumors for microsatellite instability, none of the 8 Hürthle cell carcinoma specimens were replication error positive (74). Such findings were similarly echoed by Máximo et al., who demonstrated no increase in nuclear microsatellite instability of Hürthle cell carcinoma specimens despite those having the highest frequency of mitochondrial DNA instability (66).

Poorly differentiated and anaplastic thyroid carcinoma

In contrast to well-differentiated thyroid carcinomas, anaplastic thyroid carcinomas are rare and carry a dismal prognosis (13), usually with a mean survival of less than 6 months from the time of diagnosis (75). A separate entity, with tumor biology that is somewhat intermediate from well-differentiated thyroid carcinomas and anaplastic thyroid carcinomas, has also been described, which were classified as poorly differentiated thyroid carcinomas (76, 77). Regardless, though with some histological features distinct from anaplastic thyroid carcinomas, these poorly differentiated thyroid carcinomas are often also rapidly progressive with an extremely poor prognosis (78). Mortality for poorly differentiated and anaplastic thyroid carcinomas is 38–57% and almost 100%, respectively (79–82).

There are two criteria currently employed for the diagnosis of poorly differentiated thyroid carcinomas. The Memorial Sloan-Kettering Cancer Centre (MSKCC) criteria, published in 2006, based upon the MSKCC's review of 58 patients, classifies poorly differentiated thyroid carcinomas as any thyroid carcinoma with follicular cell differentiation at a histologic and/or immunohistochemical level and yet displaying the presence of necrosis and/or ≥5 mitoses per 10 high-power fields (hpf) (79). Subsequently, in 2007, the Turin criteria, which was a consensus agreement reached by pathologists across the United States, Japan and Europe, based on 83 cases, proposes a criterion based on histopathologic features, which include (1) the presence of a solid/trabecular/insular pattern of growth; (2) the absence of conventional nuclear features of papillary carcinoma; (3) and the presence of convoluted nuclei and/or mitotic activity ≥3 × 10 hpf and/or tumor necrosis (80).

Using next-generation sequencing techniques, the genomic alterations in poorly differentiated and anaplastic thyroid carcinomas were reported (82–86). Utilizing existing knowledge gleaned from the TCGA analysis of the genomic landscape for papillary thyroid carcinoma, the genomic alterations seen in poorly and anaplastic thyroid carcinomas support a stepwise progression and dedifferentiation from well-differentiated thyroid carcinomas to eventually poorly differentiated thyroid carcinomas and finally anaplastic thyroid carcinomas (82), with increasing mutation burden as it becomes more dedifferentiated (83, 84).

Role of BRAF and RAS mutations

Like papillary thyroid carcinomas, the MAPK pathway remains one of the predominant driver mutations, with *BRAF-V600E* AND *RAS* somatic mutations being reported to occur in relatively high frequencies (82–86). Furthermore, similar to their well-differentiated thyroid cancer counterparts, *BRAF-V600E* and *RAS* mutations appear to be mutually exclusive (13). Yet, in contrast to papillary thyroid carcinomas being driven by the same MAPK pathway, there was a marked increase in mutation burden from papillary thyroid carcinoma to poorly differentiated thyroid carcinomas to anaplastic thyroid carcinomas, with a reported mutation burden of 1, 2 and 6 per tumor, respectively (83).

BRAF-V600E mutations in poorly differentiated and anaplastic thyroid cancers

BRAF-V600E mutations were reported to occur in an estimated 33% of poorly differentiated thyroid carcinomas (83) and 7–91% of anaplastic thyroid carcinomas (83, 84, 86, 87). By analyzing the tumor behavioral characteristics with these genetic driver mutations, it is likely that poorly differentiated and anaplastic thyroid carcinomas may have arisen as a result of dedifferentiation from their well-differentiated counterparts, either a papillary thyroid carcinoma or a follicular thyroid carcinoma (85). Poorly differentiated thyroid carcinomas with *BRAF-V600E* mutations exhibit behavior more closely resembling papillary thyroid carcinomas, with a higher tendency of nodal metastases and extrathyroidal extension (13, 85, 88).

Interestingly, the frequency of *BRAF-V600E* driver mutations may have geographical differences. In anaplastic thyroid carcinomas, somatic mutations in *BRAF-V600E* were exceptionally high in the Korean population, at 91% (84), in contrast to the 20–45% detected in American and European cohorts (83, 86). This finding appears to parallel the equally higher prevalence of *BRAF-V600E* mutations in papillary thyroid carcinomas in the Korean population (84), which has been increasing over the last two decades (89). The cause for such differences remains unclear, but it may be due to genetic differences or iodine deficiency (84, 89, 90).

RAS mutations in poorly differentiated and anaplastic thyroid cancers

The pattern of *RAS* mutations in poorly differentiated thyroid carcinomas and the tumor behavior suggest dedifferentiation from the follicular thyroid carcinomas as a result of increased mutational burden, similarly to *BRAF-V600E* mutations (85). *RAS* mutations are present in 28% and 24% of poorly differentiated thyroid carcinomas and anaplastic thyroid carcinomas, respectively (83). *RAS* mutants were also noted to be larger, with an increased predilection for distant metastases, similar to their follicular thyroid carcinoma counterparts (85).

Interestingly, the two definitions employed for poorly differentiated thyroid carcinomas each appears best suited at defining one particular subset of mutants. Landa et al., in their next-generation sequencing of poorly differentiated thyroid carcinomas, reported that 81% of *BRAF* mutations were found in poorly differentiated thyroid carcinomas that were defined by the MSKCC criteria, in contrast to 92% of *RAS* mutants found when the Turin criteria was employed (83). This suggests that while poorly differentiated thyroid carcinomas represent a tumor whose biology is somewhat intermediate from well-differentiated thyroid carcinomas to anaplastic thyroid carcinomas, by their molecular signatures, it may in fact be two separate entities based on its primary driver mutation and the original tumor from which it has dedifferentiated. A molecular signature-based definition of poorly differentiated thyroid carcinomas may be helpful to better allow us to understand and prognosticate this group of tumors.

Telomerase reverse transcriptase (TERT) promoter mutations

Yet, regardless of the original driver mutations and the original tumor for which poorly differentiated or anaplastic thyroid carcinomas dedifferentiated from, further stepwise mutation accumulations are necessary. The telomerase reverse transcriptase (*TERT*) promoter mutation were detected to occur in up to 40% and 73% of poorly differentiated and anaplastic thyroid carcinomas, respectively, occurring in a higher frequency than the original *BRAF-V600E* and *RAS* driver mutations (82).

The *TERT* gene, as its name implies, codes for the reverse transcriptase subunit of the enzyme telomerase (82). Telomerase is responsible for the lengthening of telomeres at the chromosomal ends, which results in cell immortality. Normally limited in somatic cells, mutations in the *TERT* promoter results in the activation of telomerase, which is an important step in tumorigenesis by preventing apoptosis. This is a crucial step in tumorigenesis, responsible for about 85% of the development of all human cancers (91). Furthermore, recent reports have also suggested that *TERT* mutations may exert oncogenic effects independent of its role in telomere elongation as well (91–94).

TERT promoter mutations confer a more aggressive tumor behavior. Even in papillary thyroid carcinomas, the presence of *TERT* promoter mutations were associated with male gender, lymph node metastases, extrathyroidal extensions, distant metastases, advanced disease stage, persistence or recurrence and mortality (95). Expectedly, in contrast to papillary (9–23%) and follicular (11%) thyroid carcinomas, TERT promoter mutations are more prevalent in poorly differentiated and anaplastic thyroid carcinomas (13).

Mutations in the *TERT* promoter results in the creation of new consensus motifs for the binding of transcription factors (82, 91) like the E-twenty-six (ETS) and T-cell factor (TCF) family (91). ETS group of transcription factors are downstream of the MAPK pathway (82), and its binding to its newly created motifs enhances *TERT* mRNA (91). The C228T point mutation in the *TERT* promoter is the more prevalent mutation in thyroid tumorigenesis (91).

In addition, *TERT* promoter mutations may coexist with *BRAF* and *RAS* mutations, which appear to have a synergistic effect on tumor aggressiveness (82). In the presence of both mutations, it predicts for increased likelihood of recurrence and mortality (96). TERT promoter mutations likely play a crucial role in dedifferentiation and transition of well-differentiated thyroid cancers to poorly differentiated and anaplastic thyroid carcinomas (82). This is best supported by the study published by Landa et al., who reported that the TERT promoter mutations were clonal in poorly differentiated and anaplastic thyroid carcinomas, rather than subclonal in papillary thyroid carcinomas (82, 83).

TP53 and other tumor suppressor gene mutations

Based on the stepwise progression model, one of the key distinguishing features between poorly differentiated and anaplastic thyroid carcinomas appears to be the frequency of mutations in tumor suppressor genes (82), with the main tumor suppressor gene in question is none other than *TP53*. *TP53* inactivating mutations were known to occur in anaplastic thyroid carcinomas for a long time (97, 98). Recent next-generation sequencing studies of poorly differentiated and anaplastic thyroid carcinomas also appear to support this finding. *TP53* somatic mutations have a reported prevalence of 10% in poorly differentiated thyroid carcinomas but occur in up to 59% of cases in anaplastic thyroid carcinomas (82–86).

The p53 protein family encodes tumor suppressor genes responsible in repair of the genome following DNA damage, in cell differentiation, control of proliferation and apoptosis. Four mechanisms of p53 inactivation have been described in thyroid cancers (99).

Firstly, increased expression of high-mobility group A factors (HMGA) can result in reduced p53 DNA-binding (99). In anaplastic thyroid carcinoma, such downregulation results in a decreased p53 binding and transcription of tumor suppressor genes, predisposing to epithelial-mesenchymal transition and cell migration (99, 100). Secondly, in anaplastic thyroid carcinoma, p53 is subjected to increased ubiquitin-based proteolysis (99). Thirdly, thyroid cancer cells possess an increased level of p53 inhibitors, such as murine double minute (MDM) family of proteins (99, 101). Lastly, alterations of proteins involved in p53 signaling also contribute to thyroid carcinogenesis (99).

In addition to *TP53*, other tumor suppressor genes also play a role in anaplastic thyroid carcinoma tumorigenesis. In contrast to poorly differentiated thyroid carcinomas, somatic mutations in other tumor suppressor genes were also more prevalent in anaplastic thyroid carcinomas. These include *ATM* (7% in poorly differentiated thyroid carcinoma vs. 13% in anaplastic thyroid carcinoma), *NF1* (0% vs. 10%), *NF2* (0% vs. 9%), *RB1* (1% vs. 8%) and *MEN1* (1% vs. 2%) (82–86).

Role of EIF1AX mutations for RAS mutants

EIF1AX was a new driver gene described in papillary thyroid carcinomas, occurring with a frequency of 1% based on the TCGA cohort (10). While its prevalence is low in papillary thyroid carcinoma, it occurs at a much higher frequency in poorly differentiated and anaplastic thyroid carcinomas, occurring in up to 11% of cases (82, 83, 86). Though described as a novel driver mutation in patients with papillary thyroid carcinoma not harboring *BRAF* or *RAS* mutations, in poorly differentiated and anaplastic thyroid carcinomas, *EIF1AX* mutations appear to coexist with *RAS* mutations (102). Up to 93% of EIF1AX mutants in poorly differentiated and anaplastic thyroid carcinomas contain a concomitant *RAS* mutation (82), and it predicts for poorer survival (82, 83, 86).

Medullary thyroid carcinoma

Medullary thyroid carcinoma is a rare malignancy, accounting for only 3–5% of all thyroid malignancies (103). They arise from the parafollicular C cells of the thyroid gland that produce calcitonin (13). They are familial in 25% of cases and sporadic in 75% (13, 103). Familial cases occur as part of multiple endocrine neoplasia type 2 (MEN 2), an autosomal dominant condition (104). Though a rare malignancy, medullary thyroid carcinomas are responsible for a significant majority of thyroid cancer mortalities (104). The main driver for medullary thyroid carcinomas is the *RET* gene, in both sporadic and hereditary cases (13). In patients with wild-type *RET*, activating mutations in *RAS* were common. In contrast to other cancers, common mutations in various tumor suppressor genes, such as *TP53* (105, 106) or oncogenes like *BRAF* (107), were extremely uncommon or absent in medullary thyroid carcinomas (104).

RET gene mutation in medullary thyroid carcinoma

The *RET* gene is the main driver for both hereditary and sporadic medullary thyroid carcinoma (13, 103, 104). As discussed previously, wild-type *RET* proto-oncogene is expressed in parafollicular C-cells of the thyroid gland (29). In contrast to *RET* gene translocations that occur in papillary thyroid carcinomas, activating mutations in *RET* occur in medullary thyroid carcinoma (104). Such activating mutations result in a ligand-independent signaling of the *RET* receptor tyrosine kinase, resulting in excessive proliferation and resistance to apoptosis (104).

In familial medullary thyroid carcinomas, germline mutations in *RET* is almost invariably present (104). Furthermore, there is a distinct correlation with the type of mutations in *RET* with the clinical MEN 2 phenotype. Mutations in exons 10 or 11 results in MEN2A phenotype while mutations in exon 16 results in MEN2B phenotype, which carries a poorer prognosis (13, 108). Up to 45% of sporadic medullary thyroid carcinomas also display somatic *RET* mutations, most of them being the M918T *RET* mutation in exon 16, commonly seen in MEN2B (13, 104). The high prevalence of M918T *RET* mutation in the sporadic group may in some way explain, in addition to other factors such as age of diagnosis (109), why sporadic group have a poorer prognosis compared to its familial counterparts.

This is further supported by a study published by Moura et al. The group analyzed the various *RET* mutations in sporadic medullary thyroid carcinomas, and further risk stratified the clinicopathological features of the cancer based on the type of *RET* mutations (110). In the study, for sporadic medullary thyroid carcinomas, the presence of exon 16 M918T mutations were present in up to 60.6% of all patients carrying a *RET* somatic mutation, followed by exon 11 point mutations or deletions, occurring in 21.2% of cases. The study group found that patients with sporadic medullary thyroid carcinomas, harboring mutations in exon 15 or 16 (which included the exon 16 M918T) mutation had a higher prevalence of lymph node metastases, multifocality and had more often persistent disease as compared to patients with other *RET* mutations (110).

RAS mutation in medullary thyroid carcinoma

In sporadic medullary thyroid carcinoma with wild-type *RET*, *RAS* mutations are critical in tumorigenesis (104). *RAS* and *RET* mutations in medullary thyroid carcinomas appear to be mutually exclusive (104), and *RET* wild-type *RAS* mutants appear to have a prognosis intermediate between the aggressive *RET* exon 15 or 16 mutants and the indolent other *RET* mutants (110).

In wild-type *RET* mutants, *HRAS* mutations were most common, occurring in 18% of the cohort, followed by *KRAS*, being present in 5% (104). These three mutations account for more than 90% of all the known driver mutations for medullary thyroid carcinoma (104) and appear to be mutually exclusive (104).

Other mutations in medullary thyroid carcinoma

In the absence of *RET* or *RAS* driver mutations, there are no other consistently mutated genes reported. Agarwal et al. proposed that this might suggest there may be no other predominant drivers for medullary thyroid carcinoma in tumors without *RET* and *RAS* mutations (104).

However, Agarwal et al. also reported the somatic mutations in mediator of DNA damage checkpoint protein 1 (*MDC1*) gene in wild-type *RAS* and *RET* tumors, possibly elucidating a role for aberrant DNA damage repair in medullary thyroid carcinogenesis. Recently, the study group by Ji et al. also described the presence of anaplastic lymphoma kinase (*ALK*) fusion genes occurring in 2% of medullary thyroid carcinomas as well (103).

Conclusion

The genomic landscaping of thyroid cancers with the use of next-generation sequencing methods have allowed for a better understanding of the various driver mutations in the stepwise carcinogenesis pathway of various thyroid carcinomas.

Such molecular mapping of the pathogenesis of thyroid carcinomas could hopefully in the future allow for precision-based medicine personalized therapy based on molecular an individual's tumor molecular signatures.

References

1. National Cancer Institute - Surveillance, Epidemiology, and End Results Program. Cancer Stat Facts: Thyroid Cancer. https://seer.cancer.gov/statfacts/html/thyro.html. Accessed 9 June 2019.
2. Shulin JH, Aizhen J, Kuo SM, Tan WB, Ngiam KY, Parameswaran R. Rising incidence of thyroid cancer in Singapore not solely due to micropapillary subtype. Ann R Coll Surg Engl. 2018; 100(4): 295–300.
3. Lee JH, Shin SW. Overdiagnosis and screening for thyroid cancer in Korea. Lancet. 2014; 384(9957): 1848.
4. Rego-Iraeta A, Pérez-Méndez LF, Mantinan B, Garcia-Mayor RV. Time trends for thyroid cancer in northwestern Spain: true rise in the incidence of micro and larger forms of papillary thyroid cancer. Thyroid. 2009; 19(4): 333–40.
5. Hussain F, Igbal S, Mehmood A, Bazarbashi S, ElHassan T, Chaudhri N. Incidence of thyroid cancer in the Kingdom of Saudi Arabia, 2000-2010. *Hematol Oncol Stem Cell Ther*. 2013; 6(2): 58–64.
6. Jayarajah U, Fernando A, Prabashani S, Fernando EA, Seneviratne SA. Incidence and histological patterns of thyroid cancer in Sri Lanka 2001-2010: an analysis of national cancer registry data. BMC Cancer. 2018; 18(1): 163.
7. Bychkov A. World Health Organization (WHO) classification. PathologyOutlines.com website. http://www.pathologyoutlines.com/topic/thyroidwho.html. Accessed June 9th, 2019.
8. Xing M. Molecular pathogenesis and mechanisms of thyroid cancer. Nat Rev Cancer. 2013; 13(3): 184–99.
9. Xing M, Westra WH, Tufano RP, Cohen Y, Rosenbaum E, Rhoden KJ, Carson KA, Vasko V, Larin A, Tallini G, Tolaney S, Holt EH, Hui P, Umbricht CB, Basaria S, Ewertz M, Tufaro AP, Califano JA, Ringel MD, Zeiger MA, Sidransky D, Ladenson PW. BRAF mutation predicts a poorer clinical prognosis for papillary thyroid cancer. J Clin Endocrinol Metab. 2005; 90(12): 6373–9.
10. Cancer Genome Atlas Research Network. Integrated genomic characterisation of papillary thyroid carcinoma. Cell. 2014; 159(3): 676–90.
11. Parameswaran R, Brooks S, Sadler GP. Molecular pathogenesis of follicular cell derived thyroid cancers. Int J Surg. 2010; 8(3): 186–93.
12. McConahey WM, Hay ID, Woolner LB, van Heerden JA, Taylor WF. Papillary thyroid cancer treated at Mayo Clinic, 1946 through 1970: initial manifestations, pathologic findings, therapy and outcome. Mayo Clin Proc. 1986; 61(12): 978–96.
13. Parameswaran R, Agarwal A (eds.), Evidence-Based Endocrine Surgery. Singapore: Springer; 2018.
14. Kimura ET, Nikiforova MN, Zhu Z, Knauf JA, Nikiforov YE, Fagin JA. High prevalence of BRAF mutations in thyroid cancer: genetic evidence for constitutive activation of RET/PTC-RAS-BRAF signalling pathway in papillary thyroid cancer. Cancer Res. 2003; 63(7): 1454–7.
15. Cohen Y, Xing M, Mambo E, Guo Z, Wu G, Trink B, Beller U, Westra WH, Ladenson PW, Sidransky D. BRAF mutation in papillary thyroid carcinoma. J Natl Cancer Inst. 2003; 95(8): 625–7.
16. Morrison DK. MAP kinase pathways. Cold Spring Harb Perspect Biol. 2012; 4(11): a011254.
17. Qi M, Elion EA. MAP kinase pathways. J Cell Sci. 118: 3569–72.
18. Shaul YD, Seger R. The MEK/ERK cascade: from signalling specificity to diverse functions. Biochim Biophys Acta. 1773; 1213–26.
19. Network CGAR. Integrated genomic characterisation of papillary thyroid carcinoma. Cell. 2014; 159(3): 676–90.
20. Durante C, Puxeddu E, Ferretti E, Morisi R, Moretti S, Bruno R, Barbi F, Avenia N, Scipioni A, Verrienti A, Tosi E, Cavaliere A, Gulino A, Filetti S, Russo D. BRAF mutations in papillary thyroid carcinomas inhibit genes involved in iodide metabolism. J Clin Endocrinol Metab. 2007; 92(7): 2840–3.
21. Lemoine NR, Mayall ES, Wyllie FS, Farr CJ, Hughes D, Padua RA, Thurston V, Williams ED, Wynford-Thomas D. Activated ras oncogenes in human thyroid cancers. Cancer Res. 1988; 48(16): 4459–63.
22. Abdullah MI, Junit SM, Ng KL, Jayapalan JJ, Karikalan B, Hashim OH. Papillary thyroid cancer: genetic alterations and molecular biomarker investigations. Int J Med Sci. 2019; 16(3): 450–60.
23. Haigis KM, Kendall KR, Wang Y, Cheung A, Haigis MC, Glickman JN, Niwa-Kawakita M, Sweet-Cordero A, Sebolt-Leopold J, Shannon KM, Settleman J, Giovannini M, Jacks T. Differential effects of oncogenic K-Ras and N-Ras on proliferation, differentiation and tumor progression in the colon. Nat Genet. 2008; 40(5): 600–8.
24. Brehar AC, Brehar FM, Bulgar AC, Dumitrache C. Genetic and epigenetic alterations in differentiated thyroid carcinoma. J Med Life. 2013; 6: 403–8.
25. Rivera M, Ricarte-Filho J, Knauf J, Shaha A, Tuttle M, Fagin JA, Ghossein RA. Molecular genotyping of papillary thyroid carcinoma follicular variant according to its histological subtypes (encapsulated vs infiltrative) reveals distinct BRAF and RAS mutation patterns. Mod Pathol. 2010 Sep; 23(9): 1191–200.
26. Takeuchi K. Discovery stories of RET fusions in lung cancer: a mini-review. Front Physiol. 2019 Mar; 10: 216. doi: 10.3389/fphys.2019.00216. PMID: 30941048; PMCID: PMC6433883.
27. Romei C, Elisei R. RET/PTC translocations and clinico-pathological features in human papillary thyroid carcinoma. Front Endocrinol (Lausanne). 2012; 3: 54.
28. Nikiforov YE. RET/PTC rearrangement in thyroid tumours. Endocr Pathol. 2002; 13: 3–16.
29. Santoro M, Rosati R, Grieco M, Berlingieri MT, D'Amato GL, de Franciscis V, Fusco A. Oncogene. 1990; 5(10): 1595–8.
30. Fusco A, Grieco M, Santoro M, Berlingieri MT, Pilotti S, Pierotti MA, Della Porta G, Vecchio G. Nature. 1987; 328(6126): 170–2.
31. Wirtschafter A, Schmidt R, Rosen D, Kundu N, Santoro M, Fusco A, Multhaupt H, Atkins JP, Rosen MR, Keane WM, Rothstein JL. Laryngoscope. 1997; 107(1): 95–100.
32. Grieco M, Santoro M, Berlingieri MT, Melillo RM, Donghi R, Bongarzone I, Pierotti MA, Della Porta G, Fusco A, Vecchio G. Cell. 1990; 60(4): 557–63.
33. Hayashi H, Ichihara M, Iwashita T, Murakami H, Shimono Y, Kawai K, Kurokawa K, Murakumo Y, Imai T, Funahashi H, Nakao A, Takahashi M. Characterisation of intracellular signals via tyrosine 1062 in RET activated glial cell line-derived neurotrophic factor. Oncogene. 2000; 19(39): 4469–75.
34. Unger K, Zurnadzhy L, Walch A, Mall M, Bogdanova T, Braselmann H, Hieber L, Tronko N, Hutzler P, Jeremiah S, Thomas G, Zitzelsberger H. RET rearrangements in post-Chernobyl papillary thyroid carcinomas with a short latency analysed by interphase FISH. Br J Cancer. 2006; 94 (10): 1472–7.
35. Hamatani K, Eguchi H, Ito R, Mukai M, Takahashi K, Taga M, Imai K, Cologne J, Soda M, Arihiro K, Fujihara M, Abe K, Hayashi T, Nakashima M, Sekine I, Yasui W, Hayashi Y, Nakachi K. RET/PTC rearrangements preferentially occurred in papillary thyroid cancer among atomic bomb survivors exposed to high radiation dose. Cancer Res. 2008; 68 (17): 7176–82.
36. Gandhi M, Dillon LW, Pramanik S, Nikiforov YE, Wang YH. Oncogene. 2010; 29(15): 2272–80.
37. Volpato CB, Martínez-Alfaro M, Corvi R, Gabus C, Sauvaigo S, Ferrari P, Bonora E, De Grandi A, Romeo G. Enhanced sensitivity of the RET proto-oncogene to ionizing radiation in vitro. Cancer Res. 2008; 68(21): 8986–92.
38. Saad A, Falciglia M, Steward DL, Nikiforov YE. Amiodarone-induced thyrotoxicosis and thyroid cancer: clinical, immunohistochemical, and molecular genetic studies of a case and review of the literature. Arch Pathol Lab Med. 2004; 128(7): 807–10.
39. Mochizuki K, Kondo T, Nakazawa T, Iwashina M, Kawasaki T, Nakamura N, Yamane T, Murata S, Ito K, Kameyama K, Kobayashi M, Katoh R. RET rearrangements and BRAF mutation in undifferentiated thyroid carcinomas having papillary carcinoma components. Histopathology. 2010; 57(3): 444–50.
40. Romei C, Ciampi R, Faviana P, Agate L, Molinaro E, Bottici V, Basolo F, Miccoli P, Pacini F, Pinchera A, Elisei R. BRAFV600E mutation, but not RET/PTC rearrangements, is correlated with a lower expression of both thyroperoxidase and sodium iodide symporter genes in papillary thyroid cancer. Endocr Relat Cancer. 2008; 15(2):511–20.
41. Lloyd RV, Osamura RY, Kloppel G, Rosai J, eds. WHO classification of Tumours of Endocrine Organs. 4th ed. Lyon, France: IARC; 2017.
42. Hsu Y, Lee J, Chien M, Chen M, Leung C, Ching S. Is papillary thyroid microcarcinoma a biologically different disease? A propensity score-matched analysis. J Surg Oncol. 2019; doi: 10.1002/jso.25670. [Epub ahead of print]
43. Parameswaran R, Hu JS, En NM, Tan WB, Yuan NK. Patterns of metastasis in follicular thyroid carcinoma and the difference between early and delayed presentation. Ann R Coll Surg Engl. 2017; 99: 151–4.
44. Raman P, Koenig RJ. Pax-8-PPAR-γ fusion protein in thyroid carcinoma. Nat Rev Endocrinol. 2014 Oct; 10(10): 616–23.

45. Liaw D, Marsh DJ, Li J, Dahia PL, Wang SI, Zheng Z, Bose S, Call KM, Tsou HC, Peacocke M, Eng C, Parsons R. Germline mutations of the PTEN gene in Cowden disease, an inherited breast and thyroid cancer syndrome. Nat Genet. 1997; 16(1): 64–7.
46. Bos JL. Ras oncogenes in human cancer: a review. Cancer Res. 1989; 49(17): 4682–9.
47. Wright PA, Williams ED, Lemoine NR, Wynford-Thomas D. Radiation-associated and "spontaneous" human thyroid carcinomas show a different pattern of ras oncogene mutation. Oncogene. 1991; 6(3): 471–3.
48. Rivera M, Ricarte-Filho J, Patel S, Tuttle M, Shaha A, Shah JP, Fagin JA, Ghossein RA. Encapsulated thyroid tumors of follicular cell origin with high grade features (high mitotic rate/tumor necrosis): a clinicopathologic and molecular study. Hum Pathol. 2010 Feb; 41(2): 172–80.
49. Wang Y, Hou P, Yu H, Wang W, Ji M, Zhao S, Yan S, Sun X, Liu D, Shi B, Zhu G, Coudouris S, Xing M. High prevalence and mutual exclusivitiy of genetic alterations in the phosphatidylinositol-3-kinase/akt pathway in thyroid tumours. J Clin Endocrinol Metab. 2007; 92(6): 2387–90.
50. Miller KA, Yeager N, Baker K, Liao XH, Refetoff S, Di Cristofano A. Oncogenic Kras requires simultaneous PI3K signalling to induce ERK activation and transform thyroid epithelial cells in vivo. Cancer Res. 2009; 69(8): 3689–94.
51. Khokhlatchev A, Rabizadeh S, Xavier R, Nedwidek M, Chen T, Zhang XF, Seed B, Avruch J. Identification of a novel Ras-regulated proapoptotic pathway. Curr Biol. 2002; 12: 253–65.
52. Praskova M, Khoklatchev A, Ortiz-Vega S, Avruch J. Regulation of the MST1 kinase by autophosphorylation, by the growth inhibitory proteins, RASSF1 and NORE1, and by Ras. Biochem J. 2004; 381: 453–62.
53. Oh HJ, Lee KK, Song SJ, Jin MS, Song MS, Lee JH, Im CR, Lee JO, Yonehara S, Lim DS. Role of tumour suppressor RASSF1A in Mstl-mediated apoptosis. Cancer Res. 2006; 66(5): 2562–9.
54. Dammann R, Li C, Yoon JH, Chin PL, Bates S, Pfeifer GP. Epigenetic inactivation of a RAS association domain family protein from the lung tumour suppressor locus 3p21.3. Nat Genet. 2000; 25: 315–9.
55. Lehtinen MK, Yuan Z, Boag PR, Yang Y, Villén J, Becker EB, DiBacco S, de la Iglesia N, Gygi S, Blackwell TK, Bonni A. A conserved MST-FOXO signalling pathway mediates oxidative-stress responses and extends life span. Cell. 2006; 125(5): 987–1001.
56. Schagdarsurengin U, Gimm O, Hoang-Vu C, Dralle H, Pfeifer GP, Dammann R. Frequent epigenetic silencing of the CpG island promoter of RASSF1A in thyroid carcinoma. Cancer Res. 2002. 62(13): 3698–701.
57. Xing M, Cohen Y, Mambo E, Tallini G, Udelsman R, Ladenson PW, Sidransky D. Early occurrence of RASSF1A hypermethylation and its mutual exclusion with BRAF mutation in thyroid tumourigenesis. Cancer Res. 2004; 64(5): 1664–8.
58. Nikiforova MN, Lynch RA, Biddinger PW, Alexander EK, Dorn GW 2nd, Tallini G, Kroll TG, Nikiforov YE. RAS point mutations and PAX8-PPAR gamma rearrangement in thyroid tumours: evidence for distinct molecular pathways in thyroid follicular carcinoma. J Clin Endocrinol Metab. 2003; 88(5): 2318–26.
59. Castro P, Rebocho AP, Soares RJ, Magalhães J, Rogue L, Trovisco V, Vieira de Castro I, Cardoso-de-Oliveira M, Fonseca E, Soares P, Sobrinho-Simões M. PAX8-PPARgamma rearrangement is frequently detected in the follicular variant of papillary thyroid carcinoma. J Clin Endocrinol Metab. 2006; 91(1): 213–20.
60. Gregory Powell J, Wang X, Allard BL, Sahin M, Wang XL, Hay ID, Hiddinga HJ, Deshpande SS, Kroll TG, Grebe SK, Eberhardt NL, McIver B. The PAX8/PPARgamma fusion oncoprotein transforms immortalized human thyrocytes through a mechanism probably involving wild-type PPARgamma inhibition. Oncogene. 2004; 23(20):3634–41.
61. Jeong SH, Hong HS, Kwak JJ, Lee EH. Analysis of RAS mutation and PAX8/PPARγ rearrangements in follicular-derived thyroid neoplasms in a Korean population: frequency and ultrasound findings. J Endocrinol Invest. 2015; 38(8): 849–57.
62. Mochizuki K, Kondo T, Oishi N, Tahara I, Inoue T, Kasai K, Nakazawa T, Okamoto T, Shibata N, Katoh R. Low frequency of PAX8-PPARγ rearrangement in follicular thyroid carcinomas in Japanese patients. Pathol int. 2015; 65(5): 250–3.
63. Bhattacharyya N. Survival and Prognosis in Hürthle Cell Carcinoma of the Thyroid Gland. Arch Otolaryngol Head Neck Surg. 2003; 129(2): 207–10.
64. Goffredo P, Roman SA, Sosa JA. Hurthle cell carcinoma: a population-level analysis of 3311 patients. Cancer. 2013; 119(3): 504–11.
65. Ahmadi S, Stang M, Jiang XS, Sosa JA. Hürthle cell carcinoma: current perspectives. Onco Targets Ther. 2016; 9: 6873–84.
66. Máximo, V, Soares, P, Lima, J, Cameselle-Teijeiro, J, Sobrinho-Simões, M. Mitochondrial DNA somatic mutations (point mutations and large deletions) and mitochondrial DNA variants in human thyroid pathology. Am J Pathol. 2002; 160(5): 1857–65.
67. Hürthle K. Beiträge zur Kenntniss des Secretionsvorgangs in der Schilddrüse [Contributions to the knowledge of the secretion process in the thyroid]. Pflüger Arch. 1894; 56(1): 1–44.
68. Sengers RC, Stadhouders AM, Trijbels JM. Mitochondrial myopathies. Clinical, morphological and biochemical aspects. Eur J Pediatr. 1984; 141:192–207.
69. Lindal S, Lund I, Torbergsen T, Aasly J, Mellgren SI, Borud O, Monstad P. Mitochondrial diseases and myopathies: a series of muscle biopsy specimens with ultrastructural changes in the mitochondria. Ultrastruct Pathol. 1992; 16:263–75.
70. Tanji K, Schon EA, DiMauro S, Bonilla E. Kearns-Sayre syndrome: oncocytic transformation of choroid plexus epithelium. J Neurol Sci. 2000; 178: 29–36.
71. Kepes JJ. Oncocytic transformation of choroid plexus epithelium. Acta Neuropathol. 1983; 62: 145–8.
72. Ohama E, Ikuta F. Involvement of choroid plexus in mitochondrial encephalomyopathy (MELAS). Acta Neuropathol. 1987; 75: 1–7.
73. Habano W, Sugai T, Nakamura SI, Uesugi N, Yoshida T, Sasou S. Microsatellite instability and mutation of mitochondrial and nuclear DNA in gastric carcinoma. Gastroenterology. 2000; 118(5): 835–41.
74. Lazzereschi D, Palmirotta R, Ranieri A, Ottini L, Verì MC, Cama A, Cetta F, Nardi F, Colletta G, Mariani-Costantini R. Microsatellite instability in thyroid tumours and tumour-like lesions. Br J Cancer. 1999; 79(2): 340–5.
75. Ain KB. Anaplastic thyroid carcinoma: behaviour, biology and therapeutic approaches. Thyroid. 1998; 8(8): 715–26.
76. Sakamoto A, Kasai N, Sugano H. Poorly differentiated carcinoma of the thyroid. A clinicopathologic entity for a high-risk group of papillary and follicular carcinomas. Cancer. 1983; 52: 1849–55.
77. Nishida T, Katayama S, Tsujimoto M, Nakamura J, Matsuda H. Clinicopathological significance of poorly differentiated thyroid carcinoma. Am J Surg Pathol. 1999; 23: 205–11.
78. Patel KN, Shaha AR. Poorly differentiated and anaplastic thyroid cancer. Cancer Control. 2006; 13(2): 119–28.
79. Hiltzik D, Carlson DL, Tuttle RM, Chuai S, Ishill N, Shaha A, Shah JP, Singh B, Ghossein RA. Poorly differentiated thyroid carcinomas defined on the basis of mitosis and necrosis: a clinicopathologic study of 58 patients. Cancer. 2006; 106(6): 1286–95.
80. Volante M, Collini P, Nikiforov YE, Sakamoto A, Kakudo K, Katoh R, Lloyd RV, LiVolsi VA, Papotti M, Sobrinho-Simoes M, Bussolati G, Rosai J. Poorly differentiated thyroid carcinoma: the Turin proposal for the use of uniform diagnostic criteria and an algorithmic diagnostic approach. Am J Surg Pathol. 2007; 31(8): 1256–64.
81. Siegel R, Ma J, Zou Z, Jemal A. Cancer statistics, 2014. CA Cancer J Clin. 2014; 64(1): 9–29.
82. Xu B, Ghossein R. Genomic landscape of poorly differentiated and anaplastic thyroid carcinoma. Endocr Pathol. 2016; 27(3): 205–12.
83. Landa I, Ibrahimpasic T, Boucai L, Sinha R, Knauf JA, Shah RH, Dogan S, Ricarte-Filho JC, Krishnamoorthy GP, Xu B, Schultz N, Berger MF, Sander C, Taylor BS, Ghossein R, Ganly I, Fagin JA. Genomic and transcriptomic hallmarks of poorly differentiated and anaplastic thyroid cancers. J Clin Invest. 2016; 126(3): 1052–66.
84. Jeon MJ, Chun SM, Kim D, Kwon H, Jang EK, Kim TY, Kim WB, Shong YK, Jang SJ, Song DE, Kim WG. Genomic alterations of anaplastic thyroid carcinoma detected by targeted massive parallel sequencing in a BRAF(V600E) mutation-prevalent area. Thyroid. 2016; 26(5): 683–90.
85. Sykorova V, Dvorakova S, Vcelak J, Vaclavikova E, Halkova T, Kodetova D, Lastuvka P, Betka J, Vlcek P, Reboun M, Katra R, Bendlova B. Search for new genetic biomarkers in poorly differentiated and anaplastic thyroid carcinomas using next generation sequencing. Anticancer Res. 2015; 35(4): 2029–36.
86. Kunstman JW, Juhlin CC, Goh G, Brown TC, Stenman A, Healy JM, Rubinstein JC, Choi M, Kiss N, Nelson-Williams C, Mane S, Rimm DL, Prasad ML, Höög A, Zedenius J, Larsson C, Korah R, Lifton RP, Carling T. Characterisation of the mutational landscape of anaplastic thyroid cancer via whole-exome sequencing. Hum Mol Genet. 2015; 24(8): 2318–29.
87. Latteyer S, Tiedje V, König K, Ting S, Heukamp LC, Meder L, Schmid KW, Führer D, Moeller LC. Targeted next-generation sequencing for TP53, RAS, BRAF, ALK and NF1 mutations in anaplastic thyroid cancer. Endocrine. 2016; 54(3): 733–41.
88. Ricarte-Filho JC, Ryder M, Chitale DA, Rivera M, Heguy A, Ladanyi M, Janakiraman M, Solit D, Knauf JA, Tuttle RM, Ghossein RA, Fagin JA. Mutational profile of advanced primary and metastatic radioactive iodine-refractory thyroid cancers reveals distinct pathogenetic roles for BRAF, PIK3CA, and AKT1. Cancer Res. 2009; 69(11): 4885–93.
89. Hong AR, Lim JA, Kim TH, Choi HS, Yoo WS, Min HS, Won JK, Lee KE, Jung KC, Park DJ, Park YJ. The frequency and clinical implications of the BRAF(V600E) mutation in papillary thyroid cancer patients in Korea over the past two decades. Endocrinol Metab (Seoul). 2014; 29(4): 505–13.
90. Kim TY, Kim WB, Song JY, Rhee YS, Gong G, Cho YM, Kim SY, Kim SC, Hong SJ, Shong YK. The BRAF mutation is not associated with poor prognostic factors in Korean patients with conventional papillary thyroid microcarcinoma. Clin Endorcinol (Oxf). 2005; 63(5): 588–93.
91. Akincilar SC, Unal B, Tergaonkar V. Reactivation of telomerase in cancer. Cell Mol Life Sci. 2016; 73(8): 1659–70.
92. Koh CM, Khattar E, Leow SC, Liu CY, Muller J, Ang WX, Li Y, Franzoso G, Li S, Guccione E, Tergaonkar V. Telomerase regulates MYC-driven oncogenesis independent of its reverse transcriptase activity. J Clin Invest. 2015; 125(5): 2109–22.
93. Li Y, Tergaonkar V. Noncanonical functions of telomerase: implications in telomerase-targeted cancer therapies. Cancer Res. 2014; 74(6): 1639–44.
94. Low KC, Tergaonkar V. Telomerase: central regulator of all of the hallmarks of cancer. Trends Biochem Sci. 2013; 38(9): 426–34.
95. Yin DT, Yu K, Lu RQ, Li X, Xu J, Lei M, Li H, Wang Y, Liu Z. Clinicopathological significance of TERT promoter mutation in papillary thyroid carcinomas: a systematic review and meta-analysis. Clin Endocrinol (Oxf). 2016; 85(2): 299–305.
96. Song YS, Lim JA, Choi H, Won JK, Moon JH, Cho SW, Lee KE, Park YJ, Yi KH, Park DJ, Seo JS. Prognostic effects of TERT promoter mutations are enhanced by coexistence with BRAF or RAS mutations and strengthen the risk prediction by the ATA or TNM staging system in differentiated thyroid cancer patients. Cancer. 2016; 122(9): 1370–9.
97. Ito T, Seyama T, Mizuno T, Tsuyama N, Hayashi T, Hayashi Y, Dohi K, Nakamura N, Akiyama M. Unique association of p53 mutations with undifferentiated but not with differentiated carcinomas of the thyroid gland. Cancer Res. 1992; 52(5): 1369–71.
98. Fagin JA, Matsuo K, Karmakar A, Chen DL, Tang SH, Koeffler HP. High prevalence of mutations of the p53 gene in poorly differentiated human thyroid carcinomas. J Clin Invest. 1993; 91(1): 179–84.
99. Manzella L, Stella S, Pennisi MS, Tirrò E, Massimino M, Romano C, Puma A, Tavarelli M, Vigneri P. New Insights in Thyroid Cancer and p53 Family Proteins. Int J Mol Sci. 2017; 18(6): 1325.
100. Chiappetta G, Valentino T, Vitiello M, Pasquinelli R, Monaco M, Palma G, Sepe R, Luciano A, Pallante P, Palmieri D, Aiello C, Rea D, Losito SN, Arra C, Fusco A, Fedele M. Oncotarget. 2015; 6(7):5310–23.

101. Marine JC, Francoz S, Maetens M, Wahl G, Toledo F, Lozano G. Keeping p53 in check: essential and synergistic functions of Mdm2 and Mdm4. Cell Death Differ. 2006; 13(6): 927–34.
102. Karunamurthy A, Panebianco F, J Hsiao S, Vorhauer J, Nikiforova MN, Chiosea S, Nikiforov YE. Prevalence and phenotypic correlations of EIF1AX mutations in thyroid nodules. Endocr Relat Cancer. 2016; 23(4): 295–301.
103. Ji JH, Oh YL, Hong M, Yun JW, Lee HW, Kim D, Ji Y, Kim DH, Park WY, Shin HT, Kim KM, Ahn MJ, Park K, Sun JM. Identification of driving ALK fusion genes and genomic landscape of medullary thyroid cancer. PLOS Genet. 2015; 11(8): e1005467.
104. Agrawal N, Jiao Y, Sausen M, Leary R, Bettegowda C, Roberts NJ, Bhan S, Ho AS, Khan Z, Bishop J, Westra WH, Wood LD, Hruban RH, Tufano RP, Robinson B, Dralle H, Toledo SP, Toledo RA, Morris LG, Ghossein RA, Fagin JA, Chan TA, Velculescu VE, Vogelstein B, Kinzler KW, Papadopoulous N, Nelkin BD, Ball DW. Exomic sequencing of medullary thyroid cancer reveals dominant and mutually exclusive oncogenic mutations in RET and RAS. J Clin Endocrinol Metab. 2013; 98(2): E364–9.
105. Herfarth KK, Wick MR, Marshall HN, Gartner E, Lum S, Moley JF. Absence of TP53 alterations in pheochromocytomas and medullary thyroid carcinomas. Genes Chromosomes Cancer. 1997; 20(1): 24–9.
106. Yana I, Nakamura T, Shin E, Karakawa K, Kurahashi H, Kurita Y, Kobayashi T, Mori T, Nishisho I, Takai S. Inactivation of the p53 gene is not required for tumourigenesis of medullary thyroid carcinoma or pheochromocytoma. Jpn J Cancer Res. 1992; 83(11): 1113–6.
107. Xing M. BRAF mutation in thyroid cancer. Endocr Relat Cancer. 2005; 12(2): 245–62.
108. American thyroid association guidelines task force, Kloos RT, Eng C, Evans DB, Francis GL, Gagal RF, Gharib H, Moley JF, Pacini F, Ringel MD, Schlumberger M, Wells SA Jr. Medullary thyroid cancer: management guidelines of the American Thyroid Association. Thyroid. 2009; 19(6): 565–612.
109. Samaan NA, Schultz PN, Hickey RC. Medullary thyroid carcinoma: prognosis of familial versus sporadic disease and the role of radiotherapy. J Clin Endocrinol Metab. 1988; 67(4): 801–5.
110. Moura MM, Cavaco BM, Pinto AE, Domingues R, Santos JR, Cid MO, Bugalho MJ, Leite V. Correlation of RET somatic mutations with clinicopathological features in sporadic medullary thyroid carcinomas. Br J Cancer. 2009; 100(11): 1777–83.

14 DIFFERENTIATED THYROID CARCINOMA

Anand Kumar Mishra

Introduction

Thyroid cancer (TC) comprises a group of tumors with strikingly different features and very good long-term prognosis. Papillary thyroid carcinoma (PTC), follicular thyroid carcinoma (FTC) and Hürthle cell carcinoma (HTC) are tumors of the thyroid follicular cell origin and collectively referred to as differentiated TC (DTC). They have similar initial management by surgery but differ in diagnosis, therapy and prognosis.

Incidence and mortality rates

TC is a relatively uncommon cancer with incidence of 1.18 people per 100,000 persons worldwide (1). It is threefold more common in females (2, 3), peaking in midlife in women, which is two decades later in comparison to men (3). In the first decade of life, its incidence is equal in boys and girls. The incidence of TC is increasing more rapidly than any other cancer in the last few decades, and the probable reasons are greater awareness among health-care providers, wide spread use of ultrasound (US) imaging of neck and effects of comprehensive and proactive screening programs in some countries leading to an earlier diagnosis. It may also be attributed to over diagnoses of micro-PTC. The incidence of PTC has been increasing. Probable reasons are exposure to ionizing radiation (5, 6), external beam irradiation and iodine prophylaxis (7). Recognition of noninvasive follicular thyroid neoplasm with papillary-like nuclear features (NIFTP) and its differentiation with PTC follicular variant by histological diagnostic criteria has also led to an increase in numbers of PTC cancers (8). In South Korea, >25% of the country population has been screened for thyroid nodules by subsidized US (9, 10). And this unselective screening has led to TC being the most commonly diagnosed cancer among both men and women in this country. In Saudi Arabia, TC is the second most common cancer in women (after breast cancer), although there is no systematic thyroid screening program (11). The reasons for this are unclear. TC is currently the fifth most-frequent cancer in US females and seventh most frequent in the US population overall (4% of all malignancies) with the incidence tripling over the past decade (9, 10).

Classification

Thyroid neoplasm can be benign or malignant. The malignant neoplasm can be primarily arising from cells of the thyroid lobe or secondary/metastatic to thyroid lobe. The most common metastasis is from renal cell cancers (Figure 14.1). Primary tumors most commonly arise from follicular cells (95%) and less commonly from parafollicular cells (3–5%) and rarely from lymphoid cells present in the thyroid parenchyma (Table 14.1). The follicular cell–derived cancers are further subdivided into well-differentiated PTC and FTC, poorly differentiated carcinoma (PDC) and anaplastic (undifferentiated) carcinoma (Figure 14.1) (12). Follicular adenoma is a benign tumor that may serve as a precursor for some follicular carcinomas. The most common TC is PTC (80–85%), followed by FTC (10–15%), HTC (3%), PDC and anaplastic (<2% each) (Figure 14.2). Table 14.1 depicts the summary of all TCs with their frequency, causative somatic mutations, route of spread and survival.

Risk factors and/or associations

Exact etiology of TC is unknown and some cancer are found to be linked to somatic or germline mutations and certain abnormalities that have been discussed in detail in the following section. Two environmental factors that are associated with the development of TC are local iodine status and exposure to radiation, especially in childhood.

Age: TC can develop at any age, but most frequently occurs after fourth or fifth decade. There are two peaks of this cancer and one is in pediatric/childhood (first and second decade) and second in adults (after fourth decade) (3, 4).

Sex: It is three to four times more prevalent in women under the age of 65 and over this age the ratio is equal. It is thought that female hormone estrogen acts as stimulus for genomic instability and causes development of TC (15).

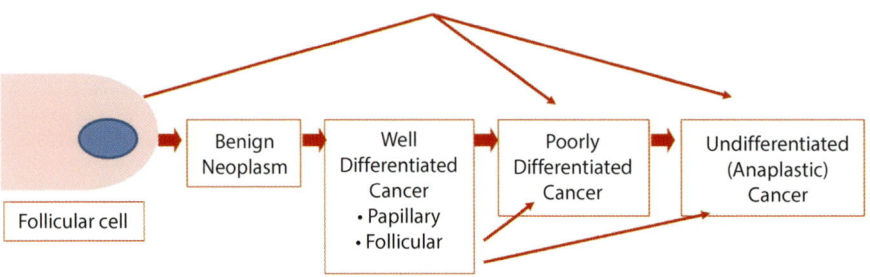

FIGURE 14.1 Stepwise differentiation of follicular cell–derived thyroid cancer.

Differentiated Thyroid Carcinoma

TABLE 14.1: Types of Thyroid Cancer with Their Characteristics

Type of Thyroid Cancer	Cell Type	Mutations (13, 14)	Prevalence in %/Familial Frequency	Main Histopathological Variants	Typical Route of Spread	10-Year Survival (%)
Papillary cancer	Follicular	BRAF (62%), predominantly BRAF V600E RAS (13%) RET-PTC (7%) TERT promoter mutation (9%)	80–85/5	Classic papillary, microcarcinoma, follicular variant, tall-cell variant, diffuse sclerosing	Lymphatic	95–98
Follicular cancer	Follicular	RAS (49%) PAX8-PPARg (30–58%) TERT promoter mutation 17%	10–15/5	Conventional type (micro and widely invasive)	Hematogenous typically to bones and lungs	90–95
Hürthle cell cancer	Follicular	Widespread chromosomal losses Alteration of mitochondrial genome RAS (9–15%) TERT promoter mutation (22–27%) TP53 mutation (7–12%)	3%	Encapsulated group of follicular cells with at least 75% Hürthle cell component	Lymphatic and hematogenous	
Poorly differentiated thyroid cancer	Follicular	BRAF 33% RAS 45% TERT promoter mutation (40%) TP53 mutation (10%)	<2/0	–	Invasive local growth, lymph-node and hematogeneous metastases	50
Anaplastic cancer	Follicular		1–2/0	–	Invasive local growth, lymph-node and hematogeneous metastases	0
Medullary cancer	C cell	Familial forms: RET > 95 Sporadic: RET (40–60%) RAS (up to 20%)	3–5/30	–	Lymph node and hematogeneous metastases	60–80

Genetics: Alteration of mitogen-activated protein kinase pathway is detected in 83% of PTC (Figure 14.3). BRAF V600E mutation is the most common (62%) overall mutation (Figure 14.4). RAS point mutations are most common (49%) in FTC. Telomerase reverse transcriptase promoter mutation (TERT) is seen more commonly in FTC compared to PTC (17 vs. 9%). HTC have widespread chromosomal losses and mitochondrial DNA mutations. RET-PTC arrangements are seen in PTC. More than ten types of RET-PTC locations have been reported; however, three are most commonly found. RETPTC 1 arrangement is associated with classic form of PTC in adults and seen in 40% of sporadic PTC. RET-PTC 2 is seen in childhood (60%) and RET-PTC 3 is

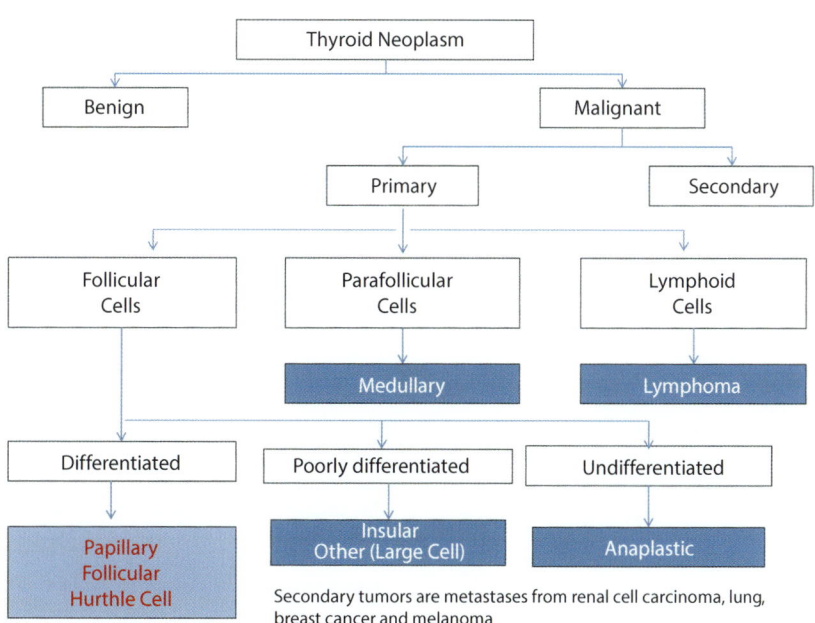

FIGURE 14.2 Classification of thyroid neoplasm.

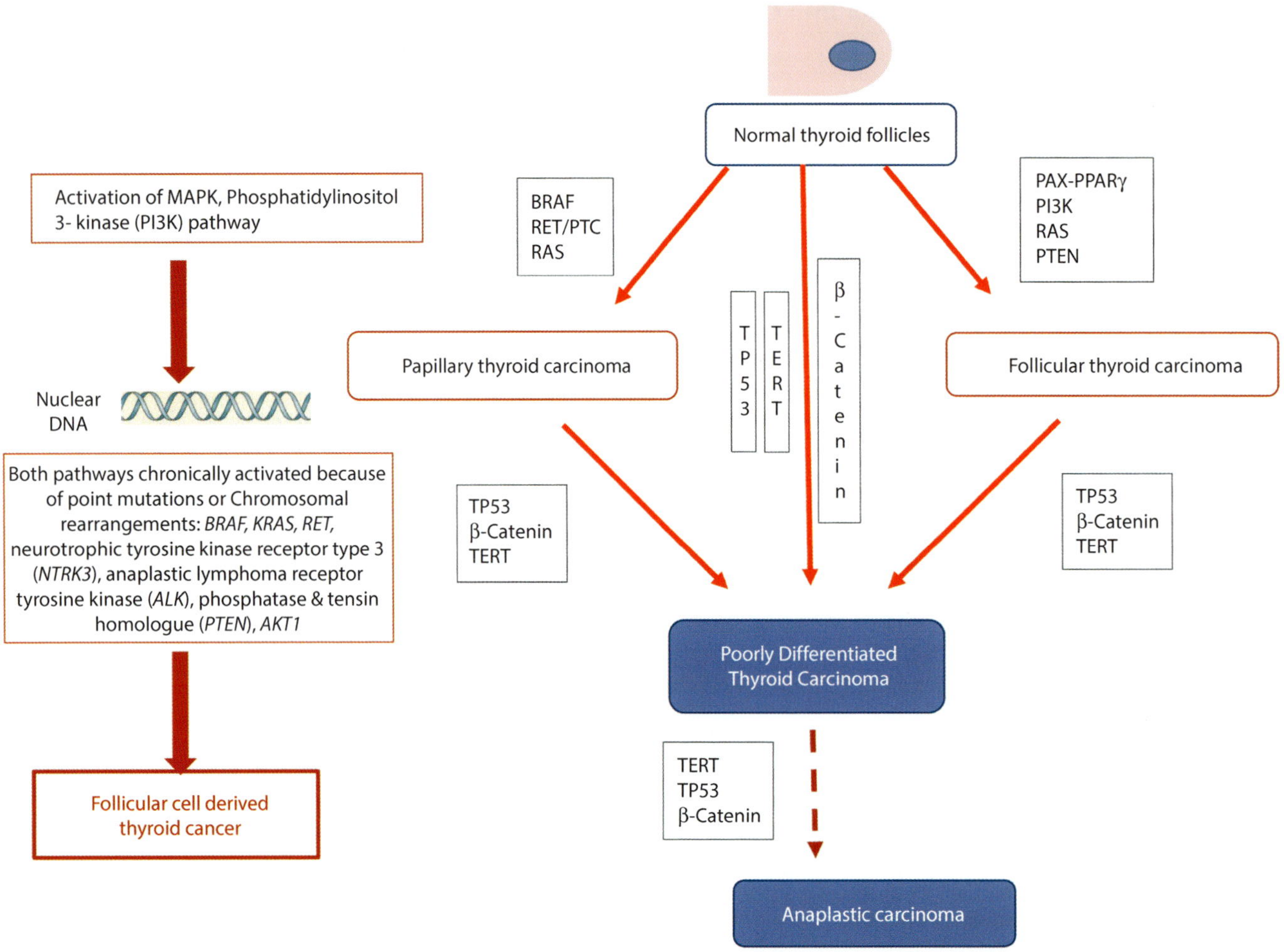

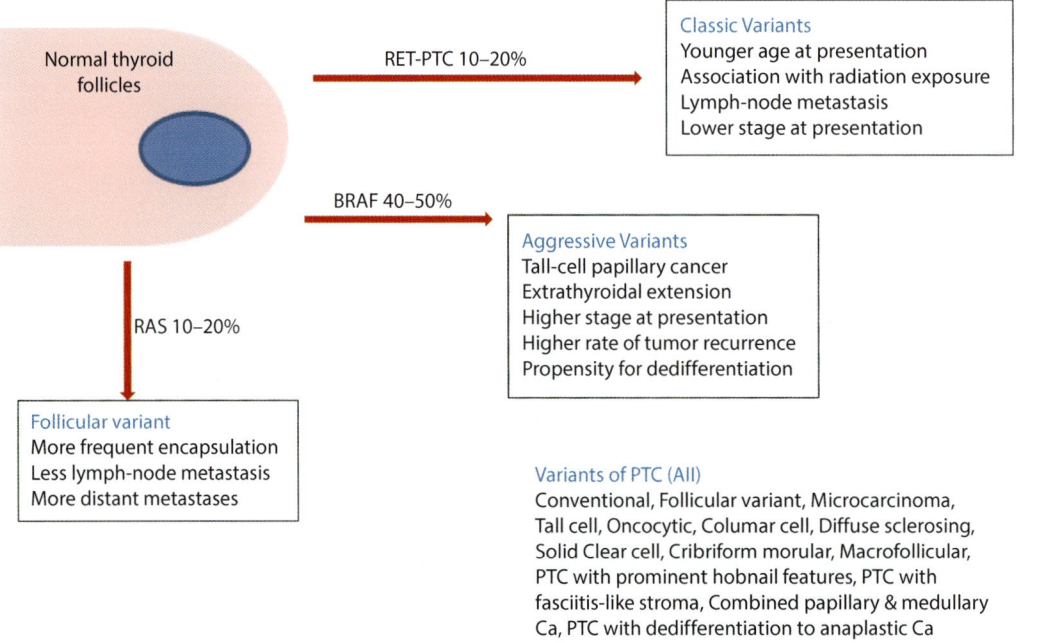

FIGURE 14.3 Pathogenesis of thyroid cancer.

FIGURE 14.4 Molecular alterations and association with variants in papillary thyroid cancer.

associated with solid variant and in children exposed to external radiation (80%). RET-PTC 3 arrangement is seen more than RET-PTC 1 in radiation-induced PTC (13, 14). Radiation-induced PTCs also have NTRK1 rearrangement (5%).

Ethnicity/race: TC is more prevalent in white populations (16).

Radiation: Ionizing radiation (RT) exposure (>10 rads) from external sources from power plant accidents or nuclear weapons or therapeutic radiotherapy to head and neck area (for acne, tonsillar hypertrophy, enlarged thymus, cervical adenitis, sinusitis and malignant disease) in childhood is a predisposing factor for development of PTC. RT-induced PTCs are multifocal. Risk for RT-induced thyroid carcinoma is greatest in pediatric age especially less than 10 years. The latency period from exposure to development of cancer varies from 10 to 20 years (up to 50 years) and maximal risk of malignancy after exposure is at 20–30 years postexposure. RT increases the risk of cancer in a thyroid nodule to 30–40% (17).

Potassium iodide prophylaxis for nuclear accidents: Radioiodine uptake by thyroid follicular cells can be blocked effectively by the administration of stable iodine in case of nuclear accidents from industry or terrorism. This can be given to the population in form of oral potassium iodide pills. The International Atomic Energy Agency recommends potassium iodide prophylaxis when thyroid dose exposure exceeds 100 mGy (18–20). In the case of a disaster, the preventive steps are:

- Pre-distribution of potassium iodide pills should be done to the whole population within a radius of ~500 km from the potential ground zero in the case a nuclear incident is expected. The lowest effective dose of potassium iodide is 15–30 mg for adults or 1–2 mg per ~4.5 kg for children, and it should be ingested within 2 hours after the incident.
- Education of the population should be done about adequate dietary iodine intake as iodine-deficient individuals are at a greater risk of developing TC after radioiodine exposure than sufficient individuals.

Endemic goiter (iodine deficiency goiter): Iodine deficiency is associated with the development of FTC and anaplastic cancer while PTC is more common in iodine-sufficient regions (3, 21). Malignant lymphomas are associated with autoimmune thyroiditis and lymphocyte infiltration in the parenchyma may be the etiological factor.

Association with nodules: Clinically palpable nodule is present in 1% of men and 5% of women and high-resolution US can detect nodules in 19–67% of unselected random population. Single nodule or nodular thyroid disease is associated with cancer in 5%. Graves's disease with a nodule that is cold on scan may have malignancy (15–38%). Nodules of size more than 4 cm may have false-negative fine needle aspiration cytology (FNAC) in 34 and 40% of indeterminate nodules (22).

Family history of thyroid nodule and cancer: Up to 9% of PTC is seen associated with a familial non medullary TC syndrome, but labeling the case as familial requires that at least three first-degree relatives are diagnosed with TC. Medullary carcinoma can be seen in familial pattern in 30% as part of multiple endocrine neoplasia II (23, 24). Other conditions can be:

1. Carney complex type 1: FTC or PTC (4%) and >60% develop mostly benign thyroid nodules.
2. Cowden disease: FTC (10%) and may also be associated with PTC or medullary thyroid cancer (MTC).
3. Familial adenomatous polyposis or Gardner syndrome: PTC (2–12%).

Clinical Presentation

A detailed history should be taken in all patients to evaluate various risk factors that may suggest malignancy. A TC patient gives history of asymptomatic lower neck mass of short duration or a progressive increase in size in a long-standing nodule. Patient may also have symptoms of compression of airway or difficulty in deglutition, recent voice change or hoarseness. The initial symptoms of compression on airway are feelings of air hunger in crowded places like stations, market. Patients later can develop a choking sensation, cough, positional discomfort or frank stridor. Some patients may present with a nodule detected on imaging done for other reasons. Clinical examination should be done to assess the features of nodules and cervical lymphadenopathy, retrosternal extension and tracheal deviation. There are certain clinical features that can suggest TC in a patient with nodular thyroid disease. The features are restricted mobility or fixity of nodule on deglutition, hard consistency, irregular, size >4 cm and associated lateral cervical lymphadenopathy (Table 14.2). Clinical examination of the neck has a variable reliability with false-positive and false-negative rates of around 20–30% (25–27). There are certain clinical features that when present require urgent referral to specialist (Table 14.3) (26–28).

Diagnostic evaluation

All patients with a thyroid nodule are evaluated by initial biochemical assessment of thyroid function. Serum thyroid-stimulating hormone (TSH) is sufficient for thyroid function status evaluation. The other investigations are neck imaging and fine needle aspiration cytology.

Imaging

Clinical evaluation of may be false positive to false negative in the range of 20–30%, and it is highly dependent on the experience of the doctor. Neck can be evaluated by US, contrast-enhanced

TABLE 14.2: Factors Suggesting the Diagnosis of Thyroid Cancer in a Patient with Nodular Thyroid Disease According to Degree of Suspicion

High suspicion	Family history of thyroid cancer, MEN or medullary thyroid cancer
	Short duration with rapid progression of nodule
	Very firm or hard nodule
	Fixed nodule
	Vocal cord paralysis
	Regional lymphadenopathy
	Distant metastases (lung or bone)
Moderate suspicion	Age <20 or >60 years
	Male sex
	Solitary nodule and diameter > 4 cm
	History of head neck radiation
	Firm nodule with restricted mobility
	Compressive symptoms: dysphagia, dysphonia or hoarseness, dyspnea, cough
Low suspicion	All others

TABLE 14.3: Clinical Features Warranting Urgent Referral

Clinical Features in Patients with Thyroid Nodules Warranting Urgent Referral
- History of increase in size (rapid growth)
- Family history of thyroid cancer
- History of previous neck irradiation
- Very young (<20) or very old (>70) patients
- Unexplained hoarseness or voice change
- Cervical lymphadenopathy
- Compression symptoms including dysphagia
- Dysphonia, hoarseness, dyspnea and cough
- Stridor
- A nodule that is very firm or hard
- Nodule fixation to adjacent structures

TABLE 14.5: Ultrasound Features Associated with Malignancy in Lymph Node (29, 30)

Sign	Sensitivity	Specificity
Microcalcification	5–69	93–100
Cystic	10–34	91–100
Round shape	37	70
Peripheral vascularity	40–86	57–93
Hyperechogenicity	30–87	43–95
Loss of hilum	100	29
Cortical medullary ratio		

computed tomography (CT), magnetic resonance imaging (MRI) or PET scan. US is the imaging study of choice for thyroid gland. Surgeon-performed US has now become an essential component of the evaluation. Surgeon-performed US should be seen as an extension of the clinical examination with objective information in the form of imaging. There are certain features that indicate a higher risk of malignancy in the nodule but one single feature is not specific (hypo echogenicity, micro-calcification, irregular or blurred margins or micro-lobulations, intranodular increased vascularity and taller than wide – Table 14.4). US has an advantage, that is, it can evaluate the lymphadenopathy from levels II to IV but it is not reliable for level VI (because of acoustic distortions), level V and superior mediastinum (Table 14.5). CT is helpful for substernal, retroclavicular, paratracheal, retrotracheal extensions, vascular, extracapsular invasions and lymphadenopathy. MRI is useful for soft tissue, muscle or tracheal invasion. It can also detect residual, recurrent and metastatic cancers. T2 sequence is useful for differentiation between tumors and fibroses in an operated neck tissue. MRI provides same imaging inferences as CT but at a higher cost. Most of the surgeons prefer CT over MRI as they can read and interpret the CT images by themselves.

Fine needle aspiration cytology

FNAC is the gold standard for the evaluation of a suspected nodule for TC. FNAC is best done under an imaging guidance as it increases the accuracy, sensitivity and specificity. In cystic lesions, the US should be used to take samples from the solid area. US-guided FNAC is specifically useful in certain situations:

1. Nonpalpable nodules of size >1 cm
2. Nodules palpable but size <1.5 cm
3. Deeply located nodules or in close vicinity to blood vessels
4. Cystic or mixed nodules, especially if a previously conventional FNAC was nondiagnostic

TABLE 14.4: Ultrasound Features Associated with Malignancy in Thyroid Nodule

Margins	Blurred, ill-defined
Halo/rim	Absent, avascular
Shape	Irregular, spherical, tall
Echo structure	Solid
Echogenicity	Hypoechoic
Calcifications	Microcalcifications, internal
Vascular pattern	Intranodular, hypervascular
Elastography	Decreased elasticity
Lymph nodes	Abnormal lymphadenopathy

5. Nodules after a nondiagnostic conventional FNAC
6. Associated nonpalpable lymphadenopathy

In 2007, Bethesda system for reporting of thyroid cytopathology was introduced. It has six categories with risk of malignancy with recommended clinical management. The categories are nondiagnostic, benign, atypia of undetermined significance/follicular lesion of undetermined significance, follicular neoplasm/suspicious for follicular neoplasm, suspicious for malignancy and malignant. In 2017, it was revised with new data available after 2010 for risk of malignancy. The risk of malignancy was also calculated when NIFTP was considered cancer and it also included molecular testing as adjunct to FNAC (31) (Table 14.6). NIFTP behave more like a premalignant condition.

Laryngoscopy

Laryngoscopy is advocated for the evaluation vocal cords preoperatively. It can be easily done by a flexible laryngoscope with topical nasal anesthetics. It is essential in cases of preexisting voice changes and TCs.

X-ray neck

X-ray neck AP and lateral view is required before surgery in all patients to see the tracheal shift, kinking, retrotracheal extension, airway narrowing, existent lung and bone metastasis and retrosternal extension. It can also show the soft tissue shadow and calcifications. Rim or eggshell pattern of calcification suggests a benign lesion, but if this rim is broken it is suggestive of cancer. Bilateral calcification in superolateral aspect of the thyroid gland indicates medullary cancer.

Blood tests

It is also recommended that serum calcium, albumin, PTH and vitamin D should be measured prior to thyroid surgery to assess hypocalcemia postoperatively and calculate PTH gradient.

Serum thyroglobulin (Tg)

Serum Tg is the most sensitive established biomarker for DTC for follow-up after total thyroidectomy (TT). Normal levels are 3.5–56 ng/mL and after TT is <2 ng/mL. It is good marker for recurrence or residual cancer after thyroidectomy. Tg should be measured when patient is hypothyroid by withholding thyroid hormone suppression or after recombinant TSH stimulation. Measurement can also be done when patient is on suppressive therapy. The presence of anti-Tg antibodies can falsely lower or elevate the Tg values so Tg and Anti-Tg both should be done simultaneously. Anti-Tg antibody is present in 25% of DTC and 10% of normal population. There are some studies that suggest that preoperative levels of anti-Tg levels are associated with more lymph node (LN) metastases.

TABLE 14.6: The Bethesda System for Reporting Thyroid Cytopathology: Implied Risk of Malignancy and Recommended Clinical Management

Diagnostic Category	Risk of Malignancy (%)			Management
	2007	2017 NIFTP Not Included	2017 NIFTP Included	
Nondiagnostic or unsatisfactory	1–4	5–10	5–10	Repeat FNAC with ultrasound guidance
Benign	0–3	0–3	0–3	Clinical + US follow-up
Atypia of undetermined significance (AUS) or follicular lesions of undetermined significance (FLUS)	5–15	6–18	10–30	Repeat FNAC Molecular testing Lobectomy
Follicular neoplasm or suspicious for a follicular neoplasm (SUSP)	15–30	10–40	25–40	Lobectomy/Hemithyroidectomy Molecular testing
Suspicious for malignancy	60–75	45–60	50–75	Lobectomy/Near total/Total thyroidectomy
Malignant	97–99	94–96	97–99	Near total/Total thyroidectomy

Abbreviation: NIFTP, noninvasive follicular thyroid neoplasm with papillary-like nuclear features.

Pathology

PTC

PTC is three times more common in women than men with mean age at presentation 34–40 years and seen in iodine sufficient areas.

Pathology: PTC appears as whitish nodules, without capsule and with ill-defined margins grossly. Microscopically, there is mixture of papillae and colloid-filled follicles. The papillae, which are lined by characteristic tumor cells, are characterized by pale, empty or ground-glass nuclei (orphan annie-eyed nuclei) with pseudo-inclusions, rare mitosis and psammoma bodies (50%) (12). Multiple foci may be seen in the same lobe or in both lobes. 'Occult' carcinoma was formally applied to all PTC less than 1.5 cm in diameter but the preferred terminology now is micro carcinoma for cancers less than 1 cm. Besides classic PTC, other variants of PTC are oxyphilic, tall cell, columnar cell, follicular variant and diffuse sclerosing. It spread through lymphatics and locally can invade airways. In these cases, the patient may present with hemoptysis, hoarse voice and dysphagia.

Regional and metastatic disease: PTC spreads to the cervical LNs. Clinically evident LN metastases are present in approximately one third; microscopic metastases are present in one half of patients at presentation. The most common site of LN involvement is central compartment (level VI). The jugular LN chains (levels II–IV) are the next most common sites. LNs in the posterior triangle of the neck (level V) may also develop metastases. Approximately 5–10% of patients develop distant metastases. Distant spread of PTC typically affects the lungs and bone.

FTC

FTC is three times more common in women than men and mean age at presentation is late in comparison to PTC with most cases present in fifth to sixth decades and seen in iodine-deficient areas.

Pathology: FTC appears macroscopically as an encapsulated mass. Microscopically tumor cells may show solid, trabecular or follicular pattern, which may invade capsule or the vascular spaces. The tumors are divided into minimally invasive and widely invasive lesions depending on the histologic evidence of capsule and vascular invasion. Local invasion can occur as PTC (12, 32).

Cervical and distant metastases: Distant spread is mainly blood–borne. Lung and bone are the most common sites.

HTC

They were previously considered a variant of FTC. They have oxyphil cell (Hürthle, Askanzy). These are large, polygonal cells with marked eosinophilic, granular cytoplasm reflective of overly abundant mitochondria. These cells should make up more than 75% of tumor population for diagnosis (12, 32). They are benign-appearing tumors but later metastasize in up to 2.5% of patients and don't concentrate radioiodine. They spread by both the hematogenous and lymphatic route. A total of 20–33% of hurtle cell neoplasm are malignant or invasive. Size of these lesions has been correlated to malignancy and 65% of lesions more than 4 cm in size are malignant.

Staging

Staging systems are needed in cancers for patient management and prognosis. There are many staging systems proposed for TC in the last 30 years from various institutes. They have their own merits but none of them are perfect (Table 14.7). Many of the elements of these staging systems are available only postoperatively (age and gender only known preoperatively) so they are of limited use for the choice of surgery. These staging systems are useful for overall prognosis. Only TNM staging system can be used

TABLE 14.7: Various Risk Classification in Thyroid Cancer (35)

EORTC,79	Gender, tumor histology type, extra-thyroidal invasion, distant metastases
AGES,88	Age, tumor grade, extrathyroidal invasion, distant metastases, tumor size
MACIS,93	Age, extrathyroidal invasion, distant metastases, completeness of resection, tumor size
AMES,88	Age, extrathyroidal invasion, distant metastases, tumor size
TNM	Size, lymph node metastases, distant metastases and age
DeGroot class	Cervical lymph node metastases, distant metastases, extrathyroidal invasion
SAG	Sex, age, grade of tumor (vascular invasion, nuclear atypia or tumor necrosis)
Mazzaferri staging	Tumor size, cervical node status, multiple tumor (>3 cm), extrathyroidal invasion, distant metastases

preoperatively but the disadvantage is that it does not include the histopathology or response of treatment, which is required for the prediction of risk of recurrence and overall prognosis (Table 14.8). The TNM system of TC is unique as it is the only cancer that takes into account the age of the patient (33, 34). Any patient with less than 55 years will be either stage I or II whatever may be the presentation. In general, 80% of DTC patients do extremely well regardless of the surgical strategy employed. Most of these staging systems use the evidence in support of the surgical procedure they perform. In contrast, 5% of patients do very badly and will die of their cancer, whatever aggressive strategy is followed. Various biological factors are inherently responsible for this poor outcome. In 15% of patients, the surgical management employed does impact their survival and here staging of cancer and risk stratification of these patients become important to plan patient-tailored management to have best outcome.

Management

TC should ideally be managed by a multidisciplinary team (MDT). The members of MDT should be an endocrinologist, a thyroid surgeon and an oncologist or a nuclear medicine physician with support from a pathologist, a radiologist. All these members should have expertise and interest in TC management. MDT should discuss all new or recurrent or persistent TC (Figure 14.5).

Initial surgical treatment

1. Nodule >4 cm: size >4 cm of a thyroid nodule, benign on FNAC (Bethesda II) was considered an indication of surgery because of problem of high false-negative rates. False-negative rates in larger nodules are highly institution, pathologist-dependent and are not significantly different from false-negative rates

TABLE 14.8: TNM Classification of Differentiated Thyroid Cancer

T1	Tumor diameter 2 cm or smaller
	T1a: ≤1 cm but limited to thyroid
	T1b: >1 cm but ≤2 cm limited to thyroid
T2	>2–4 cm, limited to thyroid
T3	T3a: >4 cm limited to the thyroid
	T3b: Gross extra-thyroidal extension to strap muscles
T4	T4a: Tumor of any size extending beyond the thyroid capsule to invade subcutaneous soft tissues, larynx, trachea, esophagus or recurrent laryngeal nerve
	T4b: Gross invasion to prevertebral fascia or encases carotid artery or mediastinal vessels
TX	Primary tumor size unknown, but without extra-thyroidal invasion
N0	No metastatic nodes
N1a	Central level VI, VII lymph nodes metastases
N1b	Lateral unilateral, bilateral, contralateral levels I–V nodes
M0	No distant metastases
M1	Distant metastases
Stage I	Age <55 Any T Any N M0
	Age ≥55 T1-2 N0 M0
II	Age <55 Any T Any N M1
	Age ≥55 T1-2 N1 M0
	T3, Any N, M0
III	Age ≥55 T4a, Any N, M0
IVA	Age ≥55 T4b Any N M0
VIB	Age ≥55 Any T, Any N, M1

in smaller nodules. With the recognition of histopathological criteria of NIFTP and its differentiation with PTC-FV (PTC follicular variant), false-negative rates will further decrease

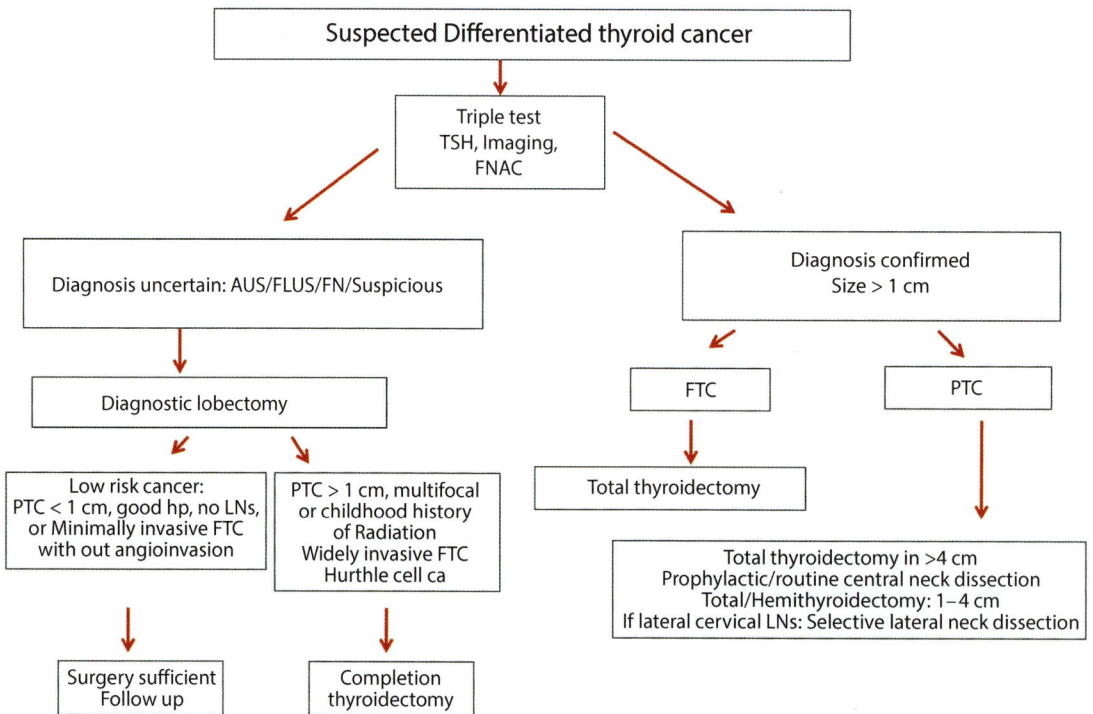

FIGURE 14.5 Management plan in differentiated thyroid cancer. AUS: Atypia of unknown significance, FLUS: follicular lesion of unknown significance, FN: follicular neoplasm, FTC: follicular thyroid cancer, hp: histopathology, PTC: papillary thyroid cancer.

in larger nodules. So, a close follow-up approach should be followed in larger nodules (36–38).

2. Low-risk PTC (≤1.5 cm) incidence has nearly tripled over the last three decades due to increased awareness, diagnostic scrutiny and better imaging opportunities. These patients should be offered a choice of surgery or active surveillance. The unfavorable tumors are those located adjacent to trachea or recurrent laryngeal nerve, high-grade malignancy on FNAC or have clinically evident LN metastases (39–41). These should be managed by surgery.

3. **TC:** Surgery is the definitive management of TC and complete surgical excision of the tumor is most important. For most patients, near TT or TT by an experienced surgeon is the procedure of choice. Table 14.9 has summary of all procedures with their indications. In selected cases, lobectomy or hemithyroidectomy can be done with same long-term results (42–51). In PTC, TT is advocated as the treatment of choice for the following reasons:
    a. Bilateral and multifocal tumours are present in 30–85% and >25% of PTC cases respectively. So, TT eliminates contralateral lobe disease.
    b. Measurement of Tg can be used for recurrence during follow-up.
    c. Radioiodine can be used for diagnostic and therapeutic purposes of metastatic disease.
    d. Lower dose of radioiodine is required for ablation.
    e. Small lesions may grow aggressively with the potential of dedifferentiation.
    f. TT reduces recurrence in all risk groups and an experienced surgeon can perform a TT with minimal or no long-term complications.
    g. Completion thyroidectomy of thyroid remnants may be associated with a higher morbidity.

Less than TT has been recommended for the following reasons:

1. Most patients have low-risk cancer and excellent prognosis and results are equally good with lobectomy/hemithyroidectomy compared with TT.
2. Role of adjuvant treatment is not defined in many patients.
3. Complications rate increase with extent of surgery.
4. Prospective randomized trials could not be possible; TC is a rare cancer with indolent course and overall good prognosis. A prospective randomized clinical trial will require 3100 patients of PTC to be recruited for randomization to see disease-specific mortality, and 12,000 patients of PTC need randomization to compare permanent complication rate with significance with a follow-up of more than 30 years.
5. Occult multicentric tumor is not clinically important and recurrence in opposite lobe is rare. There are excellent long-term outcome with lobectomy alone.
6. Most local recurrence can be treated with surgery.
7. If necessary, ablation of the thyroid remnant with radioiodine can be accomplished with no morbidity.

LN dissection in TC: The LNs levels 6 and 7 located in central compartment are the first drainage echelons for TC and lateral neck levels 4, 5, 3 and 2 are secondary drainage echelons in decreasing order of frequency. The metastases in PTC are seen in central neck in 50% and lateral neck about 30%. Dissection of level 6, 7 LNs is called as central compartment neck dissection (CND). Hürthle cell variant follicular cancer patients may develop cervical LNs metastases and it is predictor of worse outcome in this group. If metastatic LNs are identified in these patients, therapeutic neck dissection should be performed.

Therapeutic LN dissection: Therapeutic LN dissection should be performed in all patients with visibly involved nodes or there is clinical or imaging evidence of central or lateral node metastases due to the increased risk of neck recurrence and mortality (52). During thyroid surgery when opening the lateral gutter or mobilizing the thyroid lobe from trachea esophageal and carotid sheath gutter, one should inspect lateral LN and all suspected LNs should be biopsied. The compartment oriented neck dissection is indicated procedure in all PTC with clinical, radiological or histopathological evidence of LN metastases. In patients with suspicious or clearly abnormal LNs in the central neck, central dissection should be performed. Central dissection procedure

TABLE 14.9: Surgical Procedure for Differentiated Thyroid Cancer

Type of Surgery	Indications
Lobectomy/Hemithyroidectomy	Unifocal intrathyroidal thyroid ca. ≤1 cm without evidence of extra-thyroid extension in the absence of prior head and neck irradiation or radiologically or clinically involved cervical nodal metastases
	Minimally invasive (capsular only) FTC
Lobectomy or total thyroidectomy	Thyroid ca. >1 cm and <4 cm if no evidence of extra-thyroid extension
Total thyroidectomy	Thyroid ca. ≥4 cm
	FTC (minimally vascular or widely invasive)
	Hürthle cell cancer
Total thyroidectomy with LN dissection	Evidence of LN metastases
	Or PTC with evidence of gross extrathyroid extension and distant metastases
Completion thyroidectomy	Aggressive PTC variant (tall cell, columnar, diffuse sclerosing, hobnail)
	With evidence of pathological extra-thyroid extension or LN involvement or both
	FTC/Hürthle cancer after hemithyroidectomy
Lymph node dissection in DTC	Prophylactic central compartment in PTC with evidence of gross extra-thyroid extension, size >4 cm, lateral neck nodal disease and distant metastases
	Hürthle cell carcinoma
	Therapeutic neck dissection should be undertaken for macroscopic LN metastases which are clinically enlarged or H/P proven
Surgical excision of distant metastasis	Solitary and surgery accessible as excision helps reducing tumor mass and facilitate RAI therapy/RT

involves removing all fibro fatty and LNs especially in tracheoesophageal groove between two jugulars from hyoid to innominate vein.

Prophylactic LN dissection: There are views far and against routine prophylactic CND. In PTC, data suggest that about 80% patients harbor microscopic LN metastases. Clinicians do not consider microscopic LNs metastases of clinical importance and radioiodine adjuvant therapy if used will ablate these occult foci after surgery. Many authors argue against prophylactic neck dissection with purpose of removing LNs with microscopic metastases which are not clinically identifiable at the time of surgery. Prophylactic neck dissection does not improve long-term outcome and put patients at more complications than benefit.

Prophylactic CND (ipsilateral or bilateral) is advisable procedure in high risk TC including size >4 cm, tumor multifocality, extra-thyroidal invasion, gross lateral LNs metastases, anticipated radioactive iodine adjuvant therapy (high age, adverse histology, BFAF mutation, PET positivity). Routine prophylactic lateral neck dissection does not affect long-term survival (53).

Arguments in favor of performing prophylactic CND: The rationales for prophylactic CND are as follows:

- Relatively high frequency of LN metastases (50%) is seen in central compartment.
- High-resolution US that is standard preoperative study lacks accuracy in identification of central abnormal LNs and intraoperative differentiation between benign and metastatic LNs is difficult unless frozen section is used.
- Central compartment LNs metastases have a negative effect on patient overall outcome.
- Meticulous CND has a beneficial effect on subsequent course, as it allows accurate staging of the disease and decreases postoperative levels of stimulated Tg that determine the need for adjuvant postoperative radioiodine therapy.
- CND can be performed safely by experts and without extension of the surgical incision.
- Reoperation for central neck recurrence has greater morbidity.

Argument against prophylactic central dissection: includes three main concepts:

- Minority of LNs metastases progress to clinically meaningful disease.
- Lymphatic metastases have not been shown to increase overall survival.
- CND is associated with increased complication rates and reoperation for recurrent disease can be performed with acceptable morbidity by experienced surgeons.

Additional treatment

Thyroxine

Follicular cell cancers have TSH receptors and TSH stimulates tumor growth, invasion and angiogenesis. Thyroid hormone is given postoperatively for treatment of hypothyroidism and to inhibit TSH-dependent growth of residual cancer cells. After TT, these patients are advised thyroxine in suppressive doses. Thyroxine is given in a dose of 1.8–2 µg per kg body weight per day. The dose is decided by risk category of the tumor and associated comorbidities in the patient. TSH level should be measured after 6 weeks. The levels of suppression of TSH should be 0.5–2 mIU/L in low risk, 0.1–0.5 in intermediate risk and <0.1 in high risk of recurrence patients. If there is no suppression, it indicates an inadequate dose or a noncompliant patient. Before RAI treatment, patient is made hypothyroid by stopping thyroxin for 4 weeks. An alternative to thyroxine withdrawal is to administer recombinant synthetic TSH over a 48-hour period to maximize iodine uptake. Recombinant TSH is equally effective but expensive (51).

Radioiodine

Metastases are detected by scanning and treated with RAI as these differentiated malignant cells are iodine avid. RAI is taken by metastatic tissues when all normal thyroid tissue has been excised by surgery. Indication of RAI include tumors size more than 4 cm, tumor with extracapsular extension, LN disease exhibiting size >3 cm or >3 involved nodes or extranodal extension, unfavorable histological subtype (columnar cell or tall cell–variant papillary carcinoma) and distant metastasis. Individualized approach to adjuvant therapy is required in multifocal tumors, BRAF-positive tumor specimens and those with low volume nodal disease.

To increase the uptake of RAI by these cells, patients are made hypothyroid (TSH > 30). Whole body scanning is done after 6 weeks postoperatively when patient become hypothyroid (serum TSH level ≥30 µIU/mL). Diet with low iodine is advised for 2 weeks prior to whole body scanning. Alternatively, synthetic recombinant TSH may be used to stimulate uptake. The RAI treatment is indicated in patients with residual disease, local recurrence or metastatic disease, high-risk patients and in those with a rising serum Tg level during follow-up (Table 14.10). RAI (^{131}I) in dose of 30 mCi is given on outpatient as adjuvant to hypothyroid patient for successful ablation of residual thyroid tissue. It is sufficient in 80% of patients who have undergone TT. Second dose of 30 mCi ^{131}I can be repeated after 6–12 months in case all residual thyroid tissue is not successfully ablated. Whole body scan is obtained 2–5 days after ^{131}I ablation for detection of metastatic disease (51).

Potential side effects are radiation sialadenitis, xerostomia, hypogeusia, transient leucopenia, nasolacrimal duct obstruction and oligospermia. The risk of second malignancy is seen in 0.3%, patients who have received more than 500 mCi of cumulative dose of RAI. Radiation pneumonitis and fibrosis is observed after RAI treatment of pulmonary metastases. Breast feeding should be avoided after RAI treatment. Pregnancy should be avoided

TABLE 14.10: Indications for Radioactive Iodine as Adjuvant Treatment

RAI choice	Indications
RAI not required	Postoperative findings: size ≤1 cm (T1a) unifocal or multifocal both
Not routine	Postoperative findings: size >1 to <4 cm (T1b–T2) FTC with no or minimal (<4 foci) vascular invasion
Consider	Postoperative findings: size ≥4 cm (T3), microscopic extra-thyroid extension, central compartment LN metastases (N1a) or lateral neck LN metastases (N1b)
Yes indicated	Postoperative findings: FTC with extensive (>4 foci) vascular invasion Gross extra-thyroid extension (T4) Distant metastases (M1)

Differentiated Thyroid Carcinoma

TABLE 14.11: Risk Stratification for Risk of Recurrence as par American Thyroid Association

Risk Category	Recurrence (%)	
Low risk	<5	**Papillary Ca:** Intrathyroid, clinical N0 or 5 or fewer LN micro-metastases (<0.2 cm in largest diameter), V600E BRAF-mutated micro Ca
		Follicular Ca: Intrathyroid, capsular invasion and no or minimal (<4 foci) vascular invasion
Intermediate	5–20	**Papillary Ca:** Minor extra-thyroid extension, aggressive histology (tall cell, hobnail variant and columnar cell), vascular invasion
		• Clinical N1 or >5 LN metastases (0.2 to <3 cm in largest diameter)
		• V600E BRAF-mutated, intrathyroid, 1–4 cm, primary tumor
		• V600E BRAF-mutated micro Ca, multifocal with extra-thyroid extension
High	>20	**Papillary Ca:** Gross extra-thyroid extension, incomplete tumor resection, distant metastases
		• Lymph node metastasis >3 cm in largest diameter
		Follicular Ca: >4 foci of vascular invasion

from 6 to 12 months after RAI treatment as there will be risk of miscarriage and fetal malformation.

Follow-up

Few patients of DTC are at risk of recurrence and distant metastases. Patients who develop recurrence or distant metastases have higher risk of death from the disease. Patients, that is, are high risk for recurrence or distant metastases need to be identified so that they can be intensively followed. Therefore, all patients are classified for risk stratification of recurrence postoperatively on the basis of histopathology and response to treatment and other factors. Postoperative risk stratification helps in assessment of not only the risk of recurrence but also overall prognosis and risk of death. Individual tailored follow up schedules and treatment regime prepared on this basis will help in early identification of recurrences and minimize the risk of death. It will also avoid unnecessary therapies which may impact quality of life. Following factors are taken into consideration for risk stratification: age at diagnosis, histology, size of primary tumor, LN status, multifocality, vascular invasion, extra-thyroidal extension, completeness of surgical resection, presence of distant metastases and postoperative serum Tg. On these bases, patients are grouped into low intermediate or high risk for risk of recurrence (Table 14.11). Risk stratification begins with diagnosis of TC and continues after thyroid surgery and all phase of treatment and follow-up. The use of adjuvant treatment is decided by discussion with patient on this basis and it provides a balance between effective therapy and side effects of the therapy. After initial therapy, patient should be assessed for response and risks are modified as new data is available. Patients are categorized in follow-up on basis of response to therapy as having an excellent, biochemically incomplete, structurally incomplete or indeterminate response (Figures 14.6).

1. **Excellent response:** There is no clinical, biochemical or structural evidence of disease.
2. **Biochemical incomplete response:** There is no clinical or structural evidence of disease but abnormal Tg or rising anti-Tg antibody levels.
3. **Structural incomplete response:** There is persistent or newly identified loco-regional or distant metastases.
4. **Indeterminate response:** There is nonspecific biochemical or structural findings that cannot be confidently classified as either benign or malignant. These patients have stable or declining anti-Tg antibody levels without definitive structural evidence of disease.

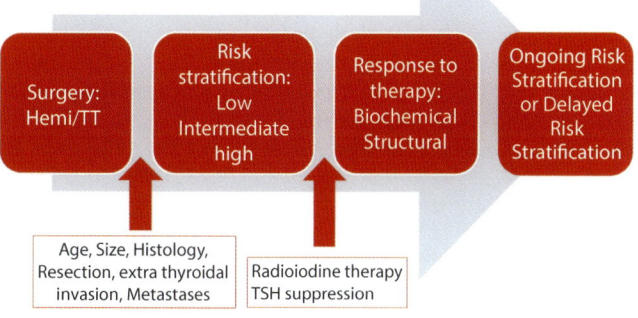

FIGURE 14.6 Follow-up plan of differentiated thyroid cancer.

The level of TSH suppression is decided category of response. Patients are generally followed up by clinical examination 3 monthly, neck US at 6–12 months and then yearly for 3–5 years. During follow-up some of the patients who were initially high risk become low risk and require fewer intensive investigations in follow-up while an intermediate risk patient may progress to high risk. This is called dynamic risk stratification (51).

There are certain prognostic factors that are beyond control while some factors are under control like surgery, adjuvant treatment, experience of the surgeon and timely treatment of the patient (54). These controllable factors should be given good consideration as they can improve the overall prognosis of the patient (Table 14.12). Factors associated with adverse prognosis are older age, distant metastases, unfavorable histology (widely invasive follicular, tall cells, columnar cells, oxyphilic cells, Hürthle cells and insular), large tumor size, extrathyroidal invasion, multicentricity, extensive LN metastases, extranodal spread, high tumor

TABLE 14.12: Prognostic Factors Associated with Thyroid Cancer

Patient Factors (No Control)	Tumor Factors (No Control)	Management Factors (Control)
Age, sex	Size, histopathology, nodal metastases in age >55 years, local invasion, distant metastases	Extent of surgery, postoperative RAI, thyroid hormone suppressive treatment Delay in treatment and experience of surgeon

TABLE 14.13: Bad Prognostic Factors

Factors Associated with Risk of Death	
Independent prognostic factors	**Other possible factors**
Size of tumor	Histology and differentiation of thyroid cancer
Extrathyroidal extension	
Presence of distant metastasis	Molecular tumor profile
Lymph node metastasis in age >45 years	Size, number and location of distant metastases (lung, bone or brain metastasis)
Age of patient	
	Effectiveness of initial therapy (surgery, RAI or radiotherapy)
Factors associated with risk of recurrence	
Presence of regional or distance metastasis	
Completeness of surgical resection	
Size of tumor	
Extrathyroidal extension	
Presence of aggressive histology (e.g., tall-cell variant, columnar cell variant and/or poor differentiation)	
Presence of RAI avid foci outside the thyroid bed	
Presence and number of vascular invasion foci	
Number, size and presence of extracapsular spread of metastatic lymph nodes	
Presence of V600E BRAF mutation	
Postoperative serum thyroglobulin level	

grade, male gender and *BRAF* (*V600E*) mutation in PTC. There are certain prognostic factors associated with risk of death and some with high recurrence. These factors are tabulated in Table 14.13.

Radio iodine refractory cancer

A subset of DTC that has resistance to RAI treatment is termed as radioiodine refractory DTC (RAIR). It is more commonly seen in older age-groups, cases of high-volume metastases, poorly differentiated histology and tumors with high 18-fluordeoxyglucose uptake on PET/CT.

There are four categories of RAIR tumors:

1. There is no uptake in the malignant or metastatic tissue except the thyroid bed during first RAI post therapy scan (**no uptake**)
2. The malignant or metastatic tissue loses the ability to concentrate RAI, which was previously RAI avid after ruling out iodine contamination (**initial yes but no**)
3. Some malignant or metastatic tissue concentrate and some do not (**mixed pattern**)
4. The malignant or metastatic tissue progress despite of RAI uptake (**uptake yes but progression**)

About 25–50% of advanced DTC are RAIR. RAIR DTC show 5- and 10-year survival rates of less than 50% and 10%, respectively (55, 56). These tumors should be imaged with PET scan (FDG PET). FDG avid lesions are associated with more cancer associated mortality. Treatment for these tumors is controversial. Initially a 100–200 mCi of ^{131}I was being given and if there was uptake then repeat therapy of RAI was given till scan became negative. There are few treatment options:

1. If a patient of RAI DTC is asymptomatic and stable on TSH suppressive therapy, only close monitoring is advised.
2. Systemic chemotherapy doxorubicin has been approved by US Food and Drug Administration (FDA) for RAIR DTC.
3. Decision of tyrosine kinase inhibitor (TKI) therapy should be based on tumor burden, volume doubling time of tumor. Patients who have slow tumor growth (less than 20%) per year should be observed (57, 58).
4. Patient who are symptomatic and vulnerable for complications should be considered for options of surgery, stereotactic radiation, external beam radiation therapy (EBRT), radiofrequency ablation, cryoablation and chemoembolization. EBRT is advisable in unresectable cervical disease, painful metastases at critical locations that may produce compression, fractures or neurological symptoms.
5. As per American Thyroid Association recommendations, TKI therapy is indicated in RAI refractory metastases that are rapidly progressive, symptomatic or immediately threatening and cannot be controlled locally by any other approach (51). TKI improve progression-free survival but don't have effect on overall survival (59). US FDA has approved sorafenib and lenvantinib on basis of DECISION and SELECT trial, respectively. The progression-free survival has improved in these trials with TKI therapy from two to six times (60, 61). US FDA has approved Sorafenib for RAIR.
6. Future drugs: MEK inhibitor (Selumetinib) has been seen to 'reverse the loss of RAI avidity in RAS mutation cancers'. Selective BRAF inhibitor (Dabrafenib) has shown higher RAI uptake in BRAF V600E mutation patients. Mammalian target of rapamycin (mTOR) inhibitor everolimus has been studied in phase II trials with promising results as mTOR is involved in the pathogenesis of DTC. Programmed cell death protein-1 (PD-1) inhibitor (pembrolizumab) is also under study.

Bone metastases respond poorly to kinase inhibitor therapy. Factors favoring kinase inhibitor therapy are:

1. Imminently threatening disease progression expected to require intervention and/or to produce morbidity or mortality in <6 months (e.g., pulmonary lesions or lymphadenopathy likely to rapidly invade airways, produce dyspnea or cause bronchial obstruction).
2. Symptomatic disease (e.g., exertional dyspnea, painful unresectable adenopathy), not adequately addressable using directed therapy.
3. Diffuse disease progression as opposed to focal progression (e.g., in multiple lung metastases, as opposed to a few growing lesions).

TKIs

There are two TKI approved for DTC by FDA for systemic treatment:

1. Sorafenib: It inhibits vaso endothelial growth factors 1–3, platelet-derived growth factor, fibroblast growth factor, KIT and RET receptors. It also inhibits RAF kinases weakly. It is approved for ^{131}I refractory DTC, renal cell carcinoma and hepatocellular carcinoma.
2. Lenvatinib: It is an antiangiogenic TKI which inhibits vaso endothelial growth factors 1–3, fibroblast growth factors 1–4, platelet-derived growth factor, KIT, RET receptors. It is approved for advanced and progressive ^{131}I refractory DTC, hepatocellular carcinoma and renal cell carcinoma.

Factors discouraging kinase inhibitor therapy:

1. Comorbidity including active or history of recent intestinal disease (e.g., diverticulitis, inflammatory bowel disease, recent bowel resection), liver disease, recent bleeding (e.g., ulcer or gastrointestinal bleed) or coagulopathy, recent cardiovascular events (cerebrovascular accident, myocardial infarction), recent tracheal radiation therapy (associated with increased risks of aerodigestive fistula with kinase inhibitor therapy)
2. Cachexia or low weight and poor nutrition
3. Poorly controlled hypertension
4. Prolonged QTc interval and history of significant arrhythmia (ventricular and bradyarrhythmias)
5. Untreated brain metastases (controversial)
6. Recent suicidal ideation (suicide has been reported in depressed patients receiving TKI)
7. Life expectancy based upon other comorbidities estimated to be too brief to justify systemic therapy

Role of chemotherapy in DTC

For TC doxorubicin was first drug to be approved by FDA in 1974. Chemotherapy regimens with doxorubicin have shown a 31–45% partial response (62–64). Chemotherapy has poor response rates with short duration of response and because of these reasons ATA does not recommend systemic adjuvant chemotherapy in DTC routinely (51).

South Asia perspective

South Asia has both iodine sufficient and deficient areas. PTC is the commonest cancer followed by FTC and HCC. Iodine-sufficient areas like coastal areas have more incidence of PTC while FTC and anaplastic cancers are more seen at referral centers in northern India. Part of places located near Himalayas, Ganga and Yamuna rivers are still iodine deficient. Like many western countries the incidence of TC has increased in India also. It may be attributed to better awareness and more use of US imaging of the neck (65). In 2014, Mathew et al. (66) reported an increase of incidence rate of TC in Thiruvananthapuram by two-fold from 2005 to 2014. They also reported that TC was seen 1 out of every 10 patients, and large numbers of these were <40 years of age. Later, this study was questioned by other study (67). In 2016, Aravindan et al. (68) reported increase in number of large TCs but with stable mortality in south India. A study done on archived specimen of TC (n = 75) from Singapore (69) reported 56% prevalence of BRAF mutation with locally advanced disease. But these patients did not have poorer survival. Rashid et al. (70) from Lucknow India reported BRAF V600E as the commonest mutation followed by p53 out of five genes tested and BRAF being more common in patients with previous history of longstanding goiter or DTC. They concluded this as an indirect evidence of neoplastic transformation of PTC to ATC. Many centers in India now have MDT for TC which has rationalized the treatment. TT is the preferred surgery for DTC in south East Asia at most centers.

Conclusion

DTC is known for good long-term prognosis; however, 10–15% of DTC behave aggressively include hurtle cell cancers, aggressive variants of PTC like tall cell, columnar cell and diffuse sclerosing variant. Patients who develop recurrences and distant metastases after initial treatment are at high risk of dying from cancer. In last few years, many controversies of DTC regarding surgery, and indications of adjuvant treatment have been resolved. Ongoing researches in the molecular genetics of DTC have made us not only wiser in understanding the behavior of these cancers but is helping us in better follow-up regimes and new treatment options such as TKI therapy, which will ultimately result in a cure for these patients.

References

1. Siegel RL, Miller KD, Jemal A. Cancer statistics, 2015. CA Cancer J Clin 2015;65:5–29.
2. Albores-Saavedra J, Henson DE, Glazer E, et al. Changing patterns in the incidence and survival of thyroid cancer with follicular phenotype—papillary, follicular, and anaplastic: a morphological and epidemiological study. Endocr Pathol 2007;18:1–7.
3. Busnardo B, De Vido D. The epidemiology and etiology of differentiated thyroid carcinoma. Biomed Pharmacother 2000;54(6):322–6. Review.
4. Gow KW, Lensing S, Hill DA, et al. Thyroid carcinoma presenting in childhood or after treatment of childhood malignancies: an institutional experience and review of the literature. J Pediatr Surg 2003;38(11):1574–80. Review.
5. Heidenreich WF, Kenigsberg J, Jacob P, et al. Time trends of thyroid cancer incidence in Belarus after the Chernobyl accident. Radiat Res 1999;151:617–25.
6. Zheng TZ, Holford TR, Chen YT, et al. Time trend and age-period-cohort effect on incidence of thyroid cancer in Connecticut, 1935–1992. Int J Cancer 1996;67:504–9.
7. Huszno B, Szybinski Z, Przybylik-Mazurek E, et al. Influence of iodine deficiency and iodine prophylaxis on thyroid cancer histotypes and incidence in endemic goiter area. J Endocrinol Invest 2003;26(2 Suppl):71–6.
8. Leenhardt L, Bernier MO, Boin-Pineau MH, et al. Advances in diagnostic practices affect thyroid cancer incidence in France. Eur J Endocrinol 2004;150(2):133–9.
9. Mao Y, Xing M. Recent incidences and differential trends of thyroid cancer in the USA. Endocr Relat Cancer 2016;23(4):313–22.
10. Kitahara C, Sosa J. The changing incidence of thyroid cancer. Nat Rev Endocrinol 2016;12:646–53.
11. Hussain F, Iqbal S, Mehmood A, Bazarbashi S, El Hassan T, Chaudhri N. Incidence of thyroid cancer in the Kingdom of Saudi Arabia, 2000-2010. Hematol Oncol Stem Cell Ther 2013;6(2):58–64.
12. Lloyd RV, Osamura RY, Kloppel G, et al. WHO classification of tumours of endocrine organs. Lyon: International Agency for Research on Cancer (IARC); 2017. Classification.
13. Xing M. Molecular pathogenesis and mechanisms of thyroid cancer. Nat Rev Cancer 2013;13(3):184–99. Genetics.
14. Haroon Al Rasheed MR, Xu B. Molecular alterations in thyroid carcinoma. Surg Pathol Clin 2019;12(4):921–30.
15. Li JJ, Weroha SJ, Lingle WL, Papa D, Salisbury JL, Li SA. Estrogen mediates Aurora – a overexpression, centrosome amplification, chromosomal instability, and breast cancer in female ACI rats. Proc Natl Acad Sci U S A 2004;101(52):18123–8.
16. Weeks KS, Kahl AR, Lynch CF, Charlton ME. Racial/ethnic differences in thyroid cancer incidence in the United States, 2007-2014. Cancer 2018;124(7):1483–91.
17. Iglesias ML, Schmidt A, Ghuzlan AA, Lacroix L, Vathaire F, Chevillard S, Schlumberger M. Radiation exposure and thyroid cancer: a review. Arch Endocrinol Metab 2017;61(2):180–7.
18. Becker DV, Zanzonico P. Potassium iodide for thyroid blockade in a reactor accident: administrative policies that govern its use. Thyroid 1997;7:193–7.
19. Franić Z. Iodine prophylaxis and nuclear accidents. Arh Hig Rada Toksikol 1999;50:223–33.
20. Braverman ER, et al. Managing terrorism or accidental nuclear errors, preparing for iodine-131 emergencies: a comprehensive review. Int J Environ Res Publ Health 2014;11:7803–4.
21. Harach HR, Escalante DA, Day ES. Thyroid cancer and thyroiditis in Salta, Argentina: a 40-yr study in relation to iodine prophylaxis. Endocr Pathol 2002;13(3):175–81.
22. McCoy KL, Jabbour N, Ogilvie JB, Ohori NP, Carty SE, Yim JH. The incidence of cancer and rate of false-negative cytology in thyroid nodules greater than or equal to 4 cm in size. Surgery 2007;142(6):837–44; discussion 844.
23. Richards ML. Familial syndromes associated with thyroid cancer in the era of personalized medicine. Thyroid 2010;20(7):707–13.
24. Nosé V. Familial thyroid cancer: a review. Mod Pathol 2011;24(Suppl 2):S19–S33.
25. Ali S, Tiwari RM, Snow GB. False-positive and false-negative neck nodes. Head Neck Surg 1985;8(2):78–82.
26. Perros P, et al. Guidelines for the management of thyroid cancer. Clin Endocrinol (Oxf) 2014;81(Suppl 1):1–122.
27. Hegedüs L. Clinical practice. The thyroid nodule. N Engl J Med 2004;351(17):1764–71.
28. Mazzaferri EL. Management of a solitary thyroid nodule. N Engl J Med 1993;328(8):553–9.
29. Xie C, Cox P, Taylor N, LaPorte S. Ultrasonography of thyroid nodules: a pictorial review. Insights Imaging 2016;7(1):77–86.
30. Liu Z, Zeng W, Liu C, et al. Diagnostic accuracy of ultrasonographic features for lymph node metastasis in papillary thyroid microcarcinoma: a single-center retrospective study. World J Surg Oncol 2017;15:32.
31. Cibas ES, Ali SZ. The 2017 Bethesda system for reporting thyroid cytopathology. Thyroid 2017;27(11):1341–6.

32. Grani G, Lamartina L, Durante C, Filetti S, Cooper DS. Follicular thyroid cancer and Hürthle cell carcinoma: challenges in diagnosis, treatment, and clinical management. Lancet Diabetes Endocrinol 2018;6(6):500–14.
33. Kim K, Kim JH, Park IS, Rho YS, Kwon GH, Lee DJ. The updated AJCC/TNM staging system for papillary thyroid cancer (8th edition): from the perspective of genomic analysis. World J Surg 2018;42(11):3624–31.
34. Lamartina L, Grani G, Arvat E, et al. 8th Edition of the AJCC/TNM staging system of thyroid cancer: what to expect (ITCO#2). Endocr Relat Cancer 2018;25(3):L7–11.
35. Lang BH, Lo CY, Chan WF, et al. Staging systems for papillary thyroid carcinoma: a review and comparison. Ann Surg 2007;245:366–78.
36. Lubitz CC, Faquin WC, Yang J, et al. Clinical and cytological features predictive of malignancy in thyroid follicular neoplasms. Thyroid 2010;20(1):25–31.
37. Choi YJ, Yun JS, Kim DH. Clinical and ultrasound features of cytology diagnosed follicular neoplasm. Endocr J 2009;56(3):383–9.
38. Raber W, Kaserer K, Niederle B, Vierhapper H. Risk factors for malignancy of thyroid nodules initially identified as follicular neoplasia by fine-needle aspiration: results of a prospective study of one hundred twenty patients. Thyroid 2000;10(8):709–12.
39. Ito Y, Kudo T, Kobayashi K, Miya A, Ichihara K, Miyauchi A. Prognostic factors for recurrence of papillary thyroid carcinoma in the lymph nodes, lung, and bone: analysis of 5,768 patients with average 10-year follow-up. World J Surg 2012;36:1274–8.
40. Pacini F. Observation for newly diagnosed micro-papillary thyroid cancer: is now the time? J Endocrinol Invest 2015;38(1):101–2.
41. Sun H, Dionigi G. Active surveillance for micro-papillary thyroid carcinoma: who are candidates, how should they be followed, when should they be treated, and what are the clinical and pathologic outcomes after delayed intervention. Surgery 2018;163(6):1325–9.
42. Hay ID, Grant CS, Taylor WF, et al. Ipsilateral lobectomy versus bilateral lobar resection in papillary thyroid carcinoma: a retrospective analysis of surgical outcome using a novel prognostic scoring system. Surgery 1988;102:1088.
43. Cady B, Rossi R. An expanded view of risk-group definition in differentiated thyroid carcinoma. Surgery 1988;104:947.
44. Hay ID, Bergstralh EJ, Goellner JR, et al. Predicting outcome in papillary thyroid carcinoma: development of a reliable scoring system in a cohort of 1779 patients surgically treated at one institution during 1940 through 1989. Surgery 1993;114:1050–8.
45. Adam MA, Pura J, Gu L, et al. Extent of surgery for papillary thyroid cancer is not associated with survival: an analysis of 61,775 patients. Ann Surg 2014;260:601–5, discussion 605–7.
46. DeGroot LJ, Kaplan EL, McCormick M, Straus FH II. Natural history, treatment and course of papillary thyroid carcinoma. J Clin Endocrinol Metab 1990;71:414–24.
47. DeGroot LJ, Kaplan EL, Straus FH II, Shukla MS. Does the method of management of papillary thyroid carcinoma make a difference in outcome? World J Surg 1994;18:123–30.
48. Mazzaferri EL, Jhiang SM. Long-term impact of initial surgical and medical therapy on papillary and follicular thyroid cancer. Am J Med 1994;97:418–28.
49. Mills SC, Haq M, Smellie WJB, Harmer C. Hürthle cell carcinoma of the thyroid: retrospective review of 62 patients treated at the Royal Marsden Hospital between 1946 and 2003. Eur J Surg Oncol 2009;35(3):230–4.
50. Arganini M, Behar R, Wu FL, et al. Hürthle cell tumors: a twenty-five-year experience. Surgery 1986;100:1108.
51. Haugen BR, Alexander EK, Bible KC, et al. 2015 American Thyroid Association management guidelines for adult patients with thyroid nodules and differentiated thyroid cancer: the American Thyroid Association Guidelines Task Force on thyroid nodules and differentiated thyroid cancer. Thyroid 2016;26:1–133.
52. Podnos YD, Smith D, Wagman LD, et al. The implication of lymph node metastasis on survival in patients with well-differentiated thyroid cancer. Am Surg 2005;71:731–4.
53. Carling T, Carty SE, Ciarleglio MM, et al. American Thyroid Association design and feasibility of a prospective randomized controlled trial of prophylactic central lymph node dissection for papillary thyroid carcinoma. Thyroid 2012;22:237–44.
54. Moosa M, Mazzaferri EL. Management of thyroid neoplasms. In: Cummings C, Fredrickson J, Harker LA, Krause CJ, Richardson MA, Schuller DE, editors. Otolaryngology Head and Neck Surgery. 3rd ed. Stuttgart: Thieme Medical; 1998. pp. 2480–518.
55. Nixon IJ, Whitcher MM, Palmer FL, et al. The impact of distant metastases at presentation on prognosis in patients differentiated carcinoma of the thyroid gland. Thyroid 2012;22:884–9.
56. Durante C, Haddy N, Baudin E, et al. Long-term outcome of 444 patients with distant metastases from papillary and follicular thyroid carcinoma: benefits and limits of radioiodine therapy. J Clin Endocrinol Metab 2006;91:2892–9.
57. Tumino D, Frasca F, Newbold K. Updates on the management of advanced, metastatic, and radioiodine refractory differentiated thyroid cancer. Front Endocrinol 2017;8:312.
58. Sabra MM, Sherman EJ, Tuttle RM. Tumor volume doubling time of pulmonary metastases predicts overall survival and can guide the initiation of multikinase inhibitor therapy in patients with metastatic, follicular cell-derived thyroid carcinoma. Cancer 2017;123:2955–64.
59. Worden F. Treatment strategies for radioactive iodine-refractory differentiated thyroid cancer. Ther Adv Med Oncol 2014;6:267–79.
60. Brose MS, Nutting CM, Jarzab B, Elisei R, Siena S, et al. Sorafenib in radioactive iodine-refractory, locally advanced or metastatic differentiated thyroid cancer: a randomised, double-blind, phase 3 trial. Lancet 2014;384:319–28.
61. Schlumberger M, Tahara M, Wirth LJ, et al. Lenvatinib versus placebo in radioiodine-refractory thyroid cancer. N Engl J Med 2015;372(7):621–30.
62. Gottlieb JA, Hill CS. Chemotherapy of thyroid cancer with adriamycin. Experience with 30 patients. N Engl J Med 1974;290:193–7.
63. Pacini F. Thyroid microcarcinoma. Best Pract Res Clin Endocrinol Metab 2012;26:381–9.
64. Droz JP, Schlumberger M, Rougier P, et al. Chemotherapy in metastatic nonanaplastic thyroid cancer: experience at the Institut Gustave-Roussy. Tumori 1990;76:480–3.
65. Veedu JS, Mathew A. Are we missing the elephant in the room? A case for thyroid cancer over diagnosis as the etiology for its increasing incidence in India. J Glob Oncol 2018;4:1–3.
66. Mathew IE, Mathew A. Rising thyroid cancer incidence in southern India: an epidemic of over diagnosis? J Endocr Soc 2017;1:480–7.
67. Pai SA. Increase in thyroid cancer incidence in Kerala-real or artificial? News from here and there. Natl Med J India 2017;30:180–1.
68. Aravindan KP. Papillary thyroid cancer: why the increase and what can be done? Indian J Cancer 2017;54(3):491–2.
69. Goh X, Lum J, Yang SP, et al. BRAF mutation in papillary thyroid cancer – prevalence and clinical correlation in a South-East Asian cohort. Clin Otolaryngol 2019;44(2):114–23.
70. Rashid M, Agarwal A, Pradhan R, et al. Genetic alterations in anaplastic thyroid carcinoma. Indian J Endocrinol Metab 2019;23(4):480–5.

15
PAPILLARY MICROCARCINOMA OF THYROID

K.M.M. Vishvak Chanthar and Sabaretnam Mayilvaganan

Introduction

Thyroid carcinoma is the most common endocrine malignancy worldwide, among which papillary thyroid carcinoma (PTC) accounts for nearly 90%. The incidence of carcinoma thyroid increased rapidly in the past four decades with mortality rate from thyroid carcinoma remaining stable. These increases is thought to be due to the introduction of thyroid cancer screening programs and increased identification of papillary thyroid microcarcinoma (PMC).

World Health Organization (WHO) Histologic Classification (1988) defined papillary microcarcinoma as PTCs with a maximum dimension ≤10 mm, irrespective of the presence or absence of aggressive malignant behavior such as vocal cord palsy, multicentricity, tumor subtype, invasiveness, risk group stratification, clinically evident lymph node metastasis and distant metastasis. WHOs' global cancer report (2014) stated that more than 50% of new-onset thyroid carcinomas are PMCs[1]. Traditionally, PMCs are classified on the basis of its detection into (i) incidental PMC – incidentally found in pathological specimen of thyroid that was operated for other causes or in imaging done for other purposes or for screening of other thyroid disorders; (ii) latent PMC – detected in autopsy of patients who died of other causes; and (iii) occult PMC – discovered as a cause of neck secondaries or distant metastasis.

Epidemiology

A total of 39–50% of all thyroid cancers are PMC[2,3–5]. PMCs were found in 5–10% of thyroidectomy specimens done for benign conditions[6] or detected in 15% at autopsy series[7] of patients who died of non-thyroid disease. Ultrasonography can readily detect latent PMC of 3–10 mm in 0.5–5.2% of the examinations[8]. A modest increase in thyroid carcinoma cases was reported over the past three decades in United States, Japan, Korea, Italy, France, England, Scotland and Australia presumably due to increased identification rate of PMC. The introduction of screening for thyroid cancer in the west has led to the overdiagnosis and sometimes overtreatment of PMC. These are usually clinically indolent, slow growing tumors with an excellent prognosis with a 10 year survival rate of 99.5%[9]. The surgery is often contemplated after disease progression. Nevertheless, 18.7% of patients present with more aggressive phenotype, including central lymph node metastasis (8%), lateral lymph node metastasis (4.4%), gross extrathyroidal extension (ETE) (0.3%) and distant metastasis (0.4%), which reiterates the need of a better understanding of the natural history of these tumors and their optimal management strategy[10].

Clinical presentation

PMCs often do not cause any symptoms, given the size of tumors is ≤1 cm. The vast majority are diagnosed incidentally from neck imaging or screening studies or while evaluation of another palpable thyroid nodule or from thyroidectomy specimen done for benign conditions (Figure 15.1).

Majority of patients are in their fourth or fifth decade with female sex preponderance in nearly 80–85%. Interestingly, male predominance was documented in autopsy series in a range of 55–58%. No association of iodine intake and PMC has been documented. Most PMCs are clinically inapparent or non-palpable; however, 15–43.8% of patients with PMC have multifocality[8] and 18–80% have lymph nodal metastasis[11–13] (Table 15.1). Central compartment lymph nodal metastasis is more common than lateral neck metastasis but is usually undetectable due to low sensitivity of ultrasound. Approximately 65% of central compartment lymph nodal metastasis and ~10% of lateral neck lymph nodal metastasis were reported in patients with PMC[14,15–17]. Preoperative predictive factors for lymph node metastasis in PMC includes multifocality, bilaterality, male gender, age <45 years, nodule size more than 5 mm and ETE[18,19]. Moreover, independent predictive factors for lateral neck lymph nodal metastasis include superior pole tumor location[20], presence of microcalcifications, Hashimoto's thyroiditis, central compartment lymph nodal metastasis, ETE and multifocality but not BRAF mutation[21,22]. High-resolution ultrasonography remains the mainstay of evaluation of a thyroid nodule. Ultrasound features of malignancy include hypoechogenicity, a taller-than-wider shape nodule (anteroposterior-to-transverse diameter ratio >1), ill-defined margin, punctuate microcalcifications within the nodule and peripheral or intra-nodular vascularity[23]. The American Thyroid Association (ATA) recommends against biopsy of thyroid nodules ≤1 cm size unless there are symptoms and ultrasonographic features of potential malignant behavior. There is no clear documentation available to forego the biopsy of the thyroid nodule harboring PMC, based on this ATA guideline[24]. The definitions for descriptive terminologies used in this context are summarized in Table 15.2.

Sugitani and Fujimoto reported a pronounced prognostic difference after surgery in patients with and without symptoms[25]. Patients with symptomatic PMC with clinically evident lymph node metastasis and/or vocal cord palsy had a recurrence rate of 30% and a cause-specific survival rate of 74.1% at 10 years, while asymptomatic PMCs without these features had a recurrence rate of 3% and 100%, respectively.

Active surveillance of PMC

PMCs have a favorable prognosis with a low progression rate even if not treated by surgery. In view of its excellent prognosis, some groups have advocated active surveillance (AS) by avoiding upfront surgery in an effort to distinguish the PMC that will eventually progress and those that will remain indolent for years. The group that proposes AS favors to delay surgery to avoid surgical complications in patients with indolent PMC, such as recurrent laryngeal nerve (RLN) injury and hypoparathyroidism. The largest prospective study on AS of PMC was initiated by Dr. Akira Miyauchi in Kuma Hospital of

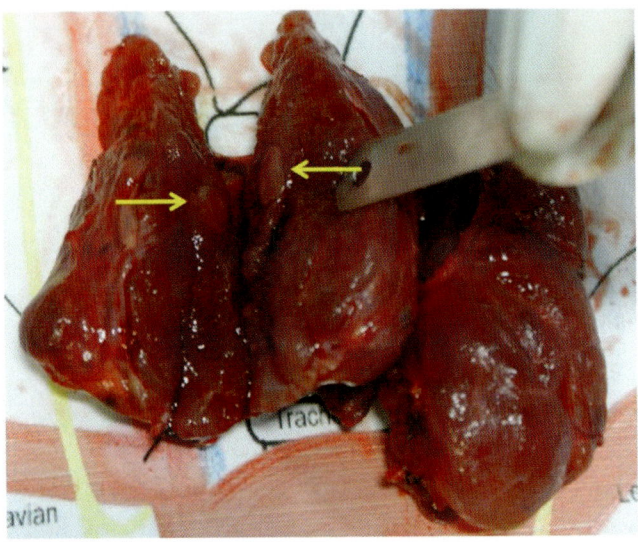

FIGURE 15.1 Incidental finding of PMC from thyroidectomy specimen operated for benign cause (arrow).

TABLE 15.1: Presenting Characteristics of Papillary Thyroid Microcarcinoma

Characteristics	Incidence (%)
Multifocality	15–43.8
Bilaterality	10–19
Central compartment lymph nodal metastasis	65
Lateral neck lymph nodal metastasis	10
Extracapsular invasion	2–38
Distant metastasis	0–3

Source: Refs. (5,11–17).

TABLE 15.2: Definitions for Descriptive Terminologies

Terminologies	Definitions
Bilaterality	Two or more pathologically proven lesions in both lobes
Multifocality	Two or more pathologically proven lesions in one lobe
Proximity to RLN	Paratracheal thyroid nodule at the level of the cricoid cartilage located posteriorly according to the axial axis on preoperative ultrasound
Proximity to trachea	Thyroid nodule in direct contact with the trachea without a visible rim of normal thyroid tissue in-between preoperative ultrasound
Extrathyroidal extension	Loss of interface between the thyroid nodule and the strap muscles, tracheal rings or esophagus
Growth/Disease progression	Tumor enlargement of ≥3 mm and/or the novel appearance of node metastasis

TABLE 15.3: Observed Age Decade-specific Disease Progression Rate at 10-Year Active Surveillance and Estimated Lifetime Probability of Disease Progression

Age at Presentation (in Decade)	Observed DP at 10-Year Surveillance (%)	Estimated Lifetime Probability of DP (%)
20s	36.9	60.3
30s	13.5	37.1
40s	14.5	27.3
50s	5.6	14.9
60s	6.6	9.9
70s	3.5	3.5

Abbreviation: DP, disease progression.

Japan in 1993[26]. Tokyo's Cancer Institute Hospital also initiated an AS study for low-risk PMC in 1995 which enrolled 300 lesions in 230 patients[27,28]. Kuma Hospital's third report of AS was published in 2014, which enrolled 1235 patients, demonstrated only 8% of patients with PMC showed an enlargement of size, and only 3.8% had novel onset of lymph nodal metastasis after 10 years of surveillance. Outside Japan, similar studies have been reported from Korea[29] and United States[30]. Till date there are scant publications on AS in PMC from south Asian countries.

Decision-making on active surveillance of PMC

The selection of patients for AS is the utmost essential strategy in the management of PMC. Patient age is an independent predictor of PMC progression. Miyauchi et al. found that young patients (<40 years) were more likely to have growth progression than those of old age-group (>60 years) and, hence, suggested low-risk PMCs in old age as the best candidate for AS[31]. The trend in DP during AS of PMC varied markedly depending on the age at presentation (summarized in Table 15.3)[32]. The estimated trend curve of DP in patients who presented in their second and third decade showed a steep increase until they reached 35 years of age, with a gradual increase thereafter. The trend curves for the patients in their 40s or older at presentation showed a more mild increase with a meager increase after 55 years (Figure 15.2). Based

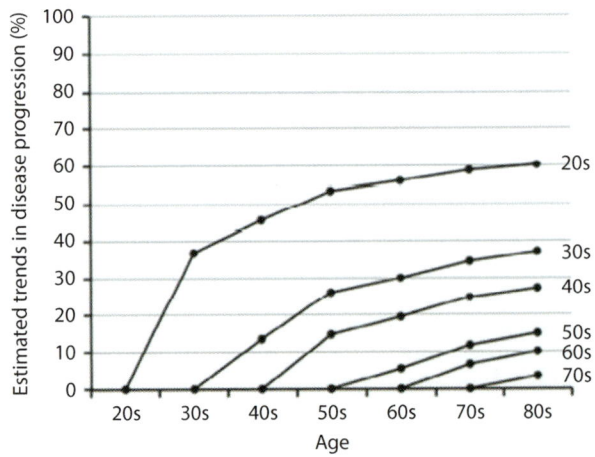

FIGURE 15.2 Estimated lifetime probability of disease progression of PMC over time of active surveillance according to the patients' ages at presentation.

TABLE 15.4: High-risk Features of PMC Associated with Biological Aggressiveness

Lymph nodal or distant metastasis
Extrathyroidal extension
High-grade cytology
Growth progression
Proximity to the RLN
Proximity to trachea

Abbreviation: RLN, recurrent laryngeal nerve.

on this estimate, it can be speculated that ≈ 40% of patients in their 20s and 63% of patients in their 30s and a vast majority of patients in their 40s or older would not require surgery in their lifetime. Sex, family history and multiplicity were less likely to be predictive of growth progression in patients with PMC[31,33].

PMC patients with high-risk features (summarized in Table 15.4) are more likely to have biological aggressiveness and, hence, are contraindicated for AS[33,34]. The decision to undertake AS more appropriately relies on the location of tumor as evident by preoperative imaging. Tumors in proximity to the trachea and/or along the course of RLN are not considered appropriate for watchful follow-up, because the aggressive behavior of such tumors is unclear. The tumor invasiveness in trachea or RLN can be better assessed by CT scan than ultrasound, and is especially suitable for tumors located in the dorsal part of thyroid lobe. Tumor size and the angle between tumor surface and tracheal cartilage serve as predictors for possible invasion into the trachea. The obtuse angle, nearly right angle or unclear angle and acute angle are considered high, intermediate and low risk for trachea invasion, respectively (Figure 15.3). Miyauchi et al. demonstrated that trachea and RLN invasion were not found in PMC size of <7 mm. Among PMCs of ≥7 mm, 24% were obtuse angled requiring segmental tracheal resection, 17% were nearly right angled or unclear angled and 2% showed an acute angle of which none required tracheal resection. Hence, if the angle formed between the tumor surface and the tracheal cartilage is acute, the patient could be considered for AS. The obtuse and nearly right/unclear angles pose risk for tracheal invasion and, hence, should be surgically treated[27].

Ultrasound/CT evidence of normal rim of thyroid interface between the tumor and the RLN course provides the possibility of 93% chance of avoiding sharp dissection along the course of RLN or resection of a part of it in low-risk PMCs. High-risk PMCs of ≥7 mm with lack of normal rim required segmental resection of RLN in 9% and sharp dissection to preserve the nerve in 23%[27].

Fukuoka et al. studied the time-dependent changes in vascularity and calcification in asymptomatic PMC. They found that tumors with macroscopic or rim calcification and poor vascularity at the index presentation had nonprogressive disease[35]. Sugitani et al.[28] at the Cancer Institute Hospital, Tokyo, and Miyauchi et al. from Kuma Hospital both demonstrated that none of the patients who underwent rescue surgery showed recurrence or died of PTC.

The Memorial Sloan Kettering Cancer Center group has framed a clinical risk stratification based on tumor ultrasound characteristics, patient factors and medical team availability and experience. Considering these three domains, they have stratified patients into three categories: ideal candidate, appropriate and inappropriate candidates according to age, sex, tumor location, multifocality, ETE and local or distant metastasis. This risk stratification may help clinicians to recognize patients who are likely to benefit from AS and to identify patients who benefit from upfront biopsy and surgical management in select patients[36].

Incidence of permanent vocal cord palsy is 0.2% even in the most experienced hands, and it would be definitely much higher in the hands of a nonexpert. The other unfavorable events after surgery such as temporary or permanent hypoparathyroidism, need for thyroxine substitution and surgical scar in neck have made some surgeons to consider AS the first-line management of low-risk PMC. The cost-effectiveness of AS is superior to that of immediate surgery, almost 4.1 times lesser than the cost of immediate surgery[37,38]. However, the patient's decision on which option to choose after being fully informed about the management options (immediate surgery or AS) should be highly respected.

Thyroid-stimulating hormone suppression in AS

The need of thyroid-stimulating hormone (TSH) suppression in patients undergoing AS is debatable. Miyauchi et al. considered TSH suppression at lower normal limit would be useful to prevent PMC progression, especially in young patients[31]. In a study by Kim et al. of 127 PMC lesions, it was reported that sustained elevation of TSH level is associated with DP. The adjusted hazard ratio (HR) of PMC progression was higher in patients with high TSH levels (HR 3.55; 95% CI, 1.22–10.28)[39]. On the contrary, Sugitani et al. demonstrated no influence of TSH suppression over the progression of PMC, provided their study population is primarily elderly, who usually have an indolent course of disease[40].

PMC surveillance in pregnancy

A total of 8% of low-risk PMC showed size enlargement of ≥3 mm during pregnancy and rescue surgery following delivery was successful. However, young females with low-risk PMC, desirous of children need not be excluded from AS. Nevertheless,

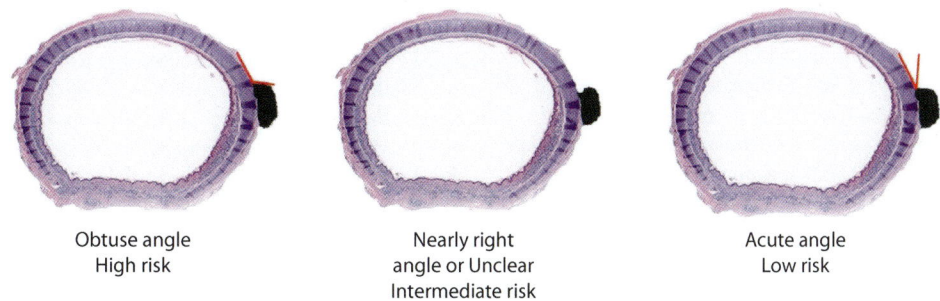

FIGURE 15.3 Schematic representation of PMC with high, intermediate and low risk for tracheal invasion.

women with PMC, even if they show tumor enlargement during pregnancy, rescue surgery after delivery would not be too late[41].

Active surveillance protocol

Patients who choose AS should be followed with ultrasound imaging at every 6 months after the diagnosis until stability is evident (usually after 2 years of serial ultrasound with no DP) and every 1–2 years thereafter. Neck lymph nodes are considered suspicious if they exhibit punctuate hyperechogenicity, cystic appearance, the absence of hilar hyperechogenicity, round shape or short axis >5 mm or color Doppler evidence of peripheral vascularization[42]. Lymph nodal metastasis can be confirmed by Fine Needle Aspiration Biopsy (FNAB) of lymph node and thyroglobulin (Tg) measurement of FNAB needle washout. Rescue surgery is recommended when there is a novel appearance of lymph nodal metastasis or tumor increase by size ≥3 mm, but if the patient prefers to continue AS, surveillance can be done until the tumor size reaches 13 mm[27].

Risk stratification of PMC

Risk profiling could be used to tailor an optimal postoperative surveillance to the individual patient's odds of developing recurrent/progressive disease. Few experts consider a relaxed follow-up for PMCs as majority have an indolent nature. But others argue that non-incidental PMC has to be followed up like classical PTC because these two groups can have no difference in terms of recurrence, ETE and angiolymphatic invasion[43,44]. A retrospective study by Noguchi et al. demonstrated that among 2070 patients with PMC, tumors of 1–5 mm recur in 3.3% while of 6–10 mm recur in 14% at 35-year follow-up period[45]. Nonetheless, it is becoming increasingly clear that tumor size cannot be used as a single criterion in risk stratification of PTC patients. A retrospective study of 312 PMC patients with long term follow up by Durante et al. reported that patients with no family history of thyroid cancer, absence of head and neck irradiation, lymph nodal metastasis, ETE, angiolymphatic invasion, aggressive histological subtype and unifocality of PMC had a very low probability of disease recurrence. Notably some of these criteria have been incorporated in the ATA guidelines.[24,46]. On the contrary, the presence of these features has been strongly associated with a high-risk phenotype.

The BRAF V600E mutation is a common genetic event in PMC that constitutes a 45–73.4% incidence[47]. The BRAF V600E mutation was found to be associated with aggressive tumor behavior such as tall-cell histological subtype, numerous cells with nuclear groove, higher invasiveness, intrathyroidal tumor spread and persistent/recurrent disease[48]. Nonetheless, Park et al.[49] and Ji et al.[47] reported that BRAF V600E mutation was not associated with age, gender, multifocality, capsular invasion, cervical lymph node metastasis or higher TNM stage. Melo et al.[50] confirmed that telomerase reverse transcriptase (TERT) promoter mutations are related to aggressive tumors and disease-specific mortality in PTC. The synergistic impact of TERT promoter mutations with BRAF V600E mutation on tumor recurrence and disease-specific mortality in patients with PMC is unknown.

Surgery

Surgical options for PMC include lobectomy, near-total thyroidectomy (NT) and total thyroidectomy (TT). Proponents of TT would argue that multifocality and postsurgery follow-up are better addressed in removing the whole thyroid gland. Contrarily, proponents of the lobectomy argue that the presence of multifocality does not influence the risk of recurrence and also spares 50–60% of patients from the need of thyroxine-replacement therapy. Moreover, the most important argument in favor of lobectomy is the lack of experienced thyroid surgeons. Vocal cord paresis and hypoparathyroidism are directly related to the extent of surgery and the experience of thyroid surgeons. A recent analysis of 1376 PMC patients treated at Mayo Clinic from 1936 to 2015 had demonstrated that 20-year locoregional recurrence rates following lobectomy were comparable to those achieved after NT/TT[51]. However, TT in the setting of PMC is recommended for patients with a history of irradiation, multicentric tumor, ETE and overt metastases.

No prospective randomized trials exist to address the need for completion thyroidectomy in patients who have had hemithyroidectomy for a benign cause and histologically reported as PMC. The consensus of data from National Thyroid Cancer Treatment Cooperative Study Group (NTCTCSG) in North America recommends against performing completion thyroidectomy for a unifocal PMC. Of course, the additional foci of tumor in contralateral lobe are unknown unless otherwise residual lobe is removed. The ATA guidelines suggest that a completion thyroidectomy can be performed only if a TT would have been indicated and if the histological findings had been known prior to the initial surgery[24]. It is best to decide after postoperative ultrasound of the contralateral lobe and fine needle aspiration (FNA) of the suspicious nodule if any.

Prophylactic central neck dissection (CND) is not advisable as a routine when surgical intervention is planned. Prophylactic CND can be performed only if enlarged lymph nodes are observed during surgery or if nodes are detected by palpation in the central neck region.

The overall prognosis for most PMC patients is excellent, with mortality well below 1%. Locoregional recurrences almost never endanger life but occur in up to 6% of patients. Most distant metastases occur in patients with bulky cervical adenopathy, and rare deaths from micropapillary cancer happen in this subset. The risk of death in most patients who do not have distant metastasis or large nodal disease is 0.1–0.2%.

Radioactive iodine remnant ablation

The rationale of radioactive iodine (RAI) remnant ablation in the setting of PMC is controversial in view of low risk of morbidity and mortality of these tumors. In several metanalysis that were conducted to assess the effectiveness of RAI ablation, it was demonstrated that the relative risk (RR) reduction for locoregional recurrence of PMC at 10-year following NT/TT is 1.15 (95% CI, 0.75–1.76; P = 0.51) or thyroid cancer-related mortality (RR 0.76; 95% CI, 0.22–2.63; P = 0.66)[52]. Thus, PMC patients treated by NT/TT would not be benefited by RAI remnant ablation for decreasing the 10-year recurrence or incidence of thyroid cancer-related mortality[53]. Instead, it would add to the cost and logistics of RAI treatment (need for RAI scan, possible withdrawal protocol and associated hypothyroid symptoms). Brito et al. from Mayo Clinic data showed that 20-year locoregional recurrence rates were not improved by the incremental RAI remnant ablation following NT/TT in 375 node-positive patients[51]. The ATA 2015 guidelines did not recommend RAI ablation following thyroidectomy in patients with unifocal/multifocal PMC in the absence of other adverse features[24].

TABLE 15.5: Summary of Pooled Data* for Efficacy of RFA, MWA and LA

Thermal Ablation	SMD of Tumor Volume Reduction	Proportion of Complete Disappearance (%)	Proportion of Complication (%)	Proportion of Recurrence (%)	Proportion of Distant Metastasis (%)
RFA	−1.35	76.2	1.7	0.01	0.0
MWA	−3.82	62.9	6.0	0.85	0.0
LA	−1.80	57.3	0.92	1.87	0.0

Abbreviations: LA, laser ablation; MWA, microwave ablation; RFA, radiofrequency ablation; SMD, standard mean difference.
Source: Adapted from Tong M et al.[54] Efficacy and safety of RFA, MWA, LA for treating PMC.

Newer management options

Percutaneous US-guided ethanol ablation

Percutaneous ethanol ablation likely represents an attractive option for patients not willing for neck surgery or who are uncomfortable with AS. This technique involves ultrasound-guided intra-tumoral injection of 95% ethanol. Hay and colleagues, as reported in the 2018 congress of European Thyroid Association, demonstrated 82% median tumor volume reduction in 16 biopsy-proven tumor foci in 14 PMC patients during a mean follow-up of 4.2 years. There was shrinkage of all tumor foci along with elimination of doppler flow. None had developed neither painful thyroiditis nor hoarseness or hypocalcemia. No significant change in serum Tg levels were observed following this procedure. This pilot study has demonstrated that ultrasound-guided percutaneous ethanol ablation can emerge as an alternative methodology to manage PMC in terms of cost-effectiveness, safety and efficacy.

Percutaneous US-guided thermal ablation

Nonsurgical therapeutic options are emerging as an attractive approach for patients who are not a candidate for surgery or to whom AS is undesirable. Several studies have reported the efficacy and safety of thermal ablations, which include radiofrequency ablation (RFA), microwave ablation (MWA) and laser ablation (LA). These techniques utilize thermal energy to ablate the tumor foci and cause a more predictable area of tumor necrosis than that caused by ethanol ablation. A recent metanalysis of 12 studies by Tong and colleagues from Dalian province of China, on efficacy and safety of thermal ablations in low-risk PMCs, has demonstrated that RFA, MWA and LA had resulted in a significant tumor volume reduction in PMC (Table 15.5)[54]. MWA showed a superior efficacy in tumor volume reduction while compared to other two ablations; however, the differences were not statistically significant. RFA has the highest proportion of complete disappearance of the tumor foci (76.2%) and the lowest proportion of recurrence (0.01%). There were no events of distant metastasis among the three ablative methods. MWA has the higher frequency of causing voice hoarseness (4.4%) among the three ablative procedures. The other minor complications include pain, bleeding, skin burn and hypothyroidism (0.9%). Thus, thermal ablations are emerging as an effective minimally invasive alternative for surgical intervention in patients with PMC. Nonetheless, currently there are no definitive guidelines available for the use of percutaneous US-guided thermal ablations to treat PMC.

South Asian perspective

Most of the patients who undergo hemithyroidectomy and have incidental PMC, in our personal experience, do well, and we follow them with Tg doubling time. However, in developing countries where follow-up is an issue, we would recommend TT as the initial procedure, so that the follow-up with Tg and if even patient is lost to follow-up after few years is reliably safe.

We have a meager experience on observation for PMC, since most of our patients have fear of carcinoma, and once the diagnosis is disclosed, they panic and most of them volunteer for surgery. In this context, as rightly said "punishment should fit the crime," and we feel in our part of the world, surgery, which might be overkill, still holds the way, and observation is theoretical. To conclude, most surgeons and patients consider surgery as the best option.

Conclusion

PTC is the most common subtype of thyroid cancer, and PTC of maximum dimension <10 mm is termed as papillary thyroid microcarcinoma. With the advent of high-resolution ultrasonography and increases in FNA of thyroid nodules, the incidence of PMC is increasing worldwide. PMCs are often inert, slowly progressive tumors with good prognosis. PMC are a heterogenous group and seem imprecise to consider a single category. Only a skilled sonographer or an endocrinologist or endocrine surgeon is likely to pick up the subtle ultrasonographic findings of PMC. A multitude of therapeutic approaches have been in practice such as surgical intervention, percutaneous US-guided ablations including AS. It is important to educate physicians, surgeons and the patients on how AS of low-risk PMC can be an excellent modality of management. Individualized treatment options should be offered to patients with PMC according to tumor biology and the clinical context and values of the patient. Shared decision-making is a treatment strategy that allows patients with PMC to be personalized.

References

1. Professional Committee on Thyroid Cancer of China Anti-Cancer Association. Chinese expert consensus on diagnosis and treatment of thyroid micropapillary carcinoma (2016 edition). Chin J Clin Oncol. 2016;43:405–411.
2. Lim H, Devesa SS, Sosa JA, Check D, Kitahara CM. Trends in thyroid cancer incidence and mortality in the United States, 1974-2013. JAMA. 2017 Apr;317(13):1338–1348.
3. Davies L, Welch HG. Current thyroid cancer trends in the United States. JAMA Otolaryngol Head Neck Surg. 2014 Apr;140(4):317–322.
4. Ahn HS, Kim HJ, Welch HG. Korea's thyroid-cancer "epidemic" – Screening and overdiagnosis. N Engl J Med. 2014 Nov;371(19):1765–1767.
5. Roti E, Rossi R, Trasforini G, Bertelli F, Ambrosio MR, Busutti L, Pearce EN, Braverman LE, Degli Uberti EC. Clinical and histological characteristics of papillary thyroid microcarcinoma: Results of a retrospective study in 243 patients. J Clin Endocrinol Metab. 2006 Jun;91(6):2171–2178.
6. Martinez-Tello FJ, Martinez-Cabruja R, Fernandez-Martin J, Lasso-Oria C, Ballestin-Carcavilla C. Occult carcinoma of the thyroid. A systematic autopsy study from Spain of two series performed with two different methods. Cancer. 1993 Jun;71(12):4022–4029.
7. Lee YS, Lim H, Chang HS, Park CS. Papillary thyroid microcarcinomas are different from latent papillary thyroid carcinomas at autopsy. J Korean Med Sci. 2014 May;29(5):676–679.
8. Ito Y, Miyauchi A. A therapeutic strategy for incidentally detected papillary microcarcinoma of the thyroid. Nat Clin Pract Endocrinol Metab. 2007 Mar;3(3):240–248.

9. Kuo EJ, Goffredo P, Sosa JA, Roman SA. Aggressive variants of papillary thyroid microcarcinoma are associated with extrathyroidal spread and lymph-node metastases: A population-level analysis. Thyroid. 2013 Oct;23(10):1305–1311.
10. Al-Qurayshi Z, Nilubol N, Tufano RP, Kandil E. Wolf in sheep's clothing: Papillary thyroid microcarcinoma in the US. J Am Coll Surg. 2020 Apr;230(4):484–491.
11. Hay ID, Hutchinson ME, Gonzalez-Losada T, McIver B, Reinalda ME, Grant CS, Thompson GB, Sebo TJ, Goellner JR. Papillary thyroid microcarcinoma: A study of 900 cases observed in a 60-year period. Surgery. 2008 Dec;144(6):980–987; discussion 987-8.
12. Mehanna H, Al-Maqbili T, Carter B, Martin E, Campain N, Watkinson J, McCabe C, Boelaert K, Franklyn JA. Differences in the recurrence and mortality outcomes rates of incidental and nonincidental papillary thyroid microcarcinoma: A systematic review and meta-analysis of 21 329 person-years of follow-up. J Clin Endocrinol Metab. 2014 Aug;99(8):2834–2843.
13. Chow SM, Law SC, Chan JK, Au SK, Yau S, Lau WH. Papillary microcarcinoma of the thyroid-Prognostic significance of lymph node metastasis and multifocality. Cancer. 2003 Jul;98(1):31–40.
14. Wada N, Duh QY, Sugino K, Iwasaki H, Kameyama K, Mimura T, Ito K, Takami H, Takanashi Y. Lymph node metastasis from 259 papillary thyroid microcarcinomas: Frequency, pattern of occurrence and recurrence, and optimal strategy for neck dissection. Ann Surg. 2003 Mar;237(3):399–407.
15. Roh JL, Kim JM, Park CI. Central cervical nodal metastasis from papillary thyroid microcarcinoma: Pattern and factors predictive of nodal metastasis. Ann Surg Oncol. 2008 Sep;15(9):2482–2486.
16. So YK, Son YI, Hong SD, Seo MY, Baek CH, Jeong HS, Chung MK. Subclinical lymph node metastasis in papillary thyroid microcarcinoma: A study of 551 resections. Surgery. 2010 Sep;148(3):526–531.
17. Kim YS. Patterns and predictive factors of lateral lymph node metastasis in papillary thyroid microcarcinoma. Otolaryngol Head Neck Surg. 2012 Jul;147(1):15–19.
18. Cheng F, Chen Y, Zhu L, Zhou B, Xu Y, Chen Y, Wen L, Chen S. Risk factors for cervical lymph node metastasis of papillary thyroid microcarcinoma: A single-center retrospective study. Int J Endocrinol. 2019 Jan;2019:8579828.
19. Zhou YL, Gao EL, Zhang W, Yang H, Guo GL, Zhang XH, Wang OC. Factors predictive of papillary thyroid micro-carcinoma with bilateral involvement and central lymph node metastasis: A retrospective study. World J Surg Oncol. 2012 May;10:67.
20. Back K, Kim JS, Kim JH, Choe JH. Superior located papillary thyroid microcarcinoma is a risk factor for lateral lymph node metastasis. Ann Surg Oncol. 2019 Nov;26(12):3992–4001.
21. Kim K, Zheng X, Kim JK, Lee CR, Kang SW, Lee J, Jeong JJ, Nam KH, Chung WY. The contributing factors for lateral neck lymph node metastasis in papillary thyroid microcarcinoma (PTMC). Endocrine. 2020 Mar 7. doi: 10.1007/s12020-020-02251-2. Epub ahead of print. PMID: 32146654.
22. Zeng RC, Li Q, Lin KL, Zhang W, Gao EL, Huang GL, Zhang XH, Zheng MH. Predicting the factors of lateral lymph node metastasis in papillary microcarcinoma of the thyroid in eastern China. Clin Transl Oncol. 2012 Nov;14(11):842–847.
23. Peng Y, Zhou W, Zhan WW, Xu SY. Ultrasonographic assessment of differential diagnosis between degenerating cystic thyroid nodules and papillary thyroid microcarcinomas. World J Surg. 2017 Oct;41(10):2538–2544.
24. Haugen BR, Alexander EK, Bible KC, Doherty GM, Mandel SJ, Nikiforov YE, Pacini F, Randolph GW, Sawka AM, Schlumberger M, Schuff KG, Sherman SI, Sosa JA, Steward DL, Tuttle RM, Wartofsky L. 2015 American Thyroid Association management guidelines for adult patients with thyroid nodules and differentiated thyroid cancer: The American Thyroid Association guidelines task force on thyroid nodules and differentiated thyroid cancer. Thyroid. 2016 Jan;26(1):1–133.
25. Sugitani I, Fujimoto Y. Symptomatic versus asymptomatic papillary thyroid microcarcinoma: A retrospective analysis of surgical outcome and prognostic factors. Endocr J. 1999 Feb;46(1):209–216.
26. Ito Y, Miyauchi A, Kudo T, Oda H, Yamamoto M, Sasai H, Masuoka H, Fukushima M, Higashiyama T, Kihara M, Miya A. Trends in the implementation of active surveillance for low-risk papillary thyroid microcarcinomas at Kuma Hospital: Gradual increase and heterogeneity in the acceptance of this new management option. Thyroid. 2018 Apr;28(4):488–495.
27. Miyauchi A, Ito Y, Oda H. Insights into the management of papillary microcarcinoma of the thyroid. Thyroid. 2018 Jan;28(1):23–31.
28. Sugitani I, Toda K, Yamada K, Yamamoto N, Ikenaga M, Fujimoto Y. Three distinctly different kinds of papillary thyroid microcarcinoma should be recognized: Our treatment strategies and outcomes. World J Surg. 2010 Jun;34(6):1222–1231.
29. Kong SH, Ryu J, Kim MJ, Cho SW, Song YS, Yi KH, Park DJ, Hwangbo Y, Lee YJ, Lee KE, Kim SJ, Jeong WJ, Chung EJ, Hah JH, Choi JY, Ryu CH, Jung YS, Moon JH, Lee EK, Park YJ. Longitudinal assessment of quality of life according to treatment options in low-risk papillary thyroid microcarcinoma patients: Active surveillance or immediate surgery (interim analysis of MAeSTro). Thyroid. 2019 Aug;29(8):1089–1096.
30. Tuttle RM, Fagin JA, Minkowitz G, Wong RJ, Roman B, Patel S, Untch B, Ganly I, Shaha AR, Shah JP, Pace M, Li D, Bach A, Lin O, Whiting A, Ghossein R, Landa I, Sabra M, Boucai L, Fish S, Morris LGT. Natural history and tumor volume kinetics of papillary thyroid cancers during active surveillance. JAMA Otolaryngol Head Neck Surg. 2017 Oct;143(10):1015–1020.
31. Ito Y, Miyauchi A, Kihara M, Higashiyama T, Kobayashi K, Miya A. Patient age is significantly related to the progression of papillary microcarcinoma of the thyroid under observation. Thyroid. 2014 Jan;24(1):27–34.
32. Miyauchi A, Kudo T, Ito Y, Oda H, Sasai H, Higashiyama T, Fukushima M, Masuoka H, Kihara M, Miya A. Estimation of the lifetime probability of disease progression of papillary microcarcinoma of the thyroid during active surveillance. Surgery. 2018 Jan;163(1):48–52.
33. Ramundo V, Sponziello M, Falcone R, Verrienti A, Filetti S, Durante C, Grani G. Low-risk papillary thyroid microcarcinoma: Optimal management toward a more conservative approach. J Surg Oncol. 2020 May;121(6):958–963.
34. Miyauchi A. Clinical trials of active surveillance of papillary microcarcinoma of the thyroid. World J Surg. 2016 Mar;40(3):516–522.
35. Fukuoka O, Sugitani I, Ebina A, Toda K, Kawabata K, Yamada K. Natural history of asymptomatic papillary thyroid microcarcinoma: Time-dependent changes in calcification and vascularity during active surveillance. World J Surg. 2016 Mar;40(3):529–537.
36. Brito JP, Ito Y, Miyauchi A, Tuttle RM. A clinical framework to facilitate risk stratification when considering an active surveillance alternative to immediate biopsy and surgery in papillary thyroid microcarcinoma. Thyroid. 2016 Jan;26(1):144–149.
37. Oda H, Miyauchi A, Ito Y, Sasai H, Masuoka H, Yabuta T, Fukushima M, Higashiyama T, Kihara M, Kobayashi K, Miya A. Comparison of the costs of active surveillance and immediate surgery in the management of low-risk papillary microcarcinoma of the thyroid. Endocr J. 2017 Jan;64(1):59–64.
38. Lang BH, Wong CK. A cost-effectiveness comparison between early surgery and non-surgical approach for incidental papillary thyroid microcarcinoma. Eur J Endocrinol. 2015 Sep;173(3):367–375.
39. Kim HI, Jang HW, Ahn HS, Ahn S, Park SY, Oh YL, Hahn SY, Shin JH, Kim JH, Kim JS, Chung JH, Kim TH, Kim SW. High serum TSH level is associated with progression of papillary thyroid microcarcinoma during active surveillance. J Clin Endocrinol Metab. 2018 Feb;103(2):446–451. Erratum in: J Clin Endocrinol Metab. 2018 May;103(5):2074.
40. Sugitani I, Fujimoto Y, Yamada K. Association between serum thyrotropin concentration and growth of asymptomatic papillary thyroid microcarcinoma. World J Surg. 2014 Mar;38(3):673–678.
41. Ito Y, Miyauchi A, Kudo T, Ota H, Yoshioka K, Oda H, Sasai H, Nakayama A, Yabuta T, Masuoka H, Fukushima M, Higashiyama T, Kihara M, Kobayashi K, Miya A. Effects of pregnancy on papillary microcarcinomas of the thyroid re-evaluated in the entire patient series at Kuma Hospital. Thyroid. 2016 Jan;26(1):156–160.
42. Leboulleux S, Girard E, Rose M, Travagli JP, Sabbah N, Caillou B, Hartl DM, Lassau N, Baudin E, Schlumberger M. Ultrasound criteria of malignancy for cervical lymph nodes in patients followed up for differentiated thyroid cancer. J Clin Endocrinol Metab. 2007 Sep;92(9):3590–3594.
43. Arora N, Turbendian HK, Kato MA, Moo TA, Zarnegar R, Fahey TJ 3rd. Papillary thyroid carcinoma and microcarcinoma: Is there a need to distinguish the two? Thyroid. 2009 May;19(5):473–477.
44. Tzvetov G, Hirsch D, Shraga-Slutzky I, Weinstein R, Manistersky Y, Kalmanovich R, Lapidot M, Grozinsky-Glasberg S, Singer J, Sulkes J, Shimon I, Benbassat C. Well-differentiated thyroid carcinoma: Comparison of microscopic and macroscopic disease. Thyroid. 2009 May;19(5):487–494.
45. Noguchi S, Yamashita H, Uchino S, Watanabe S. Papillary microcarcinoma. World J Surg. 2008 May;32(5):747–753.
46. Durante C, Attard M, Torlontano M, et al. Identification and optimal postsurgical follow-up of patients with very low-risk papillary thyroid microcarcinomas. J Clin Endocrinol Metab. 2010;95(11):4882–4888.
47. Ji W, Xie H, Wei B, Shen H, Liu A, Gao Y, Wang L. Relationship between BRAF V600E gene mutation and the clinical and pathologic characteristics of papillary thyroid microcarcinoma. Int J Clin Exp Pathol. 2019 Sep;12(9):3492–3499.
48. Tallini G, de Biase D, Durante C, Acquaviva G, Bisceglia M, Bruno R, Bacchi Reggiani ML, Casadei GP, Costante G, Cremonini N, Lamartina L, Meringolo D, Nardi F, Pession A, Rhoden KJ, Ronga G, Torlontano M, Verrienti A, Visani M, Filetti S. BRAF V600E and risk stratification of thyroid microcarcinoma: A multicenter pathological and clinical study. Mod Pathol. 2015 Oct;28(10):1343–1359.
49. Park VY, Kim EK, Lee HS, Moon HJ, Yoon JH, Kwak JY. Real-time PCR cycle threshold values for the BRAFV600E mutation in papillary thyroid microcarcinoma may be associated with central lymph node metastasis: A retrospective study. Medicine (Baltimore). 2015 Jul;94(28):e1149.
50. Melo M, da Rocha AG, Vinagre J, Batista R, Peixoto J, Tavares C, Celestino R, Almeida A, Salgado C, Eloy C, Castro P, Prazeres H, Lima J, Amaro T, Lobo C, Martins MJ, Moura M, Cavaco B, Leite V, Cameselle-Teijeiro JM, Carrilho F, Carvalheiro M, Máximo V, Sobrinho-Simões M, Soares P. TERT promoter mutations are a major indicator of poor outcome in differentiated thyroid carcinomas. J Clin Endocrinol Metab. 2014 May;99(5):E754–E765.
51. Brito JP, Hay ID. Management of papillary thyroid microcarcinoma. Endocrinol Metab Clin. 2019 Mar;48(1):199–213.
52. Hu G, Zhu W, Yang W, Wang H, Shen L, Zhang H. The effectiveness of radioactive iodine remnant ablation for papillary thyroid microcarcinoma: A systematic review and meta-analysis. World J Surg. 2016 Jan;40(1):100–109.
53. Kim HJ, Kim NK, Choi JH, Kim SW, Jin SM, Suh S, Bae JC, Min YK, Chung JH, Kim SW. Radioactive iodine ablation does not prevent recurrences in patients with papillary thyroid microcarcinoma. Clin Endocrinol (Oxf). 2013 Apr;78(4):614–620.
54. Tong M, Li S, Li Y, Li Y, Feng Y, Che Y. Efficacy and safety of radiofrequency, microwave and laser ablation for treating papillary thyroid microcarcinoma: A systematic review and meta-analysis. Int J Hyperthermia. 2019;36(1):1278–1286.

16

MEDULLARY THYROID CARCINOMA

Mithun Raam and Deepak Thomas Abraham

Introduction

Medullary thyroid carcinoma (MTC) is a rare malignancy of the thyroid gland with a neuroendocrine origin accounting for about 2% off all thyroid malignancies (1). In 1906, Jaquet first described it as a tumor of the thyroid gland that was filled with amyloid (2). Hazard et al., in 1959, described this disease entity as medullary (solid) carcinoma (3).

MTC occurs in both hereditary (25%) and sporadic forms (75%) with characteristic gain of function mutations in the REarranged during Transfection (RET) gene on chromosome 10q11.2 in both forms. Central to the management of this disease is the understanding of its genetic basis and its clinical implication.

Incidence South Asia

Thyroid cancer overall is on an increasing trend. According to GLOBOCAN 2018 data, thyroid cancer, overall, has an incidence of 29,784 cases accounting for 4207 deaths in Southeast Asia. It accounts for about 1.6% of all new cases of malignancy in India with a 5-year prevalence of 50,939 cases (4). Deshmukh et al., in a retrospective analysis of 221 patients with thyroid malignancies, showed prevalence of 4.5% of MTC (5). Mehrotra et al., in a retrospective analysis of 71 patients, showed 84.5% sporadic and 15.5% hereditary MTC (6). A retrospective analysis of MTC in our institution showed a similar prevalence of 4.45% (90 out of 2022 patients) with hereditary MTC contributing to around 35% of patients (7).

RET proto-oncogene and molecular genetics in MTC

In 1985, Takahashi et al. described a novel transfection of NIH 3T3 cells with human lymphoma cell DNA, which was thought to have been activated by recombination between unlinked human DNA segments during the process of transfection (8). This was, hence, termed as REarranged during Transfection gene. This proto-oncogene located on chromosome 10q11.2 has been identified as a central piece in our understanding of the puzzle of MTC. RET gene mutations are associated with hereditary MTC in the form of germline mutations, whereas they occur as somatic mutations in about 50% of sporadic MTC (9, 10). Apart from RET mutations, 18–80% of sporadic MTC patients were found to harbor mutations in HRAS, KRAS or NRAS gene (10).

RET gene is a 60-kb long gene with 21 exons encoding for a transmembrane receptor tyrosine kinase. This RET protein has an extracellular domain (containing four cadherin-like domains and a cysteine-rich domain), a transmembrane domain, an intracellular juxta-membrane domain and two intracellular tyrosine kinase domain (Figure 16.1) (11).

RET protein activation requires binding to GNDF (glial cell–derived neurotrophic factor) family ligands such as GDNF, artemin, persephin and neurturin mediated by ligand-specific cofactors of GDNF family receptors alpha (GFRα). This activation results in the formation of a dimeric complex including two RET proteins, two ligand molecules and two GFRα co-receptors. This causes autophosphorylation of the intracellular tyrosine kinase domain that further activates several downstream molecular signaling pathways such as Ras/ERK, P13K/Akt pathways that play a role in cell proliferation, differentiation and survival. Alternate pathways such as p38 MAPK, phospholipase C-γ, JNK and ERK5 are also activated, hence modifying cell differentiation, migration and cytokine production.

RET is expressed in multiple tissues derived from neural crest including thyroid parafollicular cells, parathyroid glands, adrenal chromaffin cells, enteric ganglia and neurons. RET signaling has been found to be essential for normal development of renal system, parasympathetic nervous system, gut-associated lymphoid tissue and enteric nervous system. However, gain-of-function germline mutations in RET proto-oncogene results in MEN syndrome.

These germline mutations have a strong genotype-phenotype correlation, which is demonstrable in their clinical aggressiveness. MEN 2A syndrome generally exhibits mutation in exons 10 and 11 within the extracellular cysteine-rich domain of RET (Codons 609, 611, 618, 620, 630, 634). The cysteine-rich domain, which stabilizes the tertiary structure of RET protein when substituted with another amino acid, results in an unpaired cysteine that may form aberrant bonds with other cysteine residues or with other abnormal RET molecule. This causes dimerization-independent persistent activation. MEN 2B syndrome, on the other hand, results from mutations in the intracellular tyrosine kinase domain of the protein. Precisely 95% of these mutations are due to the substitution of methionine with threonine at codon 918 (M918T) and 5% are due to A883F. M918T mutation causes conformational change in a region of the intracellular tyrosine kinase domain important for ATP binding causing increased affinity for ATP as compared to the wild type. Thus, these mutated proteins are highly active in both monomeric and dimeric forms.

RET mutations are associated with pathological changes in C-cells or parafollicular cells. The C-cell accounts for 0.01–0.1% of cells located centrally in the thyroid gland. They are neuroectodermal in origin and derived from the primordial cells of the neural crest that migrate to the ultimobranchial body. During development of the thyroid gland, the lateral thyroid anlages derived from the ultimobranchial body fuse with the median thyroid anlage derived from the tuberculum impar to form the lateral lobes of the thyroid. Hence, the C-cells are dispersed throughout the substance of the gland. They are round, polygonal or spindle-shaped cells that occur singly or in groups. Though they were called parafollicular cells (12), the majority of C-cells have been found to be intrafollicular. C-cells secrete the hormone calcitonin, which is a 32-amino acid linear polypeptide hormone and calcitonin gene-related peptide (CGRP). Though it increases

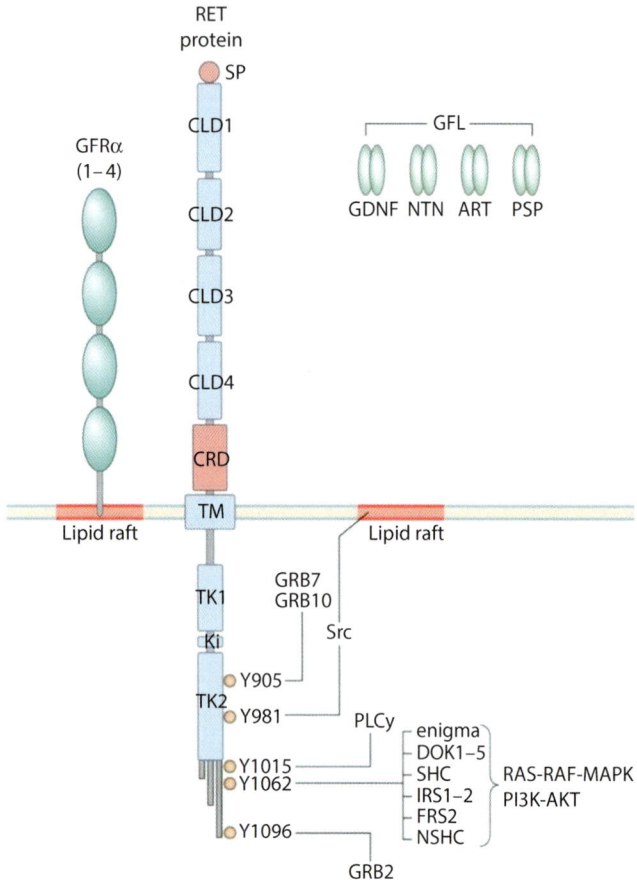

FIGURE 16.1 The RET protein.

the excretion of calcium from the renal tubules and reduces the resorption of calcium in the intestine and osteoclastic activity in the bones, its role in calcium homeostasis is insignificant as compared to calcitriol and parathyroid hormone. In hereditary MTC, RET germline mutations are associated with an increase in the size and number of C-cells causing C-cell hyperplasia, which is considered a premalignant condition (Figure 16.2).

The understanding of the molecular genetic mechanisms behind MTC has created a paradigm shift in its screening and management. This not only helps in predicting the occurrence of the disease in the future kindred but also helps in determining aggressiveness due to a strong genotype-phenotype correlation and proves to be a potential therapeutic target.

Clinical features

The commonest presentation is in the form of a solitary nodule that may present in the fourth to sixth decade in sporadic MTC vs at a much younger age in hereditary MTC, depending on the mutational genotype. It may also present as a multinodular goiter or as an incidental finding on imaging (13, 14). Lymph nodal metastases at presentation occurs in 50–70% of patients (15) and metastatic disease is the presenting feature in 10–15% (16, 17). The characteristic feature in MTC is elevated calcitonin levels due to C-cell proliferation that can be used as a diagnostic and prognostic marker. In some patients, there may be secretion of several other chemicals such as carcinoembryonic antigen, serotonin, substance P, vasoactive intestinal substance, adrenocorticotrophic hormone, corticotrophin-releasing hormone, catecholamine metabolites and calcitonin-related peptide (18). This may manifest as a paraneoplastic syndrome with symptoms such as flushing, diarrhea, ectopic Cushing's syndrome, hypercoagulability and cholestasis (19, 20).

Hereditary MTC is inherited in an autosomal dominant pattern and comprises subtypes known as Multiple Endocrine Neoplasia (MEN) 2A and 2B. These are detailed below.

Multiple endocrine neoplasia type 2

John H. Sipple first described MEN 2 syndrome in 1961 as an association of pheochromocytoma with carcinoma of the thyroid gland (21). It encompasses two distinct syndromes known as MEN 2A (currently classified as MEN2) and MEN 2B (currently classified as MEN3) (22). MEN 2A syndrome occurs due to mutations in the extracellular cysteine-rich domain in exons 10 and 11.

MEN 2A may present in the form of four clinical variants – classical MEN 2A, MEN 2A with cutaneous lichenoid amyloidosis, MEN 2A with Hirschsprung's disease and familial MTC, which are described below.

- Classic MEN 2A syndrome presents with 95% of patients presenting with MTC, about 50% patients presenting with pheochromocytoma and about 20–30% of patients presenting with primary hyperparathyroidism (PHPT) with parathyroid hyperplasia (23).
- Cutaneous lichenoid amyloidosis occurs in about 10% of MEN 2A patients and presents with a pigmented pruritic popular lesion in the scapular region corresponding to T2 to T6 dermatomes with sensory neuropathy and secondary amyloid deposition (Figure 16.3) (24,25).
- Hirschsprung's disease occurs in about 7% of patients with MEN 2A and is associated with failure of neural crest cells to migrate, proliferate and differentiate into the submucosal and myenteric plexuses (26).
- Familial MTC is a variant of MEN 2A where MTC occurs in isolation due to reduced penetrance for pheochromocytoma and PHPT (27).

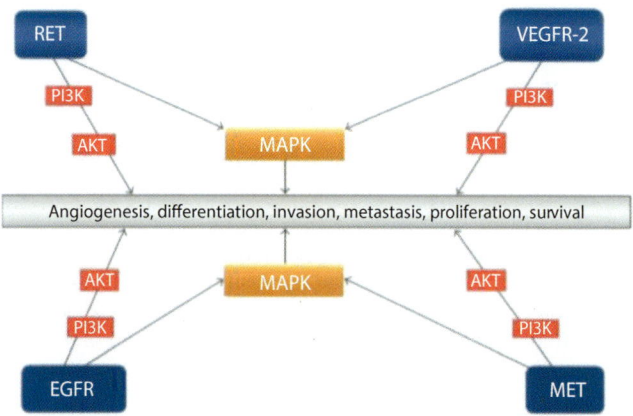

FIGURE 16.2 Tyrosine kinase and other pathways in MTC.

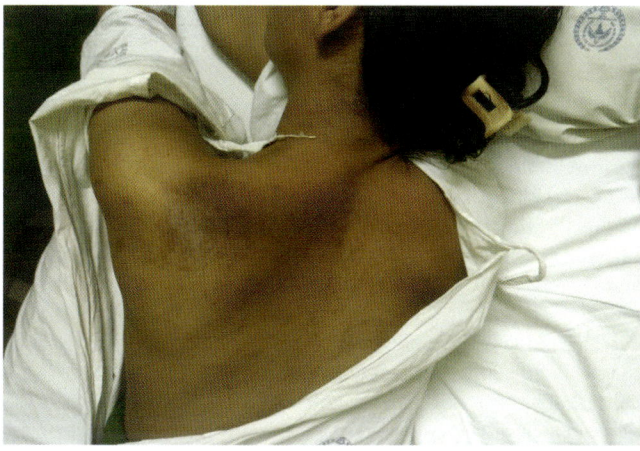

FIGURE 16.3 Patient with MEN2A syndrome with cutaneous lichenoid amyloidosis.

MEN 2B on the other hand is a syndrome with earlier onset of more aggressive disease. This occurs mostly due to the substitution of methionine with threonine at codon 918 in the intracellular tyrosine kinase domain. Almost all patients develop MTC and about 40–50% develop pheochromocytomas. These patients also have peculiar phenotypic features such as skeletal abnormalities (Marfanoid habitus, high arched palate, pectus excavatum, pes caves, etc.), mucosal ganglioneuromas in the lips, tongue, gingiva, buccal and nasal mucosa, vocal cords, conjunctiva or even in the intestinal submucosal and myenteric plexus, resulting in megacolon (Figure 16.3–16.6) (28, 29).

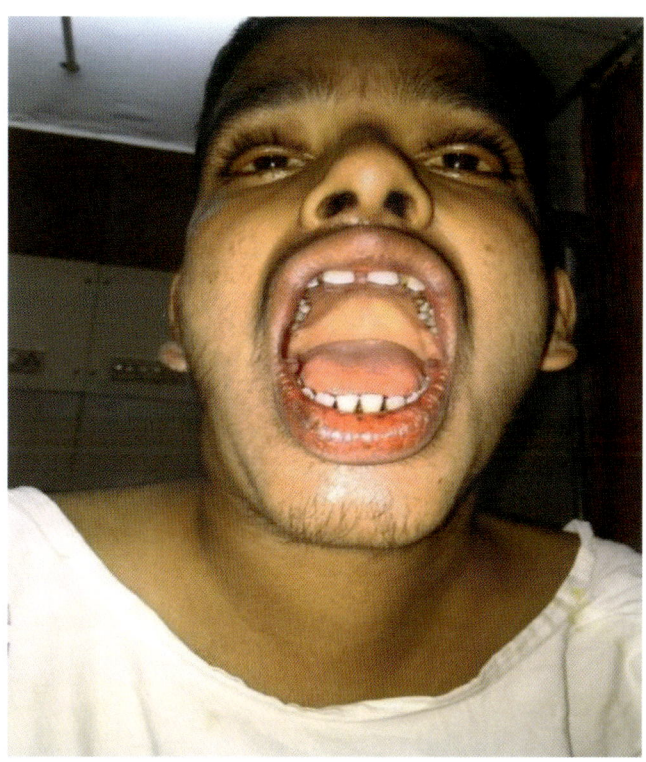

FIGURE 16.5 Patient with MEN 2B syndrome with marfanoid features (high arched palate).

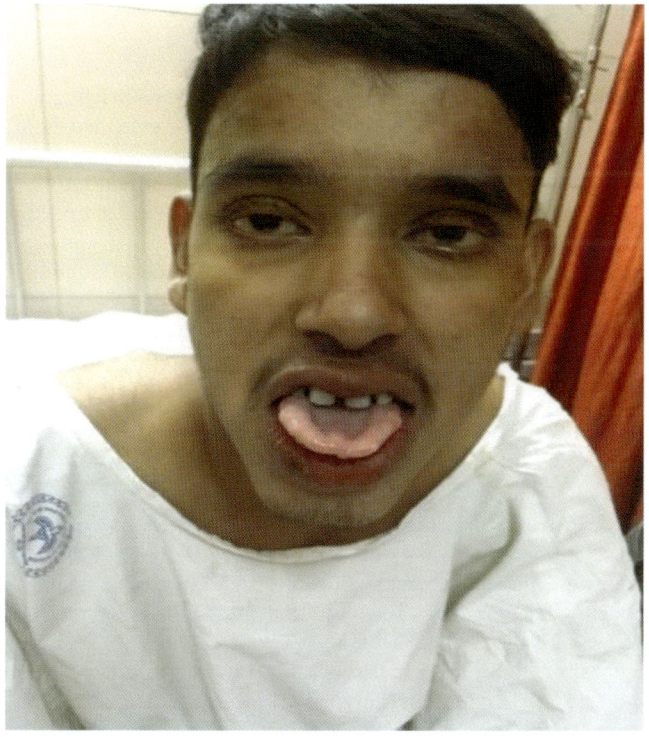

FIGURE 16.4 Patient with MEN 2B syndrome with oral ganglioneuromas.

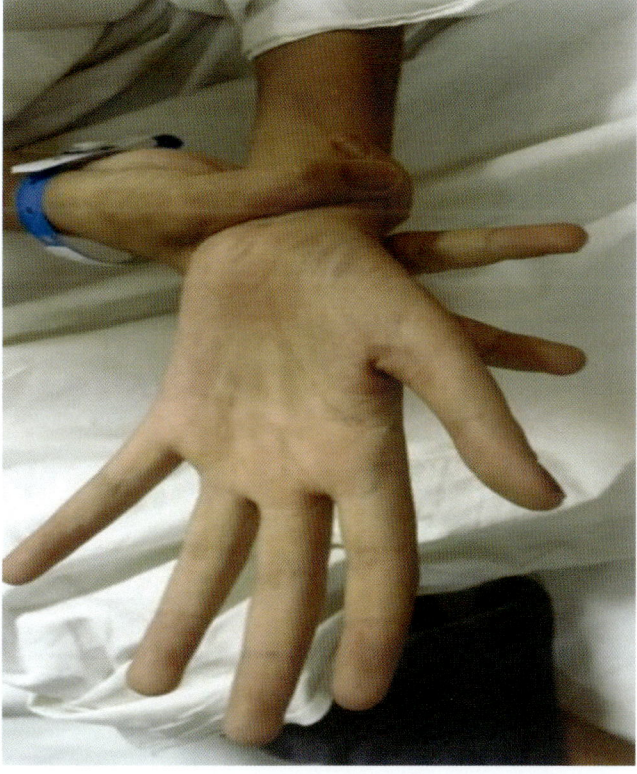

FIGURE 16.6 Patient with MEN 2B syndrome with marfanoid habitus.

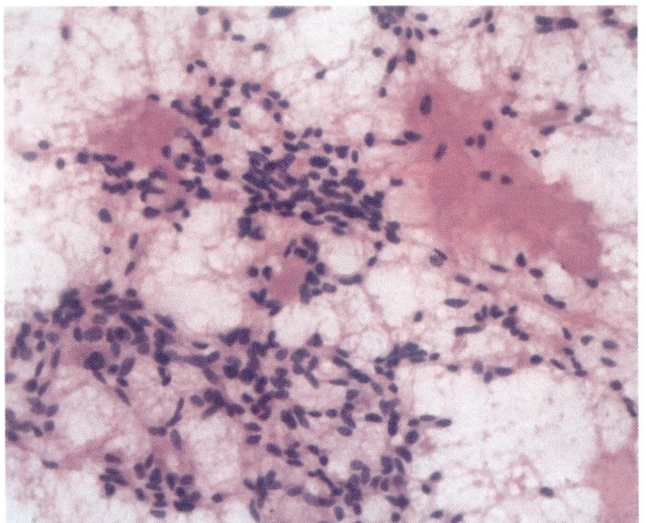

FIGURE 16.7 Loose aggregates of oval- to spindle-shaped cells with granular chromatin and clumps of amorphous eosinophilic material suggestive of amyloid (H&E ×400).

Evaluation and diagnosis

Clinical approach is done by triple assessment with clinical examination, radiological assessment and cytopathological assessment. FNAC typically shows a moderate-to-marked cellularity with spindle shaped, epithelioid or plasmacytoid cells with eccentrically placed round nuclei with fine or coarse granular chromatin (salt-pepper appearance typical of neuroendocrine tumors). There may also be present bizarre giant cells, clear cells, oncocytic cells or small cells. Amyloid is present in 50–80%, which is composed of extracellular deposits of calcitonin (Figures 16.7 and 16.8) (30). FNAC, however, has a low sensitivity in the diagnosis of MTC (31). In the setting, an indeterminate nodule measuring more than 1 cm in size, positive staining for calcitonin, CEA, chromogranin and negative staining for thyroglobulin on immunohistochemistry increases the diagnostic accuracy of FNAC (10).

Biomarkers in MTC

Serum calcitonin and carcinoembryonic antigen have been found to be of clinical relevance in aiding diagnosis, prognosticating and facilitating follow-up. Serum calcitonin has a high sensitivity to diagnose MTC (98%) (31). Serum calcitonin is elevated in MTC and correlates with its locoregional and systemic aggressiveness. It may be elevated in other conditions such as renal failure, hyperparathyroidism, thyroiditis, lung cancers, prostate cancer, mastocytosis and other neuroendocrine tumors. However, in these conditions, there is no rise in calcitonin levels after administration of calcium or pentagastrin. CEA, on the other hand, is not a specific biomarker for MTC and may not prove useful in the early diagnosis of MTC (32). However, it helps in determining disease progression and has been found to be a probable marker of dedifferentiation and, hence, predicts poorer outcomes (33).

Preoperative imaging

Ultrasonography of the neck is the primary imaging modality of choice for evaluating local disease. In patients with advanced locoregional disease in the neck or symptoms/signs of metastatic disease, cross-sectional imaging with CECT thorax, abdomen and pelvis (for mediastinal disease, lung or liver metastases) or MRI abdomen (for liver metastases) is recommended. MRI spine and bone scintigraphy may be done in suspected osseous metastases. Serum calcitonin levels, more than 500 pg/ml, warrants cross-sectional imaging irrespective of advanced locoregional disease or metastatic symptoms/signs (10, 34).

RET mutation analysis

All patients with MTC should undergo genetic counseling and *RET* mutation analysis and if positive must be extended to all first-degree relatives. Even in 1.5–7.3% of apparent sporadic MTCs, germline *RET* mutations have been identified (35, 36). Patients suspected to have MEN 2A syndrome must undergo *RET* mutation analysis in exon 10 (Codon 609, 611, 618 and 620), exon 11 (Codon 630, 634) and exons 8, 13 14, 15 and 16 (10). MEN 2B phenotype, on the other hand, should be tested for exon 16 (M918T) and exon 15 (A883F). If no mutations are discernible, the entire *RET* sequence is analyzed.

Screening for pheochromocytoma and hyperparathyroidism in MTC

Screening for pheochromocytoma and hyperparathyroidism must be done in all patients with MTC with 24-hour urinary metanephrines and normetanephrines and serum calcium, phosphorus and albumin level measurement. In hereditary MTC, screening must be done at 11 years in patients with known highest or high-risk mutations and at 16 years in patients with moderate-risk mutations. Surgical management of pheochromocytoma gains precedence over MTC or PHPT and may be done by open, laparoscopic or retroperitoneoscopic adrenalectomy (unilateral or bilateral cortical-sparing as indicated).

PHPT may be managed by subtotal parathyroidectomy with the preservation of the smallest gland or a vascularized part of it,

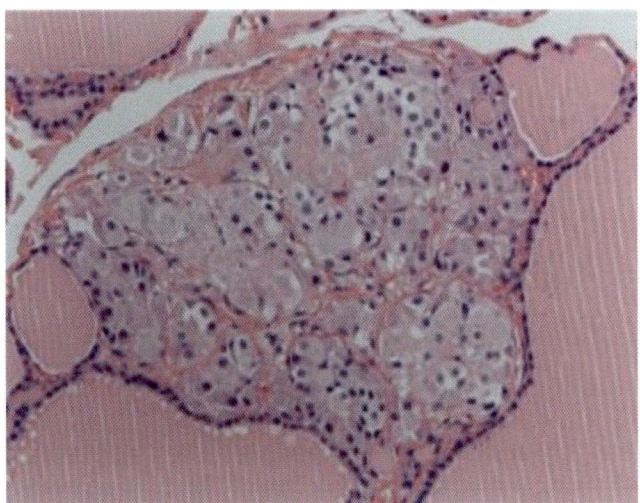

FIGURE 16.8 C-cell hyperplasia with atypical cells obliterating the follicles.

TABLE 16.1: Risk Stratification with Aggressiveness of MTC and Timing of Prophylactic Surgery

ATA Risk Level	Moderate	High	Highest
Codon mutation	321,532,533,609,611,618, 620,630,631,635,649,666, 768,790,791,804,844,891, 912	634,883	918
MTC aggressiveness	A, B	C	D
Age of onset	Adult	<5 years	First year of life
Timing of prophylactic surgery	When serum calcitonin gets elevated or earlier	Consider at <5 years. Based on serum calcitonin levels	As early as possible/first year of life (whichever is earlier)

total parathyroidectomy with heterotopic implantation of a part of the smallest gland in the nondominant brachioradialis muscle or resection of enlarged glands with intraoperative PTH monitoring.

Risk stratification by ATA MTC guidelines

Guidelines published by the American Thyroid association suggest stratification of MTC into three groups based on age at onset and aggressiveness. These are moderate risk (hereditary MTC with codon mutations other than M918T and 634), high risk (MEN 2A and codon 634, 883 mutation) and highest risk (MEN 2B and M918T mutation) (Table 16.1) (10).

Patients with the highest risk mutations are recommended prophylactic thyroidectomy within the first year or months of life. Patients with high-risk mutations are recommended prophylactic thyroidectomy within 5 years of age or when the serum calcitonin level rises (whichever is earlier) with prophylactic neck dissection in patients with calcitonin level more than 40 pg/ml or clinically/radiologically detected nodal disease. Patients with moderate risk for MTC should undergo clinical examination, USG of neck and serum calcitonin level measurement every 6 months to 1 year, lifelong and thyroidectomy may be considered when the serum calcitonin rises or at 5 years of age (if long-term follow-up is not desired). This is summarized in Table 16.1.

Surgical management of MTC

Surgical management of MTC is the most effective therapy available for MTC. As these tumors are of neuroendocrine origin, they don't take up radioactive iodine and are, hence, not amenable to radioiodine therapy. In patients with no clinical or radiological lymph nodal metastases, total thyroidectomy with central compartment lymphadenectomy (Level VI) may be done. Some authors recommend total thyroidectomy, ipsilateral central and lateral compartment lymphadenectomy (Level II–V) in the setting of serum calcitonin levels >20 pg/ml (37). In patients with clinical or radiologically positive nodal disease, total thyroidectomy, central compartment and ipsilateral lateral compartment lymphadenectomy may be recommended. In patients with serum calcitonin levels >200 pg/ml, bilateral lateral compartment lymphadenectomy may be done in addition to total thyroidectomy and central compartment dissection (37). Involvement of mediastinal nodal disease may require sternotomy and lymphadenectomy.

In patients who have undergone hemithyroidectomy with a histological surprise of MTC, completion thyroidectomy is not a necessity provided that there is no evidence of germline RET mutation, elevated calcitonin levels or radiological evidence of residual disease.

Postoperative follow up

Postoperatively, patients may be started on replacement doses of levothyroxine (1.6 µg/kg/day ideal body weight). Clinical examination and measurement of serum calcitonin and CEA levels must be done after 3 months and if normal, must be followed up every 6–12 months. If calcitonin levels are <150 pg/ml, they may be evaluated with USG of the neck, whereas values >150 pg/ml will require CECT thorax, abdomen and pelvis, bone scintigraphy, MR pelvis and spine, etc. (38). Doubling time of serum calcitonin and CEA may be calculated using serial values. Doubling time more than 24 months has been found to have better prognosis as opposed to less than 6 months (39).

Management of locoregional and metastatic disease

Patients with persistent or recurrent nodal disease in the neck must be primarily managed with compartment oriented redo central/lateral compartment neck dissection. The decision would be based on the burden of disease at the primary operation (<5 metastatic lymph nodes were removed) as well and the level of basal calcitonin (1000 pg/ml). In patients who harbor extensive disease, however, a less-aggressive approach may be considered to reduce the morbidity associated with extensive resection. A complete central compartment or lateral selective neck dissection reduces the chance of locoregional recurrence and improves survival outcomes (10).

External beam radiation therapy is used to reduce the risk of locoregional recurrence in patients with gross residual tumor, extra-thyroidal extension or extensive nodal disease. EBRT, however, does not increase the overall survival outcomes (40).

Systemic therapy in MTC is recommended in individuals with significant disease progression and metastatic disease. However, even in the setting of metastases, low volume disease, which is asymptomatic, does not require systemic therapy as the acute and chronic toxicity of the treatment regime outweigh the survival benefit provided. Treatment may be provided to palliate symptoms, hormonal excess, life-threatening events and prevent locoregional control.

Patients with isolated lung or liver metastases may benefit from metastatectomy. However, disseminated disease warrants treatment strategies such as systemic therapy or local therapy such as radiofrequency ablation or chemoembolization. Drugs such as doxorubicin, dacarbazine and 5-FU have been studied but have been shown to have short-lived low response rates. Radio-labeled molecules such as Yttrium-90 DOTA, Lutetium-177 DOTA, Indium-111 Octreotide or Iodine-131 MIBG have been studied in MTC and have shown partial response and may be tried in stabilizing disease progression.

Targeted therapy in MTC

The presence of *RET* germline mutations in virtually all familial MTC and about half of all sporadic MTC has brought targeted therapy into the limelight of management of this condition. Other important receptors such as VEGFR, EGFR and hepatocyte growth factor receptor (c-Met) are also overexpressed and, hence, are potential targets for therapy.

Different tyrosine kinase receptors are activated in MTC and, hence, inhibiting different activated tyrosine kinases has been a new strategy that has changed the face of MTC management. Vandetanib and cabozantinib have been approved by the US FDA for treatment of patients with advanced disease and may be considered first-line Tyrosine Kinase Inhibitors (TKIs).

Vandetanib, an oral 4-anilinoquinazoline, inhibits VEGFR 2, VEGFR3, RET and EGFR, VEGFR1 to a lesser extent. This docks to the ATP-binding pocket of RET, thus inhibiting it. The common adverse effects are skin rash, diarrhea, fatigue, atypical QTc prolongation, proteinuria and hypertension (41, 42). Cabozantinib inhibits MET, RET, VEGFR and CKIT, Flt-3 and Tie-2 and is administered at a dose of 140 mg daily. Adverse events include stomatitis, hypertension, diarrhea, fatigue, weight loss, Palmar-Plantar erythrodysesthesia syndrome, venous and arterial thromboembolism and rarely osteonecrosis and fistula formation (42).

Other TKIs such as sorafenib, sunitinib, lenvatinib and pazopanib have also been studied for potential use in MTC and are considered secondary TKIs Some multikinase inhibitors such as motesanib, axitinib, imatinib, gefitinib and ponatinib have been found to have limited efficacy and have not been found to be clinically useful.

Newer molecules such as nintedanib, anlotinib, regorafenib and sulfatinib are also being evaluated for their role in management of MTC. Tipifarnib is a farnesyltransferase inhibitor that blocks farnesylation of Ras proteins and may play a role in MTC with RAS mutation by blocking signal transduction. Similarly, certain statins such as lovastatin has been found to have antitumor properties in K-ras dependent thyroid tumors. Valproic acid inhibits histone deacetylase, thereby causing G2/M arrest in neoplastic cells and subsequent apoptosis. However, clinical efficacy is not yet fully understood.

Nelfinavir, a HIV protease inhibitor, has been found to target heat shock protein 90 chaperone (HSP90), which is required for folding and stability of RET mutants, and is a potential therapeutic option in the future. mTOR inhibitors such as everolimus have also been considered a therapeutic option as both RET and RAS utilize the mTOR pathway for downstream signal transduction.

Combination therapy with drugs such as temozolomide and capecitabine, sunitinib and cisplatin and cytotoxic chemotherapy with TKIs may be associated with better progression-free survival but not in overall survival. Their use, however, is limited by the toxicity profile.

Conclusion

Medullary carcinoma thyroid is a rare form of moderately differentiated carcinoma of thyroid arising from the parafollicular C-cell. Unlike WDTC, they do not take up radioactive iodine, and hence, they require aggressive surgical therapy upfront. As it is associated with a well-studied genotype-phenotype correlation with *RET* mutations, a thorough understanding of the genetic basis and molecular pathology is essential thereby making the clinician adept at offering genetic counseling and genetic testing to screen for familial disease and offer options of evolving targeted therapy.

References

1. Lim H, Devesa SS, Sosa JA, Check D, Kitahara CM. Trends in thyroid cancer incidence and mortality in the United States, 1974–2013. JAMA. 2017 Apr;317(13):1338–1348.
2. Jaquet J. Ein Fall von metastasierenden Amyloidtumoren (Lymphosarkom). Virchows Arch path Anat. 1906 Aug;185(2):251–268.
3. Hazard JB, Hawk WA, Crile G. Medullary (solid) carcinoma of the thyroid; a clinicopathologic entity. J Clin Endocrinol Metab. 1959 Jan;19(1):152–161.
4. Bray F, Ferlay J, Soerjomataram I, Siegel RL, Torre LA, Jemal A. Global cancer statistics 2018: GLOBOCAN estimates of incidence and mortality worldwide for 36 cancers in 185 countries. CA: Cancer J Clin. 2018;68(6):394–424.
5. Deshmukh A, Gangiti K, Pantvaidya G, Nair D, Basu S, Chaukar D, et al. Surgical outcomes of thyroid cancer patients in a tertiary cancer center in India. Indian J Cancer. 2018 Jan;55(1):23.
6. Mehrotra PK, Mishra A, Mishra SK, Agarwal G, Agarwal A, Verma AK. Medullary thyroid cancer: clinico-pathological profile and outcome in a tertiary care center in North India. World J Surg. 2011 Jun;35(6):1273–1280.
7. Cherian AJ, Ramakant P, Pai R, Manipadam MT, Elanthenral S, Chandramohan A, et al. Outcome of treatment for medullary thyroid carcinoma—a single centre experience. Indian J Surg Oncol. 2018 Mar;9(1):52–58.
8. Takahashi M, Ritz J, Cooper GM. Activation of a novel human transforming gene, ret, by DNA rearrangement. Cell. 1985 Sep;42(2):581–588.
9. Marsh DJ, Learoyd DL, Andrew SD, Krishnan L, Pojer R, Richardson AL, et al. Somatic mutations in the RET proto-oncogene in sporadic medullary thyroid carcinoma. Clin Endocrinol (Oxf). 1996 Mar;44(3):249–257.
10. Wells SA Jr, Asa SL, Dralle H, Elisei R, Evans DB, Gagel RF, et al. Revised American Thyroid Association Guidelines for the Management of Medullary Thyroid Carcinoma. Thyroid [Internet]. 2015 Jun [cited 2019 Jul 14]; Available from: https://www.liebertpub.com/doi/abs/10.1089/thy.2014.0335
11. Traugott AL, Moley JF. The RET protooncogene. Cancer Treat Res. 2010;153:303–319.
12. Nonidez JF. The origin of the 'parafollicular' cell, a second epithelial component of the thyroid gland of the dog. Am J Anat. 1932;49(3):479–505.
13. Saad MF, Ordonez NG, Rashid RK, Guido JJ, Hill CS, Hickey RC, et al. Medullary carcinoma of the thyroid. A study of the clinical features and prognostic factors in 161 patients. Medicine (Baltimore). 1984 Nov;63(6):319–342.
14. Kebebew E, Ituarte PH, Siperstein AE, Duh QY, Clark OH. Medullary thyroid carcinoma: clinical characteristics, treatment, prognostic factors, and a comparison of staging systems. Cancer. 2000 Mar;88(5):1139–1148.
15. Moley J, DeBenedetti M. Patterns of nodal metastases in palpable medullary thyroid carcinoma: recommendations for extent of node dissection. Ann Surg [Internet]. 1999 Jun [cited 2019 Aug 11];229(6). Available from: insights.ovid.com
16. Moley JF. Medullary thyroid carcinoma: management of lymph node metastases. J Natl Comprehensive Cancer Netw. 2010 May;8(5):549–556.
17. Simões-Pereira J, Bugalho MJ, Limbert E, Leite V. Retrospective analysis of 140 cases of medullary thyroid carcinoma followed-up in a single institution. Oncol Lett. 2016 May;11(6):3870–3874.
18. Groot JWB de, Kema IP, Breukelman H, Veer E van der, Wiggers T, Plukker JTM, et al. Biochemical markers in the follow-up of medullary thyroid cancer. Thyroid. 2006 Nov;16(11):1163–70.
19. Barbosa SL-S, Rodien P, Lebouleux S, Niccoli-Sire P, Kraimps J-L, Caron P, et al. Ectopic adrenocorticotropic hormone-syndrome in medullary carcinoma of the thyroid: a retrospective analysis and review of the literature. Thyroid. 2005 Jun;15(6):618–623.
20. Tiede DJ, Tefferi A, Kochhar R, Thompson GB, Hay ID. Paraneoplastic cholestasis and hypercoagulability associated with medullary thyroid carcinoma. Resolution with tumor debulking. Cancer. 1994;73(3):702–705.
21. Sipple JH. The association of pheochromocytoma with carcinoma of the thyroid gland. Am J Med. 1961 Jul;31(1):163–166.
22. McDonnell JE, Gild ML, Clifton-Bligh RJ, Robinson BG. Multiple endocrine neoplasia: an update [Internet]. Intern Med J. 2019 [cited 2019 Aug 14]. Available from: https://onlinelibrary.wiley.com/doi/abs/10.1111/imj.14394
23. Yip L, Cote GJ, Shapiro SE, Ayers GD, Herzog CE, Sellin RV, et al. Multiple endocrine neoplasia type 2: evaluation of the genotype-phenotype relationship. Arch Surg. 2003 Apr;138(4):409–416.
24. Nunziata V, Giannattasio R, Giovanni GD, D'armiento MR, Mancini M. Hereditary localized pruritus in affected members of a kindred with multiple endocrine neoplasia type 2a (Sipple's syndrome). Clin Endocrinol. 1989;30(1):57–63.
25. Gagel RF. Multiple endocrine neoplasia type 2a associated with cutaneous lichen amyloidosis. Ann Intern Med. 1989 Nov;111(10):802.
26. Wells SA, Pacini F, Robinson BG, Santoro M. Multiple endocrine neoplasia type 2 and familial medullary thyroid carcinoma: an update. J Clin Endocrinol Metab. 2013 Aug;98(8):3149–3164.
27. Farndon JR, Leightt GS, Dilley WG, Baylin SB, Smallridge RC, Harrison TS, et al. Familial medullary thyroid carcinoma without associated endocrinopathies: a distinct clinical entity. BJS. 1986;73(4):278–281.
28. Cohen MS, Phay JE, Albinson C, DeBenedetti MK, Skinner MA, Lairmore TC, et al. Gastrointestinal manifestations of multiple endocrine neoplasia type 2. Ann Surg. 2002 May;235(5):648–655.

29. Smith VV, Eng C, Milla PJ. Intestinal ganglioneuromatosis and multiple endocrine neoplasia type 2B: implications for treatment. Gut. 1999 Jul;45(1):143–146.
30. Khurana R, Agarwal A, Bajpai VK, Verma N, Sharma AK, Gupta RP, et al. Unraveling the amyloid associated with human medullary thyroid carcinoma. Endocrinology. 2004 Dec;145(12):5465–5470.
31. Bugalho MJM, et al. Preoperative diagnosis of medullary thyroid carcinoma: fine needle aspiration cytology as compared with serum calcitonin measurement. J Surg Oncol. [Internet]. [cited 2019 Aug 15]. Available from: https://www.ncbi.nlm.nih.gov/pubmed/15999359
32. Wells SA, Haagensen DE, Linehan WM, Farrell RE, Dilley WG. The detection of elevated plasma levels of carcinoembryonic antigen in patients with suspected or established medullary thyroid carcinoma. Cancer. 1978;42(S3):1498–1503.
33. Mendelsohn G, Wells SA, Baylin SB. Relationship of tissue carcinoembryonic antigen and calcitonin to tumor virulence in medullary thyroid carcinoma. An immunohistochemical study in early, localized, and virulent disseminated stages of disease. Cancer. 1984;54(4):657–662.
34. Machens A, Dralle H. Biomarker-based risk stratification for previously untreated medullary thyroid cancer. None. 2010 Jun;95(6):2655–2663.
35. Elisei R, Romei C, Cosci B, Agate L, Bottici V, Molinaro E, et al. RET genetic screening in patients with medullary thyroid cancer and their relatives: experience with 807 individuals at one center. None. 2007 Dec;92(12):4725–4729.
36. Eng C, Mulligan LM, Smith DP, Healey CS, Frilling A, Raue F, et al. Low frequency of germline mutations in the RET proto-oncogene in patients with apparently sporadic medullary thyroid carcinoma. Clin Endocrinol. 1995;43(1):123–127.
37. Miyauchi A, Matsuzuka F, Hirai K, Yokozawa T, Kobayashi K, Ito Y, et al. Prospective trial of unilateral surgery for nonhereditary medullary thyroid carcinoma in patients without germline RET mutations. World J Surg. 2002 Aug;26(8):1023–1028.
38. Pellegriti G, Leboulleux S, Baudin E, Bellon N, Scollo C, Travagli JP, et al. Long-term outcome of medullary thyroid carcinoma in patients with normal postoperative medical imaging. Br J Cancer. 2003 May;88(10):1537–1542.
39. Barbet J, Campion L, Kraeber-Bodéré F, Chatal J-F, GTE Study Group. Prognostic impact of serum calcitonin and carcinoembryonic antigen doubling-times in patients with medullary thyroid carcinoma. J Clin Endocrinol Metab. 2005 Nov;90(11):6077–6084.
40. Brierley J, Tsang R, Simpson WJ, Gospodarowicz M, Sutcliffe S, Panzarella T. Medullary thyroid cancer: analyses of survival and prognostic factors and the role of radiation therapy in local control. Thyroid. 1996 Aug;6(4):305–310.
41. Gómez K, Varghese J, Jiménez C. Medullary thyroid carcinoma: molecular signaling pathways and emerging therapies [Internet]. J Thyroid Res. 2011 [cited 2019 Jul 15]. Available from: https://www.hindawi.com/journals/jtr/2011/815826/
42. Priya SR, Dravid CS, Digumarti R, Dandekar M. Targeted therapy for medullary thyroid cancer: a review. Front Oncol [Internet]. 2017 Oct [cited 2019 Jul 15];7. Available from: https://www.ncbi.nlm.nih.gov/pmc/articles/PMC5635342/

# 17

POORLY DIFFERENTIATED THYROID CARCINOMA

Shreyamsa M, Anand Kumar Mishra and Kul Ranjan Singh

Introduction

Poorly differentiated thyroid carcinoma (PDTC) is a rare and heterogenous malignant lesion of the thyroid. Initially considered a variant of differentiated thyroid carcinoma, it is now classified as a separate entity (1). It was first described in 1907 by Thomas Langhans, who identified a typical nesting pattern in an epithelial thyroid malignancy and named it *"wuchernde struma"* (rampant goiter) (2). The nomenclature PDTC was coined many decades later by Granner and Buckwalter, in 1963 (3). Carcangiu in 1983 elucidated that PDTC is biologically and behaviorwise in an intermediate position, between the well-differentiated (DTC) and totally undifferentiated thyroid malignancies (4). The same year, Sakamoto and colleagues, in their landmark paper, deduced that certain tumors lost their cellular/glandular differentiation (i.e., papillary or follicular) acquiring a scirrhous or trabecular pattern instead. They also showed that this loss was associated with poor survival compared to the well-differentiated tumors (5).

Due to different diagnostic approaches and criteria, there was an uncertainty in the existence of PDTC, and the results of multiple studies varied greatly (6). It was not universally recognized till 2004, when the World Health Organization (WHO) formally accepted and introduced it in the WHO classification of endocrine tumors (7). This classification defines PDTC as "follicular-cell neoplasms with limited evidence of structural follicular cell differentiation which occupy both morphologically & behaviorally an intermediate position between differentiated and undifferentiated (anaplastic) carcinomas", emphasizing the importance of both differentiation loss, evidenced by nonglandular solid, trabecular or insular growth patterns and high-grade features (necrosis and mitoses).

Epidemiology

The incidence of PDTC varies greatly, from 0.23% in North Africa to 6.7% in Italy. Overall, it accounts for 2–3% of all thyroid cancers (8). Frequency of up to 15% has been reported previously in Northern Italy (9). The variation in incidence is due to the influence of geographic and environmental factors and genetic factors and dietary changes. Compared to DTC, PDTC generally manifests at an advanced age, mostly in the fifth or sixth decades of life (median – 59 years), and is more common in females than males (1:1.6) (10).

Risk factors

1. *Iodine deficiency*: There is increased incidence of PDTC in iodine-deficient areas and endemic goiter regions (up to 15% in Italy) compared to those sufficient in iodine (less than 1% in Japan) (9, 11).
2. *Age*: Increasing age is not only associated with higher incidence PDTC but also indicates aggressiveness and is an adverse prognostic factor (1, 10).
3. *Sex*: Although males are less affected than females, male sex is strongly associated with PDTC (1, 10).
4. *Ionizing radiation*: Evidence regarding role of radiation exposure in the genesis of PDTC is conflicting. Radiation exposure in general predisposes to thyroid malignancies and studies have noted an increased risk of PDTC among those patients (12). Large series from Chernobyl have found otherwise, with no increase in rates of PDTC (13).

Pathogenesis and molecular genetics

The genesis of PDTC is well explained by two separate models (14):

1. Partial dedifferentiation from DTC
    i. Foci of poor differentiation may be identified in a lesion diagnosed as DTC.
    ii. They can occur as recurrent lesions at sites previously resected for DTC or as metastatic lesions (15).
2. *De novo*, without the presence of a precursor lesion. This is the more common pathway of tumorigenesis.

Both the events are governed by myriad genetic changes, which play an important role in tumor progression and dedifferentiation (Figure 17.1).

Molecular profiling of PDTC demonstrates heterogeneous findings, with multiple mutations responsible for driving disease progression. Identification of these key oncogenic molecular drivers is necessary for the development of possible targeted therapies. Studies performed utilizing next-generation sequencing (NGS) have confirmed the "intermediate" position of PDTC at a molecular level. The number of mutations is significantly more than DTC, with further increase in dedifferentiation into anaplastic carcinoma (16). In PDTC, the mutation burden also carries prognostic value, with tumors exhibiting aggressive clinical, pathological features and reduced overall survival (16). The common mutations encountered in PDTC are enumerated in Table 17.1 (17–19).

Genetic alterations in follicular cells are caused by unopposed activation of either the mitogen-activated protein (MAP) kinase pathway or the phosphatidylinositol-3-kinase (PI3K)/AKT pathway (20). Similar to other types of thyroid malignancies, most common driver mutations in PDTC are mutually exclusive mutations of BRAF and RAS. BRAF-mutated PDTCs show higher rates of regional nodal metastases and RAS mutations show significantly higher rates of distant metastases, which is also seen in DTC (21). It is worth noting that lesions with BRAF mutations are also associated with a decreased capability to trap radioactive iodine (^{131}I) (14, 22). Mutations of RAS family of genes, most commonly HRAS codon 12 or 61 and NRAS at codon 13, are point mutations that occur in about 24% of all PDTCs. Unlike BRAF, which is specific to the activation of the MAP kinase pathway,

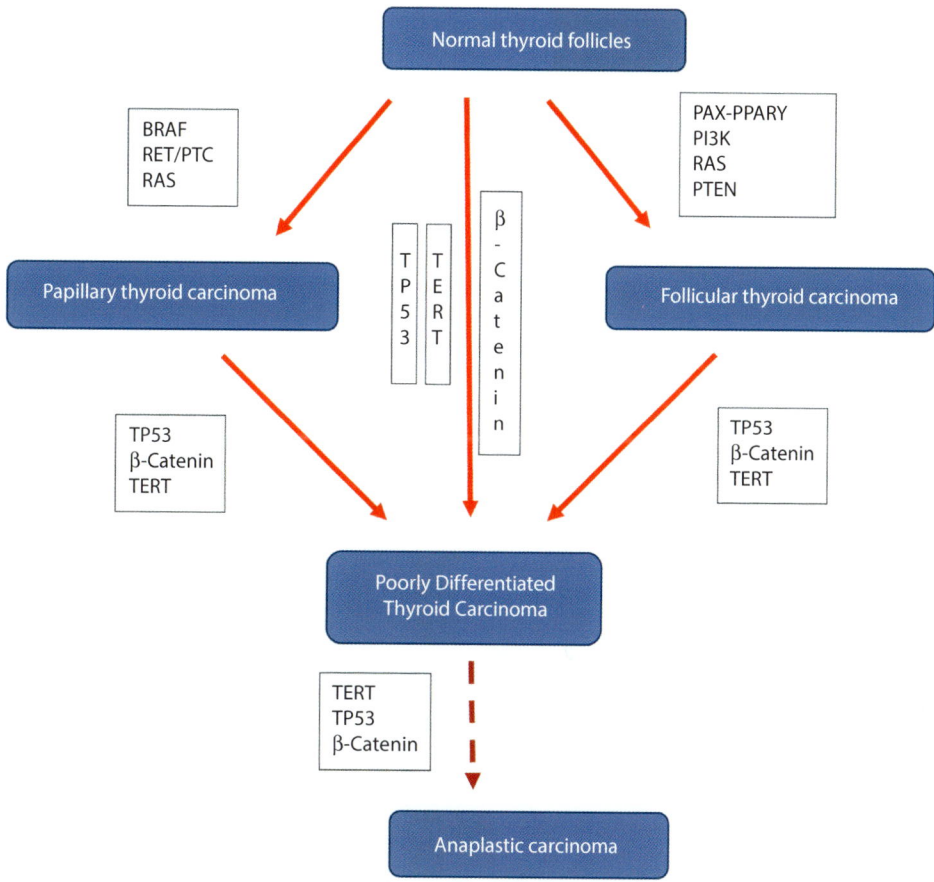

FIGURE 17.1 Pathogenesis of PDTC.

TABLE 17.1: Common Mutations Encountered in PDTC

Pathway/Type	Mutations	Percentage of Tumors (%)
TERT promoter mutation	Promoter mutation	40
RAS-RAF-MAPK	BRAFV600E	27–33
	RAS	24–28
Tumor suppressors	Tp53	8–16
	ATM	7–9
	RB1	2
	CHEK2	2
	MEN1	1
PI3K-AKT-mTOR	PTEN 4	4
	PIK3CA	3
	AKT1 and AKT3	3
Wnt	APC	4
	CDH1	3
	CTNNB1	1
STAT	JAK	3
Others	EIF1AX	11
	ABL1	4
	Histone methyltransferase	7
	RBM10	12
	MED12	15

RAS can activate both the MAP kinase pathway and the PI3K/AKT pathway. Oncogenic RAS activation is a marker of tumor dedifferentiation and adverse prognostic outcome (23). It has been observed that RAS mutations occur in up to 50% benign adenomas. Hence, it has now been established that standalone RAS mutations are less likely to result in tumorigenesis, but when combined with other mutations have a high diagnostic value (24).

BRAF-mutated papillary carcinomas show high MAPK output due to refractoriness to ERK feedback (extracellular signal-regulated kinases) and are less differentiated, whereas RAS-mutated tumors show attenuated MAPK output due to the maintained negative feedback by ERK. Hence, RAS-mutated tumors are less dedifferentiated. This phenomenon is preserved in PDTC, evident by preserved correlation of BRAF-RAS score (BRS) and thyroid differentiation scores (16, 25). This relation is lost in anaplastic carcinomas.

TERT promoter mutations are the most common alterations in PDTC. They are subclonal in DTC and clonal in PDTC and anaplastic carcinomas, which may indicate possible cell immortalization in advanced malignant lesions. TERT promoter mutations are associated with an aggressive phenotype, with increased rate of distal metastases and increased mortality (26). An association between TERT promoter mutations and BRAF/RAS is found in PDTC, with purported de novo binding elements on the mutated TERT promoter for MAPK signaling–activated transcription factors, resulting in increased aggressive behavior of the tumor (27).

TABLE 17.2: Relative Frequencies of Common Driver Mutations (16, 32, 33)

Mutation	PTC	FTC	PDTC	ATC
BRAF	45%	–	27–33%	30–45%
RAS	10–20%	36–48%	24–28%	24%
TERT	11%	17%	40%	73%
tP53	–	–	8–16%	65–73%
ATM	–	–	7–9%	9%
PTEN 4	–	–	4%	15%
PIK3CA	–	–	3%	18%

The most commonly mutated tumor suppressor gene in PDTC is TP53, albeit in lesser proportion compared to anaplastic carcinomas (20–40% vs. 65–73%) (23, 28). Mutation of ATM, another tumor suppressor gene, occurs at a similar frequency in PDTC (8%) and anaplastic carcinomas (9%) and is predictive of aggressive behavior before progression to anaplastic dedifferentiation (29). Chromosomal rearrangements are found in 10–14% of all PDTCs and include RET/PTC, PAX8-PPARG, ALK, BRAF and NTRK3. No correlation of gene fusions and clinicopathologic features was seen in PDTC (30). As these aberrations are present in lesser frequency in anaplastic carcinomas, it is proven that gene fusion–driven carcinomas do not have more potential of dedifferentiation. Several novel mutations have emerged recently, helping in identification of aggressive PDTCs. Mutation of EIF1AX, a translation initiation factor gene, occurs in about 11% and are predictive of worse survival in PDTC (31). Fatal PDTC showed a higher frequency of mutations in *TERT* promoter, MED12, RBM10, BRAF, HRAS, TP53, ATM and EIF1AX compared to nonfatal PDTC (29). Table 17.2 summarizes the relative frequencies of common driver mutations.

Epigenetic changes

miRNA profile of PDTC is well studied, and it is distinctive from that of DTC. The concept of tumor progression from DTC to PDTC reflects at the miRNA level as well (34). Several miRNAs that are upregulated in DTC like miR-221 and miR-222 are increasingly deregulated.

Clinical features

The intermediate status of PDTC is also reflected in their clinical behavior, showing biological aggressiveness of intermediate degree. At diagnosis, PDTCs typically present at an advanced stage with large tumors, features of local invasion and distant metastases. More than half the patients have extrathyroidal extension at presentation (10). Neck nodal metastases, predominantly in the central compartment, are seen in 27.8–72.4% (35). Recurrent laryngeal nerve (RLN) involvement distal metastases are common in PDTC and are seen in 48–85%, with lungs and bones being the most common sites of metastases (36).

Diagnosis

Ultrasound (US) is the investigation of choice for imaging in thyroid disorders, and it is the initial evaluation in suspected case of a thyroid cancer to assess the gland and cervical lymph nodes. Functionality of the thyroid is checked by performing thyroid function tests. Fine needle aspiration cytology (FNAC) sampling is performed for cytological analysis, which forms the mainstay of pathological confirmation. US-guided FNAC should be preferred to target solid and non-necrotic area of the nodule. In patients with clinical suspicion of PDTC, preoperative vocal cord evaluation is critical, as it is associated with high rates of involvement. When extrathyroidal extension and distant metastasis is suspected or clinically evident, further axial imaging by contrast-enhanced CT, magnetic resonance imaging (MRI) and fluorodeoxyglucose positron emission tomography (18-FDG PET) scan is recommended. Evaluation of adjacent structures in the form of endoscopies may also be required to quantify and stage the disease.

Cytopathology

Diagnosis of PDTC on FNAC samples is very challenging, due to nonspecific cytological characteristics. The rarity of the lesion, sampling errors due to poorly differentiated component in a well-differentiated lesion and overlap of cytological features with follicular neoplasms act as major confounding factors (37). Only 27–34% of all PDTCs can be correctly diagnosed on FNAC and most others are classified as follicular neoplasms (38). Features that are suggestive of PDTC are hypercellularity, presence of solid or insular architecture, high nuclear-to-cytoplasmic ratio and an increased mitotic activity.

Histopathology

To combine the different schools of thoughts of PDTC and bring about a uniform consensus for recognition and diagnosis, a group of revered thyroid experts convened in 2006 in Turin and formulated the so-called Turin criteria (39). The criteria propose a diagnostic algorithm for diagnosis of PDTC, which is now well accepted.

The Turin criteria – definition of PDTC (Figure 17.2):
A tumor with:

- Solid, trabecular or insular growth pattern (STI pattern)
- The absence of conventional nuclear features of papillary carcinoma
- The presence of either convoluted nuclei, necrosis or 3 or more mitotic activity per 10 high-power fields.

A criticism of the Turin criteria was that it did not take into consideration the measure of poorly differentiated areas within a malignant lesion required to make a diagnosis of PDTC. PDTCs are divided into focal (<10%) or diffuse PDTC (>10%) based on the proportion of the poorly differentiated component. Studies have found that focal or diffuse poor differentiation does not affect the prognosis (6, 40). Diffuse PDTC patients may have more extrathyroidal invasion and indirectly it shows the aggressive behavior locally of this tumor.

In the same year, an alternative definition was proposed based on the observations at the Memorial Sloan Kettering Cancer Center, who considered necrosis and mitotic activity of the lesion rather than the growth pattern (41). PDTC was defined as:

A tumor with follicular cell differentiation at the histologic and/or immunohistochemical levels, displaying:

- Tumor necrosis
- Five mitoses per ten high-power fields

They found that the overall survival was worse when necrosis and mitotic activity were considered for defining PDTC rather

Poorly Differentiated Thyroid Carcinoma

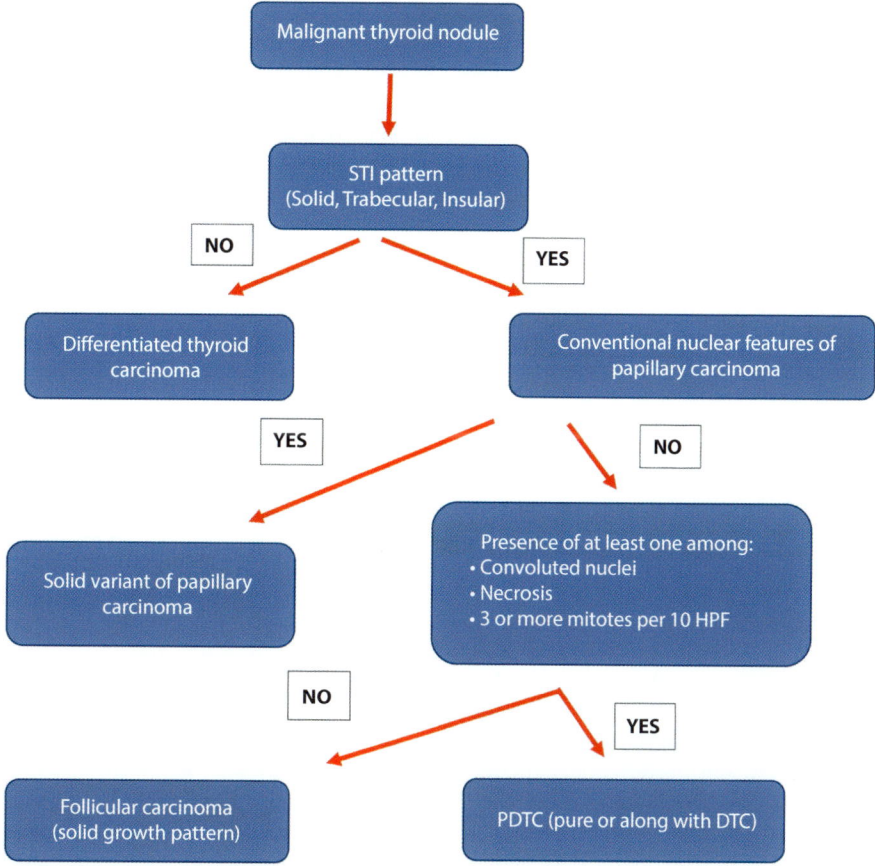

FIGURE 17.2 Diagnostic algorithm using Turin criteria.

than the growth pattern (60 and 83% at 5 years, respectively). PDTC must be differentiated from non-follicular cell–derived lesions like medullary carcinoma and metastases to thyroid usually from kidney/lung primary. Other common differential diagnosis is a solid variant of papillary cancer (42).

Immunohistochemistry (IHC)

Immunohistochemical examination is an immensely valuable tool in the diagnosis and management of thyroid tumors. There are no specific markers for PDTC, but immunohistochemistry (IHC) helps in establishing the follicular origin of the cell and/or excludes a medullary thyroid carcinoma or other differential diagnoses (43). PDTC are typically thyroglobulin positive, but the staining is focal and patchy compared to the strong and diffuse positivity shown by DTC, while anaplastic carcinomas stain mostly negatively (39, 44). E-cadherin is a cell adhesion molecule expressed in well-differentiated tumors but reduced in PDTC and not expressed in anaplastic carcinoma, indicating loss of differentiation with decreased expression (45). Loss of E-cadherin rather than mutations in β-catenin is supposed to be the key promoter of dedifferentiation. p53 staining is absent in most DTC while up to 38% PDTC and 70% anaplastic carcinomas stain positive (39). PDTC stains negative for calcitonin, carcinoembryonic antigen and chromogranin. Ki67 is a proliferation-related protein, indicating high mitotic activity. It is significantly increased in cases of dedifferentiating tumors and also portends aggressiveness (46). Immunostaining against BRAF V600E antibody is seen in PDTC and anaplastic carcinomas. This is known to be a reliable alternative for BRAF and the radioactive iodine–refractory $BRAF^{T1799}$ mutation genetic testing (47). Table 17.3 shows the differential staining of Thyroid cancers on IHC.

Imaging studies

Ultrasonography (US)

US is an indispensable tool in the management of thyroid lesions and the American Thyroid Association (ATA) guidelines endorse and recommend it in all patients with known or suspected thyroid nodules (48). There is no feature pathognomonic of PDTC, but some features may point toward malignancy/aggressiveness. Nodules are usually solid, hypoechoic, round to oval with a circumscribed margin (49). This property is lost with further dedifferentiation. PDTC appears as a distinct nest of tumor cells surrounded by a thin layer of fibrovascular stroma on histology. The area between the tumor island and the fibrovascular tissue often forms a perimeter lacking

TABLE 17.3: IHC Variance in Different Epithelial Malignancies of Thyroid

IHC Feature	DTC	PDTC	ATC
Thyroglobulin	++	+/−	−
E-cadherin	++	+/−	−
CK-19	++	+/−	−
TTF-1	++	+/−	−
p53	−	++	++
Ki67%	−	++	++
Calcitonin	−	−	−
Chromogranin	−	−	−

either typical papilla or a follicular structure (50). This may explain the appearance of a normal, circumscribed margin. Other sonological features of malignancy like irregular shape, vertical orientation, heterogeneity and microcalcification are shared with DTC and anaplastic carcinoma. Unusual findings like multiple tumors with overlapping borders have also been reported (51). US also helps in the assessment of cervical lymph nodes. Typical US features of metastatic lymph nodes include an increase in size, cystic change, hyperechogenicity, irregular margins, rounded appearance, calcifications and loss of the fatty hilum (52, 53).

Axial imaging
Further imaging using computed tomography (CT) or MRI is performed when there is a need to study the extent of the lesion, especially in cases where retrosternal extension or extrathyroidal involvement are suspected. This also aids in the operative planning. CT and MRI show similar accuracy in predicting local invasion of the aerodigestive tract and RLN (54). The key sign for aerodigestive tract invasion on CT/MRI is a mass in contact with 180° or more of the circumferences of trachea and/or esophagus. Other imaging features suggestive of tracheal involvement are deformity of the lumen, focal mucosal irregularity and intraluminal mass. Involvement of the RLN can be predicted by a finding of effacement of fatty tissue in the tracheoesophageal groove, along the course of the nerve (54, 55). Invasion of the abovementioned structures entails an extensive resection including the involved organ, while invasion of vascular and prevertebral structures usually precludes the patient from curative surgery.

Metabolic imaging
As explained by the "flip-flop phenomenon", PDTC exhibits intermediate GLUT1 (glucose transporter 1) expression and, as a result, has an FDG uptake profile that is intermediate (56). More often than not, PDTC is an FDG-PET positive tumor (57). But, owing to the difficulties concerned with the biological behavior of PDTC, further evaluations are necessary to establish the role of FDG-PET or PET/CT in PDTC. It is also useful in the detection of recurrent tumor in the setting of increased serum thyroglobulin level and negative whole-body iodine scan. Since the nodal metastases of neck are rather small, they may be missed on FDG-PET imaging, but it may detect previously unrecognized distant metastatic lesions (54).

Molecular imaging
Thyroid tumor cells in general express a variety of receptors, which makes them an attractive candidate for scintigraphic studies. Somatostatin is a ubiquitous peptide that carries out many biological functions in both endocrine and non-endocrine tissues. In addition, it is also known to regulate cell proliferation in normal and neoplastic tissues (58). ^{111}In-octreotide and ^{99m}Tc-depreotide have shown promise in this regard, especially in radioactive iodine (RAI)-resistant tumors (59). ^{99m}Tc-methoxyisobutylisonitrile (MIBI) scintigraphy has also been used for the evaluation of thyroid malignancies with variable results (60). ^{99m}Tc tetrofosmin is another useful moiety that has been used.

Treatment

Due to the rarity of disease and heterogenous diagnostic criteria, the treatment of PDTC has not been standardized unlike well-differentiated carcinomas. The TNM staging of thyroid cancer has both differentiated and undifferentiated (anaplastic) cancers, but it is lacking for PDTC. Therapeutic guidelines are mainly based on extrapolations from those of DTC. Surgical resection is the mainstay of treatment, whereby the extent of resection is determined by preoperative assessment using imaging studies and intraoperative findings. Total thyroidectomy with resection of all gross disease generally achieves satisfactory locoregional control, with 5-year disease-free survival seen in up to 81% of all patients (1, 61). A compartment-oriented lymphadenectomy of neck nodes is to be performed if there is clinical or radiological evidence of enlarged lymph nodes (62). As PDTC is known to be associated with an aggressive behavior, primary surgical resection may be more difficult and result in higher morbidity and mortality (63).

Adjuvant therapy

The indications and effectiveness of any adjuvant modalities in PDTC remain unclear and are yet to be explored. Unlike DTC, PDTC does not respond as well to the same modalities of adjuvant treatment (1). RAI avidity of PDTC is highly variable, and this may be a result of tumor heterogeneity and variable admixtures of well-differentiated and poorly differentiated tumor components. Areas of well-differentiated tumor respond excellently to RAI and areas of poor differentiation do not, resulting in persistent disease in spite of visible iodine avidity (11). It has also been observed that PDTC with lower expression of sodium iodide symporter have higher RAI resistance (64). In spite of the capacity to concentrate RAI, there is no evidence supporting improvement of survival outcomes by utilization of RAI therapy (65). The role of postoperative external beam radiation therapy (EBRT) in PDTC is equally unclear. EBRT is typically reserved for patients with aggressive forms of PDTCs or for patients with an incomplete resection of the involved thyroid/adjacent structures. EBRT is an effective adjuvant in DTC for patients with extrathyroidal extension and neck node involvement and the same has been recommended in PDTC by extrapolation (66). However, no significant survival improvement is observed in PDTC following EBRT. It may, however, be useful in high-risk settings due to a low-toxicity profile with newer techniques of radiation therapy, like the intensity-modulated radiotherapy (1). Palliative EBRT can be of utility in patients with bony pains and neurological complications (67).

Utility of cytotoxic chemotherapy in PDTC is not established and studies are extremely scarce. Most data available for the use of chemotherapy are extrapolations from studies performed for anaplastic carcinomas. It is mostly used in inoperable cases, where some locoregional control and reduction in disease progression have been observed (66). Doxorubicin-based chemotherapy has been approved for metastatic disease, but there is no improvement in overall survival (61). Studies are under progress assessing utility of cytotoxic chemotherapy in a neoadjuvant setting and the results have been encouraging, but these results await validation (68).

Targeting the various genetic mutations in PDTC has emerged as a novel avenue to bring meaningful outcomes and survival benefits in adjuvant and neoadjuvant settings. Tyrosine kinase inhibitors that block the pathogenetic molecular pathways have shown immense promise. Multikinase inhibitors *sorafenib* (RAS, BRAF, VEGF, PDGF and RET/PTC rearrangements) and *lenvatinib* (VEGF, FGF and PDGF receptors, RET and KIT mutations) are approved for use in PDTC (69). Accurate molecular characterization of patients with PDTC will be a key aspect for the future clinical management of these lesions.

Outcomes

PDTC is a more aggressive malignancy compared to DTC, regardless of focal or diffuse presence, with a higher propensity for local recurrence (1). Along the progression spectrum of follicular cell–based thyroid cancers, the prognosis of PDTC is intermediate between DTC and anaplastic carcinoma. It also holds an intermediate spot in terms of overall survival (OS) and disease-free survival (DFS). PDTC, unlike anaplastic carcinoma, is not invariably lethal and has a 5-year OS of 62–85% and a 5-year DFS of 66% (70). Resectibility of the tumor is the most important prognostic indicator, and all resectable tumors can be treated with curative-intent surgery as a first-line treatment. Age more than 45 years, higher stage at presentation (T4 disease), extrathyroidal extension, mitosis and necrosis and distant metastasis at presentation are other factors associated with poor survival (71). Matsumoto et al. have reported decreased thyrotropin receptor (TSH-R) in PDTC compared with WDTC (72), and this decreased expression has correlated with unfavorable clinical features (73). In vitro studies have demonstrated lower expression of sodium iodide symporter in PDTC cell lines (74, 75). And reduction of abovementioned differentiation markers such as TSH-R and sodium iodide symporter has been correlated with worse prognosis. Locoregional disease is the cause of death in only 18% of PDTC patients (10). However, distant control in PDTC is low, with a dismal 59% at 5 years. Metastatic disease represents the major cause of death in PDTC, accounting for up to 85% of disease-related deaths (1, 10, 70). This is particularly important since the role of current adjuvant treatment modalities in preventing systemic spread of the disease is not clear, and hence, development of new targeted therapies is necessary to improve outcomes.

Follow-up

There is scarce information regarding optimal surveillance and follow-up strategies for PDTC, due to the rarity of condition and lack of randomized trials. Most available data are again extrapolations from that of DTC. Whole-body scan with RAI can be used to visualize residual tumor tissue if the tumor is radioiodine avid. For a RAI negative tumor with increasing serum thyroglobulin levels, FDG-PET or novel molecular imaging techniques can be utilized. Clinical examinations form an invaluable part of follow-up.

South Asia perspective

Mishra et al. from Lucknow raised the question of a separate entity of insular carcinoma way back in the year 2005 as they have poor prognosis (76). Win et al. from Kuala Lumpur, Malaysia, stressed on the need of correct histopathological diagnosis of PDTC so that prognosis can be predicted. They stressed on detailed sampling of thyroid cancers, so that foci of PDTC component is not missed (77). Deshmukh et al. from Mumbai reported 2.26% (5 out of 221) of PDTC in a retrospective series of thyroid cancer. There are many isolated case reports of PDTC from various centers (78). Bichoo et al. from Lucknow concluded, in a series of thyroid cancer, which included both DTC and PDTC, that there is no difference in the outcomes of PDTC and DTC with poorly differentiated area. They had n = 27 PDTC in a series of 142 thyroid cancer during a 27-year period (79).

Conclusion

PDTC is a rare, but clinically significant entity, as it constitutes majority of deaths from follicular cell–derived non-anaplastic thyroid cancer. Patients with PDTC present with clinicopathological features associated with adverse prognosis. Initial complete surgery with resection of all gross disease is the key for tumor control, and this results in satisfactory locoregional control. However, the DFS is low (66%), and treatment failure is caused by distant metastases in majority of the cases. The role and benefits of adjuvant therapy in PDTC are inconclusive. Adjuvant RAI may be considered in patients with radioiodine avid lesions. Adjuvant EBRT can be considered in patients with gross residual locoregional disease or at high risk of recurrence, while palliative EBRT is useful for treatment of pain and compressive symptoms. Mutually exclusive mutations of *BRAF* and *RAS* are the most common driver mutations in PDTC, similar to DTC and anaplastic carcinoma. TERT and p53 mutations are associated with increased aggressiveness and mortality. With improvement of sequencing technologies, clinicopathological features will be correlated with molecular profile, leading to the development of personalized medicine, with the ultimate goal of reducing morbidity and mortality in individuals with PDTC.

References

1. Ibrahimpasic T, Ghossein R, Shah JP, Ganly I. Poorly differentiated carcinoma of the thyroid gland: current status and future prospects. Thyroid. 2019;29(3):311–321.
2. Langhans T. Über die epithelialenFormen der malignen Struma. Virchows Arch FürPatholAnatPhysiolFürKlin Med. 1907;189(1):69–152.
3. Granner DK, Buckwalter JA. Poorly differentiated carcinoma of the thyroid gland. Surg Gynecol Obstet. 1963;116:650–656.
4. Carcangiu ML, Zampi G, Rosai J. Poorly differentiated ("insular") thyroid carcinoma. A reinterpretation of Langhans' "wuchernde Struma." Am J Surg Pathol. 1984;8(9):655–668.
5. Sakamoto A, Kasai N, Sugano H. Poorly differentiated carcinoma of the thyroid. A clinicopathologic entity for a high-risk group of papillary and follicular carcinomas. Cancer. 1983;52(10):1849–1855.
6. Dettmer, MS, Schmitt, A, Komminoth, P. et al. Poorly differentiated thyroid carcinoma. Pathologe. 2019. https://doi.org/10.1007/s00292-019-0600-9
7. Delellis R, Lloyd R, Heitz P, Eng C (eds) (2004) Pathology and genetics of tumours of endocrine organs, 3rd edn. World Health Organization classificationof tumours, vol8. IARC, Lyon
8. Walczyk A, Kopczyński J, Gąsior-Perczak D, Pałyga I, Kowalik A, Chrapek M, et al. Poorly differentiated thyroid cancer in the context of the revised 2015 American Thyroid Association Guidelines and the Updated American Joint Committee on Cancer/Tumor-Node-Metastasis Staging System (eighth edition). Clin Endocrinol (Oxf). 2019;91(2):331–339.
9. Yan S, Holt S, Khan S, Nwariaku F. High-risk and poorly differentiated thyroid cancer. In: A. Mancino, L. Kim, eds., Management of Differentiated Thyroid Cancer. Cham: Springer; 2017. https://doi.org/10.1007/978-3-319-54493-9_9
10. Ibrahimpasic T, Ghossein R, Carlson DL, Nixon I, Palmer FL, Shaha AR, et al. Outcomes in patients with poorly differentiated carcinoma. J Clin Endocrinol Metab. 2014; 99(4):1245–1252.
11. Greco A, Miranda C, Borrello MG, Pierotti MA. Thyroid cancer. In: G. Dellaire, J.N. Berman, R.J. Arceci, eds., Cancer Genomics: From Bench to Personalized Medicine. Academic Press; 2014. pp. 265–280.https://doi.org/10.1016/C2011-0-06830-8
12. Yu MG, Rivera J, Jimeno C. Poorly differentiated thyroid carcinoma: 10-year experience in a Southeast Asian population. Endocrinol Metab Seoul Korea. 2017;32(2):288–295.
13. LiVolsi VA, Abrosimov AA, Bogdanova T, Fadda G, Hunt JL, Ito M, et al. The Chernobyl thyroid cancer experience: pathology. Clin Oncol R Coll Radiol G B. 2011;23(4):261–267.
14. Hannallah J, Rose J, Guerrero MA. Comprehensive literature review: recent advances in diagnosing and managing patients with poorly differentiated thyroid carcinoma. Int J Endocrinol 2013;2013:317487.
15. Baloch Z, LiVolsi VA, Tondon R. Aggressive variants of follicular cell derived thyroid carcinoma; the so called "real thyroid carcinomas." J Clin Pathol. 2013; 66(9):733–743.
16. Landa I, Ibrahimpasic T, Boucai L, Sinha R, Knauf JA, Shah RH, et al. Genomic and transcriptomic hallmarks of poorly differentiated and anaplastic thyroid cancers. J Clin Invest. 2016;126(3):1052–1066.
17. Gerber TS, Schad A, Hartmann N, Springer E, Zechner U, Musholt TJ. Targeted next-generation sequencing of cancer genes in poorly differentiated thyroid cancer. Endocr Connect. 2018; 7(1):47–55.
18. Sykorova V, Dvorakova S, Vcelak J, Vaclavikova E, Halkova T, Kodetova D, et al. Search for new genetic biomarkers in poorly differentiated and anaplastic thyroid carcinomas using next generation sequencing. Anticancer Res. 2015;35(4):2029–2036.
19. Cheng DT, Mitchell TN, Zehir A, et al. Memorial Sloan Kettering-Integrated Mutation Profiling of Actionable Cancer Targets (MSK-IMPACT): a hybridization capture-based next-generation sequencing clinical assay for solid tumor molecular oncology. J Mol Diagn. 2015;17(3):251–264.

20. Nikiforova MN, Wald AI, Roy S, Durso MB, Nikiforov YE. Targeted next-generation sequencing panel (ThyroSeq) for detection of mutations in thyroid cancer. J Clin Endocrinol Metab. 2013; 98(11):E1852–E1860.
21. Fagin JA, Wells SA. Biologic and clinical perspectives on thyroid cancer. N Engl J Med. 2016;375(11):1054–1067.
22. Nikiforov YE. Thyroid carcinoma: molecular pathways and therapeutic targets. Mod Pathol. 2008;21(Suppl2):S37–S43.
23. Penna GC, Vaisman F, Vaisman M, Sobrinho-Simões M, Soares P. Molecular markers involved in tumorigenesis of thyroid carcinoma: focus on aggressive histotypes. Cytogenet Genome Res. 2016;150(3–4):194–207.
24. Xing M. Clinical utility of RAS mutations in thyroid cancer: a blurred picture now emerging clearer. BMC Med. 2016;14:12.
25. Cancer Genome Atlas Research Network. Integrated genomic characterization of papillary thyroid carcinoma. Cell. 2014;159(3):676–690.
26. Tsou P, Wu CJ. Mapping driver mutations to histopathological subtypes in papillary thyroidcarcinoma: applying a deep convolutional neural network. J Clin Med. 2019;8(10):1675.
27. Bell RJ, Rube HT, Kreig A, et al. Cancer. The transcription factor GABP selectively binds and activates the mutant TERT promoter in cancer. Science. 2015;348(6238):1036–1039.
28. Eloy C, Ferreira L, Salgado C, Soares P, Sobrinho-Simões M. Poorly differentiated and undifferentiated thyroid carcinomas. Turk Patoloji Derg. 2015;31(Suppl 1):48–59.
29. Ibrahimpasic T, Xu B, Landa I, Dogan S, Middha S, Seshan V, et al. Genomic alterations in fatal forms of non-anaplastic thyroid cancer: identification of MED12 and RBM10 as novel thyroid cancer genes associated with tumor virulence. Clin Cancer Res. 2017;23(19):5970–5980.
30. Yakushina VD, Lerner LV, Lavrov AV. Gene fusions in thyroid cancer. Thyroid. 2018;28(2):158–167.
31. Simões-Pereira J, Moura MM, Marques IJ, Rito M, Cabrera RA, Leite V, et al. The role of EIF1AX in thyroid cancer tumourigenesis and progression. J Endocrinol Invest. 2019; 42(3):313–318.
32. Fakhruddin N, Jabbour M, Novy M, et al. BRAF and NRAS mutations in papillary thyroid carcinoma and concordance in braf mutations between primary and corresponding lymph node metastases. Sci Rep. 2017;7(1):4666.
33. Censi S, Cavedon E, Bertazza L, et al. Frequency and significance of *Ras*, *Tert* promoter, and *Braf* mutations in cytologically indeterminate thyroid nodules: a monocentric case series at a tertiary-level endocrinology unit. Front Endocrinol (Lausanne). 2017;8:273
34. Dettmer MS, Perren A, Moch H, Komminoth P, Nikiforov YE, Nikiforova MN. MicroRNA profile of poorly differentiated thyroid carcinomas: new diagnostic and prognostic insights. J Mol Endocrinol. 2014;52(2):181–189.
35. Thiagarajan, S., Yousuf, A., Shetty, R. et al. Poorly differentiated thyroid carcinoma (PDTC) characteristics and the efficacy of radioactive iodine (RAI) therapy as an adjuvant treatment in a tertiary cancer care center. Eur Arch Otorhinolaryngol. 2020. https://doi.org/10.1007/s00405-020-05898-9
36. Wong KS, Lorch JH, Alexander EK, Marqusee E, Cho NL, Nehs MA, et al. Prognostic significance of extent of invasion in poorly differentiated thyroid cancer. Thyroid. 2019;29(9):1255–1261.
37. Kane SV, Sharma TP. Cytologic diagnostic approach to poorly differentiated thyroid carcinoma: a single-institution study. Cancer Cytopathol. 2015;123(2):82–91.
38. Saglietti C, Onenerk AM, Faquin WC, Sykiotis GP, Ziadi S, Bongiovanni M. FNA diagnosis of poorly differentiated thyroid carcinoma. A review of the recent literature. Cytopathol. 2017;28(6):467–474.
39. Volante M, Collini P, Nikiforov YE, Sakamoto A, Kakudo K, Katoh R, et al. Poorly differentiated thyroid carcinoma: the Turin proposal for the use of uniform diagnostic criteria and an algorithmic diagnostic approach. Am J SurgPathol. 2007;31(8):1256–1264.
40. Akaishi J, Kondo T, Sugino K, Ogimi Y, Masaki C, Hames KY, et al. Prognostic impact of the Turin criteria in poorly differentiated thyroid carcinoma. World J Surg. 2019;43(9):2235–2244.
41. Hiltzik D, Carlson DL, Tuttle RM, Chuai S, Ishill N, Shaha A, et al. Poorly differentiated thyroid carcinomas defined on the basis of mitosis and necrosis: a clinicopathologic study of 58 patients. Cancer. 2006;106(6):1286–1295.
42. Nikiforov YE, Biddinger PW, Thompson LDR. Diagnostic Pathology and Molecular Genetics of the Thyroid: A Comprehensive Guide for Practicing Thyroid Pathology. 2nd ed. Philadelphia: LWW; 2012. 448 p.
43. Patel KN, Shaha AR. Poorly differentiated thyroid cancer. Curr Opin Otolaryngol Head Neck Surg. 2014;22(2):121–126.
44. Asioli S, Erickson LA, Righi A, Jin L, Volante M, Jenkins S, et al. Poorly differentiated carcinoma of the thyroid: validation of the Turin proposal and analysis of IMP3 expression. Mod Pathol. 2010;23(9):1269–1278.
45. Liu H, Lin F. Application of immunohistochemistry in thyroid pathology. Arch Pathol Lab Med. 2015;139(1):67–82.
46. Kakudo K, Wakasa T, Ohta Y, Yane K, Ito Y, Yamashita H. Prognostic classification of thyroid follicular cell tumors using Ki-67 labeling index: risk stratification of thyroid follicular cell carcinomas. Endocr J. 2015;62(1):1–12.
47. Ghossein RA, Katabi N, Fagin JA. Immunohistochemical detection of mutated BRAF V600E supports the clonal origin of BRAF-induced thyroid cancers along the spectrum of disease progression. J Clin Endocrinol Metab. 2013;98(8):E1414–E1421.
48. Haugen BR, Alexander EK, Bible KC, et al. 2015 American Thyroid Association Management Guidelines for Adult Patients with Thyroid Nodules and Differentiated Thyroid Cancer: The American Thyroid Association Guidelines Task Force on Thyroid Nodules and Differentiated Thyroid Cancer. Thyroid. 2016;26(1):1–133.
49. Hahn SY, Shin JH. Description and comparison of the sonographic characteristics of poorly differentiated thyroid carcinoma and anaplastic thyroid carcinoma. J Ultrasound Med. 2016;35(9):1873–1879.
50. Zhang B, Niu HM, Wu Q, et al. Comparison of clinical and ultrasonographic features of poorly differentiated thyroid carcinoma and papillary thyroid carcinoma. Chin Med J (Engl). 2016;129(2):169–173.
51. Kihara M, Amino N, Hirokawa M, Matsuzuka F, Miyauchi A. Unusual finding on ultrasonography of follicular thyroid carcinoma including poorly differentiated thyroid carcinoma. Thyroid. 2008;18(9):1021–1022.
52. Ardakani AA, Rasekhi A, Mohammadi A, Motevalian E, Najafabad BK. Differentiation between metastatic and tumour-free cervical lymph nodes in patients with papillary thyroid carcinoma by grey-scale sonographic texture analysis. Pol J Radiol. 2018;83:e37–e46.
53. Lew JI, Solorzano CC. Use of ultrasound in the management of thyroid cancer. Oncologist. 2010;15(3):253–258.
54. Hoang JK, Branstetter BF, Gafton AR, Lee WK, Glastonbury CM. Imaging of thyroid carcinoma with CT and MRI: approaches to common scenarios. Cancer Imaging. 2013 Mar;13(1):128–139.
55. Seo YL, Yoon DY, Lim KJ, Cha JH, Yun EJ, Choi CS, et al. Locally advanced thyroid cancer: can CT help in prediction of extrathyroidal invasion to adjacent structures? AJR Am J Roentgenol. 2010;195(3):W240–W244.
56. Grabellus F, Nagarajah J, Bockisch A, Schmid KW, Sheu S-Y. Glucose transporter 1 expression, tumor proliferation, and iodine/glucose uptake in thyroid cancer with emphasis on poorly differentiated thyroid carcinoma. Clin Nucl Med. 2012;37(2):121–127.
57. Treglia G, Annunziata S, Muoio B, Salvatori M, Ceriani L, Giovanella L. The role of fluorine-18-fluorodeoxyglucose positron emission tomography in aggressive histological subtypes of thyroid cancer: an overview. Int J Endocrinol. 2013;2013:856189.
58. Csaba Z, Peineau S, Dournaud P. Molecular mechanisms of somatostatin receptor trafficking. J Mol Endocrinol. 2012;48(1):R1–12.
59. Puig-Domingo M, Luque RM, Reverter JL, López-Sánchez LM, Gahete MD, Culler MD, et al. The truncated isoform of somatostatin receptor 5 (sst5TMD4) is associated with poorly differentiated thyroid carcinoma. PLOS ONE. 2014;9(1):e85527.
60. Galli F, Manni I, Piaggio G, Balogh L, Weintraub BD, Szkudlinski MW, et al. (99m) Tc-labeled-rhTSH analogue (TR1401) for imaging poorly differentiated metastatic thyroid cancer. Thyroid. 2014; 24(8):1297–1308.
61. Fat I, Kulaga M, Dodis R, Carling T, Theoharis C, Rennert NJ. Insular variant of poorly differentiated thyroid carcinoma. Endocr Pract. 2011;17(1):115–121.
62. Carling T, Ocal IT, Udelsman R. Special variants of differentiated thyroid cancer: does it alter the extent of surgery versus well-differentiated thyroid cancer? World J Surg. 2007;31:916–923.
63. Marcadis AR, Cracchiolo J, Shaha AK. Management of locally advanced thyroid cancer. In: R. Parameswaran, A. Agarwal, eds., Evidence-Based Endocrine Surgery. Singapore: Springer; 2018.
64. Underwood HJ, Shaha AR, Patel KN. Variable response to radioactive iodine treatment in poorly differentiated thyroid carcinoma. Gland Surg. 2019;8(6):589–590.
65. Walczyk A, Kowalska A, Sygut J. The clinical course of poorly differentiated thyroid carcinoma (insular carcinoma) - own observations. Endokrynol Pol. 2010;61(5):467–473.
66. Sanders EM, LiVolsi VA, Brierley J, Shin J, Randolph GW. An evidence-based review of poorly differentiated thyroid cancer. World J Surg. 2007;31(5):934–945.
67. Filetti S, Durante C, Hartl D, Leboulleux S, Locati LD, Newbold K, et al. Thyroid cancer: ESMO Clinical Practice Guidelines for diagnosis, treatment and follow-up†. Ann Oncol. 2019 01;30(12):1856–1883.
68. Besic N, Dremelj M, Schwartzbartl-Pevec A, Gazic B. Neoadjuvant chemotherapy in 13 patients with locally advanced poorly differentiated thyroid carcinoma based on Turin proposal – a single institution experience. Radiol Oncol. 2015;49(3):271–278.
69. Valerio L, Pieruzzi L, Giani C, Agate L, Bottici V, Lorusso L, et al. Targeted therapy in thyroid cancer: state of the art. Clin Oncol R Coll Radiol G B. 2017;29(5):316–324.
70. Lee DY, Won J-K, Lee S-H, Park DJ, Jung KC, Sung M-W, et al. Changes of clinicopathologic characteristics and survival outcomes of anaplastic and poorly differentiated thyroid carcinoma. Thyroid. 2016;26(3):404–413.
71. de la Fouchardière C, Decaussin-Petrucci M, Berthiller J, Descotes F, Lopez J, Lifante JC, et al. Predictive factors of outcome in poorly differentiated thyroid carcinomas. Eur J Cancer. 2018;92:40–47.
72. Matsumoto H., Sakamoto A, Fujiwara M et al., Decreased expression of the thyroid-stimulating hormone receptor in poorly-differentiated carcinoma of the thyroid. Oncol Rep. 2008;19(6):1405–1411.
73. Tanaka K., Inoue H., Miki H, et al. Relationship between prognostic score and thyrotropin receptor (TSH-R) in papillary thyroid carcinoma: immunohistochemical detection of TSH-R. Br J Cancer. 1997;76 (5):594–599.
74. Fortunati N, Catalano MG, Arena K, Brignardello E, Piovesan A, Boccuzzi G. Valproic acid induces the expression of the Na/I symporter and iodine uptake in poorly differentiated thyroid cancer cells. J Clin Endocrinol Metabol. 2004;89(2):1006–1009.
75. Furuya F., Shimura H., Miyazaki A, et al. Adenovirusmediated transfer of thyroid transcription factor-1 induces radioiodideorganification and retention in thyroid cancer cells. Endocrinology. 2004;145(11):5397–5405.
76. Mishra AK, Agawal A, Mishra SK. Insular carcinoma: subtype of thyroid cancer with aggressive clinical course. World J Surg. 2005;29(3):410; author reply 410-1.
77. Win TT, Othman NH, Mohamad I. Poorly differentiated thyroid carcinoma: a hospital-based clinicopathological study and review of literature. Indian J Pathol Microbiol. 2017;60(2):167–171.
78. Deshmukh A, Gangiti K, Pantvaidya G, Nair D, Basu S, Chaukar D, et al. Surgical outcomes of thyroid cancer patients in a tertiary cancer center in India. Indian J Cancer. 2018;55(1):23–32.
79. Bichoo RA, Mishra A, Kumari N, Krishnani N, Chand G, Agarwal G, Agarwal A, Mishra et al. Poorly differentiated thyroid carcinoma and poorly differentiated area in differentiated thyroid carcinoma: is there any difference? Langenbecks Arch Surg. 2019; 404(1):45–53.

18

ANAPLASTIC THYROID CARCINOMA

Sasi Mouli, Anand Kumar Mishra and Kul Ranjan Singh

Introduction

Thyroid cancer is a mix of good, bad and ugly prognosis tumors. Well-differentiated thyroid cancers (DTCs) are good having 20-year survival rates of more than 90% [1]. Anaplastic thyroid cancer (ATC) is ugliest with median survival of 5 months and only 20% live beyond 1 year [2]. ATC are rare cancer (1–2%) and develop as de novo or dedifferentiation in a DTC. History of goiter is present in 20–50% of patients. Patient develops a rapidly enlarging neck mass with symptoms of compression of local structures. The treatment is difficult and includes surgery, accelerated hyperfractionated external beam radiation therapy (EBRT) and chemotherapy (CT) in a localized disease and palliation in widespread disease. During last 50 years, the clinical course of ATC has not changed; however, there is now more understanding of the genetics and clinicopathology, which has risen a hope of newer treatment options.

Epidemiology

ATC comprises nearly 1–2% of all thyroid cancers. In last few decades, the incidence of DTC has risen due to iodine prophylaxis and increased incidence of micropapillary thyroid cancer (PTC) while ATC had decreased due to better treatment of DTC and iodine prophylaxis. ATC results in 20–50% of all deaths from thyroid cancer [3–5]. Incidence of ATC is approximately 1–2 per million per annum [6, 7]. In a recent study, Lin et al. analyzed surveillance, epidemiology and end results (SEER) database from 1986 to 2015, age-adjusted incidence rate was found to be 0.9 per million per annum [8]. Prevalence of ATC ranges across studies between 1.3 and 9.8% (median 3.6%). Median survival is approximately 5–6 months, 1-year survival in 20% and 10–15% live beyond 2 years [2].

ATC commonly occurs in the sixth to seventh decade of life with less than 10% in age-group below 50 years [9–11]. In a recent study, Pradhan et al., from India, found 34% of ATC occurring below 50 years [3]. Female to male ratio ranges from 1.2 to 2:1 [3,12] and in SEER database it was 1.48:1 [8].

Risk factors

The main risk factors for ATC include older age (over 65 years) with history of long-standing goiter, thyroid disorder or DTC or radiation to neck.

Morphology and histology

Grossly the tumor is usually large, tan-white, with extrathyroid involvement, and is associated with plenty of necrosis and hemorrhage [13]. Histopathology varies between patient to patient and within the same tumor. It contains three predominant histologic patterns; spindle cell (50%), pleomorphic giant cell (30–40%), squamoid cell (less than 20%), and rare variants include paucicellular and rhabdoid [14]. Spindle cell squamous carcinoma variant is a usual variant seen associated with tall cell PTC (R-52). Spindle cell variant shows a storiform pattern, and differential diagnosis is spindle cell soft tissue sarcoma. It is highly vascular and also shows resemblance with angiosarcoma. Paucicellular variant is considered as one of rare variants of spindle cell type of ATC that has low cellularity and mimics Riedel's thyroiditis. Paucicellular variant occurs in younger age-group and has a relatively indolent course [2].

Giant cell variant has bizarre cells with hyperchromatic nuclei and eosinophilic cytoplasm interspersed with occasional osteoclast-like giant cells, which are considered as fusion elements of histocyte and monocyte lineage cells giving appearance of giant cells.

Epitheloid-squamoid variant is relatively less frequent. It may be mixed with spindle variant. This variant is identified by the presence of keratin even if occasional [14] and may be confused with squamous cell carcinoma of thyroid, diffuse sclerosing variant of PTC, secondaries from neck or lung. These various subtypes ultimately do not affect the clinical management or outcome.

Macrophage infiltration

Tumor-associated macrophages (TAMs) are seen in 22–95% of ATC and they are interspersed with cancer cells [15]. TAM are of two types – activated M1 macrophages, responsible for phagocytosis in response to type 1 T-helper cytokines [16], and activated M2 macrophages [16, 17], responsible for immunosuppression and trophic activity in response to type 2 T-helper cytokines [18]. It is observed that increased TAM density is associated with decreased cancer-related survival.

Antecedent thyroid disease

ATC develops de novo or from dedifferentiation of DTC. De novo development is more common in younger age group (<50 years). The evidence in favor of this hypothesis comes from:

1. ATC patients have long history of goiter in 20–50% and coexisting DTC in 7–89% [2, 19–24]. Tall cell variant of PTC is most common synchronous DTC followed by follicular thyroid carcinoma (FTC) and Hurthle cell cancer (10%) [25]. It can also be associated with poorly differentiated carcinoma.
2. ATC and DTC share common genetic mutations (BRAF, RAS). This supports the hypothesis that ATC develops from DTC [26]. Later more mutations p53 tumor suppressor protein, 16p, catenin (cadherin-associated protein), beta 1 and PIK3CA cause ATC [27–29].

Genetics

Majority of the ATCs have a history of goiter, and a possible malignancy that goes undiagnosed [30]. The aberrations may involve somatic gene alterations or chromosomal alterations (which

TABLE 18.1: Somatic Gene Alterations and Their Percentage Across Various Studies [14,31,32]

Gene Pathway Alteration	Percentage
P53	Up to 73%
TERT	Up to 73%
CTNNB1 (Wnt-signaling pathway)	25–60%
RAS	5–50%
BRAF	Up to 25%
PTEN	4–16%
MMR	12%
ATM	9%
RB1	9%
NF2	6%
TSHR	6%
STK11	6%
CDKN2A	4.7%
EGFR	1.8%
RET/PTC	Rare

occur as gain or loss of various chromosomes). TP53 gene inactivation is implicated in progression to undifferentiated cancer from differentiated. Table 18.1 summarizes the various somatic gene mutations along with their incidence in thyroid oncogenesis.

Somatic gene alterations

As these undiagnosed thyroid malignancies dedifferentiates, there are multiple mutations that occur in ATC. The major pathway involved in thyroid cancers is MAP kinase pathway that is involved in up to 90% [14]. In ATC, MAP kinase, PIK3CA, Wnt-signaling pathways are involved with variable frequencies. Most common somatic mutations found in ATC are TP53, and B-catenin genes and both of these are rare in DTC. Other mutations are BRAF, RAS, PIK3CA and PTEN observed in 10–20% (31, 32).

Clinical features

Symptoms: The most common symptoms of ATC are local with features of mechanical compression on airway or recurrent nerve. Patient may have painful neck mass because of locally aggressive disease.

Commonest presentation is a rapidly growing neck mass (64–100%) with history of long-standing goiter (20–50%) that may be associated with erythema and edema of the overlying skin. The growth of neck mass is very rapid and it can double its volume within 3 days to a week. Other symptoms may be voice change (28–44%), dysphagia (33–40%), dyspnea with or without cough (20–33%). Hemoptysis (25%) indicates the invasion of tumor into the trachea or widespread pulmonary metastases. Other symptoms may be neck pain, stridor, chest pain, bone pain, headache, vomiting. Patient may have systemic symptoms of cancer like loss of appetite, loss of weight and shortness of breath because of pulmonary metastases [2, 3, 33]. Patients may also present with unusual features of transient hyperthyroidism (up to 20%) [34], bradycardia possibly due to compression of vagus nerve, superior vena cava syndrome, acute Horner syndrome, leucocytosis from secretion of granulocyte colony-stimulating factor from tumor, gastrointestinal symptoms, and ball-valve type respiratory obstruction. Rarely patient may present with disseminated metastasis and metastasis to skin [35].

Signs: On examination, there is presence of neck swelling in thyroid region, which usually involves both lobes of thyroid, is multinodular (may be solitary), has a hard consistency (occasionally variable), with restricted mobility, and which may or may not move with deglutition. Goiter may be fixed anteriorly to sternum that may produce fixity and/or tenderness, indicates invasion, posteriorly to the prevertebral fascia or vertebrae (Figure 18.1). Mediastinal extension causes positive Pemberton's sign (Figure 18.2) with dilated veins over neck and chest, associated with facial plethora and breathlessness [11].

Associated cervical lymphadenopathy is seen in up to 40% [11]. Tracheal deviation or invasion may give rise to luminal compromise and give rise to stridor. Severe cases may present with skin ulceration and fungation (Figure 18.3).

Spread

Loco regional spread to perithyroidal soft tissue, i.e. fatty tissue, muscle, is seen in up to 60% [2, 9, 11]. Other structures involvement includes trachea (46%), esophagus (44%), larynx (13%), internal jugular vein (IJV), carotid artery, and direct mediastinal spread [36]. Recurrent laryngeal nerve involvement is seen in up to 30%, manifesting as spontaneous vocal cord paralysis. At time of diagnosis 2–9% of ATC is intrathyroidal, 34–62% has developed local spread and distant metastases is seen in 50% of patients, and approximately 25% will develop during the course of their disease [37]. Common metastatic sites are lung (80%), bone (15%) and brain (5–13%) [22, 38]. The most frequent cause of death in patients is suffocation caused by rapid local progression of ATC [39]. Differential diagnosis of a rapidly enlarging neck mass includes poorly DTC (PDTC), and ATC, primary thyroid lymphoma, sarcoma, primary squamous cell carcinoma of thyroid, and metastatic adenopathy from poorly differentiated upper aerodigestive tract malignancies. Painful rapid enlargement of neck mass might suggest hemorrhage inside the mass.

Investigations

Diagnosis

Fine-needle aspiration cytology (FNAC) has a diagnostic yield of about 85% [40]. FNAC may reveal necrotic area, which mandates ultrasonography (US)-guided aspiration from solid area, non-necrotic tumor. Core biopsy (CB) is required as FNAC aspirate may show necrosis, inflamed issue, hemorrhage, leucocyte infiltration, extensive tumor fibrosis or coexisting DTC. CB helps in obtaining viable tissue, and helps in confirming diagnosis by routine microscopy and immunohistochemistry (IHC). CB essentially differentiates ATC from lymphoma. CB had sensitivity of 76.9% and 94.7%; positive predictive value (PPV) of 100% for ATC and thyroid lymphoma [41]. CB from the metastases can also be done if there are discrepancies [2].

Immunohistochemistry (IHC)

ATC is positive for cytokeratin (pankeratin AE1/AE3) in 40 to 100% cases [14]. Pankeratin AE1/AE3 may be positive in DTC of thyroid [2]. Paired Box Gene PAX-8 is a more specific marker for tumors arising from thyroid, including DTC, and in ATC, it may be positive in up to 79% cases, with nearly 92% of squamoid variant of ATC [14]. TP53 may be positive in squamous cell cancer (SCC) and lymphoma of thyroid, though SCCs are positive for high-molecular-weight keratin (HMWK) and lymphoma are positive for CD45 [2]. CD45 and other lymphoid markers along

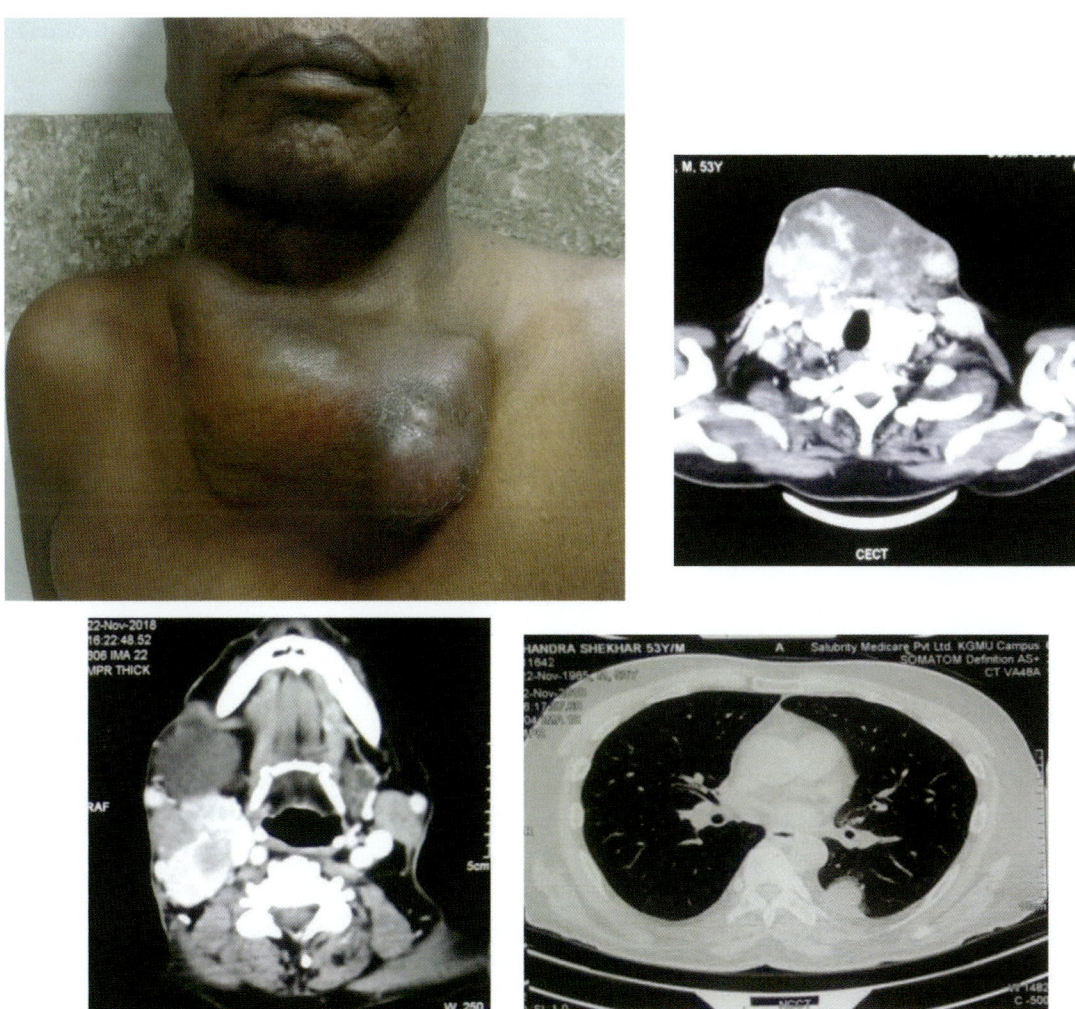

FIGURE 18.1 Top left: clinical presentation of patient malignant multinodular goiter; top right: CECT of neck showing mixed solid and cystic lesion involving predominantly right lobe with extrathyroidal extension; bottom left: bilateral cervical lymphadenopathy; bottom right: CT thorax without lung metastases patient's FNAC was PTC but after surgery, final histology revealed anaplastic thyroid carcinoma.

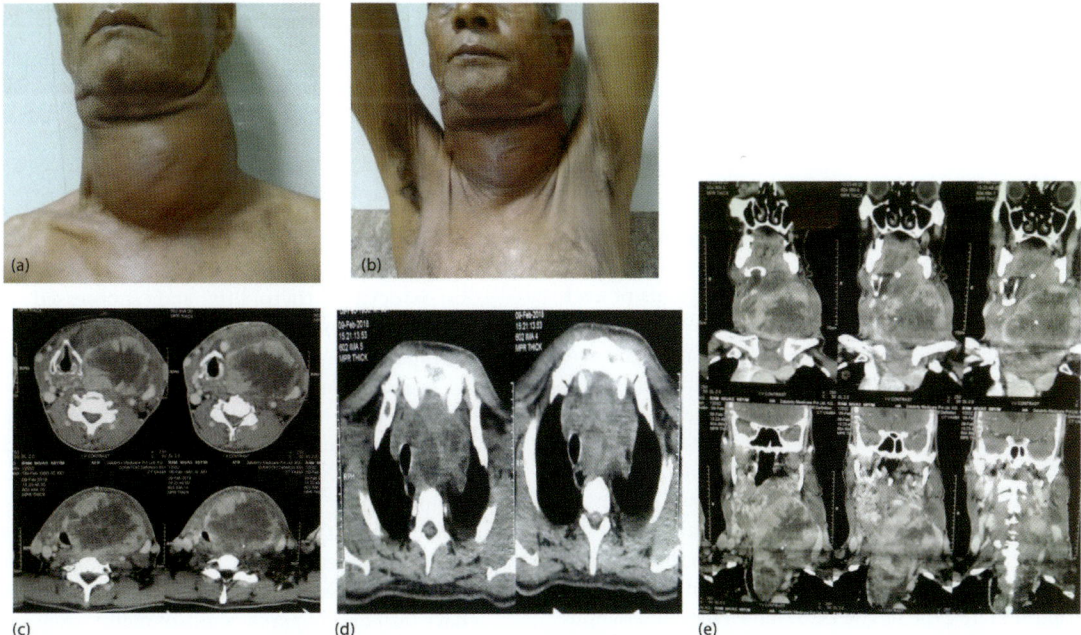

FIGURE 18.2 (a) Thyroid enlargement seen with few dilated veins over neck. (b) Patient performing Pemberton's maneuver showing increased prominence of neck veins, with facial plethora. Patient's core needle biopsy was anaplastic thyroid carcinoma! (c–e) CT scan of neck of the patient at neck, thorax and sagittal cut.

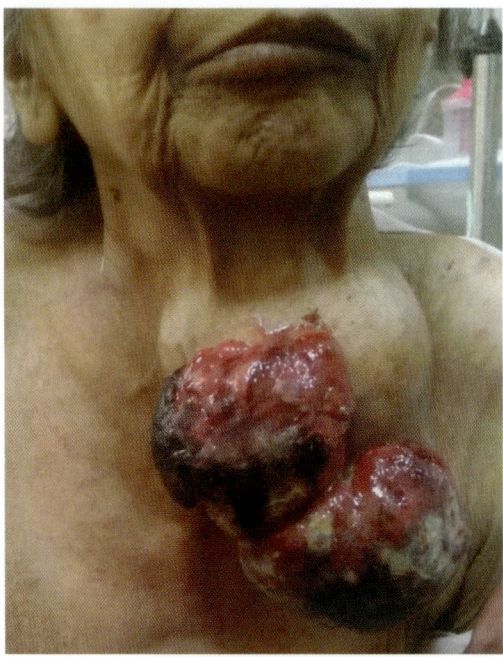
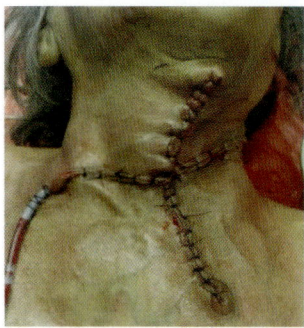
Immediate Post surgery wound
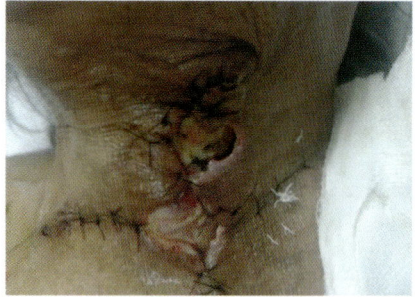
POD6- wound gaping; managed conservatively.

FIGURE 18.3 A 74-year-old female presented with multinodular goiter with ulcerated skin, fungating mass found to have anaplastic thyroid carcinoma. (i) Immediate postsurgery wound. (ii) POD6 – wound gaping; managed conservatively.

with melanocytic markers are used to exclude lymphoma and melanoma, respectively. Spindle cell variant of ATC is positive for vimentin in nearly 100%. Squamoid variant of ATC is positive for epithelial membrane antigen (EMA) in 30–50% of cases and rarely carcinoembryonic antigen (CEA) [14]. Characteristically, ATC is negative for thyroglobulin, thyroid transcription factor-1 (TTF-1), calcitonin. False-positive thyroglobulin may result from viable follicular cells entrapment in tumor cells [14].

Imaging

US is the imaging of choice in thyroid and for suspected ATC also it is the first imaging modality. There are no characteristic specific features of ATC on US but it provides information of nodule (solid, hypoechoic), margins (irregular), invasion in surrounding structures and cervical lymphadenopathy. It can be used to target solid and non-necrotic area of the nodule for FNAC. Contrast-enhanced computed tomography (CECT) imaging of neck and thorax gives a precise disease extent and local spread to adjacent structures such as great vessels of neck (39% carotid artery), esophagus (55%), trachea (69% invasion), larynx, mediastinum. More than 80% of ATC have extensive primary disease on. Solid part of ATC may show enhancement with interspersed hypodense areas that suggests necrosis (Figure 18.3). Necrosis is more common in ATC than other thyroid cancer, but it is not pathognomonic. Lee et al. found necrosis in 100% of their study on CECT [42]. Extrathyroid extension (ETE) can be seen in as high as 91% [43]. Ahmed et al. have found calcification associated within ATC in up to 62% in their cohort, coarse calcification was the commonest type, and followed by stipulated or punctuate type [43]. CECT shows regional lymphadenopathy in up to 78% [42].

Flourodeoxyglucose positron emission tomography (18-FDG PET) scan is recommended by American Thyroid Association (ATA) for metastatic work-up in ATC [2]. PET shows both locoregional spread (>75%), distant metastases (>50%) and so aids in both diagnosis of distant metastases and planning therapy [44]. Both primary and metastatic sites are widely FDG avid due to expression of glucose transporter-1 (GLUT-1) receptors [45]. Poisson et al. have also found that intensity of uptake in tumor, i.e. maximum standardized uptake value (SUV_{max}) greater than 18 and volume of FDG avid lesions >300 ml had a prognostic importance. The 6-month survival rates for SUV_{max} of >18 vs. <18 were 20 vs. 80% (p = 0.015) and FDG uptake volume for >300 ml vs. <300 ml was 10 vs. 90% (p = 0.004) [46]. However, Bogsrud et al. did not find the prognostic correlation in intensity of uptake and survival [45]. It is also is more sensitive and more efficient in detecting therapeutic response in ATC.

Other investigations

1. Thyroid-stimulating hormone (TSH) to assess thyroid function. Usually, TSH is normal but it may be high in associated thyroiditis and suppressed in transient hyperthyroidism.
2. Complete blood picture with differential counts is needed to evaluate for anemia and assess adequacy of platelets. Leucocytosis with high neutrophils may suggest infection. Low count may suggest immunodeficiency. Rare patients may have very high leucocytosis caused by tumor lymphokines.
3. Blood chemistry evaluation includes kidney and liver function tests, electrolytes. Calcium and phosphorus should be done to assess parathyroid function. Some patients may have humoral hypercalcemia of malignancy.
4. Vocal cord assessment by fiber optic or flexible laryngoscopy and bronchoscopy for airway involvement should also be done.

Anaplastic Thyroid Carcinoma

Histological differential diagnosis of anaplastic cancer includes:

- Metastatic disease to the thyroid
- Primary thyroid lymphoma
- Primary thyroid sarcoma
- Poorly differentiated thyroid carcinoma
- Squamous cell thyroid carcinoma
- Medullary carcinoma

Staging

ATC is stage as per TNM staging – the American Joint Committee on Cancer categorizes ATC as stage IV 8th edition [47, 48]. TNM staging is summarized in Table 18.2. ATC is stages into 4 A/B/C as described next.

Stage IVA: Tumors are intrathyroidal (T1–T3a) without lymph node involvement or distant metastases.

Stage IVB: Primary tumor exhibits gross ETE (any T) with lymph node metastases.

Stage IVC: Distant metastases with any T with or without any N.

Treatment

Since ATC is the most aggressive endocrine malignancy, a delay in diagnosis and treatment should be avoided. It is best considered as an oncologic emergency and requires a rapid complex integrated decision-making. The treatment should be discussed in a multidisciplinary meeting where thyroid surgeon, pathologist, radiologist, medical oncologist, radiation oncologist, palliative care expert and endocrinologist are members. Patient's clinical status and appropriate treatment pathways that are available in the hospital should be discussed thoroughly among multi-disciplinary team. Initial management of ATC involves evaluation of the airway and its stability, metastases workup (as 50% have distant metastases at diagnosis), evaluation for the resectability of the tumor and rapid test to determine whether tumor harbors a BRAF mutation. This mutation identification provides an opportunity for to use selective BRAF kinase inhibitor. It is important to define and discuss natural history, treatment options and expected outcome with the patient and family. In all ATC personalized goals of care should be established so that a therapeutic planning can be made. In all patients, risks of disease and risks of therapies should be

TABLE 18.2: TNM Staging – The American Joint Committee on Cancer Categorizes ATC as Stage IV 8th Edition

Definition of T – Tumor Staging	
T-stage	Criteria
Tx	Primary tumor cannot be assessed
T0	No evidence of tumor
T1	Tumor ≤2 cm in greatest dimension, limited to thyroid gland
T1a	Tumor ≤1 cm in greatest dimension, limited to thyroid gland
T1b	Tumor >1 cm but ≤2 cm in greatest dimension, limited to thyroid gland
T2	Tumor >2 cm but ≤4 cm in greatest dimension, limited to thyroid gland
T3	Tumor >4 cm in greatest dimension, or gross extrathyroid extension invading only strap muscles
T3a	Tumor >4 cm limited to thyroid
T3b	Gross extrathyroidal extension invading only strap muscles (sternohyoid, sternothyroid, thyrohyoid or omohyoid muscles) from a tumor of any size
T4	Includes gross extrathyroidal extension into major neck structures
T4a	Gross extrathyroidal extension invading subcutaneous soft tissue, larynx, trachea, esophagus or recurrent laryngeal nerve from a tumor of any size
T4b	Gross extrathyroidal extension invading prevertebral fascia or encasing carotid artery or mediastinal vessels from a tumor of any size

Note: All categories may be subdivided: (s) solitary tumor; (m) multifocal tumor (the largest tumor determines the classification)

Definition of Regional Lymph Node (N)	
N-Stage	Criteria
Nx	Regional lymph nodes cannot be assessed
N0	No evidence of regional lymph nodes metastasis
N0a	One or more cytological or histologically confirmed benign lymph node
N0b	No radiological or clinical evidence of locoregional lymph nodes metastasis
N1	Metastasis to regional nodes
N1a	Metastasis to level VI or VII (pretracheal, paratracheal or prelaryngeal/Delphian or upper mediastinal) lymph nodes. This can be unilateral or bilateral disease
N1b	Metastasis to unilateral, bilateral or contralateral lateral neck lymph nodes (level I, II, III, IV or V) or retropharyngeal lymph nodes

Definition of Metastasis (M)	
M-Stage	Criteria
M0	No distant metastases
M1	Distant metastases

TABLE 18.3: Overall Summary of Management

Treatment planning	Goals should be established, outcomes to be discussed with patient, relatives prior to initiation of therapy Multimodality management Discuss end life issues with all patient/relatives
Resectable disease	Surgery Extent of surgery: • Total or near-total thyroidectomy • Extrathyroidal extension: en bloc resection • No role for laryngectomy Preserve recurrent nerve, no role of debulking Adjuvant chemotherapy and radiotherapy (RT) as early as possible
Unresectable disease	Systemic therapy initially if good performance status, assess for resectability if response to systemic therapy Surgery if rendered resectable RT: aggressive/palliative Tyrosine kinase inhibitors General measures: airway, enteral nutrition
Metastatic disease	In good performance status patient, systemic therapy+RT In poor performance status – palliative RT, or HOSPICE General measures: airway, enteral nutrition Other specific measures • Bisphosphonates: bone metastasis • Steroids: brain metastasis

balanced. Treatment invariably is multimodal and depends if the disease is locoregional or metastatic. Therapy should be implemented as early as possible after diagnosis [2] and it is individualized as summarized in Table 18.3 and Figure 18.4(a) and (b): Flowchart of management.

Locoregional disease

ATC confined to thyroid gland (intrathyroidal-stage IVA) or invading surrounding structures (extrathyroidal-stage IVB), which are amenable for resection, are subjected to surgery with intent of R0/R1 resection [49, 50]. Total thyroidectomy with central neck node dissection (CNND) and lateral neck node dissection (LNND) is choice of surgery for primary [49]. The extent of resection differs in German association of endocrine surgeons practice guidelines that consider thyroid lobectomy with ipsilateral neck dissection for an intrathyroidal tumor that is confined to one lobe [50]. Aggressive resections may include the soft tissue resections of aerodigestive tract that needs expertise. Preservation of RLN should always be considered. In cases of preoperative unilateral RLN involvement, contralateral RLN should be preserved, even if mandates leaving partial thyroid tissue adjacent to nerve [2]. In unresectable tumours, BRAFV600E mutational analysis should be done and if positive, patient should be treated with targeted tyrosine kinase inhibitors (dabrafenib and trametinib). If BRAFV600E mutation is negative, other mutational analysis like ALK, NTRK and RET fusions can be done, and targeted therapy planned accordingly. Neo-adjuvant targeted tyrosine kinase and other therapies can be used to downstage disease and make it resectable.

Negative resection margins (R0) in surgical management of ATC is of utmost importance. In a large study, Goffredo et al., using the American National cancer database (NCDB), observed that in patients undergoing surgery (n = 335), overall 45.4% (n = 104) patients had R0 resection and 54.6% (n = 125) had positive resection margins (R1 + R2). Overall, stage IVA patients were found to have more R0 resections (59.8%) vs. stage IVB (30.7%) and stage IVC (36.2%). Those patients with positive resection margin had increased 30-day mortality of 16% vs. negative margins 4.8% (p = 0.007). Majority of the patients undergoing surgical intervention were of stage IVA (42.7%). Among stage IVA, R0 resection patients had a better survival compared to R1 and R2 patients (p = 0.048) [51]. R terminology is described in Table 18.4.

If an incidental ATC is found within the specimen DTC, the extent of resection varies among different centers. Some centers are conservative while others proceed with completion thyroidectomy [30]. Sugitani et al., in a retrospective study, including the Japanese database for ATC, found that the prognosis of incidentally found ATC was better than other stages with a 1-year cause-specific survival (CSS) of 57% (p < 0.001) [52].

Adjuvant therapy in the form of radiotherapy (RT), EBRT or intensity-modulated RT – IMRT) with or without systemic CT should be administered as per institutional protocols. In a retrospective study of 329 patients from South Korea, adjuvant RT, concurrent CT had improved prognosis in stage IVA, IVB (median survival 15 months) [53]. Wendler et al. have found survival benefit of multimodal therapy with surgery, RT and sequential or concurrent CT in patients of stages IVA and IVB [33].

Metastatic disease

In the setting of distant metastases (stage IVC), the intent of treatment should be palliation. If the patient is not in a condition to take a decision, a proxy should be involved who would decide regarding the best possible therapeutic option for that individual [2]. The role of surgery in metastatic setting for primary has been explained in few retrospective studies. Brignardello et al. have shown better median survival (6.57 vs. 1.54 months) with early surgery in stage IVC in 24 out of 31 patients [54]. However, Baek et al., in multicenter retrospective study of South Korean database, did not observe any benefit of aggressive management in stage IVC [53]. Wendler et al. also did not find any survival benefit of multimodality therapy in stage IVC [33]. Table 18.5 summarizes the outcome of multimodality therapy for ATC seen across various studies.

Other measures

ATC tumors grow very fast and produce symptoms of airway obstruction. Tracheotomy is best avoided and can only be thought in extreme conditions of life-threatening asphyxia. The patients who require tracheotomy have already advanced local disease with minimal long-term survival. Tracheotomy prolongs the sufferings and discomfort, can only be performed under anesthesia with preoperative intubation. It leads to all problems of maintenance like secretions management, frequent suctioning with risk of bleeding and tumor growth in the stoma. In a terminal patient whether this procedure is meaningful or not remains controversial [2, 30]. Tracheal stents are another option that can be used for mid tracheal obstruction.

Enteral feeding should always be priority as these patients are cachectic. Enteral feeding may be achieved by percutaneous endoscopic gastrostomy.

Anaplastic Thyroid Carcinoma

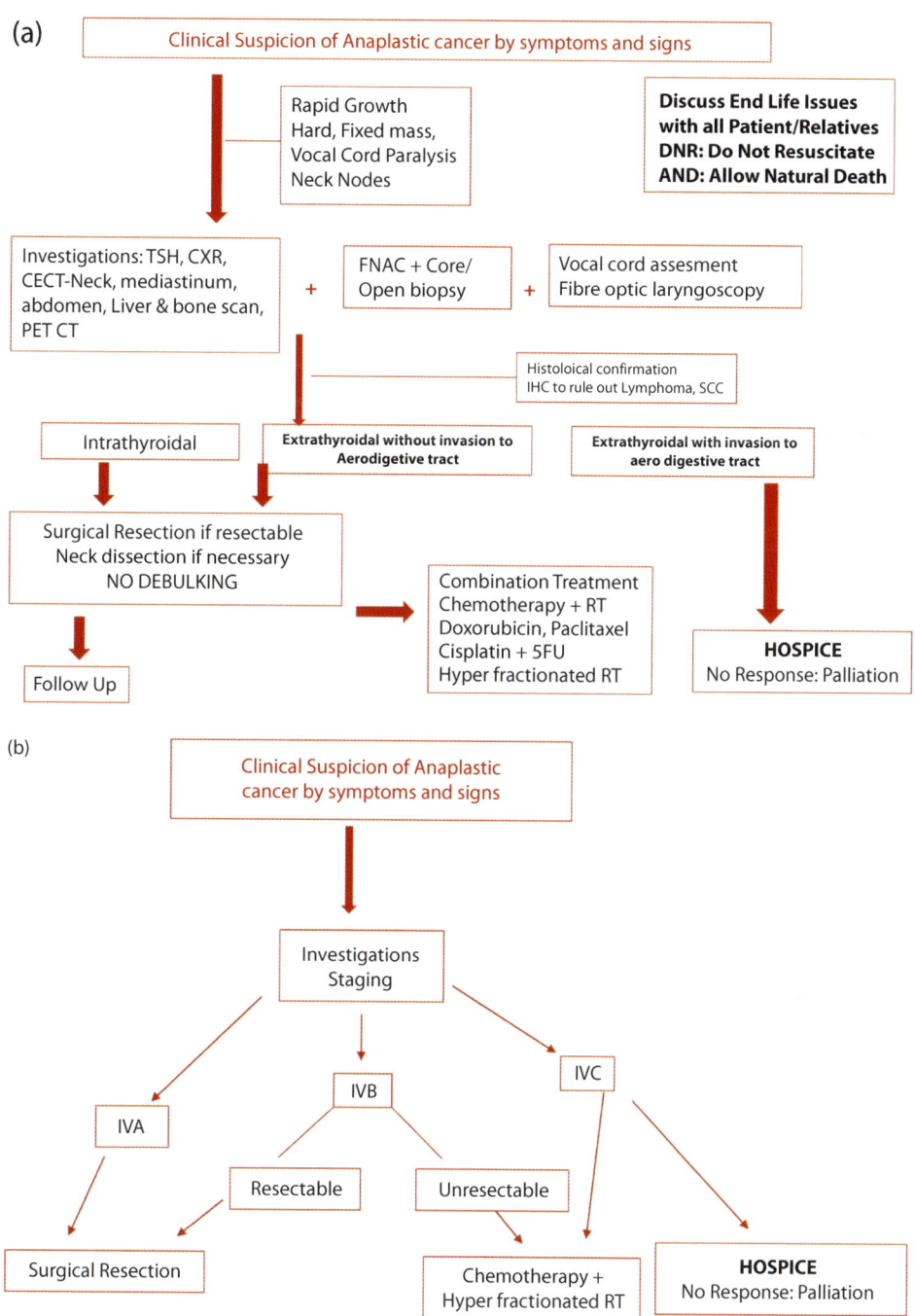

FIGURE 18.4 (a) Flowchart of management in anaplastic thyroid cancer. (b) Algorithm of initial treatment in anaplastic thyroid cancer.

TABLE 18.4: Resection Margins/Residual Tumor Definition

Terminology	Resection Margins
R0	No residual tumor
R1	Grossly no residual tumor, but residual tumor present microscopically at the resected margins
R2	Gross residual tumor

Role of radiation therapy

Adjuvant RT or concurrent chemo-RT (CCRT) has already been discussed previously. Radiation can be administered as EBRT or conformal RT or IMRT. Higher dose of radiation can be given by IMRT (more than 60 Gy) [39]. Administration of adjuvant RT is recommended at 2–3 weeks after curative surgery [2]. Adjuvant RT has been found to be beneficial in adjuvant setting with a better survival [52–54]. It has been found that the set of patients receiving >40 Gy have a better median survival of

TABLE 18.5: Studies Showing Outcome of Multimodality Therapy in ATC

Author, Year, Country [Ref]	Study Details: Duration, Type of Study	No. of Patients (n)	Study Results

Corrigan et al., 2019, United States [63]	1990–2015, retrospective	28	Median OS = 4 months
			1-year survival = 17.8%
			Survival rates better in group:
			• Surgery vs. no surgery:
			  • Median OS: 5.6 vs. 1 month
			  • 1-year survival: 25 vs. 0%
			• EBRT vs. no EBRT
			  • Median OS: 6 vs. 1 month
			  • 1-year survival: 23.8 vs. 0%
			Adjuvant chemotherapy:
			• No additional survival benefit

Lin et al., 2019, SEER database, United States [8]	1986–2015, retrospective	1567 (n = 717 for survival analysis)	Complete resection (R0) better than partial resection or subtotal resection • Median survival: 10 months vs. 5 months vs. 4 months Additional lymphadenectomy did not improve survival significantly
Huang et al., 2019, SEER database, China [64]	2004–2014, retrospective	735	R0 resection better than R1/R2 resection and no surgery: 2-year survival rate 24.6 vs. 14.4 vs. 2.4% Multimodality better than single modality: 2-year survival rates • Surgery+RT: 25.8% • Surgery alone: 7.7% • RT alone: 3%
Baek et al., 2016, Korea [53]	2000–2012, retrospective, multi-institutional	329	Surgical intervention patients had better OS than no surgery | Intervention | Median survival (months) | 1-Year survival (%) | |---|---|---| | No treatment | 2 | 8.2 | | Surgery alone | 7 | 34.6 | | Surgery+RT/CRT | 15 | 50.2 | | Surgery+CTx | 5 | 20 | | CTx alone | 3 | 0 | | RT/CRT | 5 | 15.2 | Higher dose of EBRT had better survival | Dose (Gy) | Median survival (months) | 1-Year survival (%) | |---|---|---| | ≤40 | 3 | 29.2 | | >40 | 9 | 41.2 |
Wendler et al., 2016, Germany [33]	2000–2015, retrospective, multi-institutional	100	| Intervention | Median survival (months) | 1-Year survival (%) | |---|---|---| | Stage IVA | 26 | 66 | | Stage IVB | 11 | 39 | | Stage IVC | 3 | 13 | | EBRT ≤ 40 Gy | 9 | 0 | | EBRT > 40 Gy | 50 | 38 | | No CTx | 21 | 17 | | CTx | 45 | 33 | Adjuvant EBRT in stage IVB, and CTx in stage IVC improved survival

TABLE 18.5: *(Continued)*

Author, Year, Country [Ref]	Study Details: Duration, Type of Study	No. of Patients (n)	Study Results
Goffredo et al., 2015, United States [51]	2003–2006, retrospective, National Cancer Database (NCDB)	680 (Surg – 335 and No Surg – 345)	Median survival in stages IVA, IVB, IVC were 9.7, 3.5, 1.7 months, respectively. Patients with positive resection margins had higher 30-day mortality (48%) vs. negative margins (16%). In stage IVA, R0 resection had better survival than R1/R2 ($p = 0.007$)
Brignardello et al., 2014, Italy [54]	1999–2012, retrospective, single institution surgery in locally advanced (stage IVB) and metastatic (stage IVC) ATC	55	Surgical resection in advanced ATC had improved survival

Stage	Maximum debulking (months)	Partial debulking (months)
IVB	10.94	3.02
IVC	6.5	3.25

Overall:
Median survival: 5.55 months
6-month survival: 49%
1-year survival: 19.7%

Author, Year, Country [Ref]	Study Details	n	Study Results
Aslan et al., 2014, Mexico [65]	1992–2012, retrospective	29	R0 resection and multimodality therapy has better survival ($p < 0.01$)

Stage	6 months (%)	1 year (%)	2 years (%)
IVA	59	40	40
IVB	51	25	12.5
IVC	12% at 100 days and 0% at 125 days		
Overall	37.9	21	13

Author, Year, Country [Ref]	Study Details	n	Study Results
Sugitani et al., 2012, Japan [52]	1995–2008, retrospective, Japanese multicenter registry	677	Incidental ATC had best survival ($p < 0.01$)

Type	Median survival (days)	1-year CSS (%)
Incidental	395	57
Neck node	175	30
Distant	48	0
Common	113	18

Stage IVA had a better survival rate ($p < 0.01$)

Stage	Median survival (days)	6-month CSS (%)
IVA	236	60
IVB	147	45
IVC	81	19

Surgery, RT and CTx had better survival (all $p < 0.01$)

Intervention	Median survival (days)	1-year CSS (%)
Surgery		
None	89	10
Radical	243	39
EBRT		
≤40 Gy	72	8
>40 Gy	189	31
Chemotherapy		
No	86	16
Yes	164	26

Abbreviations: ATC, Anaplastic thyroid cancer; CRT, Chemoradiotherapy; CSS, Case-specific survival; CTx, Chemotherapy; EBRT, External beam radiation therapy; OS, Overall survival; RT, Radiotherapy.

TABLE 18.6: Studies on Newer Therapeutic Agents and Their Outcomes

Author and Ref.	Agent	Phase of Trial	No. of Patients (n)	Response Rates	PFS (in Months)	Other Findings
Savvides et al. [56]	Sorafenib	II	20	PR – 2/20 (10%) SD – 5/20 (25%)	1.9	Median survival = 3.9 months 1-year survival = 20%
Sosa et al. [66]	Carboplatin and paclitaxel+fosbretabulin vs. carboplatin/paclitaxel	II	80	PR: 20 vs. 16% SD: 40 vs. 44%	3.3 vs. 3.1	OS: 5.2 vs. 4 months (NS) OS at 1 year: 25.9 vs. 8.7% Reduction in risk of death: 27%
Subbiah et al. [60]	Dabrafenib+trametinib In BRAF V600E mutations	II	16	PR: 10/16 (62.5%) CR: 1/16 (6.25) ORR: 69%	NA	Median duration of response, PFS and OS were not reached
Tahara et al. [58]	Lenvatinib	II	17	CR: 0% PR: 24% SD: 71%	7.4	OS: 10.6 months

Abbreviations: CR, Complete response; ORR, Overall response rate; OS, Overall survival; PFS, Progression-free survival; PR, Partial response; SD, Stable disease.

108 vs. 54 months than those getting <40 Gy (p < 0.0001) with a 1-year survival of 19 vs. 5% in respective groups [52].

Palliative RT can be administered to the primary in the case of unresectable advanced tumor, usually with a radio-sensitizing CT regimen using carboplatin and paclitaxel, doxorubicin with docetaxel [49]. Palliative RT in a patient with good performance status (PS) can be given at a higher dose vs. lower dose in a poor PS [2]. The dose-dependent response and survival benefit in more than 1200 patients with advanced ATC has been demonstrated by Pezzi et al. using NCDB, where the overall survival benefit was observed with an RT dosage >60 Gy as compared with <60 Gy with a 1-year survival rates of 31 vs. 16% in respective groups (p = 0.008) [55].

Systemic therapy

Systemic therapy is administered in the form of adjuvant (or radio-sensitizing) CT with doxorubicin (20 mg/m^2 weekly), other agents used are paclitaxel, cisplatin, docetaxel with doxorubicin combination. Sugitani et al. found a 1-year survival of 26% in patients undergoing adjuvant CT vs. 11% in patients not undergoing CT, with a median survival of 164 months vs. 86 months in respective groups [52]. Baek et al. found survival advantage of systemic therapy in adjuvant setting seen in patients undergoing curative resection, with CCRT as compared to surgery alone, with median survival of 15 months vs. 7 months with a 1-year survival of 50.6%, whereas in patients undergoing only adjuvant CT had median survival of 5 months vs. 7 months in patients undergoing surgery alone, and a 1-year survival of 20 vs. 34.6% in respective groups [53].

In metastatic setting, a combination of carboplatin with paclitaxel or docetaxel with doxorubicin is preferred [49]. At our institute, in a metastatic patient, we prefer paclitaxel with carboplatin 3 weekly regimen. Other agents used are single-agent paclitaxel or doxorubicin. And the newer agents shall be discussed next.

Newer therapeutic agents

These agents are used in locally advanced unresectable tumors that progress or in metastatic tumors. Tyrosine kinase inhibitors (TKIs) are the most commonly used agents. Sorafenib, a TKI with multikinase activity, had shown partial response in 2 patients with a stable disease in 5 patients enrolled in a 20-patient phase II trial [56]. Pazopanib, another multikinase inhibitor that also has inhibitory action on vascular endothelial growth factor (VEGF) has also been under study, did not have promising results in humans with a median time to progression of 62 days [57].

Lenvatinib is a newer agent with not only acts on multiple tyrosine kinase receptors but also has activity against platelet-derived growth factor receptor-α (PDGF-α), fibroblast growth factor-1 (FGF-1), VEGF, RET and KIT proto-oncogene [58]. Crizotinib is another TKI used in ALK translocation positive ATC, which showed 90% tumor reduction with a progression-free survival more than 6 months [59].

Dabrafenib is a selective BRAF kinase inhibitor and trametinib is a MEK1 and 2 kinase inhibitor. Their combination is FDA approved for the treatment of melanoma, ATC and non-small cell lung cancer if they harbor BRAF mutation. Vemurafenib, dabrafenib, trametinib have been used in patients with BRAF mutations [60]. Larotrectinib and entrectinib are molecules that are used in patients with neurotropic receptor tyrosine kinase (NTRK) fusion-positive ATCs [49, 61]. Other agents under study are everolimus (mTOR inhibitor), atezolizumab, pembrolizumab, certinib [62, 63]. Table 18.6 summarizes the newer therapeutic agents along with their response rates in ATC.

Prognostic parameters

Huang et al. from SEER data analysis on 735 patients found age <70 years, the absence of distant metastases, multimodality therapy with surgery and RT to be good prognostic factors [64]. Wendler et al. in a multicenter study observed that age >70 years, incomplete resection and the presence of distant metastasis at diagnosis were found to have poor prognosis [33]. Sugitani et al., using a multicenter Japanese registry have also found that age >70 years, tumor size >5 cm, T4b lesion, leucocytosis, the presence of distant metastasis were associated with poor overall survival [52]. The favorable prognostic factors are summarized in Table 18.7.

TABLE 18.7: Favorable Prognostic Factors for ATC

Age <65 years
Female
Tumor size <5 cm, unilateral tumors
Intrathyroidal or less extensive disease at presentation
Complete resection of tumor or R0 resection
Absence of distant metastases

South Asian perspective

The exact incidence of ATC is not available for South Asian population, but the average age of presentation is lower than the available western data. In a single-institution study by Pradhan et al., it was found that 58% of the patients were between age 41 and 60 [3], whereas patients <50 years of age comprise only 10% cases of total ATC [9–12]. The earlier presentation is probably due to higher prevalence of iodine deficiency in this region [3]. The gender ratio is almost comparable with male:female having 1:1.2 with 55% females [3] compared to almost 62.6% females in SEER database [64]. Duration of goiter is present for more than 10 years in 57% of the patients. Distant metastases are present in almost 30% of these patients. Majority present with advanced locoregional disease, as only 21% of these patients were amenable to surgical therapy. The mean size in these surgical candidates was 7.3 cm with almost 81% patients presenting with a lesion >5 cm. Other clinicopathological parameters are comparable to western data [3]. The mutations present in this South Asian population may also differ. Though there is no multicenter registry, but a recent study by Rashid et al. found that BRAF mutations were present in 29.4% of the patients presented with ATC whereas p53 mutation was present in 20.5% of the patients [34]. Multimodality treatment is the practice of choice whenever possible, with maximum benefit obtained in patients undergoing surgery with RT. The overall median survival rates are dismal with only 3 months for all the stages as compared to western population 5 months [2, 3].

Conclusion

ATC is a rare cancer and almost always fatal. The disease presents as a rapidly progressing neck swelling with associated features of locoregional invasion, and distant metastasis. Investigations to confirm should be initiated as soon as it is suspected, with the commencement of treatment without any delay. Multimodality therapy should always be administered, and carefully selected patients will benefit by aggressive surgical resection and adjuvant therapy with a meaningful survival. Therapy for patients presenting with distal metastases should be personalized. No systemic therapy has proven benefits in metastatic disease; however, newer therapeutic agents, directed against particular molecular targets are the hope for a better survival in this lethal cancer.

References

1. Ito Y, Miyauchi A, Kihara M, Fukushima M, Higashiyama T, Miya A. Overall survival of papillary thyroid carcinoma patients: a single-institution long-term follow-up of 5897 patients. World J Surg. 2018;42(3):615–22.
2. Smallridge RC, Ain KB, Asa SL, Bible KC, Brierley JD, Burman KD, et al. American Thyroid Association guidelines for management of patients with anaplastic thyroid cancer. Thyroid. 2012;22(11):1104–39.
3. Pradhan R, Agarwal A, Lal P, Kumari N, Jain M, Chand G, et al. Clinico-pathological profile of anaplastic thyroid carcinoma in an endemic goiter area. Indian J Endocrinol Metab. 2018;22(6):793–7.
4. Hundahl SA, Fleming ID, Fremgen AM, Menck HR. A National Cancer Data Base report on 53,856 cases of thyroid carcinoma treated in the U.S., 1985-1995 [see comments]. Cancer. 1998;83(12):2638–48.
5. Kitamura Y, Shimizu K, Nagahama M, Sugino K, Ozaki O, Mimura T, et al. Immediate causes of death in thyroid carcinoma: clinicopathological analysis of 161 fatal cases. J Clin Endocrinol Metab. 1999;84(11):4043–9.
6. Akslen LA, Haldorsen T, Thoresen SO, Glattre E. Incidence of thyroid cancer in Norway 1970-1985. Population review on time trend, sex, age, histological type and tumour stage in 2625 cases. Acta Pathol Microbiol Immunol Scand. 1990;98(6):549–58.
7. Burke JP, Hay ID, Dignan F, Goellner JR, Achenbach SJ, Oberg AL, et al. Long-term trends in thyroid carcinoma: a population-based study in Olmsted County, Minnesota, 1935-1999. Mayo Clin Proc. 2005;80(6):753–8.
8. Lin B, Ma H, Ma M, Zhang Z, Sun Z, Hsieh I, et al. The incidence and survival analysis for anaplastic thyroid carcinoma: a SEER database analysis. Am J Transl Res. 2019;11(9):5888–96.
9. Kebebew E, Greenspan FS, Clark OH, Woeber KA, McMillan A. Anaplastic thyroid carcinoma. Treatment outcome and prognostic factors. Cancer. 2005;103(7):1330–5.
10. Nagaiah G, Hossain A, Mooney CJ, Parmentier J, Remick SC. Anaplastic thyroid cancer: a review of epidemiology, pathogenesis, and treatment. J Oncol. 2011;2011:542358.
11. Perros P, Boelaert K, Colley S, Evans C, Evans RM, Gerrard BAG, et al. Guidelines for the management of thyroid cancer. Clin Endocrinol (Oxf). 2014;81:1–122.
12. Nehs MA, Ruan DT. 'Anapalstic Carcinoma of the Thyroid Gland' in Orlo CH. Textbook of Endocrine Surgery. 3rd ed. New Delhi: Jaypee; 2016; pp. 269–78.
13. Suh HJ, Moon HJ, Kwak JY, Choi JS, Kim E-K. Anaplastic thyroid cancer: ultrasonographic findings and the role of ultrasonography-guided fine needle aspiration biopsy. Yonsei Med J. 2013;54(6):1400–6.
14. Ragazzi M, Ciarrocchi A, Sancisi V, Gandolfi G, Bisagni A, Piana S. Update on anaplastic thyroid carcinoma: morphological, molecular, and genetic features of the most aggressive thyroid cancer. Int J Endocrinol. 2014;2014:1–13.
15. Ryder M, Ghossein RA, Ricarte-Filho JC, Knauf JA, Fagin JA. Increased density of tumor-associated macrophages is associated with decreased survival in advanced thyroid cancer. Endocr Relat Cancer. 2008;15:1069–74.
16. Mantovani A, Bottazzi B, Colotta F, Sozzani S, Ruco L. The origin and function of tumor-associated macrophages. Immunol Today. 1992;13:265–70.
17. Mosser DM. The many faces of macrophage activation. J Leukoc Biol. 2003;73:209–12.
18. Mantovani A, Sozzani S, Locati M, Allavena P, Sica A. Macrophage polarization: tumor-associated macrophages as a paradigm for polarized M2 mononuclear phagocytes. Trends Immunol. 2002;23:549–55.
19. Nel CJ, van Heerden JA, Goellner JR, et al. Anaplastic carcinoma of the thyroid: a clinicopathologic study of 82 cases. Mayo Clin Proc. 1985;60:51.
20. Aldinger KA, Samaan NA, Ibanez M, Hill CS Jr. Anaplastic carcinoma of the thyroid: a review of 84 cases of spindle and giant cell carcinoma of the thyroid. Cancer. 1978;41:2267.
21. Carcangiu ML, Steeper T, Zampi G, Rosai J. Anaplastic thyroid carcinoma. A study of 70 cases. Am J Clin Pathol. 1985;83:135.
22. Venkatesh YS, Ordonez NG, Schultz PN, et al. Anaplastic carcinoma of the thyroid. A clinicopathologic study of 121 cases. Cancer. 1990;66:321.
23. Tan RK, Finley RK 3rd, Driscoll D, et al. Anaplastic carcinoma of the thyroid: a 24-year experience. Head Neck. 1995;17:41.
24. McIver B, Hay ID, Giuffrida DF, et al. Anaplastic thyroid carcinoma: a 50-year experience at a single institution. Surgery. 2001;130:1028.
25. Chiu AC, Oliveira AA, Schultz PN, et al. Prognostic clinicopathologic features in Hürthle cell neoplasia. Thyroid. 1996;6:S29.
26. Quiros RM, Ding HG, Gattuso P, et al. Evidence that one subset of anaplastic thyroid carcinomas are derived from papillary carcinomas due to BRAF and p53 mutations. Cancer. 2005;103:2261.
27. Moretti F, Farsetti A, Soddu S, et al. p53 re-expression inhibits proliferation and restores differentiation of human thyroid anaplastic carcinoma cells. Oncogene. 1997;14:729.
28. Komoike Y, Tamaki Y, Sakita I, et al. Comparative genomic hybridization defines frequent loss on 16p in human anaplastic thyroid carcinoma. Int J Oncol. 1999;14:1157.
29. Smallridge RC, Marlow LA, Copland JA. Anaplastic thyroid cancer: molecular pathogenesis and emerging therapies. Endocr Relat Cancer. 2009;16:17.
30. Keutgen XM, Sadowski SM, Kebebew E. Management of anaplastic thyroid cancer. Gland Surg. 2015;4(1):44–51.
31. Landa I, Ibrahimpasic T, Boucai L, Sinha R, Knauf JA, Shah RH, et al. Genomic and transcriptomic hallmarks of poorly differentiated and anaplastic thyroid cancers. J Clin Invest. 2016;126(3):1052–66.
32. Cabanillas ME, Zafereo M, Gunn GB, Ferrarotto R. Anaplastic thyroid carcinoma: treatment in the age of molecular targeted therapy. J Oncol Pract. 2016;12(6):511–8.
33. Wendler J, Kroiss M, Gast K, Kreissl MC, Allelein S, Lichtenauer U, et al. Clinical presentation, treatment and outcome of anaplastic thyroid carcinoma: results of a multicenter study in Germany. Eur J Endocrinol. 2016;175(6):521–9.
34. Rashid M, Agarwal A, Pradhan R, George N, Kumari N, Sabaretnam M, et al. Genetic alterations in anaplastic thyroid carcinoma. Indian J Endocrinol Metab. 2019;23(4):480–5.
35. Lin Y-H, Jang C-S, Wu C-S, Hsu L. Unusual presentation of anaplastic thyroid carcinoma with diffuse neck and thoracic nodules and hyperthyroidism. Dermatol Sin. 2017;35(2):85–7.
36. Pasieka JL. Anaplastic thyroid cancer. Curr Opin Oncol. 2003;15(1):78–83.
37. Glaser SM, et al. Anaplastic thyroid cancer: prognostic factors, patterns of care, and overall survival. Head Neck. 2016;38(Suppl. 1):E2083–90.
38. Rossi R, Cady B, Meissner WA, Sedgwick CE, Werber J. Prognosis of undifferentiated carcinoma and lymphoma of the thyroid. Am J Surg. 1978;135:589–96.
39. Junor EJ, Paul J, Reed NS. Anaplastic thyroid carcinoma. 91 patients treated by surgery and radiotherapy. Eur J Surg Oncol. 1992;18:83–8.
40. Us-Krasovec M, Golouh R, Auersperg M, Besic N, Ruparcic-Oblak L. Anaplastic thyroid carcinoma in fine needle aspirates. Acta Cytol. 1996;40(5):953–8.
41. Ha EJ, Baek JH, Lee JH, Kim JK, Song DE, Kim WB, et al. Core needle biopsy could reduce diagnostic surgery in patients with anaplastic thyroid cancer or thyroid lymphoma. Eur Radiol. 2016;26(4):1031–6.
42. Lee JW, Yoon DY, Choi CS, Chang SK, Yun EJ, Seo YL, et al. Anaplastic thyroid carcinoma: computed tomographic differentiation from other thyroid masses. Acta Radiol Stockh Swed 1987. 2008;49(3):321–7.
43. Ahmed S, Ghazarian MP, Cabanillas ME, Zafereo ME, Williams MD, Vu T, et al. Imaging of anaplastic thyroid carcinoma. AJNR Am J Neuroradiol. 2018;39(3):547–51.
44. Marcus C, Whitworth PW, Surasi DS, Pai SI, Subramaniam RM. PET/CT in the management of thyroid cancers. Am J Roentgenol. 2014;202(6):1316–29.
45. Bogsrud TV, Karantanis D, Nathan MA, Mullan BP, Wiseman GA, Kasperbauer J, et al. 18F-FDG PET in the management of patients with anaplastic thyroid carcinoma. Thyroid. 2008;18(7):713–9.

46. Poisson T, Deandreis D, Leboulleux S, Bidault F, Bonniaud G, Baillot S, et al. 18F-fluorodeoxyglucose positron emission tomography and computed tomography in anaplastic thyroid cancer. Eur J Nucl Med Mol Imaging. 2010;37(12):2277–85.
47. Edge SB, Compton CC. The American Joint Committee on Cancer: the 7th edition of the AJCC cancer staging manual and the future of TNM. Ann Surg Oncol. 2010;17(6):1471–4.
48. Amin MB, Edge S, Greene F, Byrd DR, Brookland RK, Washington MK, et al., editors (2017). AJCC Cancer Staging Manual [Internet]. 8th ed. Springer International Publishing; [cited March 31, 2020]. Available from: www.springer.com/gp/book/9783319406176.
49. National Comprehensive Cancer Network (2019). *Thyroid Carcinoma (Version 2.2019)*. www.nccn.org/professionals/physician_gls/pdf/thyroid.pdf.
50. Dralle H, Musholt TJ, Schabram J, Steinmüller T, Frilling A, Simon D, et al. German Association of Endocrine Surgeons practice guideline for the surgical management of malignant thyroid tumors. Langenbecks Arch Surg. 2013;398(3):347–75.
51. Goffredo P, Thomas SM, Adam MA, Sosa JA, Roman SA. Impact of timeliness of resection and thyroidectomy margin status on survival for patients with anaplastic thyroid cancer: an analysis of 335 cases. Ann Surg Oncol. 2015;22(13):4166–74.
52. Sugitani I, Miyauchi A, Sugino K, Okamoto T, Yoshida A, Suzuki S. Prognostic factors and treatment outcomes for anaplastic thyroid carcinoma: ATC research consortium of Japan cohort study of 677 patients. World J Surg. 2012;36(6):1247–54.
53. Baek S-K, Lee M-C, Hah JH, Ahn S-H, Son Y-I, Rho Y-S, et al. Role of surgery in the management of anaplastic thyroid carcinoma: Korean nationwide multicenter study of 329 patients with anaplastic thyroid carcinoma, 2000 to 2012. Head Neck. 2017;39(1):133–9.
54. Brignardello E, Palestini N, Felicetti F, Castiglione A, Piovesan A, Gallo M, et al. Early surgery and survival of patients with anaplastic thyroid carcinoma: analysis of a case series referred to a single institution between 1999 and 2012. Thyroid. 2014;24(11):1600–6.
55. Pezzi TA, Mohamed ASR, Sheu T, Blanchard P, Sandulache VC, Lai SY, et al. Radiation therapy dose is associated with improved survival for unresected anaplastic thyroid carcinoma: outcomes from the National Cancer Data Base. Cancer. 2017;123(9):1653–61.
56. Savvides P, Nagaiah G, Lavertu P, Fu P, Wright JJ, Chapman R, et al. Phase II trial of sorafenib in patients with advanced anaplastic carcinoma of the thyroid. Thyroid. 2013;23(5):600–4.
57. Bible KC, Suman VJ, Menefee ME, Smallridge RC, Molina JR, Maples WJ, et al. A multiinstitutional phase 2 trial of pazopanib monotherapy in advanced anaplastic thyroid cancer. J Clin Endocrinol Metab. 2012;97(9):3179–84.
58. Tahara M, Kiyota N, Yamazaki T, Chayahara N, Nakano K, Inagaki L, et al. Lenvatinib for anaplastic thyroid cancer. Front Oncol. 2017;7. Available from: www.ncbi.nlm.nih.gov/pmc/articles/PMC5331066/.
59. Godbert Y, Henriques de Figueiredo B, Bonichon F, Chibon F, Hostein I, Pérot G, et al. Remarkable response to crizotinib in woman with anaplastic lymphoma kinase-rearranged anaplastic thyroid carcinoma. J Clin Oncol. 2015;33(20):e84–7.
60. Subbiah V, Kreitman RJ, Wainberg ZA, Cho JY, Schellens JHM, Soria JC, et al. Dabrafenib and trametinib treatment in patients with locally advanced or metastatic BRAF V600-mutant anaplastic thyroid cancer. J Clin Oncol. 2018;36(1):7–13.
61. Drilon A, Laetsch TW, Kummar S, DuBois SG, Lassen UN, Demetri GD, et al. Efficacy of larotrectinib in TRK fusion-positive cancers in adults and children. N Engl J Med. 2018;378(8):731–9.
62. Tiedje V, Stuschke M, Weber F, Dralle H, Moss L, Führer D. Anaplastic thyroid carcinoma: review of treatment protocols. Endocr Relat Cancer. 2018;25(3):R153–61.
63. Corrigan KL, Williamson H, Range DE, Niedzwiecki D, Brizel DM, Mowery YM. Treatment outcomes in anaplastic thyroid cancer. J Thyroid Res. 2019;2019:1–11.
64. Huang N, Shi X, Lei B, Wei W, Lu Z, Yu P, et al. An update of the appropriate treatment strategies in anaplastic thyroid cancer: a population-based study of 735 patients. Int J Endocrinol. 2019;2019:8428547.
65. Aslan ZA, Granados-García M, Luna-Ortiz K, Guerrero-Huerta FJ, Gómez-Pedraza A, Namendys-Silva SA, et al. Anaplastic thyroid cancer: multimodal treatment results. Ecancermedicalscience. 2014;8:449.
66. Sosa JA, Elisei R, Jarzab B, Balkissoon J, Lu S-P, Bal C, et al. Randomized safety and efficacy study of fosbretabulin with paclitaxel/carboplatin against anaplastic thyroid carcinoma. Thyroid. 2014;24(2):232–40.

19

RARE TUMORS OF THE THYROID

Murat Ozdemir and Özer Makay

Rare tumors of the thyroid

Squamous cell carcinoma

Primary squamous cell carcinoma of the thyroid (PSCCTh) are extremely rare tumors, they constitute less than 1% of all thyroid malignancies with a very poor prognosis (3). For the diagnosis of PSCCTh, all tumor cells should undergo squamous differentiation. To diagnose PSCCTh; secondary SCC (squamous cell carcinoma) spread by direct invasion from adjacent organs such as the tongue root, pharynx, larynx, upper esophagus or by metastatic spread from distant organs like lung, head and neck should be excluded. Secondary squamous cell carcinoma of the thyroid is ten times more common than primary squamous cell carcinoma (4).

It is frequently seen in elderly patients over 60 years of age. In the Surveillance, Epidemiology, and End Results Program (SEER) database analysis conducted by Yang et al., 75% of the diagnosed patients were over 60 years old. It is also more common in women than men (57.8% vs 41.2%) (5).

The diagnosis of PSCCTh is made by anamnesis, physical examination, endoscopic, radiological and histopathological evaluations. The complaints of the patients are usually a rapidly growing mass in the neck, dyspnea, dysphagia and hoarseness. Even though in most patients, it may be a local aggressive disease, it can also present with regional and distant metastases. Lungs, bones, liver, heart and kidneys are the most common targets for distant metastases. Distant metastases are present in 11% of patients at the time of diagnosis (4).

Ultrasonography (USG) shows no specific findings for PSCCTh, it shows similar findings as for other thyroid malignancies. Fine-needle aspiration biopsy (FNAB) or core needle biopsy can be performed with USG. Since PSCCThs do not use iodine, they appear as cold nodules in radionuclide imaging methods. Computed tomography (CT) is useful in showing the relationship between the mass and adjacent tissues. It may indicate airway stenosis and vascular invasion. Thoraco-abdominopelvic CT helps exclude secondary SCC. Magnetic resonance imaging (MRI) and positron emission tomography (PET) are useful for differential diagnosis of metastatic masses from distant tissues. Gastrointestinal system endoscopy, bronchoscopy, endoscopic otolaryngological evaluation should be performed. To diagnose PSCCTh, metastases from another organ should absolutely be excluded (4).

Although the diagnosis can be made by FNAB, it shows limitation between primary and metastatic carcinoma.

Macroscopically, PSCCTh's are masses that fill one or both lobes of the thyroid, while metastatic SCCs are mostly multifocal. PSCCTh are cytokeratin-19 positive; however, cytokeratin-1, -4, -11, -10/13 and -20 negative. In some cases, cytokeratin-7 and -13 positivity can be seen. Even if the tumor size is small (2–3 cm), it can invade surrounding tissue. There are various histological subtypes. Large cell, nonkeratinized tumors have a better prognosis – with a median survival time of 30 months; spindle cell and microinvasive types have the worst prognosis.

The grade of PSCCTh tumors is usually poorly differentiated. PSCCThs are PAX-8 and p53 positive, and the PAX-8 positivity is important in distinguishing primary from secondary carcinoma. BRAF mutation has also been reported in these cases. Regarding the differentiation of these tumors, frequency of good, moderate, poor and undifferentiated tumors is 7%, 21%, 51% and 21%, respectively. The median survival of T4 tumors is 3 months; and for T1-3 tumors is 18 months (6).

Factors affecting survival are age, tumor grade, tumor size (tumors larger than 5 cm have a poor prognosis), tumor subtype and T stage.

The recommended treatment for PSCCTh tumors is surgical resection with adjuvant radiotherapy. Adjuvant radiotherapy after surgical resection is the treatment method with the best prognosis. Mortality often occurs due to local complications or distant metastases. In the case of palliative treatment, interventions such as tracheostomy to maintain airway patency, percutaneous endoscopic gastrostomy (PEG) or surgical gastrostomy for nutrition of the patient may be necessary (4–6).

Mucoepidermoid carcinoma

Mucoepidermoid carcinoma (MEC) is malignant epithelial neoplasm characterized by the coexistence of epidermoid and mucin-producing cells. MEC of the thyroid is extremely rare tumor, constituting less than 0.5% of all thyroid malignancies. It was first described by Rhatigan in 1977. Nearly 50 cases have been reported to date. It is seen 1.5–2 times more in women than in men. Although it can be seen between the ages of 10 and 91, the average age of incidence is 46 (7, 8).

The origin of the thyroid MEC is controversial. There are two main theories about its development. It is thought to originate from thyroid follicular epithelial cells or from the solid cell island (solid cell nest).

MEC often presents with painless swelling in the neck. Patients are usually euthyroid. Although they can be diagnosed by FNAB, the diagnosis of MEC is made by histopathological examinations after surgery. 25% of the patients have extrathyroidal extension, 20% shows esophagus, trachea or recurrent laryngeal nerve involvement. Regional lymph node metastasis is seen in 40% of patients. Distant metastases are seen at a rate of 10%, often in lungs and bones (9, 10).

The 5-year survival of salivary gland-derived MECs is approximately 90%. Thyroid MECs also show similar properties to salivary glands.

They are usually low-grade tumors, but poorly differentiated tumors and tumors showing anaplastic transformation are associated with aggressive and poor prognosis. Death due to tumor progression occurs in 18% of patients. Death is generally seen in elderly patients and aggressive tumors showing poor or anaplastic differentiation.

Total thyroidectomy should be choice of the treatment, and the prophylactic neck dissection is controversial. Although it has been shown that radiotherapy after surgical treatment prolongs survival, all treatment methods may be insufficient in aggressive cases and recurrent disease can usually be seen in the neck region (11).

Sclerosing mucoepidermoid carcinoma with eosinophilia

Sclerosing MEC with eosinophilia (SMECE) is a malignant epithelial neoplasia showing epidermoid and glandular differentiation with eosinophilic and lymphocytic infiltration and a sclerotic stroma. It almost always develops on the basis of lymphocytic thyroiditis.

Cytokeratin, p63, CD10 and mucin are positive in the vast majority of SMECE cases. Thyroglobulin was reported as positive in 5% of patients, chromogranin and calcitonin are negative. TTF-1 and CEA were reported as positive in 47% and 75% of cases, respectively. It was first described in 1991. 62 cases have been reported to date. It is generally a low-grade, slow-progressing tumor with a survival of up to 12 years (12–14).

Patients complain of painless swelling in the neck. It had been reported in cases that were found incidentally or in patients that presented with the complaint of hoarseness. It is nine times more common in women than in men.

Cases have been reported between the ages of 26–89, the median age of incidence is 57. Average tumor size is 4.5 cm (min: 0.5, max 13 cm). The majority of cases originate from the lateral lobes of the thyroid. 2% of the reported cases originated from isthmus. Extrathyroidal spread and regional lymph node metastasis are seen in 54% and 40% of cases, respectively.

Distant metastases are rare. The most common distant metastasis site are the lungs; bones, liver, peritoneum and kidneys. Synchronous papillary carcinoma of the thyroid had been reported in 16% of cases. BRAF mutation associated with poor prognosis in thyroid carcinomas was positive in 2 SMECE cases reported by Sukumar (8). There is no clear consensus on treatment. Surgical resection is frequently performed. A clear efficacy of postoperative adjuvant radiotherapy, radioactive iodine therapy, and chemotherapy application could not be demonstrated.

Mucinous carcinoma

It is an epithelial malignant neoplasia consisting of neoplastic cell clusters surrounded by extracellular mucin deposits. Mucinous carcinoma of the thyroid was first reported by Diaz in 1976. Nine cases have been reported in the literature to date (15–17). They are extremely rare tumors with poor prognosis. There was no significant difference between both sexes. Four of the patients were male and five were female. It has been reported to be seen between the ages of 32 and 82. Its etiopathogenesis is not clear. According to some authors, this tumor originates from mucin-producing cells thought to develop from thyroglossal duct remnant or ectopic salivary glands, while according to some other authors, these tumors originate from ultimobranchial body follicles containing mucin; however, no theory has been proven. They present with a mass on the neck; almost all of the cases have lymph node metastasis at the time of presentation.

Lung metastases were reported in three cases, skin metastasis in two cases and spine metastasis in one case. In the first 4 years, six of nine cases died. Tumor diameter varies between 2.8 and 8.4 cm. It is often seen as a gelatinous nodule. Histologically, it is similar to mucinous carcinomas in other tissues. This tumor is characterized by abundant mucoid content around the trabeculae, or clusters of tumor cells that usually show large nuclei and prominent nucleoli. Often, they are thyroglobulin, TTF-1 and PAX-8 positive and calcitonin and calcitonin gene-related peptide negative. Thyroglobulin and TTF-1 can be negative in regions showing anaplastic transformation. Ki-67 is usually over 10%. Nuclear immunoreactivity is commonly seen for P53.

It should not be forgotten that mucin production may also occur in some thyroid tumors such as thyroid adenoma, papillary carcinoma, medullary carcinoma and anaplastic carcinoma. It should be kept in mind that mucinous carcinomas like ovarian cancer can also metastases to thyroid gland.

Although the available data are insufficient, thyroidectomy and lymph node dissection are recommended. Although methods such as radiotherapy, chemotherapy and TSH suppression therapy have been tried the patients have not benefited. Generally, recurrence or metastasis develops in the majority of patients and patients die due to disease-related causes. The most effective factor in long-term survival is complete resection of tumor tissue (15–17).

Ectopic thymoma

Thymomas are epithelial tumors originating from thymus gland. They are often found in the anterior superior mediastinum. These tumors are extremely rare and constitute less than 1% of all neoplasms in adults. Ectopic thymomas are thought to originate from aberrant misplacement of thymic tissue during embryological development. They are very rare. They constitute 4% of all thymomas. Ectopic thymomas are seen in the neck, posterior and middle mediastinum, trachea, pericardium, lung and pleura where ectopic thymus tissue can be found. Ectopic thymomas are very rarely found in the thyroid gland. Ectopic thymomas are organotopic thymic epithelial tumors within the thyroid gland or attached to it. Intrathyroidal thymoma shows histological features similar to mediastinal thymoma (18).

When the tumor is examined histologically, it typically forms jigsaw-like lobules separated by sclerotic septa. Almost all of the reported cases are noninvasive. CD-5 positivity is an important marker for the identification of these lesions. Ectopic thymomas are frequently seen in women and the average age of incidence is 46. Patients usually present with a mass in the neck or an enlarged thyroid gland. Thyroid function tests are in normal range. They appear as cold nodules in the radioactive iodine uptake test. Diagnosing intrathyroidal ectopic thymoma can be challenging and is usually made after surgical removal of the lesion. Apart from physical examination and USG, FNAB is usually the first step in the diagnostic examination of patients with thyroid masses.

It has been reported that ectopic cervical thymomas, which are more common, are frequently misdiagnosed as Hashimoto's thyroiditis, lymphoma or carcinoma on FNAB or frozen section examination due to their cellular composition and proximity to the thyroid gland. Ectopic thymoma can be located on either side of the thyroid lobe. In the case reported by Chan and Rosai, it was located in the isthmus. Tumor size varies between 1 and 7.3 cm. Although the follow-up periods of the reported cases are short, surgical resection seems to be sufficient for the treatment. Only one patient had recurrences in the subglottic area and right side of the neck at the 9th and 15th years after surgical resection. Recurrences were placed under control with surgery and radiotherapy.

Spindle epithelial tumor with thymus-like differentiation

Spindle epithelial cell tumor with thymus-like differentiation (SETTLE) is a rare malignant tumor of the thyroid characterized by a lobulated architecture and a biphasic cellular composition containing spindle epithelial cells combined with glandular structures. These extremely rare tumors are frequently seen in children, adolescents and young adults. The average age at diagnosis is 19. It is more common in men (19).

Unlike most thyroid cancers, no predisposing risk factors such as iodine deficiency, ionizing radiation exposure, genetic and environmental factors have been identified. It is thought to arise from branchial pouch remnants or ectopic thymus tissue showing differentiation into the embryonic thymus (thymoblastoma). Macroscopically, the tumor may be roughly encapsulated, partially confined or infiltrative. Average tumor diameter is 4.2 cm. Spindle and glandular cells produce high-molecular-weight cytokeratin and CK-7 by immunohistochemistry. Very rarely, spindle cells may show myoepithelial differentiation. Tumor cells are negative for thyroglobulin, calcitonin, CEA, TTF-1, S100 protein and CD-5 (20).

Patients appear with painless swelling and nodule formation on the neck. Rarely, they may cause a painful, tender mass in the neck and diffuse growth of the thyroid. Thyroid function tests, serum calcitonin and CEA values are generally normal. They are seen as cold nodules on radioactive iodine uptake screening. They are seen as a heterogeneous mass on USG and a structure containing heterogeneous solid and cystic formations on CT scan (21, 22).

Lymphadenopathies in the neck should also be evaluated preoperatively with the USG.

Although a full diagnosis cannot be made with FNAB, high cellular aspirate material consisting of cohesive or isolated spindle cell layers is seen in FNAB. The diagnosis is made by histopathological examinations after surgical resection.

Total thyroidectomy should be performed. It was reported that SETTLE developed in the remaining lobe in two patients who underwent lobectomy, and these cases were subsequently subjected to total thyroidectomy (23). If there are cervical lymph nodes involved, lymph node dissection should be performed in these areas. Neoadjuvant radiotherapy can be given before surgery in advanced stage and in the case of invasion to surrounding tissues. Chemotherapy or radiotherapy can be given in the presence of infiltrative local disease, vascular invasion or metastasis.

SETTLEs are slow-growing tumors. Survival at an average follow-up of 6.3 years is 86%. Although they are low-grade tumors, distant metastases can occur even years after surgical resection. During long-term follow-up, rate of 41% of distant metastasis was detected. Metastases usually occur during an average follow-up of 10 years. Distant metastasis is more likely to occur in cases with cervical lymph node metastasis. Distant metastases often develop through the bloodstream and occur in the lungs. Other than the lungs, metastases have been reported in the cervical lymph nodes, mediastinum and kidneys. Even if there is distant metastasis, a long survival time is seen after treatment (20).

Intrathyroidal thymic carcinoma

Intrathyroidal thymic carcinoma, known as a thymus-like differentiation carcinoma (CASTLE), before the WHO update in 2017, is a malignant epithelial tumor of the thyroid gland with thymic epithelial differentiation. It is the malignant counterpart of ectopic thymoma. It usually occurs in middle-aged adults in the fifth decade, and it is seen equally in men and women. It constitutes less than 0.01% of all thyroid epithelial malignancies. Most reported cases are from Asian communities. Therefore, it is thought that there may be an underlying genetic or environmental cause. Intrathyroidal thymic carcinoma is often located in the lower poles of the lateral lobes of the thyroid gland. Therefore, it is thought that it may originate from the ectopic thymus tissue or from thymus remnants found in thyroid gland or adjacent to the thyroid gland during development. The tumor shows several features of thymic differentiation (24, 25).

Intrathyroidal thymic carcinoma follows a different biological process compared to SCC and has a much better prognosis. It can be differentiated from SCC by the absence of focal squamous cells. In this type of carcinoma, the Ki-67 proliferation index is between 10% and 30%; Ki-67 is frequently more than 50% in SCC and anaplastic carcinoma. They stain positively for CD-5, p63, KIT, p53, BLC-2, calretinin, heavy-molecular-weight cytokeratin and broad-spectrum cytokeratin. They are negative for thyroglobulin, TTF-1, calcitonin. Most of the patients present with a neck mass (24, 25).

In the series of Ito (26), it was reported that 24% of the cases presented with the complaint of hoarseness due to recurrent laryngeal nerve involvement. Again, in the series of Ito, FNAB was applied to 20 patients, where only 1 patient was diagnosed with intrathyroidal thymic carcinoma in the preoperative period, while the cytology of the other 19 cases was reported as suspicious.

Lymph node metastasis is commonly seen. In the series of Ito, lymph node metastasis was found in half of 18 cases who underwent lymph node dissection.

Metastasis was detected in the central compartment in seven cases and in the lateral compartment in five cases. In 60% of cases, extension to adjacent tissues is seen. The most common site of extension is recurrent laryngeal nerve followed by trachea and esophagus. Recurrence was detected in 7 of 22 patients during follow-up. Distant metastases were detected in the lung in 3 cases, in liver in 2 cases, in bones in 2 cases, in mediastinum in 1 case and at pleura in 1 case.

The 5-year survival rate is 90% and the 10-year survival rate is 82%. In order to prevent locoregional recurrence, the entire tumor should be resected curatively. Postoperative adjuvant radiotherapy application has also been shown to be beneficial. There are reports that chemotherapeutic agents such as cisplatin and doxorubicin also keep the disease in remission in the presence of metastatic disease (26).

Paraganglioma and mesenchymal/stromal tumors

Paraganglioma: Paraganglioma is an intrathyroidal neuroendocrine tumor of paraganglionic origin. It constitutes approximately 0.5% of head and neck paragangliomas. They are frequently seen in women. Most patients present with a painless swelling mass in the neck. There is no specific finding on USG, they show similar findings of the other thyroid tumors. It is difficult to recognize them on FNAB. They can be confused with medullary carcinoma. They are also misdiagnosed during intraoperative frozen examination (27).

Tumors are usually encapsulated, but cases with invasion into surrounding tissues have been reported. Tumors are approximately 3 cm in diameter and the cross-sectional surface is pale-gray. Histologically, it is similar to other paragangliomas. It has a thin, fibrous capsule. They stain positive for Chromogranin-A and synaptophysin. Cytokeratin, calcitonin, calcitonin gene-related peptide and TTF-1 are generally negative. Locally, they most frequently spread to the cervical lymph nodes. Lung, liver, bone, skin are the most common areas of distant metastasis. Surgical resection of tumors is usually sufficient, but metastatic and recurrent cases have been reported (28, 29).

Peripheral nerve sheath tumors: Peripheral nerve sheath tumors of the thyroid gland are benign or malignant neoplasms that show Schwann cell or perineural differentiation originating from peripheral nerves in the thyroid gland. Benign neoplasms are called schwannomas and malignant neoplasms are called malignant peripheral nerve sheath tumors (MPNSTs). They are extremely rare and constitute less than 0.01% of all thyroid gland tumors. It can occur at any age, in both genders. Patients usually present with a swelling that grows in the neck. Dyspneic complaints, shortness of breath and weight loss due to airway compression have been reported in malignant peripheral margin sheath tumors. They appear as inhomogeneous low density and hypoechogenic masses on USG and CT. It is difficult to recognize them on FNAB. The diagnosis is usually made after surgery. MPNSTs are generally larger tumors than schwannomas (30).

Schwannomas are encapsulating tumors, while MPNSTs are infiltrative tumors. Necrosis can be seen in MPNSTs. Schwannomas are microscopically divided into two types: Antoni type A with palliation, compact and spindle-shaped nerve sheath cells, and Antoni type B with a sparse cellular structure with cystic degeneration or xanthomatous change. In the majority of reported cases, Antoni A and B types are seen together. Peripheral nerve sheath tumors may be associated with neurofibromatosis type 1.

MPNSTs can be associated with nerves by being gross fusiform tumors with microscopic features of spindle cells with fascicular pattern, areas of necrosis and tumor calcification, and pronounced cytological atypia or mitotic activity (31).

Schwannomas generally stain positive for S-100 protein, neuron-specific enolase, as well as actin, vimentin, cytokeratin and smooth muscle actin (SMA), distinguishing this type of tumor from other spindle cell sarcomas. In addition, the presence of the MIB1 proliferation marker can be seen and it can be used to grade the tumor and predict its prognosis. Treatment includes surgical resection. Although the prognosis for Schwannomas is near perfect, the prognosis of malignant peripheral margin sheath tumors is rather poor and the natural course of the disease results in death (30, 31).

Benign vascular tumors: Benign vascular tumors of the thyroid consist of hemangioma, cavernous hemangioma and lymphangioma. Hemangiomas are benign tumors characterized by capillary proliferation, often seen in the skin, oral cavity and liver (32). Primary thyroid hemangioma is extremely rare. Most reported cases are seen after FNAB or trauma. Therefore, it is thought that it may develop with abnormal vascular proliferation following organized hematoma or it may develop secondary to vascular changes during the development of nodular goiter. Often patients present with a growing mass in the neck. If there is bleeding into the lesion, rapidly growing or compressive symptoms may occur. Preoperative recognition is difficult with imaging methods. FNAB contains more blood than cellular components. Most of the patients are diagnosed after surgery.

Angiosarcoma: Thyroid angiosarcoma is a very rare tumor and constitutes less than 1% of all sarcomas. Thyroid angiosarcoma is a highly aggressive malignancy with poor prognosis, severe local course and rapid metastatic spread. It originates from endothelial cells. It is frequently seen in elderly patients over the age of 60; women and men are equally affected. Its etiopathogenesis is not clear. Symptoms vary depending on the size and location of the tumor.

Dyspnea, hoarseness and dysphagia can be seen frequently. Paraneoplastic syndromes such as fever, anemia and hypercalcemia can be seen. In the early period, metastasis to loco-regionel lymph nodes, lungs and bones can be seen. Metastases to soft tissues, brain, bone and skin have also been reported. Experienced cytologist can diagnose it on FNAB. It metastases early in the course, whole body scanning with CT is recommended for all patients. Histological examination usually reveals large areas of necrosis and bleeding, with the presence of freely anastomosing channels covered with typical endothelial cells (33).

A large number of both typical and atypical mitoses are found; the development nature is generally highly invasive; tumor necrosis is evident. They stain positive for CD31, CD34, FLI-1 and von Willebrand-related antigens. Results of the treatment are not satisfactory.

If possible, surgery should be performed at the earliest stage. Total thyroidectomy is the most common surgical method. Although adjuvant radiotherapy has been shown to prolong survival, its role in treatment is not clear. If surgery is not possible, radiotherapy can be applied to slow down the disease progression. In the presence of bone metastases, local radiotherapy can be applied to provide pain palliation. The results regarding chemotherapy are not clear. New generation target–focused treatment methods are being tried, but the results are not clear. Thyroid angiosarcoma has a poor prognosis. Distant metastasis and trachea or esophagus invasion are often present at the time of diagnosis. Most of the patients die a few months after the diagnosis (33, 34).

Smooth muscle tumors: Primary smooth muscle tumors of the thyroid are extremely rare tumors. Leiomyosarcomas are more common than leiomyomas. Leiomyosarcoma is the second most common sarcoma in the thyroid gland after angiosarcoma. Leiomyomas constitute less than 0.01% of all thyroid gland tumors (35). Both are thought to originate from the smooth muscles of the vascular structures within the thyroid gland. Leiomyomas occur in young and middle ages, while leiomyosarcomas are seen in older patients. Leiomyomas appear as painless, slow-growing masses. Leiomyosarcomas, on the other hand, are rapidly growing masses. In one case, hoarseness occurred due to nerve involvement. Thyroid functions are normal and appear as cold nodules (35, 36).

Leiomyosarcomas are larger than leiomyomas. While the mean tumor diameter of leiomyosarcomas is 6 cm, the mean tumor diameter of leiomyomas is 2 cm. While leiomyomas are well circumscribed, leiomyosarcomas are irregularly circumscribed. Neoplastic cells stain positive for alpha-SMA, MSA, SMA, caldesmon, calponin, desmin and vimentin. Thyroglobulin, pancytokeratin, S100, SOX10 and calcitonin are negative. Leiomyomas have a very good prognosis, surgery is sufficient; recurrence has not been reported in any case during follow-up (36).

Leiomyosarcomas have a poor prognosis. The majority of patients died within the first few months after diagnosis. Although adjuvant radiotherapy and chemotherapy are recommended after surgical resection, the results are poor (37).

Solitary fibrous tumor: Solitary fibrous tumors are tumors of mesenchymal origin, often located in the pleural cavity. They can also be found in the extra-pleural regions. Solitary fibrous tumors in the head and neck region are rare (38).

Solitary fibrous tumors of the thyroid gland are extremely rare. Nearly 30 cases have been reported in the literature so far. It is seen at the average age of 55, and it is seen equally in men and women. The tumor was malignant in only 2 of the reported cases. Malignancy criteria include the presence of hypercellularity, increased mitosis, cytological atypia, tumor necrosis and or infiltration. STAT-6 positivity is an important tumor marker. Average tumor diameter is 5.6 cm. They are slow-growing masses. It is seen as a suspicious nodule on USG, and CT is recommended if there are symptoms of airway compression. The presence of spindle cells has been reported in a case that didn't show a significant finding in FNAB. Surgical resection is treatment of choice (39).

Hematolymphoid tumors

Langerhans cell histiocytosis: Langerhans cell histiocytosis (LCH) is a rare neoplastic tumor of the Langerhans cell. The incidence rate is 4.0–5.4 per 1 million people and it is usually seen in the pediatric population (40).

Solitary disease in adults is rare and usually it is presented as a multisystem granulomatous infiltrate. The disease is confirmed by electron microscopy or immunohistochemical reactivity of histiocytes to CD1a and/or S100. It is characterized by a diffuse enlarged goiter or nodular disease. Screening is required to exclude systemic involvement. The prognosis is good in the presence of solitary involvement. The preferred surgical treatment method is hemi, subtotal or total thyroidectomy. Adjuvant chemoradiotherapy can be tried (41).

Rosai–Dorfman Disease: Rosai–Dorfman disease (RDD) was first described in 1969 by Juan Rosai and Ronald F Dorfman. It is an idiopathic, nonneoplastic, lymphoproliferative disease that is more common in men. Clinically, 95% of patients have enlarged cervical lymph nodes. This may be accompanied by enlarged inguinal and axillary lymph nodes. It is characterized by painless, bilateral cervical lymphadenopathy accompanied by fever, leukocytosis, elevated erythrocyte sedimentation rate and hypergammaglobulinemia. Malignant lymphoproliferative diseases should be excluded in the differential diagnosis. In the literature, there are cases that are diagnosed with FNAB. Surgical intervention is not required for this rare disease, which is self-limiting when diagnosed (42).

Follicular dendritic cell sarcoma: Follicular dendritic cell sarcoma (FDCS) was first described by Monda et al. based on four cases of unilateral cervical adenopathy in 1986 and is an uncommon lymph node malignancy of antigen-presenting cells of the B-cell follicles.

Thyroid involvement is extremely rare and has only been reported in five cases in the literature. Four of these cases are women and the average age is 50.2 years. Most of the cases developed on the basis of Hashimoto's thyroiditis. It manifests as a well-circumscribed swelling in the neck.

Although the diagnosis can be made with FNAB, it may be difficult to diagnose because it is rarely seen. Thyroid FDCS cells are typically positive for CD21, CD23, CD35 and vimentin; show variable positivity for CD68, CD45, S100 and epithelial membrane antigen (EMA); and are negative for cytokeratin, SMA, CD34 and CD3.

Total thyroidectomy is the treatment of choice. It can cause local recurrence and distant metastasis. Adjuvant chemoradiotherapy options can be added to the treatment (43).

Primary thyroid lymphoma: Primary thyroid lymphoma is a tumor seen in 2.1 per million and it can be confused with other malignant diseases of the thyroid. It is five times more common in women and it is a disease of advanced age (50–80). Approximately 2% of extranodal lymphoma originates in the thyroid gland and is almost always of the non-Hodgkin lymphoma type. Preexisting Hashimoto's thyroiditis is the only known risk factor for primary thyroid lymphoma and is present in approximately one-half of patients.

The vast majority of cases that are associated with non-Hodgkin lymphoma derived from B-cells, mainly including diffuse large B-cell lymphoma (DLBCL), mucosa-associated lymphoid tissue lymphoma (MALT) or a mixed type (combination of both). Patients present with the form of a rapidly growing neck mass. Symptoms may occur due to the compression of the mass. In about half of the cases, enlarged lymph nodes in the neck can also be detected. In addition to these local symptoms, lymphoma B symptoms such as weight loss, fever and night sweats can be seen in 10% of patients. Common USG sign is a hypervascular hypoechoic mass. FNAB can confirm the diagnosis of PTL in up to 70%–80% of cases.

In cases where FNAB is insufficient, incisional biopsy or core biopsy can be applied when the diagnosis is suspected (93%). Current imaging techniques (US, CT, scintigram, MRI, FDG-PET) can help define the existence of a thyroid mass as well as assistance in staging the disease. FDG-PET can be used for the initial diagnosis and monitoring the therapeutic response. Combined chemoradiotherapy is used in the treatment. The 10-year survival is about 70%.

In cases where the diagnosis can be made after surgery, adjuvant therapy should definitely be added. Surgery or only radiotherapy can be considered as treatment options for MALT lymphoma limited to the thyroid tissue (44).

Germ-cell tumors

Teratoma: Teratomas are germ-cell tumors that are characterized by three germ layers: The ectoderm, mesoderm and endoderm. Thyroid teratoma is a very rare form of germ-cell tumor. It manifests as a swelling in the neck. Hypoechoic nodule is present on the USG. Signs of compression can be seen. FNAB can differentiate between benign and malignant lesion. Surgery is an adequate treatment for benign teratomas.

Immature teratoma: Immature teratoma is extremely rare. It is difficult to differentiate it from malignant teratoma. There are not enough cases in the literature.

Malignant teratoma: Malignant teratoma of the thyroid in adults was first described by Lurje in 1908. Histologically, malignant thyroid teratomas usually show a predominance of neuroectodermal component with areas of glandular and/or squamous differentiation. Patients present clinically with a mass in the neck. They are extremely aggressive tumor and recurrence is often. Minimum treatment is total thyroidectomy and lymph node dissection. Although adjuvant treatments are used, the average survival time is 10 months (45).

Secondary tumors

Non-thyroid metastases to the thyroid gland are rare in the clinical setting and the most common primary tumor is renal cell carcinoma. The most common primary tumor in autopsy series is lung cancer. Preoperative evaluation is similar to evaluation for thyroid primary disease. Considering the presence of previous malignancy, evaluation of FNAB or core/open biopsies is helpful in diagnosis. The prognosis is related to the primary tumor. Along with triode metastasis, 30%–80% of the patients also have other metastases. Patients are mostly treated palliative. The number of patients eligible for surgery is small and the surgical criteria are unclear. Surgery can be applied in isolated thyroid metastases. Lobectomy or total thyroidectomies are among the options in surgical treatment (46).

Conclusion

Rare tumors of the thyroid are extremely rare tumors. It has been mostly reported as case reports in the literature. All of them have different biological behaviors. Due to the lack of available data, their natural course, etiopathogenesis, follow-up and treatment strategies are controversial.

Squamous cell carcinomas are tumors with poor prognosis, and there are some publications reporting that they may benefit from radiotherapy after surgical resection. MECs often have a slow course behavior similar to salivary gland-derived MECs. Eosinophilic SMECE is a slow progressing tumor containing epidermoid and glandular components and almost always develops on the basis of lymphocytic thyroiditis. In its differential diagnosis, MEC, anaplastic carcinoma, primary and secondary squamous cell carcinoma, and intrathyroidal thymic carcinoma should be considered. Mucinous carcinomas are a poor prognosis tumor characterized by neoplastic cells containing mucin. Thymomas are epithelial tumors originating from the thymus gland, their localization in the thyroid gland is extremely rare, surgical treatment is generally sufficient. Intrathyroidal thymic carcinoma is the malignant counterpart of ectopic thymoma. Paraganglioma and stromal tumors are very rare tumors originating from vascular and neural structures in the thyroid gland. It should be kept in mind when evaluating thyroid tumors, since rare tumors of the thyroid have different biological behaviors and can occur with recurrens/metastasis even after a long time.

Primary thyroid lymphoma is the most common of hematolymphoid tumors. Malignant teratoma is an extremely aggressive tumor with high mortality. In secondary tumors, the clinical course is related to the prognosis of the primary tumor.

References

1. Ricardo VL, Robert YO, Günter K, Juan R. WHO Classification of Tumours of Endocrine Organs. Lyon, France: International Agency for Research on Cancer (IARC); 2017.
2. Lam AK-y. FRCPA pathology of endocrine tumors update: World Health Organization new classification 2017—other thyroid tumors. AJSP. 2017;22(4):209–216.
3. Au JK, Alonso J, Kuan EC, Arshi A, St John MA. Primary squamous cell carcinoma of the thyroid: a population-based analysis. Otolaryngol Head Neck Surg. 2017 Jul;157(1):25–29.
4. Wang W, Ouyang Q, Meng C, Jing L, Li X. Treatment optimization and prognostic considerations for primary squamous cell carcinoma of the thyroid. Gland Surg. 2019 Dec;8(6):683–690.
5. Yang S, Li C, Shi X, Ma B, Xu W, Jiang H, Liu W, Ji Q, Wang Y. Primary squamous cell carcinoma in the thyroid gland: a population-based analysis using the SEER database. World J Surg. 2019 May;43(5):1249–1255.
6. Syed MI, Stewart M, Syed S, Dahill S, Adams C, McLellan DR, Clark LJ. Squamous cell carcinoma of the thyroid gland: primary or secondary disease? J Laryngol Otol. 2011 Jan;125(1):3–9.
7. Shah AA, La Fortune K, Miller C, Mills SE, Baloch Z, LiVolsi V, Dacic S, Mahaffey AL, Nikiforova M, Nikiforov YE, Seethala RR. Thyroid sclerosing mucoepidermoid carcinoma with eosinophilia: a clinicopathologic and molecular analysis of a distinct entity. Mod Pathol. 2017 Mar;30(3):329–339.
8. Sukumar JS, Sukumar S, Purohit D, Welch BJ, Balani J, Yan S, Hathiramani SS. Activating BRAF mutation in sclerosing mucoepidermoid carcinoma with eosinophilia of the thyroid gland: two case reports and review of the literature. J Med Case Rep. 2019 Dec;13(1):385.
9. Le QV, Ngo DQ, Ngo QX. Primary mucoepidermoid carcinoma of the thyroid: a report of a rare case with bone metastasis and review of the literature. Case Rep Oncol. 2019 Mar;12(1):248–259.
10. Warner E, Ofo E, Connor S, Odell E, Jeannon JP. Mucoepidermoid carcinoma in a thyroglossal duct remnant. Int J Surg Case Rep. 2015;13:43–47.
11. Shindo K, Aishima S, Okido M, Ohshima A. A poor prognostic case of mucoepidermoid carcinoma of the thyroid: a case report. Case Rep Endocrinol. 2012;2012:862545.
12. Wenig BM, Adair CF, Heffess CS. Primary mucoepidermoid carcinoma of the thyroid gland: a report of six cases and a review of the literature of a follicular epithelial-derived tumor. Hum Pathol. 1995 Oct;26(10):1099–1108.
13. Lai CY, Chao TC, Lin JD, Hsueh C. Sclerosing mucoepidermoid carcinoma with eosinophilia of thyroid gland in a male patient: a case report and literature review. Int J Clin Exp Pathol. 2015 May;8(5):5947–5951.
14. Iftikhar H, Awan MS, Ghaloo SK, Fatima S. Sclerosing mucoepidermoid carcinoma with eosinophilia of thyroid. BMJ Case Rep. 2019 Aug;12.
15. Bajja MY, Benassila FZ, Abada RL, Mahtar M, Chadli A. Mucinous carcinoma of the thyroid: a case report and review of the literature. Ann Endocrinol (Paris). 2017 Feb;78(1):70–73.
16. Matsuo M, Tuneyoshi M, Mine M. Primary mucinous carcinoma with rhabdoid cells of the thyroid gland: a case report. Diagn Pathol. 2016 Jun;11(1):48.
17. Wang J, Guli QR, Ming XC, Zhou HT, Cui YJ, Jiang YF, Zhang D, Liu Y. Primary mucinous carcinoma of thyroid gland with prominent signet-ring-cell differentiation: a case report and review of the literature. Onco Targets Ther. 2018 Mar;11:1521–1528.
18. Jing H, Wang J, Wei H, Liu M, Chen F, Meng Q, Tai Y. Ectopic hamartomatous thymoma: report of a case and review of literature. Int J Clin Exp Pathol. 2015 Sep;8(9):11776–11784.
19. Stevens TM, Morlote D, Swensen J, Ellis M, Harada S, Spencer S, Prieto-Granada CN, Folpe AL, Gatalica Z. Spindle epithelial tumor with thymus-like differentiation (SETTLE): a next-generation sequencing study. Head Neck Pathol. 2019 Jun;13(2):162–168.
20. Misra RK, Mitra S, Yadav R, Bundela A. Spindle epithelial tumor with thymus-like differentiation: a case report and review of literature. Acta Cytol. 2013;57(3):303–308.
21. Folpe AL, Lloyd RV, Bacchi CE, Rosai J. Spindle epithelial tumor with thymus-like differentiation: a morphologic, immunohistochemical, and molecular genetic study of 11 cases. Am J Surg Pathol. 2009 Aug;33(8):1179–1186.
22. Lee S, Kim YS, Lee JH, Hwang SH, Oh YH, Ko BK, Ham SY. Spindle epithelial tumor with thymus-like differentiation of the thyroid in a 70-year-old man. Ann Surg Treat Res. 2018 Jun;94(6):337–341.
23. Karaisli S, Haciyanli M, Gücek Haciyanli S, Tavusbay C, Gur EO, Kamer E, Arikan Etit D. Spindle epithelial tumour with thymus-like differentiation: report of two cases. Ann R Coll Surg Engl. 2020 Feb;102(2):e33–e35.
24. Sun YH, Xu J, Li M. Intrathyroid thymic carcinoma: report of two cases with pathologic and immunohistochemical studies. Int J Clin Exp Pathol. 2018 Oct;11(10):5139–5143.
25. Ren WH, Dong K, Huang XZ, Zhu YL. Intrathyroidal thymic carcinoma exhibiting neuroendocrine differentiation: case report with cytomorphology, immunocytochemistry, and review of the literature focusing on cytology. Diagn Cytopathol. 2019 Nov;47(11):1197–1202.
26. Ito Y, Miyauchi A, Nakamura Y, Miya A, Kobayashi K, Kakudo K. Clinicopathologic significance of intrathyroidal epithelial thymoma/carcinoma showing thymus-like differentiation: a collaborative study with Member Institutes of The Japanese Society of Thyroid Surgery. Am J Clin Pathol. 2007 Feb;127(2):230–236.
27. Lee SM, Policarpio-Nicolas ML. Thyroid Paraganglioma. Arch Pathol Lab Med. 2015 Aug;139(8):1062–1067.
28. Yu BH, Sheng WQ, Wang J. Primary paraganglioma of thyroid gland: a clinicopathologic and immunohistochemical analysis of three cases with a review of the literature. Head Neck Pathol. 2013 Dec;7(4):373–380.
29. Ferri E, Manconi R, Armato E, Ianniello F. Primary paraganglioma of thyroid gland: a clinicopathologic and immunohistochemical study with review of the literature. Acta Otorhinolaryngol Ital. 2009 Apr;29(2):97–102.
30. Kandil E, Abdel Khalek M, Abdullah O, Dali D, Faruqui S, Khan A, Friedlander P, Jaffe BM, Crawford B. Primary peripheral nerve sheath tumors of the thyroid gland. Thyroid. 2010 Jun;20(6):583–586.
31. Chen G, Liu Z, Su C, Guan Q, Wan F, Dong B, Bao L, Zhang W, Wang Y, Wang G. Primary peripheral nerve sheath tumors of the thyroid gland: a case report and literature review. Mol Clin Oncol. 2016 Feb;4(2):209–210.
32. Miao J, Chen S, Li Y, Fu L, Li H. A primary cavernous hemangioma of the thyroid gland: a case report and literature review. Medicine (Baltimore). 2017 Dec;96(49):e8651.
33. Kondapalli A, Redd L, DeBlanche L, Oo Y. Primary angiosarcoma of thyroid. BMJ Case Rep. 2019 Jun;12(6).
34. De Felice F, Moscatelli E, Orelli S, Bulzonetti N, Musio D, Tombolini V. Primary thyroid angiosarcoma: a systematic review. Oral Oncol. 2018 Jul;82:48–52.
35. Şahin Mİ, Vural A, Yüce İ, Çağlı S, Deniz K, Güney E. Thyroid leiomyosarcoma: presentation of two cases and review of the literature. Braz J Otorhinolaryngol. 2016 Nov–Dec;82(6):715–721.
36. Zhang Y, Tang H, Hu H, Yong X. A rare primary tumor of the thyroid gland: a new case of leiomyoma and literature review. Clin Med Insights Oncol. 2018 Nov;12.
37. Canu GL, Bulla JS, Lai ML, Medas F, Baghino G, Erdas E, Mariotti S, Calò PG. Primary thyroid leiomyosarcoma: a case report and review of the literature. G Chir. 2018 Jan-Feb;39(1):51–56.
38. Thompson LDR, Wei C, Rooper LM, Lau SK. Thyroid gland solitary fibrous tumor: report of 3 cases and a comprehensive review of the literature. Head Neck Pathol. 2019 Dec;13(4):597–605.
39. Ghasemi-Rad M, Wang KY, Jain S, Lincoln CM. Solitary fibrous tumor of thyroid: a case report with review of literature. Clin Imaging. 2019 Jan–Feb;53:105–107.
40. Pandyaraj RA, Sathik Mohamed Masoodu K, Maniselvi S, Savitha S, Divya Devi H. Langerhans cell histiocytosis of thyroid-a diagnostic dilemma. Indian J Surg. 2015 Apr;77(Suppl 1):49–51.
41. Patten DK, Wani Z, Tolley N. Solitary langerhans histiocytosis of the thyroid gland: a case report and literature review. Head Neck Pathol. 2012 Jun;6(2):279–289.
42. Chhabra S, Agarwal R, Garg S, Singh H, Singh S. Rosai-Dorfman disease: a case report with extranodal thyroid involvement. Diagn Cytopathol. 2012 May;40(5):447–449.
43. Zhang T, He L, Wang Z, Dong W, Sun W, Zhang P, Zhang H. Follicular dendritic cell sarcoma presenting as a thyroid mass: an unusual case report and literature review. J Int Med Res. 2020 Jun;48(6):300060520920433.
44. Pavlidis ET, Pavlidis TE. A review of primary thyroid lymphoma: molecular factors, diagnosis and management. J Invest Surg. 2019 Mar;32(2):137–142.
45. Vilallonga R, Zafon C, Ruiz-Marcellan C, Obiols G, Fort JM, Baena JA, Villanueva B, Garcia A, Sobrinho-Simões M. Malignant thyroid teratoma: report of an aggressive tumor in a 64-year-old man. Endocr Pathol. 2013 Sep;24(3):132–135.
46. Nixon IJ, Coca-Pelaz A, Kaleva AI, Triantafyllou A, Angelos P, Owen RP, Rinaldo A, Shaha AR, Silver CE, Ferlito A. Metastasis to the thyroid gland: a critical review. Ann Surg Oncol. 2017 Jun;24(6):1533–1539.

20

CHILDHOOD THYROID CANCERS

Emre Divarci and Ahmet Çelik

Introduction

Thyroid cancer is the most prevalent endocrine cancer in adults and children. About 2% of all thyroid cancers are diagnosed in childhood and adolescence (1). The constitute 1.5% of all pediatric cancers encountered in childhood (2, 3). The rate increases exponentially up to 8% between the ages of 15 and 19 (2, 4).

In general, 2% of children have a palpable thyroid nodule (5). Although most are benign cases such as follicular adenomas or inflammatory lesions, malignant factors are observed more frequently when compared to adults. In children, the risk of malignancy risk in thyroid nodules is higher when compared to the adults, since the thyroid gland is more sensitive to radiation and prone to carcinogenesis. The malignancy risk in nodules is 5% in adulthood, while it is about 20–25% in children (6–8). Also, lymph node metastasis and relapse in 10-year follow-up are more common in children when compared to adults. Although advanced disease is determined in diagnosis, the prognosis of thyroid cancer is much better in children when compared to adults.

Despite serious differences between pediatric and adult thyroid nodules and cancers, there were no specific diagnosis and treatment guidelines for children until 2015. In 2015, the first pediatric guideline was published by the American Thyroid Association (ATA) (9). The guideline included standard recommendations about the approach to thyroid cancer in childhood. However, there are still no multicenter, randomized, prospective studies with a high number of patients on thyroid cancer in children. Most of the previous studies include retrospective, single-center, cohort case studies. This prevents recommendations based on strong scientific evidence. In this section, the characteristics, diagnosis, and treatment approaches in pediatric thyroid cancers are discussed in detail.

Epidemiology

Although the prevalence of thyroid nodules varies based on the country of residence and even the region in a country, it is approximately 2% among the children (10). In a study conducted in Greece with large patient group, a thyroid nodule was identified in 5.8% of 5–18-year-old children in ultrasonography (USG) (11).

Although the risk of thyroid nodule malignancy is higher in children when compared to in adults, the majority of these nodules are still benign. The general malignancy risk is reported as 5% in adults, while it varies between 10 and 50% in different series among children (6–8). In general, the risk of thyroid nodule malignancy is 5% in adults, while it was reported as around 25% in children (6–8). In fact, these high rates have decreased with the addition of small-sized incidental nodules to the case series in recent studies. Similarly, thyroid nodule malignancy risk in childhood that were identified incidentally in computed tomography (CT) was 5.7%, similar to the adults (12).

The differentiated thyroid cancer (DTC) incidence has gradually increased in children in recent years. The analysis of the data for 1806 pediatric patients reported between 1973 and 2013 revealed that the incidence increased from 0.48 per 100,000 in 1973 to 1.14 per 100,000 in 2013 (13). It was suggested that both the development of diagnostic methods and the increase in the incidence may have played a role in this increase. The Surveillance, Epidemiology, and End Results (SEER) registry system reported a 3% annual increase in incidence over the same 40-year period. This has led to a higher incidence in pediatric thyroid cancers in recent years.

Pathogenesis and risk factors (Table 20.1)

Age and gender: In general, the most common age-group with the highest thyroid cancer risk is adolescent females (1). While thyroid cancer is four times more common in adult females when compared to males, the rate is more similar in prepubertal age females and males. After puberty, thyroid cancer incidence is 3–14 times more in females when compared to males (14–16).

Radiation exposure: The child thyroid gland is more susceptible to the carcinogenic effects of radiation when compared to adults. Thyroid nodule and cancer incidences are more frequent in adulthood in neck region radiotherapy patients who were treated for head and neck tumors, Hodgkin lymphoma, and leukemia (17–19). A high incidence of thyroid nodules was observed in adulthood in children who survived the Hiroshima and Nagasaki nuclear bombs (20). The risk of exposure increases after a 0.05–0.1 Gy (50–100 mGy) dose, reaching the highest rate in 45-year follow-up in individuals who were exposed at a younger age (21, 22).

Genetic disorders and family history: Several genetic syndromes could be comorbid to pediatric thyroid cancers. In multiple endocrine neoplasia (MEN) type 2, familial medullary thyroid carcinoma develops due to the mutation in the RET proto-oncogene (23). Due to its autosomal dominant inheritance, prophylactic thyroidectomy should be applied in these patients at an early age. In Gardner's syndrome, which develops due to APC (adenomatous polyposis coli) gene mutation, familial polyposis coli could accompany thyroid cancer (24). All these patients are young and female patients (25). Other genetic disorders associated with family history include Carney complex, PTEN (phosphatase and tensin homolog) hamartoma tumor syndrome, Werner's syndrome, and DICER1 syndrome (26).

Autoimmune thyroiditis: Thyroid cancer could be more frequent in patients with autoimmune thyroid diseases such as Hashimoto thyroiditis and Graves' disease (27–29).

Others: Thyroid cancer could be more prevalent in congenital goiter due to high TSH stimulation levels (30). Furthermore, certain studies reported that thyroid cancer developed on the ground of thyroglossal duct cysts (31).

TABLE 20.1: Risk Factors of Thyroid Carcinomas
Adolescence age
Female gender
Radiation exposure
Genetic inheritance and family history:
• MEN type 2
• Gardner syndrome, Carney complex, PTEN hamartoma tumor syndrome, Werner syndrome, DICER syndrome
Autoimmune thyroiditis:
• Hashimoto's thyroiditis
• Graves' disease
Congenital goiter
Thyroglossal duct cyst

TABLE 20.2: Histopathological Types of Thyroid Carcinomas
Differentiated thyroid carcinoma:
• Papillary thyroid carcinoma (83%)
• Follicular thyroid carcinoma (10%)
Medullary thyroid carcinoma (5%)
Other thyroid cancers (2%): Anaplastic carcinoma, Hurthle cell carcinoma

Histopathology and types (Table 20.2)

Thyroid gland tumors are addressed in two categories: Adenoma and carcinoma (32, 33). Adenomas are well-defined, encapsulated, benign lesions. They can enlarge over time and apply pressure on the surrounding tissues. In certain cells, malignant transformation can be observed, and they could spread to the surrounding tissues or to distant tissues through circulation (Figure 20.1).

Generally, 20–25% of the thyroid nodules diagnosed in childhood are malignant (9, 28). In a series of 1753 cases of childhood thyroid cancer published by SEER registry system in 2009, 83% of the patients were diagnosed with papillary thyroid cancer (60% papillary, 23% follicular variant), 10% with follicular thyroid cancer, 5% with medullary thyroid cancer, and 2% with other rare types (1). Thyroid cancers are classified as DTCs, medullary thyroid carcinoma (MTC), and other rare types.

Differentiated thyroid cancers (DTCs)

DTCs include papillary and follicular thyroid cancers. They originate in the thyroid follicle cells. Although more frequent invasion, metastasis, and relapse are observed in pediatric DTCs, the prognosis is much better than adults (10-year survival >95%) (2, 3, 9).

- **Papillary thyroid carcinoma (PTC)**: PTC is the most prevalent differentiated thyroid carcinoma among children and adolescents. PTC could include a wide variety of histological variants. These could be classified as classical, solid, follicular, and diffuse sclerosing type. In recent years, a new form called "noninvasive follicular thyroid neoplasm with papillary characteristics" (NIFT-P), which resembles follicular variant papillary carcinoma but identified with capsulated and noninvasive properties, was added as a new subtype (34). PTC is characterized by multifocality, bilateral location in the thyroid gland, and a local metastasis tendency to lymph nodes. Hematogenous metastasis, especially lung metastasis, could be observed in up to 20–25% of the cases (9, 35).
- **Follicular thyroid carcinoma (FTC)**: Although FTC is less prevalent when compared to PTC, it exhibits a higher rate of hematogenous and distant metastasis. Thus, unlike PTC, lung and bone metastases are more common, rather than adjacent lymph nodes.

Medullary thyroid carcinoma (MTC)

MTC originates in parafollicular C cells that secrete calcitonin. Although it is a less prevalent tumor in the general population when compared to DTCs, it exhibits autosomal dominant inheritance in familial cases with RET proto-oncogene mutation. It emerges as a MEN type-2 component and prophylactic thyroidectomy is recommended in early ages (infancy or early childhood) (36). The timing of prophylactic thyroidectomy in asymptomatic patients with positive RET oncogene is determined based on the risk group (37). The "highest risk" group patients with MEN2B based on the RET oncogene-specific mutation should undergo thyroidectomy during the first year in life.

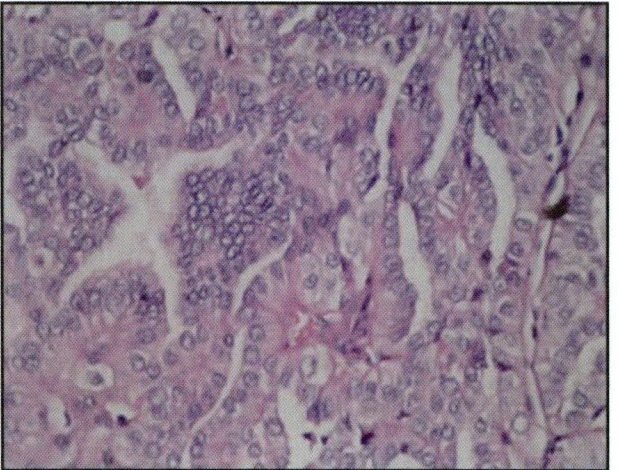
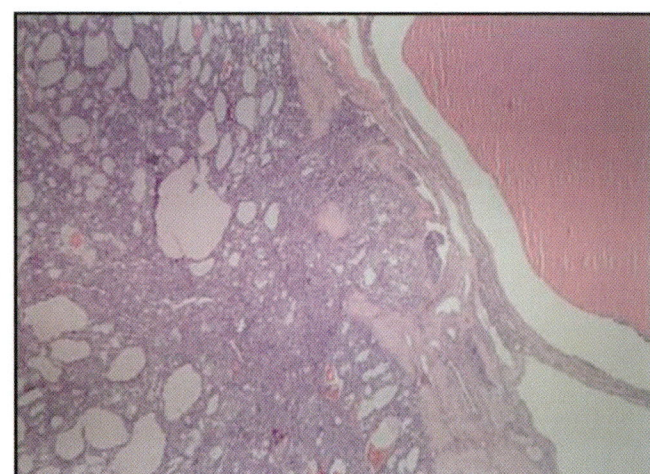

FIGURE 20.1 Microscopic images of papillary thyroid carcinoma.

Childhood Thyroid Cancers

Prophylactic thyroidectomy is recommended in the age of 5 for "high-risk" mutation-positive patients and in early childhood for the "medium-risk" group.

Anaplastic carcinoma

Anaplastic thyroid carcinoma is one of the rarest (less than 1%) but most aggressive tumor type among thyroid carcinomas.

Molecular features

Molecular changes observed in thyroid cancers should be evaluated separately in tumors that originate from follicular and parafollicular cells on a cellular basis.

Genetics in follicular cell thyroid tumors

Aberrant activations in the MAPK and/or PI3K/PTEN/AKT signal pathways are held responsible for papillary and FTCs that develop in thyroid follicle cells. Although BRAF and RAS gene mutations are the main determinants, RET and NRTK gene mutations also play a key role in carcinogenesis (38–40).

- *BRAF mutation*: It is the most common gene mutation in thyroid carcinoma. The point mutation is in the V600E gene in the majority of cases with BRAF mutation. BRAF mutation is determined in 40–80% of the PTC cases, while it is determined in 10–50% of anaplastic thyroid carcinomas with worse prognosis (38, 40). The prognostic value of the BRAF mutation is still controversial in children. Although it was reported in various publications that it was more frequently associated with extrathyroidal dissemination and local relapse, there are also publications that claimed the opposite (38, 40, 41).
- *RAS mutation*: RAS mutation is a marker for follicular thyroid lesions, and it is positive in 30–50% of FTCs, 25–45% of follicular variant papillary carcinomas, and less than 10% of PTCs (38, 40).
- *RET-PTC mutations*: These mutations often occur due to exposure to environmental or therapeutic radiation and are more frequently diagnosed in young patients with nodal metastases that exhibit aggressive clinical features (38, 40).
- *NTRK mutations*: It is diagnosed as positive in 15% of radiation-induced PTC cases (38, 40). Similar to RET-PTC mutations, NRTK mutations exhibit a worse clinical appearance.
- *Other rare mutations*: DICER1, ALK, AKT1, PPARG, TP53 gene mutations.

Genetics in parafollicular cell thyroid tumors

Parafollicular C cells in the thyroid gland are neural crest-derived cells and the medullary thyroid carcinoma may develop in these cells, making a neuroendocrine malignancy. Pediatric MTC is an autosomal dominant inheritance due to a mutation in the RET oncogene and associated with MEN types MEN2A and MEN2B. The risk of MTC development is grouped based on the type of RET mutation. The risk is higher in MEN2B, it is lower in MEN2A when compared to MEN2B (39).

Clinical presentation

The most common presenting symptom is painless swelling in the thyroid gland or neck (42). The swelling in the neck is usually due to lymph node enlargement. The thyroid gland should also be palpated, and the presence of nodules should be investigated in every patient presenting with the complaint of neck swelling due to lymph node metastasis during diagnosis (43, 44). Symptoms such as pressure on the respiratory tract, aphonia, and swallowing difficulty generally develop due to an overgrowth thyroid nodule or goiter. In advanced cases, aphonia may develop due to laryngeal recurrent nerve invasion. A hard, painless, fixed and immobile nodule in physical examination should raise a high suspicion for malignancy (42). Although lungs are the most common metastatic site in thyroid cancers in children, the presence rarely includes respiratory symptoms (45, 46). Lung metastasis may be prevalent based on miliaria aspect (Figure 20.2). Thus, lungs should be investigated for metastasis in every patient with thyroid cancer. Lung metastasis is more prevalent in prepubertal

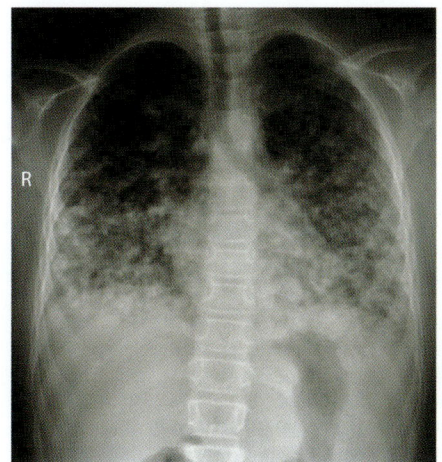

Chest X Ray
(a)

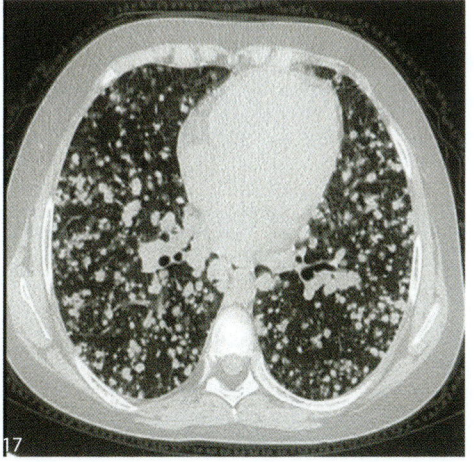

Thorax CT
(b)

FIGURE 20.2 Radiological appearance of lung metastasis in papillary thyroid carcinoma (a) Chest X-ray and (b) Thorax CT.

age bilateral tumors with invasion outside the capsule (47, 48). Abnormal findings are not encountered in most thyroid function tests in pediatric thyroid cancers, and the test lack clinical findings since they are euthyroid.

Initial evaluation and surgical strategy based on fine-needle aspiration biopsy (FNAB)

In patients diagnosed with thyroid nodules, the anamnesis should be detailed after the physical examination, and radiation exposure, iodine deficiency, genetic syndromes and thyroid diseases in the family should be investigated. Children with Hodgkin lymphoma, leukemia, and central nervous system tumors with a history of radiotherapy treatment are in the high-risk group for thyroid nodule development. Also, thyroid nodules may develop in about one-third of autoimmune thyroid diseases such as Hashimoto's thyroiditis and Graves' disease (9). After physical examination and detailed anamnesis, patients who present with thyroid nodules should be tested for TSH, T4, and thyroglobulin (Tg) blood levels and thyroid/neck USG should be conducted in the first evaluation. Thyroid scintigraphy could be conducted in only patients with suppressed blood TSH levels. Almost all pediatric thyroid cancers are euthyroid. In patients with hyperthyroidism, the characteristics of the nodule could be determined in scintigraphy.

In the approach to pediatric thyroid nodules, recommendations are made based on the ATA pediatric guideline (Figure 20.3) (9). In this guide, the first step is to investigate the TSH level in solid or solid-cystic nodules larger than 1 cm or in nodules that exhibit suspicious symptoms in USG. Suspicious nodule-specific sonographic features in USG could be listed as solid, hypoechoic, increased intralobular blood flow, irregular border, and microcalcification. Suspicious findings in lymph nodes include a round shape, peripheral blood flow, cystic areas, loss of hilum and microcalcification. If TSH level is suppressed in these nodules, initially, fine-needle aspiration biopsy (FNAB) should be conducted with USG if scintigraphy is not available.

In FNAB, pathology results are indicated as nondiagnostic or insufficient, benign, atypic or follicular lesion, follicular/Hurtle cell neoplasia, or suspicious follicular/Hurtle cell neoplasia, supporting malignant, and malignant.

If the FNAB result is benign, USG should be conducted 6–12 months later; if the nodule is stable, USG should be repeated every 1–2 years. If there is a growth in the nodule or there are suspicious changes in the findings, FNAB should be repeated or surgery should be preferred (30).

If the FNAB result is insufficient or nondiagnostic, USG and FNAB should be repeated within 3–6 months. If the nodule is stable or benign, USG should be repeated within 6–12 months.

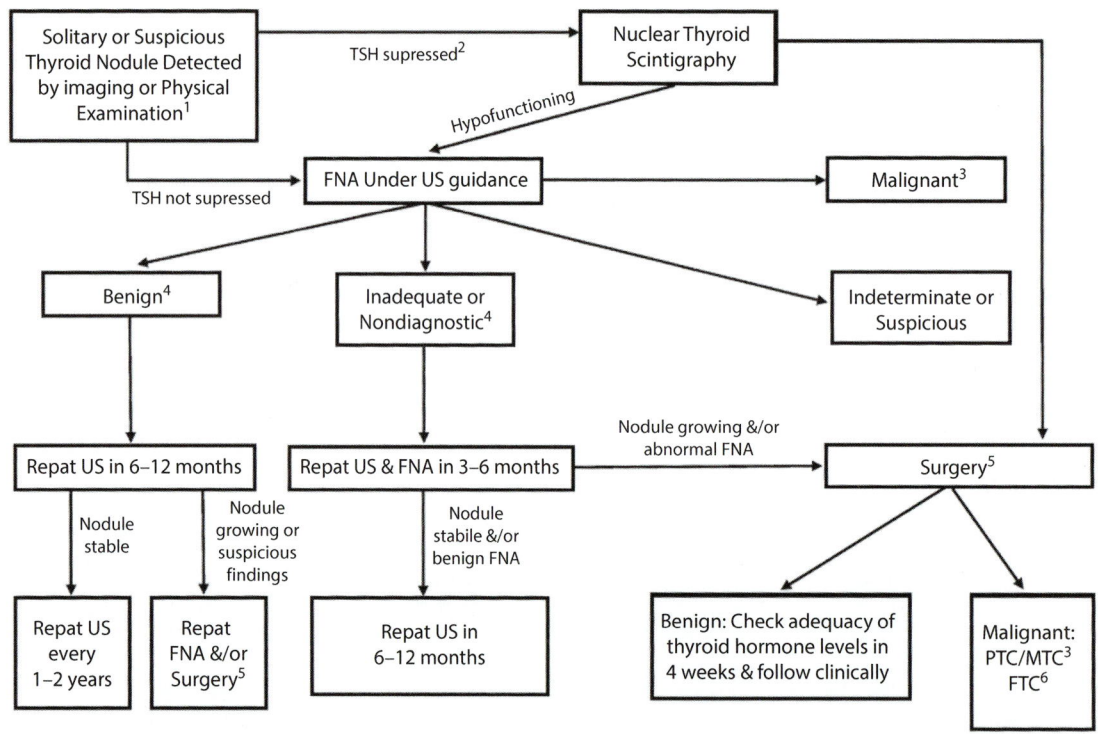

[1]Assumes a solid or partially cystic nodule ≥1 cm or a nodule with concerning ultrasonographic features in a patient without personal risk factors for thyroid malignancy. [2]A suppressed TSH indicates a value below the lower limits of normal. [3]Refer to PTC management guidelines or MTC management guidelines. [4]Surgery can always be considered based upon suspicious ultrasound findings, concerning clinical presentation, nodule size >4 cm, compressive symptoms, and/or patient/family preference. [5]Surgery implies lobectomy plus isthmusectomy in most cases. Surgery may be deferred in patients with an autonomous nodule and subclinical hyperthyroidism, but FNA should be considered if the nodule has features suspicious for PTC. Consider intraoperative frozen section for indeterminate and suspicious lesions. Can consider total thyroidectomy for nodules suspicious for malignancy on FNA. [6]Consider completion thyroidectomy – RAI versus observation – TSH suppression based upon final pathology.

FIGURE 20.3 American Thyroid Association (ATA) management guideline for pediatric thyroid nodules.

However, if the nodule is growing or the FNAB result suggests that the nodule is not benign, surgery should be preferred.

In patients with suspicious or uncertain FNAB results and require surgery, the lobe that contains the nodule should be excised with the isthmus and a frozen biopsy should be conducted, and if the result is malignant, total thyroidectomy should be performed. If the frozen biopsy result is benign or suspicious, the operation should be terminated and postponed until the definitive pathology result. Complementary thyroidectomy ± radioactive iodine (RAI) therapy ± TSH suppression may be required based on the pathology result. If the definitive pathological diagnosis is not possible within a week, the complementary surgery may be postponed for a month due to adhesions in the neck.

FNAB cannot demonstrate the relationship with the thyroid capsule. The differential diagnosis of thyroid follicular neoplasia and adenoma is based on the presence of capsule invasion. Thus, FNAB is insufficient in the differential diagnosis of follicular adenoma and neoplasia. In the case of doubt, lobectomy may be required.

The definite pathology report should be obtained in cases where cancer could not be differentiated with frozen biopsy. Complementary thyroidectomy should be conducted when cancer diagnosis is obtained within a week.

Total thyroidectomy is recommended when the thyroid nodule is larger than 4 cm, there is a familial predisposition, exposure to radiation or a bilateral disease (49).

Surgical treatment

Surgical treatment in pediatric thyroid cancers varies based on the type and clinical behavior of the cancer. In general, the surgical treatment principles should be discussed separately in DTCs and medullary thyroid carcinoma.

Surgical treatment in differentiated thyroid carcinoma

The pediatric DTC risk group is categorized in three groups according to the ATA (9):

- *Low risk*: Tumor is limited to the thyroid (usually smaller than 1 cm), there are no metastatic lymph nodes, or there are a few microscopic central compartment metastatic lymph nodes.
- *Moderate risk*: Extensive central compartment lymph node metastasis or minimal lateral lymph node metastasis.
- *High risk*: Extensive lateral compartment lymph node metastasis or aggressive local tumor exceeding the thyroid capsule, with or without distant metastasis.

Thyroid and neck USG conducted for preoperative evaluation is very important in effective planning of surgical treatment in all patients diagnosed with or suspected of DTC. In the USG examination conducted by experienced radiologists, all neck regions should be evaluated and it should be remembered that the sensitivity of USG is low in the diagnosis of malignant lymph nodes in the central neck region (level VI: peritracheal, paratracheal, prelaryngeal, and Delphian lymph nodes). The presence of regional lymph node involvement, which could not be detected in physical examination, should be investigated in USG. Thus, the risk of relapse and the need for secondary surgery could be eliminated by a thyroidectomy and lymph node dissection, if necessary, during the initial surgery. If the thyroid nodule or lymph nodes are too large, USG may be insufficient to identify the metastatic disease in deep tissues (superior mediastinum/level VII, retropharyngeal, parapharyngeal, and sub-clavicular). Cross-sectional imaging methods such as CT or magnetic resonance imaging could be employed, especially in respiratory tract or esophageal involvement. However, when using iodinated contrast material, it should be kept in mind that evaluation of RAI uptake and treatment will be delayed for 2–3 months. Since the prevalence of lung metastasis increases in patients with neck lymph node involvement, thorax CT could be conducted in addition to the plain chest X-ray.

Total thyroidectomy should be preferred in patients diagnosed with DTC. In total thyroidectomy, both isthmus and pyramidal lobes should be dissected. Since DTC is 30% bilateral and 65% multifocal in the same lobe, options such as nodulectomy, partial thyroidectomy, lobectomy, subtotal thyroidectomy, and near-total thyroidectomy should not be preferred. Total thyroidectomy decreases the need for a second surgery by reducing the risk of relapse. Total thyroidectomy is also necessary in cases that require RAI therapy after surgery for an effective treatment and to allow the use of Tg as a tumor marker in the follow-up (9).

In patients with signs of lymph node metastasis in the central or lateral neck, central neck dissection reduces the risk of persistent/recurrent local disease and increases the effectiveness of I^{131} therapy in distant metastases. Disease-free life expectancy depends on the presence of persistent/recurrent disease in children and cervical lymph node metastasis is prevalent. Thus, the prophylactic central lymph node dissection requirement should be investigated during the first surgery. There data on the findings to determine the local/regional metastasis risk are insufficient in pediatric patients. In children with thyroid cancer, the disease-specific 10-year survival chance is close to 100%. The most important factor that prolongs a life without disease is the first surgical intervention. However, there are no long-term and prospective studies that revealed the patients who benefit from aggressive surgery. Thus, the risks and potential benefits of surgical intervention should be well evaluated to prevent relapse.

In malignant cytology, in the presence of obvious extrathyroid invasion and/or local/regional metastasis in preoperative or intraoperative frozen evaluations, central lymph node dissection reduces the possibility of secondary surgery and prolongs the disease-free survival. If there is no visible extrathyroidal involvement and/or local/regional metastasis in DTC patients, central lymph node dissection should be preferred based on tumor involvement. In the presence of a unilateral tumor, central lymph node dissection is conducted on the same side, and performing the dissection on the opposite side is determined by the surgery findings.

Compartmental approach should be preferred in lymph node dissection. It is not recommended to diagnose the presence of a metastatic disease by palpation or lymph node excision with the "berry picking" method. Further studies are required to understand RAI therapy need and the effect of total thyroidectomy and central lymph node dissection on disease-free survival. Routine lateral neck dissection (level II, III, IV, V) is not recommended. Lateral neck dissection should be conducted when US data indicate the presence of a metastatic lymph node in lateral compartments and cytological data that demonstrate the presence of lateral neck metastasis. Lateral neck dissection in the presence of lateral neck metastasis reduces the risk of relapse, prolongs disease-free survival, and increases the success of postoperative radioactive I^{131} ablation therapy (50).

Although the risk of post-total thyroidectomy complications decreased in recent years, recurrent laryngeal nerve injury and permanent/temporary hypocalcemia could be observed. During dissection, the laryngeal nerve should definitely be observed and protected. In cases with laryngeal nerve involvement, the nerve should be preserved, even when residual tumor remains. Residual tumor could be cleaned with I^{131} ablation after the surgery. If the parathyroid gland blood supply is impaired during total thyroidectomy, one or two parathyroid glands should be grafted into the sternocleidomastoid muscle or the inner surface of the arm.

Lung metastasis should be investigated in the postoperative period. The prevalence of lung metastasis without lymph node involvement is about 6% in children (51). Thus, 6 weeks after total thyroidectomy, metastasis could be observed with scintigraphy imaging using I^{131}. Scintigraphy may provide false-negative results in the presence of residual thyroid tissue. To prevent this, total thyroidectomy should be ensured. TSH should be lower than 30 mIU/l for a safe iodine screening.

RAI treatment is required in the presence of local/regional disease, lymph node, and distant metastasis that could not be surgically removed are determined in postoperative iodine scanning.

In the presence of diffuse regional lymph node involvement, level VI, unilateral, bilateral, or contralateral level I, II, III, IV, V or retropharyngeal, superior mediastinal lymph node (level VII) involvement, limited tumor larger than 4 cm in the thyroid, or when the tumor extends beyond the thyroid, certain scientists recommended RAI therapy (9).

Further treatment requirements will be evaluated after I^{131} administration for each patient. The potential risks and benefits of additional treatment should be well considered.

Young age, poor histology, capsule invasion, surgical margin positivity, and lymph node and lung invasion in diagnosis increase the risk of relapse after treatment.

In the postoperative period, follow-up physical examination, USG and Tg level analysis should be conducted. Tg is a sensitive tumor marker employed in diagnosis, treatment, and long-term follow-up in DTC. Tg antibodies should be measured in all samples simultaneously. The Tg result could not be evaluated in the presence of the Tg antibody.

Surgical treatment in medullary thyroid carcinoma

Medullary thyroid cancer (MTC) is the third most prevalent thyroid cancer following DTC (papillary and follicular thyroid cancer) in children. 80% of the patients are diagnosed incidentally between the ages of 40 and 60. 20% of the incidences occur due to autosomal dominant inheritance. Hereditary MTCs are associated with a group of endocrine diseases known as MEN or familial MTC observed only in MTC.

In hereditary cases, MTC is usually multifocal and bilateral. In general, hereditary MTC starts with hyperplasia in parafollicular C cells and leads to invasive micro-cancer, followed by macroscopic disease and, if untreated, distant metastasis. Distant metastases are observed in lungs, liver, and bone in the early period, accompanied with airway obstruction and usually leading to death (52, 53). The most common symptom in severe cases is diarrhea (>10/day) and high serum calcitonin levels. Flushing could also accompany diarrhea. This is less common and was attributed to certain undetermined hormonal activities (53). MEN2A and 2B are observed in all MTC cases, albeit earlier in MEN2B. Thus, RET mutation should be determined before 5 years of age in familial cases (52). Prophylactic thyroidectomy should be performed before the age of 1 in MEN2B cases and before the age of 5 in MEN2A cases (1). If the patient is young and there is no evidence of lymph node involvement, central neck dissection is unnecessary during prophylactic thyroidectomy (51, 52).

Serum calcitonin level is a quite useful indicator in incidental MTC suspicion. All MTC cases should be examined with the United States for lymph node metastasis during the preoperative period. Central neck dissection should be conducted with the total thyroidectomy in MTC cases. Calcitonin and carcinoembryonic antigen (CEA) levels are useful in case follow-up, and increased levels indicate relapse of the disease.

Radioactive iodine therapy and TSH suppression

In the standard treatment of pediatric thyroid cancers, total or near-total thyroidectomy, followed by RAI suppression treatment with I^{131} to remove the residue thyroid tissue, and then, long-term thyroid hormone suppression therapy are included. RAI treatment (1) reduces the risk of local relapse, (2) increases the sensitivity of the whole-body scintigraphy, and (3) increases the sensitivity of Tg, which is a good marker of relapse/residual tissue in long-term follow-up (54, 55). Diagnostic whole-body scintigraphy (with I^{131} or I^{123}), serum Tg measurements, and neck USG should be performed at regular intervals during follow-up. A whole-body scan with RAI should be conducted 6 weeks after the operation and once a year to check for metastasis.

Both replacement therapy and thyroid hormone therapy for TSH suppression should be initiated after thyroidectomy and RAI suppression treatment. During the first 24 hours, the treatment is conducted with T3 with a short half-life, then long-term treatment is initiated with T4 with a half-life of 1 week. Thus, tumor tissue stimulated by TSH will be suppressed. It is recommended to keep TSH level below 0.1 mIU/ml in high-risk patients and between 0.1 and 0.5 mIU/ml in low-risk patients. Children are included in the low mortality and high relapse risk group. The effect of this treatment on bone mineral density is not yet known in children.

In the postoperative period, a Tg level above 1 ng/ml in L-thyroxine treatment and over 10 ng/ml in untreated patients is an indicator of relapse. The presence of measurable blood calcitonin operation in medullary TC in the postoperative period suggests relapse.

Around 6–8 weeks after thyroidectomy, thyroid hormone treatment is discontinued for 2 weeks, and total body scintigraphy is conducted with 1–5 mCi I^{131}. The presence of a tumor in the tumor bed is checked for distant tumor metastasis in organs such as the lungs, bones, and liver. Before scintigraphy, TSH is required to be above 35 mIU/ml. For the destruction of the residual thyroid tissue 6–8 weeks after thyroidectomy, RAI therapy is recommended, especially in papillary TC cases with multiple microscopic foci. Especially, when there is a finding such as a tumor larger than 1 cm, neck lymph node involvement, non-thyroid metastasis, postoperative "in situ" or distant disease, RAI eradication treatment is recommended (9). For a successful eradication, serum TSH level (>35 mU/l) should be high as well as maximum RAI involvement. Thus, it would be sufficient to stop thyroid hormone therapy for 3–4 weeks.

The RAI dose varies between 35 and 200 mCi. It is recommended to administer 100 mCi/m2 RAI when there is tumor residue in the tumor bed, 150 mCi/1.73 m^2 when there is regional lymph node involvement in children, and 175–200 mCi/m^2 when there is lung or other distant metastasis. It was also reported that a 30-mCi eradication dose would be sufficient in children 6 weeks after the first surgery. The recommended RAI dose for 3–5-year old children is 1.0–1.5 mCi/kg. However, pre-eradication scintigraphy is not required for these doses, but if it would be conducted, it is recommended to be conducted with I^{123}. Dosimetry should be used to suppress the bone marrow in very young children with lung invasion and require multiple RAI treatments.

Nausea, sialadenitis, xerostomia, thrombocytopenia, and leukopenia could be observed in the short term due to RAI treatment (56). In the long term, temporary increase in follicle-stimulating hormone in young males, and especially lung fibrosis in patients who received multiple doses of I^{131} for 6 months or less (57).

The absence of involvement in whole-body scintigraphy is accepted as the gold standard for prolonged treatment (i.e., a few decades) in children. In young patients, treatment is recommended until no I^{131} involvement (treatment until negativity in whole-body scintigraphy) or until a cumulative dose of 22 GBq (600-mCi). Patients should be evaluated individually when further treatment is decided in the presence of resistant disease despite the administration of the abovementioned dose. The risk of leukemia and other cancers increases over 600 mCi dose. Following stimulation with recombinant TSH, the Tg level of 2 ng/ml is important since it indicates that the disease is no longer present. Serial pediatric Tg levels of <2 ng/ml are reported to indicate the absence of the disease and useful in follow-up.

As thyroid hormone suppression continues in children who have undergone total thyroidectomy and RAI eradication, the Tg level should be at immeasurable levels (0.5 ng/ml).

It is recommended to conduct whole-body scintigraphy (2–3 mCi) with RAI and to check Tg levels at 6-month intervals during the first 18 months, and then at 3–5-year intervals. It is also considered beneficial to conduct concurrent thyroid USG. Computed thorax tomography is not recommended for children during follow-up.

The absence of disease means no finding in whole-body scintigraphy, and low or unmeasurable Tg levels. Although survival period is good in the disease, further surgery or I^{131} treatments may be required in select patients to control or eliminate metastasis.

Prognosis

In children, 90% of the first relapse after treatment occurs within 10 years. To mention the absence of persistent disease, there should be no clinical signs and imaging findings concerning the disease, and Tg levels should be immeasurable.

Tumor stage 1 or 2, a tumor mass less than 2 cm, age older than 10 years, postoperative Tg level below 2 ng/ml, and no relapse indicate low-risk group.

Although relapse incidence is higher in children, the prognosis of differentiated tumors is better when compared to adults. General survival rate varies between 89 and 98% in children. The presence of local and distant metastasis in diagnosis and a tumor volume greater than 4 cm^3 affect the prognosis badly. Pediatric patients need to be followed up for life, including the adulthood.

References

1. Hogan AR, Zhuge Y, Perez EA, Koniaris LG, Lew JI, Sola JE (2009) Pediatric thyroid carcinoma: incidence and outcomes in 1753 patients. The Journal of Surgical Research 156 (1):167–172.
2. Golpanian S, Perez EA, Tashiro J, et al. (2016) Pediatric papillary thyroid carcinoma: outcomes and survival predictors in 2504 surgical patients. Pediatric Surgery International 32 (3):201–208.
3. Dermody S, Walls A, Harley EH (2016) Pediatric thyroid cancer: an update from the SEER database 2007-2012. International Journal of Pediatric Otorhinolaryngology 89:121–126.
4. Horner MJ, Ries LA, Krapcho M, et al. SEER Cancer Statistics Review, 1975-2006. Bethesda, MD, National Cancer Institute, 2009.
5. LaFranchi S, Ross DS, Geffner ME, Hoppin AG. Thyroid Nodules and Cancer in Children, 2019. https://www.uptodate.com/contents/thyroid-nodules-and-cancer-in-children.
6. Kirkland RT, Kirkland JL, Rosenberg HS, et al. (1973) Solitary thyroid nodules in 30 children and report of a child with a thyroid abscess. Pediatrics 51:85.
7. Hung W (1999) Solitary thyroid nodules in 93 children and adolescents. a 35-years experience. Hormone Research 52:15.
8. Niedziela M (2006) Pathogenesis, diagnosis and management of thyroid nodules in children. Endocrine-Related Cancer 13:427.
9. Francis GL, Waguespack SG, Bauer AJ, et al. (2015) Management guidelines for children with thyroid nodules and differentiated thyroid cancer. Thyroid 25 (7):716–759.
10. Rallison ML, Dobyns BM, Keating FR Jr, et al. (1975) Thyroid nodularity in children. JAMA 233:1069.
11. Kaloumenou I, Alevizaki M, Ladopoulos C, et al. (2007) Thyroid volume and echostructure in schoolchildren living in an iodine-replete area: relation to age, pubertal stage, and body mass index. Thyroid 17:875.
12. Baez JC, Zurakowski D, Vargas SO, Lee EY. Incidental thyroid nodules detected on thoracic contrast-enhanced CT in the pediatric population: prevalence and outcomes. AJR: American Journal of Roentgenology 205:W360.
13. Qian ZJ, Jin MC, Meister KD, Megwalu UC (2019) Pediatric thyroid cancer incidence and mortality trends in the United States, 1973-2013. JAMA Otolaryngology–Head & Neck Surgery 145:617.
14. dos Santos Silva I, Swerdlow AJ (1993) Thyroid cancer epidemiology in England and Wales: time trends and geographical distribution. British Journal of Cancer 67 (2):330–340.
15. Farahati J, Bucsky P, Parlowsky T, Mader U, Reiners C (1997) Characteristics of differentiated thyroid carcinoma in children and adolescents with respect to age, gender, and histology. Cancer 80 (11):2156–2162.
16. Henderson BE, Ross RK, Pike MC, Casagrande JT (1982) Endogenous hormones as a major factor in human cancer. Cancer Research 42 (8):3232–3239.
17. Davies SM. (2007) Subsequent malignant neoplasms in survivors of childhood cancer: childhood Cancer Survivor Study (CCSS) studies. Pediatric Blood & Cancer 48:727.
18. Taylor AJ, Croft AP, Palace AM, et al. (2009) Risk of thyroid cancer in survivors of childhood cancer: results from the British Childhood Cancer Survivor Study. International Journal of Cancer 125:2400.
19. Sassolas G, Hafdi-Nejjari Z, Casagranda L, et al. (2013) Thyroid cancers in children, adolescents, and young adults with and without a history of childhood exposure to therapeutic radiation for other cancers. Thyroid 23:805.
20. Imaizumi M, Ohishi W, Nakashima E, et al. (2015) Association of radiation dose with prevalence of thyroid nodules among atomic bomb survivors exposed in childhood (2007-2011). JAMA Internal Medicine 175:228.
21. Lubin JH, Adams MJ, Shore R, et al. (2017) Thyroid cancer following childhood low-dose radiation exposure: a pooled analysis of nine cohorts. The Journal of Clinical Endocrinology and Metabolism 102 (7):2575–2583.
22. Iglesias ML, Schmidt A, Ghuzlan AA, et al. (2017) Radiation exposure and thyroid cancer: a review. Archives of Endocrinology and Metabolism 61 (2):180–187.
23. Lazar L, Lebenthal Y, Steinmetz A, et al. (2009) Differentiated thyroid carcinoma in pediatric patients: comparison of presentation and course between prepubertal children and adolescents. The Journal of Pediatrics 154 (5):708–714.
24. Feng X, Milas M, O'Malley M, et al. (2015) Characteristics of benign and malignant thyroid disease in familial adenomatous polyposis patients and recommendations for disease surveillance. Thyroid 25:325.
25. Uchino S, Ishikawa H, Miyauchi A, et al. (2016) Age- and gender-specific risk of thyroid cancer in patients with familial adenomatous polyposis. The Journal of Clinical Endocrinology and Metabolism 101:4611.
26. Childhood Thyroid Cancer Treatment (PDQ®)–Health Professional Version – National Cancer Institute, 2020. https://www.cancer.gov/types/thyro_d/hp/child-thyroid-treatment-pdq.
27. Corrias A, Cassio A, Weber G, et al. (2008) Thyroid nodules and cancer in children and adolescents affected by autoimmune thyroiditis. Archives of Pediatrics and Adolescent Medicine 162:526.
28. Berker D, Isik S, Ozuguz U, et al. (2011) Prevalence of incidental thyroid cancer and its ultrasonographic features in subcentimeter thyroid nodules of patients with hyperthyroidism. Endocrine 39:13.
29. Keskin M, Savas-Erdeve S, Aycan Z (2016) Co-existence of thyroid nodule and thyroid cancer in children and adolescents with Hashimoto thyroiditis: a single-center study. Hormone Research in Paediatrics 85:181.
30. Alzahrani AS, Baitei EY, Zou M, Shi Y (2006) Clinical case seminar: metastatic follicular thyroid carcinoma arising from congenital goiter as a result of a novel splice donor site mutation in the thyroglobulin gene. The Journal of Clinical Endocrinology and Metabolism 91:740.
31. Pellegriti G, Lumera G, Malandrino P, et al. (2013) Thyroid cancer in thyroglossal duct cysts requires a specific approach due to its unpredictable extension. The Journal of Clinical Endocrinology and Metabolism 98:458.

32. Dinauer C, Francis GL (2007) Thyroid cancer in children. Endocrinology & Metabolism Clinics of North America 36 (3):779–806, vii.
33. Vasko V, Bauer AJ, Tuttle RM, et al. (2007) Papillary and follicular thyroid cancers in children. Endocrine Development 10:140–172.
34. Tallini G, Tuttle RM, Ghossein RA (2017) The history of the follicular variant of papillary thyroid carcinoma. The Journal of Clinical Endocrinology and Metabolism 102:15.
35. Vali R, Rachmiel M, Hamilton J, El Zein M, Wasserman J, Costantini DL, Charron M, Daneman A (2015) The role of ultrasound in the follow-up of children with differentiated thyroid cancer. Pediatric Radiology 45 (7):1039–1045.
36. American Thyroid Association Guidelines Task Force, Kloos RT, Eng C, et al. (2009) Medullary thyroid cancer: management guidelines of the American Thyroid Association. Thyroid 19:565.
37. Wells SA Jr, Asa SL, Dralle H, et al. (2015) Revised American Thyroid Association guidelines for the management of medullary thyroid carcinoma. Thyroid 25:567.
38. Acquaviva G, Visani M, Repaci A, et al. (2018) Molecular pathology of thyroid tumours of follicular cells: a review of genetic alterations and their clinicopathological relevance. Histopathology 72 (1):6–31.
39. Bauer AJ (2017) Molecular genetics of thyroid cancer in children and adolescents. Endocrinology & Metabolism Clinics of North America 46 (2):389–403.
40. Cancer Genome Atlas Research Network (2014) Integrated genomic characterization of papillary thyroid carcinoma. Cell 159 (3):676–690.
41. Sisdelli L, Cordioli MICV, Vaisman F, et al. (2019) AGK-BRAF is associated with distant metastasis and younger age in pediatric papillary thyroid carcinoma. Pediatric Blood & Cancer 66 (7): e27707.
42. Jarzab B, Handkiewicz-Junak D, Wloch J (2005) Juvenile differentiated thyroid carcinoma and the role of radioiodine in its treatment: a qualitative review. Endocrine-Related Cancer 12 (4):773–803.
43. Bauer AJ (2014) Thyroid nodules and differentiated thyroid cancer. Endocrine Development 26:183–201.
44. Mazzaferri EL, Kloos RT (2001) Clinical review 128: current approaches to primary therapy for papillary and follicular thyroid cancer. The Journal of Clinical Endocrinology and Metabolism 86 (4):1447–1463.
45. Newman KD, Black T, Heller G, Azizkhan RG, Holcomb GW, 3rd, Sklar C, Vlamis V, Haase GM, La Quaglia MP (1998) Differentiated thyroid cancer: determinants of disease progression in patients <21 years of age at diagnosis: a report from the Surgical Discipline Committee of the Children's Cancer Group. Annals of Surgery 227 (4):533–541.
46. Schlumberger M, De Vathaire F, Travagli JP, Vassal G, Lemerle J, Parmentier C, Tubiana M (1987) Differentiated thyroid carcinoma in childhood: long term follow-up of 72 patients. The Journal of Clinical Endocrinology and Metabolism 65 (6):1088–1094.
47. Luster M, Lassmann M, Freudenberg LS, Reiners C (2007) Thyroid cancer in childhood: management strategy, including dosimetry and long-term results. Hormones 6 (4):269–278.
48. Mitsutake N, Knauf JA, Mitsutake S, Mesa C, Jr., Zhang L, Fagin JA (2005) Conditional BRAFV600E expression induces DNA synthesis, apoptosis, dedifferentiation, and chromosomal instability in thyroid PCCL3 cells. Cancer Research 65 (6):2465–2473.
49. Cooper DS, Doherty GM, Haugen BR, et al.; American Thyroid Association Guidelines Taskforce on Thyroid Nodules and Differentiated Thyroid Cancer (2009). Revised American Thyroid Association management guidelines for patients with thyroid nodules and differentiated thyroid cancer. Thyroid 19:1167–1214.
50. Karnak I, Ardicli B, Ekinci S, et al. (2011) Papillary thyroid carcinoma does not have standard course in children. Pediatric Surgery International 27:931–936.
51. Diesen DL, Skinner MA. Endocrine disorders and tumors, in Holcomb III GW, Murphy PJ, Ostlie DJ (eds): Ashcraft's Pediatric Surgery. London, Saunders/Elsevier, 2014, pp:1067–1085.
52. Piper HG, Skinner MA. Childhood diseases of the thyroid and parathyroid glands, in Coran AG, Adzick NS, Krummel TM, Laberge J-M, Shamberger RC, Caldamone AA (eds): Pediatric Surgery. USA, Saunders/Elsevier, 2012, pp:745–752.
53. Viola D, Romei C, Elisei R (2014) Medullary thyroid carcinoma in children. Endocrine Development 26:202–213.
54. Hung W, Sarlis NJ (2002) Current controversies in the management of pediatric patients with well-differentiated nonmedullary thyroid cancer: a review. Thyroid 12:683.
55. Handkiewicz-Junak D, Wloch J, Roskosz J, et al. (2007) Total thyroidectomy and adjuvant radioiodine treatment independently decrease locoregional recurrence risk in childhood and adolescent differentiated thyroid cancer. The Journal of Nuclear Medicine 48:879.
56. Kloos RT, Duvuuri V, Jhiang SM, Cahill KV, Foster JA, Burns JA (2002) Nasolacrimal drainage system obstruction from radioactive iodine therapy for thyroid carcinoma. The Journal of Clinical Endocrinology and Metabolism 87 (12):5817–5820.
57. van Santen HM, Aronson DC, Vulsma T, Tummers RF, Geenen MM, de Vijlder JJ, van den Bos C (2004) Frequent adverse events after treatment for childhood-onset differentiated thyroid carcinoma: a single institute experience. European Journal of Cancer 40 (11):1743–1751.

21

THYROID SURGERY IN SOUTH ASIA

Anand Kumar Mishra, Amit Agarwal, Rajeev Parameswaran, Soe Tin, Ranil Fernando, Khalid Alhajri, Ali Korairi, Marya Al Suhaibani and Özer Makay

Introduction

The extirpation of the thyroid gland for goiter typifies, perhaps, better than any operation the supreme triumph of the surgeon's art.

Halsted

Thyroid surgery has evolved from 40% mortality in middle of the 19th century to Theodore Kocher era when it decreased to less than 2%. Kocher propagated total thyroidectomy (TT) operation by but later on himself did not favored till there was understanding of thyroid physiology. After his era, subtotal thyroidectomy (STT) became more popular and procedure of choice for both benign and malignant disease. After the 1970s with marked improvements in understanding of thyroid pathophysiology and thyroid cancer (TC), there was shift from STT to TT. Simultaneously in next two decades, there was immense information in the field epidemiology of the disease, new developments in imaging, diagnostic techniques, which led to identification of more new thyroid nodules and TC in the population. Thyroid surgery that was rare and surgeons used to avoid because of complication now became common and there is recognition of specialist thyroid surgeons. There were four developments in the field of thyroid surgery in last five decades:

1. Epidemiological research suggested a global rise in TC incidence over the last few decades. High-resolution ultrasound availability helped in more identification and better characterization of the thyroid nodule.
2. TT became the preferred surgery.
3. Development of various surgical adjuncts which improved the overall safety and quality in thyroid surgery.
4. Development of endoscopy and robot-assisted thyroidectomy and growing patient interest in remote access thyroidectomy that eliminate anterior neck incision.

Thyroid cancer in South Asia

Epidemiological research suggests also rise in TC incidence over the last few decades in South Asian countries. South Korea database between 1999 and 2010 demonstrated an annual increase of 24.2% for TC alone (1), but it may be attributed to their aggressive national cancer screening program launched since 1999. It includes routine sonography of thyroid and positron emission tomography (PET) use as a cancer screening tool whenever needed (2). Age-standardized overall TC incidence rate was 4.2 cases per 100,000 men and 11.2 cases per 100,000 in Japan Cancer Surveillance Research Group data from 32 of 37 population-based cancer registries 2009 (3). There was a 30-fold higher TC incidence rate among populations exposed to radiation by the Fukushima plant (4). In Shanghai, China TC incidence tripled between 1983 and 2007 from 2.6 cases per 100,000 women to 11.6 cases per 100,000 women (5).

In South Indian cancer registry data of 2012–2014, TC was the most common cancer in women below the age of 40 years with linear rise in incidence from childhood to 40 years and then remained stable until 75 years (6). A retrospective study from Karachi, Pakistan reported that women (82.4%) are most commonly affected with TC with papillary histology being the most common (90.2%) (7). As the incidence is increasing in these Asian countries, the rate of thyroidectomy is also increasing.

Total thyroidectomy as preferred operation

TT eliminates all abnormal tissues to have zero recurrence rate in benign conditions. Only concern with this surgical procedure is the complication rate. And there is plenty of evidence that if TT is performed by skilled experienced surgeons, the complications rate is minimal (8, 9).

In modern day, outpatient thyroidectomy is practiced to decrease the cost of hospitalization, and it is a well-accepted procedure in appropriately selected patients using an optimized and systematic protocol. In present era, there is no concern for mortality, but all the developments are directed toward decreasing the morbidity and improve quality of life. Excellent surgeons have developed alternative access for thyroidectomy and even avoiding incision in the neck. Patients are liking this access. Modern thyroid surgery is utilizing many surgical adjuncts like electrothermal bipolar vessel sealing system along with conventional electrocautery, intraoperative nerve monitoring, assay of parathyroid hormone for predicting patients' risk of postoperative hypocalcemia. Novel minimally invasive approaches are now being offered in larger nodules. Excellent postoperative cosmesis and voice outcomes have been reported in robotic thyroidectomy. In fact, all remote access thyroidectomy techniques originated in South Asian countries, South Korea and Japan, and then they became popular in other continents. Hypocalcemia and recurrent laryngeal nerve injury are the two most dreaded complications. Morbidity in thyroid surgery is a surrogate marker of quality and safety of thyroid surgery. This will depend upon the surgeon's experience. There has been discussion on low- and high-volume thyroid surgeons regarding the safety of thyroid surgery; however, still there is no consensus on the numbers. However, everybody agrees on the concept that there has to be a minimum number of annual volumes of thyroid surgery. Surgeon should know and review his own outcomes and accordingly enhance the skills. In South Asia, there are many middle- and low-income countries, from where surgeons don't publish the morbidity data. In many South Asian countries, heath-care facilities are heterogenous. There are hospitals with world class facilities, and nearby there may be very primitive facilities. And this leads to differences in thyroid surgery outcomes in same country. In this chapter, authors from various South Asian countries will share the thyroid countries surgery experience.

Thyroid surgery in India

Thyroid surgery in India has undergone a paradigm shift in last three decades. In the last century, thyroid surgery was being performed largely by general surgeons in various medical schools of the country (>150). However, the concept of recurrent laryngeal nerve (RLN) visualization and parathyroid preservation was still unknown, and STT was the standard procedure, even in the expert hands. In the last decade of the previous century, new centers of superspecialities came up which propagated and popularized TT with emphasis on RLN and parathyroid visualization and preservation. These centers also adopted modern tools for thyroid surgery, such as neuromonitoring, energy devices for hemostasis and robotic assistance.

Goiter presents a special challenge to the endocrine/thyroid surgeon in India because of several factors. First, India has been traditionally an iodine-deficient endemic goiter belt, especially the foothills of Himalayas in the Northern part, which results in patients coming with huge goiters of long-standing duration. Understandably, surgery of large goiters is fraught with increased risk of complications like difficulty intubation, intraoperative bleeding, post-thyroidectomy tracheomalacia and profound hypocalcemia, and hence, neither the general surgeon nor the patients themselves were too keen for operation! Second, because of long-standing duration, substantial number of multinodular goiters would turn out to be harboring malignancy, and since there were never enough number of nuclear medicine centers that could offer RAI therapy, treatment of TC was suboptimal. As far as TCs are concerned, due to iodine deficiency, there was a higher incidence of FTC, and that too advanced FTC, which again presented a special challenge to the surgeons dealing with thyroid surgery.

In the last three decades, few centers of excellence in the field of endocrine/thyroid surgery have come up around different parts of the country, including various tertiary care cancer centers that offer state-of-the-art thyroid surgery with minimal complications comparable to Western figures. Not only in-patient care, these centers have become apex centers for training and teaching in the field of endocrine/thyroid surgery and are producing future/modern thyroid surgeons. Patients of TC are now being offered world class care including access to modern diagnostic tools, TT, central compartment and lateral neck dissection and minimally invasive and robotic thyroid surgery. There is now robust interaction with global leaders in the field of thyroid surgery with profound exchange of ideas leading to further standardization of surgical management of thyroid diseases especially TC. One discordant note in the harmonious development of thyroid surgery could be the potential turf war between the various care givers. The development of thyroid surgery has fuelled the long-standing dilemma as to 'Who should be operating on thyroids?'. The various stakeholders could be the Endocrine Surgeon/Thyroid Surgeon/Surgical Oncologist/Head and Neck Surgeon/ENT surgeon or the general surgeon. There is no easy answer to this dilemma. Nonetheless, perhaps anybody who has an adequate formal training in thyroid surgery, including training about the decision-making in all aspects of thyroid diseases like counseling, surgical extent of surgery, postoperative care, decisions about use of adjuvant therapy and long-term follow-up, should be allowed to deal with care of thyroid diseases.

Thyroid cancer in Singapore

The incidence of TC is rising globally (10, 11) and so is the case with Singapore (12). TC accounts for less than 1% of all cancers and is the most common endocrine malignancy. The incidence of TC is estimated to be around 0.5 to 10 per 100,000 population in the United States. In Singapore, based on the National Cancer Registry, TC is the 8th most common cancer in women and 15th most common cancer in men (13). The annual incidence reported in Singapore is about 1100 cases per year, and papillary TC accounts for most of these. The first reported study from Singapore on the incidence of TC between the years 1968 and 1977 was in 1982 (14).

Like anywhere else in the world, TC in Singapore is about three times more commonly seen in women than men (12). The reasons for such an increase in women are unknown but may correlate with the higher incidence of thyroid nodules in women. The age-standardized incidence rate (ASR) for the population increased by 224% (from 2.5/100,000 in 1974 to 5.6/100,000 in 2013). The increased incidence of TC in women was by 227% (from 3.7/100,000 in 1974 compared with 8.4/100,000 in 2013) and 180% in men (.5/100,000 in 1974 compared with 2.7/100,000 in 2013). The median age of diagnosis decreased from 64.5 years to 52 years for men, with slight increase for women from 46 to 51 years over a period of 40 years. The rising incidence of TC is higher in Malays compared to Chinese and Indians.

The histological distribution of the TCs in Singapore is as follows: 75% papillary, 17% follicular, 2% medullary, 1% anaplastic and 5% others (lymphoma and metastasis). Unlike papillary TC, the incidence of other cancers showed no change in incidence over the last four decades. Small TCs formed the higher proportion of the cases and micropapillary TC accounted for about 40% of these. While most of the increase in the incidence of TC around the world is from micropapillary TCs, in Singapore, the incidence of these lesions appeared to be the same over the last few decades, suggesting that there has been a rise in the incidence of the larger cancers as well (12). On a molecular level, there appears to be variation in BRAF mutations in PTC in Singapore (15). The prevalence varies with regions ranging from 30% to 50% in United States and Europe (16–18), 50–60% in Middle East (19) and over 60% in countries such as Japan and South Korea (20–22). In Singapore, the prevalence of BRAF mutation has been shown to be over 50% and BRAF mutation-positive tumors were associated with locally advanced disease but not poorer survival (15).

Nearly 95% of TC cases diagnosed underwent surgery with TT, and about 4% chose not to have any intervention despite best medical advice (12). About a third of patients with papillary TC present with nodal metastasis requiring nodal surgery and subsequent radioiodine ablation. Distant metastasis has been reported in 5% of PTC and 20% of patients with follicular TC, unlike other countries in Southeast Asia where higher proportions of patients present with advanced disease (23). This difference could possibly be due to the advanced health care and early detection of TCs either by screening or incidentally detected following other modalities of imaging (24). Most patients opt for TT with a diagnosis of PTC even in low risk and small TCs, despite the recommendations from ATA that hemithyroidectomy may be sufficient in such cases. In locally advanced cases, about 4% received palliative radiotherapy and 1% received chemotherapy. Despite the rise in incidence over the last four decades, the TC-specific mortality has remained at 2%.

In conclusion, Singapore has seen a rising incidence of TC, mainly small papillary TCs and the rise is more in women and Malays. About half of the papillary TCs show a BRAF mutation but locally advanced and distant metastasis is less common, possibly due to early detection. The mortality from TC is low and similar to other developed nations.

Thyroid Surgery in South Asia

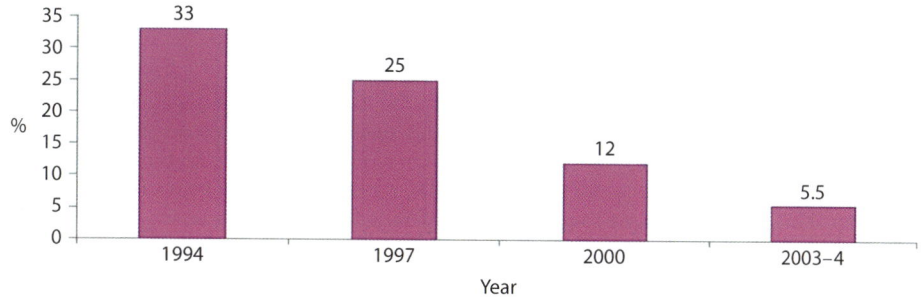

FIGURE 21.1 The national visible goiter rate in children 6–11 years in Myanmar.

Thyroid surgery in Myanmar

Epidemiology: Diseases of thyroid gland and thyroid swellings are very common in Myanmar. The goiters are more common in iodine-deficient endemic areas, especially in hilly areas such as Chin, Kachin and Shan states where iodine contents in the water is very low according to a study. There was a very high incidence of goiter in the hilly areas. The crude rate in the Chin Hills was 93.4% in males (411 of 440 examined) and 96.6% in females (255 of 264 examined). Levels in excess of 50% in males and 60% in females were found in the other areas. Though the incidence of goiter was as high in the Ywagone area, the size of the goiters was smaller, mainly Grade 1. The iodine content of the water was low in all areas, 0–1.43 µg/L in the Chin Hills, but was also extremely low in Yangon itself (0–2 µg/L). Urinary iodine excretion tests were not carried out in the Chin Hills but were moderately low in Ywagone and very low in Kayah, where one-third of the population excreted less than 25 µg/g creatinine. Low land areas of Myanmar like in Yangon division, Irrewaddy division and some other areas are regarded as sporadic goitrous areas. In other words, in Myanmar, most of the high lands are endemic goitrous areas, and most of other low land areas are sporadic goitrous areas.

Another recent study by Myanmar Micronutrient and Food Consumption Survey (MMFCS), National Nutrition Centre, Department of Public Health, Ministry of Health and Sports showed (Report on 6 Feb. 2019) that the visible thyroid swelling rate in children of 6–11 years before the National Iodized Salt Program in 1994 is 33%. In the same age group in 2003–2004 after the National Iodized Salt Program, the visible thyroid swelling rate was found to be only 5.5%, proving the efficacy of iodized salt program in the diet (Figure 21.1 and 21.2). Because of the National Iodized Salt Program, the pattern of goiter prevalence areas in the divisional regions changed a lot. Please see the map of goiter prevalence areas.

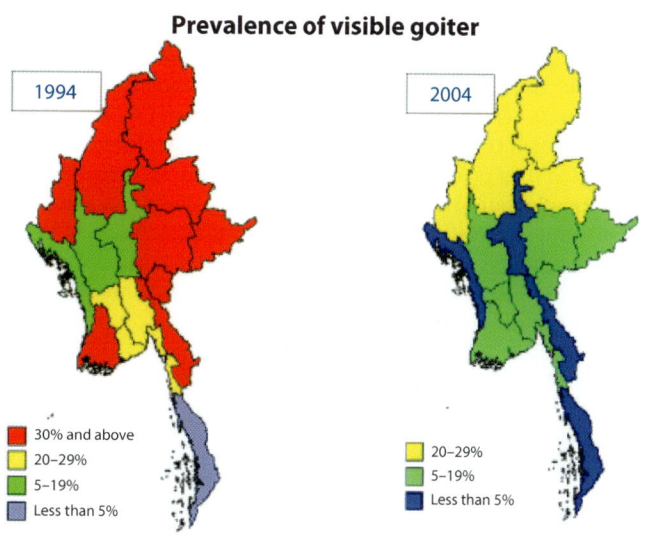

FIGURE 21.2 Prevalence of visible goiter.

Although the National Iodized Salt Program can reduce the visible goiter rates in Myanmar, the older population of above 40 years is still high as evidenced by the report by Victoria Innovative Pathological Lab. It is reported highest incidences of thyroid nodules are seen in the 40 and above age groups (Table 21.1). It means we are still dealing with the goiter endemic age, and the adult rate is still the same as pre-iodized period in Myanmar.

Many research papers from Myanmar Medical Research Department showed hypothyroidism in most of neonates in endemic areas in Myanmar. Rates of hyperthyroidism in adult population in endemic areas were high according to the studies in two high endemic and sporadic areas in Myanmar (25).

TABLE 21.1: Thyroid Cases among Age Groups at Innovative Diagnostics (Jan to Dec, 2018)

	<20 years	20–40 years	>40–60 years	>60 years	Total
MNG/Nodular goiter	2	65	144	56	267
Thyroiditis	–	25	19	9	53
Normal	–	–	1	3	4
Thyroid cyst	1	17	35	17	70
Follicular adenoma	–	25	30	11	66
Follicular carcinoma	–	3	3	6	12
Papilloma	–	1	–	1	2
Papillary carcinoma	3	13	8	9	33
Medullary carcinoma	–	1	1	2	4

Prevalence of thyroid neoplasm in Myanmar: As Myanmar is still an endemic area, the rate of thyroid neoplasm is found to be more than in Western non-endemic areas according to many reports in Myanmar (26). Incidence of differentiated TC pattern is like other countries of this region. Variation is noticed among gender, age groups and race or ethnicity. Higher rate of TC is observed in females in between 21 and 60 years. Papillary thyroid carcinoma is the more common histological type. At Yangon ORL HNS specialist hospital, overall malignant cases rate of 12% has been observed among thyroid nodules with papillary carcinoma being the commonest. In the author's series, the malignancy rate is 14 %. The overall rate of TC ranges from 12% to 34.1% among Goiters in Endemic areas of Myanmar (26).

Management: All the patients are evaluated by the standard triple test. We follow Bethesda classification of reporting of FNAC. In Myanmar, calcitonin and BRAF (V600E) studies are available but difficult and expansive as we have to send abroad. Lobectomy is the preferred choice for single-lobe lesion and TT for bilateral cases. And intraoperatively if solitary nodule has extracapsular extension then plan changes to TT. In Myanmar, recurrent nodule and completion thyroidectomies are not accepted by the patients. Therefore, we usually do TT with nerve stimulator to avoid these factors with special care for complications. Standard protocols as suggested by various guidelines are followed in Myanmar.

Thyroid surgery in Sri Lanka

Introduction

Sri Lanka has a long-standing historically documented medical practice. There have been ancient hospital sites in the towns of Anuradhapura, Polonnaruwa, Mihintale and Medirigiriya. These are believed to date back to the 9th century A.D. They were centers for the practice of ayurvedic system of medicine. It is of interest to note that thyroid disease was not recognized as problem till the late British period. It was Bennet, a British civil servant, who first described goiter in the coastal areas of Sri Lanka in 1849 (27). Goiter was considered a health problem in Sri Lanka (Ceylon) by the World Health Organization only in 1949, following the observations of Mahadeva et al. (28). However, there is no clear record of the origins of thyroid surgery in Sri Lanka. It is likely that it started in the 1950s or 1960s. By the 1970s, it was a well-established surgical procedure in Sri Lanka.

The modern era

Thyroid surgery is one of the common general surgical procedures undertaken in Sri Lanka now. It is performed mostly by general surgeons, and some ENT surgeons both in government hospitals and in the private sector hospitals.

In keeping with the world trends, the commonest surgical procedures of the thyroid undertaken in the early years (1960s–2000) were partial, subtotal or hemithyroidectomy (lobectomy). TT was performed for malignancies, especially at the national cancer institute Maharagama. This trend continued till around 2005. The concept of TT for benign disease was first introduced in 2005 (29).

Currently many surgeons would undertake TT for differentiated cancer of the thyroid and would consider undertaking TT even for benign disease. In a survey of surgeons (N-33) undertaken in 2008, 52% surgeons performed STT for multinodular goiter, 35% performed TT and 13% near TT. For toxic multinodular goiters, the figures were 42%, 35% and 22%. For Graves' disease, the figures were 35%, 35% and 13%, and 17% did not offer surgery. These figures are not very different to the figures in the literature of that era (30).

In a follow-up survey done in 2019, there was a significant change in the trends. Benign goiter was offered TT by 97% of the surgeons. Most surgeons undertake TT for benign disease now with acceptable complication rates. Surgeons who undertake thyroidectomy would perform a reasonable amount of operations; the range is 30–200 a year.

The tradition of using drains routinely in thyroid surgery is losing ground rapidly. Surgeons are happy to refrain from using drains in some thyroidectomies. Most surgeons are aware of the recent trends such as capsular dissection, nerve encountering technique, parathyroid identification, preservation and autotransplantation. These trends are being incorporated into practice. In terms of node dissection for cancer, some surgeons are comfortable with modified radical neck dissection (MRND) and practice it. There is no uniformity about the practice of central node dissection. These trends are practiced regularly at the National Cancer Institute.

Neuromonitoring is not available in Sri Lanka and is not used at present. Visual identification of nerves carefully and the use of optical loupes has kept the complication rates at a very low level. Hypocalcaemia though more prevalent is mostly of transient nature according to the data available. The reported complication rates are comparable with figures in the literature.

There was one report of an endoscopic thyroidectomy undertaken by and ENT surgeon, but the trend of endoscopic or robotic thyroidectomy has not been incorporated into the practice thyroid surgery in Sri Lanka. There are many reasons for this including the doubts about the need for these procedures and the doubts about the cost effectiveness.

Training in thyroid surgery in Sri Lanka

In the bygone era, trainees learned the technique of thyroidectomy by the apprenticeship method prevalent at that time. It was part of general surgical training. In an around 2011/2012, the board of study in surgery, Postgraduate Institute of Medicine (B.O.S. PGIM), the only postgraduate surgical educational portal of the country, introduced reforms and surgical trainees had to select a special area of interest for advanced surgical training.

The selection of an area of interest is done after completing a 38-month rigorous training stint in all aspects of surgery and passing the mid-level examination called MD surgery. One of the special areas of interest identified is endocrine surgery and the trainees will spend 3 years gaining experience in units with special interest in endocrine surgery. One year of this training is a mandatory period of training in an overseas center to broaden the experience and exposure. This gives a sound training, especially in thyroid surgery as thyroidectomy remains the main endocrine surgical procedure performed all over the world. The first surgeon with special training in endocrine surgery is practicing Sri Lanka now and two more surgeons are receiving training. This augurs well for the future.

Thyroid cancer in Saudi Arabia

Prevalence and risk factors

TC is one of the fast-growing cancers worldwide (31). TC in Saudi Arabia (SA) developed warning increase in its occurrence especially in the last decades. A report from big referral center in the capital city of SA showed the upsurge of TC incidence from 122 to 430 cases in two times period (1975–1980, 1986–1989), respectively (32). Furthermore, the annual referral rate of TC to this center is steadily increasing through 2000–2010 (33). The raising is still noticed in TC development as Saudi Cancer Registry graded it as the third common cancer in 2010 after breast and colorectal cancer (34). In King Faisal Specialist Hospital and research Center (KFSH&RC) in SA, TC was accounted for 8.8% of all cancer cases in 2010 (33). Recent data presented the incidence of TC changed from 1.6 cases per 100,000 in 2000 to 3.4 cases per 100,000 in 2017 (35). Similar to other areas in the world, TC showed female predominance in SA with male-to-female ratio of 28:100 during period of 2000–2010 (33) and 3:1 during period of 1998–2016 (36). Young age group showed the highest incidence rate in different studies with median age of 38 (33), 39 (36) and 45 (35) years old. Interestingly, TC in childhood contributed to 4.7% of all age group during 10 years period of observation (37). In addition to age and gender, multiple risk factors identified leading to TC development in SA: iodine deficiency (38) especially in mountain area (southern region of SA). Study done in southern region showed that the incidence of malignancy among all patients underwent thyroidectomy is 14% in 6 years period of time (39). Najran, which also found in the southern region, found to have the highest incidence in TC compared to other SA regions in period between 2001 and 2013 (40). Family history of thyroid diseases (41) also considered a strong risk factor for TC development. Obesity which itself showed increase in prevalence (42) may reflect increase in TC occurrence. Exposure to radiation in the war past decades is considered one of the risk factors for TC in SA according to Saudi Cancer Registry, especially in eastern region.

Symptoms

Study done in western region of SA showed that all patients with TC included in the study presented with neck mass (43). More than half of the TC patients found to have normal thyroid level in data derived from central area of SA from 2012 to 2016 (44). Hyperthyroidism was found among 70% of TC patient in a retrospective report from a university clinic, and most of the patient manifested with palpitation or tremor (45). Among pediatric age group, 26% the patients with PT complain of pressure symptoms during 10 years study period in Riyadh city, SA (47).

Types and grade

Similar to the rest of the world, papillary TC found to be the most frequent type in SA. Among 600 cases of TC during the period of 2004–2005, 77% were of classical papillary type and 17.3% with others subtypes of papillary TC such as T-cell and follicular variant (46). A report from rural central area of SA during 2012–2016 showed that papillary TC diagnosed in more than half of the patients with TC followed by follicular type (44). Anaplastic, medullary types and lymphoma found in 1.7%, 1.2% and 2% among TC patients, respectively, during 18 years study period in western region of SA (45). Most of the TC patients in SA presented in early stages which may be explained by availability of health facilities in the country. A big referral hospital in central area of SA reported that during 2000–2010, 48% of the patient presented in localized stage with no lymphatic invasion or extrathyroidal tissue extension (43). During the period of 2004–2005, study included 600 patients diagnosed with TC showed that only 13.3% of the patients had distant metastasis and 69.4% staged as stage I according to TNM classification (46). Twenty patients out of 100 TC patients had lymph node involvement at time of operation reported from eastern region in SA (43). Another report among pediatric patients with TC showed 26.1% extrathyroidal extension (47).

Management and prognosis

A retrospective review of 10 years surgical practice among TC patients showed that 60% received combination of surgery, radiation and hormonal therapy and 0.8% received only radiotherapy with no surgical intervention (33). A total of 3.3% of reported cases died due to TC in a large report from central area of SA compared to 53.3% with excellent response (36). The prognosis also is promising in pediatric age group as only one child had recurrence postsurgical management in a study conducted among 23 pediatric patients with TC in university hospital in SA (37).

Thyroid surgery practice in Turkey

Turkey, situated in the most western part of Asia, also known as 'Asia Minor', has more than 82 million inhabitants (46). The geographical pattern of the country may show enormous differences from region to region, which may reflect on cultural habits. Since the last two decades, Turkey has mostly solved the problem regarding iodine deficiency. The legal iodination of table salts has a major impact on this. According to cancer statistics, the rise of TC is the one that has the steepest ascent and has positioned as the second most common cancer in the female population (47, 48). Incidentally, compared to other countries in Asia, Turkey is one of the countries with the highest age-standardized rate (49).

The sum of general surgeons in Turkey reaches 3900. Nearly all of them are a member of the Turkish Society of Surgery. This is the main roof for general surgeons. The number of hospitals is 1536 in total. Nearly a thousand are state hospitals and less than a hundred are university hospitals. This reflects also on the number of surgeries, where state hospitals are the centers that carries out the highest number of surgeries in total (50). Practice of thyroid surgery is taken care of by general surgeons and otolaryngologists. The difference between general surgeons and otolaryngologists is that thyroid surgery is in the routine practice in every educational setting, besides being in the curriculum. Turkish Association of Endocrine Surgery is the body of endocrine surgeons that forms under the roof of the Turkish Society of Surgery. This society has more than 300 members and acts actively on the scientific and educational platform (51–53). Next year, in 2021, the society will organize its 10th National Congress, with international participation. Besides, very recently it has published a report consisting Covid-19 recommendations of the society for endocrine surgery patients (54). According to our previous report, a search of Turkish general surgery clinics revealed 497 international publications, between 1976 and 2012. The rates of thyroid, parathyroid, adrenal tissue and neuroendocrine tumors related publications were 69%, 10%, 15% and 6%, respectively. The contribution of Turkish general surgeons to world science is apparent when evaluated in terms of publications related to endocrine surgery. Particularly, since 2002, with the increase in the number of publications in the field of endocrine surgery, there has been an increase in Turkey's importance on the international platform (55).

According to the statistics of the national health care system, yearly nearly 60,000 thyroidectomies are performed in Turkey. About 75% of these cases are covered by the national care system. The remaining ones are those cases operated in a private setting. In the year 2015, we had carried out a national survey wondering the perspective of endocrine surgery practice in Turkey. The distribution of surgeons according 'region' was homogeneous. Nearly 50% of surgeons responded that they performed 10–50 thyroidectomies a year. Central neck dissection and/or lateral neck dissection rates were less than five in more than 60% of the surgeons. The rate of endocrine surgery in their daily surgical practice was reported between 1 and 24% in nearly 70% of general surgeons.

Technical advances have been integrated in surgical practice in Turkey, also for thyroid surgery. The use of energy based devices is a standard in the operating room nationwide. Intraoperative nerve monitoring is used increasingly but still has not reached the high rates of Germany, where nerve monitoring is used in more than 90% of cases. Nerve monitoring has to be counted into the standards of modern thyroid surgery. Problems regarding the reimbursement of the process have to be solved on the national platform. Scientific forensic reports on Turkish national level point out the importance of the use of nerve monitoring during thyroid surgery (56). The transoral endoscopic thyroidectomy program has started in 2017 and recently has reached more than 300 cases in experienced centers. We also have created educational platforms for innovative approaches on the national and international level. Robotic surgery is carried out as well in some centers. Turkey owns nearly 40 robotic surgical units. A few of these have been used also for practice in thyroid surgery.

Other Asian countries

An et al. in a study from Korea on trends of use of robot in different diseases in their country concluded that robotic surgery got popularized only in in thyroid diseases in last 10 years (57). Altaf et al. in a study on thyroid surgery from a tertiary care center in Pakistan in a retrospective review concluded that better understanding of thyroid techniques and use of newer surgical adjuncts have helped in decreasing the complication rate at their center (58). Han et al. from China stressed on TT as the minimal surgery in all TC of size larger than 1 cm (59). Li et al. reported the increasing trend of TC in East Asian countries (60).

Conclusion

Safe thyroid surgery is a surgical art, which can be practiced and reproduced with proper training. Modern-day adjuncts definitely help not only in reducing the operation time but also in safe thyroid surgery. The above chapter is a monograph from authors on thyroid surgery who are well known experts in field of thyroid surgery in their country.

References

1. Jung K-W, et al. Cancer statistics in Korea: incidence, mortality, survival, and prevalence in 2012. Cancer Res Treat. 2015;47:127–141.
2. Lee JW, et al. Cancer screening using 18F-FDG PET/CT in Korean asymptomatic volunteers: a preliminary report. Ann Nucl Med. 2009;23:685–691.
3. Hori M, et al. Cancer incidence and incidence rates in Japan in 2009: a study of 32 population-based cancer registries for the monitoring of cancer incidence in Japan (MCIJ) project. Jpn J Clin Oncol. 2015;45:884–891.
4. Tsuda T, Tokinobu A, Yamamoto E, Suzuki E. Thyroid cancer detection by ultrasound among residents ages 18 years and younger in Fukushima, Japan: 2011 to 2014. Epidemiology. 2016;27:316–322.
5. Wang Y, Wang W. Increasing incidence of thyroid cancer in Shanghai, China, 1983–2007. Asia Pac J Public Health. 2015;27:NP223–NP229.
6. Jagathnath Krishna KM, Sebastian P. Cancer incidence and mortality: district cancer registry, Trivandrum, South India. Asian Pac J Cancer Prev. 2017;18:1485–1491.
7. Bukhari U, Sadiq S, Memon J, Baig F. Thyroid carcinoma in Pakistan: a retrospective review of 998 cases from an academic referral center. Hematol Oncol Stem Cell Ther. 2009;2:345–348.
8. Delbridge L, Guinea AI, Reeve TS. Total thyroidectomy for bilateral benign multinodular goiter: effect of changing practice. Arch Surg. 1999;134(12):1389–1393.
9. Delbridge L. Total thyroidectomy: the evolution of surgical technique. ANZ J Surg. 2003 Sep;73(9):761–768. PMID: 12956795.
10. Cramer JD, Fu P, Harth KC, Margevicius S, Wilhelm SM. Analysis of the rising incidence of thyroid cancer using the Surveillance, Epidemiology and End Results national cancer data registry. Surgery. 2010;148(6):1147–1153.
11. Kitahara CM, Sosa JA. The changing incidence of thyroid cancer. Nat Rev Endocrinol. 2016;12(11):646–653.
12. Shulin JH, Aizhen J, Kuo SM, Tan WB, Ngiam KY, Parameswaran R. Rising incidence of thyroid cancer in Singapore not solely due to micropapillary subtype. Ann Royal Coll Surg Engl. 2018;100(4):295–300.
13. Office NRoD. Singapore Cancer Registry Annual Registry Report 2015. Health Promotion Board Singapore; 2017.
14. Lee Y-S. Thyroid cancers in Singapore 1968-77. Trop Geograph Med. 1982;34(4):303–308.
15. Goh X, Lum J, Yang SP, Chionh SB, Koay E, Chiu L, et al. BRAF mutation in papillary thyroid cancer—prevalence and clinical correlation in a South-East Asian cohort. Clin Otolaryngol. 2019;44(2):114–123.
16. Xing M, Westra WH, Tufano RP, Cohen Y, Rosenbaum E, Rhoden KJ, et al. BRAF mutation predicts a poorer clinical prognosis for papillary thyroid cancer. J Clin Endocrinol Metab. 2005;90(12):6373–6379.
17. Kebebew E, Weng J, Bauer J, Ranvier G, Clark OH, Duh Q-Y, et al. The prevalence and prognostic value of BRAF mutation in thyroid cancer. Ann Surg. 2007;246(3):466.
18. Fugazzola L, Mannavola D, Cirello V, Vannucchi G, Muzza M, Vicentini L, et al. BRAF mutations in an Italian cohort of thyroid cancers. Clin Endocrinol. 2004;61(2):239–243.
19. Abubaker J, Jehan Z, Bavi P, Sultana M, Al-Harbi S, Ibrahim M, et al. Clinicopathological analysis of papillary thyroid cancer with PIK3CA alterations in a Middle Eastern population. J Clin Endocrinol Metabol. 2008;93(2):611–618.
20. Kim SK, Woo J-W, Lee JH, Park I, Choe J-H, Kim J-H, et al. Role of BRAF V600E mutation as an indicator of the extent of thyroidectomy and lymph node dissection in conventional papillary thyroid carcinoma. Surgery. 2015;158(6):1500–1511.
21. Kim TY, Kim WB, Song JY, Rhee YS, Gong G, Cho YM, et al. The BRAFV600E mutation is not associated with poor prognostic factors in Korean patients with conventional papillary thyroid microcarcinoma. Clin Endocrinol. 2005;63(5):588–593.
22. Ito Y, Yoshida H, Maruo R, Morita S, Takano T, Hirokawa M, et al. BRAF mutation in papillary thyroid carcinoma in a Japanese population: its lack of correlation with high-risk clinicopathological features and disease-free survival of patients. Endocrine J. 2009;56(1):89–97.
23. Lo TEN, Uy AT, Maningat PDD. Well-differentiated thyroid cancer: the Philippine General Hospital experience. Endocrinol Metabol. 2016;31(1):72–79.
24. Morris LGT, Sikora AG, Tosteson TD, Davies L. The Increasing Incidence of Thyroid Cancer: The Influence of Access to Care. Thyroid (New York, NY). 2013;23(7):885–891.
25. Yee AA, Oo KM, Swe SM, Win YY, Maw AA. Comparison of thyroid hormones profiles in people residing in Yangon and Muse. Myanmar Health Research Congress. 2011; p. 18–19.
26. Htwe TT. Thyroid malignancy among goitrous thyroid lesions: a review of hospital-based studies in Malaysia and Myanmar. Singapore Med J. 2012;53(3):159–163.
27. Bennet M - Ceylon and it's Capabilities. London WM H. Allen AND CO., 7 Leadenhall Street 1849- National Archives of Sri Lanka.
28. Mahadeva K, Shanmuganathan ss. Problem of goitre in Sri Lanka. Br J Nutr. 1967;21(2):341–352.
29. Siriwardana PN, Fernando R. Total thyroidectomy in benign disease of the thyroid. Ceylon Med J. 2005; 50(Supplement 1):56 http://repository.kln.ac.lk/handle/123456789/9947
30. Pinto MDP, Sandhakumari GS, Nimeshi WA, Fernando R. overview of current trends in thyroid surgery in Sri Lanka. Abstracts annual sessions college of surgeons of Sri Lanka August 2019.
31. Siegel RL, Miller KD, Jemal A. Cancer statistics, 2016. CA: Cancer J Clin. 2016;66(1):7–30.
32. Ahmed M, Al Saihati B, Greer W, et al. A study of 875 cases of thyroid cancer observed over a 15-year period (1975-1989) at the King Faisal Specialist Hospital and Research Centre. Ann Saudi Med 1995;15:579–584.
33. Hussain F, Iqbal S, Mehmood A, Bazarbashi S, ElHassan T, Chaudhri N. Incidence of thyroid cancer in the Kingdom of Saudi Arabia, 2000–2010. Hematol/Oncol Stem Cell Ther. 2013 Jun;6(2):58–64.
34. Alhozali A, Al-Ghamdi A, Alahmad J. Pattern of thyroid cancer at King Abdulaziz University Hospital, Jeddah: a 10-year retrospective study. Open J Endocrine Metabol Dis. 2016;6:121–125.
35. Aljabri KS, Bokhari SA, Al Shareef MA, Khan PM. An 18-year study of thyroid carcinoma in the western region of Saudi Arabia: a retrospective single-center study in a community hospital. Ann Saudi Med. 2018 Sep;38(5):336–343.
36. Alzahrani AS, Alomar H, Alzahrani N. Thyroid cancer in Saudi Arabia: a histopathological and outcome study. Int J Endocrinol. 2017.
37. Alsaif AA. Differentiated thyroid carcinoma in paediatric and adolescent age group: 10-year experience in a university hospital in Saudi Arabia. J Health Specialties. 2015 Jul;3(3):179.
38. Al-Nuaim AR, Al-Mazrou Y, Kamel M, Al-Attas O, Al-Daghari N, Sulimani R. Iodine deficiency in Saudi Arabia. Ann Saudi Med. 1997;17(3):293–297.
39. Banzal S, Singhai A, Shekhawat B, Raman PG. Pattern of thyroid carcinoma in Gizan region of Saudi Arabia. Thyroid Res Pract. 2014 Sep;11(3):108.
40. Alshehri B. Descriptive epidemiological analysis of thyroid cancer in the Saudi population (2001-2013). Asian Pac J Cancer Prev. 2017;18(5):1445.
41. Schulten HJ, Salama S, Al-Mansouri Z, et al. BRAF mutations in thyroid tumors from an ethnically diverse group. Hered Cancer Clin Pract. 2012;10(1):10.
42. Aljabri K, Bokhari S. High prevalence of obesity in a Saudi community. J Obes Manage. 2014;1:1–10.

43. Al-Amri AM. Pattern of thyroid cancer in the eastern province of Saudi Arabia: university hospital experience. J Cancer Ther. 2012 Jun;3(03):187.
44. Aljarbou A, Morgan A, Alshaalan F, Alshehri D, Alshathri M, Alsayyali K. The patterns of surgically treated thyroid disease in central rural region of Saudi Arabia. Egypt J Hosp Med. 2018 Jan 70;(6):1066–1071.
45. Abdelrazik M, Okash WA, Rahman A, Alenazi M, Alanazi FS, Alanzi AA. Pattern of thyroid disease in Alkharj Province, Saudi Arabia. Int J Adv Res. 2017;5(1):2986–2998.
46. https://www.tuik.gov.tr
47. https://hsgm.saglik.gov.tr/depo/birimler/kanser-db/istatistik/2009kanseraporu-1.pdf
48. www.globocan.iarc.fr
49. www.ci5.iarc.fr
50. www.rapor.saglik.gov.tr
51. www.endokrincerrahisi.org
52. Makay Ö, Özdemir M, Şenyürek YG, Tunca F, Düren M, Uludağ M, et al. Surgical approaches for papillary microcarcinomas: Turkey's perspective. Turk J Surg. 2018;34(2):89–93.
53. Enver N, Doruk C, Sormaz IC, Makay O, Uludag M. Awareness of thyroid surgeons on voice and airway complications: an attitude survey in Turkey. J Voice. 2019;S0892-1997(19):30216–30214.
54. Aygun N, Iscan Y, Ozdemir M, Soylu S, Aydin OU, Sormaz IC, et al. Endocrine surgery during the COVID-19 Pandemic: recommendations from the Turkish Association of Endocrine Surgery. Sisli Etfal Hastan Tip Bul. 2020;54(2):117–131.
55. Demir B, Alçı E, Hasanov R, Mulailua K, Makay Ö, Koçak S. Turkish endocrine surgery publications in international scientific journals. Ulus Cerrahi Derg. 2015;31(2):81
56. Karakaya MA, Koç O, Ekiz F, Ağaçhan AF, Göret NE. Analysis of the Istanbul Forensic Medicine Institute expert decisions on recurrent laryngeal nerve injuries due to thyroidectomy between 2008-2012. Ulus Cerrahi Derg. 2015;32(1):43–46.
57. An L, Hwang KS, Park SH, Kim YN, Baek SJ, Park S, et al.; Korean Association of Robotic Surgeons (KAROS) Study Group. Trends of robotic assisted surgery for thyroid, colorectal, stomach and hepatopancreaticobiliary cancer-10 year Korea trend investigation. Asian J Surg. 2020 Jun:S1015-9584(20)30164–0.
58. Altaf S, Mehmood Z, Baloch MN, Javed A. Experience of thyroid surgery at a tertiary care hospital in Karachi, Pakistan. Open J Thyroid Res. 2019;2(1):009–014.
59. Han L, Li W, Li Y, Wen W, Yao Y, Wang Y. Total thyroidectomy is superior for initial treatment of thyroid cancer. Asia Pac J Clin Oncol. 2020 Aug. doi: 10.1111/ajco.13379. Epub ahead of print. PMID: 32757466.
60. Li R, Wang Y, Du L. A rapidly increasing trend of thyroid cancer incidence in selected East Asian countries: Joinpoint regression and age-period-cohort analyses. Gland Surg. 2020 Aug;9(4):968–984.

22
THYROIDECTOMY

Anand Kumar Mishra and Kul Ranjan Singh

Introduction

Operations on the thyroid gland were never popular in eighteenth century and in fact before 1850 thyroidectomy was banned by French academy of surgeons because of near 100% mortality. Samuel Gross, one of the respected surgeon in 1866 said that thyroid surgery is butchery*. Later after 10 years, Theodor Kocher, considered as 'Father of thyroid surgery' propagated 'capsular dissection' a technical principle of thyroid surgery which is followed in present day and it dramatically reduced the mortality and complication rate. In 1909, Kocher was awarded Nobel Prize for Medicine, the first surgeon ever to receive it. Other principles proposed by him for safe thyroid surgery were proper understanding of surgical anatomy, handling of important adjacent structures and emphasis on meticulous homeostasis. And these are basic principles of modern surgery in terms of prevention of complications and safety. In Theodor Kocher words, thyroid surgery depicts 'Supreme Triumph' of the surgeon (1–3).

> * 'Can the thyroid gland when in the state of enlargement be removed with a reasonable hope of saving the patient? Experience emphatically answers, no! If a surgeon should be so fully **foolhardy** as to undertake it. Every step he takes will be environed with difficulty, every stroke of his knife will be followed by a torrent of blood, and lucky will it be for him if his victim live **long enough** to enable him to finish his horrid **butchery**. No honest and sensible surgeon would ever engage in it'.

Surgical excision of part or whole of thyroid gland is defined as thyroidectomy. It encompasses bilateral (subtotal, total or near-total thyroidectomy [TT]) and unilateral (lobectomy, hemithyroidectomy) surgical procedures. Sub-TT is not uncommonly practiced in present era because of risk of recurrent disease and high morbidities associated with repeat surgery. Decisions regarding the extent of resection depend on pathology.

Types of thyroid operations

Following are the definitions of various surgical procedures associated:

Lobectomy: It is removal of one lobe of thyroid gland. It is the minimum surgery indicated (Figure 22.1).

Hemithyroidectomy (HT): It is removal of one lobe, isthmus and pyramidal lobe if present. Most of time during surgery in asymmetrical nodule the isthmus is absent. So lobectomy and HT is used interchangeably in these cases.

Sub-TT: It is incomplete excision of both lobes and isthmus, leaving about 4–6 g of thyroid tissue on either side. The left thyroid tissue obliterates the trachea-esophageal (TO) groove on either side. The aim of leaving thyroid tissue is to prevent injury to parathyroid glands and recurrent laryngeal nerve (RLN) and achieve normal thyroid function (Figure 22.2).

Dunhill operation: It is defined as complete lobectomy on one side and subtotal lobectomy on other side with excision of the isthmus (Figure 22.2).

Near-TT: It is excision of both lobes with isthmus and leaving one to 2 g of thyroid tissue near entry of RLN.

TT: It is excision of all visible thyroid tissue which include both lobes, isthmus, pyramidal lobe and thyrothymic rests if present (Figure 22.3).

Clinical indications for thyroidectomy

The indications for thyroid surgery include the following 5 "C" mnemonic:

1. *C*ancer – Solitary thyroid nodule usually with fine needle aspiration (FNA) indicative of a suspicious lesion or cancer;
2. *C*ompression – Multinodular goiter with continued enlargement and symptoms ranging from stridor, dysphagia or obstructive sleep apnea etc.;
3. *C*ardiac – Definitive management for toxic goiter, particularly if radioiodine ablation or antithyroid medications are contraindicated.
4. *C*osmesis – Patient's preference for surgery for cosmetic concerns.
5. *C*omeback – Recurrent thyroid cancer

Preoperative evaluation and preparation

Patients planned for thyroid surgery are evaluated by detailed history, physical examination and investigations. In the following paragraphs, the various aspects of the history, examination and investigations are summarized and highlighted to revisit before surgery.

1. **History and physical examination**:
   a. Nodule growth rate, duration and mode of onset should be noted.
   b. Presence of dysphagia, dyspnea, dysphonia or hypo, hyperthyroidism symptoms should be noted.
   c. Information regarding family history of cancer, endocrine disease, radiotherapy to neck or previous neck, thyroid surgery
   d. A thorough physical examination of neck, and cervical nodes should be performed.

Thyroidectomy

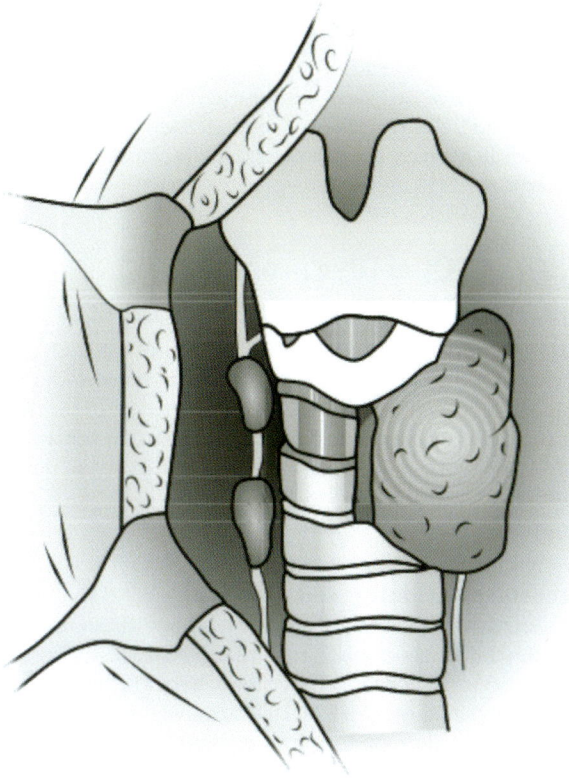

FIGURE 22.1 Unilateral operation – right lobectomy.

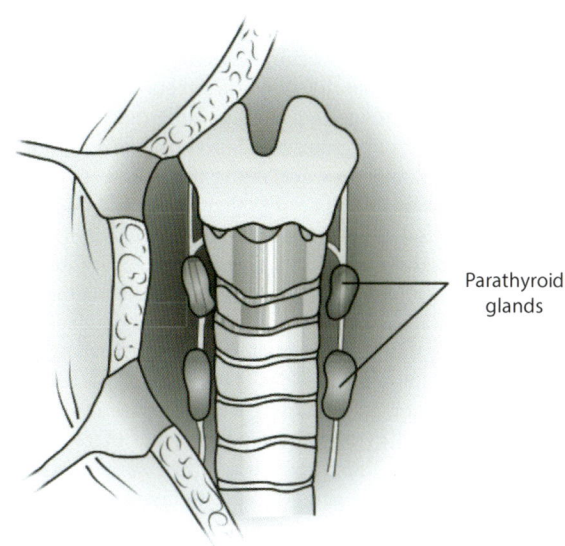

FIGURE 22.3 Total thyroidectomy.

e. Symptoms of upper respiratory tract infection like cough or sneezing should not be there.
f. Evaluation of neck for should be done for a crease in which incision is planned. An evaluation of difficulty of intubation should be assessed by thyromental distance, mouth opening and tracheal shift.
g. Allergy to the medication should be reviewed.

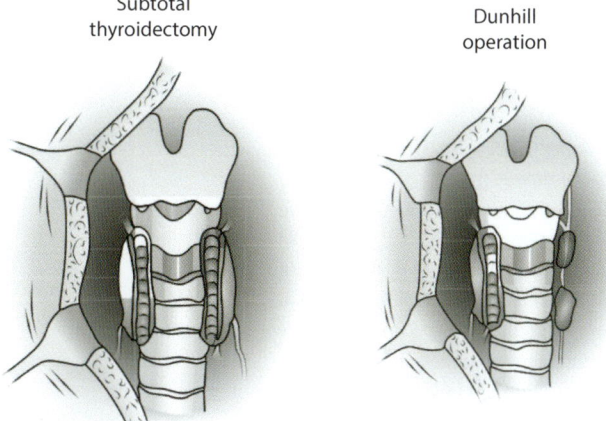

FIGURE 22.2 Bilateral subtotal operation.

2. **Investigations**:
   The following investigations should be reviewed before planning for surgery.
   a. TSH: It should be in normal range. In hyperthyroid patients, TSH remains suppressed even after patient achieves euthyroidism. So, in these patients, free T4 levels should be checked.
   b. Blood investigations: Hemoglobin, total and eosinophil counts, liver function tests, kidney functions, blood sugar, calcium, phosphorus (if TT is planned) should be checked. If patient is diabetic then HbA1c should be checked.
   c. Preoperative PTH is done to calculate the PTH gradient after surgery for prediction of hypocalcemia.
   d. Vitamin D (25-hydroxy) levels should be checked and if low should be corrected before surgery if TT is planned.
   e. Thyroglobulin estimation does not have any role and calcitonin estimation is indicated only when suspicion of hereditary syndromes, family history of thyroid cancer, medullary thyroid cancer or suspicion of the same is there.
   f. Imaging (high-resolution ultrasound) should be reviewed and the finding will decide whether unilateral or bilateral procedure has to be done. If unilateral procedure then side should be noted. Also it will help in taking a decision of central or lateral lymph node dissection in cases of thyroid cancer. Other imaging like CT scan or MRI is indicated in presence of compressive symptoms, malignancy, lymph nodes, local infiltration, or there is suspicion of retrosternal component. PET CT is only indicated in suspicion of recurrence of thyroid cancer. Thyroid scan is indicated in hyperthyroidism and in case of solid nodule with undetermined cytology where hyperfunction nearly rules out malignancy.

g. FNAC is usually not indicated in nodule less than 1 cm unless ultrasound has suspicious features. It should be reported by Bethesda system. The FNAC report will decide about the extent of thyroidectomy.
h. Laryngoscopy: It confirms the mobility of the vocal cord. Nowadays at some centers, it is routine to perform it preoperatively while others use it selectively. Laryngoscopy is indicated in patients with history of neck, thyroid surgery and presence of dysphonia or recent change in voice, malignant nodule or suspicion of invasion. Vocal cord evaluation should also be done in benign conditions like retrosternal goiter, goiter with compression or tracheal displacement and whenever intraoperative nerve monitoring is planned (4, 5).
i. Reoperative thyroid surgery: It is technically challenging and if not performed properly have more than double the complications of nerve injury and hypoparathyroidism. In situations when reoperative surgery is performed by different surgeon and different hospital than the primary place where first surgery was done, roadmap of the surgery needs to be planned to be safe. Review of detailed operative record, pathology report, imaging of thyroid to know the residual mass, side are important prerequisite. Reoperative or completion thyroidectomy can be done in 7–10 days of the operation or after 6 weeks once inflammation has subsided. This surgery should be done by experienced surgeon.
j. Blood cross-match if extensive dissection is being planned.
k. Tetanus vaccination is not required.

Previous evening patient should take normal light diet and adequate sleep. There should be 4–6 hours fasting as per institute protocol if surgery is being planned under general anesthesia. Patient should be allowed to have antihypertensive drug, antithyroid and beta-blockers medication with sips of water as indicated on the morning of surgery.

In the operation theater:

1. Incision marking in neck crease in sitting position should be done for the best cosmetic results.
2. Antibiotic prophylaxis: Single-dose antibiotic which should cover gram-positive cocci (streptococci species, negative coagulase staphylococcus, staphylococcus aureus).
3. Anti-thrombolytic prophylaxis: It is usually not needed.

4. Frozen section requirement: It is not useful in follicular neoplasm and reserved only for cases having suspicion of malignancy on FNAC. It is indicated for metastatic lymph nodes confirmation and their differentiation from parathyroids. However, if of is planned then pathologist should be informed for the same.
5. Intraoperative neuromonitoring (IONM): In most of the centers in India, it is not used routinely. Most of the departments do not have the equipment. If it is planned, the anesthetist needs to inform (6).

Operative procedure

Lobectomy is the minimum procedure in thyroid gland and if isthmus is removed along lobe, it is HT. Lobectomy on both sides along with isthmus removal becomes TT. So a surgeon who can perform a safe lobectomy can always perform safe TT as there is only repetition of the same surgical steps on the other side. Table 22.1 summarizes the thyroid techniques in vogue during last century.

Following are operative steps of lobectomy:

Anesthesia, positioning and draping

Almost universally, patients receive general anesthesia for thyroidectomy while some groups have utilized local anesthesia with superficial cervical block for HT. In cases where RLN monitoring is demanded by the surgeon – EMG (electromyographic) endotracheal tubes with neuromonitoring apparatus is used. These tubes are specialized in having electrodes near the cuff which come in contact with true vocal cords while intubation and hence record their electrical activity when RLN is stimulated by a probe. Long-acting muscle relaxants are avoided in such surgeries for correct documentation. In large goiters and invasive thyroid cancers, nasogastric tube should be placed so that esophagus can be palpated during retrotracheal dissection.

Patient preparation

The patient is placed in supine position and extension of the neck is achieved with a roll or sand bag under shoulders. A padded ring under the head is placed 15–30 degree up (Figure 22.4). The appropriate amount of extension is individually modified for each patient. In female patients with high BMI, big breasts can be taped inferiorly to improve access to the surgical site. Both the arms of the patient are placed on the sides and taped.

TABLE 22.1: Evolution of Surgical Technique

	Last 100 Years Till the 1980s	Today
Surgical technique	Lateral dissection and tying the inferior thyroid trunk	Capsular dissection – tying the tertiary branches of ITA on the capsule of the thyroid
Parathyroid gland	Preservation	Identification by indocyanine green dye Preservation with pedicle After surgery: if color tan or dusky – knife test Autotransplantation of ischemic or risky glands
Recurrent laryngeal nerve	Inferior thyroid artery main trunk was tied	Nerve identification and use of intraoperative nerve monitoring
External branch of superior laryngeal nerve	No concept and course not defined Mass ligation of vessels near the upper pole	Nerve anatomy defined Identification and intra operative nerve monitoring use
Completeness of resection	Subtotal thyroidectomy was common	Better understanding of embryological remnants like pyramidal lobe, tubercle of Zuckerkandl, thyrothymic thyroid rests and complete resection of gland in all bilateral thyroid disease (total thyroidectomy)

Thyroidectomy

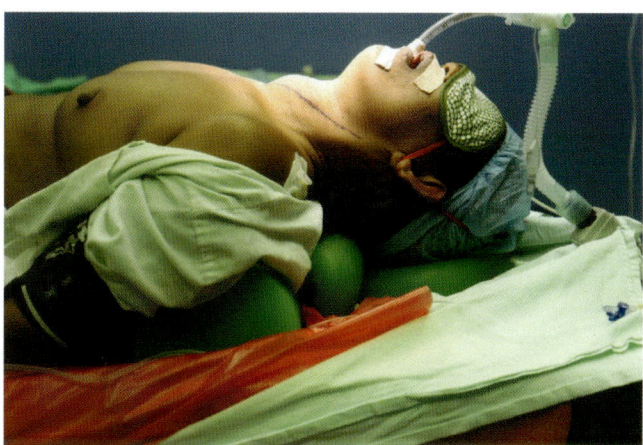

FIGURE 22.4 Patient is positioned with hyperextended neck and with silicon head ring and silicon roll under neck and beneath shoulders (flexometallic endotracheal tube in situ).

The neck (from the chin to at least 4 cm below the clavicles and laterally to the trapezius) is prepared with Savlon and Betadine scrub or as per institutional protocol.

Incision and exposure

Skin incision is placed in a neck crease and lies between two heads of sternocleidomastoid muscle. It is usually 4–6 cm in length but depends on size of the gland, pathology and procedure. Some surgeons mark it after positioning with a silk thread or marking pen (Figure 22.5). Local infiltration with 1–2% xylocaine with adrenaline can be done to facilitate homeostasis and dissection. Incision is given by blade and subcutaneous tissue is divided. The next layer is platysma and as it is cut it retracts.

Subplatysmal flaps and gland exposure

Subplatysmal flaps are created by help of monopolar cautery by having superior traction by assistant and surgeon puts pressure inferiorly on the strap muscles. The plane of dissection is below platysmal muscle in avascular areolar tissue. Anterior jugular vein if present can be identified and injury should be prevented. If injured, it can be tied with absorbable sutures. Blunt dissection should be avoided to create flaps. The extent of flap is from thyroid cartilage superiorly to suprasternal notch inferiorly (Figures 22.6–22.8).

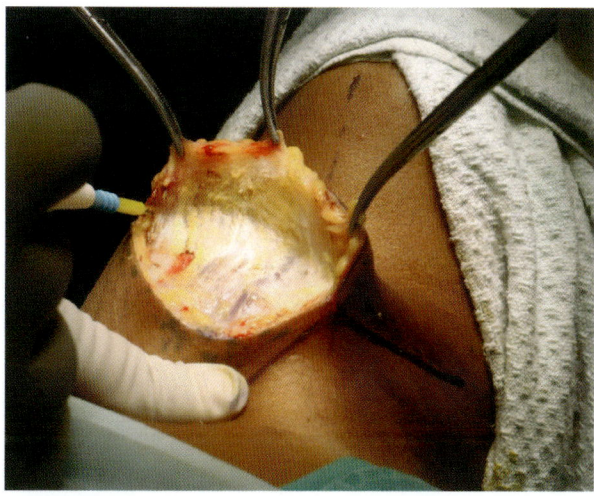

FIGURE 22.6 After skin incision, platysma being cut with monopolar cautery.

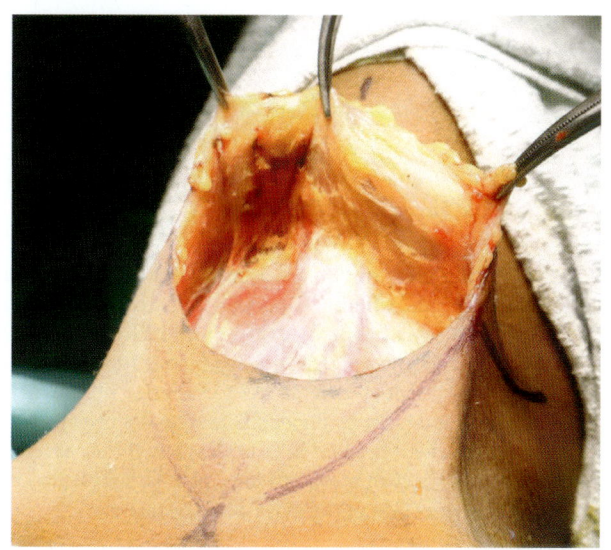

FIGURE 22.7 Superior subplatysmal flap being raised.

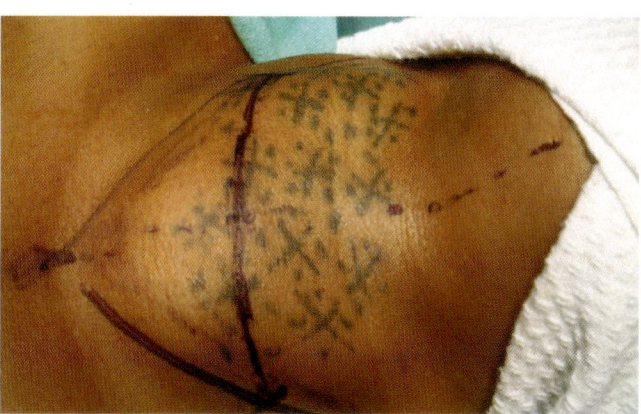

FIGURE 22.5 Incision marked in natural neck crease with other surface markings.

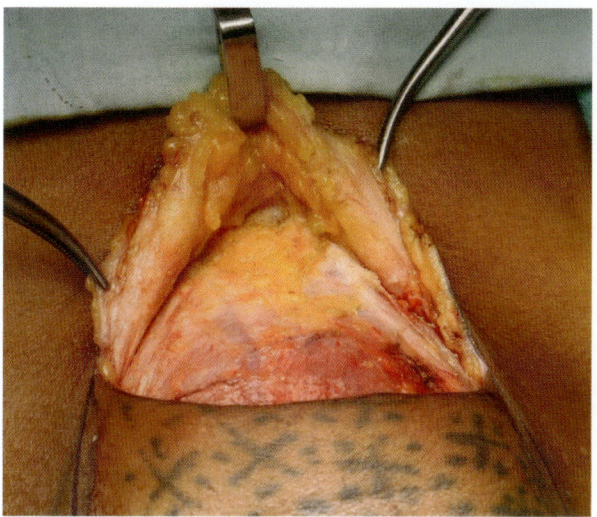

FIGURE 22.8 Inferior subplatysmal flap raised till suprasternal notch.

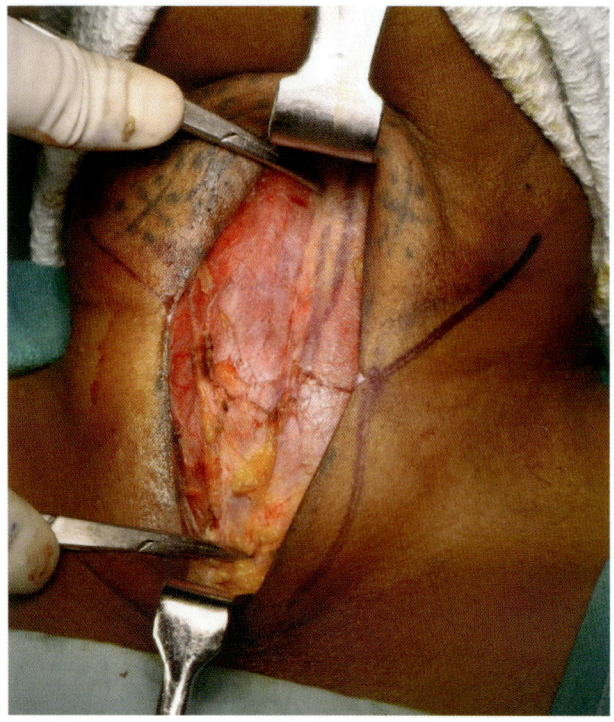

FIGURE 22.9 Straps midline identified and held with two small hemostatic forceps before division.

Next step is to define midline, avascular plane between strap muscles of either side. Midline is opened and strap muscles are retracted laterally by assistant (Figures 22.9 and 22.10). This gives exposure of isthmus and anterior trachea below. In large goiters or in short-neck patients where access to superior poles will be difficult, strap muscle can be divided transversally to gain additional exposure either on one side or both sides. If the thyroid is invading into the anterior strap muscles, plan should be to perform an en-bloc resection of the mass with the muscle.

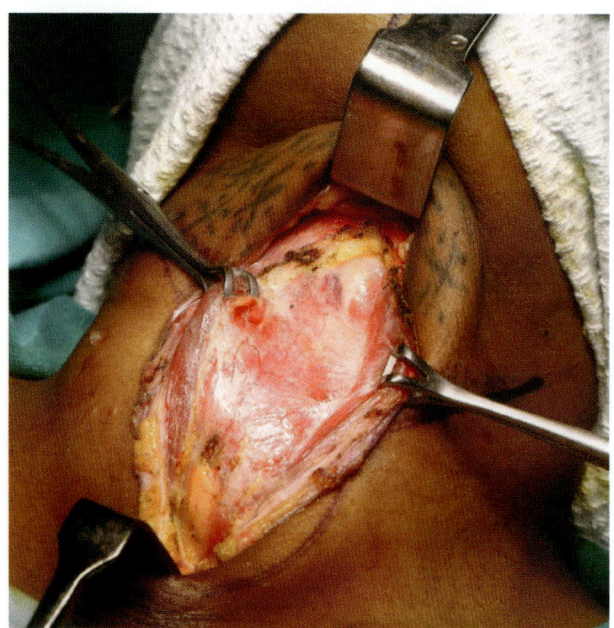

FIGURE 22.10 Straps being divided in midline.

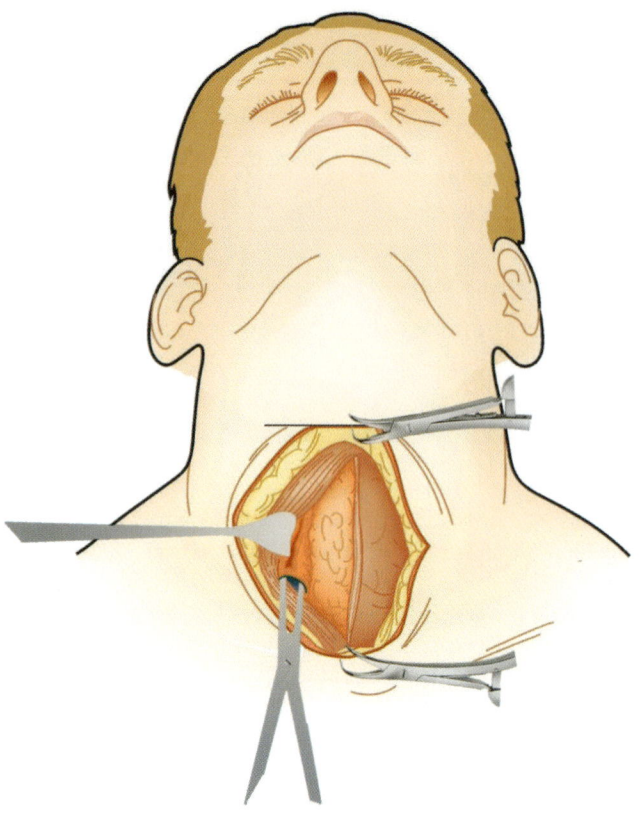

FIGURE 22.11 Lateral dissection on lobe to identify the middle thyroid veins.

Lateral dissection
Dissection on anteromedial surface of lobe is started and this continues laterally (Figure 22.11). When surgical plan is TT, dissection is started on the side with the greatest pathology. The lobe is retracted anteromedially by nondominant hand of the surgeon and strap muscles are retracted laterally. This can be done at lower pole and then lobe can be even delivered from TO groove (Figures 22.11–22.13). After delivering the lobe medially, dissection is continued in the plane between strap muscles

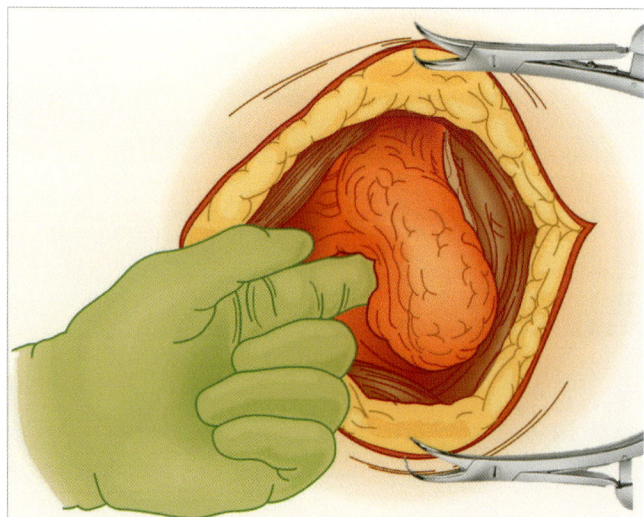

FIGURE 22.12 Right lobe delivered/dislodged from TO groove.

Thyroidectomy

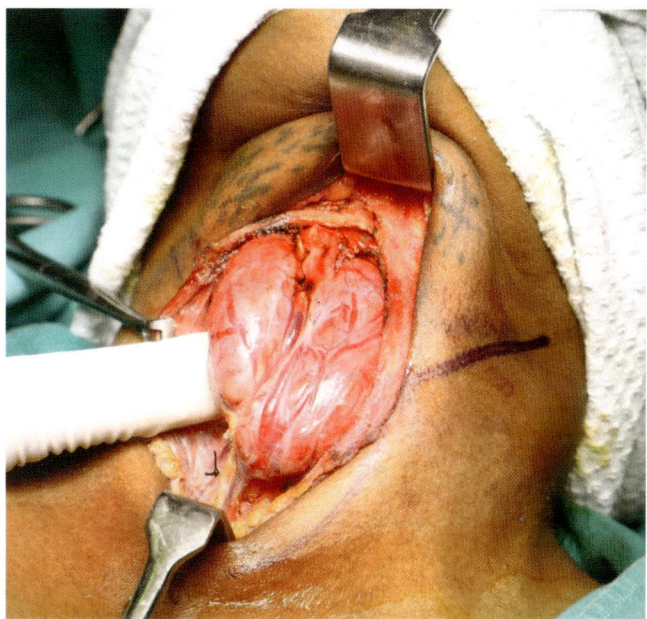

FIGURE 22.13 Right lobe delivered/dislodged from TO groove.

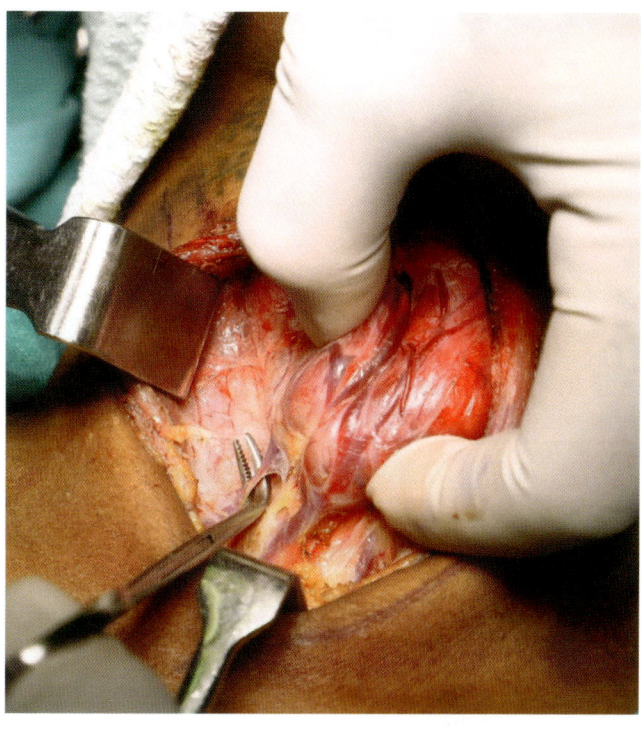

FIGURE 22.14 Middle thyroid vein, right side near lower pole.

and the thyroid gland until the carotid sheath has been reached and then superiorly till the lateral surface of the superior pole. Some surgeons at this stage divide the isthmus in large goiters or retrosternal goiters.

Middle thyroid vein (MTV) division: The lobe cannot be delivered completely out of TO groove till MTVs are ligated and cut close to the carotid sheath. MTV are short, thin-walled vessels draining into internal jugular vein and one to three in numbers. They are sometimes absent. The vessel hemostasis can be done by traditional suture ligation, or bipolar cautery, or newer energy devices electrothermal bipolar vessel sealing system, or LigaSure, harmonic scalpel (Figure 22.14).

Superior pole dissection

The avascular space medial to superior pole between the pole and cricothyroid muscle, known as space of Reeves/Clark/Jolle is opened. The pole is retracted inferiorly and laterally by the help of a clamp or suture, so that this space gets opened more. External branch of the superior laryngeal nerve (EBSLN) is looked for. If EBSLN is identified in this space, it can be confirmed with the help of IONM (Figure 22.15). The superior

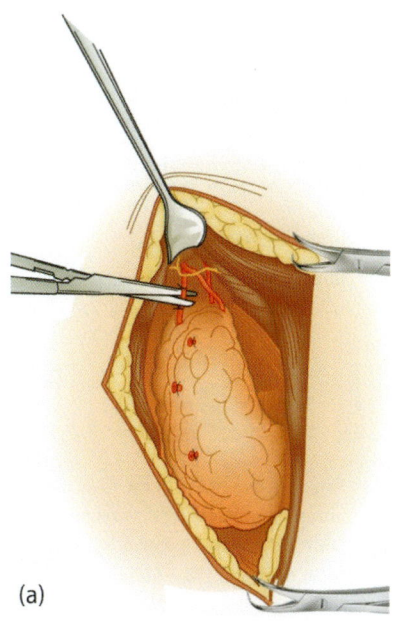
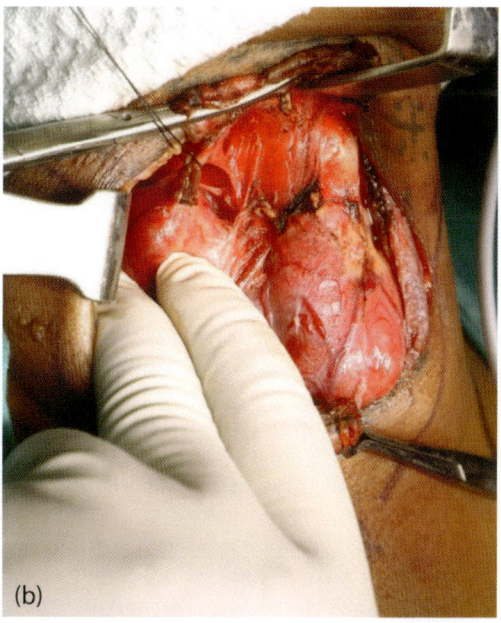

FIGURE 22.15 Creation of medial space and latelization of superior pole vessels, EBSLN seen in space. (a) Pictorial view of medial space with superior pole vessels. (b) Intraoperative view.

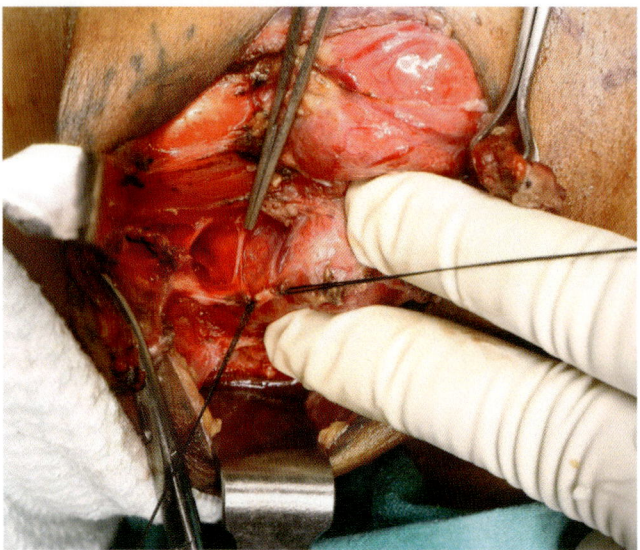

FIGURE 22.16 Right superior pole vessels individual ligation, EBSLN in medial space.

thyroid artery and vein are ligated individually as close to the gland as possible in a medial to lateral direction to minimize the risk of injury to the EBSLN (Figure 22.16). Mass ligation of the pedicle is not done as previously practiced. Superior parathyroid glands are located posterior to superior pole. They should be dissected carefully from thyroid capsule with intact blood supply and viability.

Recurrent laryngeal nerve identification

Identification of the RLN is essential for prevention of the injury. RLN runs in TO groove and enters the larynx at the inferior cornu of the thyroid cartilage. The possibility of a nonrecurrent nerve must be considered if there are difficulties in identification. First three landmarks should be identified – trachea and TO groove, inferior thyroid artery branches or trunk, inferior cornua of thyroid cartilage. There are three approaches for identification of RLN (Table 22.2).

1. Superior approach
2. Lateral approach
3. Inferior approach

During dissection in the TO groove no linear structure should be divided, ligated or clamped till RLN has been identified. The aggressive traction or medial rotation of the lobe should be avoided as it can cause traction injury to RLN. Bipolar cautery and local pressure are used to control bleeding during dissection in TO groove. RLN runs posterior to the tubercle of Zuckerkandl, posterior to the inferior parathyroid gland and anterior to the superior parathyroid gland. If several branches of the RLN become evident, follow the most medial/anterior branch (motor branch). All branches of the RLN should be preserved. Palpation of RLN as firm linear structure can be done with tip of index finger in the TO groove. The dissection should be perpendicular to the RLN to avoid confusing areolar tissue and fibrous tissue with the RLN (Figures 22.17–22.20). RLN is identified as 'Pearly white tubular structure in TO groove' with overlying 'Vasa nervorum'. The anterior branch is commonly the motor branch to the larynx. Most vulnerable point for RLN injury is at entry into the larynx when it is related to Berry's ligament. RLN is wrapped around by the two fibrous sheets of this ligament. There is usually an unnamed vessel running over it. The ligament of Berry should always be tied or cauterized with bipolar diathermy. Any attempt to cauterize bleeding vessels on it or near this area may burn the nerve. Nerve monitoring can identify injuries of RLN intraoperatively. If still RLN is not identified because of central compartment lymph nodes, and in reoperative surgery due to inflammation and fibrosis, leave a cuff of thyroid remnant behind to avoid injuring the RLN (6–8).

Capsular dissection

It is division of the terminal branches of the inferior thyroid artery on the capsule of the thyroid. Inferior parathyroid glands

TABLE 22.2: Advantages and Disadvantages of Three Approaches to the Recurrent Laryngeal Nerve

Approach of RLN Dissection	Advantages	Disadvantages
Lateral	Identifies the RLN in its course or mid portion Approach familiar to all surgeons RLN is related to inferior thyroid artery main trunk or its branches Tubercle of Zuckerkandl if present can help in identification as 'pointer to the nerve' It may travel on the posterolateral surface of lobe RLN is related to the ligament of Berry	Injury by ligatures or clamp possible
Inferior	Identifies the RLN at the level of its exit from the thorax Helpful in reoperative thyroidectomy Permits identification it divides into branches	Requires dissection of the RLN over a long distance and increases the risk of devascularization of nerve and inferior parathyroid glands
Superior	Identifies RLN at level of its entry into larynx This approach is indicated for large or retrosternal goiters	Most common place for injury of RLN Dissection is sometimes difficult due to possible adhesions between the RLN and ligament of Berry

Thyroidectomy

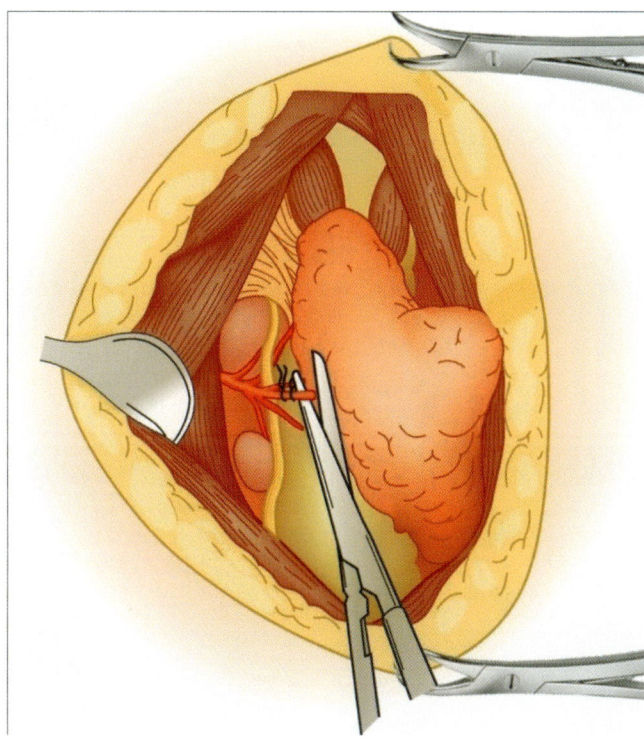

FIGURE 22.17 Relation of inferior thyroid artery branches and RLN on right side.

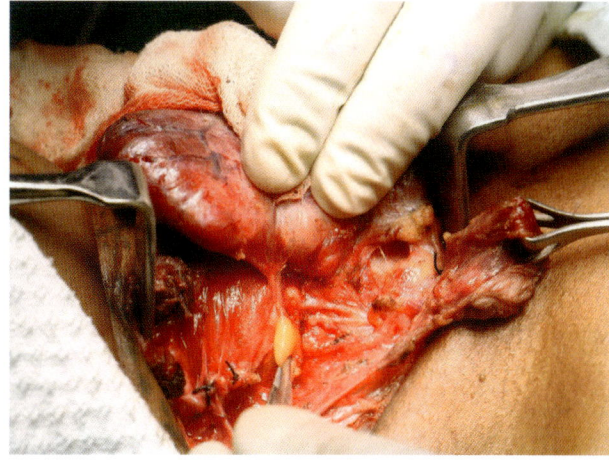

FIGURE 22.19 Ligament of Berry.

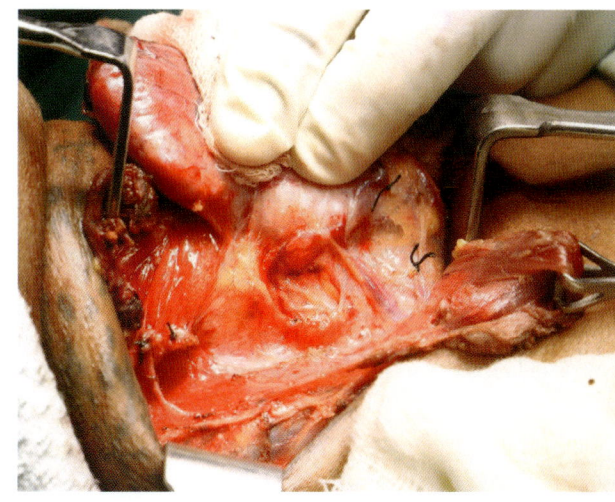

FIGURE 22.20 Left TO groove, RLN two branches with superior parathyroid gland.

are located anterior to RLN on the capsule in inferior pole area. It is meticulously and gently dissected away from thyroid lobe. Blood vessels coming directly out of the thyroid gland are identified and divided away from the inferior parathyroid gland. The inferior pedicle is skeletonized and then ligated as close to the gland as possible (Figure 22.21).

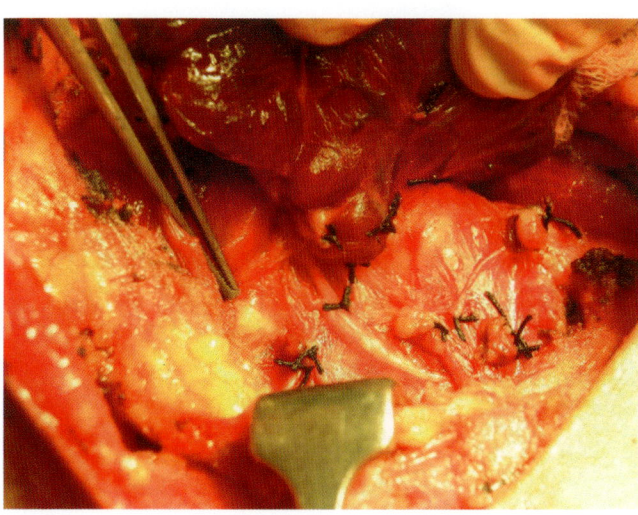

FIGURE 22.18 RLN and tubercle of Zuckerkandl.

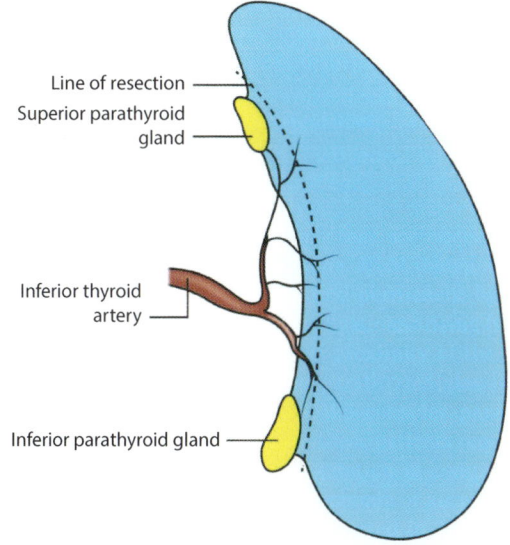

FIGURE 22.21 Capsular dissection (tying the tertiary branches of inferior thyroid artery on the capsule).

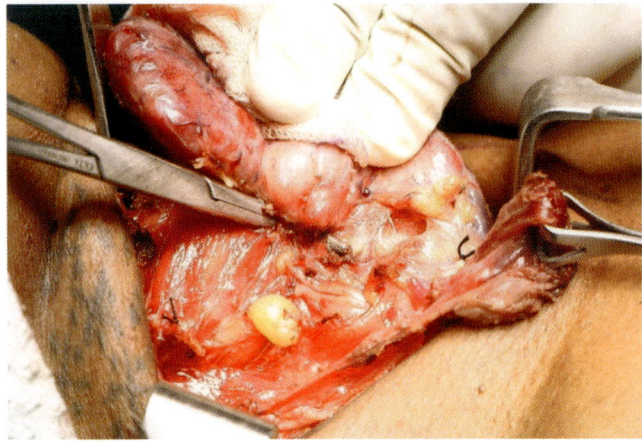

FIGURE 22.22 Ligament of Berry dissection with hemostat.

Removing thyroid off trachea

The posterior surface of thyroid gland now remains attached to the tracheal anterior surface by the ligament of Berry (Figures 22.22 and 22.23). Lobe is lifted and dissected off trachea by using bipolar or monopolar cautery (Figure 22.4). HT operation is completed by including isthmus also. For TT, same steps of lobectomy are repeated on contralateral side to complete the procedure. After removing the thyroid specimen, it should be meticulously examined for any inadvertently excised parathyroid gland. If there is a pyramidal lobe, it is mobilized and included with the specimen (Figure 22.24). If TT is planned the same steps are repeated on the opposite side and the operation is completed (Figure 22.25).

Closure

Thyroid bed is irrigated with water and suctioned on gauze to avoid suction injury to parathyroids and RLN. Thyroid bed, ligated inferior and superior poles vessels are inspected. Hemostasis is confirmed by performing a sustained Valsalva maneuver. Integrity of RLN and viability of parathyroid gland is checked by knife test. If an

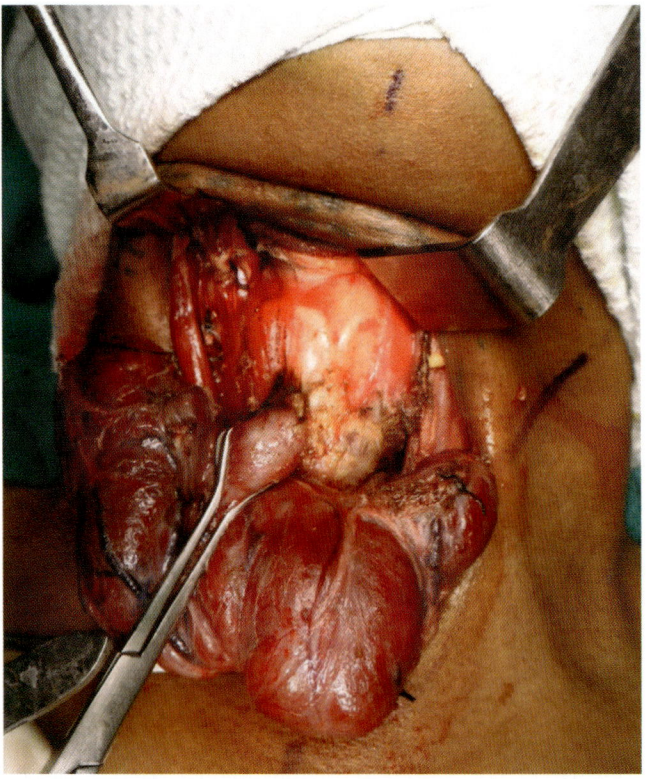

FIGURE 22.24 Pyramidal lobe.

incision is given on the capsule of parathyroid gland, a viable gland will bleed while devascularized gland will have dark tan look and will not bleed. Usage of drains depends on the surgeon's preference. Straps are reapproximated with interrupted absorbable sutures, leaving an opening caudally of about 1–1.5 cm (Figure 22.26). The platysma is reapproximated with interrupted absorbable sutures

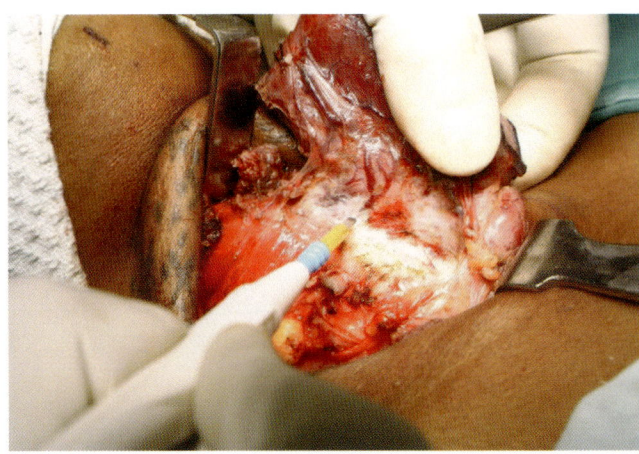

FIGURE 22.23 Right lobe lifted off from tracheal surface.

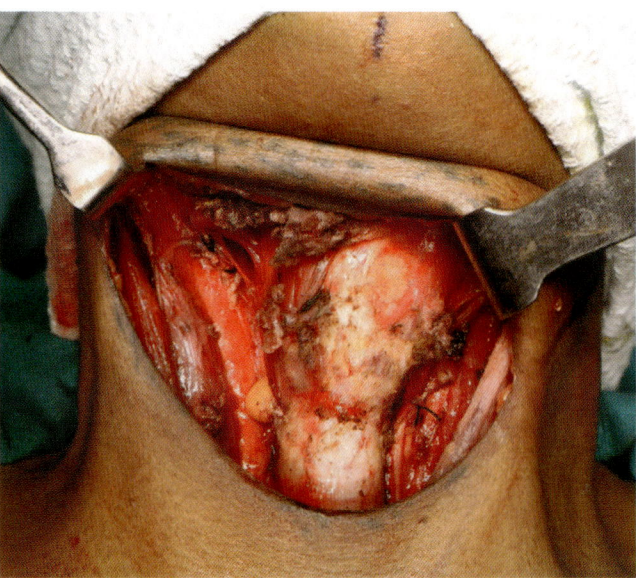

FIGURE 22.25 Total thyroidectomy bed.

Thyroidectomy

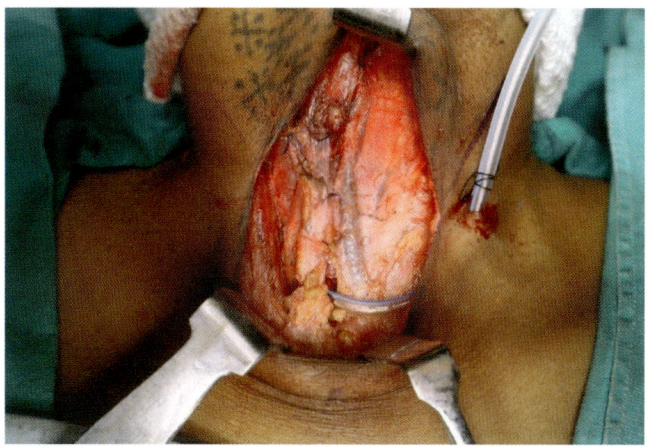

FIGURE 22.26 Midline closed with weeping holes in caudal portion, drain placed.

(Figure 22.27), and the skin is closed using a subcutaneous running closure (Figure 22.28).

Postoperative management

All patients generally are kept under observation overnight after TT for development of hematoma. Signs and symptoms of hypocalcemia, and calcium levels are checked in the postoperative period after bilateral surgery of thyroid. Calcium supplementation is often required in cases of symptomatic hypocalcemia. Immediate or 4–6 hours PTH levels post-operatively can predict hypocalcemia (less than 10 pg/mL). If preoperative PTH is available, pre- and post-operative PTH values are compared and PTH gradient is calculated. A PTH gradient of more than 65–70% is predictive of hypocalcemia. HT patients may be discharged on same or next day. Thyroid hormone replacement is initiated in TT patients in a dose of 1.6–2 µg/kg/day as per institutional protocol. TSH levels maybe checked 4–6 weeks after surgery, with titration of thyroid hormone replacement as necessary.

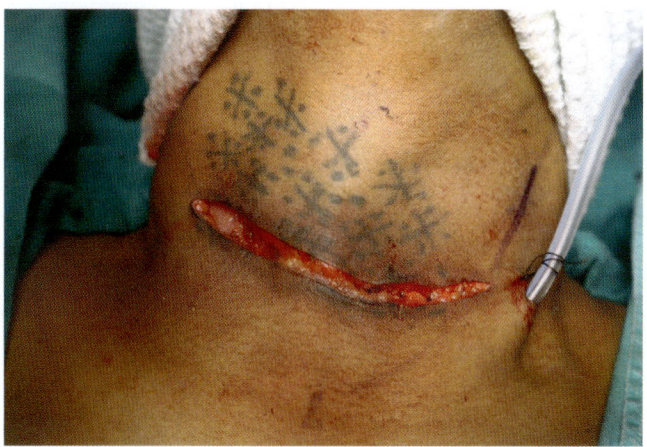

FIGURE 22.27 Platysma closed with absorbable suture.

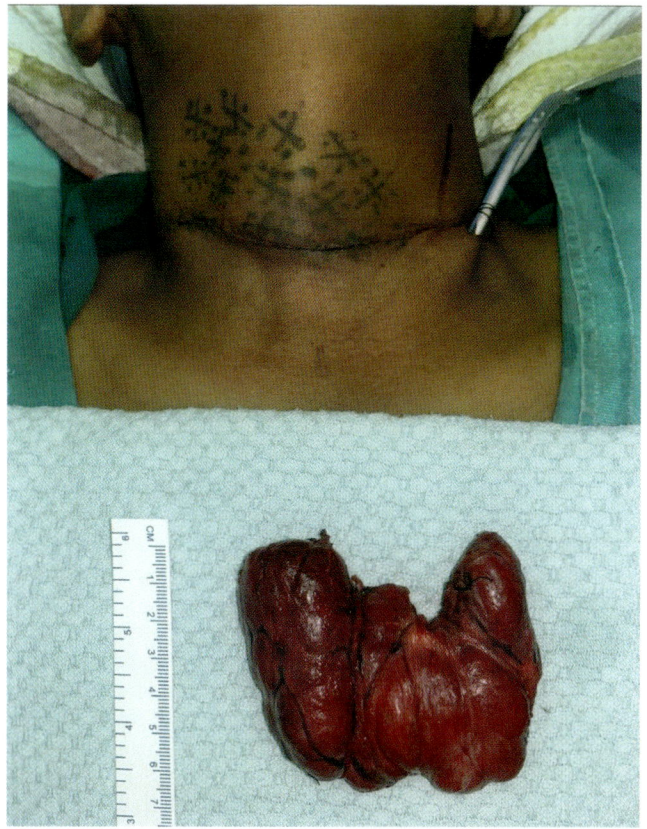

FIGURE 22.28 Incision after complete subcuticular closure and drain in situ.

Complications of thyroidectomy

Following are the risk factors described in the literature responsible for complications in thyroid surgery (9–11):

1. Patient-related factors (previous cervical surgery)
2. Procedure-related factors (associated central compartment lymph-node dissection, retrosternal goiter, reoperative surgery)
3. Thyroid pathology (thyroiditis, cancer)
4. Surgical volume of thyroid
5. Surgeon experience

There are five major complications that are observed after thyroid procedures – wound hematoma, RLN injury, injury to EBSLN, postoperative hypocalcemia and permanent hypoparathyroidism (12–17). Two classical complications arising from two anatomic structures which lie in close proximity of the thyroid gland are RLN or EBSLN injury and parathyroid glands injury resulting in various manifestations. We consider parathyroid injury more dreaded complications as these patients require lifelong calcium and vitamin D supplementation in comparison to nerve injury patients who have only dysphonia or air way issues.

Temporary hypoparathyroidism is reported in 20–30% while permanent in 1–4%.

Hematoma: If patient develops hematoma, drains do not help. Patient develop discomfort in postoperative period and a swelling with bulge of the wound can be noticed which is quickly followed by respiratory impairment. Incidence of postoperative hematoma in the published series is reported from 0% to 3%. Adequate homeostasis and valsalva maneuver at the end of procedure are the steps to prevent post-op hemorrhage and hematoma. Recognition of this situation is an emergency as it is potentially fatal. If there is suspicion of a postoperative hematoma, the neck sutures must be immediately removed, wound opened and evacuation of the hematoma should be performed immediately at bedside. Bedside emergency tracheotomy or cricothyroidotomy is usually not required, and the patient is resuscitated with fluids humidified oxygen and shifted to operation theater for inspection of the surgical bed under general anesthesia. The bleeding vessel can be ligated in a careful and more comfortable manner under optimal sterile conditions with good lighting in the operating room

Respiratory distress: Respiratory difficulty after thyroidectomy can be because of hemorrhage and hematoma causing compression on airway or laryngeal edema, excessive wound edema causing pressure on the airway, larynx and surrounding tissues, traumatic intubation, nerve injury (RLN or EBSLN), hypocalcemia and tracheomalacia in long-standing large goiters. Use of ice packs on the neck after thyroidectomy reduces wound edema. In case of distress, neck should be raised and oxygen supplemented, suction can be if secretions are present. Signs of hypocalcemia are checked and immediate bedside surgical drainage is done if bleeding is suspected.

RLN injury: Temporary dysphonia is reported in 5–11% while permanent in 1–3.5%. RLN nerve is vulnerable for injury especially in following areas: near Berry's ligament at nerve entry to larynx, near Zuckerkandl's tubercle if present, TO groove, inferior thyroid poles and during central compartment dissections. Injuries to the RLN occur in 1–4% of thyroid operations in most series. RLN injury can be caused by the six mechanisms: transection (intentional or inadvertent), clamp, stretch, electrothermal, ligature entrapment and ischemia. In retrosternal goiters, RLN identification may be difficult due to large size or it may be stretched over thyroid mass in an unusual manner, adherent to post capsule of thyroid, displaced medially or anteriorly. RLN supplies both abductors and adductors muscle and after injury abductors muscles are affected before adductors. Semon's law (1881) states that the abductors and adductors lie in separate bundles in RLN. In an advancing lesion, the abductors which are phylogenetically younger are paralyzed first and cord lies in paramedian position. Then the adductors which are phylogenetically older are paralyzed and cord lies in lateral (cadaveric) position. Semon's law actually predicts that the affected vocal fold would shift laterally over time. Wegner and Gross Man theory (1897) states, that if there is pure RLN paralysis the cord lies in paramedian position because the intact cricothyroid muscle adducts the cord and if there is combined RLN and superior laryngeal nerve paralysis, the cord lies in lateral position because of the loss of adductive force. In unilateral RLN injury, nonfunction of the intrinsic muscles of the larynx on the affected side (loss of abduction with intact adduction by cricothyroid) causes the vocal cord to assume a paramedian position. The voice is breathy but compensation occurs, though rarely back to normal. The airway is adequate and may become compromised only with exertion. In bilateral RLN, injury cords lie in paramedian position, voice is good, but patient has variable degree of stridor. In unilateral RLN injuries, the voice becomes husky because the vocal cords do not approximate one another. Bilateral injury of the RLN s may result in paralysis of both vocal cords thus both vocal cords may assume a medial or paramedian position and cause airway obstruction, which would require reintubation and possibly tracheostomy due to airway compromise.

Constricting and clamping injury happens when tying a vessel too closely to nerve. Inadvertent clamping can injure in bifurcated RLN, during troublesome oozing at the region of Berry's ligament. Reanastomosis in an acutely transected RLN should be done or not is a controversial issue; however, several patients have some return of function after immediate reanastomosis. Many have noted adverse functional results, including airway obstruction resulting from paradoxical motion, return of adductor but not abductor function and poor voice. Fundamental problem is that when nerve regenerates, many axons reinnervate wrong muscles. At present, reanastomosis of an acutely transected nerve seems reasonable, because it will maximize amount of reinnervation. Doing nothing could also be justified, as some reinnervation will occur and there would be less chance of dysfunction. Alternatively, one may anastomose a branch of the ansa cervicalis to the distal stump of the nerve. This would restore resting tone, but no useful motion, and carries the least risk of synkinesis. Permanent surgical rehabilitation of U/L paralysis should usually be deferred for 6–12 months to allow for optimal recovery or accommodation. Treatment options in unilateral injury are voice therapy alone or in combination with vocal fold augmentation, laryngoplastic phonosurgery like medialization thyroplasty, arytenoid adduction or laryngeal reinnervation – nerve to nerve anastomosis, nerve to muscle transfer. This is indicated when there is breathy voice, chronic aspiration, diminished cough.

Treatment options in bilateral injury are tracheostomy (valved), arytenoid abduction procedure, thyrotomy, arytenoidectomy with laryngeal stent, nerve muscle pedicle reinnervation techniques, lateral fixation of vocal cord by endoscopy, CO_2 laser endoscopic arytenoidectomy and cordectomy.

Injury to EBSLN: EBSLN innervates ipsilateral cricothyroid muscle and is a tensor of vocal cord. EBSLN may be stretched by retractor, or transected when these vessels are divided. Incidence of EBSLN unknown (0–28%). Loss of sensation to the supraglottic larynx can cause subtle symptoms such as frequent throat clearing, paroxysmal coughing, voice fatigue, vague foreign body sensations. Loss of motor function to cricothyroid muscle can cause a slight voice change, which patient usually interprets as hoarseness. Most common finding is diplophonia (with decreased range of pitch, most noticeable when trying to sing). Symptoms are hoarseness (slight), voice fatigue, reduced range of pitch volume in singers, professional speakers, lecturers/teachers. Methods to safeguard the nerve are accurate dissection in cricothyroid space, skeletonization and individual ligation of vessels, identification of the nerve before ligation if possible and confirmation by nerve stimulator if the facility is available (14).

Postoperative hypocalcemia: Hypocalcemia is defined as a total serum calcium level less than 2 mM/L (8.0 mg/dL) or an ionized calcium level less than 1.1 mM/L (0.275 mg/dL). Incidence varies from 2% to 83% depending on the definition. Hypocalcemia can be symptomatic, asymptomatic or biochemical hypocalcemia. Temporary or transient hypocalcemia is considered a sequelae of TT while permanent hypocalcemia (more than 1 year) is a complication of thyroidectomy. In circulation, about 50% of total serum calcium is in ionized, 40% is albumin-bound and 10% is complexed to phosphate or citrate. It is therefore advisable to 'correct' the measurement of total calcium using the following formula: 'corrected calcium' (mg/dL) = total calcium/0.8

(4 − albumin level [g/dL]). Postoperative PTH or PTH gradient is a better predictor of hypocalcemia than an isolated calcium level. In a metanalysis by Grodski et al., undetectable PTH at 4 hours postoperatively was predictive of hypocalcemia with sensitivity 48.5%, specificity of 96.7% (15). A metanalysis by Noordzij et al. reported PTH gradient of >65% from basal PTH 6 hours postoperatively predictive of hypocalcemia with sensitivity 96.4%, specificity of 91.4% (16).

The risk of postoperative hypocalcemia several factors depend on several factors:

1. As parathyroid gland are supplied by end arteries, so saving gland with pedicle is most important.
2. Difficult of identification of glands in large goiters particularly inferior glands, leading to incidental parathyroidectomy (6–21%).
3. Extremely large goiter, Graves' disease or thyroid cancer
4. Extensive central compartment nodal metastases requiring bilateral dissection.
5. Reoperative thyroid surgery increasing risk of devascularizing the parathyroid glands
6. Young age and female sex
7. Preoperative vitamin D deficiency

Biochemical hypocalcemia is treated by oral calcium (1–3 g) and vitamin D calcitriol (0.5 μg) and high calcium diet. Symptomatic hypocalcemia (paresthesias, signs of neuromuscular excitability) may require bolus of calcium gluconate injections 1–2 vials or continuous infusion (1–2 mg/kg body weight) with oral calcium (1–3 g) and vitamin D calcitriol (1–2 μg). IV calcium is tapered over 3–4 days gradually. The salts used are calcium carbonate, calcium citrate maleate (preferable as better tolerated and bioavailability). Oral calcium and vitamin D doses should be modified on weekly basis depending upon measurement of calcium and phosphate levels until biological equilibrium is reached. Magnesium deficiency, which can cause resistance to PTH, must be diagnosed and treated (1.5 g of magnesium/day) (Figure 22.29).

Thyroid insufficiency: Hypothyroidism is seen following lobotomy or hemi or TT. After HT thyroid function assessment should be done after 3 months. A total of 15–30% patients require thyroid hormone supplementation after HT. Risk factors for developing hypothyroidism after HT are age, sex, preoperative TSH level >1.5, lower free T4 levels, presence of antithyroid antibodies, autoimmune thyroiditis in the excised lobe and volume of remnant thyroid lobe. Various factors which influence the dose of thyroid hormone supplementation after surgery are body weight, age, sex, body mass index, preoperative TSH, iron supplementation and vitamin-mineral supplementation. After TT, dose of levothyroxine (LT4) is 1.6 μg/kg body weight. Table 22.3 shows various schemes proposed for the estimation of LT4 requirements after thyroidectomy. In malignancy, the thyroid hormone dose depends on thyroid cancer risk stratification whether low risk or high risk.

Recent technical advances in thyroid surgery

There have been several technical advancements with a purpose of reducing complications in thyroid surgery over the past decade. Following is a brief list:

1. Devices developed for surgical dissection which help in hemostasis and reduced heat transfer resulting in less direct or collateral tissue damage (Table 22.4).
2. Intraoperative nerve monitoring devices (IONM): The use of IONM has become recently popular in many institutions. The monitoring can continuous or intermittent. The equipment consists of a PVC endotracheal tube with inbuilt two pairs of electrodes which are positioned along the true vocal cords. An electrical arc is created from electrodes to vocalis muscle RLN and nerve stimulator. A 1-mA current is delivered through probe to RLN and a waveform is seen on screen with auditory signal when the arc is completed. So basic principle is that whenever the nerve is stimulated there is EMG signals produced and which are detected on monitor as waveform. Visual identification of the nerve remains the gold standard; however, IONM is useful in reoperative surgery, advanced cancers, in patients with one side paresis or paralysis. It has been seen to be more useful in EBSLN injury prevention (8).
3. Parathyroid hormone assays for early detection of hypocalcemia (15, 16)

South Asia Practice of thyroidectomy

Thyroidectomy operation in India and other South Asian countries is practiced by specialist endocrine surgeons' and by many other specialties like ENT, general and oncosurgeons. There is no watershed line between these specialties. The major part of surgery is still done by ENT or general surgeons; however, in last decades the major cities have specialist surgeons. The emergence

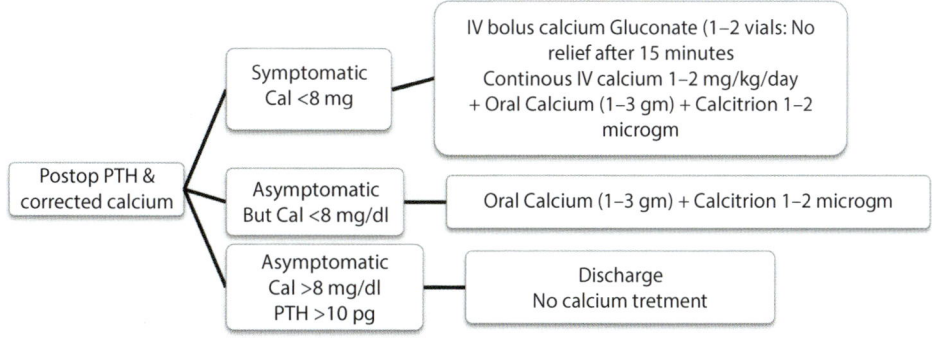

FIGURE 22.29 Management of hypocalcemia.

TABLE 22.3: Methods in the Literature for the Estimation of LT4 Requirements after Thyroidectomy

Author/Location	Formula or Scheme			
Cunningham et al. (18)	LT4 dose (μg/day) = 3.4 × LBM − 11			
	LBM (male) = (79.5 − 0.24 × weight − 0.15 × age) × weight/73.2			
	LBM (female) = (69.8 − 0.26 × weight − 0.12 × age) × weight/73.2			
Olubowale et al. (19)	LT4 dose (μg/day) = 100 if weight <53			
	= 125 if 53 ≤ weight ≤ 86			
	= 150 if 86 < weight ≤ 108			
	= 175 if weight >108			
Sukumar et al. (20)	Body surface area 2.04 μg/kg/day			
Mistry et al. (21)	LT4 dose (μg/day) = (0.943 × weight) + (−1.165 × age) + 125.8			
Ojomo et al. (22)	LT4 dose (μg/day) = (−0.018 × BMI + 2.13) × weight			
Jin et al. (23)	LT4 dose (μg/day) = 1.5 × weight			
Di Donna et al. (24)	LT4 dose (μg/kg/day) BMI	≤23	23–28	>28
	Age			
	≤40	1.8	1.7	1.6
	>40–55	1.7	1.6	1.5
	>55	1.6	1.5	1.4
Elfenbein et al. (25)	LT4 dose (μg/kg/day)		Male	Female
	BMI			
	<21		2.1	1.8
	22–26		1.9	1.7
	27–32		1.7	1.6
	33–40		1.5	1.4
	>40		1.3	1.2
Chen et al. (26)	Poisson regression dosing scheme using machine learning			

Abbreviations: LBM, Lean Body Mass; BMI, Body Mass Index; LT4, Levothyroxine.

TABLE 22.4: Hemostasis Devices: Advantages and Disadvantages (27, 28)

Methods/Device for Homeostasis	Advantage	Disadvantages
Suture ligation		• Risk of slippage, time consuming and cumbersome in closed spaces
		• Suture granuloma (foreign body reaction)
Vascular clips		• Risk of slippage, cost
		• Interfere with CT, MRI
Electrocautery — Monopolar		• High temperature at tip, >400°C
		• Hazardous near parathyroid glands and nerve
		• Lateral spread of heat 15 mm^3
Electrocautery — Bipolar	Good for smaller vessel, near nerves, parathyroids Lateral spread heat 1–6 mm^3	At 1 second the tip is cooler in comparison to monopolar but at 2 seconds the tip temperature is more
Electrothermal bipolar vessel sealing system – LigaSure • Enhancement of bipolar electrocautery which uses computer-controlled impedance monitoring • Hemostasis by tissue coagulation • Radiofrequency bipolar energy high current (4 A), low voltage (<200 V) to denature collagen, elastin and form a coagulative sealant	• Lateral spread of heat within 3 mm • Decreased transient hypocalcemia, reduce surgical time by 10–29 minutes in studies • Seal up to 7 mm vessels (FDA)	• Cost of the device and handpiece • No decrease in complication rates
Harmonic scalpel • Mechanical energy produces by ultrasound vibration of a blade at 55 kHz over distance of 80 denatures proteins by cleaving hydrogen bonds	• Less heat than electrocautery (60–80°C) • Lateral spread up to 2.2 mm • No current transmitted to patient • Coagulate and cut tissues simultaneously • Efficient dissection, produce less smoke, charring • Seal up to 5 mm vessels (FDA)	• Cost of the device • Connecting cable for specific number of cases • Handpiece (focus) use in specific number of cases • No decrease in complication rates

of the specialities has led to more standard operation and decrease in complications rate. The specialist surgeons believe in visualization of RLN while many old timer general surgeons still believe in not dissecting the nerve. IONM is practiced only in few centers. Most of the surgeons are moving from sub-TT to TT in case of benign multi nodular goiters. Suture less thyroidectomy is being done at many centers.

Conclusion

Thyroidectomy is indicated in established thyroid malignancy, suspicious of malignancy on history, clinical examination or investigation, in benign goiters with compressive symptoms, retrosternal extension and definitive therapy of hyperthyroidism and sometimes for diagnostic purposes in suspicious cases on FNAC. Preoperative counseling about the possible risks and complications of surgery like bleeding, voice changes and hypocalcemia should be discussed with patients and attendants. Nodulectomy or less than lobectomy is not a standard operation and minimum thyroid operation is lobectomy. Hypocalcemia and RLN injury are the two most common postthyroidectomy complications. Postoperative PTH and PTH gradient is used for predication of hypocalcemia. Hypocalcemia management depend on presentation whether biochemical or clinical and managed by administration of calcium plus vitamin D. Prevention of RLN injury depends on meticulously careful dissection and visualization of the nerves. In today's era with experienced surgeon and development of anesthesia techniques and modern surgical gadgets, thyroid surgery has become a very safe procedure.

References

1. Hannan SA. The magnificent seven: a history of modern thyroid surgery. Int J Surg. 2006;4(3):187–91.
2. Tröhler U. Towards endocrinology: Theodor Kocher's 1883 account of the unexpected effects of total ablation of the thyroid. J R Soc Med. 2011;104(3):129–32.
3. Rogers-Stevane J, Kauffman GL Jr. A historical perspective on surgery of the thyroid and parathyroid glands. Otolaryngol Clin North Am. 2008;41:1059.
4. Sinclair CF, Bumpous JM, Haugen BR, et al. Laryngeal examination in thyroid and parathyroid surgery: an American Head and Neck Society consensus statement: AHNS Consensus Statement. Head Neck. 2016;38:811.
5. Steurer M, Passler C, Denk DM, et al. Advantages of recurrent laryngeal nerve identification in thyroidectomy and parathyroidectomy and the importance of preoperative and postoperative laryngoscopic examination in more than 1000 nerves at risk. Laryngoscope. 2002;112:124.
6. Cirocchi R, Arezzo A, D'Andrea V, et al. Intraoperative neuromonitoring versus visual nerve identification for prevention of recurrent laryngeal nerve injury in adults undergoing thyroid surgery. Cochrane Database Syst Rev. 2019;1:CD012483.
7. Hayward NJ, Grodski S, Yeung M, Johnson WR, Serpell J. Recurrent laryngeal nerve injury in thyroid surgery: a review. ANZ J Surg. 2013;83(1–2):15–21.
8. Wong KP, Mak KL, Wong CK, Lang BH. Systematic review and meta-analysis on intraoperative neuro-monitoring in high-risk thyroidectomy. Int J Surg. 2017;38:21–30.
9. Adkisson CD, Howell GM, McCoy KL, et al. Surgeon volume and adequacy of thyroidectomy for differentiated thyroid cancer. Surgery. 2014;156:1453.
10. Adam MA, Thomas S, Youngwirth L, et al. Is there a minimum number of thyroidectomies a surgeon should perform to optimize patient outcomes? Ann Surg. 2016;265(2):402–407.
11. Haugen BR, Alexander EK, Bible KC, et al. 2015 American Thyroid Association management guidelines for adult patients with thyroid nodules and differentiated thyroid cancer: the American Thyroid Association Guidelines Task Force on thyroid nodules and differentiated thyroid cancer. Thyroid. 2016;26:1.
12. Erbil Y, Ozluk Y, Giriş M, et al. Effect of Lugol solution on thyroid gland blood flow and microvessel density in the patients with Graves' disease. J Clin Endocrinol Metab. 2007;92:2182.
13. Oltmann SC, Brekke AV, Schneider DF, et al. Preventing postoperative hypocalcemia in patients with Graves' disease: a prospective study. Ann Surg Oncol. 2015;22:952.
14. Mishra AK, Tamidari H, Singh N, Mishra SK, Agarwal A. External branch of superior laryngeal nerve in thyroid surgery: no more neglected nerve. Indian J Med Sci. 2007;61(1):3–8.
15. Grodski S, Serpell J. Evidence for the role of perioperative PTH measurement after total thyroidectomy as a predictor of hypocalcemia. World J Surg. 2008;32(7):1367–73.
16. Noordzij JP, Lee SL, Bernet VJ, et al. Early detection of hypocalcemia after thyroidectomy using parathyroid hormone: an analysis of pooled individual patient data from nine observational studies. J Am Coll Surg. 2007;205:748–54.
17. Agarwal A, Mishra AK, et al. High incidence of tracheomalacia in long-standing goiters: experience from an endemic goiter region. World J Surg. 2007;31(4):832–7.
18. Cunningham JJ, Barzel US. Lean body mass is a predictor of the daily requirement for thyroid hormone in older men and women. J Am Geriatr Soc. 1984;32:204–7.
19. Olubowale O, Chadwick DR. Optimization of thyroxine replacement therapy after total or near-total thyroidectomy for benign thyroid disease. Br J Surg. 2006;93:57–60.
20. Sukumar R, Agarwal A, Gupta S, et al. Prediction of LT4 replacement dose to achieve euthyroidism in subjects undergoing total thyroidectomy for benign thyroid disorders. World J Surg. 2010;34:527–31.
21. Mistry D, Atkin S, Atkinson H, et al. Predicting thyroxine requirements following total thyroidectomy. Clin Endocrinol (Oxf). 2011;74:384–7.
22. Ojomo KA, Schneider DF, Reiher AE, et al. Using body mass index to predict optimal thyroid dosing after thyroidectomy. J Am Coll Surg. 2013;216:454–60.
23. Jin J, Allemang MT, McHenry CR. Levothyroxine replacement dosage determination after thyroidectomy. Am J Surg. 2013;205:360–4.
24. Di Donna V, Santoro MG, de Waure C, Ricciato MP, Paragliola RM, Pontecorvi A, et al. A new strategy to estimate levothyroxine requirement after total thyroidectomy for benign thyroid disease. Thyroid. 2014;24:1759–64.
25. Elfenbein DM, Ojomo KA, Schaefer S, Shumway C, Chen H, Sippel RS, et al. Prospective intervention of a novel levothyroxine dosing protocol based on body mass index after thyroidectomy. J Am Coll Surg. 2014;219:S125.
26. Chen SS, Zaborek NA, Doubleday AR, et al. Optimizing levothyroxine dose adjustment after thyroidectomy with a decision tree. J Surg Res. 2019;244:102–6.
27. Becker AM, Gourin CG. New technologies in thyroid surgery. Surg Oncol Clin N Am. 2008;17(1):233–48.
28. Manouras A, Markogiannakis HE, Kekis PB, Lagoudianakis EE, Fleming B. Novel hemostatic devices in thyroid surgery: electrothermal bipolar vessel sealing system and harmonic scalpel. Expert Rev Med Dev. 2008;5(4):447–66.

23
POSTTHYROIDECTOMY HYPOCALCEMIA

Loreno E. Enny, Faraz Ahmad, Kul Ranjan Singh and Anand Kumar Mishra

Introduction

Hypocalcemia is the most common complication and cause of prolonged hospital stay following thyroid surgery (1). Total serum calcium levels less than the given normal reference range is known as biochemical hypocalcemia. Clinical hypocalcemia is defined as symptomatic hypocalcemia characterized by one or more of perioral/fingertip tingling and numbness, positive Trousseau's or Chvostek sign in the setting of biochemical hypocalcemia.

The reported incidence of postthyroidectomy hypocalcemia ranges from 13% to 49% (2, 3). A review of 114 observation studies pegged the median incidence of temporary and permanent hypocalcemia at 27% (19–38%) and 1% (0–3%), respectively. (4) Hypocalcemia occurring up to 6 months postsurgery defines transient/temporary hypocalcemia. Transient hypocalcemia may normalize spontaneously after the recovery of parathyroid glands. It may sometimes reflect dynamic changes in electrolyte and state of hydration rather than true hypocalcemia. Any hypocalcemia persisting beyond 6 months is permanent and it causes significant impairment to patient's quality of life requiring lifelong supplementation (5).

Although various causes of hypocalcemia have been described, including excessive loss of calcium in urine due to stress of surgery, vitamin D deficiency, hyperphosphatemia, hypercalcitonemia and hungry bone syndrome due to hyperparathyroidism. Postthyroidectomy hypocalcemia occurs due to inadvertent damage/removal of all four parathyroids and disturbance of blood supply to parathyroids (6). Knowledge of parathyroid anatomy along with meticulous surgery is needed to avert postoperative hypocalcemia.

Calcium homeostasis

Calcium in serum is present in three distinct fractions that are in equilibrium. Ionized and complexed calcium together account for 50% each. A total of 40–50% of the calcium is protein bound, of which 80% is bound to albumin and 20% to globulin; therefore, hypoalbuminemia can significantly lower the total serum calcium. A measured ionic calcium value is more accurate than total calcium or estimated ionic calcium. A corrected calcium value taking into consideration the albumin should ideally be used for management of patient.

$$\text{Corrected Calcium} = \text{Measured Calcium (mg/dL)} + 0.8(4 - \text{serum albumin (g/dL)})$$

Calcium regulation is executed by the synchronized action of parathyroid hormone (PTH), vitamin D and calcitonin at bone, kidney and intestine. Changes in ionized component of extracellular calcium are sensed by calcium sensing receptor (CaSR) present on parathyroid cell surface. Activations of these receptors by small increase in ionized calcium results in inhibition of PTH secretion whereas deactivation of this receptors results in increase in PTH secretion. The cascading effects of PTH are shown in Figure 23.1. PTH secretion and receptor activation require the presence of magnesium (7).

Clinical sign and symptoms

Presentation of hypocalcemia depends on the severity and rate of development of hypocalcemia. A rapid fall causes neuromuscular excitability and cardiac electrical instability but chronic hypocalcemia may remain asymptomatic or manifest by renal function derangements, premature cataracts, ectopic calcifications, convulsions, abnormal teeth and psychiatric symptoms (8). Paresthesia along with tingling and numbness more pronounced in perioral region and fingers are common early symptoms. Patient may appear confused and delirious. Sustained muscle contraction may lead to life-threatening bronchospasm or laryngospasm. Myocardial contractility may be depressed, and patients may present with heart failure or arrhythmias due to QT prolongation.

Signs of hypocalcemia include observed or elicited tetany. It is usually observed if ionized calcium level falls below 1 mmol/l. Sever hypocalcemia causes increase in neuronal permeability of sodium. Classic sign of hypocalcemia includes the following. All these signs should be tested before surgery to avoid false positives.

1. *Trousseau's sign (T-sign)* – manifested by hyperflexion of the wrist and metacarpophalangeal joints, hyperextension of the fingers and flexion of the thumb on raising the sphygmomanometer cuff 10 mmHg above the systolic blood pressure for 1 minute. T sign has a sensitivity of 94% for detecting hypocalcemia.
2. Chvostek sign is elicited by tapping the facial nerve 2 cm in front of the tragus of the ear. A positive sign results in abnormal contraction of the facial muscles. This sign is present in 25% of normal and up to 25% of hypocalcemic patients may not elicit this sign (9).
3. Hyperventilation induced.

Risk factors

Several risk factors predisposing to postthyroidectomy hypocalcemia have been described, including female sex, increased age at surgery, surgery for large volume goiter, recurrent goiter,

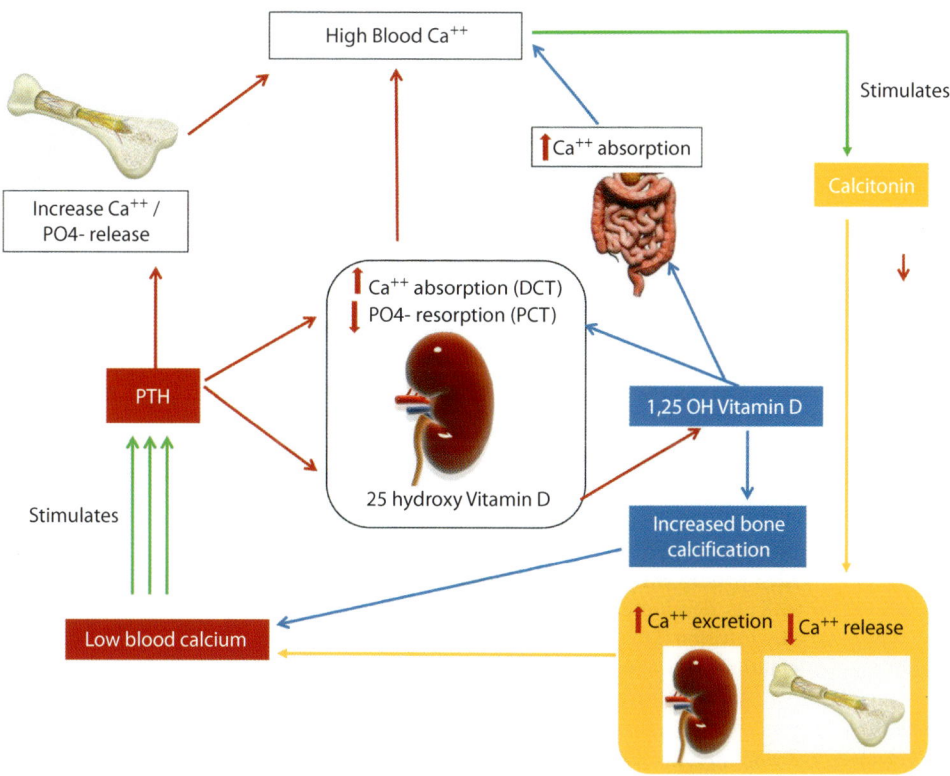

FIGURE 23.1 Calcium metabolism. *Abbreviations:* DCT: Distal convoluted tubule, PCT: Proximal convoluted tubule.

retrosternal extension, advanced cancer, hyperthyroidism and experience of the surgeons (10–13) (Table 23.1). Studies have contrasting views on many factors.

TABLE 23.1: Potential Risk Factors Predisposing Postthyroidectomy Hypocalcemia

Risk Factor	Variables
Patient factors	Female sex
	Pregnancy
	Lactation
	Age
Perioperative biochemistry	Serum calcium
	PTH
	Vitamin D
	Magnesium
	Alkaline phosphatase
Surgical related	Parathyroid identification
	Large volume thyroid
	Surgery for recurrent goiter
	Advanced thyroid cancer
	Total thyroidectomy
	Autoimmune thyroid disease (Graves' disease, thyroiditis)
	Central compartment lymph node
	Low volume thyroid surgeon
	Longer duration of surgery
	Substernal goiter
	Malabsorptive state
	Simultaneous thyroid and parathyroid surgery

Predictors of postthyroidectomy hypocalcemia

A number of biochemical- and surgical-related factors have been debated as predictors of hypocalcemia.

Biochemical predictors
Serum calcium

The association of preoperative/early postoperative low calcium level with postoperative hypocalcemia remains unclear. A recent metanalysis, including 2,439 patients, found association between low preoperative calcium and transient hypocalcemia and postoperative calcium <1.88 mmol/l at 24 hours with permanent hypocalcemia (4). However, in a large multicentric study, Bergenflez et al. in 2008, including 3,660 patients, found that a lower level of preoperative calcium level was associated with increased risk of postoperative hypocalcemia. (14) After thyroidectomy, a positive calcium slope at 6 and 12 hours or a negative calcium slope but normal calcium at 12 hours helps predict the development of hypocalcemia and feasibility of early discharge (15). Pattou et al. studied the predictors of hypocalcemia in 1.071 patients of subtotal or total thyroidectomy. They found that in patient receiving calcium supplementation at 1–3 weeks postsurgery, serum calcium of ≤2 mmol/l was significantly associated with increased risk of permanent hypocalcemia (16).

Serum PTH

Postoperative serum PTH is considered one of the most accurate predictors of hypocalcemia. Many centers use perioperative PTH measurements to predict postoperative hypocalcemia. Studies have shown that absolute PTH estimated at various stages or a negative pre-op to post-op PTH-gradient hypocalcemia (4, 17, 18). The absolute cutoff of PTH value or gradient and time frame varies from center to center and same needs to be standardized. Nowadays, most advanced centers use postoperative PTH and calcium level-based protocols to take decision regarding calcium/ Vit D supplementation and early discharge.

Vitamin D
Vit D levels as a sole predictor for hypocalcemia remains controversial. Studies have given conflicting results pertaining to preoperative Vit D levels and incidence of postoperative hypocalcemia (19–21).

Magnesium
Several retrospective and prospective studies have found a significant association between low magnesium level and postoperative hypocalcemia (22–24). Hypomagnesemia occurs commonly in postoperative period after thyroidectomy. In up to 1/3 patients, hypomagnesemia may coexist with hypocalcemia. Magnesium levels need to be monitored in patients developing hypocalcemia and same corrected by oral or I/v infusion if hypocalcemia is unresponsive to calcium supplementation

Alkaline phosphatase
It's a marker of bone turnover and high preoperative levels have been found in patients developing postthyroidectomy patients with normal PTH. This association was stronger after surgery performed for Graves' disease (25).

Surgery and patient-related factors
Parathyroid gland
Routine identification of parathyroid glands with preservation of delicate vasculature has been advocated for best outcomes during thyroid surgery is still a controversy. A large retrospective study, including 5,846 patients, found that identification of <2 parathyroid glands was 1.4 times more likely to develop temporary hypocalcemia and 4.1 times more likely to developed permanent hypocalcemia (26). However, contrary to this, Sheahan et al. found that patients having <2 PGs identified had lower incidence of hypocalcemia as compared to identification of 3–4 glands (27). Routine identification of parathyroids during surgery has been found to increase the rates of temporary hypocalcemia but significantly reduces the rates of permanent hypocalcemia (28).

Several agents help predict the viability of anatomically preserved parathyroid glands. Indocyanine green, aminolevulinic acid hydrochloride (5-ALA), methylene blue, parathyroid gland near-infrared fluorescence imaging (29–32).

Parathyroid autotransplantation is associated with a higher incidence of temporary hypocalcemia, but it is likely to reduce/not impact permanent hypocalcemia rates (4, 33). A large Australian study by Palazzo et al. examined the clinical outcomes after autotransplantation of 0,1, 2 or 3 parathyroid glands and found that the incidence of temporary hypocalcemia increased with increase in number of parathyroid glands autotransplanted but the number of glands auto transplanted did not impact permanent hypocalcemia rates (34).

Central neck dissection (CND)
Central neck dissection impacts hypocalcemia rates but its impact varies across difference studies. A metanalysis of 5 studies involving 1.132 patients noted that for every 7.7 central neck dissection performed with total thyroidectomy, there was one extra case of temporary hypocalcemia, but no significant difference was evident for permanent hypocalcemia. (35) Similar view were echoed in another metanalysis of 15 observational studies and 1 RCT.(36) South Korean national database of 192,333 patients found that thyroidectomy combined with CND was associated with greater risk of permanent hypocalcemia as compared to total thyroidectomy alone (5.4% vs. 4.6%, p < 0.001) (37).

Surgical volume
Surgeon volume has a significant impact in outcome of thyroid surgery. Volumes inversely correlated with complication rates, duration of hospital stays and total cost in many studies. A prospective study by Gonzalez et al. analyzed the relationship between surgeon volume and morbidity in patients operated by dedicated endocrine surgeons and those operated by general surgeons. The study found that rate of hypocalcemia (both temporary and permanent) was significantly higher in those patients operated by general surgeon (<5 surgery per surgeon per year) than those operated by endocrine surgeons (>40 surgery per surgeon per year) (38). In contrast to this study, however, Thomusch et al. found no link between surgical volume (<10 and 10–50 compared to >50 per year) and temporary and permanent hypocalcemia (26).

Other surgical-related factors found to be potential predictors for permanent hypocalcemia are longer duration of surgery and surgery for recurrent goiter (39, 40).

Patient factors
Factors relating to age, female gender, surgery for cancers, hyperthyroidism and retrosternal goiter have been found to predictors for developing hypocalcemia (41–43).

Treatment of hypocalcemia

The treatment of hypocalcemia depends on the severity and underlying cause. For example, asymptomatic hypocalcemia may not require therapy, while severe hypocalcemia (i.e. total corrected serum calcium level of <7.5 mg/dl or ionized calcium concentration <0.9 mmol/l) or acute symptomatic hypocalcemia merits urgent medical attention.

Postoperative prophylaxis

Meticulous surgery preserving delicate parathyroid blood supply is the best prophylaxis for preventing hypocalcemia. Despite preserving the parathyroid glands, hypocalcemia has been reported to occur after 10–20% of thyroid surgery and can be increased up to 30% or more after surgery for hyperthyroidism and cancer (44).

Empirical prophylactic postoperative management of hypocalcemia is to start oral calcium routinely with or without calcitriol immediately after surgery without testing for serum calcium and PTH level. Routine calcium supplementation has been found to be cost-effective and also has both advantages of early discharge of the patients and preventing postoperative hypocalcemia symptoms. Several oral and parenteral calcium preparations are used for treatment of hypocalcemia, including oral calcium carbonate, citrate maleate, phosphate, acetate and parenteral calcium gluconate, chloride and lactate (Table 23.2), of which oral calcium carbonate is the most widely available and least expensive and also provides the highest amount of elemental calcium. It is given

TABLE 23.2: Calcium Preparations

Calcium Formulations	% of Elemental Calcium	Notes
Oral calcium formulations		
Calcium carbonate	40	Small, frequent dosing, requires acidic environment for absorption; best taken in between meals
Calcium citrate	21	Preferred option for patients on proton pump inhibitor, achlorhydria
Calcium phosphate	31–38	Solubility is less than that of calcium carbonate
Calcium acetate	25	Preferred choice in CRF with hyperphosphatemia
Parenteral formulations		
Calcium gluconate	9	Dose to be individualized and frequent calcium monitoring (preferably ionic)
Calcium chloride	27.3	Tissue toxicity is high and, hence, better infused through central line

TABLE 23.4: Prophylactic Postoperative Management

Preparations	Dose
Calcium salts	
Calcium carbonate	1000–3000 mg/day
Calcium citrate maleate	1000–3000 mg/day
Vitamin D	
1,25-Dihydoxycholecalciferol (calcitriol)	0.5–2 µg/day
25 Hydroxycholecalciferols	50,000 IU/week × 8–12 weeks

at a dose 500–1000 mg (one to three times a day) (Table 23.4). Calcium salt selection also depends on the availability, cost, patient tolerance and surgeon preference. Routine administration of oral calcium has been reported to reduce postoperative hypocalcemia (45).

A decision to add Vitamin D can be based on the preoperative vitamin D level if available. Several preparations of vitamin D include cholecalciferol, calcitriol, ergocalciferol, calcifediol, alfacalcidol and dihydrotachysterol (Table 23.3). Adding calcitriol, usually in a dose of 0.5–1 µg/day increases the effectiveness oral calcium (44, 46, 47). Calcitriol increases the intestinal absorption of calcium. The half-life of calcitriol is 5–8 hours whereas half-life of cholecalciferol is weeks to months. However, this aggressive approach may be sometimes associated with serious risk of overshooting and causing hypercalcemia and potential renal injury. Therefore, patients given prophylaxis should be monitored for rebound hypercalcemia and/or vitamin D toxicity as appropriate.

Treatment of early/mild-to-moderate hypocalcemia

Postoperative calcium supplementation should be considered if postsurgery PTH <15 pg/ml and corrected calcium <8.5 mg/dl or ionized calcium of < 1 mmol/l, The recommended dose of calcium carbonate 1–3 g/day or calcium citrate 2–6 g/day with the addition of calcitriol of 0.25–0.5 µg two times a day in patients who are symptomatic and if serum calcium level is declining on sequential measuring or remaining below 7 mg/dl. Magnesium oxide at a dose of 400 mg once or twice daily to be added if serum magnesium level is <1.6 mg/dl. Calcium level should be measured at least every 24 hourly or more frequently if there is decline in serial calcium level or if patient become symptomatic. The management of hypocalcemia is summarized in Table 23.5.

Treatment of progressive/symptomatic hypocalcemia

If severe symptomatic hypocalcemia develops despite oral calcium and calcitriol supplementation or patient develops trousseaus sign, parenteral infusion is indicated. Calcium gluconate is the preferred salt despite lower calcium content compared to calcium chloride. A 12 lead ECG, corrected QT interval should also be measured. Initial one or three doses of calcium is given by intravenous (i.v.) bolus of 1–2 g of calcium gluconate in 50 ml of 5% dextrose infused over 20 minutes. Up to 3 g of calcium gluconate can be infused over 30–90 minutes to control severe symptoms. Thereafter, a continuous infusion of calcium will be required at a rate of 1–1.5 mg/kg/h and should not exceed 1–2 mg/min. Oral therapy should be instituted as soon as possible and the infusion tapered slowly (over a period of 24–48 hours or longer). Serum calcium levels should be monitored frequently during infusion.

If the serum magnesium level is low, 2–4 g of magnesium sulfate is added every 8 hours.

In spite of all these efforts and treatment, if the calcium level remains low, thiazide diuretics may be considered. It enhances calcium absorption from distal renal tubules thereby decreasing the urinary calcium excretion. It is given at a dose of 12.5–50 mg/day but may be titrated to avoid hypotension.

Once the patient is stable enough to be discharged on oral calcium and vitamin D, calcium level should be monitored at least twice weekly and dose of oral calcium plus vitamin D to be slowly tapered off. Some few patients, especially those operated for Graves' disease, are at risk of developing 'Hungry bone syndrome' (profound, rapid and chronic hypocalcemia with

TABLE 23.3: Vitamin D Preparations

Preparations	Dosing Information	Onset of Action	Notes
D_2 (ergocalciferol) D_3 (cholecalciferol)	2000–100,000 IU OD	10–14 days	Serum calcium, phosphorus and creatinine to be monitored
Calcifediol	20–200 µg/day	5–10 days	Used in patient with hepatic failure with intact renal function
Alfacalcidol	0.5–3 µg/day	1–2 days	Rapidly conversion to active 1,25-dihydroxyvitamin D_3
1,25-Dihydroxyvitamin D_3	0.25–1 µg once or twice daily	1–2 days	Does not require renal conversion
Dihydrotachysterol	0.2–1 mg/day	4–7 days	Active D metabolite

TABLE 23.5: Recommendation for Management of Hypoparathyroidism (5)

Setting	Indication	Oral Calcium	Oral Vitamin D_3	I.V. Calcium	Magnesium
Early/mild to moderate	PTH <15 pg/ml or Serum calcium <8.5 mg/dl or ionized calcium <1.1 mmol/l	1–3 g BID-TID	Calcitriol 0.25–0.5 µg BID (Symptomatic hypocalcemia and serum calcium level that is declining on sequential measurements or remaining below 7 mg/dl	N/A	400 mg once or twice daily (if serum magnesium level is <1.6 mg/dl
Progressive/ symptomatic	• Symptoms and sign of hypocalcemia progress • Serum calcium remains below 7 mg/dl	3–4 g daily in divided doses BID-QID	Calcitriol 0.25–1 mcg BID	i.v. bolus of 1–2 g calcium gluconate followed by i.v. infusion	• Intravenous magnesium sulfate (2–4 g) every 8 hours • Oral magnesium

hypomagnesemia and hypophosphatemia due to rapid influx of calcium from blood to bone after surgery) and, therefore, should be monitored closely.

Management of chronic hypocalcemia

Therapy is individualized to keep patient asymptomatic and maintain the serum calcium level slightly below the normal reference range or in the normal range, to maintain the calcium phosphate product to below 55 mg^2/dl^2, to prevent hypercalciuria, renal/dystrophic calcifications.

Conventional management options for patients with chronic hypocalcemia include dietary calcium and oral calcium supplements with dose ranging up to 3500 mg of elemental calcium per day. Calcitriol is usually recommended, with most patient requiring 0.25 µg/day (0.25–4.0 µg/day). Vitamin D2 (ergocalciferol) and vitamin D3 (cholecalciferol) are occasionally used for long-term management.

Hydrochlorothiazide in a dose of 12.5–50 mg/day can be added to prevent hypercalciuria. Phosphate binders with low phosphate diet may occasionally be required.

Monitoring guidelines on conventional therapy

The frequency of monitoring should be individualized based on dose requirement and patient's conditions (48) Parameters to be monitored are serum calcium, phosphate, magnesium, BUN/creatinine, 24 hours urinary along with urinary calcium. Extraskeletal calcification and bone mineral density should be monitored as clinically indicated (48)

Acute episodes in chronic hypocalcemia

Even after the patient is stabilized on oral calcium and vitamin D supplements, certain predisposing factors including acute illness, sepsis, stress, dehydration, pregnancy, lactation, intestinal surgeries and vitamin D deficiency may cause episodes of hypocalcemia or hypercalcemia. There are no controlled data on the use of calcitriol in human pregnancy and caution is to be exercised. Calcitriol use is also not recommended during lactation because it is presumed to pass into breast milk. Thus, if it is used during breastfeeding, serum calcium levels of both mother and infant should be monitored (5).

Newer therapies – synthetic PTH

Recombinant PTH (1–84) (rhPTH [1–84]) has revolutionized management of patients with refractory hypoparathyroidism. rhPTH reduced the requirement of calcium and vitamin D supplementation by 50% and an associated decrease in urinary calcium along with improvement of bone density (49–51).

Indication for considering the use of rhPTH (1–84) should not be limited to biochemical hypocalcemia or requirement of large doses of calcium and vitamin D to maintain normal calcium levels. The formation of renal stones, nephrocalcinosis, reduced creatinine clearance and hypercalciuria merit rhPTH therapy. A calcium phosphate product >55, malabsorptive states or compromised quality of life, should prompt rhPTH therapy (48)

Teriparatide acetate [rhPTH (1–34)] introduced for the treatment of osteoporosis holds promise as an alternative for treatment for postoperative hypoparathyroidism (52, 53).

South Asian perspective

The reported incidence of post thyroidectomy hypocalcemia is similar to that of western countries. Technological advances along with improved access to endocrine surgery facilities is likely to improve the outcomes further.

Summary

Post total thyroidectomy hypocalcemia causes significant short- and long-term morbidity. Meticulous surgery preserving delicate parathyroid vasculature remains the best prophylaxis of post-thyroidectomy hypocalcemia. There are several predictors of postoperative hypocalcemia and knowledge of these predictors in individualizing early discharge and monitoring. The treatment of hypocalcemia depends on the severity and underlying cause of hypocalcemia.

References

1. Hauch A, Al-Qurayshi Z, Randolph G, Kandil E. Total thyroidectomy is associated with increased risk of complications for low- and high-volume surgeons. Ann Surg Oncol 2014; 21: 3844–52.
2. Wingert DJ, Friesen SR, Iliopoulos JI, et al. Post-thyroidectomy hypocalcemia. Incidence and risk factors. Am J Surg 1986; 152: 606–10.
3. Wiseman JE, Mossanen M, Ituarte PH, et al. An algorithm informed by the parathyroid hormone level reduces hypocalcemic complications of thyroidectomy. World J Surg. 2010; 34: 532–7.
4. Edafe O, Antakia R, Laskar N, Uttley L, Balasubramanian SP. Systematic review and meta-analysis of predictors of post-thyroidectomy hypocalcaemia. Br J Surg 2014; 101: 307–20.

5. Orloff LA, Wiseman SM, Bernet VJ, et al. American thyroid association statement on postoperative hypoparathyroidism: diagnosis, prevention, and management in adults. Thyroid. 2018 Jul;28(7):830–841.
6. Bilezikian JP, Khan A, Potts JT Jr, Brandi ML, Clarke BL, Shoback D et al. Hypoparathyroidism in the adult: epidemiology, diagnosis, pathophysiology, target-organ involvement, treatment, and challenges for future research. J Bone Miner Res. 2011; 26: 2317–233.
7. Tong GM, Rude RK, magnesium deficiency in critical illness. J Intensive Care Med. 2006; 20(1): 3–17.
8. Underbjerg L, Sikjaer T, Mosekilde L, et al. Postsurgical hypoparathyroidism–risk of fractures, psychiatric diseases, cancer, cataract, and infections. J Bone Miner Res 2014; 29: 2504–10.
9. Fonseca, OA, Calverley JR. Neurological manifestations of hypoparathyroidism. Arch Intern Med. 1967; 120(2): 202–6.
10. Del Rio, Rossini M, et al. Postoperative hypocalcemia: analysis of factors influencing early hypocalcemia development following thyroid surgery. BMC Surg. 2019; 18(suppl 1): 25.
11. Thomusch O, Machens A, Sekulla C, et al. Multivariate analysis of risk factors for postoperative complications in benign goiter surgery: prospective multicenter study in Germany. World J Surg. 2000; 24: 1335–41.
12. Zambudio AR, Rodríguez J, Riquelme J, Soria T, Canteras M, Parrilla P. Prospective study of postoperative complications after total thyroidectomy for multinodulargoiters by surgeons with experience in endocrine surgery. Ann Surg. 2004; 240: 18–25.
13. Wingert DJ, Friesen SR, Iliopoulos JI, Pierce GE, Thomas JH, Hermreck AS. Post-thyroidectomy hypocalcemia. Incidence and risk factors. Am J Surg. 1986; 152: 606–10.
14. Bergenfelz A, Jansson S, Kristoffersson A, et al. Complications to thyroid surgery: results as reported in a database from a multicenter audit comprising 3,660 patients. Langenbecks Arch Surg 2008; 393: 667–73.
15. Nahas et al. A safe and cost-effective short hospital stay protocol to identify patients at low risk for the development of significant hypocalcemia after total thyroidectomy. Laryngoscope. 2006 Jun; 116(6): 906–10.
16. Pattou F, Combemale F, Fabre S, et al. Hypocalcemia following thyroid surgery: incidence and prediction of outcome. World J Surg. 1998; 22: 718–24.
17. Lecerf P, Orry D, Perrodeau E, et al. Parathyroid hormone decline 4 hours after total thyroidectomy accurately predicts hypocalcemia. Surgery. 2012; 152: 863–8.
18. Schlottmann F, Arbulú AL, Sadava EE, et al. Algorithm for early discharge after total thyroidectomy using PTH to predict hypocalcemia: prospective study. Langenbecks Arch Surg. 2015; 400: 831–6.
19. Al-Khatib T et al. Severe vitamin D deficiency: a significant predictors of early hypocalcemia after total thyroidectomy. Otolaryngol-Head Neck Surg. 2014;152(3):424–31.
20. Cherian AJ, Ponraj S, Gowri SM, et al. The role of vitamin D in post-thyroidectomy hypocalcemia: still an enigma. Surgery. 2016; 159: 532–8.
21. Lee GH, Ku YH, Kim HI, et al. Vitamin D level is not a predictor of hypocalcemia after total thyroidectomy. Langenbecks Arch Surg. 2015; 400: 617–22.
22. Garrahy A, Murphy MS, Sheahan P. Impact of postoperative magnesium levels on early hypocalcemia and permanent hypoparathyroidism after thyroidectomy. Head Neck. 2016; 38: 613–9.
23. Chincholikar SP, Ambiger S. Association of hypomagnesemia with hypocalcaemia after thyroidectomy. Indian J Endocr Metab. 2018; 22: 656–60.
24. Cherian AJ, Gowri M, Ramakant P, et al. The role of magnesium in post-thyroidectomy hypocalcemia. World J Surg. 2016; 40: 881–8.
25. Miah MS, Mahendran S, Mak C, et al. Pre-operative serum alkaline phosphatase as a predictive indicator of post-operative hypocalcaemia in patients undergoing total thyroidectomy. J Laryngol Otol. 2015; 129: 1128–32.
26. Thomusch O, Machens A, Sekulla C, et al. The impact of surgical technique on postoperative hypoparathyroidism in bilateral thyroid surgery: a multivariate analysis of 5846 consecutive patients. Surgery. 2003; 133: 180–5.
27. Sheahan P, Mehanna R, Basheeth N, et al. Is systematic identification of all four parathyroid glands necessary during total thyroidectomy? a prospective study. Laryngoscope. 2013; 123: 2324–8.
28. Puzziello A, Rosato L, Innaro N, et al. Hypocalcemia following thyroid surgery: incidence and risk factors. A longitudinal multicenter study comprising 2,631 patients. Endocrine. 2014; 47: 537–42.
29. Sound S, Okoh A, Yigitbas H, Yazici P, Berber E. Utility of indocyanine green fluorescence imaging for intraoperative localization in reoperative parathyroid surgery. Surg Innov. 2019 Dec;26(6):774–779.
30. Tummers QR, Schepers A, Hamming JF, et al. Intraoperative guidance in parathyroid surgery using near-infrared fluorescence imaging and low-dose methylene blue. Surgery. 2015; 158: 1323–30.
31. McWade MA, Sanders ME, Broome JT, Solorzano CC, Mahadevan-Jansen A. Establishing the clinical utility of autofluorescence spectroscopy for parathyroid detection. Surgery 2016; 159: 193–202.
32. Galvez-Pastor S, et al. Prediction of hypocalcemia after total thyroidectomy using indocyanine green angiography of parathyroid glands: a simple quantitative scoring system. Am J Surg. 2019 Nov; 218(5): 993–9.
33. Lo CY, Lam KY. Routine parathyroid autotransplantation during thyroidectomy. Surgery. 2001; 129: 318–23.
34. Palazzo FF, et al. Parathyroid autotransplantation during total thyroidectomy – does the number of glands transplanted affect outcomes? World J Surg. 2005; 29: 629–31.
35. Chisholm EJ, Kulinskaya E, Tolley NS. Systematic review and meta-analysis of the adverse effects of thyroidectomy combined with central neck dissection as compared with thyroidectomy alone. Laryngoscope. 2009; 119: 1135–9.
36. Lang BH, Ng SH, Lau LL, et al. A systematic review and meta-analysis of prophylactic central neck dissection on short-term locoregional recurrence in papillary thyroid carcinoma after total thyroidectomy. Thyroid. 2013; 23: 1087.
37. Seo, GH Chai, YJ et al. Incidence of permanent hypocalcaemia after total thyroidectomy with or without central neck dissection for thyroid carcinoma: a nationwide claim study. Clin Endocrinol. 2016 Sep; 85(3): 483–7.
38. González-Sánchez C, Franch-Arcas G, Gómez-Alonso A. Morbidity following thyroid surgery: does surgeon volume matter? Langenbecks Arch Surg. 2013; 398: 419–22.
39. Hallgrimsson P, Nordenstrom E, Almquist M, et al. Risk factors for medically treated hypocalcemia after surgery for Graves' disease: a Swedish multicenter study of 1,157 patients. World J Surg. 2012; 36: 1933–42.
40. Cappellani A, Di Vita M, Zanghi A, et al. The recurrent goiter: prevention and management. Ann Ital Chir. 2008; 79: 247–53.
41. Vitalijus E, Algridas S, et al. Predictors of postoperative hypocalcaemia occurring after a total thyroidectomy: result of a prospective multicentric study. BMC Surg. 2018; 18: 55
42. Erbil Y, Barbaros U, Temel B, et al. The impact of age, vitamin D(3) level, and incidental parathyroidectomy on. Am J Surg. 2009; 197: 439–46.
43. Testini M, Gurrado A, Avenia N, et al. Does mediastinal extension of the goiter increase morbidity of total thyroidectomy? A multicenter study of 19,662 patients. Ann Surg Oncol. 2011; 18: 2251–9.
44. Karakas E, Osei-Agyemang T, Schlosser K, et al. The impact of parathyroid auto transplantation during bilateral surgery for Graves' disease on postoperative hypocalcemia. Endocr Regul. 2008;42:39–44.
45. Arer M, Kus M, et al. Prophylactic oral calcium supplementation therapy to prevent early post thyroidectomy hypocalcemia and evaluation of postoperative parathyroid hormone levels to detect hypocalcemia: a prospective randomized study. Inter J Surg. 2017; 38: 9–14.
46. Alhefdhi A, Mazeh H, Chen H. Role of postoperative vitamin D and/or calcium routine supplementation in preventing hypocalcemia after thyroidectomy: a systematic review and meta-analysis, Oncologist. 2013; 18(5): 533–42.
47. Stack BC, et al. AACE and ACE disease state clinical review: postoperative hypoparathyroidism - definitions and management. Endocrine Pract. June 2015; 21(No. 6): 674–85.
48. Brandi ML, et al. Management of hypoparathyroidism: summary statement and guidelines. J Clin Endocrinol Metabol. 2016; 101(6): 2273–83.
49. Sikjaer T, Rejnmark L, Rolighed L, Heickendorff L, Mosekilde L, Hypoparathyroid Study Group. The effect of adding PTH(1-84) to conventional treatment of hypoparathyroidism: a randomized, placebo-controlled study. J Bone Miner Res. 2011; 26: 2358–70.
50. Cusano NE, Rubin MR, McMahon DJ, et al. Therapy of hypoparathyroidism with PTH (1-84): a prospective four-year investigation of efficacy and safety. J Clin Endocrinol Metab. 2013; 98: 137–44.
51. Mannstadt M, Clarke BL, Vokes T, et al. Efficacy and safety of recombinant human parathyroid hormone (1-84) in hypoparathyroidism (REPLACE): a double-blind, placebo-controlled, randomised, phase 3 study. Lancet Diabetes Endocrinol. 2013; 1: 275–83.
52. Shah M, Bancos I, Thompson GB, et al. Teriparatide therapy and reduced postoperative hospitalization for postoperative hypoparathyroidism. Otolaryngol Head Neck Surg. 2015; 141: 822–27.
53. Palermo A, Mangiameli G, Tabacco G, et al. PTH(1-34) for the Primary Prevention of Postthyroidectomy Hypocalcemia: The THYPOS Trial. J Clin Endocrinol Metab. 2016 Nov; 101(11): 4039–45.

24

NECK DISSECTIONS IN THYROID CANCER

Chintamani

Introduction

...Technically challenging that is synonymous with killing a mosquito with a gun ... the irony is ... this unique cancer with long term survival is a boon for patients and bane for researchers as the controversies remain unresolved in the absence of any substantial prospective data ...

Anonymous

With the rising incidence of thyroid cancers and particularly the differentiated thyroid cancer (DTC), more and more surgeons would be operating on thyroid in future. According to the Surveillance and End Results Program (SEER), there will be 62,450 new cases of thyroid cancer and estimated 1950 deaths estimated in 2015. The overall 5-year survival rate, however, has been stable at around 98% in the last couple of decades [1, 2].

So, it continues to be a good and relatively benign cancer with a good outcome, and in DTCs, one may be talking about 20-year survival. The other significant difference from cancers of other sites is the availability of a very effective adjunct in the form of radioiodine (RAI) therapy. Therefore, if thyroidectomy alone also is performed in clinically node negative patients, one can achieve a similar outcome. Does that justify an inadequate surgery? Certainly not, and no amount of RAI therapy is a compensation for suboptimal surgery.

In view of such good outcomes many believe, an extra aggressive approach may sometimes amount to *killing a mosquito with a gun*. With such excellent outcomes, the associated and lasting morbidity may not be justifiable even in a minority of cases. At the same time, the flip side thinking could be this is one cancer where one can offer cure, and therefore, an aggressive approach still makes sense, at least in selected cases. But it is also mandatory and justifiably so to consider the associated morbidity especially with low volume surgeons and centers. The key, therefore, lies in tailoring the therapy to the patient, tumor, center and the surgeon.

The very high incidence, heterogenous nature and sporadic pattern make prospective randomized controlled trials (RCTs) in these cancers an obvious challenge. So, whatever data or recommendations that are available are based on observational trials and retrospective studies. This could be a problem as such studies always involve some biases. The handicap is the nonfeasibility and, therefore, nonavailability of any prospective RCTs for this cancer. This would not only apply to the extent of optimum surgery for the primary but also to the extent of neck dissections in these cancers. According to various studies, it is estimated that some prerequisites must be met before contemplating an RCT in thyroid cancer to get a statistically significant outcome. A total of 5840 patients will have to be included, it will have to be a 7-year study with 4 years enrolment and at least 5 years of average follow-up will be needed.

It is also interesting that the AJCC 8th staging system for head and neck squamous cell cancers (HNSCC) emphasizes on the status of cervical lymph nodes – their presence, size, number have considerable significance, and thus, their management remains the cornerstone in surgery for these cancers. The same, however, is not true for DTCs, and most studies indicate that involvement of cervical lymph nodes does not have a great prognostic impact on outcome of DTCs. This also reflects in the staging system that gives more importance to the primary tumor while neck nodes are indicated only as absent or present with no mentioning of their size or number.

There is also a continuous debate about our knowledge regarding the biological behavior of this disease in the absence of any prospective randomized controlled trials. The biological nature of thyroid cancer is heterogenous and so is its distribution. At one end of the spectrum are DTCs with an indolent clinical course, excellent prognosis and reasonably good outcome and at the others are the deadliest of all cancers like anaplastic carcinomas with a lethal outcome.

It has been known for a long time now that presence of lymph nodes may not affect the overall survival, although the recurrence-free survival may be affected. Therefore, the extent and type of neck dissection should not make a difference. So how much is the optimum surgery for thyroid cancers continues to be a subject that is still debated, although for an oncologist and endocrine surgeon, oncological clearance of any cancer regardless of its nature would be an inherent tendency.

The primary goal in a cancer surgery is to save life and provide disease or recurrence-free survival. However, thyroid cancer is unique in this regard because of very low mortality rates and very long survival irrespective of the treatment provided. Hence, it becomes rather necessary to tailor and set our goals in context of the nature and behavior of thyroid cancer.

The goals of treatment in thyroid cancers are:

- Improving survival
- Decreasing rate of recurrence
- Minimizing morbidity

Is anything that is not worth doing, worth doing well?

Most thyroid surgeons including the author would mostly complete central neck dissection along with total thyroidectomy because as they say *"since it is there and we are there might as well do it"*. It is well known that the morbidity of reexploring the neck is definitely much higher and lower recurrence rates do affect the outcome in some way. The flip side being the fact that overall survival being reasonably good in patients with DTCs irrespective of the treatment, there is not much to gain on that account. The primary goal of treatment in thyroid cancer is, therefore, to have a prolonged "recurrence-free" survival because with recurrence there is likelihood of dedifferentiation changing the biology and, thus, the outcome. One may, therefore, consider neck dissection either as an ***essential evil or an overkill***. There is also an improvement in the accuracy of staging (upstaging), but this won't necessarily translate in to any survival benefit.

Like it has happened in case of breast cancer, axillary lymph node dissection once used to be a staging procedure, but now it will be considered an overkill in an N0 disease. The addressal of drainage basin, in this case axilla, is now being done with sentinel lymph node biopsy and/or other sampling techniques. The recent advances in imaging modalities with dedicated breast radiologists, one can hit the target most of the times. But the same has not been achieved in cases of thyroid cancer. Imaging modalities, although have got better, still lack the sensitivity and specificity to be able to confirm the presence or absence of metastatic nodes in the neck preoperatively. High-resolution USG with Doppler or elastography have made it much better and more sensitive but besides being operator dependent are still not the gold standard in detecting the nodal metastases.

In some studies, 40% of node negative patients had positive central nodes on histopathology and in a recent study where patients were subjected to routine systematic node dissection, 80% of pathologically positive nodes were found have been misjudged by the operating surgeon as being clinically negative. This certainly can translate into high "long term recurrence rates" (15–30%) which is the main concern in clinically node-negative (cN0) patients. This definitely supports the argument in favor of routine prophylactic central neck dissection (pCND) [3, 4].

Incidence of positive nodes in thyroid cancers

According to SEER database-2014 registry, the distribution of these nodes is as follows:

- Ipsilateral central compartment – 42–86%
- Ipsilateral lateral groups – 32–68%
- Contralateral lateral groups – 12–24%
- Mediastinal group – 3–20%

Since majority of these cancers can present or are detected early (following some routine ultrasound scanning of neck), most of the may not have any lymph nodes warranting attention. There is, however, an issue with the occult lymph node metastases (*or laboratory metastases*), and it has been found in many studies that they may be present in 50–60% cases, although their clinical or prognostic significance is debatable, and in a large majority, they may not become clinically apparent as macro-metastases [1, 5].

Surveillance and follow-up of microscopic disease

It has been observed on following up these cases that only 10% of recurrent thyroid bed nodules are observed in low-risk DTC that increase substantially in size and nearly 15% disappear [6].

Risk factors for the presence and prediction of lymph node metastases (central compartment) in thyroid cancers especially DTC [1]:

- T-size
- Extrathyroidal extension
- Aggressive histology
- Male gender
- Extremes of age

The current status and significance nodal disease in thyroid cancers

The current AJCC 8th edition does not make any distinction between whether central or the lateral group of lymph nodes is involved. Besides the age criteria (< or >55 years), presence or absence of lymph node metastases divides the stages between N0 and N1 (stages I and II), unlike the 7th edition where a distinction was made between central compartment nodal involvement (N1a) and lateral nodal involvement (N1b). In many cases, it may be difficult to differentiate clearly between level-VI (N1a) and VII (which was staged as N1b).

Is the lymphatic spread predictable (skip metastases and their significance)?

Although the pattern of lymphatic spread is fairly predictable in DTCs, there are studies indicating that the usually accepted pattern of first central compartment (level VI) and then downward and lateral spread (levels III and IV) may not be observed in some percentage of patients that may actually have skip metastases (Figure 24.1). These if neglected/missed during dissection may be associated with local recurrence [7].

Likely predictors of skip metastases

- Age >55 years
- Unilateral tumors (bilateral tumors have a higher incidence of central compartment nodal involvement while unilaterality has been associated with skip metastases to lateral groups)
- Extrathyroidal extension [8, 9]
- Tumors confined to the superior portion of thyroid (24.6% probably the lymphatic drainage following the blood supply and drainage from superior thyroid pedicle and lateral nodes may be the first echelon in these tumors)

Some authors have developed a prediction model for skip metastases and recommend tailoring of neck dissection based on this model especially in papillary thyroid cancers [7].

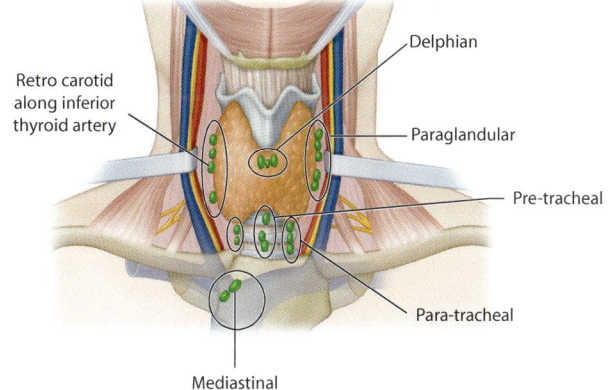

FIGURE 24.1 The lymphatic drainage of thyroid gland. The boundaries of the central compartment of neck extend from hyoid bone superiorly, innominate vein inferiorly and internal jugular veins on either side. The first echelon of spread is the central compartment nodes. Some including the author consider Delphian node as a sentinel node for the central compartment and lateral nodes spread. Retrocarotid nodes are an important group that lie along the inferior thyroid vessels posterior to common carotid artery are important site for recurrence. Therefore, they must be dissected meticulously.

Pre-laryngeal node (Delphian) and its significance

There is a special significance attached to the pre-laryngeal node (Delphian node), and many believe it to be the sentinel node in DTC. This node is often associated with **an aggressive histology, extrathyroidal extension (ETE), central and lateral nodes involvement.** It is recommended to sample this node as a sentinel node for predicting involvement of central and lateral compartment [1, 10].

Indications for neck dissections in thyroid cancers with node positive necks

1. All patients of **DTC** would undergo lateral neck dissections (ipsilateral) in the form of selective neck dissection (SND), modified radical neck dissection (MRND-III) or functional neck dissection. There is rarely an indication to perform routine clearance of levels I, Va and IIb.
2. For all **medullary thyroid cancers (MTC) that are N0**, all patients should undergo total thyroidectomy along with central neck dissection (levels VI, VII), i.e., Delphian node, pre- and paratracheal nodes, nodes along inferior thyroid artery under the carotid vessels. The lower limit being innominate vessel (Figure 24.1)
3. In **MTC > 4 cm** in size that are N0 or if the neck has positive nodes, ipsilateral MRND-III or SND along with removal of levels I–V nodes and preservation of extra-lymphatic structures (SAN, IJV, SCM) may have to be done.

Prophylactic (pCND) or elective central neck dissection in thyroid cancers

Prophylactic central neck dissection (pCND) is defined as the complete excision of level VI (a and b) and rarely level-VII lymph nodes (*based on the recognized anatomic continuity from the neck and superior mediastinum*) in patients with no evidence of nodal involvement. It will be useful to note that in DTC, lymph node metastases rate ranges from 20% to 50% with a micro-metastases (size <2 mm) rate being as high as 90% with a subsequent locoregional recurrence rate of 15–30%, the central compartment recurrence rate ranges between 5% and 20% in 5–10 years. However, in node negative patients, the median risk of recurrence is only 2% [11]. Patients who underwent TT without pCND presented a low risk of locoregional recurrence, although it may not change the overall prognosis. Lower recurrence rates and improved staging seem appear to be the only two benefits favoring pCND while the risk of causing postoperative complications, upstaging the disease and administration of high-dose RAI ablation are points against the routine pCND. If lateral nodes are positive, there are 80% chances that central nodes will be positive and *vice versa*. If they the lateral nodes are clinically negative, 80% chances are that they will be histologically negative. Similarly, if central nodes are positive, it is better to perform ipsilateral modified radical neck dissection or at least SND because chances of them being positive are quite high and first time is the best time. Central neck should be ideally be assessed using cross-sectional imaging, which is preferred to ultrasound, particularly for the mediastinal component (level VII). Nodal disease (macroscopic) has been found to be associated with increased risk of recurrence, and the impact of "microscopic" metastases on recurrence and survival is, however, less clear as mentioned earlier in the chapter.

Arguments "for" pCND [12–14]

- LN metastases have a negative effect on outcome in terms of recurrence.
- Ultrasonography (USG) might undervalue smaller lymph nodes (*40% negative ultrasound [USG] and positive CND [false negatives], sensitivity 30–95%, specificity 86–90%, operator dependent* [4] *giving high false-negative results*).
- Reoperation for central node recurrence is associated with higher rate of severe complications such as recurrent laryngeal nerve injury and hypoparathyroidism. Dissecting this compartment after total thyroidectomy is technically challenging due to fibrosis and desmoplastic reaction. Also, recurrence is not the same disease. It may dedifferentiate and be more aggressive with a poorer outcome.
- The proponents of pCND often cite that it should be performed in cN0 patients to avoid the locoregional recurrence and to provide pathological evidence for rationalizing adjuvant RAI treatment.
- CN metastases cannot be reliably identified on operation table. Intraoperative detection is not accurate, regardless of experience.
- CND can be performed safely in experienced hands as this compartment is, as it is exposed during thyroidectomy.
- Improves accuracy in staging patients with thyroid cancer and planning adjuvant treatment.
- Shown to decrease postoperative thyroglobulin (Tg) levels. If Tg levels are undetectable, RAI may not be required.
- Shown to reduce the amount of I-131 needed if nodes come out to be negative. Although the flip side is that presence of even micro-metastasis (laboratory cancers) will upstage the disease exposing the patient to high dose of RAI therapy [13].

Arguments "against" pCND

- More surgical morbidity in the immediate postoperative period [15]
- Identical locoregional recurrence observed with or without CND [16, 17]
- Metanalysis of retrospective studies on prophylactic CND and local recurrence in Papillary thyroid cancer (PTC) comprising 1264 patients undergoing TT with or without CND indicated no difference in the risk of recurrence of thyroid cancer 1.05 (0.48–2.31) between the two groups [14].
- Upstages the disease and adds RAI in adjuvant setting [13].
- Improved resolution of imaging modalities and utilization of multidisciplinary tools have assisted in clinical evaluation such as genetic assessment, incorporation of tumor biology into screening and standardized TIRADS classification system etc.
- Increasing sensitivity of Tg assays. It is possible to detect very small volume, persistent and/or recurrent disease.
- An over kill for a cancer that does well regardless. According to ATA 2015 guidelines, "No" pCND for smaller DTC (T1–T2 cN0)
- Increased complications for little or no gain in terms of survival. It was, however, observed to the contrary in a metanalysis by Wang et al. including 11 studies with total of 2318 patients there was no statistical difference in permanent hypocalcemia or vocal cord palsy with or without CND after total thyroidectomy [14].

- Should be considered (*weak recommendation*) in case of a laterocervical lymph node involvement (cN1b), of a T3–T4 tumor.

"Opposite of a true statement is a false statement and opposite of a true statement may well be another profound truth" (Niels Bohr). We must try and strike a balance between the potential risks and the benefits involved and find a middle path. Such a situation generally demands individualization of the treatment approach according to various prognostic factors related to the disease, patient and the surgeon. Not being too complacent and not being too feverish is the key toward optimum management. Various international bodies have different recommendation for prophylactic central neck dissection:

- *Japanese Society of Thyroid Surgeons* – They recommend pCND routinely and perform unilateral or bilateral prophylactic central lymph node dissections with parathyroid autotransplantation in all cases of papillary thyroid cancer at the time of total thyroidectomy.
- *American Thyroid Association* – The recommendation is only for T3 or T4 lesions.
- *British Thyroid Association* – Recommendation for age >55 years, male patients, with tumor >4 cm and extracapsular or ETE.
- *National Cancer Comprehensive Network* – Their guidelines favor pCND in patients <15 years and >55 years, with history of radiation therapy, tumor >4 cm, with ETE, aggressive variant, bilateral nodularity or distant metastasis.
- *American Association of Clinical Endocrinologists* – Do not recommend it routinely.
- *Consensus report of the European Society of Endocrine surgeons (ESES)* suggests that pCND should be risk stratified and indicated in T3, T4 tumors, age less than 45 years or more than 15 years, in males, bilateral or multifocal tumors.

Extent of optimum pCND

Besides the controversy regarding pCND itself, the guidelines for optimum extent of performing this procedure are also not established. Studies reveal 46% unilateral and 25% bilateral central LN positivity. According to many studies, the complication rates do not differ between the two groups [18]. In a study by Koo et al., the rate of occult contralateral central lymph node metastasis was found to be relatively high (34.3%) based on which the study insisted on bilateral central neck dissection, especially in cases of multifocal primary tumors and positive lateral group of lymph node [19]. Retrospective analysis of pattern of nodal metastases in surgical specimens by Moo et al. concluded that ipsilateral dissection is sufficient in tumors <1 cm and those >1 cm require bilateral CND based on the high incidence of contralateral central neck disease [20].

Work up and surgical approach

It is mandatory to subject all thyroid patients to a classical quadruple test including through history and clinical examination followed by high-resolution ultrasound followed by thyroid function tests, especially TSH, to exclude hyperthyroidism before doing the FNAC (fine needle aspiration cytology) and a gene panel in *high risk cases for BRAF^{v600v} mutation*. There are studies to suggest a correlation between the presence of mutation and the risk of lymph node metastases. But there is no robust evidence (*the evidence is mixed*) suggesting a strong predictive value of this mutation for recurrence. This, therefore, should not form the basis of prophylactic central neck dissection [1].

Preoperative ultrasound (especially the high-resolution ultrasound) is considered by most as an extension of clinical examination and is mandatory to preoperatively stage the disease accurately. Ultrasound can pick up even subcentric nodes in the central as well as lateral compartments [21, 22]. There is an additional advantage of adding color Doppler and elastography to further find out if the node is likely to be metastatic. Suspicious nodes must be subjected to FNAC. CT scan is indicted in recurrent or remnant disease or in the presence of lateral nodes.

Surgical technique (salient features)

The lymphatic drainage of the thyroid gland is fairly constant and is first mainly to the central compartment and later it proceeds down wards and laterally to involve the lower lateral lymph nodes (levels III, IV and V[b]). It is only later that it may spread to the upper lateral level II. It has been observed by some authors that the lymphatic drainage from the superior part of the gland may proceed directly to the level II, bypassing the central compartment (skip metastases). This is explained by the drainage happening along the superior thyroid pedicle. The surgical anatomy and the lymphatic drainage of the thyroid is depicted in Figures 24.1 and 24.2.

- *"Always is always wrong in surgery and never is never right"* one has to tailor the surgical approach.
- Maintaining ability to go medial to lateral or lateral to medial is important. A lot of surgeons prefer to go lateral to medial to get control of the pedicles and clearing the levels II, III and IV in the process.

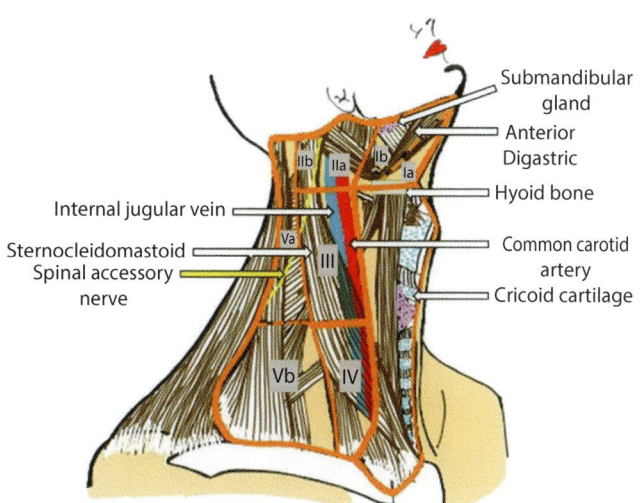

FIGURE 24.2 (Ia) All levels of lymph nodes levels can be seen. In most DTCs while dissecting the neck levels-I (both a and b), (II-b) and (V-a) may not be dissected unless there is an evidence of node positivity. This is to protect the spinal accessory nerve (SAN) and marginal mandibular nerve.

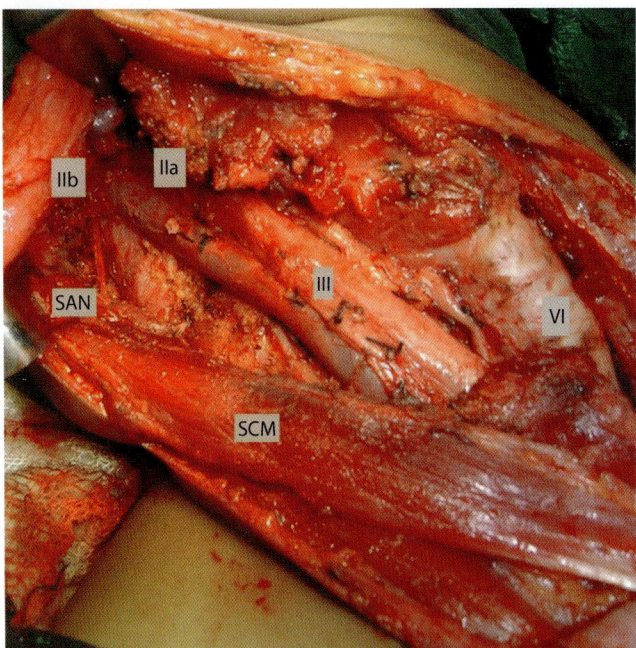

FIGURE 24.3 The MRND (type III) and CLND completed. The spinal accessory nerve can be seen coming out nearly 2 cm above the Erb's point.

- The strap muscles may be divided to get an adequate exposure but sternocleidomastoid muscles may not need to be transected unless directly infiltrated by the tumor especially when one is performing lateral dissection along with CND although may not be necessary (Figure 24.3).

Steps

Positioning

The classical position for thyroidectomy with a little tilt of head to the contralateral side (*which is helpful in exposing all triangles optimally*) is done for a classical neck dissection. The head of the table is in reverse Trendelenburg position with extension of the neck. One may use a Dunhill pillow or a thin but comfortable sand bag under the shoulders to achieve a reasonable extension of neck. The purpose of keeping the reverse Trendelenburg position is to reduce venous congestion. Ligation in continuity is a technique that the author employs while dealing with a vessel especially a vein. Bipolar diathermy is the energy source of preference by the author.

Incision

In most cases, it is possible to use the classical thyroidectomy incision without extension for clearance. The standard "collar incision" may be tailored according to the build of the patient size and extent of the tumor and whether or not lateral neck dissection is also contemplated. In such cases, the author prefers the utility incision (Figure 24.4) which is essentially an extension of the collar incision in a natural skin crease with an extension on the ipsilateral side toward the mastoid process. This may make dissection of level-V easier; however, the author only uses this incision in cases taken up for second surgery or recurrence.

The recurrent laryngeal nerves must be identified, and the author likes to trace them from their entry in the neck right up to their destination close to ligament Berry. This allows for a complete clearance of the lymphatic tissue. It is mandatory to identify and preserve all the parathyroid glands. The superior gland is by and large constant in location, and the inferior may go places as it develops along with the thymus. It is essential to preserve the blood supply of these otherwise hardy glands and only the capsular branches of the inferior thyroid are to be ligated. If the parathyroid gland is devascularized, it should be autotransplanted. The thyroidectomy specimen along with central compartment dissection can be removed in continuity (Figure 24.5).

There are studies to suggest that one gland may routinely be autotransplanted as a protocol to prevent ischemic damage during CND. However, there are others, including the author, who believe that this may not be necessary. The author also recommends autotransplantation of only the devascularized glands. It is often possible for these glands to recover after some cold saline dripping. The best site for the creating a pocket for autotransplantation is sternocleidomastoid muscle.

Neck dissection in proven lateral neck disease

SND is the procedure of choice. Since level I is rarely involved in thyroid cancers, its routine dissection is not recommended. There is also recommendation against routine IIb and V(a) and also because they are rarely involved. They may be spared unless there is an evidence (ultrasound based) of their involvement. So classically the lateral neck dissection would involve removal of levels IIa and Vb. It is possible to use the unextended thyroidectomy

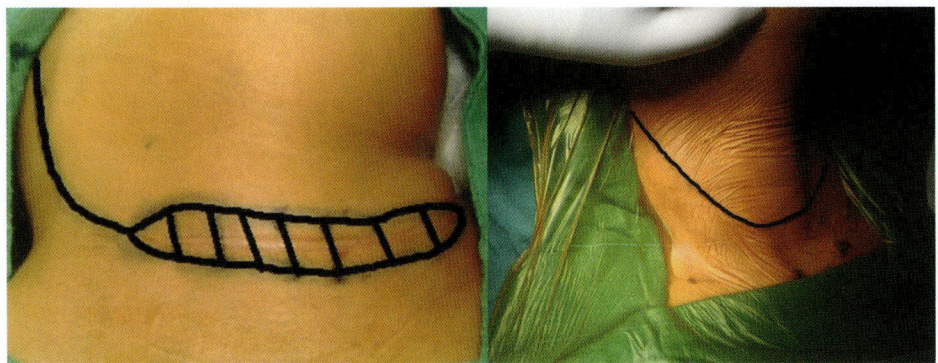

FIGURE 24.4 Utility incision being utilized for a recurrent thyroid cancer. To be oncologically safe, and especially while performing lateral dissection, utility incision may be more useful.

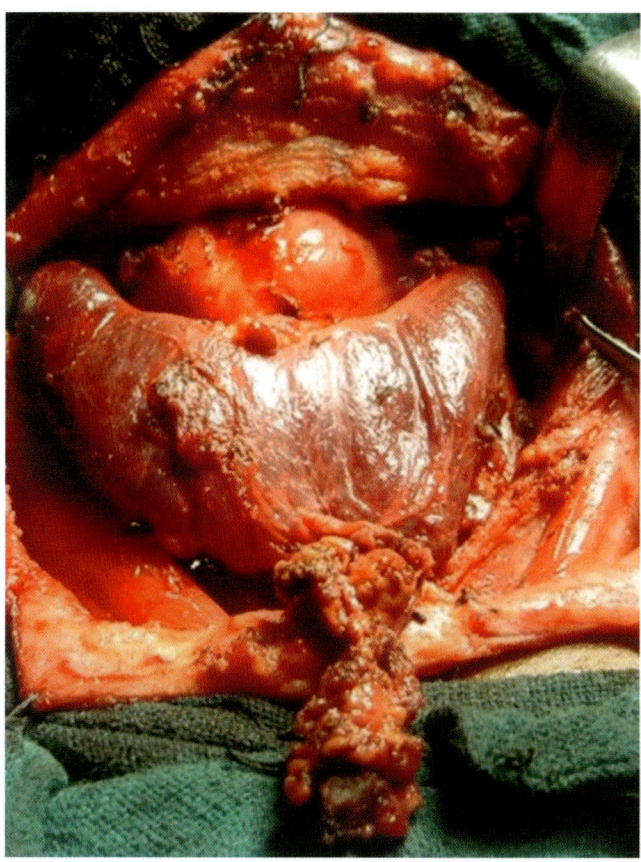

FIGURE 24.5 The specimen of total thyroidectomy, bilateral central compartment dissection.

incision for the purpose. One has to be extra cautious to avoid injury to thoracic duct on the left side. If identified (although difficult in fasting patient), it must be ligated. The chyle leak in the postoperative period can be a challenge to manage [9, 23].

Complications of neck dissection [1]

Intraoperative: In high-volume centers and with high-volume surgeons, the risk of any complication is only 5–7%, and usually these are minor. Major complications are seen in less than 1%. Intraoperative complications are hemorrhage, pneumothorax, air embolism, phrenic nerve/brachial plexus injury, tracheal injury and rarely esophageal injury, laryngotracheal injury, injury to hypoglossal, spinal accessory, thoracic duct injury.

Postoperative: Postoperative complications are hematoma, airway issues, facial edema, carotid blow out, wound infection, chyle leak, wound-related complications, Horner's syndrome, electrolyte imbalances and hypoesthesia of skin.

Follow-up and recurrence in the neck

Recurrence is defined as local or regional disease requiring treatment 6 months after the initial standard operation. It must be diagnosed by ultrasound-guided FNAC [7]. Regional recurrence is not rare, and literature reports its incidence to be around 30% [24]. The most common site for recurrence is in the central compartment. Known risk factors for recurrent nodal disease especially in the lateral compartment are extra nodal spread or extension of lymph node metastases and the number of positive nodes out of the total nodes excised during the initial dissection [25]. For early detection of recurrences, regular surveillance is needed for a patient who has undergone surgery for thyroid cancer regardless of whether the neck was addressed or not. Stimulated Tg, unstimulated Tg, ultrasound examination is required and ultrasound-guided FNAC can confirm the nodal recurrence [26–30]. It may be difficult to differentiate the recurrence in central compartment from recurrence in thyroid bed. In this scenario, cross-sectional imaging is, therefore, indicated. Computed tomography and magnetic resonance imaging (MRI) are indicated as imaging modality in recurrent nodal disease. Fluorodeoxyglucose positron emission tomography (FDGPET) is useful only in poorly differentiated cancers as they are less radioactive iodine avid [6, 31].

Management of recurrence in the neck

Every recurrent nodule in the neck does not need to be excised and a large number may be followed up with serial high-resolution ultrasound [26, 27]. According to the "Thyroid Cancer Care Collaborative", recurrent nodal disease in thyroid cancer can be managed more conservatively in select patients of DTC as long as one can comprehend a life-long surveillance of recurrent nodal disease [28]. Surgery with curative intent is the treatment of choice for recurrent disease confined to neck. There is no place for SND due to distorted anatomy and minimum of MRND-III or functional neck dissection is recommended in recurrences. An experienced thyroid surgeon is required to get an oncologically safe outcome with minimal or no morbidity [32, 33]. Ultrasound guided percutaneous ethanol ablation have been tried at various centers across Europe and the United States including centers like Mayo Clinic and they recommend its usage in limited neck metastases [34].

"In theory there is no difference between theory and practice but in practice there is"....

JA Snepschant

Conclusions

The clinical significance of lymph node metastases in DTC is variable and has a wide spectrum. Routine prophylactic central neck dissection is advised in suspected or proven lymph node disease in central compartment or locally advanced tumors (T3, T4) and lateral lymph node dissection in suspected or proven lateral lymph node disease. Serial ultrasound is the most useful modality for follow-up of lymph nodes in lateral neck along with Tg (may provide false-negative results in less than 10% cases with anti-Tg antibodies). The decisions must be made in multidisciplinary meetings with patient in the center taking in to account not only the clinical and surgical aspects but also the patients understanding of treatment and the associated morbidity.

Acknowledgments

With lots of joy and pride, I would like to acknowledge the efforts made in the writing of this chapter by arguably my best student Dr Sukriti. She was involved in the compiling of this chapter. She has assisted me in all my academic endeavors, data keeping and recording of events as they happened, has a great future and will make an outstanding surgeon, excelling at both the science and art of surgery. As a *guru*, I am proud of my *shishya* who is going to be an open book that will make this world richer and better with all her hard work, values, compassion and dedication.

References

1. Mizrachi, A, Shaha, A. Neck Dissection for Thyroid Cancer. Imaging Radionucl Ther 2017;26(Suppl 1):10–5.
2. Bethesda, MD. November 2014 SEER Data Submission, Posted to the SEER Web Site, April 2015.
3. Noguchi S, Noguchi A, Murakami N. Papillary Carcinoma of the Thyroid. Developing Pattern of Metastasis. Cancer 1970;26:1053–60.
4. Noguchi S, Murakami N. The Value of Lymph-Node Dissection in Patients with Differentiated Thyroid Cancer. Surg Clin N Am 1987;67:251–61.
5. Haugen Bryan R, Alexander EK, Bible KC, Doherty G, Mandel SJ, Nikiforov YE, Pacini F, Randolph G, Sawka A, Schlumberger M, Schuff KG, Sherman SI, Sosa JA, Steward D, Tuttle RMd, Wartofsky L. 2015 American Thyroid Association Management Guidelines for Adult Patients with Thyroid Nodules and Differentiated Thyroid Cancer: what is new and what has changed? Cancer 2017;123(3):372–381.
6. Robenshtok E, Fish S, Bach A, Dominguez JM, Shaha A, Tuttle RM. Suspicious Cervical Lymph Nodes Detected after Thyroidectomy for Papillary Thyroid Cancer Usually Remain Stable over Years in Properly Selected Patients. J Clin Endocrinol Metab 2012;97:2706–13.
7. Hu D, Lin H, Zeng X, et al. Risk Factors for and Prediction Model of Skip Metastasis to Lateral Lymph Nodes in Papillary Thyroid Carcinoma. World J Surg 2020;44:1498–505.
8. Lim YC, Koo BS. Predictive Factors of Skip Metastases to Lateral Neck Compartment Leaping Central Neck Compartment in Papillary Thyroid Carcinoma. Oral Oncol 2012;48:262–5.
9. Khanna J, Chintamani, Mohil RS, Bhatnagar D. Is the Routine Drainage after Surgery for Thyroid Necessary? A Prospective Randomized Clinical Study [ISRCTN63623153]. BMC Surg 2005;5:11.
10. Iyer NG, Shaha AR. Central Compartment Dissection for Well Differentiated Thyroid Cancer and the Band Plays On. Curr Opin Otolaryngol Head Neck Surg 2011;19:106–12.
11. Zetoune T, Keutgen X, Buitrago D, Aldailami H, Shao H, Mazumdar M, Fahey TJ 3rd, Zarnegar R. Prophylactic Central Neck Dissection and Local Recurrence in Papillary Thyroid Cancer: A Meta-Analysis. Ann Surg Oncol 2010;17(12):3287–93.
12. Lang BH, Ng SH, Lau L, Cowling B, Wong KP, Wan KY. A Systematic Review and Meta-Analysis of Prophylactic Central Neck Dissection on Short-Term Locoregional Recurrence in Papillary Thyroid Carcinoma after Total Thyroidectomy. Thyroid 2013;23(9):1087–98.
13. Hughes DT, White ML, Miller BS, Gauger PG, Burney RE, Doherty GM. Influence of Prophylactic Central Lymph Node Dissection on Postoperative Thyroglobulin Levels and Radioiodine Treatment in Papillary Thyroid Cancer. Surgery 2010;148:1100–6.
14. Wang TS, Cheung K, Farrokhyar F, Roman SA, Sosa JA. A Meta-Analysis of the Effects of Prophylactic Central Neck Dissection on Locoregional Recurrence Rates in Patients with Papillary Thyroid Cancers. Ann Surg Oncol 2013;20:3477–83.
15. Shan CX, Zhang W, Jiang DZ, Zheng XM, Liu S, Qiu M. Routine Central Neck Dissection in Differentiated Thyroid Carcinoma: A Systematic Review and Meta-Analysis. Laryngoscope 2012;122:797–804.
16. Gyorki DE, Untch B, Tuttle RM, Shaha AR. Prophylactic Central Neck Dissection in Differentiated Thyroid Cancer: An Assessment of the Evidence. Ann Surg Oncol 2013;20:2285–9.
17. Wang TS, Cheung K, Farrokhyar F, et al. A Meta-Analysis of the Effect of Prophylactic Central Compartment Neck Dissection on Locoregional Recurrence Rates in Patients with Papillary Thyroid Cancer. Ann Surg Oncol 2013;20:3477–83.
18. Yoo HS, Shin MC, Chang YBJ, Seung MS. Optimal Extent of Prophylactic Central Neck Dissection for Papillary Thyroid Carcinoma: Comparison of Unilateral versus Bilateral Central Neck Dissection. Asian J Surg 2018;41(4):363–369.
19. Koo BS, Choi EC, Yoon YH, et al. Predictive Factors for Ipsilateral or Contralateral Central Lymph Node Metastasis in Unilateral Papillary Thyroid Carcinoma. Ann Surg 2009;249:840–4.
20. Moo TA, Umunna B, Kato M, et al. Ipsilateral versus Bilateral Central Neck Lymph Node Dissection in Papillary Thyroid Carcinoma. Ann Surg 2009;250:403–8.
21. Hwang HS, Orloff LA. Efficacy of Preoperative Neck Ultrasound in the Detection of Cervical Lymph Node Metastasis from Thyroid Cancer. Laryngoscope 2011;121:487–91.
22. Mizrachi A, Feinmesser R, Bachar G, Hilly O, Cohen M. Value of Ultrasound in Detecting Central Compartment Lymph Node Metastases in Differentiated Thyroid Carcinoma. Eur Arch Otorhinolaryngol 2014;271:1215–8.
23. Ito Y, Higashiyama T, Takamura Y, Miya A, Kobayashi K, Matsuzuka F, Kuma K, Miyauchi A. Risk Factors for Recurrence to the Lymph Node in Papillary Thyroid Carcinoma Patients without Preoperatively Detectable Lateral Node Metastasis: Validity of Prophylactic Modified Radical Neck Dissection. World J Surg 2007;31:2085–91.
24. Shaha AR. Recurrent Differentiated Thyroid Cancer. Endocr Pract 2012;18:600–3. Thyroid carcinoma.
25. Ahmadi N, Grewal A, Davidson BJ. Patterns of Cervical Lymph Node Metastases in Primary and Recurrent Papillary Thyroid Cancer. J Oncol 2011;2011:735678.
26. Chéreau N, Buffet C, Trésallet C, Tissier F, Leenhardt L, Menegaux F. Recurrence of Papillary Thyroid Carcinoma with Lateral Cervical Node Metastases: Predictive Factors and Operative Management. Surgery 2016;159:755–62.
27. Baek SK, Jung KY, Kang SM, Kwon SY, Woo JS, Cho SH, Chung EJ. Clinical Risk Factors Associated with Cervical Lymph Node Recurrence in Papillary Thyroid Carcinoma. Thyroid 2010;20:147–52.
28. Urken ML, Milas M, Randolph GW, Tufano R, Bergman D, Bernet V, Brett EM, Brierley JD, Cobin R, Doherty G, Klopper J, Lee S, Machac J, Mechanick JI, Orloff LA, Ross D, Smallridge RC, Terris DJ, Clain JB, Tuttle M. Management of Recurrent and Persistent Metastatic Lymph Nodes in Well-Differentiated Thyroid Cancer: A Multifactorial Decision-Making Guide for the Thyroid Cancer Care Collaborative. Head Neck 2015;37:605–14.
29. Mazzaferri EL, Robbins RJ, Spencer CA, Braverman LE, Pacini F, Wartofsky L, Haugen BR, Sherman SI, Cooper DS, Braunstein GD, Lee S, Davies TF, Arafah BM, Ladenson PW, Pinchera A. A Consensus Report of the Role of Serum Thyroglobulin as a Monitoring Method for Low-Risk Patients with Papillary Thyroid Carcinoma. J Clin Endocrinol Metab 2003;88:1433–41.
30. Pacini F, Sabra MM, Tuttle RM. Clinical Relevance of Thyroglobulin Doubling Time in the Management of Patients with Differentiated Thyroid Cancer. Thyroid 2011;21:691–2.
31. Schlüter B, Bohuslavizki KH, Beyer W, Plotkin M, Buchert R, Clausen M. Impact of FDG PET on Patients with Differentiated Thyroid Cancer Who Present with Elevated Thyroglobulin and Negative ^{131}I Scan. J Nucl Med 2001;42:71–6.
32. Clayman GL, Shellenberger TD, Ginsberg LE, Edeiken BS, El-Naggar AK, Sellin RV, Waguespack SG, Roberts DB, Mishra A, Sherman SI. Approach and Safety of Comprehensive Central Compartment Dissection in Patients with Recurrent Papillary Thyroid Carcinoma. Head Neck 2009;31:1152–63.
33. Yehuda MN, Freeman JL. Revision Central Compartment Surgery: Indications, Management and Outcomes in 60 Consecutive Patients. Annual Meeting of the American Head and Neck Society; San Diego, California, 2007.
34. Hay ID, Charboneau JW. The Coming of Age of Ultrasound-Guided Percutaneous Ethanol Ablation of Selected Neck Nodal Metastases in Well-Differentiated Thyroid Carcinoma. J Clin Endocrinol Metab 2011;96:2717–20.

25

EXTENT OF SURGERY IN THYROID CANCER

Anand Kumar Mishra and Kul Ranjan Singh

Introduction

Palpable thyroid nodule disease is present in 1% men and 5% women in iodine-sufficient regions (1, 2). High-resolution ultrasound can detect thyroid nodules in 19–67% of randomly selected population, with higher frequencies in elderly people and females (3). Five to fifteen percent of thyroid nodules harbour malignancies depending upon age, sex, radiation exposure, family history and other factors (4, 5). A 2.4-fold increase in thyroid cancer has been observed from 1973 to 2002. It had increased from 3.6 per lakh population in 1973 to 8.7 per lakh in 2002. This increase in number is attributed to extensive use of high-resolution ultrasound and early diagnosis and treatment (6). The observed increase in thyroid cancer is mainly attributed to papillary thyroid carcinoma, which has increased by 2.9 folds from 1998 to 2002. There has been an increase of 49% in 1 cm or less tumors and 87% increase in 2 cm or less tumors (7).

Differentiated thyroid cancers (DTC) are characterized by indolent and aggressive subtypes. Incidence and presentation of thyroid cancer varies in different practice settings, regions and countries. It probably reflects distinct genetic, epidemiological and environmental risk factors. Countries differ in public awareness, screening programs, infrastructure, health facilities and policies. Total thyroidectomy (TT) and adjuvant radioactive iodine (RAI) ablation was a nearly universal paradigm for all DTC, but recent trend is toward a more conservative and individualized treatment philosophy. Philosophy of treatment is that indolent disease should not be over-treated and aggressive disease is not under treated. Treatment should be tailored to the individual clinical scenario based on balanced analysis of these factors. All thyroid cancer should be managed by multidisciplinary care teams, and treatment decisions are to be based upon dynamic risk stratification.

Extent of thyroidectomy

Extent of surgery in thyroid cancer determines overall survival, hence it should be planned meticulously. The aim of surgery is to remove "complete thyroid cancer" from neck with minimal complications and sequelae. Preoperative decision is based on meticulous history, physical examination and result of triple test (TSH, ultrasound with fine needle aspiration cytology assessment) in all patients and computed tomography or magnetic resonance imaging in select cases. Age >45 years, tumor size >4 cm, major extrathyroidal extension, poor histology and presence of distant metastasis are independent prognostic factors associated with mortality risk. Factors associated with increased risk of clinically significant persistent or recurrent disease are presence of more than three palpable lymph node (LN) metastases, metastatic LN size >3 cm and extracapsular nodal spread. There are patient (medical history, anatomy, lifestyle factors, performance index, finances, residence and literacy) and physician factors (experience, available resources at hospital) that also influence the treatment decisions. There are two schools of thoughts and one belief in lobectomy or hemithyroidectomy for low-risk TT in high-risk tumors. Retrospective data of papillary thyroid carcinoma (PTC) and follicular cancer suggested that any tumor of size >1 cm with or without evidence of locoregional or distant metastases should be treated by TT for better survival and decrease recurrences (8–11). TT would allow routine use of RAI remnant ablation and facilitate early detection of recurrent disease during follow-up in all these patients. Papers published in last two decades have suggested that in properly selected patients, less than TT can have similar clinical outcomes (11–15). RAI adjuvant therapy was the major advantage after TT, but patients with less than TT can be very well followed with neck ultrasonography and serial serum Tg measurements.

Proponents of TT argue that complete resection allows the use of RAI for treatment of residual or metastatic disease and facilitates the use of serum thyroglobulin as a tumor marker to detect residual and recurrent disease (16, 17). TT removes undetected multifocal disease in the contralateral lobe (18). Lobectomy proponents argue that papillary thyroid carcinoma is an indolent disease with an excellent prognosis, and all patients should not be subjected to risks for TT-related complications without a clear survival benefit (19) (Table 25.1).

In DTC, TT is advocated as the treatment of choice for the following reasons:

1. Bilateral and multifocal PTC is seen in 30–85% and >25% patients respectively. So, TT eliminates contralateral lobe disease.
2. Thyroglobulin can be used as tumor marker for the recurrence during follow-up.
3. Radioiodine can be used for the treatment of residual, recurrent and metastatic disease and can also be used to diagnose metastatic disease.
4. A lower dose of radioiodine is required for ablation.
5. Small lesions may grow aggressively with the potential of dedifferentiation.
6. TT reduces recurrence in all risk groups, and experienced surgeon can perform a TT with minimal or no long-term complications.
7. Completion thyroidectomy of thyroid remnants may be associated with a higher morbidity.

Less than TT has been recommended for the following reasons:

1. Most patients have low-risk cancer and excellent prognosis, and results are equally good with lobectomy/hemithyroidectomy compared with TT.
2. Role of adjuvant treatment is not defined in many patients.
3. Complications rate increase with extent of surgery.
4. Prospective randomized trials are not be possible as thyroid cancer is a rare cancer with indolent course and

TABLE 25.1: Comparison of Arguments for Hemithyroidectomy and Total Thyroidectomy

Factors	Lobectomy/Hemithyroidectomy	Total Thyroidectomy
Bilateral and multifocality	No relevance of multifocality in PTC	PTC is bilateral (30–85%) and multifocal (>25%) TT eliminates contralateral lobe disease
Thyroglobulin as tumor marker in follow-up	No need and can be followed with neck ultrasound	Yes
Radioiodine	Can be used even for ablation of left lobe. It is not needed in all patients as adjuvant therapy	Diagnostic for metastatic disease and therapeutic for residual and recurrent disease
Complications of surgery	Hypoparathyroidism and Recurrent laryngeal nerve injury can be avoided as they increase with extent of surgery	TT can be safely done with minimal complications by experienced surgeons
Completion surgery	Can be done whenever needed later	Completion thyroidectomy has two- to fourfold higher overall complications
Overall survival	No survival advantage with extent of surgery and properly selected patients can have similar outcomes	Improves overall survival in all groups
Thyroxine	No need for thyroid hormone supplementation	Thyroid hormone can be used as suppressive therapy

overall good prognosis. A prospective randomized clinical trial will require 3100 patients of PTC to be recruited for randomization to see disease-specific mortality, and 12,000 patients of PTC need randomization to compare permanent complication rate with significance with a follow-up of more than 30 years.

5. Occult multicentric tumor is not clinically important, and recurrence in opposite lobe is rare. There is excellent long-term outcome with lobectomy alone.
6. Most local recurrence can be treated with surgery.
7. If necessary, ablation of the thyroid remnant with radioiodine can be accomplished with no morbidity.

Retrospective data from Bilimoria et al. and other series (20–22) suggested that TT is required in all DTC for better overall survival and outcomes, and it led to the recommendation in 2009 that clinicians should consider TT for all DTC nodules >1 cm (23). Bilimoria et al.'s paper was based on national cancer data analysis of 52,173 PTC patients of whom 43,227 underwent TT and 8946 lobectomies from 1988 to 1998 and concluded that statistically significant differences in survival and recurrence were seen for all sizes >1 cm based on the extent of initial surgery. The criticism for this paper is that it has not calculated the overall survival with extrathyroidal extension or completeness of resection or other comorbid conditions, and all these factors could have had a major impact on survival and recurrence risk (20). Later on, an updating of National Cancer Database (1998–2006) published by Adam et al. on analysis of 61,775 PTC patients, out of which 54,926 underwent TT and 6849 lobectomies, concluded no survival advantage associated with TT (24). And similar conclusion was available from other series (25–28) (Table 25.2). This led to a shift in extent of surgery in 2015 ATA guidelines. The 2015 ATA guidelines consider lobectomy or TT both a reasonable option for DTC measuring between 1 and 4 cm (29).

Choice of procedure: The following procedures are suggested for patients with papillary or follicular cancer (Table 25.3).

- **Tumor <1 cm without extrathyroidal extension and no LNs:** For unilateral intrathyroidal DTC <1 cm without history of head and neck radiation, strong family history of thyroid cancer lobectomy is the preferred approach.
- **Tumor 1–4 cm without extrathyroidal extension and no LNs:** For intrathyroidal tumors between 1 and 4 cm, initial surgical procedure can either be a TT or thyroid lobectomy. The extent of surgery will depend upon patient preference, clinical parameters, imaging ultrasonographic abnormalities in the contralateral lobe (nodules, thyroiditis in the contralateral lobe or nonspecific lymphadenopathy), local surgical team belief and protocols and treatment team decision of radioiodine use postoperatively as adjuvant therapy or during follow-up.
- **Tumor ≥4 cm, extrathyroidal extension or metastases:** TT is surgical procedure of choice for all tumors of 4 cm or larger. It is also recommended in all tumors with extrathyroidal extension, or LNs metastases or distant metastases.
- **Any tumor size and history of childhood head and neck radiation:** TT should be the surgical procedure of choice for all tumors in patients with history of childhood exposure to ionizing radiation of head and neck.
- **Multifocal papillary microcarcinoma (fewer than five foci):** Hemithyroidectomy is an appropriate surgery in patients with pathology reports, subsequently showing multifocal papillary microcarcinomas with fewer than five foci.
- **Multifocal papillary microcarcinoma (more than five foci):** In multifocal papillary cancer, with more than five foci preoperatively on imaging; especially if foci are of size 8–9 mm, TT should be performed". So in any patient with large number of microcarcinoma, TT is the choice of surgery, and if initial surgery was hemithyroidectomy in such a patient and pathology shows multifocal papillary microcarcinomas with more than five foci, completion thyroidectomy should be done.

LN dissection in thyroid cancer: The LNs levels 6 and 7 located in central compartment are the first drainage echelons for thyroid cancer, and lateral neck levels 4, 5, 3 and 2 are secondary drainage echelons in decreasing order of frequency. The metastases in PTC are seen in central neck in 50% and lateral neck about 30%. Dissection of levels 6 and 7 LNs is called central compartment neck dissection (CND). Hürthle cell variant follicular cancer patients may also develop cervical LNs metastases, and is predictor of worse outcome in this group. If metastatic LNs are identified in these patients, therapeutic neck dissection should be performed (30).

Therapeutic LN dissection: Therapeutic LN dissection should be performed in all patients with visibly involved nodes, or there

TABLE 25.2: Comparison of Studies Regarding Extent of Surgery (Hemithyroidectomy and TT) in Terms of Outcome

Study	Methods	Result	Comment
Favoring TT in DTC			
Bilimoria et al., Ann Surg. 2007 (20) National Cancer Data Base (1985–1998) analysis of 52,173 PTC patients (43,227 receiving TT, 8946 undergoing lobectomy)	<1 cm extent of surgery did not impact recurrence or survival For tumors > or = 1 cm, lobectomy resulted in higher risk of recurrence and death (P = 0.04, P = 0.009) 10-year relative overall survival for TT as opposed to thyroid lobectomy (98.4% vs. 97.1%, respectively, P < 0.05) and a slightly lower 10-year recurrence rate (7.7% vs. 9.8%, respectively, P < 0.05)	TT results in lower recurrence rates and improved survival for PTC > or = 1.0 cm compared with lobectomy Data on extrathyroidal extension, completeness of resection and other comorbid conditions, which could have had a major impact on survival and recurrence risk, were not available	Survival benefit
Grant et al., Surgery. 1988 (21) Single center	963 PTC patients underwent unilateral (15%), bilateral subtotal/near-total (69%) or TT (16%) from 1946 through 1975 at the Mayo Clinic	AGES scoring system used	Higher local recurrence with unilateral operation and higher mortality in local recurrence group
Hay et al., Surgery. 1998 (22) Single center	1685 patients initially treated during 1940 through 1991 and followed for up to 54 postoperative years at Mayo Clinic	AMES criteria low-risk PTC patients	Significantly higher locoregional recurrence with unilateral operation and bilateral operation is probably a preferable initial surgical operation in low-risk PTC
Not Favoring TT in All DTC			
Adam et al., Ann Surg. 2014 (24) National Cancer Data Base (1998–2006)	Analysis of 61,775 PTC patients, 54,926 underwent TT and 6849 lobectomy TT patients had more nodal (7% vs. 27%), extrathyroidal (5% vs. 16%) and multifocal disease (29% vs. 44%) (all P < 0.001)	Multivariate analysis revealed overall survival similar in patients of TT and lobectomy (size 1.0–4.0 cm). Older age, male sex, black race, lower income, tumor size and presence of nodal or distant metastases were independently associated with compromised survival (P < 0.0001)	No survival benefit by extent of initial surgery
Haigh et al., Ann Surg Oncol. 2005 (28) SEER database PTC patients	4402 (81%) low-risk and 1030 (19%) high-risk patients; 84.9% underwent total thyroidectomy		No survival benefit by extent of initial surgery
Mendelsohn et al., Arch Otolaryngol Head Neck Surg. 2010 (27) SEER database PTC patients	22,724 PTC patients diagnosed between 1998 and 2001 (16,760 with TT 5964 with lobectomy)	Among lobectomy 1.6% received external beam radiation therapy, 16% had extrathyroidal extension, 9% of tumors were >4 cm and 20% received RAI ablation	No survival benefit by extent of initial surgery
Barney et al., Head Neck. 2011 (26) SEER database, 23,605 papillary or follicular thyroid cancer from 1983 to 2002	12,598 with TT 3266 with lobectomy	No difference in 10-year overall survival (90.4% for TT vs. 90.8% for lobectomy) or 10-year cause-specific survival (96.8% for TT vs. 98.6% for lobectomy)	No survival benefit by extent of initial surgery
Matsuzu et al., World J Surg. 2014 (25) Retrospective, single center	1088 PTC patients with lobectomy at Ito Hospital from 1986–1995	Lobectomy is a valid alternative to TT in PTC in <45 years, size 4 cm or less without LN metastasis and extrathyroidal invasion	Unilateral operation is valid option in <4 cm tumors

Abbreviations: LN, Lymph node; SEER, Surveillance, epidemiology and end results; TT, Total thyroidectomy.

is clinical or imaging evidence of central or lateral node metastases due to the increased risk of neck recurrence and mortality (31, 32). During thyroid surgery, when opening the lateral gutter or mobilizing the thyroid lobe from trachea esophageal and carotid sheath gutter, one should inspect lateral LN, and all suspected LNs should be biopsied. Lateral dissection involves removal of all LN and soft tissues in levels IIA (most commonly level IIB nodes not involved), III, IV and V, usually with preservation of the internal jugular vein, carotid artery, vagus nerve, phrenic nerve, sternocleidomastoid muscle and spinal accessory nerve. The dissection is called compartment-oriented neck dissection, and it should be the indicated procedure in all PTC with clinical, radiological or histopathological evidence of LN metastases. There are views for and against routine prophylactic CND. In patients with suspicious or clearly abnormal LNs in the central neck, central dissection should be performed. Central dissection procedure involves removing all fibro-fatty LNs, especially in tracheoesophageal groove between two jugulars from hyoid to innominate vein (31, 33, 34).

Prophylactic LN dissection: There are views for and against routine prophylactic CND. Preoperative cervical ultrasound

TABLE 25.3: Summary of Surgical Procedure with Indication for Differentiated Thyroid Cancer

Type of Surgery	Indications
Lobectomy/Hemithyroidectomy	Unifocal intrathyroidal thyroid ca. ≤1 cm without evidence of extrathyroid extension in the absence of prior head and neck irradiation or radiologically or clinically involved cervical nodal metastases
	Minimally invasive (capsular only) FTC
Lobectomy or total thyroidectomy	Thyroid ca. >1 cm and <4 cm if no evidence of extrathyroid extension
Total thyroidectomy	Thyroid ca. ≥4 cm
	FTC (minimally vascular or widely invasive)
	Hürthle cell cancer
Total thyroidectomy with LN dissection	Evidence of LN metastases
	Or PTC with evidence of gross extrathyroid extension and distant metastases
Completion thyroidectomy	Aggressive PTC variant (tall cell, columnar, diffuse sclerosing, hobnail)
	With evidence of pathological extrathyroid extension or LN involvement, or both
	FTC/Hürthle cancer after hemithyroidectomy
Lymph node dissection in DTC	Prophylactic central compartment in PTC with evidence of gross extrathyroid extension, size >4 cm, lateral neck nodal disease and distant metastases
	Hürthle cell carcinoma
	Therapeutic neck dissection should be undertaken for macroscopic LN metastases which are clinically enlarged or H/P proven
Surgical excision of distant metastasis	Solitary and surgery accessible as excision helps reducing tumor mass and facilitate RAI therapy/RT

can detect clinically nonpalpable, metastatic nodes in up to 20% of patients with papillary cancer, including those with primary tumors <1 cm in diameter (35). In PTC, data suggest that about 80% patients harbor microscopic LN metastases. Clinicians do not consider microscopic LNs metastases of clinical importance and radioiodine adjuvant therapy if used will ablate these occult foci after surgery. Many authors argue against prophylactic neck dissection with purpose of removing LNs with microscopic metastases that are not clinically identifiable at the time of surgery. Prophylactic neck dissection does not improve long-term outcome and put patients at more complications than benefit (36–38). Prophylactic CND (ipsilateral or bilateral) is advisable procedure in high-risk thyroid cancer including size >4 cm, tumor multifocality, extrathyroidal invasion, gross lateral LNs metastases, anticipated RAI adjuvant therapy (high age, adverse histology, BFAF mutation, PET positivity). Routine prophylactic lateral neck dissection does not affect long-term survival (39, 40).

Arguments in favor of performing prophylactic CND: The rationales for prophylactic CND are as follows.

- Relatively high frequency of LN metastases (50%) is seen in central compartment.
- High-resolution ultrasound which is standard preoperative study lacks accuracy in identification of central abnormal LNs and intraoperative differentiation between benign and metastatic LNs is difficult unless frozen section is used.
- CND LNs metastases have a negative effect on patient overall outcome.
- Meticulous CND has a beneficial effect on subsequent course, as it allows accurate staging of the disease and decrease postoperative levels of stimulated thyroglobulin which determines need for adjuvant postoperative radioiodine therapy.
- CND can be performed safely by experts and without extension of the surgical incision.
- Reoperation for central neck recurrence has greater morbidity.

Argument against prophylactic central dissection includes three main concepts:

- Minority of LNs metastases progress to clinically meaningful disease.
- Lymphatic metastases have not been shown to increase overall survival.
- CND is associated with increased complication rates, and reoperation for recurrent disease can be performed with acceptable morbidity by experienced surgeons.

Invasive thyroid cancer: In invasive thyroid cancer, goal of surgical intervention is resection of all visible gross tumors, and every attempt should be made to preserve normal organ function whenever possible. Conservative procedures like vertical hemilaryngectomy for unilateral laryngeal cartilage invasion or circumferential tracheal resection for subglottic invasion and total laryngectomy for extensive intraluminal invasion can be performed. A functioning recurrent nerve should be preserved as adjuvant RAI will take care of residual or microscopic tumor left on the nerve.

Surgery of metastases: Distant metastases in a DTC patient increase morbidity and mortality; and long-term prognosis depends upon age, histology of primary tumor, number, sites of metastasis (e.g., brain, bone and lung), tumor burden, 18-FDG and RAI avidity. Whenever feasible, the isolated bony or brain metastases should be resected as it will facilitate a lower RAI dose requirement (Figure 25.1(a) and (b), preoperative and postoperative).

Extent of surgery in micropapillary thyroid cancer

Risk stratification of micro-PTC

Majority of patients with micro-PTC (PMC) have an indolent nature. Criterion for the risk stratification of PMC patients are tumor size, family history of thyroid cancer, history of neck irradiation, lymph nodal metastasis, extrathyroidal extension,

Extent of Surgery in Thyroid Cancer

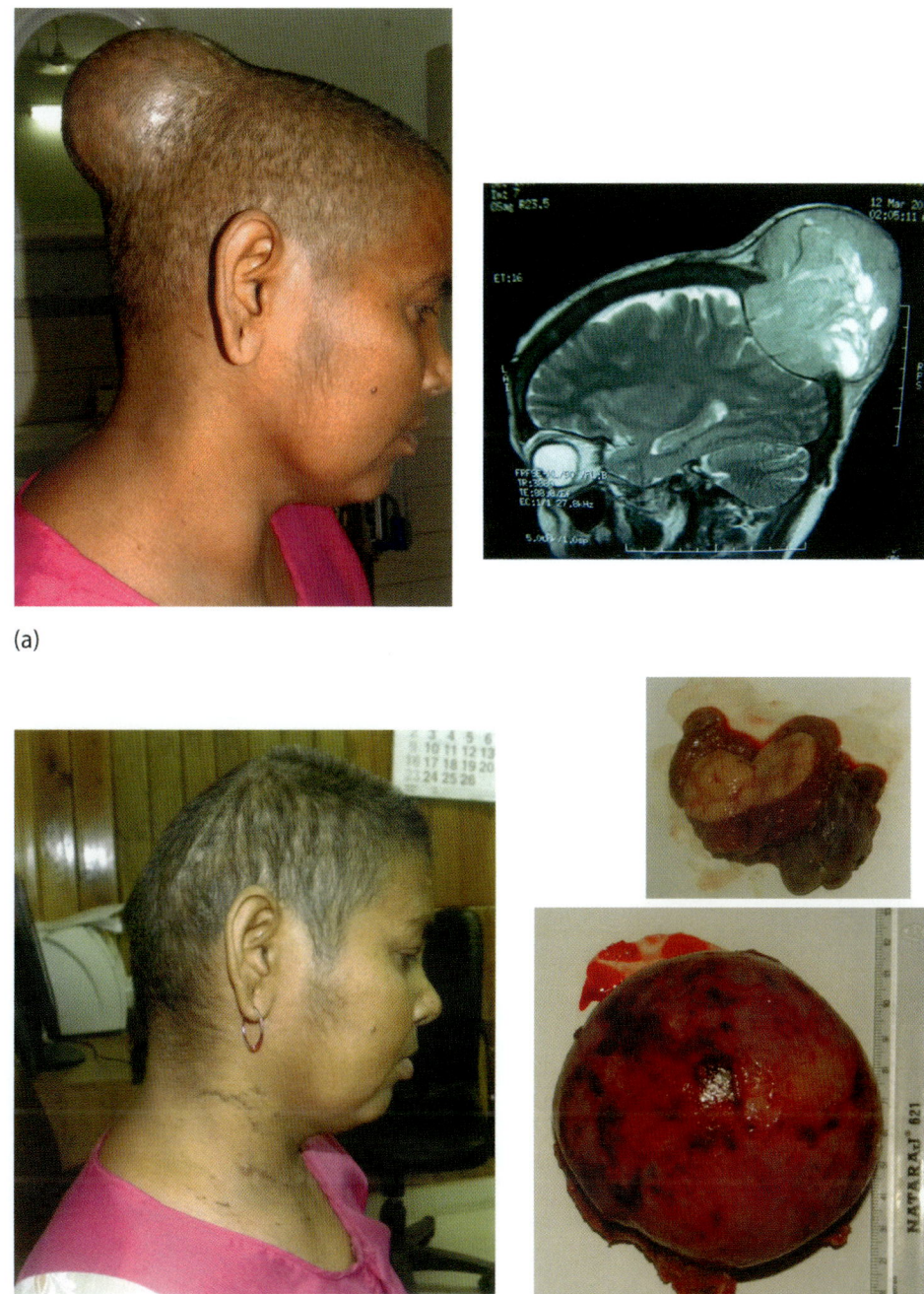

FIGURE 25.1 (a) Follicular neoplasm with scalp mass. (b) Postoperative clinical photograph with specimen picture of scalp mass and total thyroidectomy.

angiolymphatic invasion, multifocality, aggressive histological subtype (29, 41). The BRAF V600E mutation is seen in 45–73% cases (42). A total of 4% PMC was found to be associated with aggressive tumor behavior such as tall cell histological subtype, numerous cells with nuclear groove, higher invasiveness, intrathyroidal tumor spread and persistent/recurrent disease (43). Telomerase reverse transcriptase (TERT) promoter mutations are related to aggressive tumors and disease-specific mortality in PTC (44). The synergistic impact of TERT promoter mutations with BRAF V600E mutation on tumor recurrence and disease-specific mortality in patients with PMC is unknown.

Surgery

Surgical options for PMC include lobectomy, near-total thyroidectomy (NT) and TT. Proponents of TT would argue that multifocality and postsurgery follow-up are better addressed in removing the whole thyroid gland. Contrarily, proponents of the lobectomy argue that the presence of multifocality does not influence the risk of recurrence and also spares 50–60% of patients from the need for thyroxine replacement therapy. Analysis of 1376 PMC patients treated from Mayo Clinic between 1936 and 2015 had demonstrated that 20-year locoregional recurrence rates following lobectomy were comparable to near-total/TT (45). TT is recommended in PMC patients with history of irradiation, multicentric tumor, ETE and overt metastases. Prophylactic central neck dissection is not advisable as a routine and can be performed only if enlarged LNs are observed while in surgery or if nodes are detected by palpation in the central neck region.

Comparison of various international guidelines

Most of the guidelines agree that all high-risk thyroid cancer irrespective of size should undergo TT. Hemithyroidectomy is indicated only in low-risk cases that are less than 1 cm in size, unifocal, without extrathyroidal extension, without LN or distant metastases and with favorable histology. Any patient who comes under intermediate risk factors like age more than 55 or family history of thyroid cancer, history of childhood radiation to neck, extrathyroidal extension with size less than 4 cm or LN metastases or distant metastases should also undergo TT (29, 46–49) (Table 25.4).

South Asian perspective

Hemithyroidectomy is practiced at many centers for low-risk tumors defined by ATA criteria as smaller tumors less than 4 cm. However, many centers in India prefer TT for all the DTC size more than 1 cm.

Conclusion

Extent of surgery in thyroid cancer determines overall survival, hence is an important element of management and follow-up plan. The aim of surgery is to remove "complete thyroid cancer" from neck with minimal complications and sequelae. Preoperative decision is based on meticulous history, physical examination and result of triple test (TSH, ultrasound with fine needle aspiration cytology assessment) in all patients and computed tomography or magnetic resonance imaging in select cases.

TABLE 25.4: Comparison of Major Thyroid Cancer Guidelines

	American Thyroid Association (ATA 2015)	NCCN 2016	British Thyroid Association (BTA 2014)	German Association of Endocrine Surgeons (GAES 2013)	Japan Association of Endocrine Surgeons (JAES 2010, with 2014 Update)
Active surveillance	Low-risk thyroid tumors – micropapillary (PMC) without invasion, M0, no evidence of aggressive histology or High surgical risk or Comorbidities with limiting lifespan	No comment	No comment	No comment	Low-risk PMC, N0, M0, no extrathyroidal disease
Hemithyroidectomy	T < 1 cm and 1–4 cm + no FH + no RT + no E + unifocal + LN0 Completion if aggressive histology	T < 4 cm, +no FH + no RT + no E + LN0 + M0 Completion if T > 4 cm, E+, M1 or N1, margins+, B/L, poor differentiation, multifocal or vascular invasion	Individual decision T < 4 cm, age <45, no E, N0, M0	PTMC, no E, N0, unifocal, classical subtype PTC, FTC without vascular invasion	T < 4 cm, age <45, N0, M0, no E
Total thyroidectomy	T > 4 cm, or any of following: E+, N1, M1	T > 4 cm, or any of following: RT+, E+, N1, M1, B/L, poor differentiation	T > 4 cm, or any of following: multifocal, B/L, E+, FH+, N1, M1	T > 1 cm, one of the following: N1, M1, E+ widely invasive FTC	T > 4 cm, any of following: N1, M1, E+ to trachea or esophagus widely invasive FTC
Central neck dissection	LN in levels 6 and 7 Prophylactic in T3–4, lateral neck nodes or further RAI adjuvant plan	LN in levels 6 and 7 Prophylactic in T3–4, lateral neck nodes	N1, unclassical histology, age > 45, multifocal, T > 4 cm, E+ Prophylactic: individual decision	LN+	Clinically apparent LN in levels 6 and 7 Prophylactic: decision on merits and demerits
Lateral neck dissection	Clinically apparent lateral compartment disease	Clinically apparent lateral compartment disease	Clinically apparent lateral compartment disease	Clinically apparent lateral compartment disease	Clinically apparent lateral compartment disease

Abbreviations: B/L, Bilateral; E, Extrathyroidal extension; FH, Family history of thyroid cancer; M, Metastasis stage; N, Nodal disease; RT, Positive radiation history in childhood to head and neck; T, Tumor stage.

Extent of Surgery in Thyroid Cancer

Age >45 years, tumor size >4 cm, major extrathyroidal extension, poor histology and presence of distant metastasis are independent prognostic factors associated with mortality risk. Factors associated with increased risk of clinically significant persistent or recurrent disease are presence of more than three palpable LN metastases, metastatic LN size >3 cm and extracapsular nodal spread. There are patient (medical history, anatomy, lifestyle factors, performance index, finances, residence and literacy) and physician factors (experience, available resources at hospital) that also influence the treatment decisions. Hemithyroidectomy and TT are two accepted approaches for thyroid cancer. Recent trend is toward a more conservative and individualized treatment philosophy. Philosophy of the treatment is that indolent disease is not overtreated and aggressive disease is not under treated. Treatment avenues should be tailored to the individual clinical scenario based on balanced analysis of above factors. All thyroid cancer should be managed by multidisciplinary care teams, and treatment decisions should be based upon dynamic risk stratification with avoidance of overtreatment.

References

1. Tunbridge WMG, Evered DC, Hall R, Appleton D, Brewis M, Clark F, Evans JG, Young E, Bird T, Smith PA 1977 The spectrum of thyroid disease in a community: the Whickham Survey. Clin Endocrinol (Oxf) 7:481–493.
2. Vander JB, Gaston EA, Dawber TR 1968 The significance of nontoxic thyroid nodules. Ann Intern Med 69:537–540.
3. Tan GH, Gharib H 1997 Thyroid incidentalomas: management approaches to nonpalpable nodules discovered incidentally on thyroid imaging. Ann Intern Med 126:226–231.
4. Hegedus L 2004 Clinical practice. The thyroid nodule. N Engl J Med 351:1764–1771.
5. Mandel SJ 2004 A 64-year-old woman with a thyroid nodule. JAMA 292:2632–2642.
6. Leenhardt L, Bernier MO, Boin-Pineau MH, Conte DB, Marechaud R, Niccoli-Sire P, Nocaudie M, Orgiazzi J, Schlumberger M, Wémeau JL, Chérié-Challine L, De Vathaire F 2004 Advances in diagnostic practices affect thyroid cancer incidence in France. Eur J Endocrinol 150:133–139.
7. Davies L, Welch HG 2006 Increasing incidence of thyroid cancer in the United States, 1973–2002. JAMA 295:2164–2167.
8. Grant CS, Hay ID, Gough IR, Bergstralh EJ, Goellner JR, McConahey WM 1988 Local recurrence in papillary thyroid carcinoma: is extent of surgical resection important? Surgery 104:954–962.
9. Hay ID, Grant CS, Bergstralh EJ, Thompson GB, van Heerden JA, Goellner JR 1998 Unilateral total lobectomy: is it sufficient surgical treatment for patients with AMES low-risk papillary thyroid carcinoma? Surgery 124:958–964.
10. Mazzaferri EL, Kloos RT 2001 Clinical review 128: current approaches to primary therapy for papillary and follicular thyroid cancer. J Clin Endocrinol Metab 86:1447–1463.
11. Matsuzu K, Sugino K, Masudo K, Nagahama M, Kitagawa W, Shibuya H, Ohkuwa K, Uruno T, Suzuki A, Magoshi S, Akaishi J, Masaki C, Kawano M, Suganuma N, Rino Y, Masuda M, Kameyama K, Takami H, Ito K 2014 Thyroid lobectomy for papillary thyroid cancer: long-term follow-up study of 1,088 cases. World J Surg 38:68–79.
12. Barney BM, Hitchcock YJ, Sharma P, Shrieve DC, Tward JD 2011 Overall and cause-specific survival for patients undergoing lobectomy, near-total, or total thyroidectomy for differentiated thyroid cancer. Head Neck 33:645–649.
13. Mendelsohn AH, Elashoff DA, Abemayor E, St John MA 2010 Surgery for papillary thyroid carcinoma: is lobectomy enough? Arch Otolaryngol Head Neck Surg 136:1055–1061.
14. Haigh PI, Urbach DR, Rotstein LE 2005 Extent of thyroidectomy is not a major determinant of survival in low- or high-risk papillary thyroid cancer. Ann Surg Oncol 12:81–89.
15. Nixon IJ, Ganly I, Patel SG, Palmer FL, Whitcher MM, Tuttle RM, Shaha A, Shah JP 2012 Thyroid lobectomy for treatment of well differentiated intrathyroid malignancy. Surgery 151:571–579.
16. DeGroot LJ, Kaplan EL, McCormick M, et al. 1990 Natural history, treatment, and course of papillary thyroid carcinoma. J Clin Endocrinol Metab 71:414–424. [PubMed: 2380337].
17. Kebebew E, Clark OH 2000 Differentiated thyroid cancer: "complete" rational approach. World J Surg 24:942–951. [PubMed: 10865038].
18. Pasieka JL, Thompson NW, McLeod MK, et al. 1992 The incidence of bilateral well-differentiated thyroid cancer found at completion thyroidectomy. World J Surg 16:711–716, discussion 716–717. [PubMed: 1413840].
19. Shaha AR 2010 Extent of surgery for papillary thyroid carcinoma: the debate continues: comment on "surgery for papillary thyroid carcinoma". Arch Otolaryngol Head Neck Surg 136:1061–1063. [PubMed: 21079157].
20. Bilimoria KY, Bentrem DJ, Ko CY, Stewart AK, Winchester DP, Talamonti MS, Sturgeon C 2007 Extent of surgery affects survival for papillary thyroid cancer. Ann Surg 246(3):375–378.
21. Grant CS, Hay ID, Gough IR, Bergstralh EJ, Goellner JR, McConahey WM 1988 Local recurrence in papillary thyroid carcinoma: is extent of surgical resection important? Surgery 104:954–962.
22. Hay ID, Grant CS, Bergstralh EJ, Thompson GB, van Heerden JA, Goellner JR 1998 Unilateral total lobectomy: is it sufficient surgical treatment for patients with AMES low-risk papillary thyroid carcinoma. Surgery 124:958–964, discussion 964–956.
23. Cooper DS, Doherty GM, Haugen BR, Kloos RT, Lee SL, Mandel SJ, Mazzaferri EL, McIver B, Pacini F, Schlumberger M, Sherman SI, Steward DL, Tuttle RM 2009 Revised American Thyroid Association management guidelines for patients with thyroid nodules and differentiated thyroid cancer. Thyroid 19(11):1167–1214.
24. Adam MA, Pura J, Gu L, Dinan MA, Tyler DS, Reed SD, Scheri R, Roman SA, Sosa JA 2014 Extent of surgery for papillary thyroid cancer is not associated with survival: an analysis of 61,775 patients. Ann Surg 260(4):601–605, discussion 605–607.
25. Matsuzu K, Sugino K, Masudo K, et al. 2014 Thyroid lobectomy for papillary thyroid cancer: long-term follow-up study of 1,088 cases. World J Surg 38:68–79.
26. Barney BM, Hitchcock YJ, Sharma P, Shrieve DC, Tward JD 2011 Overall and cause-specific survival for patients undergoing lobectomy, near total, or total thyroidectomy for differentiated thyroid cancer. Head Neck 33:645–649.
27. Mendelsohn AH, Elashoff DA, Abemayor E, St John MA 2010 Surgery for papillary thyroid carcinoma: is lobectomy enough? Arch Otolaryngol Head Neck Surg 136:1055–1061.
28. Haigh PI, Urbach DR, Rotstein LE 2005 Extent of thyroidectomy is not a major determinant of survival in low- or high-risk papillary thyroid cancer. Ann Surg Oncol 12:81–89.
29. Haugen BR, Alexander EK, Bible KC, Doherty GM, Mandel SJ, Nikiforov YE, Pacini F, Randolph GW, Sawka AM, Schlumberger M, Schuff KG, Sherman SI, Sosa JA, Steward DL, Tuttle RM, Wartofsky L 2016 2015 American Thyroid Association Management Guidelines for adult patients with thyroid nodules and differentiated thyroid cancer: the American Thyroid Association Guidelines Task Force on thyroid nodules and differentiated thyroid cancer. Thyroid 26(1):1–133.
30. Stojadinovic A, Ghossein RA, Hoos A, et al. 2001 Hürthle cell carcinoma: a critical histopathologic appraisal. J Clin Oncol 19:2616.
31. Haugen BR, Alexander EK, Bible KC, Doherty GM, Mandel SJ, et al. 2016 2015 American Thyroid Association Management Guidelines for adult patients with thyroid nodules and differentiated thyroid cancer: the American Thyroid Association Guidelines Task Force on thyroid nodules and differentiated thyroid cancer. Thyroid 26:1–133.
32. Mazzaferri EL, Jhiang SM 1994 Long-term impact of initial surgical and medical therapy on papillary and follicular thyroid cancer. Am J Med 97:418.
33. Podnos YD, Smith D, Wagman LD, et al. 2005 The implication of lymph node metastasis on survival in patients with well-differentiated thyroid cancer. Am Surg 71:731–734.
34. Carling T, Carty SE, Ciarleglio MM, et al. 2012 American Thyroid Association design and feasibility of a prospective randomized controlled trial of prophylactic central lymph node dissection for papillary thyroid carcinoma. Thyroid 22:237–244.
35. Kouvaraki MA, Shapiro SE, Fornage BD, et al. 2003 Role of preoperative ultrasonography in the surgical management of patients with thyroid cancer. Surgery 134:946.
36. Tuttle RM, Fagin JA 2009 Can risk-adapted treatment recommendations replace the 'one size fits all' approach for early-stage thyroid cancer patients? Oncology (Williston Park) 23:592, 600–603.
37. Zetoune T, Keutgen X, Buitrago D, et al. 2010 Prophylactic central neck dissection and local recurrence in papillary thyroid cancer: a meta-analysis. Ann Surg Oncol 17:3287.
38. Shan CX, Zhang W, Jiang DZ, et al. 2012 Routine central neck dissection in differentiated thyroid carcinoma: a systematic review and meta-analysis. Laryngoscope 122:797.
39. Randolph GW, Duh QY, Heller KS, et al. 2012 The prognostic significance of nodal metastases from papillary thyroid carcinoma can be stratified based on the size and number of metastatic lymph nodes, as well as the presence of extranodal extension. Thyroid 22:1144.
40. Sippel RS, Chen H 2009 Controversies in the surgical management of newly diagnosed and recurrent/residual thyroid cancer. Thyroid 19:1373.
41. Durante C, Attard M, Torlontano M, et al. 2010 Identification and optimal postsurgical follow-up of patients with very low-risk papillary thyroid microcarcinomas. J Clin Endocrinol Metab 95(11):4882–4888.
42. Ji Y, Xie H, Wei B, Shen H, Liu A, Gao Y, Wang L 2019 Relationship between BRAF V600E gene mutation and the clinical and pathologic characteristics of papillary thyroid microcarcinoma. Int J Clin Exp Pathol 12(9):3492–3499.
43. Tallini G, de Biase D, Durante C, Acquaviva G, Bisceglia M, Bruno R, Bacchi Reggiani ML, Casadei GP, Costante G, Cremonini N, Lamartina L, Meringolo D, Nardi F, Pession A, Rhoden KJ, Ronga G, Torlontano M, Verrienti A, Visani M, Filetti S 2015 BRAF V600E and risk stratification of thyroid microcarcinoma: a multicenter pathological and clinical study. Mod Pathol 28(10):1343–1359.
44. Melo M, da Rocha AG, Vinagre J, Batista R, Peixoto J, Tavares C, Celestino R, Almeida A, Salgado C, Eloy C, Castro P, Prazeres H, Lima J, Amaro T, Lobo C, Martins MJ, Moura M, Cavaco B, Leite V, Cameselle-Teijeiro JM, Carrilho F, Carvalheiro M, Máximo V, Sobrinho-Simões M, Soares P 2014 TERT promoter mutations are a major indicator of poor outcome in differentiated thyroid carcinomas. J Clin Endocrinol Metab 99(5):E754–65.
45. Brito JP, Hay ID 2019 Management of papillary thyroid microcarcinoma. Endocrinol Metab Clin 48(1):199–213.
46. National Comprehensive Cancer Network (NCCN) 2016 Clinical practice guidelines in oncology, thyroid carcinoma. www.nccn.org.
47. British Thyroid Association 2007 Royal College of Physicians. Guidelines for the management of thyroid cancer. In: Perros P, editor. Report of the thyroid cancer guidelines update group. 2nd ed. London: Royal College of Physicians.
48. Dralle H, Musholt TJ, Schabram J, et al. 2013 German Association of Endocrine Surgeons practice guideline for the surgical management of malignant thyroid tumors. Langenbecks Arch Surg 398:347–375.
49. Takami H, Ito Y, Okamoto T, Onoda N, Noguchi H, Yoshida A 2014 Revisiting the guidelines issued by the Japanese Society of Thyroid Surgeons and Japan Association of Endocrine Surgeons: a gradual move towards consensus between Japanese and western practice in the management of thyroid carcinoma. World J Surg 38:2002–2010.

26

ADJUVANT TREATMENT AND FOLLOW-UP OF THYROID CANCERS

Hian Liang Huang, Kelvin Loke Siu Hoong, Sumbul Zaheer and David Ng Chee Eng

Introduction

Radioactive iodine in the setting of adjuvant therapy for thyroid cancer commonly refers to the beta- and gamma-emitting isotope of iodine, Iodine-131 (I-131). It has been used for approximately seven decades in the treatment of well-differentiated thyroid carcinoma (DTC). I-131 leverages the innate ability of well differentiated thyroid cells to concentrate iodine via the sodium iodide cotransporter. The beta emission from I-131 causes single-strand DNA breaks to occur and with sufficient damage induction of apoptosis.

The absorption of I-131 also depends on various factors, including blood supply, presence of sodium iodide symporter receptors and having sufficient thyroid stimulating hormone (TSH) elevation to drive uptake into the target cells. This will be further elucidated in the section on practical aspects of therapy. Whilst the side effects are limited to sodium iodide expressing tissues or other local effects from beta radiation, in general poorly differentiated thyroid cancer, which has lost the ability to concentrate I-131, should not be treated using I-131.

Post radioiodine therapy, patients are followed up mainly by serum thyroglobulin assays and by neck ultrasonography (US) complementing low dose diagnostic whole body radioiodine scans. If there is suspicion of radioiodine negative or refractory disease, other advanced hybrid imaging modalities such as [^{18}F] fluorodeoxyglucose (FDG) PET/CT scanning may be warranted, and other options of therapy, including targeted therapies with tyrosine kinase inhibitors (TKIs) such as sorafenib and lenvantinib can be considered.

Risk stratification for adjuvant therapy

The AJCC/TNM staging system for thyroid carcinoma (8th edition)[1] uses patient data accumulated in the preoperative, intraoperative and immediate 4 months following thyroid surgery to define initial nodal (N) and metastasis (M) status. It is particularly useful in determining an individual patient's overall (OS) and disease specific survival (DSS) rates after thyroid surgery.

There are several changes to the staging system over the seventh edition, namely, raising the age cut-off at diagnosis from 45 to 55 years (for the purpose of assigning the stage) and reclassifying the stages. The effect of these would be to downstage a significant proportion of patients.

Separate from the AJCC/TNM staging system, there is risk stratification of the postsurgical patient into low, intermediate and high-risk categories based on various types of risk assessment, e.g., the American Thyroid Association System is based on patient factors, surgical findings and postoperative histopathological features and appears to be good at predicting the risk of persistent or recurrent structural disease in thyroid cancer patients. In general, these would include patients who have a more aggressive histology; more numerous and bulky nodal disease involvement; more extensive locoregional extension and incomplete surgical excisions.

This risk categorization aids the treating nuclear medicine physician in deciding which patient would benefit from radioiodine treatment and if so, the subsequent administered dose activities for radioiodine remnant ablation (RRA) and adjuvant radioactive iodine therapy.

RRA is not routinely recommended in very low risk patients. These would include patients with ≤1 cm unifocal or multifocal well DTC (classical papillary, follicular variant of papillary thyroid carcinoma and follicular carcinoma) which may be minimally invasive but demonstrate no angioinvasion or invasion of the thyroid capsule and with a postoperative unstimulated thyroglobulin (Tg) <1.0 ng/mL in the absence of detectable anti-thyroglobulin antibodies. For all other patients, RRA and/or therapy would be selectively or typically recommended. Whilst the postoperative assessment of thyroid cancer patients, prior to RRA or radioiodine therapy, using diagnostic I-123 scanning can be helpful in clinical decision making regarding the need for further radioiodine treatment and dose activity selection; this practice within South Asia is varied. In most instances, estimation of remnant thyroid tissue volume and disease burden via such diagnostic iodine scanning is not commonly performed due to the unavailability of I-123 and the possible stunning effect from I-131. These limitations also make pretreatment dosimetry and personalized radioiodine therapy challenging but not impossible.

In the absence of large randomized clinical trials on radioactive iodine therapy and the long indolent period of recurrent disease, the latest guidelines published by the American Thyroid Association (ATA) in 2015, British Thyroid Association (BTA) in 2014 and National Comprehensive Cancer Network (NCCN) in 2019 have incorporated this patient risk categorization with regards to the use of I-131 in the post-op patient. The dose activity selected would depend on the aim and intention of radioiodine. Low- and intermediate-risk category patients can receive a lower activity of I-131 (1110–1850 MBq) for the purpose of RRA. Lower administered activities have been shown to be non-inferior to higher activities. Selective adjuvant therapy doses of 1850–3700 MBq can also be considered in patients who are deemed to have higher risks. High-risk patients may receive higher activities of radioiodine within suggested activity ranges of 3700–7400 MBq. Radioiodine therapy with activities ≥3700 MBq (or activities adjusted according to dosimetry) can be considered for empirical treatment of patients who have recurrent metastatic disease. The final decision regarding the administered activity should be undertaken by the treating nuclear medicine physician taking all patient factors into consideration.

Where technically feasible, pretreatment tumor dosimetry to determine administered dose activity should be considered especially in the at-risk patient population. Dosimetry with radioiodine has been described[2]. Whilst this might be logistically challenging, dosimetry is a more scientifically sound methodology of prescribing personalized I-131 to thyroid cancer patients. This applies especially to special categories of patients such as pediatric patients, patients with pulmonary metastases and in patients who have renal impairment. In this way, I-131 can be prescribed within safe dose limits, ensuring delivery of adequate radiation absorbed dose to remnant thyroid tissue and diseased tissues whilst minimizing potential side effects of treatment.

Practical aspects of radioiodine therapy

In accordance to most countries' national radiation protection agencies requirements, high activity I-131 is generally carried out as an inpatient procedure. The definition of what constitutes high activity can vary, and in certain countries, all patients are hospitalized regardless[3]. In some national jurisdictions in Asia, activities more than 1110 MBq are generally considered high and patients receiving these are hospitalized until their radiation exposure at 1 m measures less than 80 mSv/h[4]. Hydration is encouraged along with laxatives to increase clearance of radioactivity. End-stage renal failure is not a contraindication to radioiodine therapy, as it can be cleared in the dialysate.

Patients need to take low iodine diet for 1–2 weeks prior to therapy[5]. To allow for adequate concentration of I-131 in target tissue, there is iatrogenic elevation of TSH levels, either by withdrawal of levothyroxine in the post total thyroidectomy patient, or by intramuscular injection of recombinant human TSH (rhTSH, Genzyme®). Generally, a TSH level of more than 30 IU/mL is accepted as adequate elevation. Withdrawal of levothyroxine can be used in patients who are younger and more able to tolerate the symptoms of hypothyroidism[6]. In the setting of known metastatic disease, there is currently insufficient evidence to support rhTSH use, and therefore, thyroxine withdrawal is recommended[7]. The advantage of rhTSH would be preventing symptomatic hypothyroidism, especially in the elderly or frail population[8]. In patients who cannot mount a TSH response (possibly due to functional metastases or hypopituitarism) rhTSH is also a viable option.

Post-radioiodine therapy scans are typically done between 3 and 14 days later. The relatively long 8-day physical half-life of I-131 allows for delayed sequential imaging to be performed to reduce false-positive and -negative scan results[9]. Patients are advised to avoid prolonged close contact, especially with children below the age of 5 and pregnant women. Sleeping in a separate room is recommended for a few days. Because I-131 is excreted in the sweat and saliva, radiation protection efforts would include laundry arrangements, cooking, eating utensils and strict personal hygiene. Keeping the toilet clean with flushing twice helps clearance of radioactive urine.

It is generally advised to wait before attempting pregnancy after radioiodine treatment (usually at least 4 months for males and 6–12 months for females) because of the concern of iatrogenic hypothyroidism of the newborn and effects on sperm quality. As I-131 may be transmitted in the breastmilk, breastfeeding should be stopped before receiving RAI and should not be resumed. However, breastfeeding is unaffected for subsequent childbirths[10].

Side effects of radioiodine therapy

I-131 therapy is generally well tolerated; however, knowledge of the potential adverse effects of I-131 is of importance in the informed consent process.

As with all side effects, these can be divided into acute (up to 3 months post treatment) and subacute. They can also be divided into side effects from the preparation for I-131 therapy and those as a direct result of the therapy.

Early complications include gastrointestinal symptoms[11], ageusia[12], sialadenitis/xerostomia, lacrimal gland dysfunction, transient male gonadal and transient female gonadal dysfunction as well as radiation thyroiditis[13]. Salivary gland swelling, pain and dysfunction are more common with doses in excess of 3700 MBq. Sour candy or lemon juice have been recommended to increase salivation-stimulation after I-131 administration to reduce retention of radiation in salivary glands. Fortunately, these complications tend to be limited and well managed with supportive measures such as analgesia and antiemetics.

Patients were prone to developing pain or swelling of neck with low pretreatment TSH levels while severe gastrointestinal symptoms were more commonly noted in patients with high pretreatment TSH levels. This may be related to the amount of remnant thyroid tissue in the neck being ablated and thereby more symptomatic, although this is less likely currently due to the practice of total thyroidectomy.

Increasing incidence and severity of adverse effects following I-131 therapy were in general associated with increasing administered cumulative I-131 activity[14]; hence, there is renewed emphasis on patient selection and risk stratification, as with any other medication use.

Late complications include secondary cancers (ranging from 0% to 8% as quoted in the literature), pulmonary fibrosis (if presence of pulmonary metastases and radiation dose to the lungs exceeds 80 mCi), permanent bone marrow suppression (rare with low cumulative doses) and permanent xerostomia.

As it is an efficacious form of treatment, I-131 therapy remains the principal mode of adjuvant treatment for patients with DTC but patient selection and appropriate risk stratification for dose selection is paramount in improving the therapeutic index of I-131.

Follow-up of thyroid cancer patients

The posttreatment follow-up of patients with differentiated thyroid cancer (DTC) falls into two broad categories, early management after initial therapy and long-term management.

Early management after initial therapy

A key aspect of early management for clinicians is deciding the appropriate degree of TSH suppression. Both 2015 ATA[15] and the 2014 BTA[16] guidelines advocate a risk adjusted titration of TSH suppression.

DTC mostly retains expression of TSH receptors on the cell membrane and responds to TSH stimulation by increasing production of several thyroid specific proteins (for example, thyroglobulin and the sodium iodide symporter) and by increasing the rates of cell growth[17]. Suppression of TSH, using supra-physiologic doses of levothyroxine, is, therefore, logically used for patients with thyroid cancer to decrease the risk of symptomatic disease recurrence[18–22] and delay the need for further intervention.

The degree of TSH suppression should depend on the risk stratification and response assessment of the individual patient. Both retrospective and prospective studies showed that TSH suppression below 0.1 mU/L may improve outcomes in high-risk thyroid cancer patients[23], though not in low-risk patients.

On the flip side, adverse effects of overzealous TSH suppression may include subclinical thyrotoxicosis, exacerbation of angina, increased risk for atrial fibrillation in older patients[24], and increased risk of osteoporosis in postmenopausal women[25]. Thus, there is a need for using clinical judgment to get the balance of TSH suppression and symptoms just right, by taking into consideration the patient as a whole, not merely paying attention to numbers. We typically review these patients approximately 3–4 months post-radioiodine ablation to check on symptoms and adequacy of TSH suppression. Risk stratification and need for RAI after initial surgery are summarized in Figure 26.1.

Long-term management

The broad aims of long-term follow-up are for early detection of recurrence, monitoring adequacy of TSH suppression and further management of disease recurrences and complications.

It is now increasingly recognized that the risk of recurrence in thyroid cancer is a spectrum dependent on patient and disease specific factors, as well as the initial response to treatment. There are various risk stratification systems published by various thyroid associations, which provides a valuable tool for predicting recurrence.

Given that many patients initially classified as intermediate or high risk of recurrence can be reclassified as having a subsequent low risk of recurrence based on having an excellent response to initial therapy[26,27], there is hope even for those initially deemed to have high risk, and our therapies aim to achieve this favorable outcome.

Validated dynamic risk stratification systems are, therefore, recommended. The ATA guidelines are among the most commonly used, and we have adopted several of their recommendations for risk stratification in our practice. The concept and initial validation of the four response to therapy categories presented in the ATA guidelines were described by Tuttle et al. and modified in Vaisman et al.[28]. As originally conceived, these clinical outcomes described the best response to initial therapy during the first 2 years of follow-up, but they are now being used to describe the clinical status at any point during follow-up.

The dynamic risk stratification categories are:

Excellent response: No evidence of disease on clinical examination, blood tests or imaging

Biochemical incomplete response: Abnormal thyroglobulin (Tg) or rising anti-thyroglobulin antibody (TgAb) levels, but the disease cannot be localized on imaging.

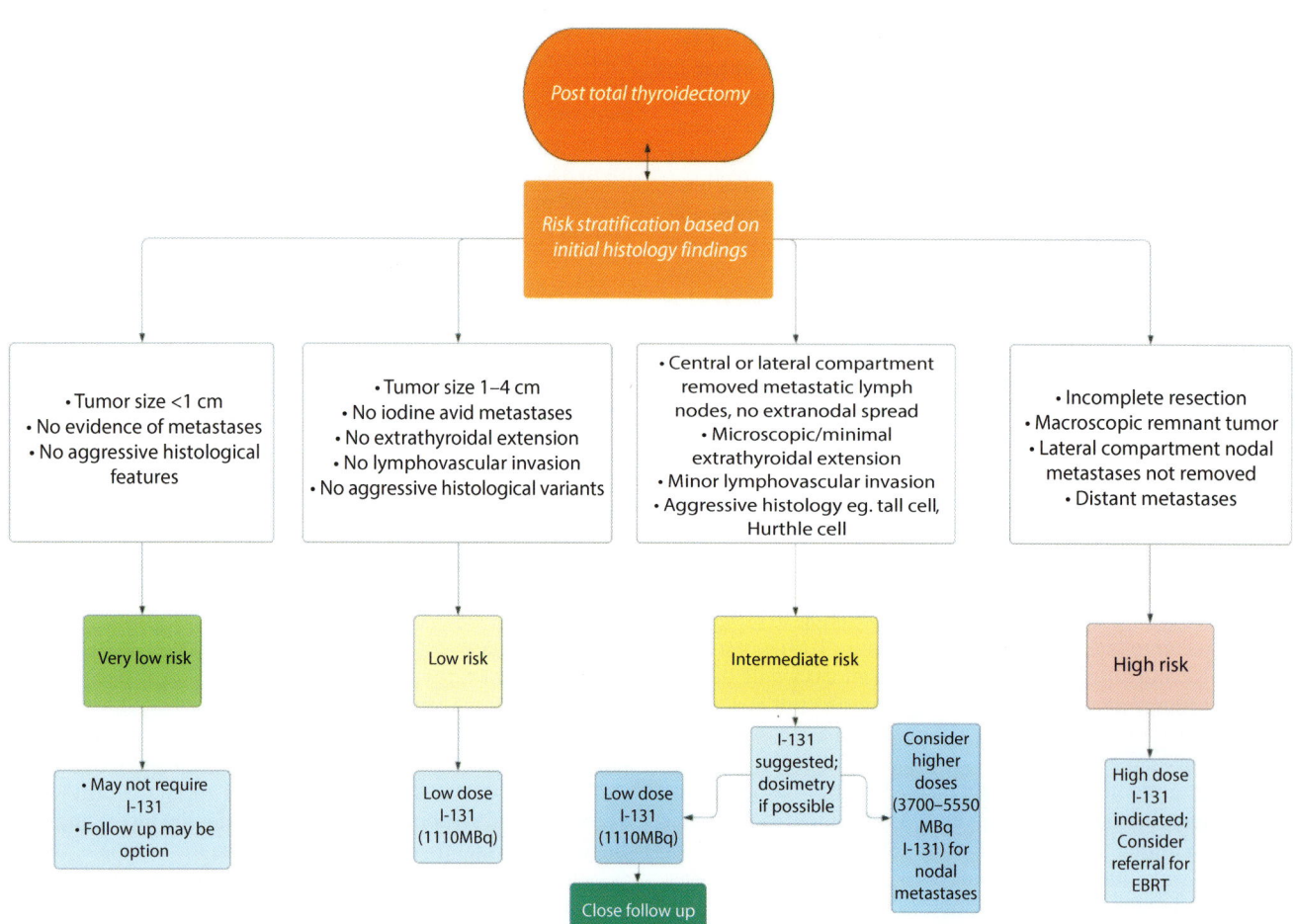

FIGURE 26.1 Suggested approach to risk stratification and I-131 treatment of patients post total thyroidectomy, based on surgical, histological and preoperative imaging findings.

Structural incomplete response: There is presence of locoregional or distant metastases that are either newly discovered or known but persistent.

Indeterminate response: A catch all category for patients who don't meet the other criteria. For example, patients with stable or declining anti-thyroglobulin antibody levels without definitive structural evidence of disease.

Based on these categories, a personalized strategy for the level of TSH suppression, frequency of follow-up visits, blood tests and imaging, can be devised. Clearly, the worst prognosis would belong to those with structural incomplete response and these may be monitored more closely, and conversely those with excellent response may be better served by a less stringent level of monitoring. Dynamic stratification and approach is outlined in Figure 26.2.

The following investigations are usually performed in the follow-up of DTC patients:

Serum Tg and TgAb

Serum Tg is a key laboratory test in the follow-up of DTC patients. Tg is usually only elevated in the presence of functioning thyroid cells, hence the utility of trending the levels of Tg as an indication of the disease course. Note that normal thyroid remnant tissue may also give a measurable level of Tg, depending on the level of TSH; hence, there is benefit of thyroid remnant ablation with radioiodine to give a minimal baseline level of Tg for ease and accuracy of follow-up.

A rising serum Tg with adequate levels of TSH suppression is highly suggestive of tumor recurrence or progression and should prompt further evaluation for such. However, endogenous TgAb and other unidentified factors may interfere with the measurement of serum Tg and cause unnecessary patient concern. Therefore, measurement of TgAb is valuable in interpreting the serum Tg result and in our practice TgAb is automatically included in the laboratory order set for Tg.

Initially, serum Tg is recommended to be measured every 6–12 months. More frequent Tg measurements may be appropriate for high-risk patients with the hope of catching aggressive disease and instituting further curative therapy early on.

The highest sensitivity for serum Tg are noted with higher levels of serum TSH[29], which may be obtained by thyroxine withdrawal or by administration of recombinant human TSH (rhTSH). However, it should be noted that serum Tg may fail to identify patients with relatively small amounts of residual tumor[12,30–32]. These minimal amounts of residual disease are often located in the neck. Given that this may not cause any prognostic significance and the recent trend toward reducing the doses of radioiodine given, there should be a discussion with the patient and the

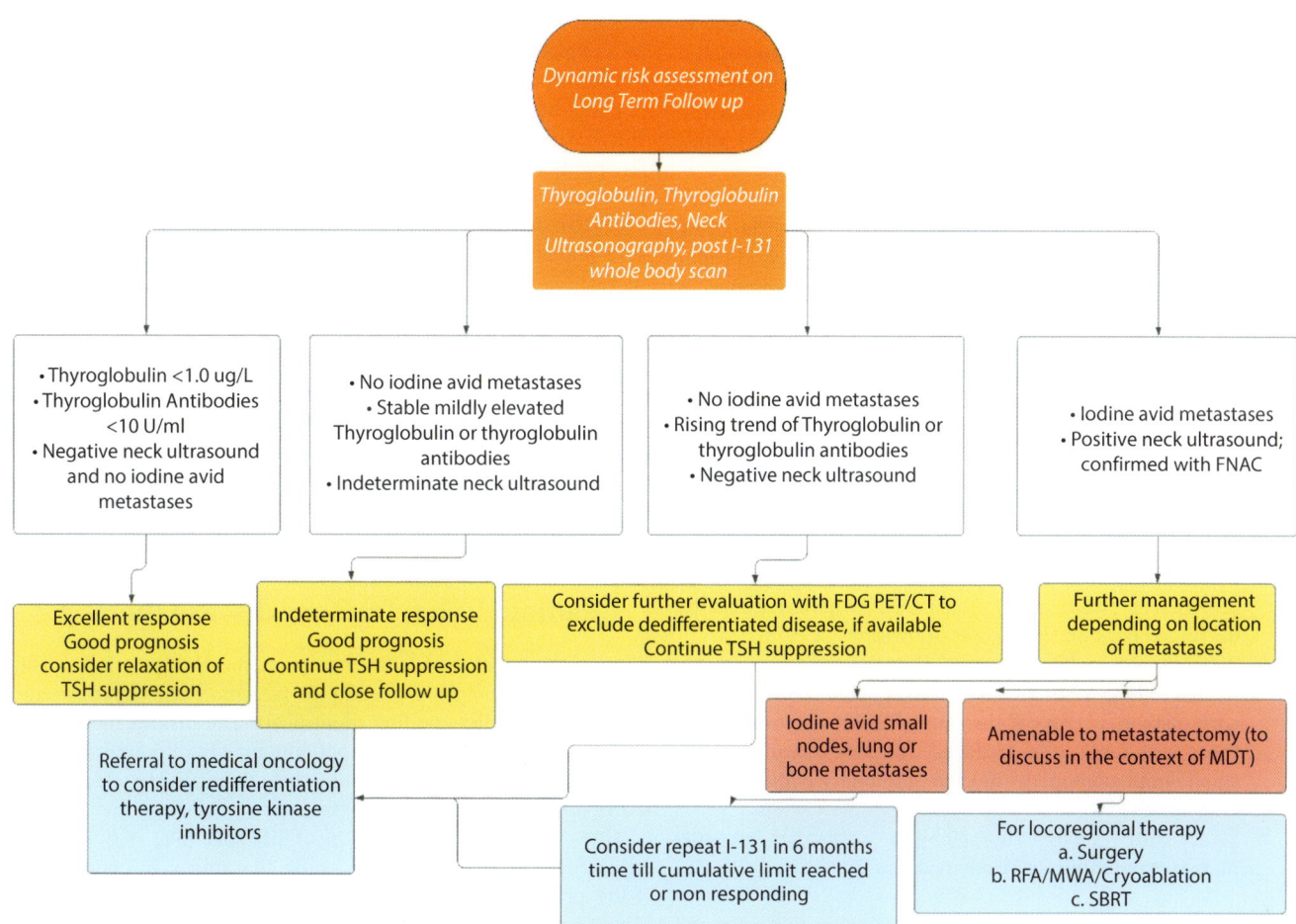

FIGURE 26.2 Suggested approach to patient assessment and dynamic risk assessment in follow-up clinics for the long-term management of thyroid cancer patients, based on serum tumor markers, neck ultrasonography, I-131 scan findings.

multidisciplinary team about the need to carry out stimulated Tg measurements, as these may involve side effects and potentially a period whereby the growth of tumor is stimulated by elevation of TSH. Performing neck US in these patients may be considered as one of the more sensitive modalities for finding these small amounts of residual tumor[33], but the impact on management of finding these may be questionable as well.

Anti-Tg antibodies occur in approximately a quarter of thyroid cancer patients[34], some even in the absence of disease, and they are a potential confounder, as explained above[35].

Neck ultrasonography (US)

We would recommend neck US to evaluate the thyroid bed and central and lateral cervical nodal compartments at approximately 6–12 months and thereafter depending on the patient's risk for recurrent disease and Tg levels. Suspicious lesions may then be considered for fine needle aspiration biopsy. Measurement of the Tg level in the biopsy aspirate fluid helps to increase specificity, especially in lymph nodes.

Diagnostic whole-body radioiodine scan, preferably with SPECT/CT (I-123 or I-131) or rarely PET/CT (I-124) imaging

With the advent of hybrid imaging techniques such as SPECT or PET/CT, the inherent sensitivity of the radionuclide technique can be improved by adding the specificity and anatomical localization capabilities of CT.

If available, it would be preferable to use isotopes of iodine (I-123 and I-124) which do not emit any beta-particulate radiation, so as to avoid potential for stunning (which is a debatable topic currently) and also to allow better imaging characteristics. These isotopes also have shorter half-lives than I-131 and allow faster imaging, for greater patient convenience.

If unavailable, the need to justify the use of I-131 for purely diagnostic purposes becomes paramount, especially if the same information may be obtained by using neck US which is cheaper and lacks ionizing radiation. This is less so for other isotopes. In general, the radiation dose from these is much less than for I-131, and therefore, smaller amounts of I-131 can be injected, limiting the imaging characteristics further.

A diagnostic iodine scan may be considered in four primary clinical settings, in decreasing order of importance:

1. Patients with suspicious findings on conventional imaging, where knowledge of the sodium iodide symporter expression has impact on management
2. Patients with abnormal uptake outside the thyroid bed on post-therapy whole body scan (WBS), where it would be useful to check on the success of therapy
3. Patients with high uptake of I-131 in the neck, presumably related to large remnants (an arbitrary cut off of >2% of the administered activity at the time of WBS, also consider in those with large 'star' artifacts) that may obscure nearby small lymphadenopathy or even pulmonary nodules in the lung apices and
4. Significantly raised thyroglobulin antibodies as this increases potential for falsely-negative Tg levels.

Diagnostic WBS may be performed following thyroid hormone withdrawal or rhTSH. If found to be positive, further therapeutic doses of I-131 can be planned, as there is now evidence of iodine-avid disease. Knowledge of the normal and benign variants of iodine uptake is, however, essential to avoid overtreatment, and here the experience of the nuclear medicine physician combined with the anatomical information from the CT can increase specificity.

As with all hybrid imaging techniques, the CT portion of the examination should also be carefully scrutinized to ensure that incidental anatomical findings and indeed iodine-negative metastases are not missed, as these may have significant impact on patient outcomes.

FDG PET/CT scanning

FDG-PET/CT is a growing modality worldwide. It promises increased sensitivity over conventional imaging, given that in general malignant cells have increased metabolism and, therefore, uptake of FDG, a glucose analogue. However, there are minor drawbacks of cost and increased radiation exposure. Again, the risk/benefit ratio should be considered, but there is evidence to suggest a complementary role of FDG PET/CT with iodine WBS. In general, we would recommend using FDG PET/CT in high-risk DTC patients with elevated stimulated serum Tg (generally >10 ng/mL) but have negative I-131 imaging (the so-called Thyroglobulin Elevated, Negative Iodine Scintigraphy [TENIS] syndrome). This would be to detect the macroscopic but non-iodine-avid foci of disease, that further potentially curative therapy (surgery or local ablation techniques) can be instituted. In a metanalysis of 25 studies that included 789 patients, the sensitivity of FDG-PET/CT was 83% (ranging from 50% to 100%) and the specificity was 84% (ranging from 42% to 100%) in non-iodine-avid DTC[36].

Like in most malignancies, FDG-PET is more sensitive in patients with more aggressive histological subtypes. Because of this fact, FDG uptake in metastatic DTC patients is a major negative predictive factor for response to I-131 treatment and an independent prognostic factor for survival[37,38]; therefore, it would be useful to identify these foci of more aggressive disease and institute potentially curative treatment early on before the disease metastasizes and the patients prognosis worsens.

CT and MRI scanning

These modalities may be considered in special settings such as when neck ultrasound is felt to be inadequately visualizing possible neck nodal disease, but in general, their use is fairly limited at the current time. It should also be noted that CT should be done without iodinated contrast if radioiodine use is being considered in the near future, given potential reduction in uptake given the high iodine load.

Radioiodine refractory disease therapy

One of the benefits of I-131 therapy is the ability to follow the theranostic principle, especially in patients with distant metastatic disease, allowing first identification of distant metastases and thereafter therapy. These patients may have poorer prognosis, but if these metastases demonstrate the ability to concentrate I-131 they have potential to be treated.

However, a small proportion of patients (5%) may become refractory to I-131, either by losing the ability to concentrate I-131 or by lack of response to repeated courses of therapy[39]. These patients have the worst prognosis (10% 10-year survival)[40]. They should be uniformly on TSH suppression (target TSH < 0.1 mU/L) and monitored for symptoms, leading to focal treatment of metastases where necessary. If the disease can be surgically resected or debulked, it should be considered (for example, wedge resection of pulmonary metastases), and other locoregional therapies from ethanol ablation to RF ablation may also be applied. External beam radiotherapy may be of benefit in this situation. In patients with bone metastases, antiresorptive agents such as bisphosphonates or denosumab may be of benefit[41]. A multidisciplinary approach is, therefore, essential. Traditional systemic chemotherapy has poor response rates and significant toxicities. Especially in the TENIS syndrome, FDG PET/CT may have a key role in identifying potentially treatable disease and, if negative, may give some degree of reassurance to the patients who can then be followed up closely with serial Tg measurements and neck US.

In recent years, a number of TKIs have been approved for the treatment of I-131 refractory/progressive disease. There is phase III data available showing benefit of lenvatinib and sorafenib, with phases I and II studies for a variety of other TKIs.

Unfortunately the use of TKIs can be associated with significant side effects ranging from hypertension to Hand Foot syndrome, and this may limit their early usage in this clinical context. In general, those with rapidly progressing disease (1–2 cm increase in size of metastases in 3 months, or rapid doubling time of Tg) or larger burden of disease by size or symptoms would be candidates to receive TKI therapy[42].

There are also recent efforts to use retinoic acid, MEK inhibitors (selumetinib) or BRAF inhibitors (dabrafenib) to reinduce I-131 uptake[43]. There are also anecdotal reports of the use of peptide receptor radionuclide therapy (PPRT) with lutetium-177 or yttrium-90 radiolabelled somatostatin receptor analogues in papillary[44] and follicular[45] thyroid carcinomas, if somatostatin receptor expression has been confirmed with the use of octreotide scintigraphy[46] or Ga-68 somatostastin receptor analogue PET/CT, although the clinical efficacy of these is not conclusively proven.

Conclusion

In conclusion, the adjuvant therapy and follow-up of DTC is an ever-evolving field necessitating a multidisciplinary approach, in which advanced imaging and therapeutic modalities are available.

References

1. Tuttle M, Morris LF, Haugen B, Shah J, Sosa JA, Rohren E, Subramaniam RM, Hunt JL, Perrier ND 2017 Thyroid-Differentiated and Anaplastic Carcinoma (Chapter 73). In: Amin MB, Edge SB, Greene F, Byrd D, Brookland RK, Washington MK, Gershenwald JE, Compton CC, Hess KR, Sullivan DC, Jessup JM, Brierley J, Gaspar LE, Schilsky RL, Balch CM, Winchester DP, Asare EA, Madera M, Gress DM, Meyer LR, (eds) AJCC Cancer Staging Manual. 8th ed. Springer International Publishing, New York City.
2. Chlumberger, Martin, Bogdan Catargi, Isabelle Borget, Désirée Deandreis, Slimane Zerdoud, Boumédiène Bridji, Stéphane Bardet, et al. "Strategies of Radioiodine Ablation in Patients with Low-Risk Thyroid Cancer." New England Journal of Medicine 366, no. 18 (May 3, 2012): 1663–73.
3. Klerk, J M de. "131I Therapy: Inpatient or Outpatient?" Journal of Nuclear Medicine: Official Publication, Society of Nuclear Medicine 41, no. 11 (November 1, 2000): 1876–78.
4. "Radiation Protection (Ionising Radiation) Regulations - Singapore Statutes Online," 2001. https://sso.agc.gov.sg/SL/RPA1991-RG2?DocDate=20000201#pr44-.
5. Chung, Jae Hoon. "Low Iodine Diet for Preparation for Radioactive Iodine Therapy in Differentiated Thyroid Carcinoma in Korea." Endocrinology and Metabolism (Seoul, Korea) 28, no. 3 (September 2013): 157–63.
6. Kim, Jahae, Sang-Geon Cho, Sae-Ryung Kang, Seong Young Kwon, Dong-Hyeok Cho, Jin-Seong Cho, and Ho-Chun Song. "Preparation for Radioactive Iodine Therapy Is Not a Risk Factor for the Development of Hyponatremia in Thyroid Cancer Patients." Medicine 96, no. 5 (February 2017): e6004.
7. Haugen, Bryan R, Erik K Alexander, Keith C Bible, Gerard M Doherty, Susan J Mandel, Yuri E Nikiforov, Furio Pacini, et al. "2015 American Thyroid Association Management Guidelines for Adult Patients with Thyroid Nodules and Differentiated Thyroid Cancer The American Thyroid Association Guidelines Task Force on Thyroid Nodules and Differentiated Thyroid Cancer." Thyroid 26, no. 1 (2016): 1–133.
8. Sager, Sait, Esra Hatipoglu, Burcak Gunes, Sertac Asa, Lebriz Uslu, and Kerim Sönmezoğlu. "Comparison of Day 3 and Day 5 Thyroglobulin Results after Thyrogen Injection in Differentiated Thyroid Cancer Patients." Therapeutic Advances in Endocrinology and Metabolism 9, no. 6 (June 2018): 177–83.
9. Fatourechi, Vahab, Ian D. Hay, Brian P. Mullan, Gregory A. Wiseman, Gulti Z. Eghbali-Fatourechi, Linda M. Thorson, and Colum A. Gorman. "Are Posttherapy Radioiodine Scans Informative and Do They Influence Subsequent Therapy of Patients with Differentiated Thyroid Cancer?" Thyroid 10, no. 7 (July 30, 2000): 573–77.
10. Luster, M, S E Clarke, M Dietlein, M Lassmann, P Lind, W J G Oyen, J Tennvall, and E Bombardieri. "Guidelines for Radioiodine Therapy of Differentiated Thyroid Cancer." Accessed July 3, 2019. doi:10.1007/s00259-008-0883-1.
11. Lu, Liyan, Fengling Shan, Wenbin Li, and Hankui Lu. "Short-Term Side Effects after Radioiodine Treatment in Patients with Differentiated Thyroid Cancer." BioMed Research International 2016 (February 17, 2016): 1–5.
12. Nostrand, Douglas Van. "The Benefits and Risks of I-131 Therapy in Patients with Well-Differentiated Thyroid Cancer." Thyroid 19, no. 12 (December 14, 2009): 1381–91.
13. Fard-Esfahani, Armaghan, Alireza Emami-Ardekani, Babak Fallahi, Pezhman Fard-Esfahani, Davood Beiki, Arman Hassanzadeh-Rad, and Mohammad Eftekhari. "Adverse Effects of Radioactive Iodine-131 Treatment for Differentiated Thyroid Carcinoma." Nuclear Medicine Communications 35, no. 8 (August 1, 2014): 808–17.
14. Clement, S.C., R.P. Peeters, C.M. Ronckers, T.P. Links, M.M. van den Heuvel-Eibrink, E.J.M. Nieveen van Dijkum, R.R. van Rijn, et al. "Intermediate and Long-Term Adverse Effects of Radioiodine Therapy for Differentiated Thyroid Carcinoma – A Systematic Review." Cancer Treatment Reviews 41, no. 10 (December 2015): 925–34.
15. Bryan R. Haugen et al., "2015 American Thyroid Association Management Guidelines for Adult Patients with Thyroid Nodules and Differentiated Thyroid Cancer: The American Thyroid Association Guidelines Task Force on Thyroid Nodules and Differentiated Thyroid Cancer," Thyroid 26, no. 1 (January 2016): 1–133.
16. Petros Perros et al., "Guidelines for the Management of Thyroid Cancer," Clinical Endocrinology 81 Suppl 1 (July 2014): 1–122,
17. G. Brabant, "Thyrotropin Suppressive Therapy in Thyroid Carcinoma: What Are the Targets?," The Journal of Clinical Endocrinology & Metabolism 93, no. 4 (April 1, 2008): 1167–69.
18. D. S. Cooper et al., "Thyrotropin Suppression and Disease Progression in Patients with Differentiated Thyroid Cancer: Results from the National Thyroid Cancer Treatment Cooperative Registry," Thyroid: Official Journal of the American Thyroid Association 8, no. 9 (September 1998): 737–44.
19. Jacqueline Jonklaas et al., "Outcomes of Patients with Differentiated Thyroid Carcinoma Following Initial Therapy," Thyroid: Official Journal of the American Thyroid Association 16, no. 12 (December 2006): 1229–42.
20. Nayahmka J. McGriff et al., "Effects of Thyroid Hormone Suppression Therapy on Adverse Clinical Outcomes in Thyroid Cancer," Annals of Medicine 34, no. 7–8 (2002): 554–64.
21. Stefanie Diessl et al., "Impact of Moderate vs Stringent TSH Suppression on Survival in Advanced Differentiated Thyroid Carcinoma," Clinical Endocrinology 76, no. 4 (April 2012): 586–92.
22. Bernadette Biondi and David S. Cooper, "Benefits of Thyrotropin Suppression versus the Risks of Adverse Effects in Differentiated Thyroid Cancer," Thyroid: Official Journal of the American Thyroid Association 20, no. 2 (February 2010): 135–46.
23. P. Pujol et al., "Degree of Thyrotropin Suppression as a Prognostic Determinant in Differentiated Thyroid Cancer," The Journal of Clinical Endocrinology and Metabolism 81, no. 12 (December 1996): 4318–23.
24. C. T. Sawin et al., "Low Serum Thyrotropin Concentrations as a Risk Factor for Atrial Fibrillation in Older Persons," The New England Journal of Medicine 331, no. 19 (November 10, 1994): 1249–52.
25. Iwao Sugitani and Yoshihide Fujimoto, "Effect of Postoperative Thyrotropin Suppressive Therapy on Bone Mineral Density in Patients with Papillary Thyroid Carcinoma: A Prospective Controlled Study," Surgery 150, no. 6 (December 2011): 1250–57.
26. R. Michael Tuttle et al., "Estimating Risk of Recurrence in Differentiated Thyroid Cancer after Total Thyroidectomy and Radioactive Iodine Remnant Ablation: Using Response to Therapy Variables to Modify the Initial Risk Estimates Predicted by the New American Thyroid Association Staging System," Thyroid: Official Journal of the American Thyroid Association 20, no. 12 (December 2010): 1341–49.
27. Fernanda Vaisman et al., "Spontaneous Remission in Thyroid Cancer Patients after Biochemical Incomplete Response to Initial Therapy," Clinical Endocrinology 77, no. 1 (July 2012): 132–38.
28. Fernanda Vaisman et al., "Initial Therapy with Either Thyroid Lobectomy or Total Thyroidectomy without Radioactive Iodine Remnant Ablation Is Associated with Very Low Rates of Structural Disease Recurrence in Properly Selected Patients with Differentiated Thyroid Cancer," Clinical Endocrinology 75, no. 1 (July 2011): 112–19.
29. C. F. A. Eustatia-Rutten et al., "Diagnostic Value of Serum Thyroglobulin Measurements in the Follow-up of Differentiated Thyroid Carcinoma, a Structured Meta-Analysis," Clinical Endocrinology 61, no. 1 (July 2004): 61–74.
30. Luca Giovanella et al., "Undetectable Thyroglobulin in Patients With Differentiated Thyroid Carcinoma and Residual Radioiodine Uptake on a Postablation Whole-Body Scan," Clinical Nuclear Medicine 36, no. 2 (February 2011): 109–12.
31. Anne Bachelot et al., "Neck Recurrence from Thyroid Carcinoma: Serum Thyroglobulin and High-Dose Total Body Scan Are Not Reliable Criteria for Cure after Radioiodine Treatment," Clinical Endocrinology 62, no. 3 (March 2005): 376–79.
32. Martin H. Cherk et al., "Incidence and Implications of Negative Serum Thyroglobulin but Positive I-131 Whole-Body Scans in Patients with Well-Differentiated Thyroid Cancer Prepared with RhTSH or Thyroid Hormone Withdrawal: Negative Thyroglobulin Positive I-131 Body Scans Thyroid Cancer," Clinical Endocrinology 76, no. 5 (May 2012): 734–40.

33. Andrea Frasoldati et al., "Diagnosis of Neck Recurrences in Patients with Differentiated Thyroid Carcinoma," Cancer 97, no. 1 (January 1, 2003): 90–6.
34. C.A. Spencer et al., "Detection of Residual and Recurrent Differentiated Thyroid Carcinoma by Serum Thyroglobulin Measurement," Thyroid 9, no. 5 (May 1999): 435–41.
35. Carole A. Spencer, "Challenges of Serum Thyroglobulin (Tg) Measurement in the Presence of Tg Autoantibodies," The Journal of Clinical Endocrinology & Metabolism 89, no. 8 (August 1, 2004): 3702–4.
36. Sophie Leboulleux et al., "The Role of PET in Follow-up of Patients Treated for Differentiated Epithelial Thyroid Cancers," Nature Clinical Practice. Endocrinology & Metabolism 3, no. 2 (February 2007): 112–21.
37. Richard J. Robbins et al., "Real-Time Prognosis for Metastatic Thyroid Carcinoma Based on 2-[18F]Fluoro-2-Deoxy-D-Glucose-Positron Emission Tomography Scanning," The Journal of Clinical Endocrinology and Metabolism 91, no. 2 (February 2006): 498–505.
38. D. Deandreis et al., "Do Histological, Immunohistochemical, and Metabolic (Radioiodine and Fluorodeoxyglucose Uptakes) Patterns of Metastatic Thyroid Cancer Correlate with Patient Outcome?," Endocrine-Related Cancer 18, no. 1 (February 2011): 159–69.
39. Tumino, D, F Frasca, and K Newbold. "Updates on the Management of Advanced, Metastatic, and Radioiodine Refractory Differentiated Thyroid Cancer." Frontiers in Endocrinology 8 (2017): 312.
40. Schlumberger, Martin, Makoto Tahara, Lori J. Wirth, Bruce Robinson, Marcia S. Brose, Rossella Elisei, Mouhammed Amir Habra, et al. "Lenvatinib versus Placebo in Radioiodine-Refractory Thyroid Cancer." New England Journal of Medicine 372, no. 7 (February 12, 2015): 621–30.
41. Gild, Matti L., Duncan J. Topliss, Diana Learoyd, Francis Parnis, Jeanne Tie, Brett Hughes, John P. Walsh, Donald S.A. McLeod, Roderick J. Clifton-Bligh, and Bruce G. Robinson. "Clinical Guidance for Radioiodine Refractory Differentiated Thyroid Cancer." Clinical Endocrinology 88, no. 4 (2018): 529–37.
42. Pacini, Furio, and Martin Schlumberger. "S3-SELECTION OF PATIENTS FOR TKI TREATMENT." Accessed August 11, 2019. https://pdfs.semanticscholar.org/44c9/dfa85de1fb9a30754c15a9ecfa27e608785d.pdf.
43. Brown, Sarah R, Andrew Hall, Hannah L Buckley, Louise Flanagan, David Gonzalez De Castro, Kate Farnell, Laura Moss, et al. "Investigating the Potential Clinical Benefit of Selumetinib in Resensitising Advanced Iodine Refractory Differentiated Thyroid Cancer to Radioiodine Therapy (SEL-I-METRY): Protocol for a Multicentre UK Single Arm Phase II Trial." Accessed August 11, 2019. doi:10.1186/s12885-019-5541-4.
44. Budiawan, Hendra, Ali Salavati, Harshad R Kulkarni, and Richard P Baum. "Peptide Receptor Radionuclide Therapy of Treatment-Refractory Metastatic Thyroid Cancer Using (90)Yttrium and (177)Lutetium Labeled Somatostatin Analogs: Toxicity, Response and Survival Analysis." American Journal of Nuclear Medicine and Molecular Imaging 4, no. 1 (2013): 39–52.
45. Society of Nuclear Medicine (1953-), Vikas, Hendra Budiawan, Ali Salavati, Dieter Hoersch, C. Zachert, and Richard Baum. The Journal of Nuclear Medicine : JNM. Journal of Nuclear Medicine. Vol. 51. Society of Nuclear Medicine, 2010. http://jnm.snmjournals.org/content/51/supplement_2/1157.
46. Stokkel, Marcel P.M., Robbert B. Verkooijen, and Jan W.A. Smit. "Indium-111 Octreotide Scintigraphy for the Detection of Non-Functioning Metastases from Differentiated Thyroid Cancer: Diagnostic and Prognostic Value." European Journal of Nuclear Medicine and Molecular Imaging 31, no. 7 (July 26, 2004): 950–57.

27

RECURRENT GOITER

Surabhi Garg, Kul Ranjan Singh and Anand Kumar Mishra

Introduction

Thyroid nodules (TNs), both benign and malignant, are common endocrine disorders worldwide with ever increasing incidence. The prevalence of TN ranges from 3 to 7% and 19 to 67% by palpation and sonography, respectively, amongst general population (1). With the improvement in training and operative techniques over time along with the substitution of total thyroidectomy (TT) for subtotal thyroidectomy (STT)/nodulectomy, surgeons are becoming more proficient at excising the diseased gland in toto with reduced complications. This would translate into lower recurrence rates. However, when recurrence occurs, it represents a unique clinical and surgical challenge. Redo completion thyroidectomy is fraught with potential morbidity. Understanding of embryology and anatomy along with the meticulous surgery is likely to improve outcomes of surgery in the setting of recurrent goiter (RG).

Prevalence

RG is defined as regrowth of thyroid tissue after initial thyroidectomy. They may be seen in the setting as both benign and malignant pathologies. Recurrence in a malignant background may not be completely avoidable as it's multifactorial. However, RG should be prevented or kept to a bare minimum after surgery is performed for benign thyroid diseases. RG can be seen in 2–39% after any procedure less than TT. The recurrence rates are seen to go up to 70% without thyroxine replacement (2, 3). RG may constitute up to 12% of all thyroid surgeries performed (4). The shift from STT to TT has translated into declining recurrence rates. However, the time to recurrence has also showed a corresponding increase.

Etiopathogenesis

The pathogenesis of RG is not well understood and is likely to be multifactorial. However, the following may contribute to the recurrence of benign goiter (4, 5):

1. Inadequate/incomplete surgery
2. Residual embryological remnants (ER)
3. Malignant transformation of residual tissue

Inadequate/incomplete surgery

The surgeon may be faced with the following circumstances that have led to the recurrence of goiter:

1. A dominant nodule in multinodular goiter (MNG) treated by hemithyroidectomy.
2. Nodulectomy or STT performed for diffuse thyroid disease.
3. After an apparent TT. The recurrence occurs from the microscopic remnant, though benign has an aggressive biology. Tissue continues to grow despite suppressive LT4.

Initial lobectomy for a dominant nodule

Lobectomy for MNG with dominant nodule is acceptable and justified. Fear of post-TT complications and inherent aversion to replacement of LT4 make patient choose lobectomy over TT. Careful patient selection will minimize the risk of recurrence. Patients taken up for lobectomy should have predominantly unilateral growth with no or minimal involvement of the opposite side. Surgery for recurrence will be required in approximately 12% of such patients (4). Lobectomy on the opposite side for RG has minimal risk of complications.

Initial inadequate resection

Most endocrine surgeons advocate either hemithyroidectomy (HT) or TT as primary procedures for most thyroid pathologies. Unconventional thyroid surgeries like isthmusectomy, nodule enucleation, subtotal lobectomy or STT increase the risk of RG (6). Freedom from the replacement of LT4 and averting potential RLN and parathyroid-related complications have been advocated as deterrents of TT for dominant nodule by proponents of lobectomy (7). To the contrary, recent evidence shows that STT is not significantly safer for RLN and parathyroids compared to TT, and STT is associated with the recurrence rate ranging from 2.5 to 42% (8).

Also, incidentally detected carcinoma was seen in 3–16.6% of resected specimens. These results were further reinforced by metanalysis by Li et al. (9), which did not see any statistical differences in complications between STT and TT.

Aggressive benign multinodular disease

Female gender, younger age, euthyroid MNG, genetic factors and large size of remnant have been seen as factors associated with a higher risk of recurrence (10–12). Recurrence after apparent excision of the entire diseased gland has been attributed to polyclonal genesis of TN or morphologically and functionally independent aggregates of varying growth potential being present in the thyroid (13, 14). Hence, RG has been thought to arise from the proliferation of different groups of thyrocytes with exaggerated growth rates. It has been postulated that growth factors like EGF and IGF have been involved in the cascade of recurrence (15).

Embryological remnants (ER)

ER are documented sources of RGs. Embryogenesis of thyroid involves medial and lateral anlages followed by their descent and fusion (16, 17). In this descent, there are several anomalies that give rise to clinical conditions. In addition, there are some remnants of this embryological process, which have critical significance in thyroidectomy. There are four ER that are recognized and are very important in thyroidectomy (17):

- Thyroglossal duct remnants (TGDR)
- Pyramidal lobe
- Tubercle of Zuckerkandl (TZ)
- Thyrothymic remnants/rests

TABLE 27.1: Grades of Thyrothymic Remnants (20)

Grades	Description	
I	Protrusion of thyroid tissue	80%
II	Attached to thyroid by a narrow pedicle of thyroid tissue	
III	Attached to thyroid by a fibrovascular band	
IV	Completely separate from thyroid gland	20%

Pyramidal lobe and thyroglossal duct remnants

The pyramidal lobe is of various shapes and is found only in 28 and 55% of individuals (18). If not looked for during surgery, a pyramidal lobe in part or toto may be left behind. It's the most common site of recurrent disease. Though excision of RG arising from pyramidal lobe is straightforward, a scarred and thin cricothyroid membrane may be pierced and larynx entered inadvertently (19).

Thyrothymic remnants/rests

Small rests or protuberances of thyroid tissue located below the inferior pole in the line of thyrothymic descent constitute thyrothymic rests. These are found in almost 50% of individuals and confused with lymphoid tissue or inferior parathyroids. These rests are best classified by a system proposed by Sackett et al. (Table 27.1) (20). Close to 88% of these are subcentimetric, predisposing them to be left behind, if not meticulously looked for and excised during surgery (20).

Tubercle of Zuckerkandl (TZ)

TZ, described by Zuckerkandl in the early twentieth century as the "processus posterior glandulae thyroidea" is a poorly understood but important landmark responsible for the fraction of recurrent cases (21). The presence of dual tissue planes around the thyroid helps minimize the risk of RLN damage when TZ is lifted off the thyroid bed and preserve the vascularity of superior parathyroid glands (22, 23). A tubercle is identified in 63–80% of patients during thyroidectomy at least on one side. More than half of goiters have nodularity in TZ. These are classified based on their size (Table 27.2) (24). The significance of nodular enlargement of the tubercle lies in the fact that the nodular change may be primarily retro-esophageal and not appreciated at the initial surgery, leading to the recurrence. This makes subsequent surgery more difficult and puts the nerve at greater risk than primary surgery due to scarring and altered anatomy.

Development of malignancy in remnant

The incidence of development of carcinoma in a thyroid remnant left behind at primary surgery is speculated to vary from 11 to 22%, and the prevalence of occult carcinoma thyroidectomy for presumed benign disease is 3–16% (6). Such patients with residual thyroid tissue may be at higher risk of recurrence, especially if LT4 suppression or radioactive iodine has been curtailed.

TABLE 27.2: Grades of Zuckerkandl Tubercles

Grades	Size (cm)
0	Unrecognizable
I	<0.5
II	0.5–1
III	>1

TABLE 27.3: Indications of Recurrent Thyroid Surgery

Benign disease
- Bleeding or hematoma
- Recurrent thyrotoxicosis

Recurrent Graves' disease after subtotal thyroidectomy
- Recurrent compressive symptoms for an MNG

Thyroid nodularity after initial thyroid lobectomy
Recurrent thyroid nodularity after the previous subtotal thyroidectomy for nodular goiter
- New pathology (hyperparathyroidism)

Recurrent or inadequately treated malignant pathology
- Completion surgery for cancer
- Locoregional cancer recurrence

Reoperations for nodal disease
- Lateral neck nodes (either clinically palpable or seen on ultrasound)
- Surgical exploration for persistent hypercalcitonemia after initial surgery for medullary thyroid cancer

Presentation of recurrent nodular goiter

Patients may remain totally asymptomatic or present with severe compressive features along with hypo/hyperthyroidism. Progressive decrease in thyroxine supplementation should alert the physician to look for a recurrence. Those under periodical follow-up are likely to be picked up with no or minimal symptoms. RGs are told to have higher incidence and intensity of compressive symptoms for a given size of goiter due to fibrosis resulting from the previous surgery further resulting in a compartment syndrome–like scenario. The strap muscles adhere to the trachea medially, preventing the free anterior expansion of goitrous enlargement and disproportionate compressive features (25). Table 27.3 summarizes the indications of recurrent thyroid surgery.

Preoperative workup

Diagnostic assessment and protocols are similar to those for de novo TN (26). Detailed clinical history should be elicited with the documentation of the type of the previous surgery, and a review of previous surgical and pathological records is very important and it should be done in all cases whenever possible. Physical examination may reveal a firm, immobile mass due to dense scarring and fibrotic tissue occasionally mimicking a carcinoma. Post-lobectomy patients may present with contralateral recurrence.

Thyroid functions are routinely evaluated before surgery. Hyperthyroid patients are made euthyroid prior to proper antithyroid medication before surgery.

All patients should undergo comprehensive imaging of the neck. A high-resolution ultrasound may be adequate in most cases; however, in cases of suspicion or malignancy, a computed tomography scan of the neck may be undertaken (Figure 27.1). Some suggest a thyroid scan in all patients to delineate all functional thyroid tissues. A combination of anatomical and functional imaging will provide the maximum information about residual tissues if the patient has been operated on at some other centers, and the details of the operative notes would be missed. Fine needle aspiration cytology is a must to rule out malignancy in the recurrent lesion. Preoperative serum calcium and PTH

Recurrent Goiter

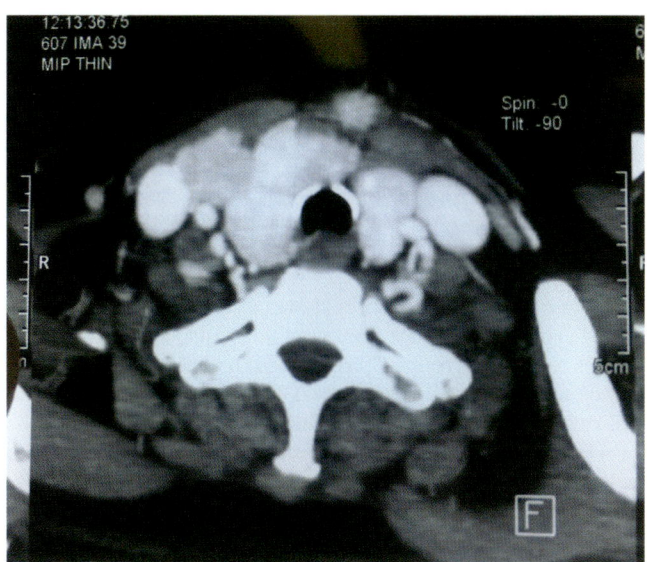

FIGURE 27.1 CT scan picture of recurrent multinodular goiter.

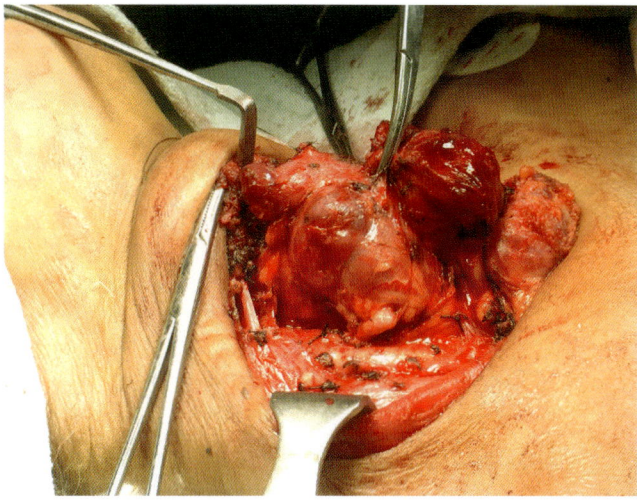

FIGURE 27.2 Intraoperative picture of the same patient. Multiple nodules can be appreciated (left head end and right-side foot end of the patient).

levels are measured, and some have even suggested the measurement of PTH before and during surgery, with samples retrieved from the lower part of internal jugular vein to ascertain the functionality of ipsilateral parathyroids. (27). However, most centers don't do this and visual identification with or without adjuncts remains the gold standard during re-exploration.

A normal voice does not rule out vocal cord (VC) palsy arising from initial operation. Preoperative VC assessment is mandatory in all patients before reoperative surgery (26). One out of five patients presenting with RG may have compromised VC function, thus presenting with recurrent disease (28).

Operative strategy

Reoperative surgery aims at providing relief from compressive features with optimal cosmesis. A completion TT should be performed to keep chances of future recurrence to a bare minimum.

Not all patients are subjected to surgery as the risk of complications is higher for primary surgery. Suspicion of malignancy and compressive symptoms are rare absolute indications for a surgical management. Hyperthyroid RG patients who are poor surgical candidates may be subjected to RAI therapy.

The extent and approach of surgical intervention is guided by the type and completeness of primary surgery. An RG is best approached from a virgin plane. A lateral approach has been advocated for prior isthmusectomy and nodulectomy. Post-hemithyroidectomy RG may not pose much of a challenge, but the ipsilateral RLN and parathyroids should be thought to be the only functional and caution exercised.

Repeat surgery in those having undergone STT or TT is challenging. Identification of anatomic landmarks away from the thyroid bed facilitates safe dissection and has been advocated for optimal outcome.

Surgery starts with the excision of scar and flap raising in a standard fashion. Proper exposure of surgical field is a must. The lateral approach is most commonly used for redo surgeries; however, this approach may not be required in certain cases like pyramidal lobe recurrences. The dissection is first carried out laterally hitherto untouched. Sternocleidomastoid muscle is mobilized and retracted laterally to expose the carotid sheath. Posterior dissection continues to the prevertebral fascia and then medially to the region of the esophageal groove. Caution is to be exercised as the RLN may be misplaced ventrally and adhered to the strap muscles. Trachea is then identified in the midline. The anatomical landmarks are now clear medially and laterally, and one can proceed with the dissection (Figure 27.2). (25).

RLN can be identified and preserved by conventional "lateral/backdoor approach", "inferior approach" and "medial superior pole approach" (25). The lateral approach involves dissection along the sternocleidomastoid as described above. The inferior approach can be utilized when there is extensive lateral scarring, wherein the trachea-esophageal grove is approached at a lower level. Failing this strategy, the medial superior pole approach can be used, in which an avascular plane is identified between the thyroid and cricothyroid muscle followed by dissection inferiorly along the laryngotracheal groove. This nerve is then identified as it pierces the cricopharyngeus muscle (Figures 27.3 and 27.4).

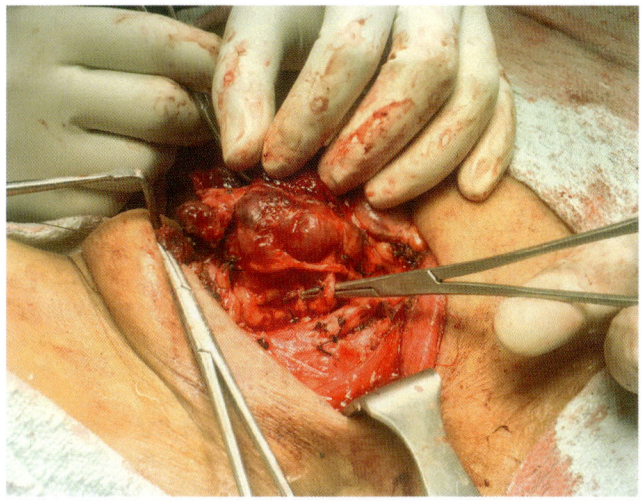

FIGURE 27.3 Right recurrent laryngeal nerve and inferior thyroid artery relation in the same patient.

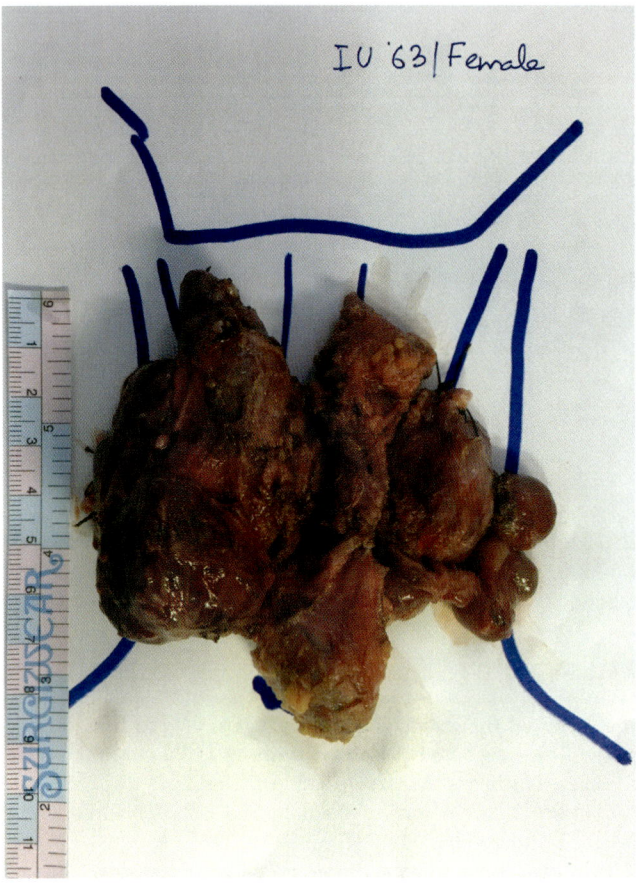

FIGURE 27.4 Thyroidectomy specimen of the patient.

Parathyroid preservation is accomplished by capsular dissection, keeping a watchful search for any parathyroid tissue. It needs to be emphasized that in situ parathyroid preservation is difficult due to the alteration of parathyroid vascular anatomy during the previous surgery. Hence, whenever parathyroid vascular supply is of question, autotransplantation should be routinely done (25). Surgery can be eased and made safer by the use of intraoperative adjuncts like intraoperative neuromonitoring, magnifying loops or operating microscopes and parathyroid localization by dyes/fluorescence.

Postoperative complications

Redo surgery for recurrent nodular goiter is associated with higher morbidity than primary surgery. This has been attributed to likely alteration in tissue architecture, which makes dissection difficult and compromises the vascularity of parathyroids.

The incidence of RLN injury is reported to be five times higher in redo surgeries, even when primary and secondary surgeries are performed by the same team. Hypoparathyroidism occurs more frequently after redo surgeries as compared to primary surgery (0.5–9.5% compared to 1.5%) (6). Moalem et al. reviewed the complication rates across ten studies following recurrent benign thyroid and concluded that both temporary and permanent RLN injury rates were higher in the completion surgery compared to the first surgery (0–22% versus 0.5–18%) and (0–13% versus 0–4%), respectively. No difference was noted for the incidence of temporary hypocalcemia (0–25% versus 1–27%), but permanent hypoparathyroidism was seen in 0–22% compared to 0–4% for primary surgery (4).

Postoperative management for prevention of further recurrence – Role of TSH suppression

Conventionally, TSH suppression has been used to prevent or delay recurrence. Proponents of this popular strategy cite data by Feldkamp et al. suggest that this is the only available method in preventing MNG recurrence (29). TSH suppression resulted in beneficial effects across two other studies but their methodological flaws make them unfit for making practice recommendations (30, 31). However, because of methodologic inconsistencies, these studies cannot be grouped and be used to make practice recommendations. However, Hegedüs et al. did not find any advantage of LT4 suppression in an RCT involving 202 patients followed up for 1–14 years (median 10 years) (32). Autonomy of recurrent nodules owing to their polyclonality is likely the reason for failed suppressive therapy. Currently, the deleterious effects of suppressive LT4 therapy on bone health and cardiovascular system have deterred clinicians from relying on this approach for reducing recurrence. (33). Presently, there is no clear consensus on the use of TSH suppression for the prevention of recurrent nodular goiter.

South Asian perspective

In spite of hemithyroidectomy and TT being propagated as the standard procedures for thyroid pathologies, a large number of nodulectomies and subtotal thyroidectomies are still performed for benign diseases in these countries. Socioeconomic conditions, inconsistent follow-up for TSH monitoring, inadequate training of surgeons and unjustified fear of complications result in STT and nodulectomies. Increased awareness and training along with specialized endocrine surgery training are likely to reverse the trend.

Conclusion

Carefully planned and meticulously carried out complete primary surgery is the best prevention against RGs. Special attention should be paid to the embryonic remnants during primary surgery. In the event of recurrence, there is higher risk of nerve injury and permanent hypoparathyroidism. Intraoperative adjuncts, like neuromonitoring, may help reduce the prevalence of nerve injuries. TSH suppression postoperatively has a controversial role in preventing recurrences.

References

1. Jiang H, Tian Y, Yan W, Kong Y, Wang H, Wang A, et al. The prevalence of thyroid nodules and an analysis of related lifestyle factors in Beijing communities. Int J Environ Res Public Health. 2016 Apr;13(4):442.
2. Kraimps JL, Marechaud R, Gineste D, Fieuzal S, Metaye T, Carretier M, et al. Analysis and prevention of recurrent goitre. Surg Gynecol Obstet. 1993 Apr;176(4):319–322.
3. Abdella MR, Al-Ahmer MMH, Khidr HM. Recurrent nodular goitre: predictors of recurrence and outcome after reoperation. Al-Azhar Assiut Med J. 2014; 12(1):194–209.
4. Moalem J, Suh I, Duh Q-Y. Treatment and prevention of recurrence of multinodular goitre: an evidence-based review of the literature. World J Surg. 2008 Jul;32(7):1301–1312.
5. Fernando R. Recurrent goitres. World J Endocr Surg. 2019 Apr;11(1):15–18.
6. Cappellani A, Di Vita M, Zanghì A, Lomenzo E, Cavallaro A, Alfano G, et al. The recurrent goitre: prevention and management. Ann Ital Chir. 2008 Jul;79:247–253.
7. Rolle der totalen Thyreoidektomie im primären Therapiekonzept der benignen Knotenstruma [Internet]. springermedizin.de. [cited 2020 Nov 30]. Available from: https://www.springermedizin.de/rolle-der-totalen-thyreoidektomie-im-primaeren-therapiekonzept-d/8015546
8. Agarwal G, Aggarwal V. Is total thyroidectomy the surgical procedure of choice for benign multinodular goitre? An evidence-based review. World J Surg. 2008 Jul;32(7):1313–1324.

9. Li Y, Li Y, Zhou X. Total thyroidectomy versus bilateral subtotal thyroidectomy for bilateral multinodular nontoxic goitre: a meta-analysis. ORL. 2016;78(3):167–175.
10. Gibelin H, Sierra M, Mothes D, Ingrand P, Levillain P, Jones C, et al. Risk factors for recurrent nodular goitre after thyroidectomy for benign disease: case-control study of 244 patients. World J Surg. 2004 Nov;28(11):1079–1082.
11. Scerrino G, Cocorullo G, Paladino N, Salamone G, Gulotta G. Quantification of the risk of relapses after thyroid loboisthmusectomy for benign thyroid nodules. Ann Ital Chir. 2005 Jul;76:321–328; discussion 328.
12. Yoldas T, Makay O, Icoz G, Kose T, Gezer G, Kismali E, et al. Should subtotal thyroidectomy be abandoned in multinodular goitre patients from endemic regions requiring surgery? Int Surg. 2015 Jan;100(1):9–14.
13. Harrer P, Broecker M, Zint A, Schatz H, Zumtobel V, Derwahl M. Thyroid nodules in recurrent multinodular goitres are predominantly polyclonal. J Endocrinol Invest. 1998 Jun;21(6):380–385.
14. Seiler CA, Schäfer M, Büchler MW. [Surgery of the goitre]. Ther Umsch Rev Ther. 1999 Jul;56(7):380–384.
15. Maiorano E, Ambrosi A, Giorgino R, Fersini M, Pollice L, Ciampolillo A. Insulin-like growth factor 1 (IGF-1) in multinodular goitres: a possible pathogenetic factor. Pathol Res Pract. 1994 Nov;190(11):1012–1016.
16. Rosen RD, Sapra A. Embryology, thyroid. In: StatPearls [Internet]. Treasure Island (FL): StatPearls Publishing; 2020 [cited 2020 Nov 30]. Available from: http://www.ncbi.nlm.nih.gov/books/NBK551611/
17. Fernando R. Embryological descent, remnants and implications for thyroid surgery. J Anat Soc Sri Lanka. 2017 Oct 1;volume I:Editorial.
18. Kim DW, Jung SL, Baek JH, Kim J, Ryu JH, Na DG, et al. The prevalence and features of thyroid pyramidal lobe, accessory thyroid, and ectopic thyroid as assessed by computed tomography: a multicenter study. Thyroid. 2013 Jan;23(1):84–91.
19. Snook KL, Stalberg PLH, Sidhu SB, Sywak MS, Edhouse P, Delbridge L. Recurrence after total thyroidectomy for benign multinodular goitre. World J Surg. 2007 Mar;31(3):593–598.
20. Sackett WR, Reeve TS, Barraclough B, Delbridge L. Thyrothymic thyroid rests: incidence and relationship to the thyroid gland. J Am Coll Surg. 2002 Nov;195(5):635–640.
21. Irkorucu O. Zuckerkandl tubercle in thyroid surgery: Is it a reality or a myth? Ann Med Surg. 2016 Apr;7:92–96.
22. Jw S. New operative surgical concept of two fascial layers enveloping the recurrent laryngeal nerve. Ann Surg Oncol. 2010 Feb;17(6):1628–1636.
23. Fernando R, Rajapaksha A, Ranasinghe N, Gunawardana D. Embryological remnants of the thyroid gland and their significance in thyroidectomy. World J Endocr Surg. 2014 Dec;6(3):110–112.
24. Hisham AN, Aina EN. Zuckerkandl's tubercle of the thyroid gland in association with pressure symptoms: a coincidence or consequence? Aust N Z J Surg. 2000 Apr;70(4):251–253.
25. Randolph GW. Surgery of the Thyroid and Parathyroid Glands E-Book: Expert Consult Premium Edition - Enhanced Online Features. Amsterdam: Elsevier Health Sciences; 2012. 900 p.
26. Haugen BR, Alexander EK, Bible KC, Doherty GM, Mandel SJ, Nikiforov YE, et al. 2015 American Thyroid Association management guidelines for adult patients with thyroid nodules and differentiated thyroid cancer: The American Thyroid Association Guidelines Task Force on Thyroid Nodules and Differentiated Thyroid Cancer. Thyroid. 2016 Jan;26(1):1–133.
27. Cranshaw IM, Moss D, Whineray-Kelly E, Harman CR. Intraoperative parathormone measurement from the internal jugular vein predicts post-thyroidectomy hypocalcaemia. Langenbecks Arch Surg. 2007 Mar;392(6):699–702.
28. Culp JM, Patel G. Recurrent laryngeal nerve injury. In: StatPearlss [Internet]. Treasure Island (FL): StatPearls Publishing; 2020 [cited 2020 Nov 30]. Available from: http://www.ncbi.nlm.nih.gov/books/NBK560832/
29. Feldkamp J, Seppel T, Becker A, Klisch A, Schlaghecke R, Goretzki PE, et al. Iodide or l-thyroxine to prevent recurrent goitre in an iodine-deficient area: prospective sonographic study. World J Surg. 1997 Jan;21(1):10–14.
30. Koc M, Ersoz HO, Akpinar I, Gogas-Yavuz D, Deyneli O, Akalin S. Effect of low- and high-dose levothyroxine on thyroid nodule volume: a crossover placebo-controlled trial. Clin Endocrinol (Oxf). 2002 Nov;57(5):621–628.
31. Wémeau J-L, Caron P, Schvartz C, Schlienger J-L, Orgiazzi J, Cousty C, et al. Effects of thyroid-stimulating hormone suppression with levothyroxine in reducing the volume of solitary thyroid nodules and improving extranodular nonpalpable changes: a randomized, double-blind, placebo-controlled trial by the French Thyroid Research Group. J Clin Endocrinol Metab. 2002 Nov;87(11):4928–4934.
32. Hegedüs L, Nygaard B, Hansen JM. Is routine thyroxine treatment to hinder postoperative recurrence of nontoxic goitre justified? J Clin Endocrinol Metab. 1999 Feb;84(2):756–760.
33. Low Serum Thyrotropin Concentrations as a Risk Factor for Atrial Fibrillation in Older Persons | NEJM [Internet]. [cited 2020 Nov 30]. Available from: https://www.nejm.org/doi/full/10.1056/nejm199411103311901
34. Bauer DC, Ettinger B, Nevitt MC, Stone KL; Study of Osteoporotic Fractures Research Group. Risk for fracture in women with low serum levels of thyroid-stimulating hormone. Ann Intern Med. 2001 Apr;134(7):561–568.

28

RETROSTERNAL GOITER

Kul Ranjan Singh, Anand Kumar Mishra and Pooja Ramakant

Introduction

Retrosternal goiters (RSG) described way back 1749 have continued to challenge endocrine surgeons despite improvements in diagnostics and surgical techniques (1). There remains a dearth of consensus on terminology, pathophysiology and surgical techniques of RSG. Varied terminologies have been and are being used for goiters, the lower border of which cannot be felt during clinical examination. Retrosternal, substernal, thoracic or mediastinal goiters are the terms used for goiters that are in part or whole within the thorax.

There has been no universal definition for retrosternal goiters, and the spectrum ranges from a goiter, the lower border of which cannot be palpated even on hyperextension of the neck or during the act of deglutition to more objective definitions. Commonly RSG are defined as goiters with >50% of the mass below thoracic inlet (2). The definition of RSG takes into context the concerned surgeon and the findings of clinical and imaging (3).

Epidemiology

The exact incidence of RSG remains obscure due to absence of consensus on diagnostic criteria and ranges between 0.2% and 45% (4). There are 10 or more different definitions of RSG (clinical, Hsu, Kocher's, Torre's, Eschapase's, Lahey's, Lindskog's, Crile's, Katlics's, subcarinal) (4). The fall out of varied criteria in vogue will prevent estimation of true incidence. This is evident from a study by Antonio Rios et al. in which of the 201 patients categorized as having RSG by clinical definition, only 12 met the diagnostic criteria of subcarinal definition if RSG. (4) This study also concluded that clinical definition is best adopted as it is easiest to use and most of them overlap. RSG are most commonly encountered during the fifth to sixth decade of life, and women are more likely to be affected (5, 6). However, there seems to be regional differences between its incidence rates among males and females (7).

Clinical features

The clinical features may range from being totally asymptomatic to patients presenting with respiratory distress in emergency. They may be picked up incidentally on imaging. But most patients have a history of long-standing goiter (3). Up to one-third of the patients with RSG don't have an easily palpable goiter with a major bulk being in the chest (5). Compressive features related to one or more of trachea, esophagus and recurrent laryngeal nerve (RLN) are present in majority of patients. Compressive features are more common in RSG compared to a goiter localized to the neck, and respiratory symptoms are commoner then symptoms due to esophageal compression (8). Up to 9 out of 10 patients report some degree of respiratory symptoms (1, 9). Compression on the trachea manifests as upper airway obstruction which translates to compromise of inspiratory capacity primarily (10). Breathlessness, obstructive pneumonia, obstructive sleep apnea may be presenting feature, and many a times, RSG are misdiagnosed and treated as asthma (11). Alteration of esophageal anatomy characterized by deviation and compression is seen in 14% and 8%–27%, respectively. This impairment increases with volume and degree of retrosternal component (12). A growing goiter can impede SVC drainage due to a rigid thoracic inlet, and patients present with signs of SVC syndrome in up to 5% of RSG (13). Thin-walled SVC and brachiocephalic veins are compressed easily and result in congestion of face, neck and upper extremity. Though SVC syndrome is usually seen after malignant infiltration, benign RSG are encountered commonly (9). Latent SVC syndrome can be made manifest by performing Pemberton's maneuver, which is explained by the conventional "cork effect" or recently conceptualized "nut cracker effect" (14). RSG in elderly may present with thyrotoxicosis (8). Inability to palpate the lower border on clinical examination or chest X-ray suggestive of displaced and/or compressed trachea in region of superior and anterior mediastinum should followed by a CT scan. Horner's syndrome and diaphragmatic palsy are occasionally seen in RSG (9).

Pathophysiology and relevant anatomy

The continued growth of thyroid faces obstruction from surrounding structures and it grows inferiorly due to the negative intrathoracic pressure, act of swallowing and assisted by the force of gravity (15). The brachiocephalic veins, SVC, aortic arch and its branches offer resistance to continued progression, and hence, a posterior mediastinal goiter is more likely to be right sided. The retrosternal component usually has its vascular supply from the neck. The thyroid ima artery present in 3%–10% (more commonly encountered in Asians) has a variable anatomy but can be taken care of in the neck as it travels upward to insert into the isthmus (16). A primary intrathoracic goiter (IG) originates from ectopic thyroid rests and receives the blood supply from mediastinal vessels. IG account for less than 1% of RSG (17). Most IGs are located in superior and anterior mediastinum. A total of 15% are located in middle and posterior mediastinum, and their diagnosis and management is more demanding (17).

Investigations

Appropriate and adequate preoperative investigations including clinical examination, biochemical appropriate imaging and pathology should be carried out in all patients. Additional thyroid function tests are required only if TSH is abnormal.

Scintigraphy of RSG is often suboptimal due to poor relative vascularity, high proportion of calcification and possible interference of gamma emission by chest wall tests (10). A good imaging helps plan and execute the surgery safely. Examination of vocal cords using a mirror or fiber-optic laryngoscope should be done in all patients. This helps confirm the function of VC and also preempt intubation difficulties and take necessary precautions (3).

CT imaging is mandatory for evaluation of RSG as the retrosternal component cannot be assessed by sonography. It defines the size and extent of goiter. CT may delineate necrosis, infiltrative margins, invasion, calcification and lymphadenopathy raising the suspicion of malignancy. Though CT does not accurately help predict the need of a thoracic approach in all cases, it does in some cases suggest that a thoracic approach would be mandatory and also helps decide the ideal thoracic approach (2).

Though a cytological/histopathological evaluation of the retrosternal component of all RSG is not required, it helps characterize the tissue of origin and the nature of mass lesion in which there is a doubt. CT- or US-guided cytology and/or histopathology are safe and highly effective tool that can be made use of (18).

Classification

As with the definition of RSG, there are many classification systems in literature. Most of these systems aim at trying to predict the ideal surgical approach in a given situation. All these systems are based on CT images that delineate the supero-inferior, anteroposterior and lateral extents and the relation of goiter with trachea and esophagus (19).

A simple method to classify RSG is primary RSG (primary IG or aberrant goiter) and secondary RSG (cervical portion connected/continuous with the mediastinal part). Porzio et al. proposed a classification based on the location of goiter in right, left, anterior or posterior (20).

The CT scan cross-sectional imaging classification (CT-CSI) by Mercante et al classifies RSG as: grades 1, 2, 3 (above, at and below the level of aortic arch, respectively); types A, B, C (prevascular, retrovascular-paratracheal and retrotracheal, respectively) and laterality as mono-/bilateral (21).

Huins et al. proposed a classification based on the systematic review of complications and management of RSG surgery of 2426 patients across 34 publications. It took into account the cranio-caudal extent of goiter, grades 1, 2, 3 (above aortic arch, aortic arch to pericardium and below right atrium), and suggested cervical/manubriotomy and full sternotomy for their extirpation (22).

TABLE 28.1: Classification of Retrosternal Goiter on Coronal CT Images Based on Cvasciuc et al.

Grade	Shape	Surgical Approach
Type A	Pyramidal with its apex pointing downward	Cervical
Type B	Pyramidal with its apex pointing up	Cervical ± manubriotomy/sternotomy or thoracotomy
Type C	Bilobed goiter with a narrow neck or pedicle	Cervical ± manubriotomy/sternotomy
Type D	Ectopic or remnants not connected to thyroid in neck	Sternotomy ± thoracotomy

Cvasciuc et al. based their classification on shape of goiter on coronal CT images which is summarized in Table 28.1(23). Another classification offered by Shahhian et al. provides useful surgical information that has been used extensively and is of help in surgical planning (Table 28.2) (7).

Management

The choice of therapy should be individualized based on the symptomatology, rate of progression, thyroid function, risk of malignancy, patient performance status and choice.

Thyroid malignancy may be more prevalent in retrosternal component (8). However, metanalysis has concluded that it's no higher than cervical goiters, and the risk factors for suspecting malignancy are common to both types (5). Conventionally, surgery has been advocated for all RSG, but conservative approach with observation can be an option for asymptomatic patients in whom malignancy has been ruled out (5, 10). At total of 5%–37% of surgeries for RSG are due to a persistent or recurrent thyroid disease. The initial surgery was likely to be a subtotal thyroidectomy or hemithyroidectomy (5, 15). A substernal tracheal compression of >35% usually merits thyroidectomy (24).

Technique of intubation remains a matter of debate. Some anesthetists prefer intubation after anesthesia, whereas few are comfortable with awake fiber-optic intubation. Laryngotracheal trauma during intubation may exacerbate obstruction leading to airway trauma necessitating prompt securing of airway. The intubation should be done by a senior anesthetist avoiding trauma and consequent acute airway-related emergency. Direct laryngoscopy, video laryngoscopy or a combined use of video laryngoscope and fiber-optic laryngoscopy makes securing the airway easy and minimizes risks (25, 26). These techniques also help secure the electrodes of neuromonitoring tube in place.

TABLE 28.2: Classification of Retrosternal Goiter Based on Location, Anatomy and Surgical Approach Based on Shahhian et al.

Type	Type	Location	Anatomy	Approach
1		Anterior mediastinum	Anterior to great vessels, trachea and RLN	Transcervical, sternotomy only of retrosternal diameter > thoracic inlet diameter
2		Posterior mediastinum	Posterior to great vessels, trachea and RLN	
	A	Ipsilateral extension		
	B	Contralateral extension	B1 – Posterior to both trachea and esophagus	B2 – Sternotomy or posterolateral thoracotomy
			B2 – Between trachea and esophagus	
3		Isolated mediastinal		Sternotomy

Nevertheless, prior multidisciplinary approach helps in safe airway management.

Most RSG are removed via the neck incision avoiding potential subsequent complications of various thoracic incisions. The lobe that is higher up is tackled first. In most cases, the inferior pole is mobilized gradually by gentle traction and blunt finger dissection and delivered in the neck. Traction using sutures/sharp instruments is used but attendant complication like hemorrhage/rupture should be kept in mind and avoided. The authors have noted that ligation of the arteries supplying the thyroid up front makes the goiter shrink considerably and makes subsequent delivery easy. Various maneuvers have been described to avoid a median sternotomy or thoracotomy. Cervical leverage making use of a right angle retractor may aid removal of large retrosternal component (27). Marzouk procedure involves an incision through the second intercostal space and extrapleural mobilization of the retrosternal component and delivery via the standard neck incision (28). Transclavicular approach involving the breaking of continuity of ipsilateral clavicle near its sternoclavicular joint widens the thoracic inlet. Though invasive, it avoids a sternotomy and additional incision, and cosmetic outcome is said to be good without compromise of function (29). A simple maneuver described by Welman et al. involves delivery of retrosternal component with "spoon technique" that is said to provide better protection to RLN (Figures 28.1 and 28.2) (30).

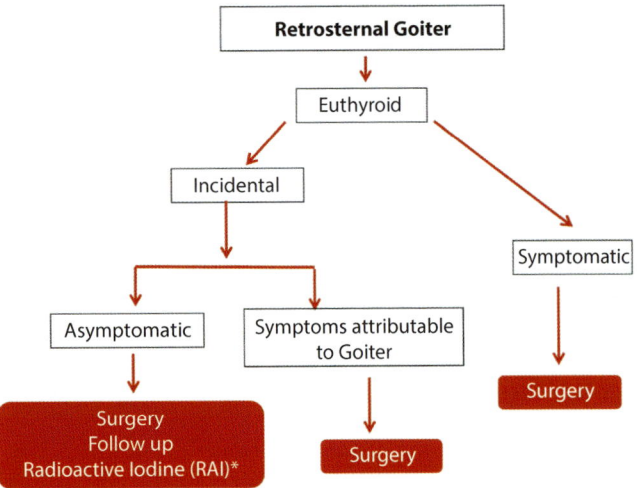

FIGURE 28.1 Management plan in retrosternal goiter. *Upto 30%–40% shrinkage on RAI.

Identification and dissection of recurrent laryngeal nerve may pose as a challenge. A goiter in the posterior mediastinum and connected to the cervical thyroid can cause anterior displacement of the RLN, making it prone to injury (3). A higher

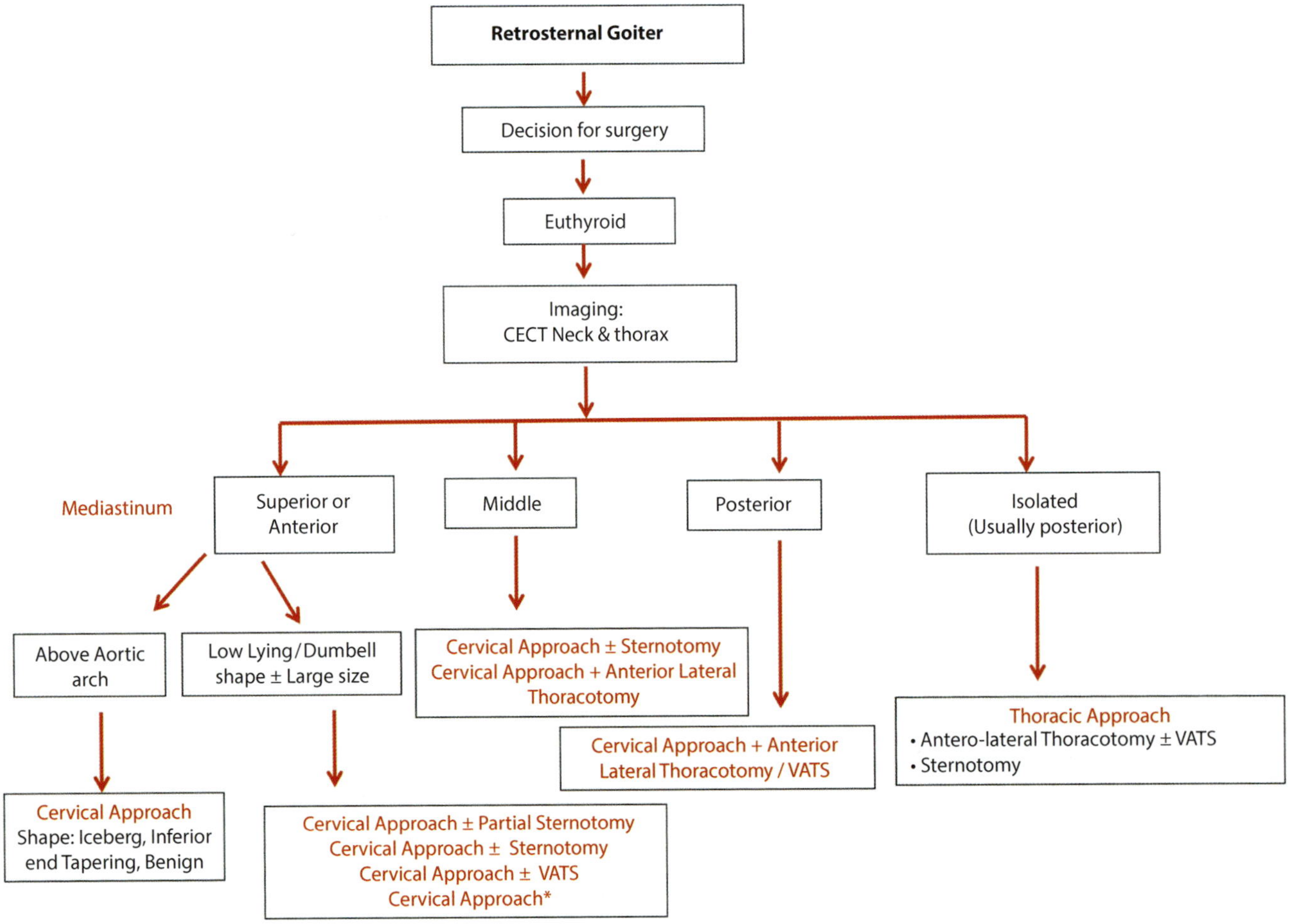

FIGURE 28.2 Management plan in retrosternal goiter. *Spoon technique, *Cervical leverage, *Clavicular traction action.

incidence of RLN injury has been recorded in thyroidectomy for RSG compared to cervical goiter alone (5). EBSLN impairment after RSG surgery has not been addressed adequately. Intraoperative neuromonitoring (IONM) has been advocated for high-risk thyroid surgery. Though studies and metanalysis evaluating use of IONM in setting of RSG surgery are underpowered, it has been shown to be of benefit though insignificant (31–33). Increased surgeon confidence and improved safety have been cited as common reasons for ever-increasing employment of IONM during routine and high-risk thyroid surgery (34).

Need for sternal split/thoracotomy

Most RSG (>90%–95%) felt in the neck can be removed via the cervical incision; however, all preparations should be made for a possible sternotomy (5, 35–37). A recurrent substernal goiter, having undergone previous thoracic surgery, a high likelihood of advanced malignancy, retrotracheal extension, retrosternal component with width more than thoracic inlet, coexistent thyroiditis posterior mediastinal location and a substernal goiter that reaches the subcarina are likely to require a sternotomy (3–5, 28, 36, 38, 39). Extension of goiter to carina or below, vascular anatomy, anticipated bleeding and coexisting lymphadenopathy in presence of suspected malignancy may suggest upfront thoracic approach (15). Size alone is not a criterion for thoracic approach. The requirement of sternotomy is best predicted by applying the Katlics's definition of RSG (at least 50% of the goiter is retrosternal) (4). A total of 10.6% of patients with more than 50% of the goiter being retrosternal and 45% of goiters reaching the aortic arch ultimately require some form of thoracic approach (2). The shape of goiter can predict the need of thoracic approach. An iceberg-shaped RSG is 60 times more likely to require an extracervical approach compared to an oval-shaped one (36). An RSG having been present for more than 160 months is in itself a predictor of sternotomy (38). These patients may require a multidisciplinary approach, specialized gadgets and good postoperative care, and hence, its best carried out in specialized centers. Thoracic approach improves the access and securing hemostasis is made easier. A formal sternotomy is not a solution for all RSGs requiring thoracic approach. Right-sided RSG may better be managed by an anterolateral thoracotomy (15). A sternotomy provides compromised access to middle and posterior compartments, and goiters in these locations are best dealt with high thoracotomy. A partial sternotomy up to second intercostal space can be a less morbid procedure that provides sufficient access up to innominate vessels and pericardium and morbid and potentially lethal complications like sternal dehiscence and mediastinitis (40).

A hybrid procedure of cervicotomy and thoracoscopy can be performed for RSG, especially those growing deep into the mediastinum and middle of posterior mediastinum. This procedure is safe with comparable results while preventing pulmonary complications and reduced pain (40, 41). The advent of robotic surgery is likely to make the hybrid procedure more popular in future (42).

Though there seems to be a consensus that medical management is ineffective for RSG, periodical follow-up and radioactive I-131 with or without rhTSH may be a valid alternative to surgery in some with large goiters with or without retrosternal extension (10). It should be kept in mind that RSG can present as a life-threatening emergency due to a sudden increase in size due to intratumoral bleeding or malignant transformation (43).

Complications

Bleeding is the commonest intraoperative complication and is usually from a retracted inferior thyroid vein. It should be secured well. Postthyroidectomy hemorrhage is usually encountered within 24 hours in 90% (44). Drains are an independent risk factor for postthyroidectomy hematoma, but same is advocated by most and should be kept in place for at least 48 hours. Tracheomalacia is a dreaded complication, but it's rarely encountered even in RSG. It's more likely to be present when an RSG has been present for more than 5 years with a significant tracheal compression (5). Leak test and or palpation of trachea should be performed before wound closure to rule out tracheomalacia in cases of large, long-standing RSGs. If tracheomalacia is anticipated, the trachea may be buttressed. Occasionally a tracheostomy is performed, which is removed after 5–7 days. However, most patients can be extubated safely but need to be closely monitored in the postoperative period and positive pressure ventilation be provided. Most patients stabilize in 5–7 days. Continued intubation and mechanical ventilation in the postoperative and gradual extubation provide a stenting function and process of sclerosis and fibrosis of peritracheal tissue stabilizes it (15). Parathyroid gland identification may also pose a challenge due its adherence to thyroid capsule or displacement. Transient and permanent hypocalcemia occurs at a higher rate for RSG compared to cervical goiters and can be source of significant morbidity. Elderly patients with RSG are likely to have more complications than their young counterparts, but age alone should not withhold the benefits of surgery among the aged (45).

South Asian perspective

The incidence of RSG is said to be higher in regions endemic to goiter (7). A higher rate of RSE, airway compromise, difficult intubation and tracheomalacia is encountered in Indian subcontinent (46). Though specialized endocrine surgery centers are limited, the outcome of thyroid surgery including RSG in India seems to match Western results.

Conclusion

RSG are encountered commonly in endocrine surgery practice. There remains a dearth of consensus regarding universal terminology, and hence, published literature is difficult to analyze and interpret. RSG merit a comprehensive workup, meticulous well-planned surgery for optimal outcome. Most RSG can be delivered via cervical incision. The need of thoracic approach should be anticipated and preparation made for same beforehand.

References

1. Newman, E and ARS. Substernal goiter. J Surg Oncol. 1995;60(3):207–212.
2. Qureishi A, Garas G, Tolley N, Palazzo F, Athanasiou T, Zacharakis E. Can preoperative computed tomography predict the need for a thoracic approach for removal of retrosternal goitre? Int J Surg [Internet]. 2013;11(3):203–208.
3. Shaha AR. Substernal goiter: what is in a definition? Surgery [Internet]. 2010; 147(2):239–240.
4. Ríos A, Rodríguez JM, Balsalobre MD, Tebar FJ, Parrilla P. The value of various definitions of intrathoracic goiter for predicting intra-operative and postoperative complications. Surgery. 2010;147(2):233–238.
5. White ML, Doherty GM, Gauger PG. Evidence-based surgical management of substernal goiter. World J Surg. 2008;32(7):1285–1300.
6. Lin YS, Wu HY, Lee CW, Hsu CC, Chao TC, Yu MC. Surgical management of substernal goitres at a tertiary referral centre: A retrospective cohort study of 2,104 patients. Int J Surg [Internet]. 2016;27(5):46–52.

7. Abdelrahman H, Al-Thani H, Al-Sulaiti M, Tabeb A, El-Menyar A. Clinical presentation and surgical treatment of retrosternal goiter: a case series study. Qatar Med J. 2020;2020(1):1–8.
8. Hegedüs L, Bonnema SJ, Bennedbæk FN. Management of simple nodular goiter: current status and future perspectives. Endocr Rev. 2003;24(1):102–132.
9. Anders HJ. Compression syndromes caused by substernal goitres. Postgrad Med J. 1998;74(872):327–329.
10. Hegedüs L, Bonnema SJ. Approach to management of the patient with primary or secondary intrathoracic goiter. J Clin Endocrinol Metab. 2010;95(12):5155–5162.
11. Rodrigues J, Furtado R, Ramani A, Mitta N, Kudchadkar S, Falari S. A rare instance of retrosternal goitre presenting with obstructive sleep apnoea in a middle-aged person. Int J Surg Case Rep [Internet]. 2013;4(12):1064–1066.
12. Sorensen JR, Bonnema SJ, Godballe C, Hegedüs L. The impact of goiter and thyroid surgery on goiter related esophageal dysfunction. A systematic review. Front Endocrinol (Lausanne). 2018;9(November):1–9.
13. Giulea C, Enciu O, Nadragea M, Badiu C, Miron A. Pemberton's sign and intense facial edema in superior vena cava syndrome due to retrosternal goiter. Acta Endocrinol (Copenh). 2016;12(2):227–229.
14. De Filippis EA, Sabet A, Sun MRM, Garber JR. Pemberton's sign: explained nearly 70 years later. J Clin Endocrinol Metab. 2014;99(6):1949–1954.
15. Polistena A, Sanguinetti A, Lucchini R, Galasse S, Monacelli M, Avenia S, et al. Surgical approach to mediastinal goiter: an update based on a retrospective cohort study. Int J Surg [Internet]. 2016;28:S42–S46.
16. Toni R, Della Casa C, Mosca S, Malaguti A, Castorina S, Roti E. Anthropological variations in the anatomy of the human thyroid arteries. Thyroid. 2003;13(2):183–192.
17. Foroulis CN, Rammos KS, Sileli MN PC. Primary intrathoracic goiter: a rare and potentially serious entity. Thyroid. 2009;19(3):213–218.
18. Petkov R, Minchev T, Yamakova Y, Mekov E, Yankov G, Petrov D. Diagnostic value and complication rate of ultrasound-guided transthoracic core needle biopsy in mediastinal lesions. PLOS ONE [Internet]. 2020;15(4):1–11.
19. Perincek G, Avci S, Celtikci P. Retrosternal goiter: a couple of classification methods with computed tomography findings. Pakistan J Med Sci. 2018;34(6):1494–1497.
20. Porzio S, Marocco M, Oddi A, Lombardi V, Porzio O, Calvelli C, et al. Endothoracic goitre: anatomoclinical and therapeutic considerations. Chir Ital. 2001;53(4):453–460.
21. Mercante G, Gabrielli E, Pedroni C, Formisano D, Bertolini L, Nicoli F, Valcavi RBV. CT cross-sectional imaging classification system for substernal goiter based on risk factors for an extracervical surgical approach. Head Neck. 2010;33(6):792–799.
22. Huins CT, Georgalas C, Mehrzad H, Tolley NS. A new classification system for retrosternal goitre based on a systematic review of its complications and management. Int J Surg. 2008;6(1):71–76.
23. Cvasciuc IT, Fraser S, Lansdown M. Retrosternal goitres: a practical classification. Acta Endocrinol (Copenh). 2017;13(3):261–265.
24. Stang MT, Armstrong MJ, Ogilvie JB, Yip L, McCoy KL, Faber CN, Carty SE. Positional dyspnea and tracheal compression as indications for goiter resection. Arch Surg. 2012;147(7):621–626.
25. Kim SM, Kim HJ. Successful advancement of endotracheal tube with combined fiberoptic bronchoscopy and videolaryngoscopy in a patient with a huge goiter. SAGE Open Med Case Reports. 2020;8:2050313X2092323.
26. Heinz E, Quan T, Nguyen H, Pla R. Intubation of a patient with a large goiter: the advantageous role of videolaryngoscopy. Case Rep Anesthesiol. 2019;2019(Figure 1):1–4.
27. Naraynsingh V, Ramarine I, Cawich SO, Maharaj R, Dan D. Cervical leverage: a new procedure to deliver deep retrosternal goitres without thoracotomy. Int J Surg Case Rep [Internet]. 2013;4(11):992–996.
28. Rathinam S, Davies B, Khalil-Marzouk JF. Marzouk's procedure: a novel combined cervical and anterior mediastinotomy technique to avoid median sternotomy for difficult retrosternal thyroidectomy. Ann Thorac Surg. 2006;82(2):759–760.
29. Picardi N, Di Rienzo M, Annunziata A, Bartolacci M, Relmi F. Transclavicular approach for delivery of intrathoracic giant goiter. An alternative surgical option. Ann Ital Chir. 1999;70(5):741–748.
30. Welman K, Heyes R, Dalal P, Hough S, Bunalade M, Anikin V. Surgical treatment of retrosternal goitre. Indian J Otolaryngol Head Neck Surg. 2017;69(3):345–350.
31. Wong KP, Mak KL, Wong CKH, Lang BHH. Systematic review and meta-analysis on intraoperative neuro-monitoring in high-risk thyroidectomy. Int J Surg [Internet]. 2017;38:21–30.
32. Choi SY, Son YI. Intraoperative neuromonitoring for thyroid surgery: the proven benefits and limitations. Clin Exp Otorhinolaryngol. 2019;12(4):335–336.
33. Wang JJ, Lu IC, Chang PY, Wu CW, Wang LF, Huang TY, et al. Peculiar anatomic variation of recurrent laryngeal nerve and EMG change in a patient with right substernal goiter and pre-operative vocal cord palsy-case report. Gland Surg. 2020;9(3):802–805.
34. Schneider R, Machens A, Lorenz K, Dralle H. Intraoperative nerve monitoring in thyroid surgery – shifting current paradigms. Gland Surg. 2020;9(Suppl 2):S120–S128.
35. Wang X, Zhou Y, Li C, Cai Y, He T, Sun R, et al. Surgery for retrosternal goiter: cervical approach. Gland Surg. 2020;9(2):392–400.
36. Tikka T, Nixon IJ, Harrison-Phipps K, Simo R. Predictors of the need for an extracervical approach to intrathoracic goitre. BJS Open. 2019;3(2):174–179.
37. Brenet E, Dubernard X, Mérol JC, Louges MA, Labrousse M, Makeieff M. Assessment and management of cervico-mediastinal goiter. Eur Ann Otorhinolaryngol Head Neck Dis [Internet]. 2017;134(6):409–413.
38. McKenzie GAG, Rook W. Is it possible to predict the need for sternotomy in patients undergoing thyroidectomy with retrosternal extension? Interact Cardiovasc Thorac Surg. 2014;19(1):139–143.
39. Casella C, Molfino S, Cappelli C, Salvoldi F, Benvenuti MR, Portolani N. Thyroiditis process as a predictive factor of sternotomy in the treatment of cervico-mediastinal goiter. BMC Surg. 2019;18(Suppl 1):1–7.
40. Brichkov I, Chiba S, Lagmay V, Shaw JP, Harris LJ, Weiss M. Simultaneous unilateral anterior thoracoscopy with transcervical thyroidectomy for the resection of large mediastinal thyroid goiter. J Thorac Dis. 2017;9(8):2484–2490.
41. Gupta P, Lau KKW, Rizvi I, Rathinam S, Waller DA. Video assisted thoracoscopic thyroidectomy for retrosternal goitre. Ann R Coll Surg Engl. 2014;96(8):606–608.
42. Tsilimigras DI, Patrini D, Antonopoulou A, Velissaris D, Koletsis E, Lawrence D, et al. Retrosternal goitre: the role of the thoracic surgeon. J Thorac Dis. 2017;9(3):860–863.
43. Rugiu MG, Piemonte M. Surgical approach to retrosternal goitre: do we still need sternotomy? Acta Otorhinolaryngol Ital [Internet]. 2009;29(6):331–338.
44. Salem FA, Bergenfelz A, Nordenström E, Dahlberg J, Hessman O, Lundgren CI, et al. Evaluating risk factors for re-exploration due to postoperative neck hematoma after thyroid surgery: a nested case-control study. Langenbeck's Arch Surg. 2019;404(7):815–823.
45. Huang WC, Huang CH, Hsu HS, Hsieh CC, Hsu WH, Tsai TH, et al. Intrathoracic goiter in elderly patients. Int J Gerontol [Internet]. 2013;7(1):8–12.
46. Agarwal A, Agarwal S, Tewari P, Gupta S, Chand G, Mishra A, et al. Clinicopathological profile, airway management, and outcome in huge multinodular goiters: an institutional experience from an endemic goiter region. World J Surg. 2012;36:755–760.

29

HISTORY OF PARATHYROID SURGERY

Poongkodi Karunakaran

The text of this chapter is available online at www.routledge.com/9781032136509.

ANATOMY AND PATHOLOGY OF THE PARATHYROID GLAND

Rajeev Parameswaran and Sheeja Sainulabdeen

Introduction

The parathyroid glands (from Lat. *glandulae parathyroideae*) are endocrine glands that secrete the parathyroid hormone (PTH) and regulate the levels of calcium and phosphorus levels in the body. The gland was discovered by Ivor Sandström in 1880 (1). The parathyroid glands are usually four in number with superior pair located on the middle third of the posterolateral border of the thyroid gland and the inferior pair along the inferior pole of the thyroid gland, in proximity to the inferior thyroid artery. However, multiple parathyroid glands have been described in the literature (2, 3). The color of the glands is usually described to be tan brown; however, the color varies from brown to yellow, depending on fat content, and this in turn depends on the age, nutrition and activity of the individual. The blood supply of both the superior and inferior parathyroid glands is from the inferior thyroid artery. Embryologically, the parathyroid glands develop from the branchial clefts with the upper pair arising from the fourth branchial cleft, and the lower pair arises from the third branchial cleft. The parathyroid glands are usually symmetrically distributed as a mirror image of the place occupied by a gland (4). Aberrations in the embryological descent in the embryonic life lead to the parathyroid glands being placed in anomalous positions in the neck or mediastinum (5–8).

Normal histology

The parathyroid glands are normally the size of a grain and have a thin connective tissue capsule. The main component of the parathyroid glands is the **chief cell** and usually measures about 6–8 μm in diameter with a centrally located nucleus and pale granular cytoplasm. The chief cells contain a variable amount of glycogen (9) and droplets of neutral lipids (10). The cells are usually arranged in a solid pattern surrounded by capillary network, with the presence of stromal fat, trabeculation occurs and forms round to angular nests.

The second type of cell seen in the parathyroid glands is the **oxyphil cell** that has a polygonal shape with abundant eosinophilic granular cytoplasm, with higher amount of mitochondria but fewer organelles and granules than chief cells (11, 12). The oxyphilic cells are often present in the form of nodular collections. Other types of cells are the **transitional oxyphil cells** (have an appearance that is intermediate between chief cells and oxyphil cells) and **water-clear cell** (have abundant clear cytoplasm). The cytoplasmic granules in the chief cells contain the **PTH**, which regulates the blood calcium levels by acting on three target organs, namely, the bone, kidney and the intestines. Besides PTH the parathyroid glands also synthesize chromogranin A (13, 14), cytokeratins and parathyroid hormone–related protein (PTHrP) (14, 15).

With increasing age, more than half the chief cells are replaced with adipocytes, and also in patients with chronic diseases (16). Parathyroid cells have a low proliferation activity as shown on Ki-67 immunohistochemistry (17, 18). Rarely, microcystic structures, scars or fibrous hyalinizing tissue, bone marrow and salivary gland remnants have been reported in parathyroid tissues (9, 19).

Physiology of the parathyroid gland

Ionized serum calcium acts as the major regulator of PTH secretion, along with vitamin D which plays a minor role, and both can increase or decrease the synthesis of PTH. PTH is a linear polypeptide hormone which contains 84 amino acid residues, has a molecular weight of 9.5 kDa and a short half-life of about 4 minutes (20, 21). The hormone is transcribed as a prepro-PTH of 115 amino acids, which is truncated to a 90-amino acid polypeptide proPTH. A further 6 amino acid residues are removed from the amino terminal of proPTH in the Golgi apparatus to form the final 84 amino acid product, which is packaged in secretory granules. The biological activity is contained in the 34 N-terminal amino acids that are rapidly hydrolyzed, especially in the kidney.

The three primary target organs for PTH activity are the kidneys, intestines and bones. PTH causes increased renal excretion of phosphate, increased renal tubular reabsorption of calcium, increased formation of 1,25-dihydroxycholecalciferol, and this increases intestinal absorption of calcium. In the bone, there is an increase in the number of osteoblasts, osteoclasts and their phagocytic activity, which results in increased resorption of bone tissue. At a cellular level, the parathyroid cell membrane carries a Ca^{2+}-sensing receptor (CaSR), a member of the G protein-coupled receptor (GPCR) family that binds Ca^{2+} in a saturable manner, with an affinity profile that is similar to the concentration dependence for PTH secretion. Besides this there are two other PTH receptors – one that binds PTHrP and known as the hPTH/PTHrP receptor (22) and the other receptor, PTH2 (hPTH2-R), that does not bind PTHrP and is found in the brain, placenta and pancreas (23).

Hyperparathyroidism

Increased activity of the parathyroid glands due to an intrinsic tumor or cancer or hyperplasia leads to increased hypercalcemia, resulting in primary hyperparathyroidism (24, 25). It is the most common cause of hypercalcemia and treated by removing the pathological gland. In contrast, secondary hyperparathyroidism occurs as a result of renal disease and hypocalcemia leading to four-gland hyperplasia. The condition is predominantly treated medically with bisphosphonates and calcimimetics. In patients

Anatomy and Pathology of the Parathyroid Gland

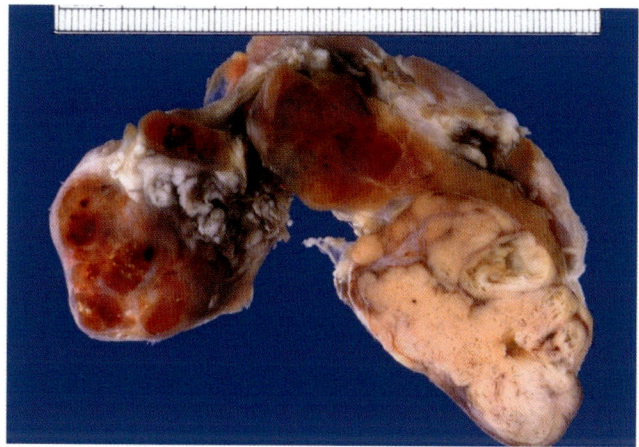

FIGURE 30.1 Gross appearance of a case of parathyroid carcinoma (top right) with adjacent thyroid gland. Fleshy pale tan appearance with slightly irregular borders.

with failed medical treatment, surgery may be necessary in the form of total parathyroidectomy plus *autotransplantation* or subtotal parathyroidectomy (26).

Parathyroid adenoma

It is estimated that 90–95% of primary hyperparathyroidism is caused by parathyroid adenoma. Adenomas are usually solitary, but double and multiple adenomas can occur. The incidence is highest in the age group of 50–60 years, with a slight female preponderance (F:M – 3:1). Most adenomas involve a single gland, usually in the inferior parathyroid (75%), but may arise from the superior glands (15%). In about 10% of the patients, the adenomas can be located in ectopic sites such as mediastinum, in thymic tissue or eutopically in the intrathyroidal tissue or soft tissue of esophagus.

On gross examination, adenomas are soft and encapsulated with smooth consistency and a rim of normal parathyroid gland at the periphery (Figure 30.1). Larger and long-standing adenomas show areas of hemorrhage and cystic degeneration. Size and weight of the adenomas can vary considerably, weighing anywhere between 300 mg and several grams. The size of the adenoma ranges from less than 1 cm to more than 3 cm. Microadenomas are tumors with weight less than 0.1 g and are usually nonencapsulated and missed on surgical exploration and on frozen sections (27).

On microscopic examination, the adenomas are composed mainly of chief cells arranged within a delicate capillary network. Cells are arranged in lobules, nests and sheets, and sometimes nodules formations are seen. Stromal fat is usually absent. Most adenomas disclose a normal rim or even atrophic parathyroid tissue in the periphery. The absence of a rim does not exclude the diagnosis of adenoma because large tumors may have overgrown the preexisting normal gland, or the rim may have been lost during processing. The cells in adenoma are round with small, uniform, densely stained nuclei, which are larger than those present in the nonneoplastic parathyroid tissue at the rim or periphery. Bizarre multinucleated cells with dark, wrinkled nuclei can be seen focally which are thought to be of degenerative change rather than malignant or premalignant change. The other glands have a normal morphological appearance or even may be atrophic. *The presence of a microscopically normal parathyroid gland in the presence of an adenoma is the best evidence of the presence of adenoma rather than hyperplasia.*

There are three variants of parathyroid adenoma and the differences are highlighted in Table 30.1.

Parathyroid hyperplasia

Parathyroid hyperplasia is seen in 5–10% of patients with hyperparathyroidism and is seen when all the four glands are abnormal. This may arise in the context of primary gene abnormality as in the case of familial endocrine syndromes and is called as primary hyperplasia. Both multiple endocrine neoplasias (MEN) type 1 and 2 and nonfamilial MEN develop polyglandular disease (28, 29). The various familial endocrinopathies leading to hyperparathyroidism is shown in Table 30.2.

Based on the cellular content of the parathyroid, hyperplasia may be classified as **chief cell hyperplasia** or **water clear cell hyperplasia**. Primary chief cell hyperplasia is a constant finding in patients with MEN syndromes (types 1 and 2a) (18), whereas only seen in a mild form in MEN 2B (30). In primary chief cell hyperplasia, all the glands are asymmetrically enlarged, with the superior glands being larger than the inferior glands; however, in some cases, all four glands may be morphologically normal, but histological evaluation shows hyperplasia (31). In chief cell hyperplasia of secondary cause, the parathyroids all gradations of sizes are seen, from normal sized to large glands. There is an inverse correlation between the size of the gland and the mean serum calcium level (32).

Distinguishing between the two types of chief cell hyperplasia can be quite difficult based on morphology alone (33).

TABLE 30.1: Variants of Parathyroid Adenoma and Their Features

	Oxyphil Adenoma	Lipoadenoma or Hamartoma	Water Clear Adenoma
Incidence	8% of all adenomas	Rare	0.4% of adenomas
Histology	Composed of at least 90% of cells with abundant granular eosinophilic cytoplasm with regular central nuclei and prominent nucleolus	Few parenchymal cells (chief cells and oncocytes) intimately admixed with variable amount of mature adipose tissue and fibrous stroma	Consists of large polygonal cells with abundant clear cell cytoplasm; nuclei are small and hyperchromatic and are located either in the center of the cell or toward its periphery
Arrangement	Arranged in trabecular, solid or glandular patterns	Are arranged in thin, branching, cord-like patterns	Fibrotic and adherent; can mimic parathyroid carcinoma
Symptoms	Very symptomatic	Less symptoms	Symptomatic

TABLE 30.2: Familial Hyperparathyroid Disorders with Genetics and Associated Pathologies

Disorder	Mode of Inheritance	Gene Involved	Chromosome Loci	Parathyroid Pathology	Associated Tumors
MEN 1	AD	Menin	11q13	MGD	Pituitary, EPT, adrenocortical carcinoid
MEN 2A	AD	RET	10q21	Adenoma/MGD	MTC, pheochromocytoma
HPT-JT	AD	HRPT2	1q21-q32	Cystic parathyroid tumors Parathyroid carcinoma	Jaw tumors, renal lesions
FIHPT	AD	HRPT2	1q21-q32	Adenoma/MGD	
ADMH	AD	CASR	3q13-21	Adenoma/MGD	
FHH	AD	CASR	3q13-21	Hyperplasia mild	
NSHPT	AR/AD	CASR	3q13-21	Severe hyperplasia	

Abbreviations: MEN, multiple endocrine neoplasia; *HPT-JT*, hereditary hyperparathyroidism-jaw tumor syndrome; *FIHPT*, familial isolated hyperparathyroidism; *ADMH*, autosomal dominant mild hyperparathyroidism; *FHH*, familial hypocalciuric hypercalcemia; *NSHPT*, neonatal severe hyperparathyroidism; *AD*, autosomal dominant; *AR*, autosomal recessive; *EPT*, endocrine pancreatic tumors; *MTC*, medullary thyroid carcinoma.

In the primary form of hyperplasia nodularity, fibrous septation, acinar formation and giant nuclei are more common, whereas in the secondary form, the number of oxyphil cells is higher. The distinction between hyperplasia and adenoma can also be difficult as well based on morphology alone and even proliferative index (18). **Currently the only definite criteria to distinguish adenoma from hyperplasia is the presence of normal rim of parathyroid tissue and presence of at least one normal parathyroid gland**, but both of these pathologies may represent different morphology of the same process (34).

Atypical parathyroid adenoma

Atypical parathyroid adenomas are a group of neoplasms that demonstrate some features of parathyroid carcinoma but lack overt characteristics for malignant behavior like infiltrative growth, vascular invasion or metastasis at presentation. These neoplasms are also known as tumors of uncertain malignant potential (35). They usually have a smaller dimension, weight and volume compared to carcinomas and occur at an early age group. The microscopic features include banding, fibrosis (with or without associated hemosiderin deposition), adherence to (but not invasion of) contiguous structures, presence of tumor within the surrounding capsule, solid or trabecular growth patterns, nuclear atypia and prominent nucleoli and mitotic activity. However, none of these features alone or in combination is diagnostic of malignancy. Atypical parathyroid neoplasms are less likely to have coagulative tumor necrosis. Atypical adenoma can be sporadic or as a part of hereditary syndromes. The molecular pathogenesis of these neoplasms is still unknown. However, few studies have shown that that the phenotypes p27(+), bcl2(+), Ki-67(–) and mdm2(+) were present in 29% of atypical adenomas, respectively, and in no cases of carcinoma (36).

Atypical parathyroid adenoma may represent a precancerous or early-stage parathyroid cancer (37). Most patients with atypical adenomas have a benign clinical course; however, close follow-up for longer interval is mandatory as recurrences can occur. CDC73 immunoreactivity has proven to be a useful to predictor for recurrence. Recurrences in these tumors have not been documented in any CDC73-positive cases, whereas it recurred in 10% of CDC73-negative tumors. In contrast, in parathyroid carcinomas, recurrence was documented in both CDC73-positive (36%) and -negative tumors (38%) (38).

Parathyroid carcinoma

Parathyroid carcinoma is the least common endocrine malignancy representing only 0.005% and is responsible for less than 1% of cases of primary hyperparathyroidism (39, 40). Most of parathyroid carcinoma are functional presenting with clinical features of primary hyperparathyroidism, but 10% patients are nonfunctional. There is no gender preponderance in parathyroid cancer unlike in adenomas and hyperplasia, where there is a female preponderance. Parathyroid carcinoma tends to be seen in the younger age group. Most patients present with clinical and biochemical manifestations of severe hyperparathyroidism, including severe hypercalcemia, significantly elevated PTH level as well as renal and osseous complications (41). A palpable neck mass may be present in 30–76% of patients. A preoperative diagnosis of parathyroid carcinoma is made very rarely. Most parathyroid cancers arise sporadically but are also seen in association with familial forms of parathyroid disease such as familial isolated primary hyperparathyroidism (42), hyperparathyroidism-jaw tumor syndrome (HPT-JT) (43) and MEN (44).

Preoperative diagnosis of parathyroid cancer is difficult as they often present with the same symptoms as patients with benign, sporadic primary hyperparathyroidism. The key tests used for preoperative demonstration of increased cancer risk are measurement of blood calcium levels, tumor size and the PTH assay ratio, known as the rule of 3s (41). Fine needle aspiration of primary lesion is not recommended because of the risk of seeding of the tumor cells through needle track (45, 46). The only indication for a fine needle cytology is in confirming suspected metastatic parathyroid carcinoma with the aid of PTH immunostaining for PTH and parafibromin on cell block material.

Intraoperative identification of parathyroid cancer is also difficult, but malignant nature is suspected when a firm solid gray large mass is seen involving adjacent structures (Figure 30.2). The two absolute diagnostic criteria is **extensive invasion of adjacent tissues** and **metastatic spread**. The treatment choice is open excision of the tumor with en-bloc excision of the ipsilateral thyroid lobe and other tissues if there is evidence of local invasion (41, 47). Lymphadenectomy is performed if there is evidence of lymph nodes involvement, whereas prophylactic neck dissection is not recommended (41, 48). Intraoperative frozen section to establish a definitive diagnosis of carcinoma is somewhat controversial because of the overall difficulty in providing a diagnosis. It is useful to confirm the parathyroid origin of the lesion,

Anatomy and Pathology of the Parathyroid Gland

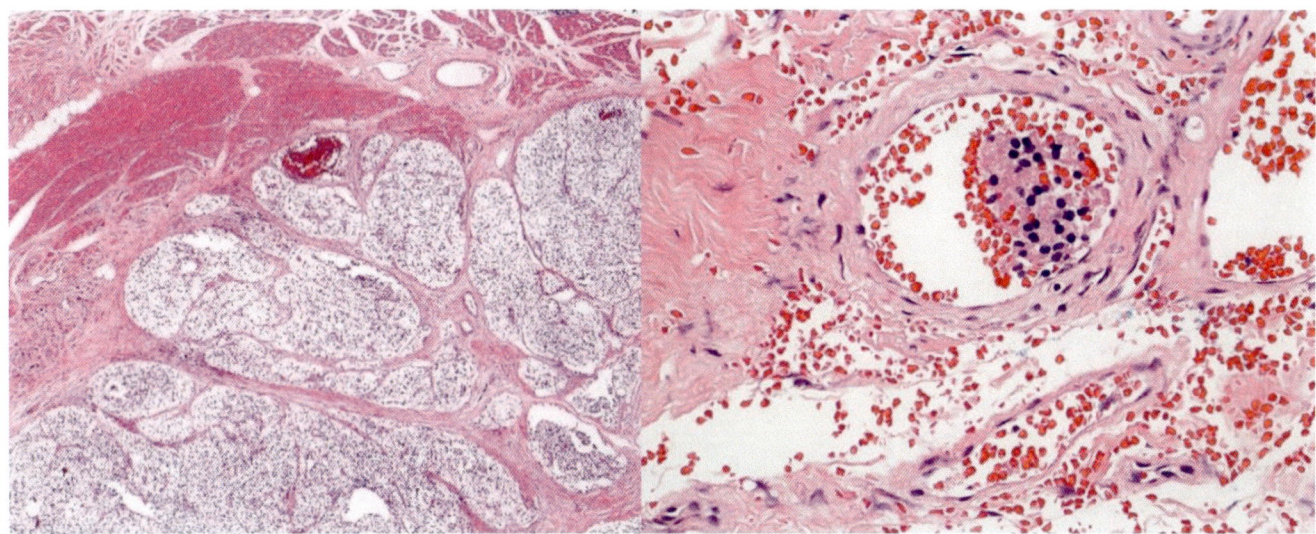

FIGURE 30.2 Left: Low power photomicrograph of a case of parathyroid carcinoma, showing the coarse nodularity. The tumor directly abuts the surrounding skeletal muscle tissue (top left corner). Original magnification ×20. Right: Parathyroid carcinoma showing vascular invasion (tumor embolus within a vessel, associated with some fibrin). The vessel is outside the confines of the tumor. Original magnification ×200.

but distinction between adenoma, hyperplasia and carcinoma is often difficult.

Parathyroid cancers are generally large, lobulated, irregular, grayish-white, firm to hard tumors and often tethered to the adjacent tissues (49, 50) (Figure 30.1). The mean tumor size is approximately 3 cm (range 1–7 cm), and the average weight is 3 g; however, larger cancers as much as 100 g have been described (51). Local invasion commonly occurs into the ipsilateral strap muscles and thyroid lobe, recurrent laryngeal nerve, esophagus and trachea (52). Up to 20% of patients may present with lymph node metastasis (53) and metastases may be 7.5 times more likely in patients with tumors ≥3 cm than those with tumors <3 cm (54). Distant metastasis occurs in about 3–4% of patients (55, 56).

The histological diagnosis can be difficult and challenging as some of the features exhibited by carcinomas may also be seen in benign adenomas as well as hyperplastic parathyroid lesions (57). Schantz and Castleman, in 1973, established a set of criteria for the pathological diagnosis of this malignancy based on their analysis of 70 parathyroid cancers (58). Table 30.3 highlights the histological features that are associated with a higher risk of malignant behavior.

A histologic diagnosis of malignancy can only be made if there is histologic evidence of invasion into capsular or extracapsular vessels, adjacent extracapsular structures in the neck (without prior instrumentation) or metastases. Other features such as coarse nodularity with fibrous bands are seen more frequently in malignancy but may occasionally occur in benign lesions which have undergone fibrous scarring due to degenerative changes. Cytologic atypia (enlarged nuclei with macronucleoli) is described more frequently in carcinoma; however, these features alone are insufficient for a histologic diagnosis of malignancy (Figures 30.2 and 30.3). Even mitotic counts show significant overlap between benign and malignant lesions and are an unreliable indicator of malignancy (60).

Where the distinction between cancer and atypical adenoma is difficult, immunostaining with parafibromin appears to be helpful in cases with complete absence of nuclear staining (61, 62). Ki-67 cell proliferative marker has been used as a marker to identify parathyroid cancers (63) but, as a single-modality marker, is unreliable in differentiating these from benign adenomas due to significant overlap between the two entities.

TABLE 30.3: Histological Features of Parathyroid Carcinoma

Most definitive features

- Capsular invasion with growth into adjacent tissues
- Vascular invasion (vessels in capsule or surrounding tissue)
- Perineural invasion

Non-definitive features that may be seen in malignancy

- Band-forming fibrosis
- Solid growth pattern
- Coagulative necrosis*
- Mitotic activity >5 figures per 50 high-power fields*
- Macronucleoli*

*When seen together, this triad of features is associated with malignant behavior (59).

Molecular pathogenesis of parathyroid tumors

There has been a steady and substantial increase in the knowledge of the genetic profile of parathyroid tumors over the past few decades. Formation of tumors and hyperplasia involve multiple different mechanisms such as activation of oncogenes, inactivation of tumor suppressor genes, imbalance between growth factors and proteins involved in cell regulation and epigenetic alterations. The various genetic and molecular events seen in

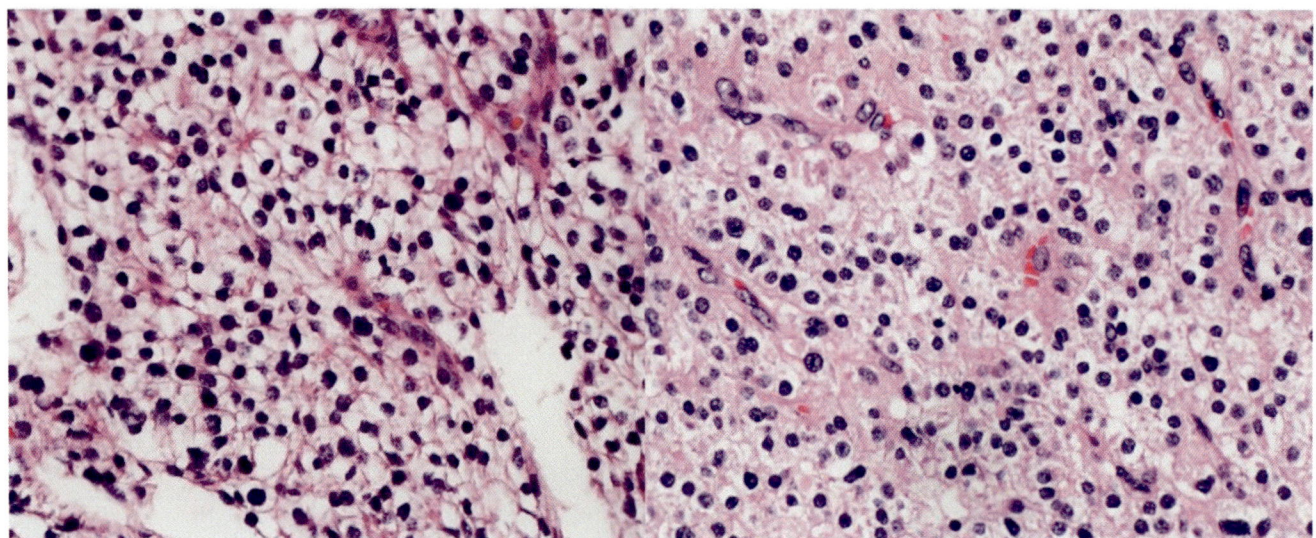

FIGURE 30.3 Left: Parathyroid carcinoma – high-power photomicrograph showing sheets of cells with slightly raised nuclear:cytoplasmic ratios. Marked nuclear pleomorphism is not apparent. Original magnification ×400. Right: Parathyroid adenoma – high-power photomicrograph showing nests of cells with mild variation in nuclear size. Compare with parathyroid carcinoma. Original magnification ×400.

parathyroid adenoma, hyperplasia and carcinoma are summarized in Table 30.4.

Parathyroid cysts

Parathyroid cysts are uncommon and are usually asymptomatic, with majority of them being nonfunctional. Most commonly they arise from the inferior glands but may be seen in the mediastinum (92, 93). The cysts are usually lined by columnar epithelial cells with some parathyroid tissue on the wall. Parathyroid cysts that are functional are thought to arise from cystic degeneration of normal glands or existing adenomas (94), whereas the non-functioning cysts may represent an embryologic remnant of a branchial cleft (95), the persistence of the Kürsteiner canals of the fetal parathyroids (96) or retention cysts of the parathyroid (94).

Intraoperative assessments of parathyroid and frozen section

To identify the parathyroid glands, both normal and abnormal, one should clearly have an understanding of the embryology and attention to detail at surgery. An experienced surgeon is the best modality of identification of the parathyroids (97). Parathyroid glands have a distinct appearance in comparison to a thyroid nodule, fat or lymph node. One of the techniques used intraoperatively is the ***gliding sign***, wherein the parathyroid gland demonstrates a discrete gliding motion within the fat. "The absence of capsular fixation permits an impression of mobility uniquely characteristic of the parathyroid" as described by Wang (98). Where one is uncertain, frozen section may be performed to confirm the presence of parathyroid tissue with an accuracy of over 99% (99, 100). Imprints using polychrome methylene blue can also be useful with a short turn over from the laboratory to the operating theatre without having to wait long for the confirmatory tests (101, 102).

To a pathologist, distinction between an adenoma, hyperplasia and carcinoma can be difficult on frozen section and the impression given usually is that of cellular parathyroid tissue, especially if the biopsy is from a single gland only. The diagnosis is that of an adenoma if only one gland is enlarged and cellular, but this requires biopsies of all the other glands which should morphologically be small and low to normal cellularity. However, this scenario can be avoided using intraoperative PTH assay to confirm successful resection of the parathyroid gland (103, 104). Cases of water-clear cell hyperplasia and parathyroid cancers may be identified on frozen section if there is evidence of local invasion.

Asian perspective

The incidence of primary hyperparathyroidism is similar in the West and the East, but the clinical presentation appears to be different. In the West, there has been a striking change in the presentation from symptomatic to asymptomatic hyperparathyroidism, with most cases detected on incidental biochemical screening (105, 106). However, in Asia, patients still present with classic florid skeletal and renal manifestations, including in India (107–109). Patients have significant skeletal symptoms (fractures in more than 50% and brown tumors), renal stone disease and palpable neck mass in up to 30% (109–115). Another significant difference between the developed nations and Asia is the weight of the glands, with tumors excised in Asia showing significant higher weight of the glands (1.25–102 g) in comparison to 2–4 g in the West (110, 116, 117). Another interesting fact is that the incidence of parathyroid cancer appears to be higher (2–6%) in comparison to 1–2% in the Western world (107, 110, 117).

The incidence of renal hyperparathyroidism requiring surgery in Asia is also significantly higher than the West. Factors that contribute to higher need for surgery in renal hyperparathyroidism in Asia is due to lack of funding and costs associated with cinacalcet therapy, lack of access to renal transplant and higher

Anatomy and Pathology of the Parathyroid Gland

TABLE 30.4: The Various Genetic and Molecular Events Leading to Adenoma, Hyperplasia and Carcinoma Formation

	Adenoma	Secondary Hyperplasia	Carcinoma	References
Oncogenes				
MEN1N				
Loss of allele	25–40%	Rare or not seen	Rare or not seen	(44, 64)
Inactivating mutation	40–50%	Not seen	Not seen	
RET	27–54% Adenoma and hyperplasia		Rare	(65, 66)
CDC73/HRPT2 loss or inactivation caused by LOH or mutation of the gene	Rare (1%)	Not seen	15–20%	(67, 68)
CDKN1B germline and somatic mutations	Low frequency	Not seen	Not seen	(69, 70)
CASR in FIHPT Somatic mutations	Common	Not seen	Not seen	(71, 72)
Cell-cycle regulators				
Rb gene loss of heterozygosity and inactivating mutations	Not seen	Not seen	Common	(73)
Cyclin D1				
Amplification	20–40%	30%	90%	(44, 64, 74)
Overexpression	8%	Not seen	Not seen	
CDK inhibitor 1B (P27)	Not reported	Not reported	Decreased expression	(75)
CDK inhibitor 1A (P21)				
Ki-67	Very low	Very low	Frequent	(76, 77)
Proliferating cell nuclear antigen (PCNA)	Frequent	Frequent	Rare	(77, 78)
Growth factors				
Vascular endothelial growth factor (VEGF) Proangiogenic effect	Seen	Seen	Seen	(79)
Basic fibroblast growth factor (bFGF, FGF-2) proangiogenic effect	Seen	Seen	Seen	(80, 81)
Transforming growth factor beta (TGF-b) pro-proliferative	Seen	Seen	Seen	(82)
Insulin-like growth factor (IGF-1) stimulates cell proliferation and promotes S-phase	Seen	Seen	Seen	(83)
Factors involved in apoptosis				
TNF-related apoptosis-inducing ligand (TRAIL; CD253) overexpression	Seen	Seen	Not seen	(84)
FAS receptor overexpression	High	Highest	Not seen	(84)
BCL-2				(84)
Anti-apoptotic BCL-X(L) and BCL-W	Highest	High	Low	
Pro-apoptotic members BIM and BOK	Lowest	Low	Low	
Mouse double minute 2 homolog (MDM2, E3 ubiquitin-protein ligase)	High	High	None	(84)
Other factors				
Galectin-3	None	None	High	(84, 85)
Adenomatous polyposis coli (APC)	None	None	High	(86)
Cytokeratin-8 or keratin-8 (CK-8)	None	None	Present	(84)
E-cadherin expression	High	High	None	(87)
Snail and twist	High	High	Limited	(87)
Synaptophysin	High	High	Limited	(84)
Protein gene product 9.5 (PGP9.5)	None	None	High	(88)
Human telomerase reverse transcriptase (hTERT)	Low	Low	High	(89)
Loss of heterozygosity and comparative genomic hybridization	50–73%		30–40%	(90, 91)

incidence of chronic renal disease from diabetes and other nephropathic conditions requiring long-term dialysis. Vitamin D deficiency is also higher and of longer duration, and there is some speculation that longstanding vitamin D deficiency may progress to secondary and tertiary hyperparathyroidism (118), along with the spectrum of bony disease as well from acquired pseudohypoparathyroidism (hypocalcemia with normal phosphate) at one end through typical osteomalacia (normal or low serum calcium with low phosphate) (119).

Conclusion

Parathyroid glands control calcium in the body by PTH. These glands are located usually in the neck and rarely in mediastinum. Parathyroid tumors lead to hyperparathyroidism that can be asymptomatic or very symptomatic as seen in Asia. Parathyroid tumors and hyperplasias develop either sporadically or as a result of genetic mutations or aberrations in molecular pathways involved in tumorigenesis.

References

1. Carney JA. The glandulae parathyroideae of Ivar Sandström. Contributions from two continents. Am J Surg Pathol. 1996;20(9):1123–1144.
2. Barczyński M, Bränström R, Dionigi G, Mihai R. Sporadic multiple parathyroid gland disease – A consensus report of the European Society of Endocrine Surgeons (ESES). Langenbecks Arch Surg. 2015;400(8):887–905.
3. Mohebati A, Shaha AR. Anatomy of thyroid and parathyroid glands and neurovascular relations. Clin Anat. 2012;25(1):19–31.
4. Akerstrom G, Malmaeus J, Bergstrom R. Surgical anatomy of human parathyroid glands. Surgery. 1984;95(1):14–21.
5. Hu J, Ngiam KY, Parameswaran R. Mediastinal parathyroid adenomas and their surgical implications. Ann R Coll Surg Engl. 2015;97(4):259–261.
6. Harach HR, Vujanic GM. Intrathyroidal parathyroid. Pediatr Pathol. 1993;13(1):71–74.
7. Herrold KM, Rabson AS, Ketcham AS. Aberrant parathyroid gland in pharyngeal submucosa. Arch Pathol. 1961;71:60–62.
8. Lack EE, Delay S, Linnoila RI. Ectopic parathyroid tissue within the vagus nerve. Incidence and possible clinical significance. Arch Pathol Lab Med. 1988;112(3):304–306.
9. Gilmour JR. The normal histology of the parathyroid glands. J Pathol Bacteriol. 1939;48(1):187–222.
10. Dufour DR. Evaluation of parathyroid gland lesions. JAMA. 1982;247(12):1694–1695.
11. Cinti S, Sbarbati A, Morroni M, Carboni V, Zancanaro C, Lo Cascio V, et al. Parathyroid glands in primary hyperparathyroidism: An ultrastructural morphometric study of 25 cases. J Pathol. 1992;167(3):283–290.
12. Roth SI, Capen CC. Ultrastructural and functional correlations of the parathyroid gland. Int Rev Exp Pathol. 1974;13(0):161–221.
13. Khan A, Tischler AS, Patwardhan NA, DeLellis RA. Calcitonin immunoreactivity in neoplastic and hyperplastic parathyroid glands: An immunohistochemical study. Endocr Pathol. 2003;14(3):249–255.
14. Kitazawa R, Kitazawa S, Fukase M, Fujita T, Kobayashi A, Chihara K, et al. The expression of parathyroid hormone-related protein (PTHrP) in normal parathyroid: Histochemistry and in situ hybridization. Histochemistry. 1992;98(4):211–215.
15. Miettinen M, Clark R, Lehto VP, Virtanen I, Damjanov I. Intermediate-filament proteins in parathyroid glands and parathyroid adenomas. Arch Pathol Lab Med. 1985;109(11):986–989.
16. Dufour DR, Wilkerson SY. The normal parathyroid revisited: Percentage of stromal fat. Hum Pathol. 1982;13(8):717–721.
17. Wang W, Johansson H, Kvasnicka T, Farnebo LO, Grimelius L. Detection of apoptotic cells and expression of Ki-67 antigen, Bcl-2, p53 oncoproteins in human parathyroid adenoma. APMIS. 1996;104(11):789–796.
18. Loda M, Lipman J, Cukor B, Bur M, Kwan P, DeLellis RA. Nodular foci in parathyroid adenomas and hyperplasias: An immunohistochemical analysis of proliferative activity. Hum Pathol. 1994;25(10):1050–1056.
19. Edwards PC, Bhuiya T, Kahn LB, Fantasia JE. Salivary heterotopia of the parathyroid gland: A report of two cases and review of the literature. Oral Surg Oral Med Oral Pathol Oral Radiol Endod. 2005;99(5):590–593.
20. Truszkowski R, Blauth-Opieńska J, Iwanowska J. Parathyroid hormone. Biochem J. 1939;33(6):1005–1011.
21. Mihai R, Farndon JR. Parathyroid disease and calcium metabolism. Br J Anaesth. 2000 July;85(1):29–43.
22. Gensure RC, Gardella TJ, Juppner H. Parathyroid hormone and parathyroid hormone-related peptide, and their receptors. Biochem Biophys Res Commun. 2005;328(3):666–678.
23. Dobolyi A, Dimitrov E, Palkovits M, Usdin TB. The neuroendocrine functions of the parathyroid hormone 2 receptor. Front Endocrinol (Lausanne). 2012;3:121.
24. Bilezikian JP, Bandeira L, Khan A, Cusano NE. Hyperparathyroidism. Lancet. 2018;391(10116):168–178.
25. Thakker RV. Multiple endocrine neoplasia type 1 (MEN1). Best Pract Res Clin Endocrinol Metab. 2010;24(3):355–370.
26. Rajeev P, Lee KY, Tang XJ, Goo TT, Tan WB, Ngiam KY. Outcomes of parathyroidectomy in renal hyperparathyroidism in patients with No access to renal transplantation in Singapore. Int J Surg. 2016;25:64–68.
27. Liechty RD, Teter A, Suba EJ. The tiny parathyroid adenoma. Surgery. 1986;100(6):1048–1052.
28. Thakker RV. Multiple endocrine neoplasia type 1 (MEN1) and type 4 (MEN4). Mol Cell Endocrinol. 2014;386(1–2):2–15.
29. Wells SA, Jr., Pacini F, Robinson BG, Santoro M. Multiple endocrine neoplasia type 2 and familial medullary thyroid carcinoma: An update. J Clin Endocrinol Metab. 2013;98(8):3149–3164.
30. Carney JA, Roth SI, Heath H, 3rd, Sizemore GW, Hayles AB. The parathyroid glands in multiple endocrine neoplasia type 2b. Am J Pathol. 1980;99(2):387–398.
31. Black WC, Haff RC. The surgical pathology of parathyroid chief cell hyperplasia. Am J Clin Pathol. 1970;53(5):565–579.
32. Roth SI, Marshall RB. Pathology and ultrastructure of the human parathyroid glands in chronic renal failure. Arch Intern Med. 1969;124(4):397–407.
33. Roth SI. Pathology of the parathyroids in hyperparathyroidism. Discussion of recent advances in the anatomy and pathology of the parathyroid glands. Arch Pathol. 1962;73:495–510.
34. Black WC, 3rd, Utley JR. The differential diagnosis of parathyroid adenoma and chief cell hyperplasia. Am J Clin Pathol. 1968;49(6):761–775.
35. Ippolito G, Palazzo FF, Sebag F, De Micco C, Henry JF. Intraoperative diagnosis and treatment of parathyroid cancer and atypical parathyroid adenoma. Br J Surg. 2007;94(5):566–570.
36. Stojadinovic A, Hoos A, Nissan A, Dudas ME, Cordon-Cardo C, Shaha AR, et al. Parathyroid neoplasms: Clinical, histopathological, and tissue microarray-based molecular analysis. Hum Pathol. 2003;34(1):54–64.
37. Levin KE, Galante M, Clark OH. Parathyroid carcinoma versus parathyroid adenoma in patients with profound hypercalcemia. Surgery. 1987;101(6):649–660.
38. Guarnieri V, Battista C, Muscarella LA, Bisceglia M, de Martino D, Baorda F, et al. CDC73 mutations and parafibromin immunohistochemistry in parathyroid tumors: Clinical correlations in a single-centre patient cohort. Cell Oncol (Dordr). 2012;35(6):411–422.
39. Shane E. Clinical review 122: Parathyroid carcinoma. J Clin Endocrinol Metab. 2001;86(2):485–493.
40. Rawat N, Khetan N, Williams DW, Baxter JN. Parathyroid carcinoma. Br J Surg. 2005;92(11):1345–1353.
41. Schulte KM, Talat N. Diagnosis and management of parathyroid cancer. Nat Rev Endocrinol. 2012;8(10):612–622.
42. Hannan FM, Nesbit MA, Christie PT, Fratter C, Dudley NE, Sadler GP, et al. Familial isolated primary hyperparathyroidism caused by mutations of the MEN1 gene. Nat Clin Pract Endocrinol Metab. 2008;4(1):53–58.
43. Cristina E-V, Alberto F. Management of familial hyperparathyroidism syndromes: MEN1, MEN2, MEN4, HPT-Jaw tumour, Familial isolated hyperparathyroidism, FHH, and neonatal severe hyperparathyroidism. Best Pract Res Clin Endocrinol Metab. 2018;32(6):861–875.
44. Westin G, Bjorklund P, Akerstrom G. Molecular genetics of parathyroid disease. World J Surg. 2009;33(11):2224–2233.
45. Spinelli C, Bonadio AG, Berti P, Materazzi G, Miccoli P. Cutaneous spreading of parathyroid carcinoma after fine needle aspiration cytology. J Endocrinol Invest. 2000;23(4):255–257.
46. Agarwal G, Dhingra S, Mishra SK, Krishnani N. Implantation of parathyroid carcinoma along fine needle aspiration track. Langenbecks Arch Surg. 2006;391(6):623–626.
47. Owen RP, Silver CE, Pellitteri PK, Shaha AR, Devaney KO, Werner JA, et al. Parathyroid carcinoma: A review. Head Neck. 2011;33(4):429–436.
48. Givi B, Shah JP. Parathyroid carcinoma. Clin Oncol (R Coll Radiol). 2010;22(6):498–507.
49. Wang CA, Gaz RD. Natural history of parathyroid carcinoma. Diagnosis, treatment, and results. Am J Surg. 1985;149(4):522–527.
50. Kebebew E. Parathyroid carcinoma. Curr Treat Options Oncol. 2001;2(4):347–354.
51. Wynne AG, van Heerden J, Carney JA, Fitzpatrick LA. Parathyroid carcinoma: Clinical and pathologic features in 43 patients. Medicine (Baltimore). 1992;71(4):197–205.
52. Koea JB, Shaw JH. Parathyroid cancer: Biology and management. Surg Oncol. 1999;8(3):155–165.
53. Schulte KM, Talat N, Miell J, Moniz C, Sinha P, Diaz-Cano S. Lymph node involvement and surgical approach in parathyroid cancer. World J Surg. 2010;34(11):2611–2620.
54. Hsu KT, Sippel RS, Chen H, Schneider DF. Is central lymph node dissection necessary for parathyroid carcinoma? Surgery. 2014;156(6):1336–1341; discussion 41.
55. Lee PK, Jarosek SL, Virnig BA, Evasovich M, Tuttle TM. Trends in the incidence and treatment of parathyroid cancer in the United States. Cancer. 2007;109(9):1736–1741.
56. Busaidy NL, Jimenez C, Habra MA, Schultz PN, El-Naggar AK, Clayman GL, et al. Parathyroid carcinoma: A 22-year experience. Head Neck. 2004;26(8):716–726.
57. Delellis RA. Challenging lesions in the differential diagnosis of endocrine tumors: Parathyroid carcinoma. Endocr Pathol. 2008;19(4):221–225.
58. Schantz A, Castleman B. Parathyroid carcinoma. A study of 70 cases. Cancer. 1973;31(3):600–605.
59. Bondeson L, Sandelin K, Grimelius L. Histopathological variables and DNA cytometry in parathyroid carcinoma. Am J Surg Pathol. 1993;17(8):820–829.
60. Obara T, Fujimoto Y. Diagnosis and treatment of patients with parathyroid carcinoma: An update and review. World J Surg. 1991;15(6):738–744.
61. Tan MH, Morrison C, Wang P, Yang X, Haven CJ, Zhang C, et al. Loss of parafibromin immunoreactivity is a distinguishing feature of parathyroid carcinoma. Clin Cancer Res. 2004;10(19):6629–6637.
62. Gill AJ, Clarkson A, Gimm O, Keil J, Dralle H, Howell VM, et al. Loss of nuclear expression of parafibromin distinguishes parathyroid carcinomas and hyperparathyroidism-jaw tumor (HPT-JT) syndrome-related adenomas from sporadic parathyroid adenomas and hyperplasias. Am J Surg Pathol. 2006;30(9):1140–1149.

63. Abbona GC, Papotti M, Gasparri G, Bussolati G. Proliferative activity in parathyroid tumors as detected by Ki-67 immunostaining. Hum Pathol. 1995;26(2):135–138.
64. Costa-Guda J, Arnold A. Genetic and epigenetic changes in sporadic endocrine tumors: Parathyroid tumors. Mol Cell Endocrinol. 2014;386(1–2):46–54.
65. Howe JR, Norton JA, Wells SA, Jr. Prevalence of pheochromocytoma and hyperparathyroidism in multiple endocrine neoplasia type 2A: Results of long-term follow-up. Surgery. 1993;114(6):1070–1077.
66. Schuffenecker I, Virally-Monod M, Brohet R, Goldgar D, Conte-Devolx B, Leclerc L, et al. Risk and penetrance of primary hyperparathyroidism in multiple endocrine neoplasia type 2A families with mutations at codon 634 of the RET proto-oncogene. Groupe D'etude des Tumeurs a Calcitonine. J Clin Endocrinol Metab. 1998;83(2):487–491.
67. Carpten JD, Robbins CM, Villablanca A, Forsberg L, Presciuttini S, Bailey-Wilson J, et al. HRPT2, encoding parafibromin, is mutated in hyperparathyroidism-jaw tumor syndrome. Nat Genet. 2002;32(4):676–680.
68. Shattuck TM, Valimaki S, Obara T, Gaz RD, Clark OH, Shoback D, et al. Somatic and germ-line mutations of the HRPT2 gene in sporadic parathyroid carcinoma. N Engl J Med. 2003;349(18):1722–1729.
69. Pellegata NS, Quintanilla-Martinez L, Siggelkow H, Samson E, Bink K, Hofler H, et al. Germ-line mutations in p27Kip1 cause a multiple endocrine neoplasia syndrome in rats and humans. Proc Natl Acad Sci USA. 2006;103(42):15558–15563.
70. Lauter KB, Arnold A. Mutational analysis of CDKN1B, a candidate tumor-suppressor gene, in refractory secondary/tertiary hyperparathyroidism. Kidney Int. 2008;73(10): 1137–1140.
71. Giusti F, Cavalli L, Cavalli T, Brandi ML. Hereditary hyperparathyroidism syndromes. J Clin Densitom. 2013;16(1):69–74.
72. Frank-Raue K, Leidig-Bruckner G, Haag C, Schulze E, Lorenz A, Schmitz-Winnenthal H, et al. Inactivating calcium-sensing receptor mutations in patients with primary hyperparathyroidism. Clin Endocrinol (Oxf). 2011;75(1):50–55.
73. Cryns VL, Thor A, Xu HJ, Hu SX, Wierman ME, Vickery AL, Jr., et al. Loss of the retinoblastoma tumor-suppressor gene in parathyroid carcinoma. N Engl J Med. 1994;330(11):757–761.
74. Arnold A, Kim HG, Gaz RD, Eddy RL, Fukushima Y, Byers MG, et al. Molecular cloning and chromosomal mapping of DNA rearranged with the parathyroid hormone gene in a parathyroid adenoma. J Clin Invest. 1989;83(6):2034–2040.
75. Szende B, Arvai K, Petak I, Nagy K, Vegso G, Perner F. Changes in gene expression in the course of proliferative processes in the parathyroid gland. Magy Onkol. 2006;50(2):137–140.
76. Alo PL, Visca P, Mazzaferro S, Serpieri DE, Mangoni A, Botti C, et al. Immunohistochemical study of fatty acid synthase, Ki67, proliferating cell nuclear antigen, and p53 expression in hyperplastic parathyroids. Ann Diagn Pathol. 1999;3(5):287–293.
77. Yamaguchi S, Yachiku S, Morikawa M. Analysis of proliferative activity of the parathyroid glands using proliferating cell nuclear antigen in patients with hyperparathyroidism. J Clin Endocrinol Metab. 1997;82(8):2681–2688.
78. Ohta K, Manabe T, Katagiri M, Harada T. Expression of proliferating cell nuclear antigens in parathyroid glands of renal hyperparathyroidism. World J Surg. 1994;18(4):625–628; discussion 8-9.
79. Ferrara N, Gerber HP, LeCouter J. The biology of VEGF and its receptors. Nat Med. 2003;9(6):669–676.
80. Lambert D, Eaton CL, Harrison BJ. Fibroblast growth factors and their receptors in parathyroid disease. World J Surg. 1998;22(6):520–525.
81. Wilkie AO, Morriss-Kay GM, Jones EY, Heath JK. Functions of fibroblast growth factors and their receptors. Curr Biol. 1995;5(5):500–507.
82. Schuster N, Krieglstein K. Mechanisms of TGF-beta-mediated apoptosis. Cell Tissue Res. 2002;307(1):1–14.
83. Tanaka R, Tsushima T, Murakami H, Shizume K, Obara T. Insulin-like growth factor I receptors and insulin-like growth factor-binding proteins in human parathyroid tumors. World J Surg. 1994;18(4):635–641; discussion 41-2.
84. Arvai K, Nagy K, Barti-Juhasz H, Petak I, Krenacs T, Micsik T, et al. Molecular profiling of parathyroid hyperplasia, adenoma and carcinoma. Pathol Oncol Res. 2012;18(3):607–614.
85. Wang O, Wang CY, Shi Z, Nie M, Xia WB, Li M, et al. Expression of Ki-67, galectin-3, fragile histidine triad, and parafibromin in malignant and benign parathyroid tumors. Chin Med J (Engl). 2012;125(16):2895–2901.
86. Svedlund J, Auren M, Sundstrom M, Dralle H, Akerstrom G, Bjorklund P, et al. Aberrant WNT/beta-catenin signaling in parathyroid carcinoma. Mol Cancer. 2010;9:294.
87. Fendrich V, Waldmann J, Feldmann G, Schlosser K, Konig A, Ramaswamy A, et al. Unique expression pattern of the EMT markers Snail, Twist and E-cadherin in benign and malignant parathyroid neoplasia. Eur J Endocrinol. 2009;160(4):695–703.
88. Howell VM, Gill A, Clarkson A, Nelson AE, Dunne R, Delbridge LW, et al. Accuracy of combined protein gene product 9.5 and parafibromin markers for immunohistochemical diagnosis of parathyroid carcinoma. J Clin Endocrinol Metab. 2009;94(2):434–441.
89. Osawa N, Onoda N, Kawajiri H, Tezuka K, Takashima T, Ishikawa T, et al. Diagnosis of parathyroid carcinoma using immunohistochemical staining against hTERT. Int J Mol Med. 2009;24(6):733–741.
90. Kytola S, Farnebo F, Obara T, Isola J, Grimelius L, Farnebo LO, et al. Patterns of chromosomal imbalances in parathyroid carcinomas. Am J Pathol. 2000;157(2):579–586.
91. Erickson LA, Jalal SM, Harwood A, Shearer B, Jin L, Lloyd RV. Analysis of parathyroid neoplasms by interphase fluorescence in situ hybridization. Am J Surg Pathol. 2004;28(5):578–584.
92. Clark OH. Parathyroid cysts. Am J Surg. 1978;135(3):395–402.
93. Rogers LA, Fetter BF, Peete WP. Parathyroid cyst and cystic degeneration of parathyroid adenoma. Arch Pathol. 1969;88(5):476–479.
94. Turner A, Lampe HB, Cramer H. Parathyroid cysts. J Otolaryngol. 1989;18(6):311–313.
95. Wang C, Vickery AL, Jr., Maloof F. Large parathyroid cysts mimicking thyroid nodules. Ann Surg. 1972;175(3):448–453.
96. Armstrong J, Leteurtre E, Proye C. Intraparathyroid cyst: A tumour of branchial origin and a possible pitfall for targeted parathyroid surgery. ANZ J Surg. 2003;73(12):1048–1051.
97. Faquin WC, Roth SI. Frozen section of thyroid and parathyroid specimens. Arch Pathol Lab Med. 2006;130(9):1260.
98. Wang C. The anatomic basis of parathyroid surgery. Ann Surg. 1976;183(3):271–275.
99. Anton RC, Wheeler TM. Frozen section of thyroid and parathyroid specimens. Arch Pathol Lab Med. 2005;129(12):1575–1584.
100. Westra WH, Pritchett DD, Udelsman R. Intraoperative confirmation of parathyroid tissue during parathyroid exploration: A retrospective evaluation of the frozen section. Am J Surg Pathol. 1998;22(5):538–544.
101. Shidham VB, Asma Z, Rao RN, Chavan A, Machhi J, Almagro U, et al. Intraoperative cytology increases the diagnostic accuracy of frozen sections for the confirmation of various tissues in the parathyroid region. Am J Clin Pathol. 2002;118(6):895–902.
102. Wong NACS, Mihai R, Sheffield EA, Calder CJ, Farndon JR. Imprint cytology of parathyroid tissue in relation to other tissues of the neck and mediastinum. Acta Cytol. 2000;44(2):109–113.
103. Inabnet WB. Intraoperative parathyroid hormone monitoring. World J Surg. 2004;28(12):1212–1215.
104. Chen L-S, Singh RJ. Niche point-of-care endocrine testing – Reviews of intraoperative parathyroid hormone and cortisol monitoring. Crit Rev Clin Lab Sci. 2018;55(2):115–128.
105. Clark OH. How should patients with primary hyperparathyroidism be treated? J Clin Endocrinol Metab. 2003;88(7):3011–3014.
106. The American Association of Clinical Endocrinologists and the American Association of Endocrine Surgeons position statement on the diagnosis and management of primary hyperparathyroidism. Endocr Pract. 2005;11(1):49–54.
107. Kapur MM, Agarwal MS, Gupta A, Misra MC, Ahuja MM. Clinical & biochemical features of primary hyperparathyroidism. Indian J Med Res. 1985;81:607–612.
108. Mishra SK, Agarwal G, Kar DK, Gupta SK, Mithal A, Rastad J. Unique clinical characteristics of primary hyperparathyroidism in India. Br J Surg. 2001;88(5):708–714.
109. Bhansali A, Masoodi SR, Reddy KS, Behera A, das Radotra B, Mittal BR, et al. Primary hyperparathyroidism in north India: A description of 52 cases. Ann Saudi Med. 2005;25(1):29–35.
110. Gopal RA, Acharya SV, Bandgar T, Menon PS, Dalvi AN, Shah NS. Clinical profile of primary hyperparathyroidism from western India: A single center experience. J Postgrad Med. 2010;56(2):79–84.
111. Biyabani SR, Talati J. Bone and renal stone disease in patients operated for primary hyperparathyroidism in Pakistan: Is the pattern of disease different from the west? J Pak Med Assoc. 1999;49(8):194–198.
112. Younes NA, Al-Trawneh IS, Albesoul NM, Hamdan BR, Sroujieh AS. Clinical spectrum of primary hyperparathyroidism. Saudi Med J. 2003;24(2):179–183.
113. Pradeep PV, Jayashree B, Mishra A, Mishra SK. Systematic review of primary hyperparathyroidism in India: The past, present, and the future trends. Int J Endocrinol. 2011;2011:921814–921817.
114. Chan FK, Tiu SC, Choi KL, AuYong TK, Tang LF. Primary hyperparathyroidism in Hong Kong: An analysis of 44 cases. Hong Kong Med J. 1998;4(2):229–234.
115. Hamidi S, Soltani A, Hedayat A, Kamalian N. Primary hyperparathyroidism: A review of 177 cases. Med Sci Monit. 2006;12(2):Cr86–Cr89.
116. Mack LA, Pasieka JL. Asymptomatic primary hyperparathyroidism: A surgical perspective. Surg Clin North Am. 2004;84(3):803–816.
117. Goyal A, Chumber S, Tandon N, Lal R, Srivastava A, Gupta S. Neuropsychiatric manifestations in patients of primary hyperparathyroidism and outcome following surgery. Indian J Med Sci. 2001;55(12):677–686.
118. Priya G, Jyotsna VP, Gupta N, Chumber S, Bal CS, Karak AK, et al. Clinical and laboratory profile of primary hyperparathyroidism in India. Postgrad Med J. 2008;84(987):34–39.
119. Stanbury SW, Torkington P, Lumb GA, Adams PH, de Silva P, Taylor CM. Asian rickets and osteomalacia: Patterns of parathyroid response in vitamin D deficiency. Proc Nutr Soc. 1975;34(2):111–117.

31

SYMPTOMS AND NATURAL HISTORY OF PRIMARY HYPERPARATHYROIDISM

K.M.M. Vishvak Chanthar and Gaurav Agarwal

Introduction

Primary hyperparathyroidism (PHPT) is a common endocrine disorder, next only to diabetes mellitus and thyroid disorders. The disease began to emerge as a severe disorder of "stones, bones and groans" as described by Fuller Albright and others in the 1930s (1). With the advent of the automated serum chemistry autoanalyzer in the early 1970s, the recognition of asymptomatic PHPT became much more common, with a four- to five-fold increase in incidence (2). In India and many other developing countries, the number of PHPT patients diagnosed remains comparatively low in absence of routine biochemical screening for calcium. Almost all patients are, thus, diagnosed due to symptomatic manifestations or complications of PHPT (3). A small proportion of PHPT, <10% in most countries occur in familial setting, as part of MEN-1, MEN-2a and other familial or genetic forms, which are addressed in other chapters of this book.

In the developed world, symptomatic PHPT is now the exception rather than the rule, with more than three-fourths of patients having no symptoms attributable to the disease. Similarly, there has been a changing trend in the profile of PHPT manifestation in developing countries over the past three decades (4–7). Majority of manifestations of PHPT are on account of the damage hyperparathyroidism does to various target organs, including the musculoskeletal system, kidneys and GIT. This chapter describes the clinical spectrum of PHPT as it is present today in India and other South Asian countries, natural course of untreated PHPT and the course of recovery of target-organ manifestations following surgical cure.

PHPT incidence, demographics and diagnosis

Since the classical description of PHPT by Fuller Albright, there had been an apparent increase in the incidence of disease in most European countries. Before the advent of multichannel autoanalyzer, a frequency of 7.8 cases per 100,000 persons was reported in Rochester, Minnesota. With the introduction of serum autoanalyzer, this rate rose to 51.1 cases per 100,000 in the same community. The incidence declined to 27 per 100,000 persons per year once all the prevalent cases were diagnosed. Since the mid-1970s, there has been a declining trend in the incidence of PHPT in Rochester (8).

Until very recently, PHPT patients in India and other South Asian countries were almost entirely diagnosed with the symptomatic disorder with marked skeletal, renal and metabolic manifestations. A change in the clinical and biochemical profile of PHPT has been observed in the last two decades, with a rising trend of asymptomatic cases and a significant decrease in patients presenting with severe bone disease (6, 7). In a study by Yadav SK et al. between January 1990 and December 2016 from India, patients had milder symptoms of the disease in recent two decades, reflecting a similar evolution of this disease, as has been noted in the West (6). In Asian countries, majority of patients still presents with the classical symptomatic phenotype.

PHPT currently has a prevalence of 1–4 per 1000 population in the western countries. There is no robust data on its incidence or prevalence in Indian population. The disease predominantly affects females (9, 10). As per data from the Indian PHPT registry, the mean age at presentation in India is two decades earlier (40 ± 14 years) than that reported in the West, with a female-to-male ratio of 2.4:1 (11). Similar age of presentation at 15–20 years earlier than that in West was reported from other developing Asian countries (12). Often, the diagnosis of PHPT in India and other developing countries is missed, resulting in a long duration of symptoms and severe disease manifestations. In one of the studies, the mean duration of symptoms was reported as 84 ± 56.7 months (13).

Clinical presentation and symptomatology of PHPT

The clinical manifestations of PHPT can be on account of the following:

1. Metabolic effects of parathyroid hormone excess and hypercalcemia
2. Target organ/organ system damage due to hyperparathyroidism/hypercalcemia
3. Local tumor effects, which are seen rarely, due to large and/or invasive tumor

PHPT is characterized by inappropriately elevated serum-intact parathormone (PTH) levels along with high serum total or ionized calcium. It is sporadic in 90% and most commonly due to a solitary benign adenoma (85–90%). Symptomatic disease is still the most contemporary presentation in developing countries. In a recent systemic review of 17 studies from 10 developing countries, 79.6% are symptomatic (12). The mean serum PTH (668.6 ± 539 pg/ml), serum total calcium (11.9 ± 1.4 mg/dl) and mean alkaline phosphatase (619 ± 826.9 IU/l) levels were high in developing countries from what was reported in West. The mean value of vitamin D in patients of few Asian countries has been reported as 22.0 ± 22.6 ng/ml (insufficient category) (12). The majority of symptoms are due to the target organs involvements, which are discussed here on. Palpable parathyroid tumors are often seen as indicative of a malignant disease in the literature from western countries. In Indian and South Asian experience, many PHPT patients with benign parathyroid tumors too are often palpable (3, 6, 12).

Musculoskeletal manifestations of PHPT

Musculoskeletal manifestations have been described in different literatures of the West, ranging from 13 to 93% of patients with

PHPT (14). In developing countries, musculoskeletal disease constitutes 52.9% of overall clinical presentation (12). Symptomatic disease is often picked up late in the developing countries after a series of management for fractures and renal stones. While there is no paucity of literature from Indian and other developing country centers reporting common musculoskeletal manifestations of PHPT, only a few studies from the western countries report significant musculoskeletal disease. Bone pain and proximal muscle weakness are the most common manifestations. Other musculoskeletal manifestations include back pain, chest/rib cage pain, arthralgia, gout, pseudo-gout, muscle weakness, paraplegia, myotonic dystrophy, jaw tumors as well as radiological findings of osteitis fibrosa cystica (OFC), apatite deposition and osteopenia. The most common articular features reported in PHPT are chondrocalcinosis and arthralgia. Arthralgia usually affects the hands, wrists, knees and hip joints, which may, however, appear normal radiologically. The course of chondrocalcinosis is independent of parathyroid activity, and patients with pseudogout may continue to experience such attacks many years after parathyroidectomy (PTx) (15). There have been studies that reported an association of apatite crystals and monosodium urate crystal deposits in PHPT (16). The prevalence of bone involvement and other overall presentation of PHPT in the Indian subcontinent and other developing countries is summarized in **Table 31.1** (3,4,6,7,12,13,17,18).

OFC is the classical skeletal manifestation of PHPT, characterized by the presence of osteoporosis/osteopenia due to cortical bone loss, fibrosis and cysts formation mostly in the cortical bones (3, 18). Such overt bone disease is still seen in patients managed in India and other South Asian countries but has become unusual, being seen in less than 5% of patients with PHPT in the western countries. Large, multiple brown tumors causing deformity and spontaneous fracture were a more conventional presentation two decades ago. The proximal tibia and pubic rami are the most common sites of fractures and brown tumors, while the vertebral body, iliac crest, hard palate and ribs are the unusual sites (3). Severe osteoporosis in vitamin D–deficient PHPT patients can lead to the *"syndrome of disappearing bones"* on skeletal radiographs – an interesting observation reported for the first time by Agarwal G et al. Equally startling is the early and remarkable remineralization of the bony lesions at 3 months after successful parathyroid surgery, as reported by us (18). Facial involvement of brown tumor is rare and when present, mandible is the most common site, although rare cases of maxillary bone involvement were reported (**Figure 31.1**). Radiological manifestation of OFC (**Figure 31.2**) includes diffuse demineralization associated with cystic bone lesions, lytic lesions, subperiosteal bone resorption affecting clavicles, medial phalanges and long bones, demineralization of the skull causing "salt and pepper" or "pepper in the pot" appearance, thinning of the dipole, absence of lamina dura in teeth. Histologically, OFC is characterized by the presence of increased osteoblastic and osteoclastic activity, peritrabecular fibrous tissue deposition with numerous multinucleated osteoclasts seen in the scalloped areas on the surface of bone (Howship's lacunae).

TABLE 31.1: Clinical Manifestations of Primary Hyperparathyroidism in Developing Countries

Clinical Presentation	% Affected*
Overall symptomatic	79.6
Musculoskeletal disease	52.9
Osteitis fibrosa cystica	72.9
Osteoporosis (t score < −2.5)	58.9
Fractures	17.8–50.8
Crippled (due to multiple fractures)	13.7–30.5
Bone deformity/brown tumors	19.6–52.9
Proximal muscle weakness	41–62.7
Syndrome of disappearing bone	7.8
Renal disease	34.9
Combined bone and kidney disease	36
Gastrointestinal disease:	
Acid peptic disease	50
Pancreatitis	15
Neuropsychiatric symptoms	8.9
Palpable neck mass	5–33
Asymptomatic disease	5.6

Source: Data taken from references (3,4,6,7,12,13,17 and 18).
*Denominator differs for the various manifestations listed as reported in different series.

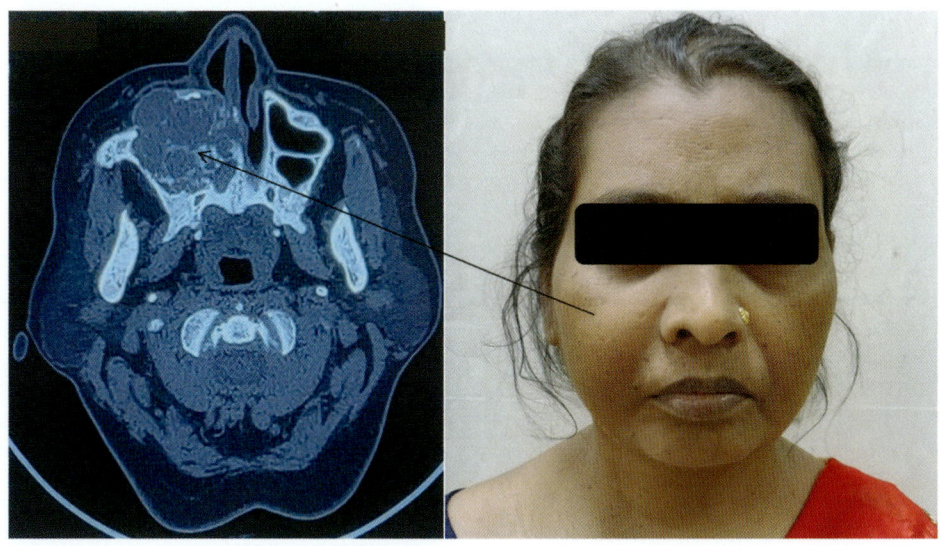

FIGURE 31.1 Right maxillary brown tumor, seen clinically and on CT scan.

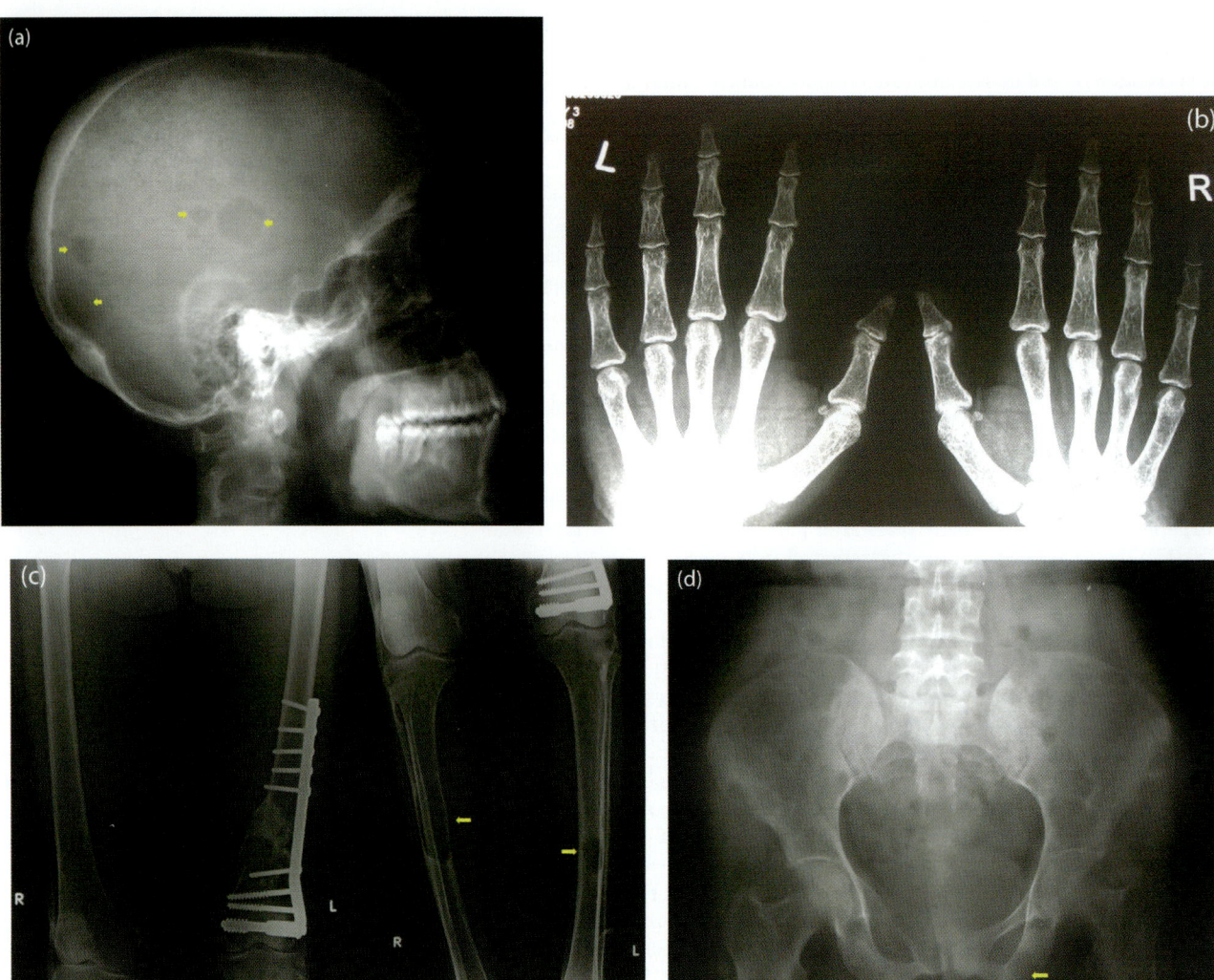

FIGURE 31.2 Radiological appearances in PHPT. (a) X-ray skull with salt and pepper appearance, loss of outer table with hair on end appearance and lytic lesions (arrows); (b) X-ray hand with subperiosteal resorption in phalanges and tunneling with trabecularization; (c) X-ray long bones showing internal fixation of distal femur with thinned out cortex in tibia and cystic lesions (arrows); and (d) X-ray pelvis showing osteopenia in bilateral iliac bone, coarse trabecular pattern, thinning of cortex and cystic bone lesion in left inferior pubic ramus (arrow).

A decrease in bone mineral density, as commonly seen on bone mineral densitometry (BMD) by dual-energy absorptiometry (DEXA), is a relatively more common manifestation of bone involvement in patients with PHPT. PHPT mainly affects cortical bone (e.g., at distal radius), while cancellous bone (e.g., at lumbar vertebrae) density decreases in more advanced disease at a later stage of disease progression (18). With the advent of trabecular bone score and high-resolution peripheral quantitative computed tomography (HRpQCT), newer insights in the assessment of trabecular microstructure have evolved. These noninvasive technologies demonstrated trabecular deterioration, especially at the radius and tibia, despite preserved bone mineral density by DEXA scan. The detrimental trabecularization of bone poses an increased risk of vertebral fractures observed in PHPT patients (19, 20).

Renal manifestations of PHPT

A 34.9% prevalence of renal disease was found in patients with PHPT in developing countries (12). Renal manifestations of PHPT are described in **Table 31.2**. Indian PHPT data registry reported that the frequency of nephrolithiasis and nephrocalcinosis in India varies from 20 to 47.2% and 10 to 30%, respectively. Renal calculi may be a presenting complaint in 15.1% of patients with PHPT and recurrent renal calculi in 21% (21, 22). In a series of 294 patients with PHPT, Tassone et al. found that 17% of them

TABLE 31.2: Renal Manifestations of Primary Hyperparathyroidism

Hypercalciuria

Nephrolithiasis and nephrocalcinosis

Decreased glomerular filtration rate

Impaired urinary concentrating ability (polyuria)

Low tubular maximum phosphate reabsorbtion

Increased urinary excretion of magnesium

Proximal/distal renal tubular acidosis

Simple renal cysts

Source: Adapted from Lila et al. (26).

Symptoms and Natural History of Primary Hyperparathyroidism

had an estimated glomerular filtration rate of <60 ml/minute (23). Occult urolithiasis in asymptomatic PHPT was reported in 36% by Cipriani et al. (24).

PTH excess damages the integrity of renal tubular epithelium and hampers the acidification of urine. PHPT mostly affects proximal renal tubules by causing inhibition of bicarbonate reabsorption and thus tends to result in metabolic acidosis (proximal renal tubular acidosis [RTA]). However, longer duration of illness can cause medullary nephrocalcinosis (**Figure 31.3**) and predispose to distal RTA (25). The presence of hypokalemia and fasting urine pH >5.5 in a patient with nephrolithiasis should always arouse the suspicion of distal RTA.

Renal manifestations in hereditary hyperparathyroidism-jaw tumor syndrome include renal cysts (two-thirds of cases), Wilms tumor, hamartomas and renal cell carcinoma. Simple renal cysts are usually related to the effect of chronically elevated PTH level on tubular cells and are considered as a benign renal complication of PHPT (26).

Cardiovascular manifestation of PHPT

The cardiovascular (CV) system is affected by PHPT in more than one ways. The hypercalcemia of PHPT results in ectopic calcification, which may manifest with valvular calcifications and premature atherosclerosis. Besides, PTH is considered a cardiotoxic agent, causing a direct myocardial insult, which can be seen manifesting with subtle rise in the titers of serum NT-proBNP, a humoral marker to myocardial function, to overt cardiomyopathy (17). The spectrum of CV manifestation ranges from hypertension, left ventricular (LV) hypertrophy (LVH), myocardial, interventricular septal and valvular calcifications, diastolic dysfunction, arrhythmias, intimal and medial calcification in coronary artery, premature atherosclerosis (17). PHPT patients are more likely to have tunica media sclerosis resulting in impaired carotid and coronary distensibility. The prevalence of cardiac manifestation in PHPT is summarized in **Table 31.3** (17,27–30).

The association of PHPT and hypertension was initially elaborated by Hellström in 1958. Lafferty revealed that hypertension was twice more common in PHPT patients than in the general population (31). The prevalence of hypertension in PHPT patients ranges from 21 to 65% in several reported series (17, 31, 32). Hypertension in PHPT is heterogeneous in origin, probably weak relation between PTH and plasma rennin activity exists (33). PHPT patients have higher circulating levels of vasopressors such as renin, angiotensin, aldosterone and norepinephrine resulting in more potent vasoconstriction, which could be an attributed mechanism for hypertension. LV hypertrophic effect is due to the direct activation of parathormone related peptide (PTHrP) receptors by PTH.

PHPT patients in South Asian countries with long duration of disease, and with severe hypercalcemia and hyperparathyroidism, even at a relatively young age when compared to the West are more likely to have CV dysfunction. The degree of hypercalcemia (34) and serum PTH titers (17) are predictors of CV mortality. The degree of LVH correlates to serum levels of PTH and vitamin D, rather than serum calcium or hypertension (17).

Gastrointestinal manifestation of PHPT

PHPT is not so uncommonly associated with peptic ulcer disease and pancreatitis, although there are conflicting data concerning constipation (35). Peptic ulcer disease is often identified in patients with MEN1 or MEN4 syndromes, who can develop gastrin-producing tumors (36). The proposed higher incidence of pancreatitis in association with PHPT in India (12–16%) could be due to a high number of patients with symptomatic hyperparathyroidism and severe hypercalcemia. The possible mechanisms

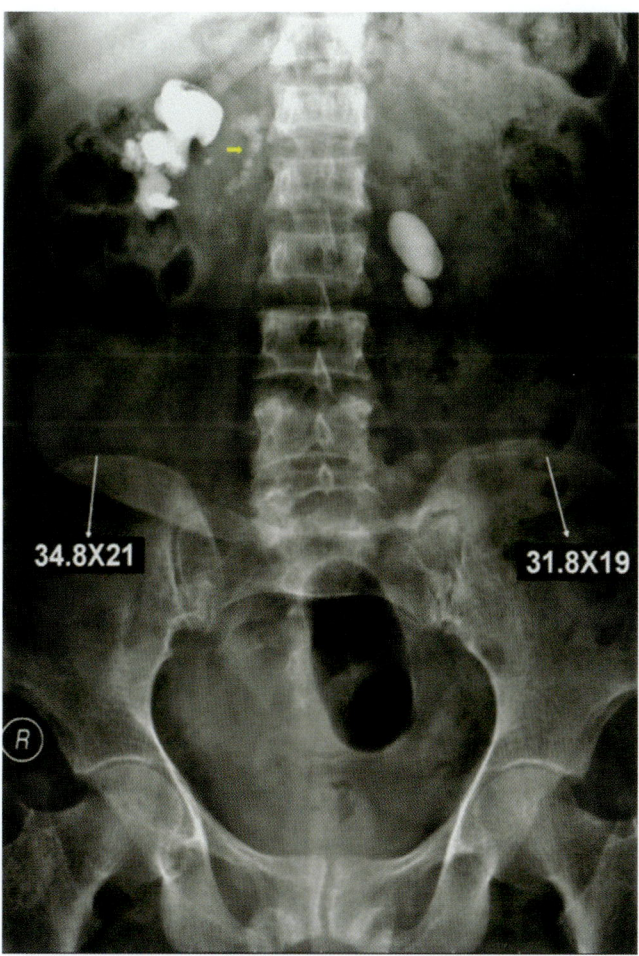

FIGURE 31.3 X-ray KUB region showing bilateral nephrocalcinosis with pancreatic duct calcification (short wide arrow).

TABLE 31.3: Prevalence of Cardiovascular Manifestations in PHPT

Agarwal et al. (17); n = 56	Left ventricular hypertrophy – 68%
	Myocardial, valvular calcification – 28%
	Diastolic dysfunction – 53.5%
	Hypertension – 37.5%
	Extremely high NT-proBNP (> 300 pg/ml) – 21%
Bondeson et al. (27); n = 300	Coronary artery disease – 44%
Längle et al. (28); n = 132	Left ventricular hypertrophy – 48%
	Coronary artery disease – 12.8%
Niederle et al. (29); n = 54	Hypertension – 27%
	Aortic valve calcification – 63%
	Mitral valve calcification – 49%
	Myocardial calcification – 69%
Stefenelli et al. (30); n = 64	Aortic calcification – 63%
	Mitral calcification – 49%
	Myocardial calcification – 69%

of pancreatitis in PHPT are deposition of calcium-phosphate in pancreatic ducts (**Figure 31.3**), calcium-mediated activation of trypsinogen to trypsin, increased permeability of pancreatic duct due to hypercalcemia and direct effect of PTH on pancreas (21).

Neuropsychiatric manifestation of PHPT

Subjective psychiatric and cognitive symptoms were described as early as the 1940s and included lethargy, confusion, depression, anxiety, disturbance of thought content, loss of memory, neurasthenia, lassitude, sleep disturbance, diminished quality of life, paranoid ideation, delusions, hallucinations, senile dementia, delirium and organic brain syndrome with altered sensorium. These symptoms develop irrespective of serum calcium levels. Peterson reported the correlation of serum calcium level with the severity of psychiatric symptoms. Personality changes and affective disorder were associated with serum calcium 12–16 mg/dl, paranoid ideation and hallucinations were observed at 16–19 mg/dl level (37). Other studies could not demonstrate a significant association between the severity of symptoms and serum calcium/PTH levels.

Cognitive-psychiatric disturbances and older age have been reported to be significantly correlated, more so compared with correlation of age with bone and kidney disease (38). Psychiatric and behavioral symptoms are mostly vague and nonspecific in geriatric patients and are often neglected. Hallucination and delusion have been noted in 10% of patients who have psychiatric symptoms. Serious depression is observed in 10% of patients with PHPT and may be associated with headache. High serum PTH increases the permeability of blood-brain barrier and enhances cerebrospinal fluid (CSF) calcium concentration, which in turn influences the central neurotransmitter activity attributed to psychological disturbance. After PTx, CSF calcium concentration decreases and demonstrates a significant improvement in cognitive and psychological performance.

In the 1990s, more studies focused on the health-related quality of life in patients with PHPT, which employed specialized, validated testing of psychiatric and cognitive function. Burney et al. first used the Medical Outcomes Short Form 36 (SF-36) health survey in 1999, studying 155 patients to determine mental health, emotional and social function (39). He noted a functional decline in social, physical, emotional, energy and health perception. Pasieka and Parsons developed a visual analog scale questionnaire-based outcome tool, measuring 13 disease-specific items such as forgetfulness, weakness, bone pain and energy level in patients with PHPT (40). They found that these patients had more symptoms of pain, weakness and forgetfulness.

Others manifestations of PHPT

The other manifestations in PHPT include visual changes, band keratopathy due to corneal calcification, conjunctivitis and pruritus. Corneal calcification could be present but may not be a related feature.

Influence of vitamin D status on the clinical profile of PHPT

PHPT patients who are vitamin D deficient present with severe musculoskeletal manifestations (3, 18). Young PHPT patients with severe vitamin D deficiency present with a dramatic clinical syndrome, with crippling, a condition called as "parathyroid cripple" by us (41). A significant negative correlation exists between vitamin D and serum PTH, alkaline phosphatase (ALP) levels and bone mineral density in PHPT. Widely prevalent vitamin D deficiency in South Asian countries is known to influence the clinical profile of PHPT patients and result in severely symptomatic disease and large parathyroid tumors (41). Most PHPT patients with vitamin D deficiency are younger and present with classic OFC, one or multiple fractures and with specific manifestations of vitamin D deficiency such as generalized bone pain, profound proximal muscle weakness, extreme fatigability and association of rickets with PHPT (18, 41). These patients had become symptomatic earlier than the vitamin D–sufficient PHPT patients because of the severity of the bone disease. The percentage fall in the intra operative parathormone (IOPTH) is steeper in patients with lower vitamin D levels and larger parathyroid tumors (42). Most of these patients develop prolonged symptomatic hypocalcemia after PTx requiring parenteral calcium along with high doses of oral calcium and an active form of vitamin D. Postoperatively, 75% of patients have persistent vitamin D deficiency that impact in slow and prolonged BMD recovery and renal recovery (43). Therefore, the vitamin D store replenishment has to be ensured for early skeletal and renal recovery. Extracellular calcium levels inversely regulate parathyroid cellular proliferation and PTH secretion. Low extracellular calcium stimulates PTH secretion and PTH gene expression, whereas high extracellular calcium inhibits secretion. As the median dietary calcium in developing countries has been reported to be low, this could increase PTH secretion/PTH gene expression and stimulate cellular proliferation.

PHPT in special situations

Hypercalcemic crisis

Markedly elevated serum calcium value above 14 mg/dl, associated with symptoms and signs of hypercalcemia is recognized as hypercalcemic crisis, an endocrine emergency, also known as parathyroid crisis or parathyrotoxicosis. Hypercalcemic crisis was first described by Hanes in 1939 and is recognized as an endocrine emergency. Though the prevalence of hypercalcemic crisis reported in western literature was between 1.6 and 6%, its incidence in India and South Asian countries is upto 21%, perhaps due to the high number of markedly symptomatic cases and delayed diagnosis (44). Acute manifestation predominantly includes gastrointestinal (GI) symptoms such as recurrent vomiting, dyspepsia, epigastric pain, anorexia, constipation and renal symptoms like polydipsia, polyuria, dehydration, oliguria and anuria, which may become fatal. Acute pancreatitis in PHPT is mostly associated with mean serum calcium of 13.2 mg/dl in the Indian population (44). Cardiac manifestation may include tachyarrhythmia, which may be life-threatening.

The most common histopathological finding in hypercalcemic crisis is solitary parathyroid adenoma. As such parathyroid carcinoma in PHPT is <2%, but it contributes to 5% in hypercalcemic crisis. The unique histopathological feature of extensive hemorrhage and/or intracytoplasmic vacuoles within a parathyroid gland is considered as precipitating factors (lysis of PTH filled vacuoles) of hypercalcemic crisis (45).

PHPT in children

As per data retrieved from the Indian PHPT registry, nearly 13% of PHPT patients are young with slight female preponderance (46). PHPT is unusual between 0 and 10 years of life and is encountered in less than 5% in this subset. The incidence of familial PHPT ranges between 5 and 15% in young patients. Majority of patients are symptomatic with bone pain as the most common clinical presentation. The widely prevalent vitamin D deficiency in South Asian countries contributes to greater bone involvement in young PHPT patients. The frequency of renal stones was much less when compared to the adult group. Shah VN et al. reported in a study involving young PHPT patients, the prevalence of renal stone, gall stone disease were lower and ALP level was higher in the young patient group when compared to adults (47). Parathyroid adenoma is the most predominant pathology in this cohort, with median tumor weight greater than that noted in western literature due to the presence of coexisting vitamin D deficiency or relatively more prolonged duration of disease.

PHPT in pregnancy

Pregnant patients had predominantly GI symptoms (36%) and higher serum Ca and serum PTH levels than those of nonpregnant patients (48). Acute pancreatitis is the most serious GI complications of PHPT in pregnancy and has been reported to affect 7–13% pregnant PHPT patients, which is a much higher incidence than that of both nonpregnant PHPT patients (1–2%) and healthy pregnant women (0.02–0.1%) (49). Pregnancy changes of increased glomerular filtration rate and intestinal-calcium absorption may lead to an increase in urinary calcium excretion, particularly in the third trimester. There is a trend of higher 24-hour urinary calcium levels in pregnant PHPT patients. Higher urinary calcium levels can lead to the formation of urinary calculi. Some studies reported urinary calculi as the most common clinical manifestation of PHPT during pregnancy, with the incidence ranging from 24 to 36% (50), which is significantly higher than its incidence in healthy pregnancy (0.02–0.5%). The physiological changes of pregnancy, such as hemodilution and hypoalbuminemia, would underestimate the severity of hypercalcemia when evaluated by total serum-calcium levels. Until now, only a total of six cases of PHPT-inducing hypercalcemic crisis related to pregnancy had been reported in the literature; three cases occurred during pregnancy and three developed immediately after delivery. Of these six patients, two resulted in maternal death, two resulted in infant death and two resulted in neonatal seizures (51, 52).

PHPT due to parathyroid carcinoma

Carcinoma parathyroid constitutes less than 2% of cases with PHPT overall, but literature from the developing countries reported higher prevalence (2.6–6%) (3, 41). Series from the developed world reported a decade earlier presentation of parathyroid carcinoma than adenoma, with a mean age of 45 years for carcinoma and 55 years for adenomas (53). However, in developing countries, the average age of PHPT patients with benign and malignant pathology is comparable, reflecting an overall earlier age of PHPT patients in these countries (41). The warning signs of parathyroid carcinoma are simultaneous symptomatic skeletal and renal manifestations in young, palpable parathyroid mass, serum calcium level >14 mg/dl, high serum PTH level, tumor invasion into strap muscles, thyroid lobe, other adjacent structures and high tumor weight. Nevertheless, Indian patients do not differ in these clinical, biochemical, pathological characteristics among patients with adenoma, hyperplasia and carcinoma, except for significantly higher tumor weight in malignant pathology. The average tumor weight in developed countries was 2–4 g, while in Indian patients, it ranges from 1.25 to 102 g (41). This behavior in developing countries could be attributed to the presentation of PHPT at late symptomatic stage and more prevalence of vitamin D deficiency causing severe skeletal manifestations (54). We have reported an isolated small recurrent parathyroid carcinoma in the subcutaneous plane, occurring along the initial fine needle aspiration track, 5 years after surgical management of the primary tumor revealing the limitation of fine needle aspiration cytology (FNAC) as a diagnostic modality in the management of parathyroid pathologies (55).

Asymptomatic PHPT

In Indian centers, the reported prevalence of asymptomatic PHPT is 5.6% (13), unlike in western countries where most PHPT patients are asymptomatic. Literature evaluating the prevalence of asymptomatic PHPT in the developing world is very scarce. The exact cause of asymptomatic sporadic PHPT is unknown. Presuming its etiology similar to that of classical PHPT, it was postulated that exposure to neck irradiation and genetic abnormality could be a cause (56). These patients typically have serum calcium levels within 1 mg/dl above the upper end of limit and a PTH level <2 times above the upper assay limit. The term "asymptomatic" is more of a misnomer since these patients have milder forms of constitutional and neuropsychiatric symptoms with or without subclinical end-organ damage (20). Patients who are on follow-up generally have mild hypercalcemia with stable disease, although nearly 25% may progress to symptoms requiring surgery, such as osteoporosis, over 15 years (57). Similarly, the relative risk of developing nephrolithiasis and renal failure are 4.6 and 19.3%, respectively, over follow up of 2.9 years (26).

Normocalcemic PHPT and normohormonal PHPT

Normocalcemic variant is recognized as a distinct entity of PHPT after the consensus of 3rd and 4th International Workshops on the Management of Asymptomatic PHPT held in 2009 and 2013, respectively (58, 59). Patients of normocalcemic hyperparathyroidism have consistently normal calcium (total and ionized) level along with elevated PTH level. The prevalence rate ranges from 0.5 to 16% in various series of studies (60). Though recognized as an early form of classical disease, it is essential to exclude the secondary causes of elevated PHPT such as vitamin D deficiency, renal failure, hypercalciuria, malabsorption, thiazide and lithium medications. Little is known about the natural history, utility of imaging and operative guideline due to scarce literature. Lowe et al. have demonstrated that these patients have a history of renal stones (14%), trivial trauma fractures (11%) and osteoporosis (57%) (61). The most significant feature in normocalcemic PHPT is smaller adenoma weight compared to the classical entity and is the reason for operative complexity, warranting bilateral exploration (62).

Normohormonal variant consisted of patients with repeatedly normal PTH and high serum calcium. The incidence is 7.4–9%, consistent with most series (63). Applewhite et al. demonstrated 22.5% incidence of normohormonal variant in his study of 516 patients (64). The single gland disease dominance (90.9%) is the most significant feature of this variant and perhaps attribute to straightforward operative treatment.

Natural history of PHPT

This section of the book chapter will address the natural history of untreated PHPT and the course of disease, specifically the target organ damage recovery following successful surgical treatment.

With the advent of autoanalyzers in the 1970s, routine biochemical screening for hypercalcemia became a common practice. This led to a large number of predominantly asymptomatic PHPT cases being identified, and the endocrinology fraternity was faced with the vital question of which of those needed active surgical management. Studies on the natural history of untreated PHPT and the benefit derived from surgical and nonsurgical treatment options led to the formulation of guidelines for the management of asymptomatic or mild PHPT. Prospective studies on the natural history of asymptomatic PHPT demonstrated 27% disease progression at 10 years and 37% disease progression at 15 years follow–up, respectively, with increased hypercalcemia, worsened hypercalciuria and decrease in bone mass (57, 65).

Musculoskeletal disease

The musculoskeletal disease due to untreated PHPT has been reported to worsen over a period of time in majority of patients. Common manifestations including bone pain, muscle weakness, generalized osteopenia, one or more appendicular skeleton fracture, crippled owing to fracture or muscle weakness, clinically evident brown tumors and bony deformities are identified with increasing frequency during follow-up of untreated PHPT patients. A long-term follow-up study on natural course of PHPT by Rubin et al. demonstrated stable biochemical values for 12 years, stable BMD for 8–10 years, loss of bone mineral density at cortical sites after 9–10 years of follow up, while 37% showed disease progression after 15 years, meeting the indication for surgery (57). Overall, 60% of patients on follow-up lost more than 10% of BMD in 15 years of observation. PHPT patients typically demonstrate preferential loss of cortical bone with relative preservation of cancellous bone in early stages. Reduction in cortical bone is more pronounced in the ultradistal third of the radius and may be most evident in postmenopausal women. The relative sparing of vertebral bone mass in postmenopausal women with PHPT despite estrogen deficiency is because of the anabolic activity of PTH at cancellous bones. Patients with overt skeleton manifestation were found to have bone mineral reduction up to an average z score of −4.8 at the distal radius and −3.9 at the lumbar spine. A newer method for assessment of bone involvement, such as HRpQCT has revealed trabecular bone mass reduction. The risk for fracture in vertebrae, forearm and distal leg is two- to three-fold higher than the healthy individuals. The upper end of tibia is the most common site of fracture and the other sites are neck/shaft of femur and humerus. The most common site of brown tumor is the upper end of tibia and the other sites are femur, hip, mandible, ribs and vertebrae. It was demonstrated nearly 9–40% of patients develop chondrocalcinosis. A total of 25% of those who had chondrocalcinosis developed acute arthritis (pseudogout) (66). Arthritis is precipitated by the deposition of calcium pyrophosphate dihydrate crystals in the synovial joint fluid, and episodes of acute attacks may be influenced by the concentration of serum calcium. Unlike gout, pseudogout most commonly affects knee, elbow and wrist.

PTx had shown a consistent improvement in serum calcium, PTH, vitamin D level and 24-hour urinary calcium. Few patients may have high serum PTH despite normal serum calcium for upto 3 months post-surgery. Interestingly, improvement in bone pain and regaining muscle strength have been observed within 1 week after successful PTx (18). Patients with OFC had hypocalcemia in the immediate postoperative period requiring parenteral calcium infusion for 36–168 hours (18). These patients also had low serum phosphorus and magnesium, which could be attributed to the hungry bone syndrome. The markers of bone formation such as serum ALP and osteocalcin were found to be increased in most patients initially after PTx and normalized in 6–9 months. Urinary type-I collagen specific peptides, marker of bone resorption decreases as early as 1 week and normalizes in 3 months. The effect of PTx is demonstrated by a remarkable early increment in BMD at the lumbar spine and femoral neck (more at cancellous than the cortical bone sites), with sustained BMD beyond 1 year. The rate of increment in BMD at the hip and lumbar spine with mean +166 and +101% change, respectively, from preoperative BMD at 6 months after PTx hint at skeleton recovery (18). Substantial and continued increments in bone density at spine and hip have been documented for upto 10 years (67) and seem to stabilize until 15 years (57). Fractures healed promptly, but the sites of bone cysts, fractures, brown tumors appeared abnormally hyperdense on radiographs within 3 months of PTx. Patients with chondrocalcinosis were found to develop acute arthritis in the postoperative days 1–10, triggered by hypocalcemia (14).

Renal disease

The etiology of renal stones in PHPT is multifactorial. Serum phosphorus found to be in the lower end of normal range, whereas 25% have frank hypophosphatemia (65). Mean urinary calcium excretion remains at the upper range of normal limits with frank hypercalciuria seen in 40% of patients (66). Reduction of creatinine clearance occurs in one-third of patients. A prospective study of patients with asymptomatic PHPT by Scholz and Purnell revealed 10% of patients with an increase in serum calcium, 8% with decreased renal function and 6% with active renal stone disease at 10 years follow up (68). Kidney stones are common in younger men and correlation exists with higher serum calcium and nonoperated patients are at risk for recurrent stone disease. Vitamin D levels tend to be in the lower range of normal limit.

Nephrocalcinosis progression is remarkably reversible after PTx. Over 90% of patients with renal stones do not form recurrent nephrolithiasis after parathyroid surgery (69). Diminished glomerular filtration rate consequent to renal parenchymal damage may not recover following successful PTx. Decline in renal function in PHPT can be due to progressive hypertension and perhaps that could be attributed to the failure of improvement of renal impairment after PTx (70). Nevertheless, urinary calcium excretion and rate of stone formation after PTx is comparable to idiopathic stone formers.

Cardiovascular disease

CV disease worsens over time if PHPT is left untreated. The degree of hypercalcemia and serum PTH titers worsen in a substantial proportion of untreated PHPT patients over a period of time, and these are correlated negatively with various indices of cardiac and vascular function. The association of PHPT and hypertension poses a high risk for CV disease and cerebrovascular events. Hypertension failed to improve in 92% following PTx (31). Hypercalcemia induces arterial stiffness in peripheral and coronary arteries due to intimal and medial calcification. In our study, flow-mediated vasodilatation (FMD), a sensitive marker of arterial wall compliance was found to be impaired in patients with PHPT, which was perhaps a reflection of premature atherogenesis consequent to elevated PTH or calcium-mediated endothelial dysfunction (17). The calcium deposit in the vessel wall in patients with PHPT does not reverse after PTx and this was evident by modest improvement in FMD after surgery (17).

CV complications are the most common cause of mortality in PHPT. The cardiac-specific cause of mortality in PHPT patients is shown in **Table 31.4** (71, 72). PTH levels predicted the risk of CV mortality rather than serum calcium level. Increased risk of death has been documented in moderate to severe PHPT, while the risk

TABLE 31.4: Cause Specific Cardiovascular Mortality in PHPT

	Death Due to Cardiovascular Disease	Specific Cause of Mortality
Hedbäck et al. (71); n = 896	53%	Myocardial infarction – 32%
		Heart failure – 34%
		Stroke – 28%
		Atherosclerosis – 6%
Ronni-Sivula (72); n = 34	68%	Myocardial infarction, heart failure – 53%
		Stroke – 12%
		Mesentric artery thrombosis – 3%

disappeared in lower serum calcium level (17). The fact that LVH was independent of the effect of hypertension was evident by the development of LVH in normotensive patients (17). Several series revealed an association of LV mass with increased PTH levels, low vitamin D levels and may be a strong predictor of CV morbidity and mortality. Though hypertension failed to normalize after PTx, LVH was found to regress after surgery. Our study reported a lower prevalence of myocardial and valvular calcifications in Indian patients with PHPT compared to western literature. It correlated this to the low calcium-phosphorus product, consequent to dietary calcium, phosphorus and vitamin D deficiency (17).

PTx consistently causes a 50–60% reduction in LV mass postoperatively and confers its sustained reduction at 6 months (17). Reduction in LV mass leads to progressive improvement in diastolic relaxation from 3 to 6 months after parathyroid surgery, which brings about an optimal reduction in left ventricle end diastolic dimension (LVEDD), improvement in left ventricle end systolic volume (LVESV), thereby enhanced stroke volume and left ventricle ejection fraction (LVEF). Overall, patients with worse CV indices at baseline had more marked improvement in systolic and diastolic functions after PTx. Serum NT-proBNP titers showed a marked decline to a greater extent in hypertensive PHPT patients than the normotensive ones. The myocardial and valvular calcifications did not regress after PTx up to 6-month follow-up.

Neuro-psychiatric disease

Worsening of subjective psychiatric and cognitive symptoms is reported in untreated PHPT patients. Longer the duration of illness, less likely these symptoms will recover after PTx. Joborn et al. demonstrated improvement in dementia for patients with a duration of mental symptoms less than 2 years. Pasieka et al. recognized a marked improvement in cognitive performance, depressive mood, anxiety and somatic symptoms after PTx (40). The most recent studies utilized SF-36 or Hopkins symptom checklist (HSCL-56) scores, reported improvement in psychopathologic and neurocognitive symptoms with enhanced health-related quality of life after PTx (73, 74). Neuro-cognitive assessment of Indian patients with PHPT by Ramakant et al. has shown that these patients had higher preoperative PAS and SF-36 scores and PTx resulted in improvement of neuropsychiatric symptoms as early as 1-week postoperatively (75). Clinical manifestations of Indian PHPT and their recovery after successful PTx is summarized in **Table 31.5**.

TABLE 31.5: Clinical Manifestations of Indian PHPT and Their Recovery after Successful Parathyroidectomy

Clinical Presentation	Affected (%)	Recovery (%)	Mean Duration of Recovery
Musculoskeletal disease (n = 51) (18)			
Bone pain	upto 90%	Improved in 70.5%	1 week
Osteopenia	62.7	Increment in BMD of +166% at hip +101% at lumbar spine	6 months
Proximal muscle weakness	62.7	Improved in 100%	1 week
Crippled	13.7	85.7% became ambulated	>3 months
Bone deformity/brown tumors	52.9	Regressed in 22.2%	
Fracture	64.7	Healed in 100%	3 months
Syndrome of disappearing bones	7.8	Bony outline became visible in 100%	3 months
Renal disease (n = 82) (43)		**Follow Up Range**	
Nephrocalcinosis, hydronephrosis, pelvic renal stones	40	Symptom free in 74%	2–13 years follow up
		Progressed to ESRD in 9%	
		Required renal transplantation in 3%	
Gastrointestinal disease			
Pancreatitis (n = 82) (43)	8.5	Resolution of pancreatitis in 71.4%	1–9 years follow up
Acid peptic disease (n = 56) (17)	50	Reduction in peptic ulcer in 95%	
Cardiovascular disease (n = 56) (17)	**Preoperative Value**	**Postoperative Value**	**Mean Duration of Recovery**
LVEDD, mm	45.4 ± 7.0	41.6 ± 7	6 months
LVESV, ml	25.1 ± 11.8	21.8 ± 11.1	
LVEF, (%)	61 ± 9	68 ± 11	
LV Mass, g	204.2 ± 68.6	146.1 ± 59.1	
Sr. NT-proBNP, pg/ml	406 ± 1135	127 ± 253	
FMD	10 ± 9	13 ± 17	
Neuropsychiatric Symptoms (n = 42) (75)	**Mean Preoperative PAS Score** 430.87 ± 215.61	**Mean Postoperative PAS Score** 293.65 ± 118.31	**Mean Duration of Recovery** 1 week

Symptoms and natural history of PHPT – A South Asian perspective

PHPT is one of the most common endocrine disorders managed in South Asian countries. There is only a very limited data available from South Asia regarding the incidence and prevalence of this disease. Unlike the industrialized or developed countries, most South Asian countries do not have a policy of routine biochemical screening for serum calcium. Hence, majority of PHPT patients diagnosed in most South Asian countries have overt manifestations. The diagnosis of PHPT is often delayed in the developing world, and so many patients are managed with advanced manifestations on one or more target organs/organ systems of PTH, or their complications. The musculoskeletal disease accounts for most of the presentation of PHPT in South Asian countries. Many patients present with overt bone disease such as OFC, brown tumors, deformities, fragility fracture(s) and proximal muscle weakness. Even such patients who do not have overt bone disease have substantial loss of BMD. Renal manifestations are also common and are often present with skeletal disease. Many have extremely high serum PTH levels and palpable parathyroid tumor. Nutritional deficiency of vitamin D and calcium, which is common in South Asian countries, contributes to marked parathyroid enlargement and may be palpable even though benign, pathogenesis of parathyroid bone disease, and severe osteopenia on BMD. Indian patients with benign parathyroid tumors do not differ in their clinical, biochemical and pathological features from those with malignant pathology. Left untreated, PHPT patients in South Asian countries progress to have severe osteoporosis, complications of musculoskeletal disease such as fractures, deformities, brown tumors and even crippling. Once treated with successful PTx, PHPT patients with severe manifestations show early, remarkable and sustained improvement in their bone pain, BMD and muscle strength. The renal disease too may progress and result in renal functions impairment, and even end stage renal disease, which may not be entirely reversible after a successful PTx.

Conclusion

PHPT, since its first description from 1930, has been extensively studied about its clinical manifestations and sequelae. The earliest descriptions point to a progressive, crippling and fatal metabolic bone disease. Currently, there appears a changing trend in its presentation in South Asian countries toward the milder form of disease. Several variants of PHPT presentation are possible, such as classical, asymptomatic, normocalcemic, normohormonal and hypercalcemic crisis. Insidious effects of PHPT occur in bone, renal function, CV and metabolic profile. The skeleton remains the most common target organ in PHPT. The bone involvement becomes more evident after 8 years of observation in patients followed without being treated surgically. The CV effect of PHPT remains the most common cause of morbidity and mortality. There are no robust predictors of disease progression available in patients followed up without surgery. Hypertension and impairment in renal function may not improve after PTx. Vitamin D deficiency is common in South Asian countries, which is associated with more severe bone disease and enhanced parathyroid growth. Continued effort of observing patients with PHPT from different parts of the world will provide more insights into this ever-changing disease.

References

1. Albright F, Reifenstein EC. Clinical hyperparathyroidism. In: Mt. Royal and Gullford Aves, eds., The Parathyroid Glands and Metabolic Bone Disease. Baltimore (MD): Williams & Wilkins; 1948.
2. Mundy GR, Cove DH, Fisken R. Primary hyperparathyroidism: Changes in the pattern of clinical presentation. Lancet. 1980 Jun;1(8182):1317–1320.
3. Mishra SK, Agarwal G, Kar DK, Gupta SK, Mithal A, Rastad J. Unique clinical characteristics of primary hyperparathyroidism in India. Br J Surg. 2001 May;88(5):708–714.
4. Sridhar CB, Ram BK, Sunder AS, Bhargava SB, Prakash A, Kapoor MM, Ahuja MM. Primary hyperparathyroidism – A clinical, biochemical and radiological profile with emphasis on geographical variations. Australas Radiol. 1973 Jun;17(2):199–204.
5. Kapur MM, Agarwal MS, Gupta A, Misra MC, Ahuja MM. Clinical & biochemical features of primary hyperparathyroidism. Indian J Med Res. 1985 Jun;81:607–612.
6. Yadav SK, Mishra SK, Mishra A, Mayilvagnan S, Chand G, Agarwal G, Agarwal A, Verma AK. Changing profile of primary hyperparathyroidism over two and half decades: A study in tertiary referral center of North India. World J Surg. 2018 Sep;42(9):2732–2737.
7. Shah VN, Bhadada S, Bhansali A, Behera A, Mittal BR. Changes in clinical & biochemical presentations of primary hyperparathyroidism in India over a period of 20 years. Indian J Med Res. 2014 May;139(5):694–699.
8. Wermers RA, Khosla S, Atkinson EJ, Hodgson SF, O'Fallon WM, Melton LJ 3rd. The rise and fall of primary hyperparathyroidism: A population-based study in Rochester, Minnesota, 1965-1992. Ann Intern Med. 1997 Mar;126(6):433–440.
9. Agarwal G, Singh KR, Chand G. Update on surgical management of primary hyperparathyroidism. In: Puneet, ed., Recent Advances in Surgery. India: Jaypee Bros; 2018.
10. Jha S, Jayaraman M, Jha A, Jha R, Modi KD, Kelwadee JV. Primary hyperparathyroidism: A changing scenario in India. Indian J Endocrinol Metab. 2016 Jan-Feb;20(1):80–83.
11. Bhadada SK, Arya AK, Mukhopadhyay S, Khadgawat R, Sukumar S, Lodha S, Singh DN, Sathya A, Singh P, Bhansali A. Primary hyperparathyroidism: Insights from the Indian PHPT registry. J Bone Miner Metab. 2018 Mar;36(2):238–245.
12. Yadav SK, Johri G, Bichoo RA, Jha CK, Kintu-Luwaga R, Mishra SK. Primary hyperparathyroidism in developing world: A systematic review on the changing clinical profile of the disease. Arch Endocrinol Metab. 2020 Apr;64(2):105–110.
13. Pradeep PV, Jayashree B, Mishra A, Mishra SK. Systematic review of primary hyperparathyroidism in India: The past, present, and the future trends. Int J Endocrinol. 2011;2011:921814.
14. Pappu R, Jabbour SA, Reginato AM, Reginato AJ. Musculoskeletal manifestations of primary hyperparathyroidism. Clin Rheumatol. 2016 Dec;35(12):3081–3087.
15. Glass JS, Grahame R. Chondrocalcinosis after parathyroidectomy. Ann Rheum Dis. 1976 Dec;35(6):521–525.
16. Grahame R, Sutor DJ, Mitchener MB. Crystal deposition in hyperparathyroidism. Ann Rheum Dis. 1971 Nov;30(6):597–604.
17. Agarwal G, Nanda G, Kapoor A, Singh KR, Chand G, Mishra A, Agarwal A, Verma AK, Mishra SK, Syal SK. Cardiovascular dysfunction in symptomatic primary hyperparathyroidism and its reversal after curative parathyroidectomy: Results of a prospective case control study. Surgery. 2013 Dec;154(6):1394–1403; discussion 1403-4.
18. Agarwal G, Mishra SK, Kar DK, Singh AK, Arya V, Gupta SK, Mithal A. Recovery pattern of patients with osteitis fibrosa cystica in primary hyperparathyroidism after successful parathyroidectomy. Surgery. 2002 Dec;132(6):1075–1083; discussion 1083-5.
19. Vu TD, Wang XF, Wang Q, Cusano NE, Irani D, Silva BC, Ghasem-Zadeh A, Udesky J, Romano ME, Zebaze R, Jerums G, Boutroy S, Bilezikian JP, Seeman E. New insights into the effects of primary hyperparathyroidism on the cortical and trabecular compartments of bone. Bone. 2013 Jul;55(1):57–63.
20. Walker MD, Bilezikian JP. Primary hyperparathyroidism: Recent advances. Curr Opin Rheumatol. 2018 Jul;30(4):427–439.
21. Gopal RA, Acharya SV, Bandgar T, Menon PS, Dalvi AN, Shah NS. Clinical profile of primary hyperparathyroidism from western India: A single center experience. J Postgrad Med. 2010 Apr-Jun;56(2):79–84.
22. Bhansali A, Masoodi SR, Reddy KS, Behera A, das Radotra B, Mittal BR, Katariya RN, Dash RJ. Primary hyperparathyroidism in north India: A description of 52 cases. Ann Saudi Med. 2005 Jan-Feb;25(1):29–35.
23. Tassone F, Gianotti L, Emmolo I, Ghio M, Borretta G. Glomerular filtration rate and parathyroid hormone secretion in primary hyperparathyroidism. J Clin Endocrinol Metab. 2009 Nov;94(11):4458–4461.
24. Cipriani C, Biamonte F, Costa AG, Zhang C, Biondi P, Diacinti D, Pepe J, Piemonte S, Scillitani A, Minisola S, Bilezikian JP. Prevalence of kidney stones and vertebral fractures in primary hyperparathyroidism using imaging technology. J Clin Endocrinol Metab. 2015 Apr;100(4):1309–1315.
25. Muthukrishnan J, Hari Kumar KV, Jha R, Jha S, Modi KD. Distal renal tubular acidosis due to primary hyperparathyroidism. Endocr Pract. 2008 Dec;14(9):1133–1136.
26. Lila AR, Sarathi V, Jagtap V, Bandgar T, Menon PS, Shah NS. Renal manifestations of primary hyperparathyroidism. Indian J Endocrinol Metab. 2012 Mar;16(2):258–262.
27. Bondeson AG, Thompson NW, Santinga J. Coronary artery disease in primary hyperparathyroidism. Abstracts presented at the 34th World Congress of Surgery, Stockholm, Sweden; 1991.
28. Längle F, Abela C, Koller-Strametz J, Mittelböck M, Bergler-Klein J, Stefenelli T, Woloszczuk W, Niederle B. Primary hyperparathyroidism and the heart: Cardiac abnormalities correlated to clinical and biochemical data. World J Surg. 1994 Jul-Aug;18(4):619–624.
29. Niederle B, Roka R, Woloszczuk W, Klaushofer K, Kovarik J, Schernthaner G. Successful parathyroidectomy in primary hyperparathyroidism: A clinical follow-up study of 212 consecutive patients. Surgery. 1987 Dec;102(6):903–909.
30. Stefenelli T, Mayr H, Bergler-Klein J, Globits S, Woloszczuk W, Niederle B. Primary hyperparathyroidism: Incidence of cardiac abnormalities and partial reversibility after successful parathyroidectomy. Am J Med. 1993 Aug;95(2):197–202.

31. Lafferty FW. Primary hyperparathyroidism. Changing clinical spectrum, prevalence of hypertension, and discriminant analysis of laboratory tests. Arch Intern Med. 1981 Dec;141(13):1761–1766.
32. Nelson JA, Alsayed M, Milas M. The role of parathyroidectomy in treating hypertension and other cardiac manifestations of primary hyperparathyroidism. Gland Surg. 2020 Feb;9(1):136–141.
33. Bernini G, Moretti A, Lonzi S, Bendinelli C, Miccoli P, Salvetti A. Renin-angiotensin-aldosterone system in primary hyperparathyroidism before and after surgery. Metabolism. 1999 Mar;48(3):298–300.
34. Wermers RA, Khosla S, Atkinson EJ, Grant CS, Hodgson SF, O'Fallon WM, Melton LJ 3rd. Survival after the diagnosis of hyperparathyroidism: A population-based study. Am J Med. 1998 Feb;104(2):115–122.
35. Ragno A, Pepe J, Badiali D, Minisola S, Romagnoli E, Severi C, D'Erasmo E. Chronic constipation in hypercalcemic patients with primary hyperparathyroidism. Eur Rev Med Pharmacol Sci. 2012 Jul;16(7):884–889.
36. Bilezikian JP, Cusano NE, Khan AA, Liu JM, Marcocci C, Bandeira F. Primary hyperparathyroidism. Nat Rev Dis Primers. 2016 May;2:16033.
37. Petersen P. Psychiatric disorders in primary hyperparathyroidism. J Clin Endocrinol Metab. 1968 Oct;28(10):1491–1495.
38. Casella C, Pata G, Di Betta E, Nascimbeni R. Neurological and psychiatric disorders in primary hyperparathyroidism: The role of parathyroidectomy. Ann Ital Chir. 2008 May-Jun;79(3):157–161; discussion 161-3. Italian.
39. Burney RE, Jones KR, Peterson M, Christy B, Thompson NW. Surgical correction of primary hyperparathyroidism improves quality of life. Surgery. 1998 Dec;124(6):987–991; discussion 991-2.
40. Pasieka JL, Parsons LL. A retrospective analysis on the change in symptoms resulting from hyperparathyroidism following surgical intervention: Allowing for the validation of a prospective surgical outcome study questionnaire. World Cong Surg. 1995:338–383.
41. Agarwal G, Prasad KK, Kar DK, Krishnani N, Pandey R, Mishra SK. Indian primary hyperparathyroidism patients with parathyroid carcinoma do not differ in clinicoinvestigative characteristics from those with benign parathyroid pathology. World J Surg. 2006 May;30(5):732–742.
42. Agarwal G, Sadacharan D, Ramakant P, Shukla M, Mishra SK. The impact of vitamin D status and tumor size on the intraoperative parathyroid hormone dynamics in patients with symptomatic primary hyperparathyroidism. Surg Today. 2012 Dec;42(12):1183–1188.
43. Pradeep PV, Mishra A, Agarwal G, Agarwal A, Verma AK, Mishra SK. Long-term outcome after parathyroidectomy in patients with advanced primary hyperparathyroidism and associated vitamin D deficiency. World J Surg. 2008 May;32(5):829–835.
44. Singh DN, Gupta SK, Kumari N, Krishnani N, Chand G, Mishra A, Agarwal G, Verma AK, Mishra SK, Agarwal A. Primary hyperparathyroidism presenting as hypercalcemic crisis: Twenty-year experience. Indian J Endocrinol Metab. 2015 Jan-Feb;19(1):100–105.
45. Starker LF, Björklund P, Theoharis C, Long WD 3rd, Carling T, Udelsman R. Clinical and histopathological characteristics of hyperparathyroidism-induced hypercalcemic crisis. World J Surg. 2011 Feb;35(2):331–335.
46. Mukherjee S, Bhadada SK, Arya AK, Singh P, Sood A, Dahiya D, Ram S, Saikia UN, Behera A. Primary hyperparathyroidism in the young: Comparison with adult primary hyperparathyroidism. Endocr Pract. 2018 Dec;24(12):1051–1056.
47. Shah VN, Bhadada SK, Bhansali A, Behera A, Mittal BR, Bhavin V. Influence of age and gender on presentation of symptomatic primary hyperparathyroidism. J Postgrad Med. 2012 Apr-Jun;58(2):107–111.
48. Carella MJ, Gossain VV. Hyperparathyroidism and pregnancy: Case report and review. J Gen Intern Med. 1992 Jul-Aug;7(4):448–453.
49. Inabnet WB, Baldwin D, Daniel RO, Staren ED. Hyperparathyroidism and pancreatitis during pregnancy. Surgery. 1996 Jun;119(6):710–713.
50. Yilmaz BA, Altay M, Değertekin CK, Çimen AR, Iyidir ÖT, Biri A, Yüksel O, Töruner FB, Arslan M. Hyperparathyroid crisis presenting with hyperemesis gravidarum. Arch Gynecol Obstet. 2014 Oct;290(4):811–814.
51. Matthias GS, Helliwell TR, Williams A. Postpartum hyperparathyroid crisis. Case report. Br J Obstet Gynaecol. 1987 Aug;94(8):807–810.
52. Bronsky D, Weisberg MG, Gross MC, Barton JJ. Hyperparathyroidism and acute postpartum pancreatitis with neonatal tetany in the child. Am J Med Sci. 1970 Sep;260(3):160–164.
53. DeLellis RA. Parathyroid carcinoma: An overview. Adv Anat Pathol. 2005 Mar;12(2):53–61.
54. Rao DS, Agarwal G, Talpos GB, Phillips ER, Bandeira F, Mishra SK, Mithal A. Role of vitamin D and calcium nutrition in disease expression and parathyroid tumor growth in primary hyperparathyroidism: A global perspective. J Bone Miner Res. 2002 Nov;17 Suppl 2:N75–N80.
55. Agarwal G, Dhingra S, Mishra SK, Krishnani N. Implantation of parathyroid carcinoma along fine needle aspiration track. Langenbecks Arch Surg. 2006 Nov;391(6):623–626.
56. Bart L. Clarke (2019). Asymptomatic Primary hyperparathyroidism. In: Brandi ML, ed., Parathyroid disorders. Focusing on Unmet needs (vol 51). Basel, Karger: Front Horm Res. pp. 13–22.
57. Rubin MR, Bilezikian JP, McMahon DJ, Jacobs T, Shane E, Siris E, Udesky J, Silverberg SJ. The natural history of primary hyperparathyroidism with or without parathyroid surgery after 15 years. J Clin Endocrinol Metab. 2008 Sep;93(9):3462–3470.
58. Bilezikian JP, Khan AA, Potts JT Jr; Third International Workshop on the Management of Asymptomatic Primary Hyperthyroidism. Guidelines for the management of asymptomatic primary hyperparathyroidism: Summary statement from the third international workshop. J Clin Endocrinol Metab. 2009 Feb;94(2):335–339.
59. Silverberg SJ, Clarke BL, Peacock M, Bandeira F, Boutroy S, Cusano NE, Dempster D, Lewiecki EM, Liu JM, Minisola S, Rejnmark L, Silva BC, Walker MD, Bilezikian JP. Current issues in the presentation of asymptomatic primary hyperparathyroidism: Proceedings of the Fourth International Workshop. J Clin Endocrinol Metab. 2014 Oct;99(10):3580–3594.
60. Cusano NE, Silverberg SJ, Bilezikian JP. Normocalcemic primary hyperparathyroidism. J Clin Densitom. 2013 Jan-Mar;16(1):33–39.
61. Lowe H, McMahon DJ, Rubin MR, Bilezikian JP, Silverberg SJ. Normocalcemic primary hyperparathyroidism: Further characterization of a new clinical phenotype. J Clin Endocrinol Metab. 2007 Aug;92(8):3001–3005.
62. McCoy KL, Chen NH, Armstrong MJ, Howell GM, Stang MT, Yip L, Carty SE. The small abnormal parathyroid gland is increasingly common and heralds operative complexity. World J Surg. 2014 Jun;38(6):1274–1281.
63. Kiriakopoulos A, Petralias A, Linos D. Classic primary hyperparathyroidism versus normocalcemic and normohormonal variants: Do they really differ? World J Surg. 2018 Apr;42(4):992–997.
64. Applewhite MK, White MG, Tseng J, Mohammed MK, Mercier F, Kaplan EL, Angelos P, Vokes T, Grogan RH. Normohormonal primary hyperparathyroidism is a distinct form of primary hyperparathyroidism. Surgery. 2017 Jan;161(1):62–69.
65. Silverberg SJ, Shane E, Jacobs TP, Siris E, Bilezikian JP. A 10-year prospective study of primary hyperparathyroidism with or without parathyroid surgery. N Engl J Med. 1999 Oct;341(17):1249–1255. Erratum in: N Engl J Med 2000 Jan;342(2):144.
66. Pak CY, Oata M, Lawrence EC, Snyder W. The hypercalciurias. Causes, parathyroid functions, and diagnostic criteria. J Clin Invest. 1974 Aug;54(2):387–400.
67. Abdelhadi M, Nordenström J. Bone mineral recovery after parathyroidectomy in patients with primary and renal hyperparathyroidism. J Clin Endocrinol Metab. 1998 Nov;83(11):3845–3851.
68. Scholz DA, Purnell DC. Asymptomatic primary hyperparathyroidism. 10-year prospective study. Mayo Clin Proc. 1981 Aug;56(8):473–478.
69. Yadav SK, Mishra SK, Mishra A, Mayilvagnan S, Chand G, Agarwal G, Agarwal A, Verma AK. Surgical management of primary hyper parathyroidism in the era of focused parathyroidectomy: A study in tertiary referral centre of North India. Indian J Endocrinol Metab. 2019 Jul-Aug;23(4):468–472.
70. Salahudeen AK, Thomas TH, Sellars L, Tapster S, Keavey P, Farndon JR, Johnston ID, Wilkinson R. Hypertension and renal dysfunction in primary hyperparathyroidism: Effect of parathyroidectomy. Clin Sci (Lond). 1989 Mar;76(3):289–296.
71. Hedbäck G, Tisell LE, Bengtsson BA, Hedman I, Oden A. Premature death in patients operated on for primary hyperparathyroidism. World J Surg. 1990 Nov-Dec;14(6):829–835; discussion 836.
72. Ronni-Sivula H. Causes of death in patients previously operated on for primary hyperparathyroidism. Ann Chir Gynaecol. 1985;74(1):13–18.
73. Sheldon DG, Lee FT, Neil NJ, Ryan JA Jr. Surgical treatment of hyperparathyroidism improves health-related quality of life. Arch Surg. 2002 Sep;137(9):1022–1026; discussion 1026-8.
74. Weber T, Eberle J, Messelhäuser U, Schiffmann L, Nies C, Schabram J, Zielke A, Holzer K, Rottler E, Henne-Bruns D, Keller M, von Wietersheim J. Parathyroidectomy, elevated depression scores, and suicidal ideation in patients with primary hyperparathyroidism: Results of a prospective multicenter study. JAMA Surg. 2013 Feb;148(2):109–115.
75. Ramakant P, Verma AK, Chand G, Mishra A, Agarwal G, Agarwal A, Mishra SK. Salutary effect of parathyroidectomy on neuropsychiatric symptoms in patients with primary hyperparathyroidism: Evaluation using PAS and SF-36v2 scoring systems. J Postgrad Med. 2011 Apr-Jun;57(2):96–101.

32

LOCALIZATION STUDIES IN PARATHYROID DISEASES

Alka Ashmita Singhal

Introduction

Parathyroid imaging is a valuable tool in the surgical management of hyperparathyroidism (HPT) and a good diagnostic study allowing focused parathyroidectomy over bilateral neck exploration for most single-gland diseases. Localization of abnormal parathyroids in cases of HPT still remains a diagnostic challenge in most cases across the globe including Southeast Asia. Various diagnostic modalities are utilized, each having its own sensitivity and specificity. Factors of cost and availability of the modality in the region of Southeast Asia is an important factor. Ultrasound imaging with color Doppler to localize the abnormal parathyroid nodules is a cost effective and convenient tool with great sensitivity and specificity in experienced hands. Technetium 99m sestamibi scan is a functional imaging and has been used as a reference imaging for localization of parathyroids. It can demonstrate lesions well within the mediastinum, which are beyond the access of conventional ultrasound imaging. Contrast enhanced computed tomography (CT) (CECT) neck or four-dimensional CT (4D-CT) where scans in different vascular phases are utilized to localize the parathyroids as rapidly enhancing areas and with early wash out in the corresponding anatomical location. Ultrasound and parathyroid scintigraphy with methoxyisobutylisonitrile (Technetium 99m sestamibi) are the dominant imaging techniques used; CT and MRI are generally used as an additional imaging for ectopic mediastinal adenomas or for failed surgeries. The chapter aims to provide a pictorial review of the common localization studies in parathyroid disorders in a simple well illustrative manner, easy to understand by surgeons, physicians and radiologists.

Hyperparathyroidism

HPT has a prevalence is 1–2 per 1000 population; however, prevalence of subclinical HPT may be 5–10 per 1000 population [1]. Female preponderance is noted in the ratio of 2:1 or 3:1. Majority patients are over 50 years or middle aged. It is less common in pediatric age group with the incidence being 2–5 per 100,000 [2,3]. Primary HPT (PHPT) results due to overactivity of the parathyroid glands resulting in elevated serum calcium levels or hypercalcemia. It is diagnosed biochemically in a symptomatic individual presenting with hypercalcemia and its sequelae or may present with incidental hypercalcemia along with elevated parathyroid hormone (PTH) levels. Mean range of normal serum calcium levels in adult population range from 8.5 mg/dl to 10.2 mg/dl [4]. The range of normal serum PTH levels in adult population range from 10 pg/ml to 65 pg/ml. Serum parathyroid levels are elevated in majority of cases of HPT; however, serum PTH levels may be normal in some cases of HPT. Diagnosis is confirmed when the serum PTH level is "inappropriately high" for the corresponding serum calcium level. Clinically patients may present with the classic signs such as renal stones, pancreatitis, bone pain and psychiatric symptoms or with vague symptoms of fatigue and lethargy. Secondary HPT (SHPT) results when a cause outside the parathyroid glands stimulates hyperactivity and enlargement of the parathyroid glands, as commonly seen in chronic renal failure and vitamin D deficiency. Parathyroid hyperplasia is often seen in these cases. In long-standing cases, HPT may persist even after the cause which initially stimulated it has been corrected, this condition is known as tertiary HPT (THPT).

Clinical history and laboratory parameters must be reviewed carefully to aid in understanding the spectrum of HPT and whether to expect a single- or multiglandular disease [5]. Family history, age of patient, clinical symptoms and association with other endocrine abnormalities needs to be considered when suspecting a familial predisposition as in multiple endocrine neoplasia (MEN). Very highly elevated serum calcium levels along with highly elevated serum PTH levels arouse suspicion of parathyroid carcinoma.

Parathyroid glands: Anatomy

Anatomy forms the fundamental basis of diagnostic imaging. An understanding of the anatomy of the parathyroid glands including the vascular anatomy is important to identify the parathyroid glands on imaging and to differentiate them from thyroid nodules and lymph nodes. Normal parathyroid glands are usually four in number, two on each side, superior and inferior parathyroids embedded on the posterior surface of the thyroid gland [6]. They are tiny pea sized glands, measuring less than 5 mm in diameter. They contain glandular fat and the chief cells which secrete the PTH. Color of parathyroid glands vary from yellow due to fat content and pinkish red due to increased vascularity as in case of an adenoma. The two superior parathyroids are usually located behind the mid pole of thyroid, just around (within 2-cm radius) and above the level of crossing of recurrent laryngeal nerve and inferior thyroid artery. The inferior parathyroid glands are usually located around the posterior aspect of the lower pole of thyroid gland.

Parathyroid glands: Vascular supply

The main arterial supply to both superior and inferior parathyroids is mainly from the inferior thyroid artery (77%–90% cases) [7]. Less often they are supplied by superior thyroid artery (in 10%–15% cases) and by anastomosis of both superior and inferior thyroid arteries in about 5%–8% cases. The feeding artery reaches one pole of the gland and then forms an arc around the pole and divides into vessels to supply the gland. This polar feeding artery is seen as a dominant vessel seen on imaging. Identification of this characteristic vascular pattern is important to help confirm an enlarged parathyroid gland. This vascular pattern is maintained and well identified even in intrathyroidal parathyroids. Venous outflow and lymphatic drainage accompany the tributaries of the supplying arteries.

Parathyroid glands: Embryology

Embryology of the parathyroid glands is closely related to that of the thyroid gland and thymus, and any variations in the origin and migration of these glands leads to substantial anatomical variation in the location of parathyroids in the neck and mediastinum.

Parathyroid glands arise from the dorsal aspect of third and fourth branchial pouches. The inferior parathyroid glands arise from the more cranial third pharyngeal pouch in close relation to thymus glands. The superior parathyroids arise from the fourth pharyngeal pouch along with the lateral lobes of thyroid gland. The parathyroid glands are ectopic in location in about 16% cases. Ectopic parathyroids [8] may occur due to abnormalities of descent leading to undescended parathyroids located high up in the neck or over descended parathyroids which may reach into the anterior mediastinum. The ectopic superior parathyroids may be retroesophageal or in the tracheoesophageal groove or in the retropharyngeal space and may descend further into posterosuperior mediastinum. The superior parathyroids are usually deeper and more posteriorly located as compared to the inferior parathyroids. Rarely the superior parathyroids may be undescended and may be found at the angle of mandible [9] just lateral to the submandibular glands or near the upper border of thyroid gland. The inferior parathyroids, also called the parathymus glands descend caudally along with the thymus in the anterior part of the neck. Owing to their longer descent, inferior parathyroids are more likely to be ectopic in location as compared to superior parathyroids. Most common ectopic location of the inferior parathyroids is along the thymothymic tract (25% of ectopic parathyroids) in the lower anterior neck or in the anterior mediastinum. Undescended ectopic inferior parathyroids may be located as high as anterior to carotid bulb or in the carotid sheath or in the posterior triangle of neck. Over descended inferior parathyroids may be seen in the mediastinum posterior to esophagus, at the carina or in the aorto pulmonary window.

Parathyroid glands may be intrathyroidal [10,11] if they become trapped within the thyroid at the time of fusion of median and lateral anlage during the embryological development. In these cases, the parathyroid gland is seen surrounded by the thyroid tissue and the thyroid capsule. Supernumerary parathyroids are known to exist in about 13% cases at autopsy and are often seen in the thymic region. These are more likely in cases of familial HPT such as MEN and often may be the cause of refractory or persistent HPT [12].

Radionuclide scintigraphy

Technetium 99m sestamibi scan [13–15] is a functional study and has been considered as a reference standard for localization of parathyroid nodules in HPT. A standard dose of 10 mCi of Technetium 99m sestamibi is injected intravenously and early images are obtained at 30-minute interval. Delayed images are taken at 2 hours (Figure 32.1). SPECT images are taken after the early images in orthogonal planes to give three-dimensional localization. The field of view included extends from the level of ears to the level of diaphragm, as to include the eutopic as well as all likely ectopic sites for parathyroids. Early images show uptake by thyroid, parathyroid and salivary glands. The two sets of planar images (early and delayed) are inspected for any focal areas of increased uptake, which show either a relative progressive increase over time or a fixed uptake which persists on delayed

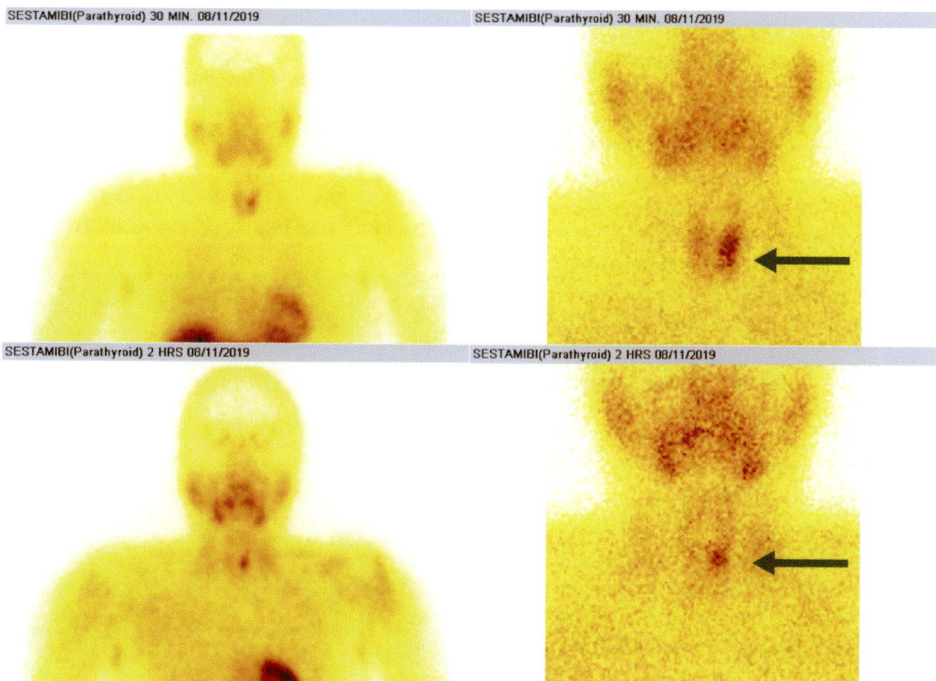

FIGURE 32.1 Nuclear scintigraphy with methoxyisobutylisonitrile (Technetium 99m sestamibi scan or MIBI scan) in a 45-year-old woman with clinical hyperparathyroidism (serum calcium 12.5 mg/dl and serum PTH 433.2 mg/dl). Early images taken at 30 minutes and delayed images taken at 2 hours post injection of tracer. Images zoomed for the area of interest. Early images showing uniform uptake of the tracer by the thyroid gland and the salivary glands, with increased uptake along the left thyroid (arrow). Delayed images show retention of the tracer along the left thyroid (arrow) suggestive of left parathyroid adenoma.

imaging, these are considered to be pathological hyperfunctioning parathyroid glands.

Technetium 99m is taken up by the tissues having high mitochondrial activity and the sensitivity of Technetium 99m sestamibi (MIBI) depends on the increased number of mitochondria within the abnormal parathyroids. The sensitivity and positive predictive value of MIBI scintigraphy has been reported in literature to be 81% and 89%, respectively, in patients with single-glandular disease and 37% and 100%, respectively, in patients with multiglandular disease [16]. Thyroid follicular adenomas also show increased mitochondrial activity and may show false positive results. False negative results are commonly seen in cystic parathyroids or in very small parathyroid nodules less commonly due to p glycoprotein expressing adenomas [17]. Nuclear scintigraphy is often negative in multiglandular disease. The two main reasons for failed surgery are ectopic parathyroid glands and multiglandular disease. Scintigraphy results should be confirmed with another imaging modality, ultrasound or CT. Hybrid SPECT/CT are helpful in localization studies. Combined interpretation of scintigraphy with ultrasound or with CT improves patient management outcomes [18].

Ultrasound imaging

Ultrasound neck is often the first investigation performed for anatomical localization of the parathyroid glands in HPT due to its wider availability, convenience and cost effectiveness, whilst without the harmful effects of any ionizing radiation. Ultrasound assessment for localization of parathyroids in HPT begins with a careful review of clinical and lab parameters which might give important clues to whether single- or multiglandular disease is expected. The serum calcium and serum PTH values are recorded in the clinical details section on the report. Note is made of any previous neck investigations and surgeries. A brief history of thyroid clinical status is obtained to assess whether patient is euthyroid, hypothyroid or hyperthyroid. Patients with long-standing hypothyroidism on thyroid supplement medication often have very small and atrophic thyroid. Patients with hyperthyroidism or thyroiditis may have a diffusely enlarged and a hypoechoic thyroid gland, limiting the comparative assessment of the relative echotexture of thyroid gland and parathyroid adenoma. Patients with large multinodular goiter pose a challenge as the parathyroid glands may be difficult to identified amidst nodules of varying echogenicity and anatomical distortion of the gland. This is especially a challenge in the region of Southeast Asia where large multinodular goiters are endemic in certain areas [18]. A thorough ultrasound evaluation of the complete thyroid gland precedes the search and localization of parathyroids. The ultrasound examination is then extended to include the whole neck area from the angle of mandible, jaw line and inferiorly up to the supraclavicular regions and sternal angle. Any associated thyroid gland or other neck pathology is recorded. Cases of MEN and other familial syndromes may have associated thyroid gland and other endocrine abnormalities. The sensitivity, specificity and positive predictive value of sonography for identifying abnormal parathyroid glands as per reported studies has been 74%, 96% and 90%, respectively [19]. Ultrasound being an operator-dependent modality, the sensitivity and specificity data vary largely due to the variable expertise and experience of the operator in various studies. Ultrasound assessment also allows for concomitant evaluation of the thyroid, lymph nodes and other neck structures for any associated pathology. An ultrasound guided fine needle aspiration from target areas may be combined if needed. A PTH washout of the target area may be attempted in equivocal cases. In large multinodular goiters and for ectopic parathyroids extending into the mediastinum, ultrasound is limited and further imaging by contrast enhanced CT (4D-CT) is recommended.

Ultrasound technique and transducer selection

The basic principle of ultrasound imaging is to use the highest available transducer frequency to penetrate the required depth of imaging, to give the best possible resolution.

For most scans, 7–12-MHz transducer is chosen to begin the scan; however, lower frequency transducer may be needed to penetrate in cases of large multinodular goiter. A higher frequency transducer, up to 14 MHz or more gives better resolution of superficial nodules. Availability of small foot print transducers such as the "hockey stick probe" is helpful in scanning around the narrow spaces along the bones and cartilage such as in tracheo-esophageal groove, sternal angle and angle of mandible.

Patient position is usually supine with a pillow under the shoulders to allow for mild extension of the neck. The examination may be performed alternatively in a sitting position. Patient is advised to limit swallowing and talking during the scan. The whole neck area is scanned thoroughly in transverse and longitudinal planes, with both conventional gray scale and color Doppler ultrasound. Ultrasound elastography may be applied to associated thyroid, lymph node and other lesions. An extended field of view or panoramic view is used to represent a larger pathology or a larger area in one image, thereby attempting to give a complete pictorial orientation of relevant anatomy and pathology (Figure 32.2).

Typical ultrasound appearances of a parathyroid adenoma

A typical parathyroid adenoma on ultrasound appears as a discrete, oval homogenously hypoechoic nodule (Figure 32.3) located posterior or posteromedial to the thyroid gland, anterior to the longus colli muscles and usually medial or posteromedial to the carotid vessels. Various shapes of parathyroid nodules have been described such as ovoid, tear drop shape, rounded,

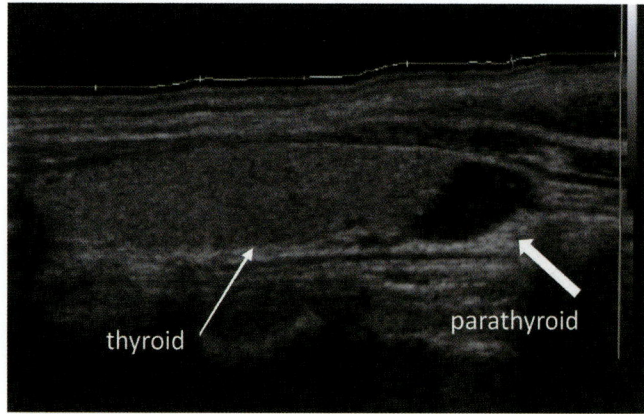

FIGURE 32.2 Panoramic view of longitudinal gray scale ultrasound in a patient with hyperparathyroidism showing a typical hypoechoic nodule (thick arrow) at the lower pole of thyroid suggestive of an inferior parathyroid adenoma. The normal thyroid gland with its smooth homogenous hyperechoic echoes is seen in the upper part (thin arrow).

Localization Studies in Parathyroid Diseases

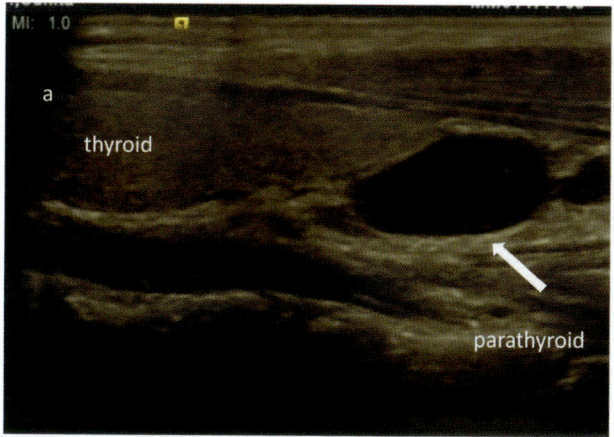 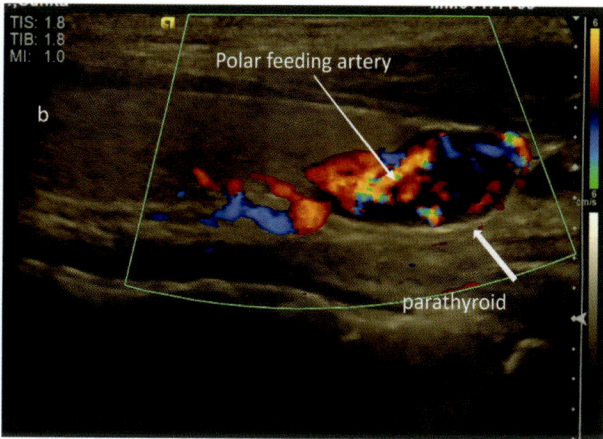

FIGURE 32.3 (a) and (b) Typical inferior parathyroid adenoma. Image (a) Longitudinal gray scale ultrasound showing a well-defined ovoid to tear-drop shaped homogenously hypoechoic nodule located posteroinferior to the lower pole of right thyroid gland. Image (b) showing the characteristic polar feeding artery on color Doppler scan.

elongated, elliptical, flattened and bilobed [13]. The hypoechoic echotexture of the parathyroid gland is compared relative to the thyroid gland and any altered echotexture of the thyroid gland due to any preceding diffuse thyroid disorder may limit the same. A thin echogenic line representing the compressed thyroid capsule, that separates the thyroid gland from the enlarged parathyroid gland can usually be seen and helps in differentiating between a thyroidal or an extrathyroidal lesion. An indentation may be noted at the adjacent thyroid due to the parathyroid adenoma. Larger adenomas are more likely to have cystic change, lobulations, increased echogenicity due to fatty deposition and occasional calcifications. The parathyroid nodule shape may be lobulated and margins ill-defined and merging with thyroid and the adjacent neck structures as in case of parathyroid carcinoma.

Color Doppler findings of parathyroid adenoma

Parathyroid adenomas tend to be hypervascular lesions (Figure 32.4) and the increased vascularity is well demonstrated in most cases on color Doppler ultrasound.

The vessel is usually a branch off the inferior thyroidal artery (80%–90% cases) or from the superior thyroid artery (10%–20% cases). It usually enters the parathyroid gland at one of the poles. The feeding artery tends to branch around at the periphery of the gland before penetration leading to a characteristic eccentric arc or rim of vascularity (Figures 32.5, 32.6(a)–(c) and 32.7(a)–(d)). Internal vascularity is also seen in a peripheral distribution. Adjacent thyroid parathyroid may show asymmetric hypervascularity that may give a clue in localizing parathyroid nodule.

Parathyroid adenoma may undergo changes in cellularity and may at times show slightly nonhomogeneous echotexture on gray scale imaging; however, the eccentric vascular arc on color Doppler still remains to be a characteristic feature and helps

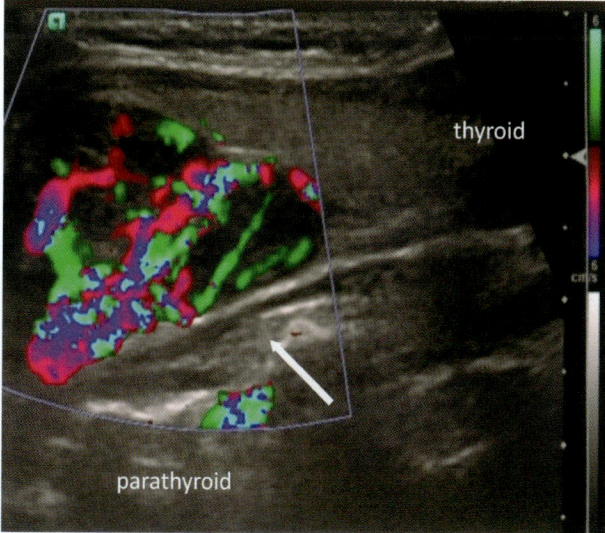 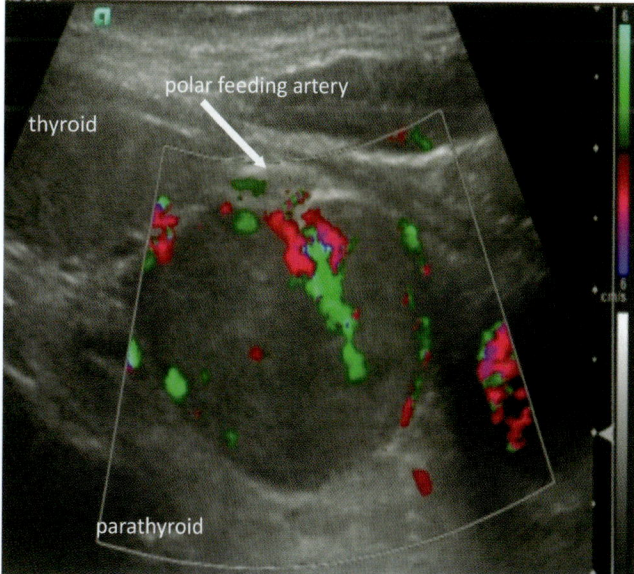

FIGURE 32.4 Longitudinal scan at the upper pole of a 43-year-old man with PHPT showing a hypoechoic nodule posterior to the upper pole of thyroid (arrow) with increased vascularity on color Doppler.

FIGURE 32.5 Color Doppler demonstrates the characteristic dominant parathyroid artery (arrow) conforming to the surface of the parathyroid adenoma. Note the parathyroid artery entering an inferior parathyroid adenoma from an anterosuperior direction.

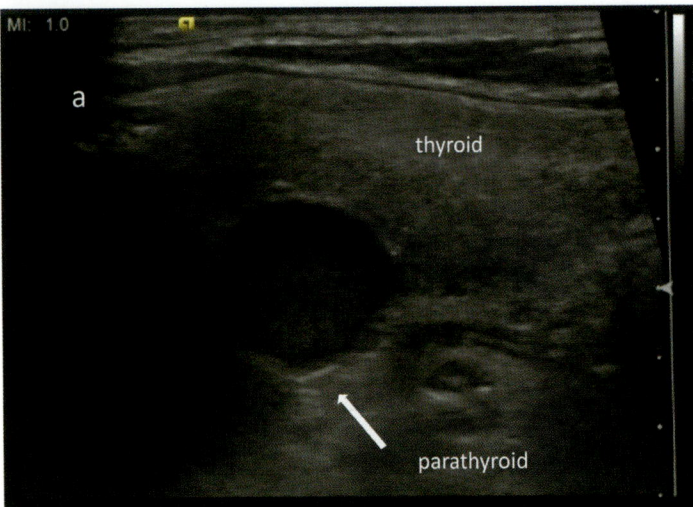
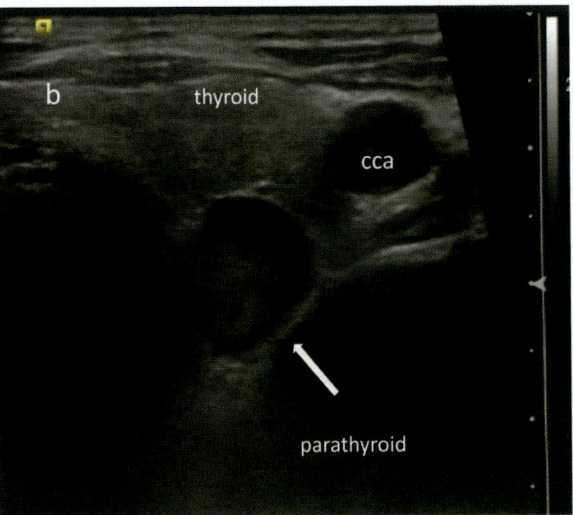
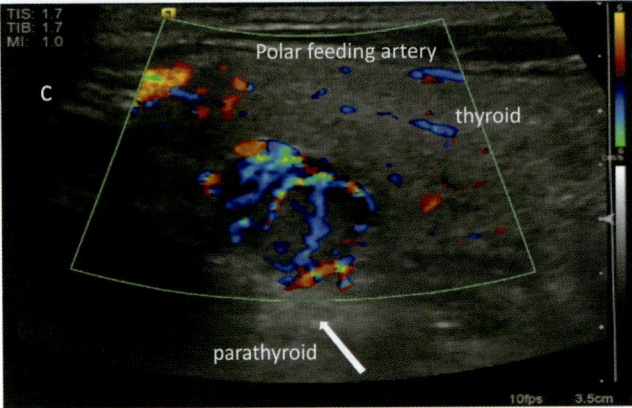

FIGURE 32.6 (a)–(c) Longitudinal and transverse scans with color Doppler showing a 13 mm × 9 mm × 12 mm typical left superior parathyroid adenoma as a well-defined hypoechoic rounded nodule (arrow) located posterior to the upper part of left thyroid. Note the characteristic polar feeding vessel entering the parathyroid nodule at its inferomedial aspect and then branching out to supply the gland. (Patient of CKD with serum calcium 8.10 mg/dl, PTH 1838 pg/ml. The left inferior and right superior parathyroid glands were also prominent in this case—not shown here. Patient underwent three and a half parathyroidectomy.)

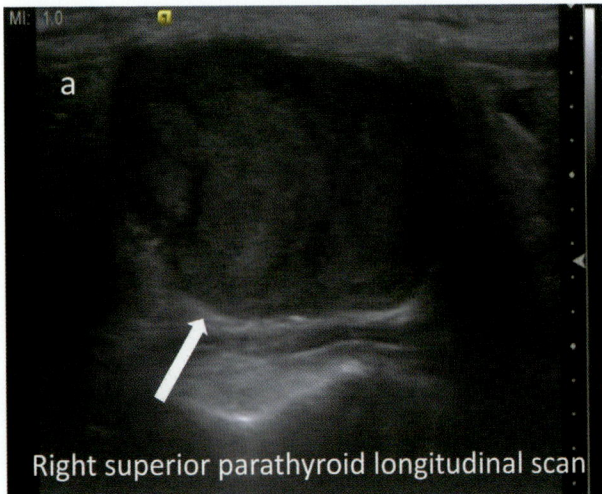
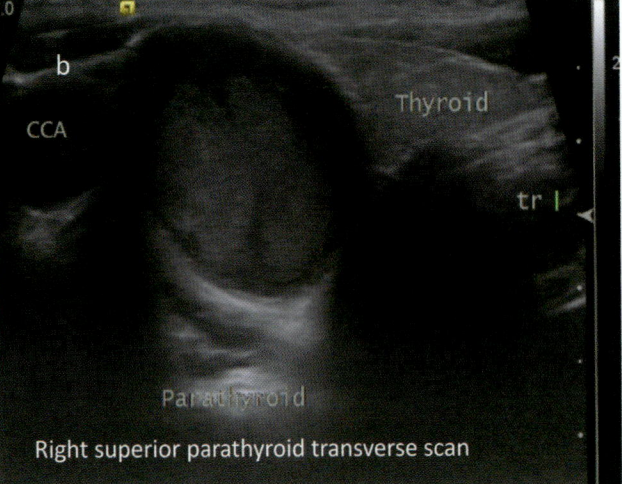

FIGURE 32.7 (a)–(d) Longitudinal and transverse scans with color Doppler showing a 17 mm × 16 mm × 17 mm typical left superior parathyroid adenoma as a well-defined hypoechoic rounded nodule (bold arrow) located posterior to the upper part of left thyroid. Not the characteristic polar feeding vessel (thin arrow) entering the parathyroid nodule at its inferomedial aspect and then branching out to supply the gland. (Patient of CKD under dialysis with serum calcium 11.5 mg/dl, PTH 380 pg/ml.)

Localization Studies in Parathyroid Diseases

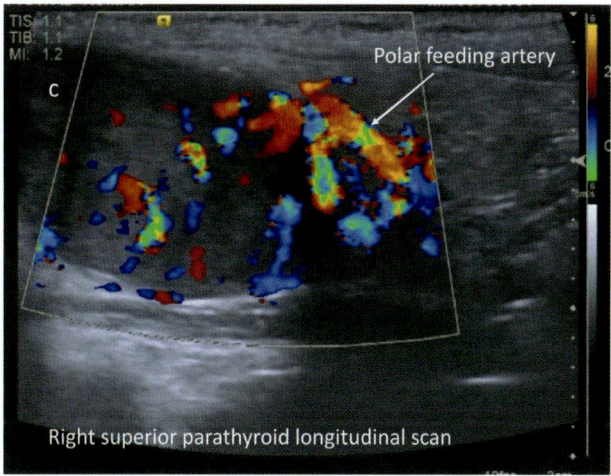
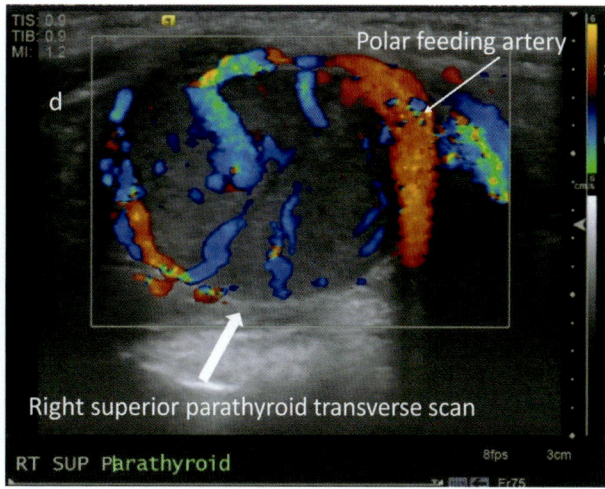

FIGURE 32.7 *(Continued)*

in diagnosis (Figure 32.8(a)–(c)). Correlation with bio-clinical parameters along with MIBI scan findings must be done when available (Figure 32.9(a)–(e)).

Thyroid follicular adenomas and lymph nodes are a common differential diagnosis as both can appear as homogenous hypoechoic nodules; however, the extrathyroidal location of a parathyroid adenoma combined with the demonstration of typical polar feeding vessel helps in establishing the diagnosis. Thyroid follicular adenomas may also show intense hypervascularity; however, the pattern is usually peripheral vascularity which may be combined

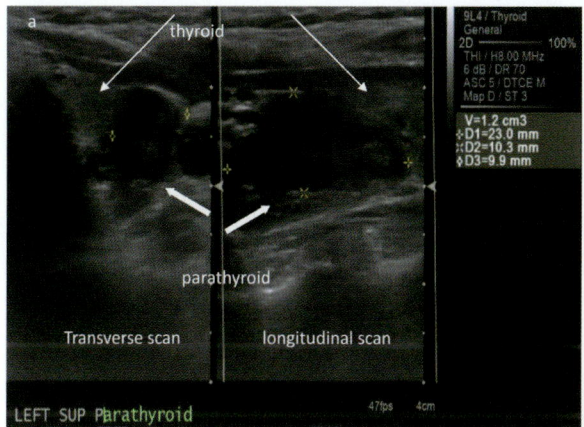
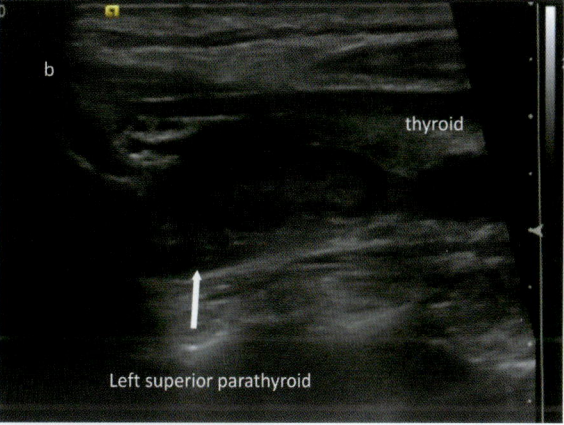
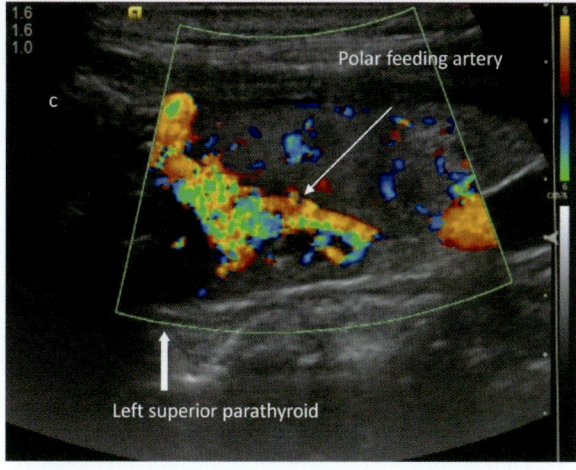

FIGURE 32.8 (a)–(c) Gray scale ultrasound shows a 23 mm × 10 mm × 19 mm, slightly heterogenous hypoechoic superior parathyroid adenoma (bold arrow) located posterior to the upper part of left thyroid gland. On color Doppler the arc rim vascularity (thin arrow) is seen along the inferomedial aspect of the parathyroid gland adjoining the thyroid parenchyma. (Serum calcium 12.8 mg/dl, PTH 76.1 pg/ml.)

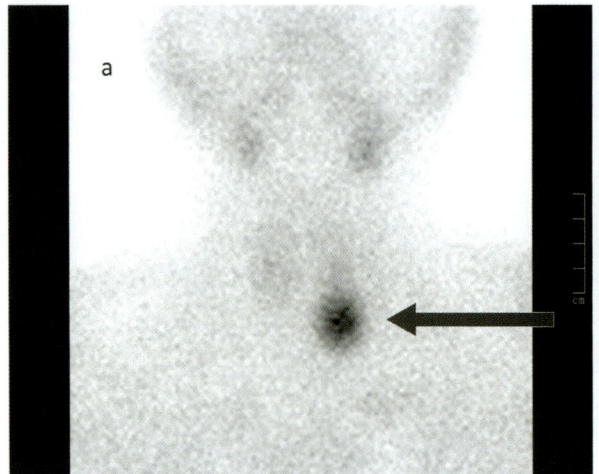
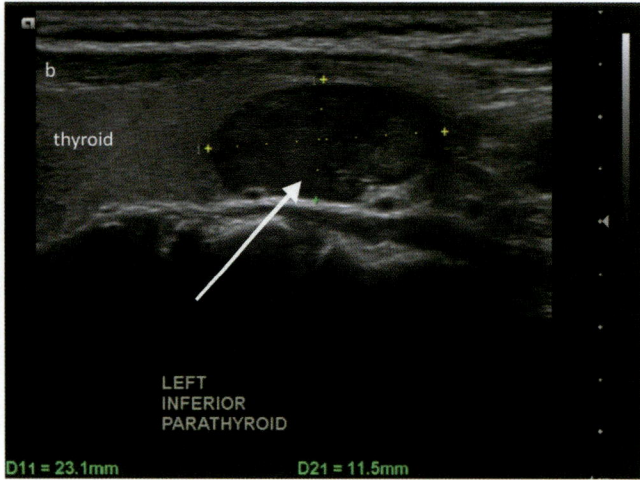
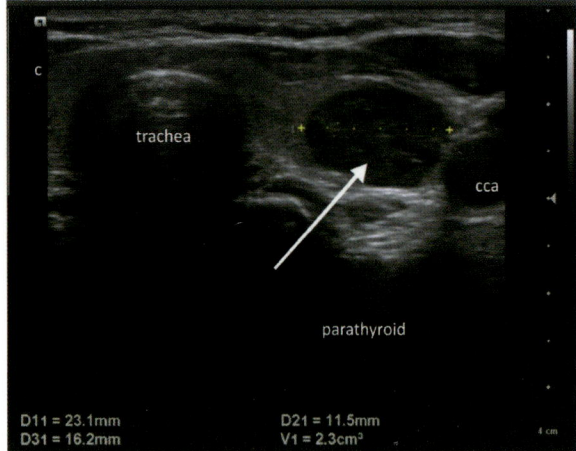
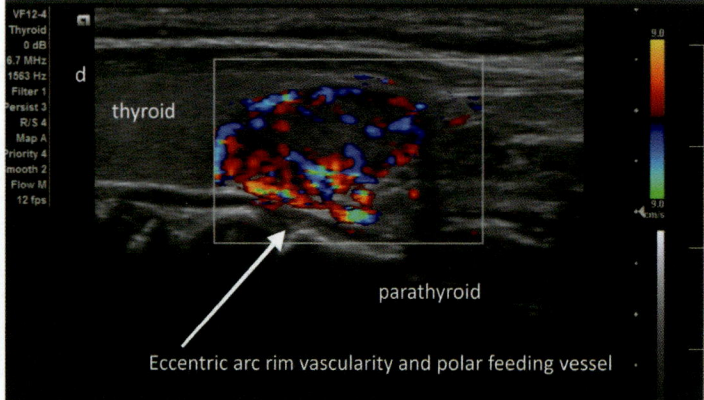
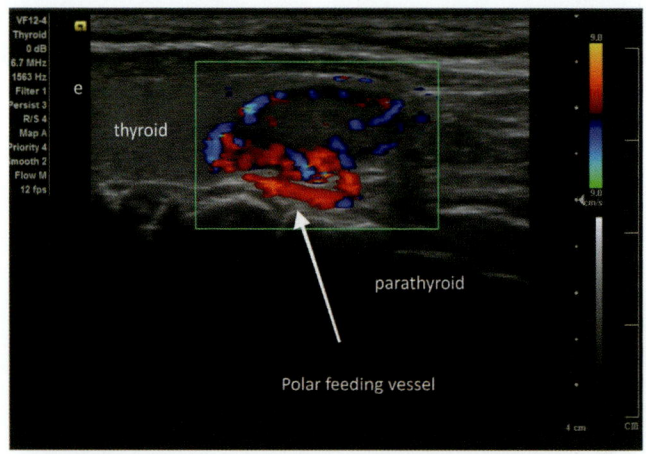

FIGURE 32.9 (a)–(e) A 48-year-old woman with serum calcium 11.6 mg/dl and PTH 1070 pg/ml revealing a typical left inferior parathyroid adenoma: MIBI and ultrasound correlation. Image (a) Technetium 99m sestamibi scan delayed image showing retention of the tracer at the lower pole of left thyroid (black arrow). Images (b)–(e) ultrasound showing a 23 mm × 11 mm × 16 mm, well-defined ovoid hypoechoic nodule (white arrow) along the lower pole of left thyroid which shows the diagnostic poplar feeding vessel and arc rim vascularity on color Doppler.

Localization Studies in Parathyroid Diseases

with central vascularity. Inflammatory lymph nodes typically show hilar vascularity.

Parathyroids with large cystic change and other atypical features may not show the characteristic vascular pattern and often require further confirmation with alternative imaging as CT. Demonstration of the diagnostic features on Doppler ultrasound is an operator-dependent technique and largely varies with the skill and experience of the operator along with equipment sensitivity and appropriate Doppler settings The overall sensitivity, specificity and accuracy of color Doppler ultrasound in diagnosis of parathyroid lesions in primary HPT and SHPT is 97%, 100%, 98.6% and 62%, 100% and 83%, respectively [20–22].

Tiny parathyroid nodules

The size of the parathyroid adenomas varies greatly. They may often be as small as tiny sub centimeter nodules. These are often negative on Technetium 99m sestamibi scan and CECT neck. These pose a diagnostic challenge and reliance is placed entirely on a detailed ultrasound scan by an experienced professional, which often points to the diagnosis. These patients may include those with subclinical HPT or may be suffering with symptoms of HPT. These tiny parathyroid adenomas show the same typical gray scale features and the characteristic Doppler flow pattern on ultrasound; however, great skill and experience is required to demonstrate the same (Figures 32.10(a)–(c), 32.11(a)–(c), 32.12(a) and (b) and 32.13(a)–(d))

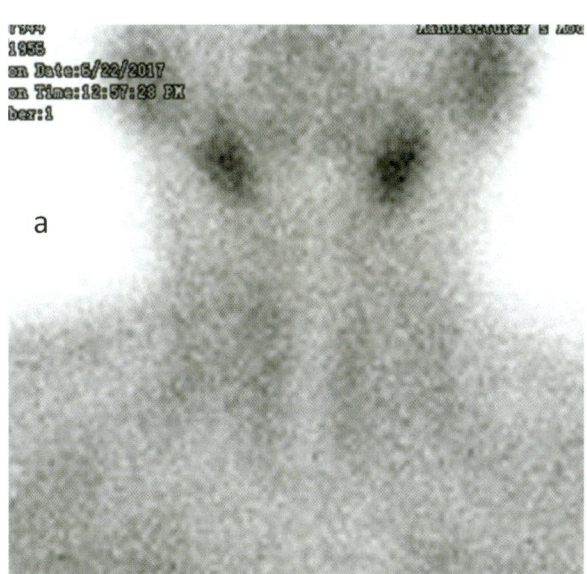
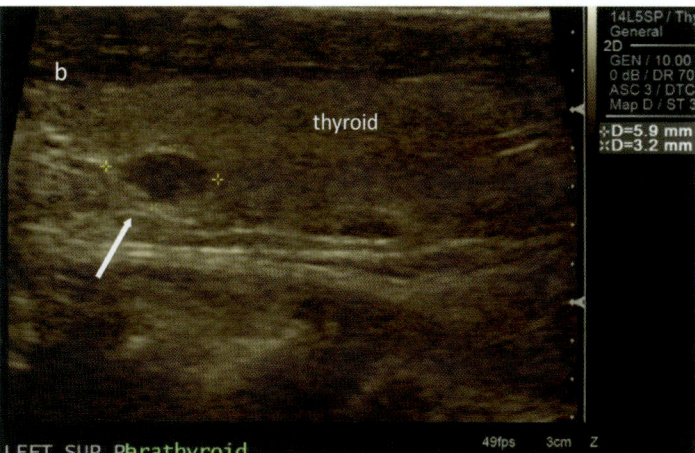
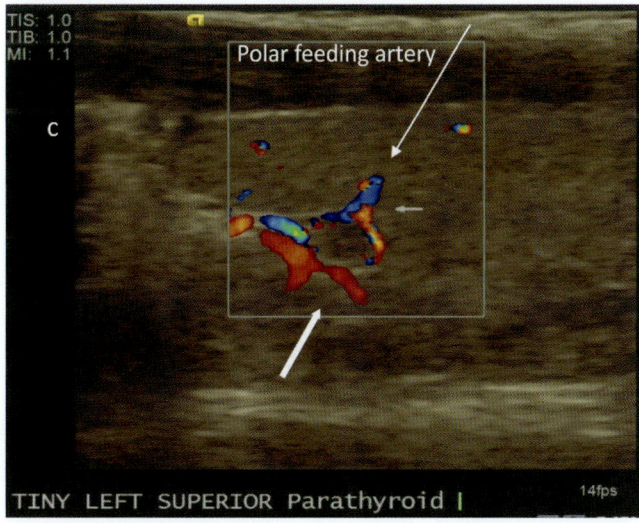

FIGURE 32.10 (a)–(c) (a) Tc99m sestamibi scan and (b) and (c) ultrasound with color Doppler scan of a patient with PHPT (serum calcium 10.5 mg/dl and serum PTH 168 pg/ml). Technetium 99m sestamibi scan showing no uptake on delayed scan suggesting negative scan for parathyroid adenoma. Ultrasound neck demonstrates a well-defined small 6 mm × 3 mm hypoechoic nodule at upper pole of thyroid with the characteristic polar feeding vessel on Doppler scan. Findings confirmed at surgery, parathyroidectomy performed and subsequent histopathology confirmed parathyroid adenoma.

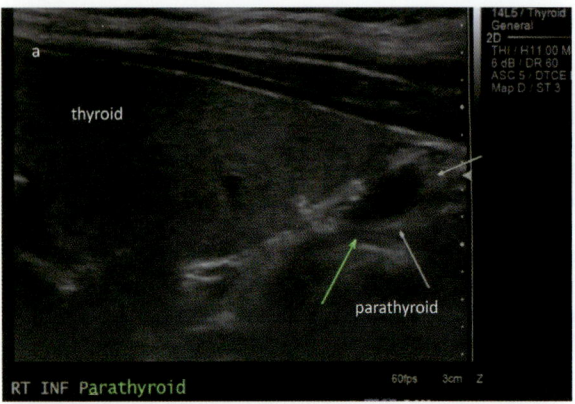
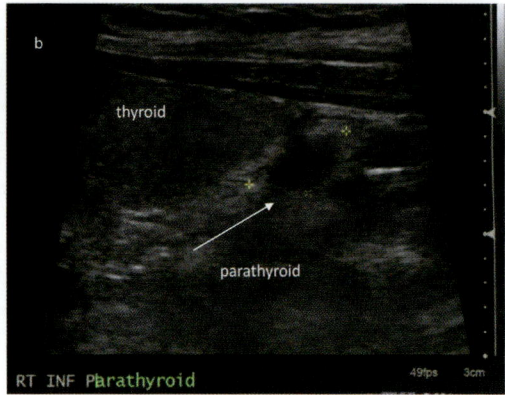
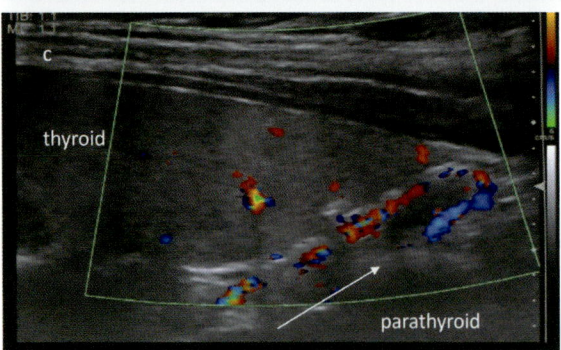

FIGURE 32.11 (a)–(c) MIBI negative tiny inferior parathyroid demonstrated on ultrasound as a 6 mm × 3 mm hypoechoic nodule posterior to the lower pole of thyroid with the polar feeding vessel leading to it as seen on color Doppler. Focused parathyroidectomy was performed and parathyroid adenoma confirmed at histopathology.

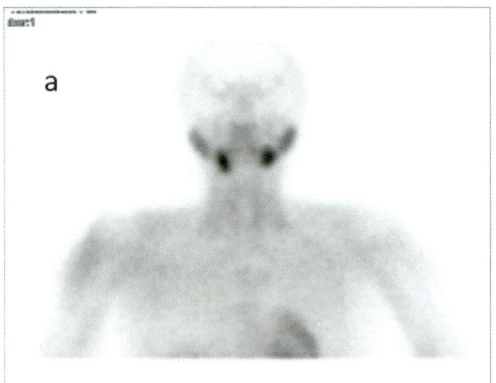
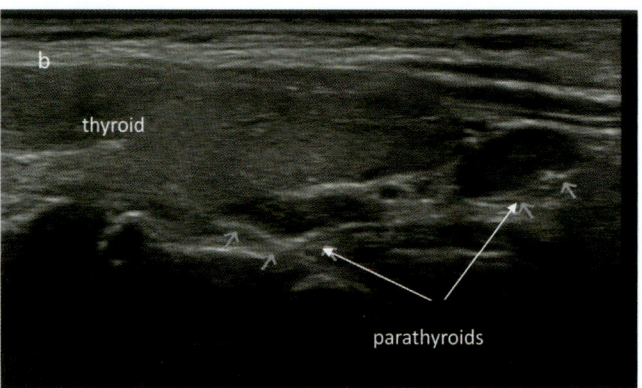

FIGURE 32.12 (a) and (b) (a) Tc 99m sestamibi scan and (b) ultrasound of a 41-year-old woman with PHPT (serum calcium 10.6 mg/dl, serum PTH 298 pg/ml and clinical history of pain in legs and knees). Tc99m sestamibi scan showing as negative scan for parathyroids, ultrasound showed two left parathyroid nodules in the lower part, findings confirmed at surgery.

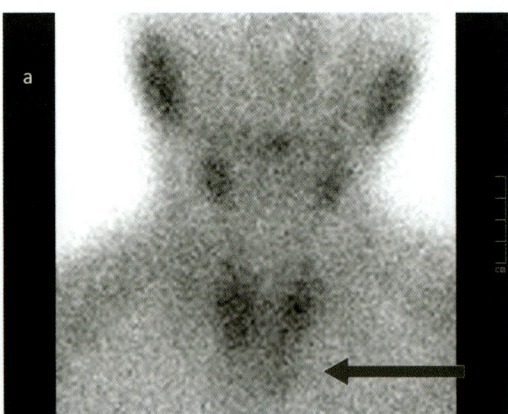
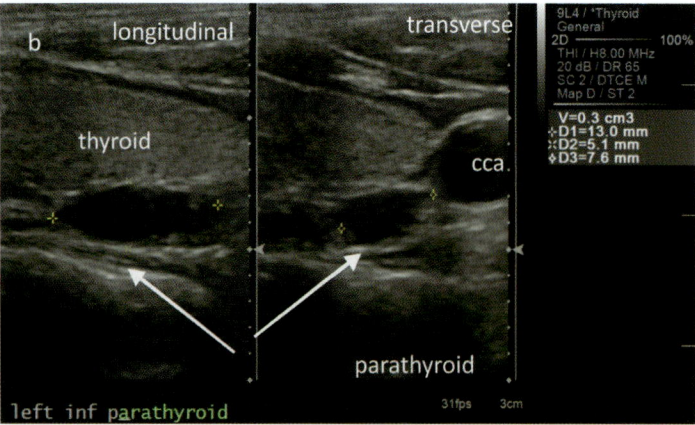

FIGURE 32.13 (a)–(d) A 31-year-old man with PHPT (serum calcium 11.2 mg/dl, PTH 183.2 pg/ml). Image (a) Technetium 99m sestamibi scan showing marginal retention of the tracer on delayed scan along the left thyroid suggesting possible left parathyroid adenoma. Images (b)–(d) ultrasound neck demonstrated a corresponding well-defined small 13 mm × 7 mm hypoechoic nodule posterior to the mid pole of left thyroid with the characteristic polar feeding vessel on Doppler scan. Findings confirmed at surgery, parathyroidectomy performed and subsequent histopathology confirmed parathyroid adenoma.

Localization Studies in Parathyroid Diseases

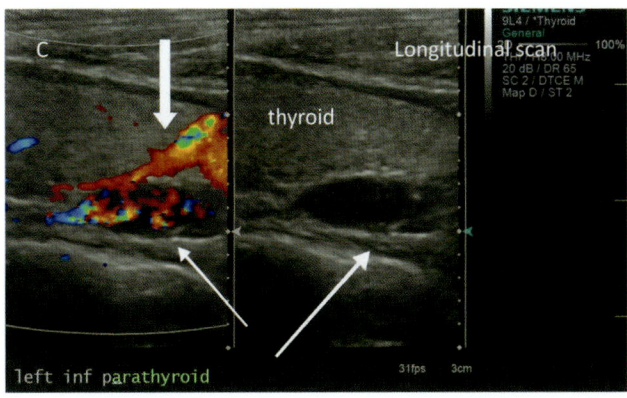 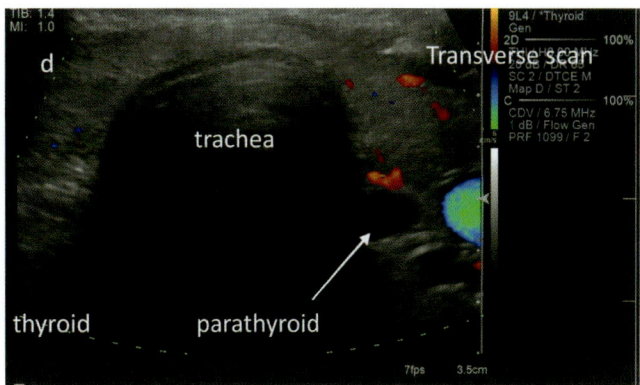

FIGURE 32.13 *(Continued)*

Large parathyroid nodules

Larger or mid-sized parathyroid nodules measuring more than 15 mm in longest diameter are usually well identified on ultrasound (Figure 32.14(a)–(c)); however, differentiation between thyroid nodules and other neck lesions must be considered. These parathyroid nodules are usually localized on Technetium 99m sestamibi scan, and the role of ultrasound imaging is as an adjunct to confirm and to give a precise anatomical localization, whilst excluding any additional nodules and other neck pathology.

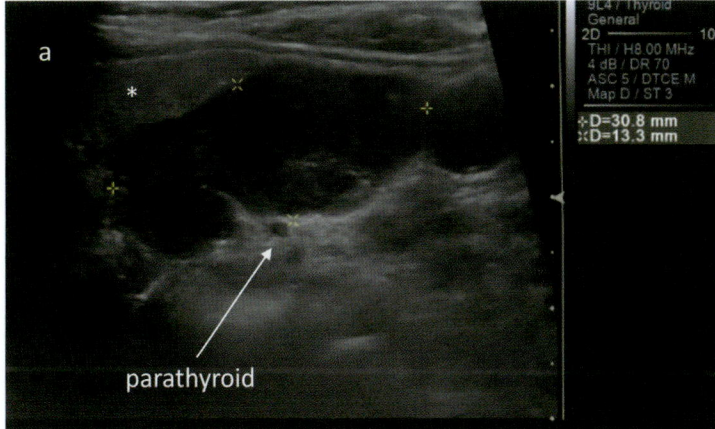 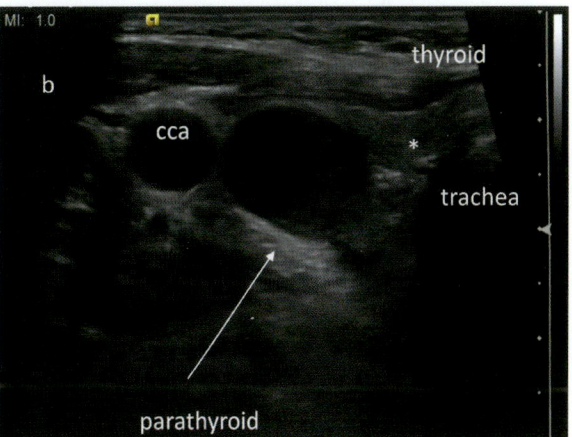

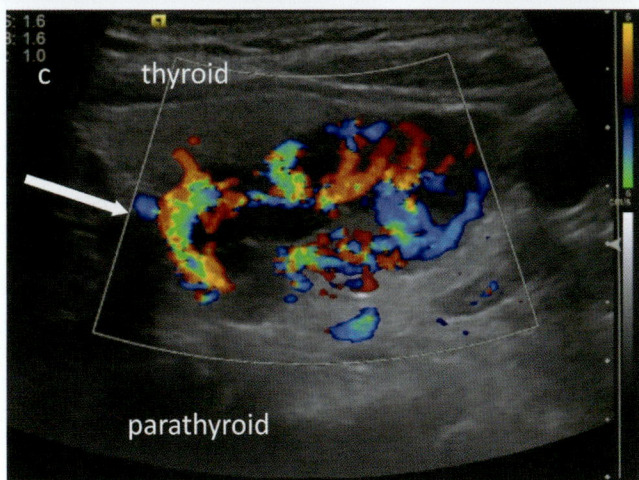

FIGURE 32.14 (a)–(c) Longitudinal and transverse scans with color Doppler showing a hypoechoic nodule (thin arrow) measuring 30 mm × 13 mm located postero-inferior to the lower part of left thyroid suggestive of left inferior parathyroid adenoma. Note the characteristic polar feeding vessel (bold arrow) entering the parathyroid nodule at its superomedial aspect and then branching to supply the gland.

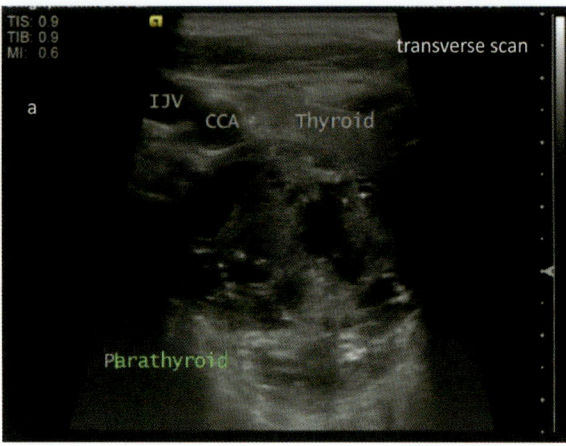
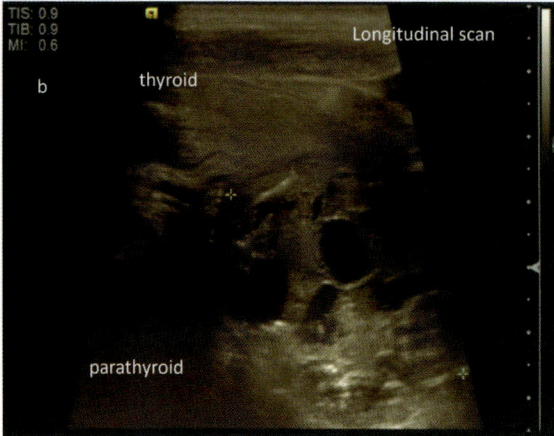

FIGURE 32.15 (a) and (b) A 56-year-old man with PHPT: Transverse and Longitudinal and scans showing a large 39 mm × 30 mm × 47 mm heterogenous hypoechoic nodule with small cystic changes located posterior inferior to the lower part of right thyroid gland suggestive of right inferior parathyroid adenoma. (serum calcium 11.0 mg/dl, PTH 265 pg/ml.)

Parathyroid adenomas with a large cystic component may only show subtle uptake on Technetium 99m sestamibi scan, depending on the number of active mitochondria available to bind with the tracer. In these cases, the role of ultrasound imaging to further demonstrate the complete extent of the lesion cannot be overemphasized (Figures 32.15, 32.16 and 32.17(a)–(c)).

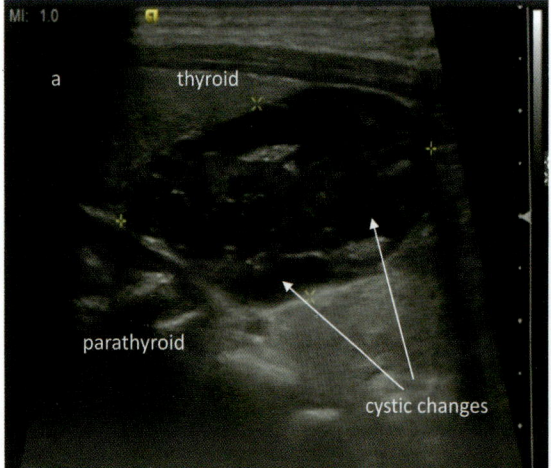
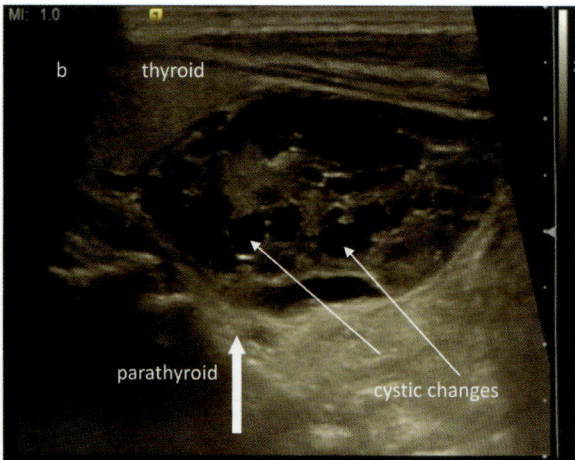
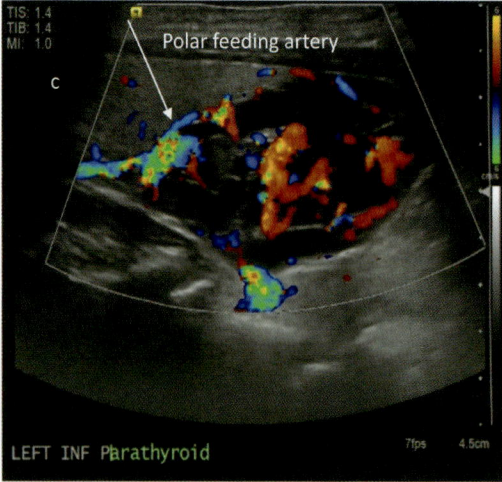

FIGURE 32.16 (a)–(c) Gray scale and color Doppler showing a hypoechoic nodule measuring 30 mm × 13 mm, located inferior and adjacent to the lower part of left thyroid suggestive of left inferior parathyroid adenoma. Note the cystic changes within the nodule as marked (thin arrows). The characteristic polar feeding vessel is seen entering the parathyroid nodule at its superomedial aspect. (Patient of CKD under dialysis with serum calcium 10.1 mg/dl, PTH 4170 pg/ml.)

Localization Studies in Parathyroid Diseases

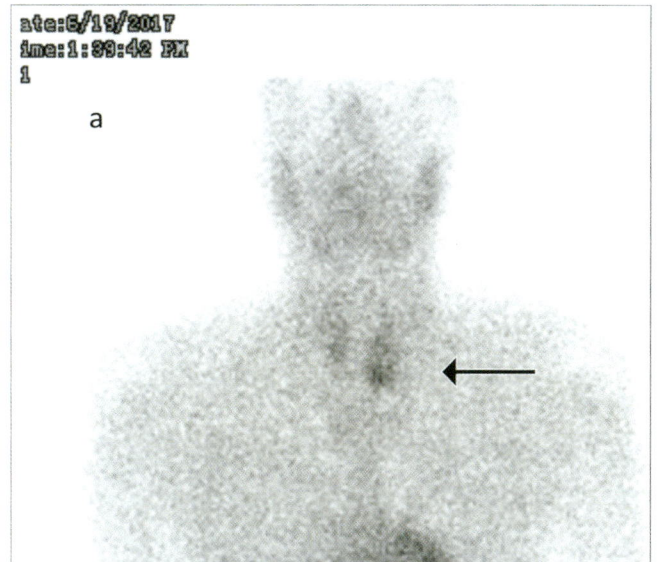
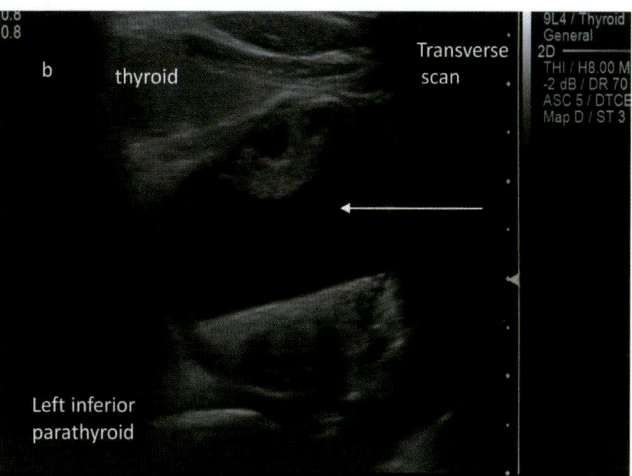
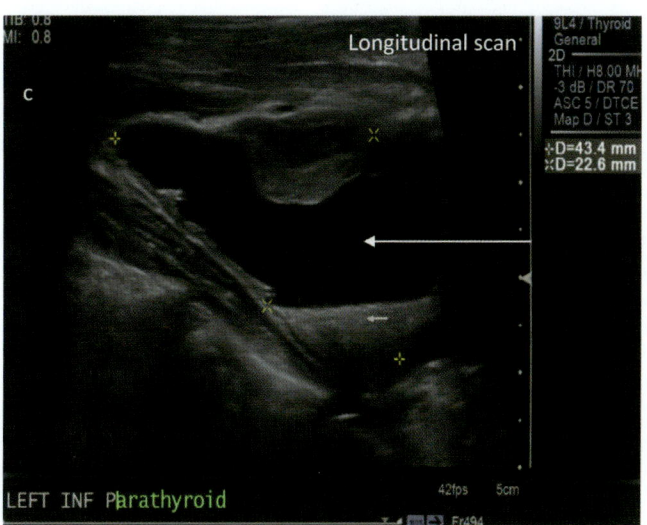

FIGURE 32.17 (a)–(c) A 52-year-old man with chronic pancreatitis diagnosed as PHPT. Image (a) Technetium 99m scan delayed scan showing a faint tracer retention (black arrow) at the lower pole of left thyroid. Corresponding ultrasound images (b) and (c), transverse and longitudinal scan showing a large (43 mm × 22 mm) predominantly cystic left inferior parathyroid adenoma, located deep into the posterior neck. Note the large cystic change in the adenoma as marked by the white arrow.

Parathyroid adenomas can be of a large size, at times being almost that of the whole of thyroid gland or even larger (Figures 32.18(a)–(d) and 32.19(a)–(c)). In these cases, care must be taken not to misinterpret a parathyroid adenoma as a thyroid gland. The thyroid gland may often be compressed in these cases. Diagnostic dilemma often ensues in cases of patients with long landing thyroid supplement medication where the thyroid gland may be small and atropic.

Ultrasound measurement of the size of each of the enlarged parathyroid nodule in three orthogonal planes and detailed anatomical orientation and relation with adjacent neck structures helps the surgeon in planning the optimum surgical approach.

Ectopic parathyroids

The parathyroid glands develop from the endoderm of the third and fourth pharyngeal pouches beginning at the fifth week of embryonic life [23,24] along with the thyroid and thymus and then descend into the neck. Variations in the descent lead to ectopic location of parathyroids in about 16% cases [25,26].

The superior parathyroid glands arise from the endoderm of the fourth pharyngeal pouch. During the sixth week of embryonic development they descend along with the thyroid, usually in a close relation to the posterior aspect of mid thyroid lobe.

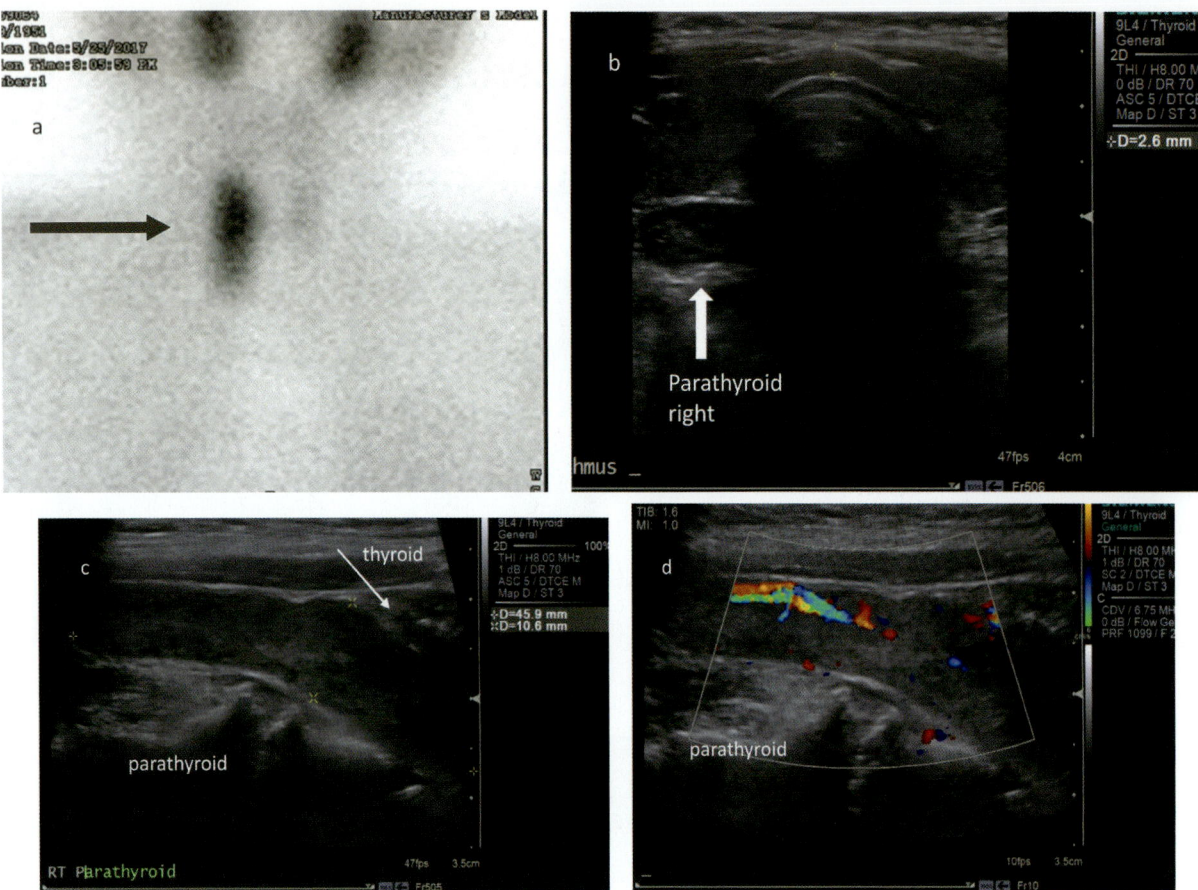

FIGURE 32.18 (a)–(d) A 65-year-old woman, known case of carcinoma breast had serum calcium 12.6 mg/dl and serum PTH of 193 pg/ml. Image (a) Technetium 99m delayed scan showing tracer retention (black arrow) along the right thyroid gland. Corresponding ultrasound images (b) and (c), transverse and longitudinal scan showing a large (45 mm × 11 mm × 24 mm) hypoechoic elongated right inferior parathyroid adenoma. The compressed thyroid parenchyma is seen along the medial part. Note the arc rim vascularity on color Doppler. Patient had a history of hypothyroidism on thyroid hormone supplements for past 25 years.

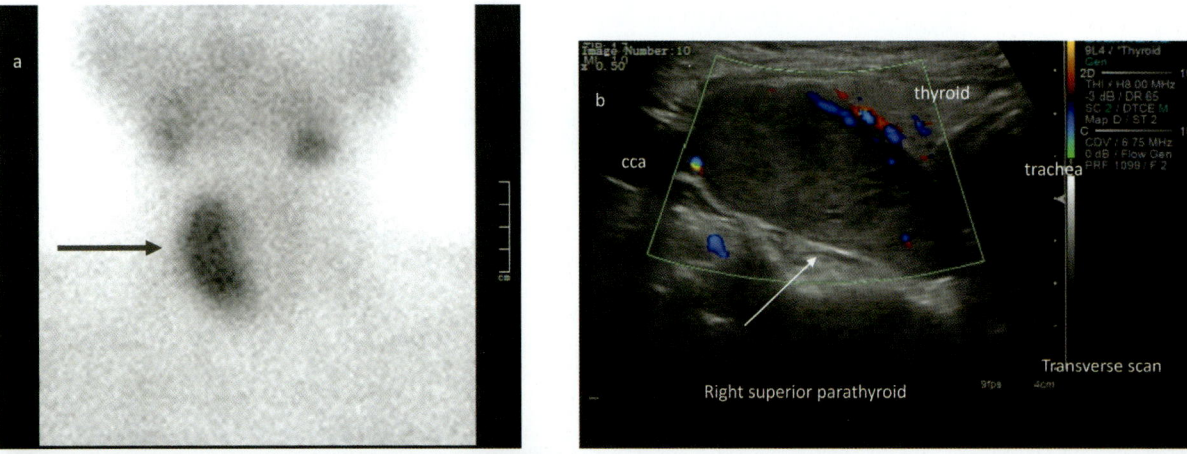

FIGURE 32.19 (a)–(c) Patient with PHPT. Image (a) Technetium 99m sestamibi delayed scan showing tracer retention (black arrow) along the right thyroid gland. Corresponding ultrasound images (b) and (c), transverse and longitudinal scan showing a large (43 mm × 18 mm) hypoechoic ovoid right superior parathyroid adenoma. The compressed thyroid parenchyma is seen along the medial part. Note the arc rim vascularity on color Doppler.

Localization Studies in Parathyroid Diseases

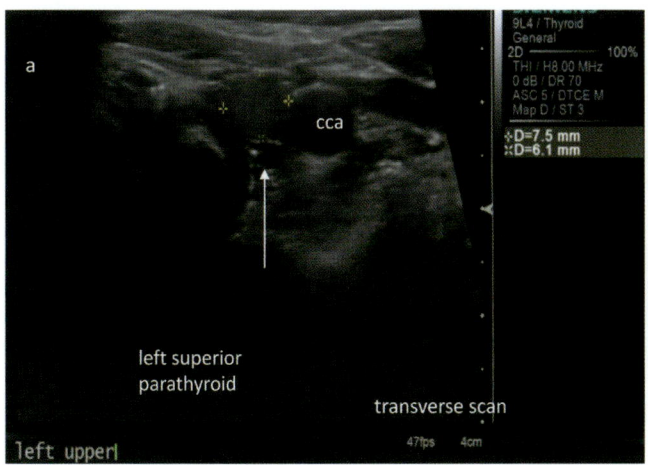
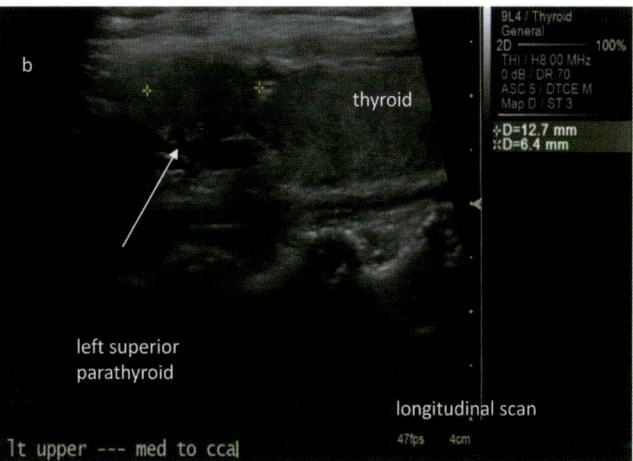

FIGURE 32.20 (a) and (b) Transverse and longitudinal gray scale ultrasound in patient with PHPT showing a well-defined rounded hypoechoic nodule (arrow) located just above the upper pole of left thyroid gland suggestive of left superior parathyroid adenoma. The nodule is located just medial to the carotid artery as noted on the transverse scan.

The typical location of superior parathyroids is just above or within a centimeter radius of the crossing of the inferior thyroid artery and the recurrent laryngeal nerve on the posterior mid surface of the thyroid. As the superior parathyroids have a smaller descent as compared to inferior parathyroids, they are less likely to show anatomical variability of locations. The commonest ectopic location of superior parathyroids is behind the upper pole of thyroid (Figure 32.20(a) and (b)) seen in about 2% cases. Superior parathyroids are very rarely seen beyond the superior pole of thyroid gland.

Ectopic parathyroids may be intrathyroidal in location (Figure 32.21(a)–(e)). Differentiating an intrathyroidal

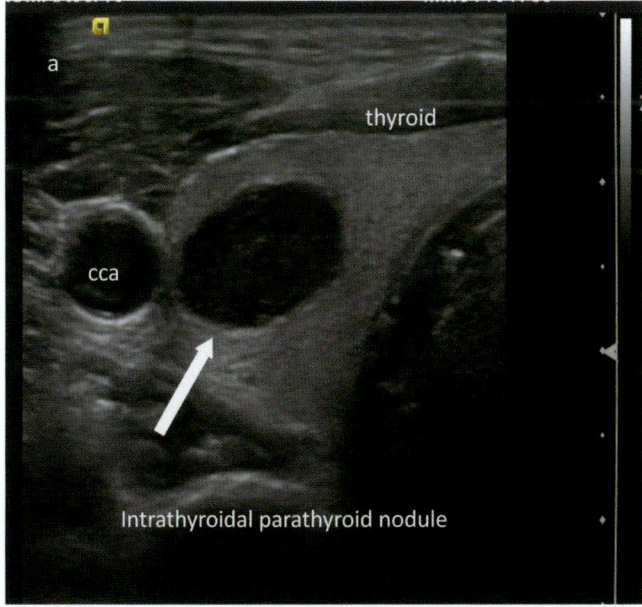
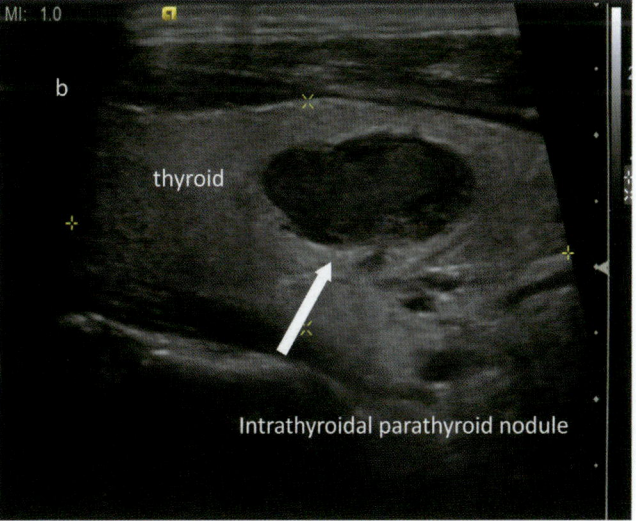

FIGURE 32.21 (a)–(e) Intrathyroidal parathyroid adenoma (serum calcium: 12.6 mg/dl, PTH 1316.0 pg/ml). Ultrasound right thyroid transverse and longitudinal scans showing a 20 mm × 9 mm × 11 mm, well-defined homogenously hypoechoic nodule within the upper pole of right thyroid, which shows arc rim vascularity along with the characteristic polar feeding vessel well demonstrated on Doppler scan. Image of MIBI scan showing retention of tracer at the upper pole of right thyroid. In this patient of PHPT findings are suggestive of intrathyroidal parathyroid adenoma. The patient underwent ipsilateral hemithyroidectomy, PTH values returned within normal limits and subsequent histopathology confirmed parathyroid embedded in the thyroid.

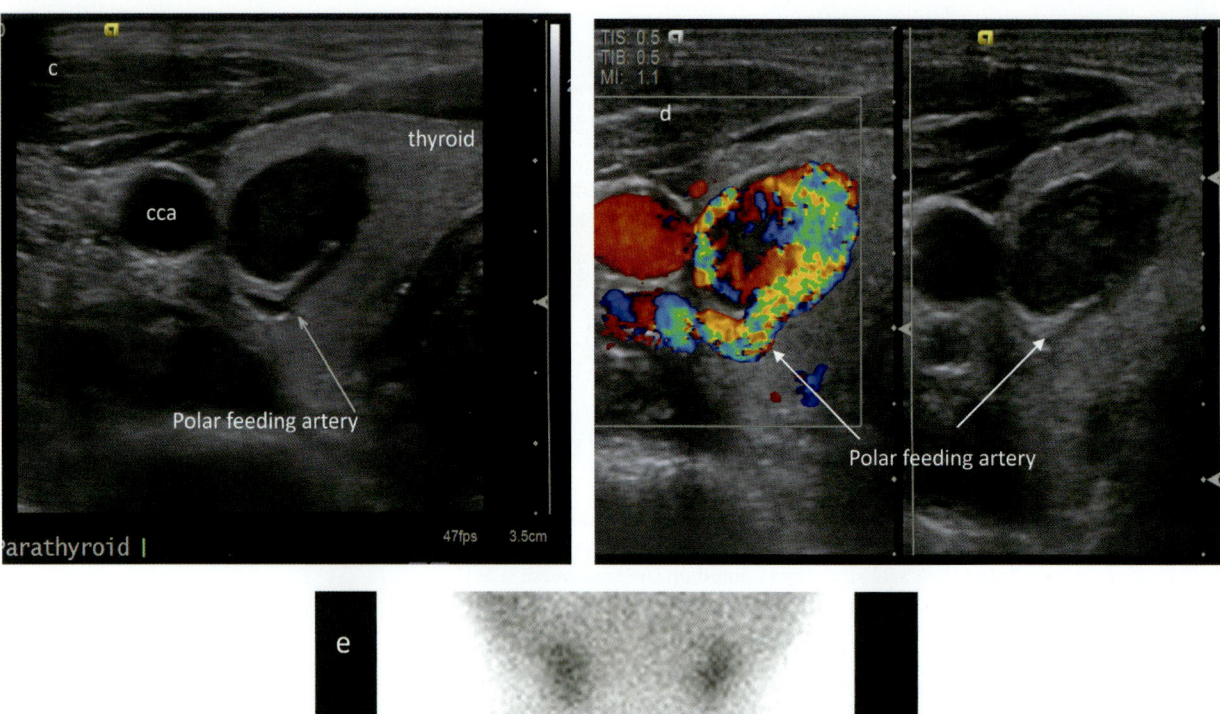

FIGURE 32.21 *(Continued)*

parathyroid adenoma from a thyroid nodule on ultrasound can be a challenge as both can appear as similarly looking hypoechoic nodules. Doppler ultrasound recognition of the characteristic polar feeding vessel and eccentric arc rim vascularity supports the diagnosis of parathyroid adenoma located within the thyroid gland.

The inferior parathyroid glands arise from the endoderm of the third pharyngeal pouch along with the thymus and descent together inferomedially toward the upper mediastinum. The inferior parathyroids separate from the thymus before it enters into the mediastinum and usually localize close to the lower pole of the thyroids. However, any aberration to their separation and descent accounts for the significant anatomical variability in their localization. They could be undescended, overdescended or trapped within the thyroid gland. Ectopic inferior parathyroids may be located as high up as the angle of jaw, in the carotid sheath, or intrathyroidal or overdescended along the thymothymic tract (Figures 32.22–32.24).

Ectopic parathyroids may be found in parapharyngeal or paraesophageal (Figure 32.25), retropharyngeal or retroesophageal locations or may be pushed down the tracheoesophageal groove. They may be located in the mediastinum, where they are usually

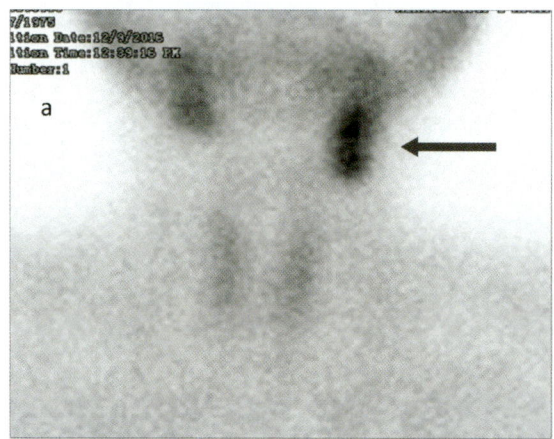

FIGURE 32.22 Ectopic undescended parathyroid. Technetium 99m sestamibi scan-delayed image showing tracer retention at the angle of left mandible in a patient with PHPT suggesting an undescended left parathyroid. Patient underwent parathyroidectomy for the same, which normalized the PTH values, histopathology confirmed parathyroid adenoma.

Localization Studies in Parathyroid Diseases

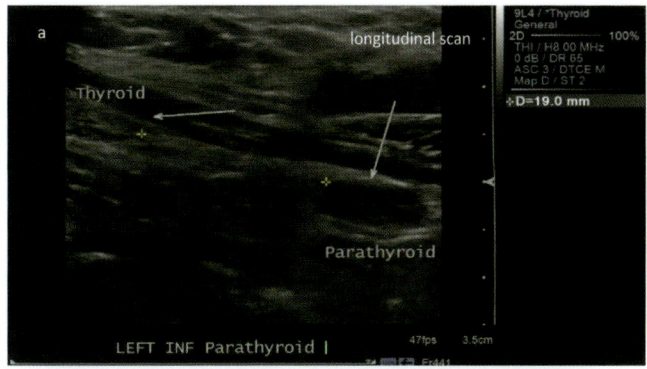
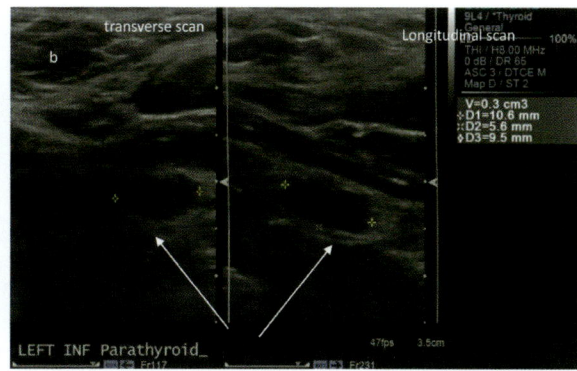
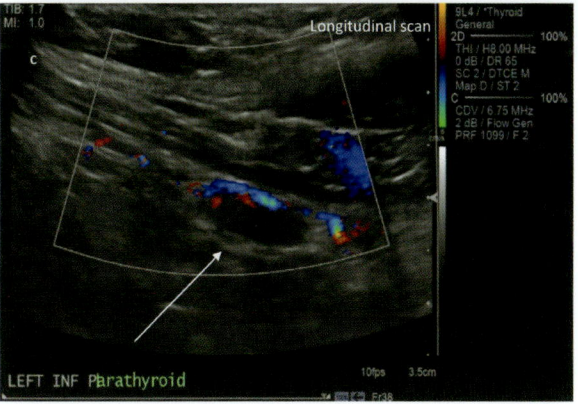

FIGURE 32.23 (a)–(c) Ultrasound neck – longitudinal and transverse ultrasound below the lower pole of left thyroid reveals a typical parathyroid adenoma located approximately 2 cm below the lower pole of left thyroid gland. The nodule measured 10 mm × 9 mm × 5 mm. Note the arc rim vascularity on color Doppler. Findings were confirmed at surgery.

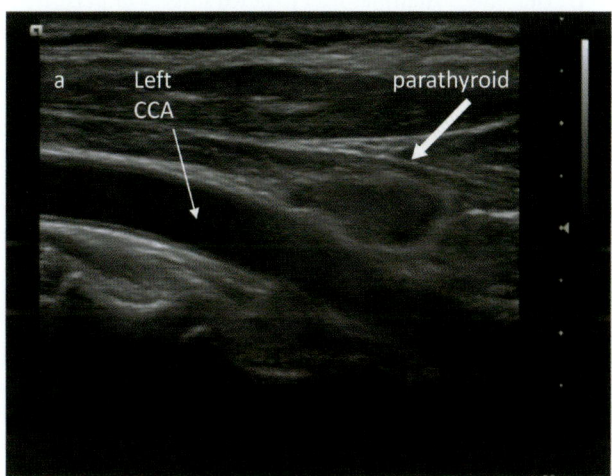
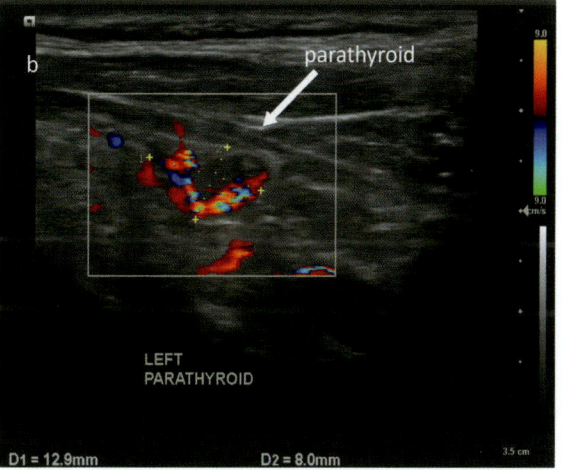
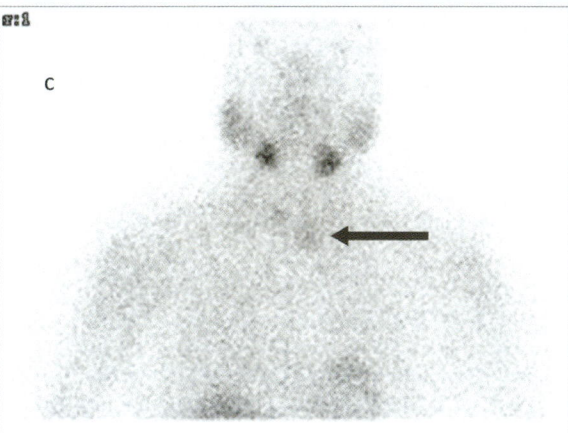

FIGURE 32.24 (a)–(c) A 53-year-old woman with PHPT (serum calcium: 10.3 mg/dl, PTH 100.9 pg/ml). Images (a) and (b) Neck ultrasound with color Doppler showing a small 12 mm × 8 mm hypoechoic nodule suggestive of ectopic parathyroid adenoma (bold arrow) in relation to the carotid sheath. The common carotid artery is marked by thin arrows. Note the characteristic arc rim vascularity on color Doppler. Technetium 99m sestamibi scan in image (c) did not show any appreciable uptake on delayed scan.

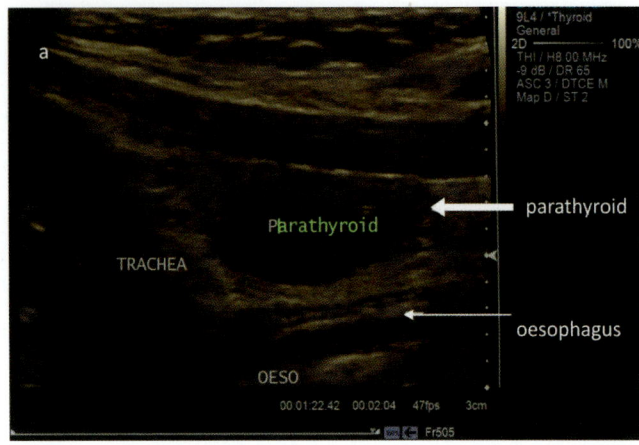 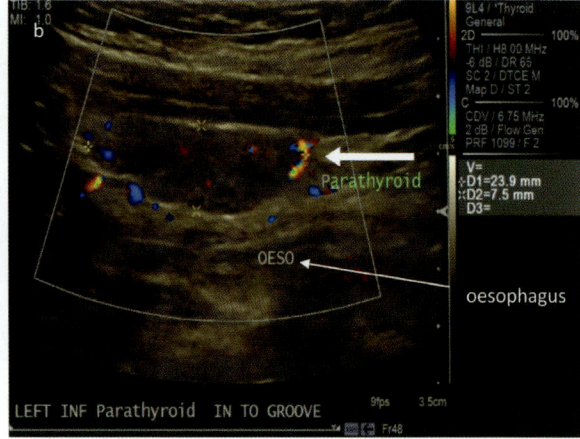

FIGURE 32.25 (a) and (b) Gray scale and color Doppler ultrasound neck in a 55-year-old woman with PHPT (serum calcium 10.2 mg/dl and serum PTH 99 pg/ml) showing an ectopic parathyroid adenoma located in tracheoesophageal groove. Note the esophagus visualized as a luminal structure located posterior to the parathyroid adenoma.

found in the anterior mediastinum (Figure 32.26) just below the manubriosternal junction [27,28]. Further imaging by CECT is required to evaluate deeper and posteriorly located nodules and for those in the mediastinum where ultrasound may have limited access.

The parathyroid glands show contralateral symmetry of location, with superior parathyroid glands in 80% cases, and inferior parathyroids in only 70% cases.

The superior and inferior parathyroid gland nomenclature is based on the embryologic origin of the parathyroid and not by their level of location in the neck. The inferior parathyroid gland may be located at the same or higher level than the superior parathyroid (in case of undescended ectopic inferior parathyroids).

Supernumerary parathyroids

Supernumerary parathyroids [29] are very rare and have been reported in some series to be up to 12.2% in cases of MEN type 1 (MEN1) syndromes. They may lead to failed surgery or persistent HPT.

Four-dimensional computed tomography (4D-CT)

4D-CT is valuable in preoperative localization of both eutopic and ectopic locations, especially those beyond the reach of ultrasound as for the ectopic parathyroid nodules located in the mediastinum. 4D-CT [30,31] provides superior spatial resolution and has the ability to evaluate contrast enhancement patterns when compared to other imaging modalities such as nuclear scintigraphy or ultrasound. The protocol for parathyroid localizations involves scanning in four phases – plain, arterial, venous and delayed phases. The characteristic contrast pattern of a parathyroid adenoma is low attenuation on the non-contrast-enhanced images, peak enhancement on the arterial phase and washout of contrast material from the arterial to delayed phase (Figures 32.27(a) and (b) and 32.28(a)–(d)). CT for parathyroids is often used as a second-line investigation or for patients undergoing repeat surgery. It offers a unique combination of detailed cross-sectional imaging and basic perfusion information. After axial acquisition, coronal and sagittal reformations are made. 4D-CT accurately localizes single-gland adenomas in more than 90% of cases and shows a high specificity for the detection of multiglandular disease.

Multiglandular disease

HPT is most commonly caused by a single-glandular disease in about 85% cases. Incidence of multiglandular disease varies from being sporadic to familial cases and is in the range of

FIGURE 32.26 Mediastinal parathyroid: Tc 99m sestamibi scan in a PHPT patient showing an area of retention of tracer in the left upper mediastinum (arrow) suggestive of ectopic left over descended parathyroid adenoma.

Localization Studies in Parathyroid Diseases

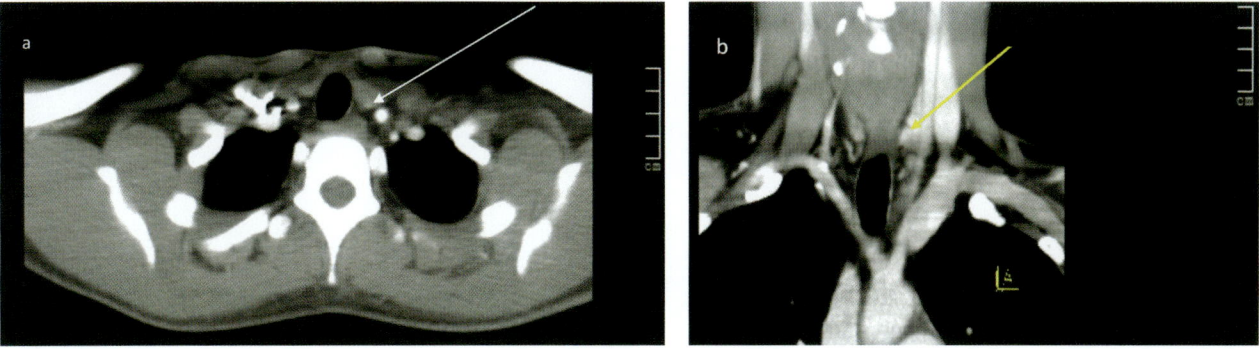

FIGURE 32.27 (a) and (b) Contract enhanced computed tomography: Axial and coronal images showing a lesion posterior to the superior part of left thyroid (arrows), with early arterial enhancement. Patient underwent parathyroidectomy and subsequent histopathology confirmed parathyroid adenoma.

7–23% [32,33]. Patients with multiglandular disease may have a double adenoma or hyperplasia of three or all four parathyroid glands. Whilst PHPT caused by single-glandular disease can be treated by focused parathyroidectomy, multiglandular disease requires bilateral neck exploration is associated with its increased operative risk and morbidity. Accurate preoperative localization studies help in preoperative patient counseling and surgical planning.

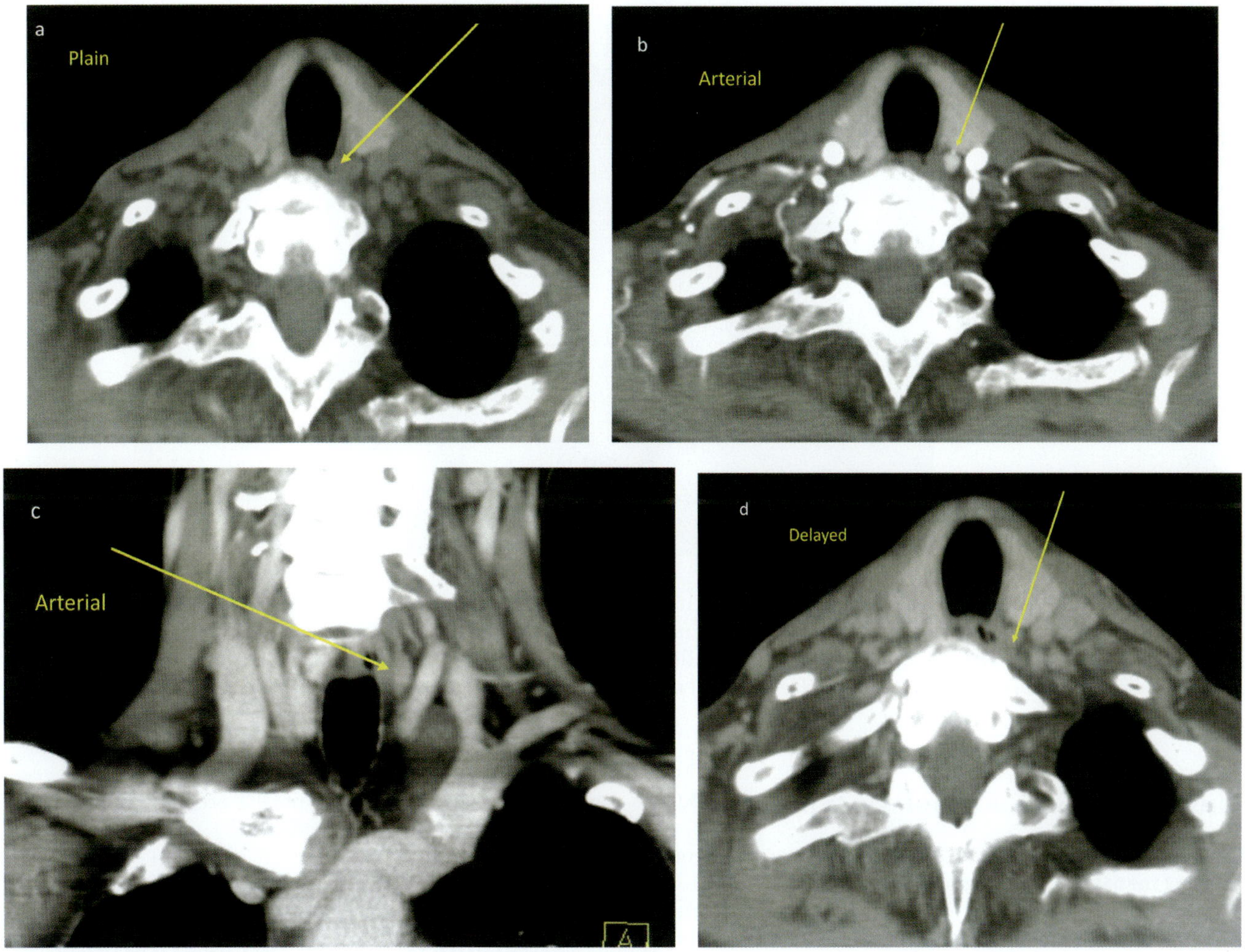

FIGURE 32.28 (a)–(d) Contract enhanced computed tomography – 4D-CT Scan: Axial and coronal images showing a small relatively rounded discrete 5.5 mm arterially enhancing lesion with corresponding decrease in enhancement in the sequential scans seen closely abutting the inferomedial aspect of the left lobe of thyroid suggestive of left inferior parathyroid adenoma. Patient underwent parathyroidectomy and subsequent histopathology confirmed parathyroid adenoma.

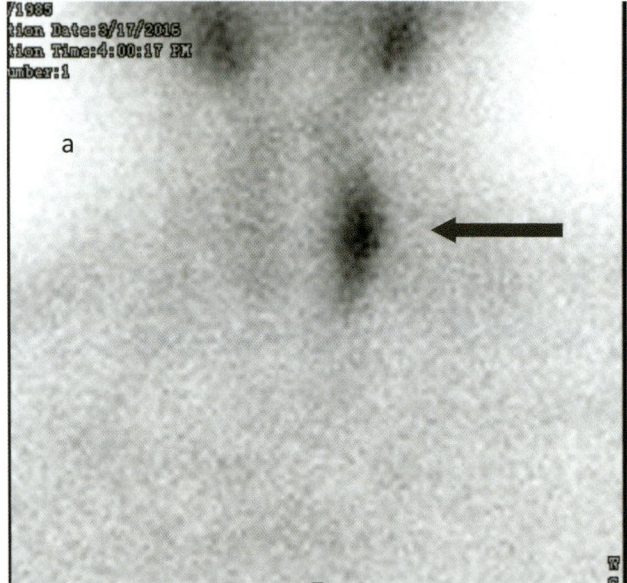
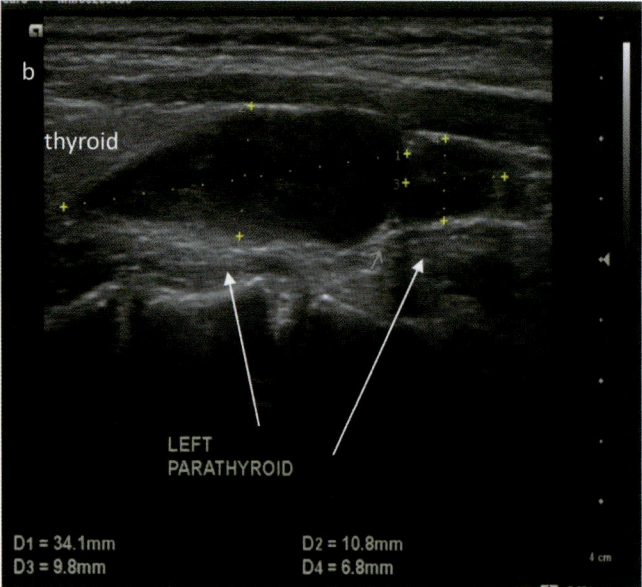
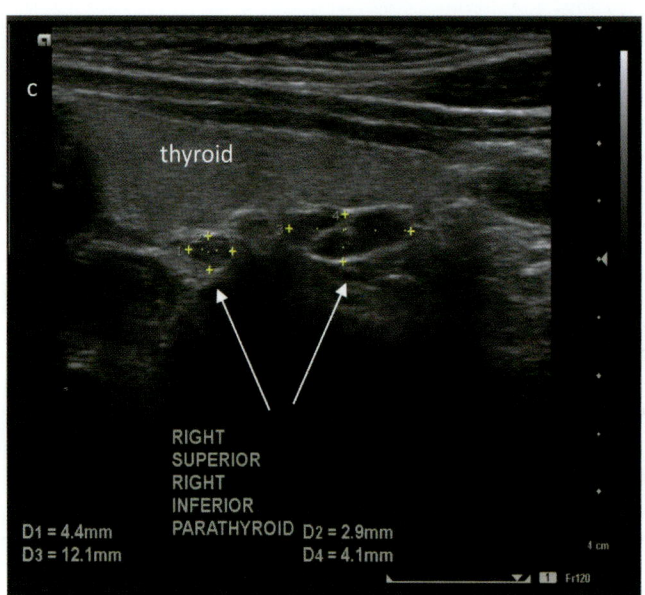

FIGURE 32.29 (a)–(c) A 31-year-old woman with PHPT: Image (a) Tc 99m sestamibi scan – delayed scan showing retention of the tracer in the region of upper pole of left thyroid. Ultrasound neck, longitudinal thyroid view demonstrating four enlarged parathyroid glands (arrows), two larger ones on the left side and two smaller ones on the right side. (Clinically patient had hyperinsulinemic hypoglycemia, pancreatic neuroendocrine tumor and left adrenal nodule (serum calcium: 10.3 mg/dl, PTH 435 pg/ml.)

Multiple endocrine neoplasia type 1 (MEN1)

MEN1, originally known as Wermer syndrome, has tumors involving the parathyroids (Figures 32.29(a)–(c) and 32.30(a)–(d)) and endocrine tissue of pancreas and anterior pituitary gland. MEN1 is called familial when it associated with an affected first degree relative with tumors in any of three glands (parathyroid, pancreas or pituitary) or a first degree relative with a positive MEN1 gene mutation. Genetic testing to detect MEN1 gene mutation is recommended to identify asymptomatic adults in the family and for prenatal diagnosis of MEN1. Age of onset being second or third decade, any case of HPT presenting at young age is highly suspicious of MEN1 syndrome.

Hyperparathyroidism-jaw tumor syndrome (HPT-Jaw tumor syndrome)

HPT-jaw tumor syndrome is an autosomal dominant disorder that occurs due to a mutation in CDC73 gene and presents in late adolescence or early adulthood as hypercalcemia and its symptoms due to primary HPT. PHPT may be due to parathyroid

Localization Studies in Parathyroid Diseases

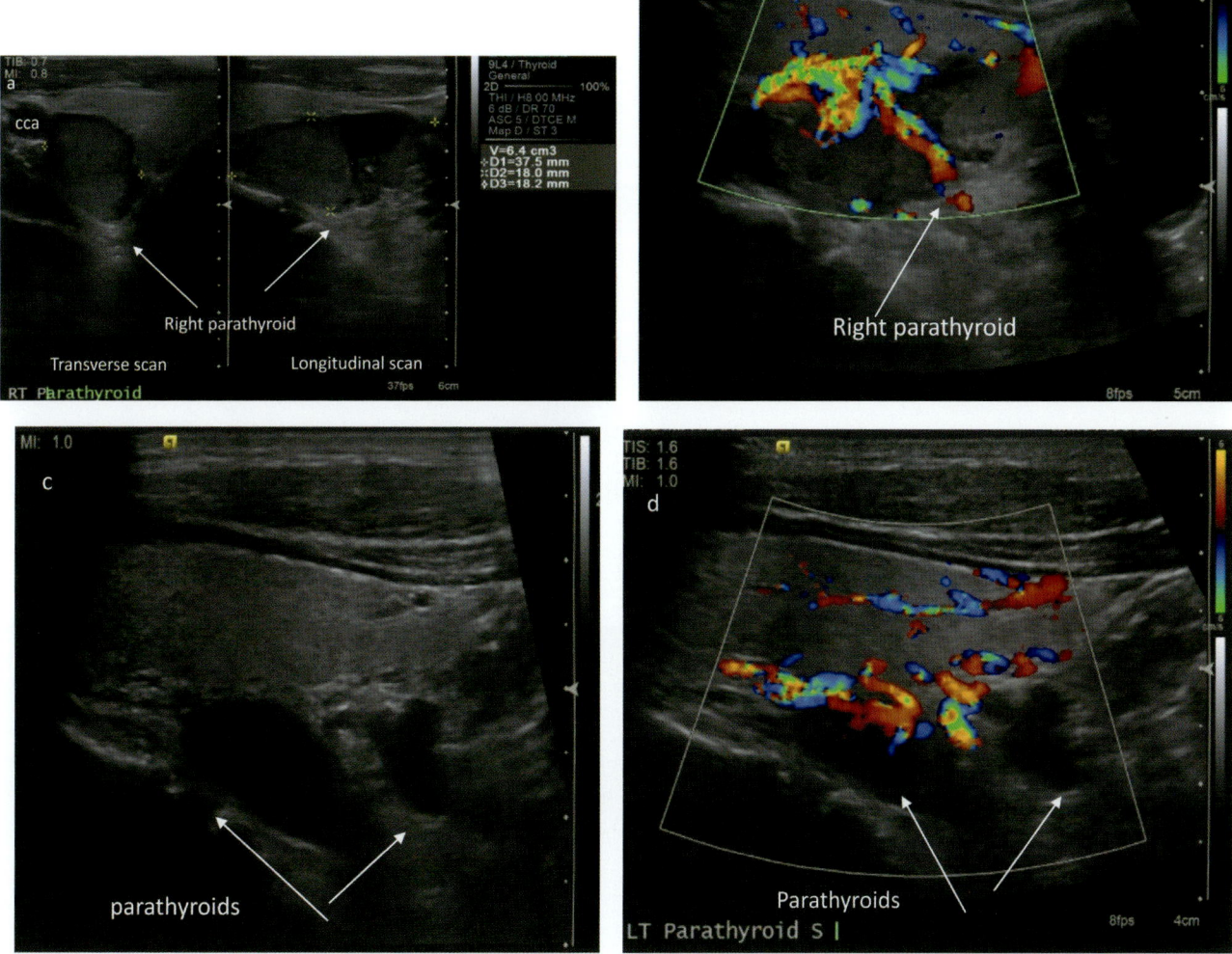

FIGURE 32.30 (a)–(d) Ultrasound longitudinal thyroid view of a patient with MEN1 demonstrates four enlarged parathyroid glands (arrows), two larger ones on the right side and a larger and a smaller on the left side. Note the typicla homogenous hypoechoic appearance of a parathyroid adenoma and the characteristic vascularity on color Doppler.

adenoma or carcinoma. It is associated with benign and malignant tumors, such as non-ossifying fibromas in mandible and maxilla (in 30%–40% cases) and Wilms' tumor (in 20% cases), uterine tumors are seen in females.

Parathyroid hyperplasia

Parathyroid hyperplasia is enlargement of all four parathyroid glands and accounts for approximately 4% cases of primary HPT and about 15% cases of secondary and THPT. Parathyroid hyperplasia may be sporadic or a part of familial syndromes such as MEN1), MEN type 2A (MEN2A) and isolated familial HPT. MEN1 is associated with tumors in the pituitary gland and pancreas. MEN2A is associated with tumors in adrenal and thyroid glands. Sporadic cases of parathyroid hyperplasia occur secondary to other medical diseases commonly being chronic kidney disease and vitamin D deficiency. Clinical presentation and symptoms depend on level and duration of hypercalcemia. Increased association of neurocognitive symptoms with parathyroid hyperplasia has been reported in literature [34]. All the four parathyroid glands are affected; however, enlargement of the glands is asymmetric with usually one or two predominantly enlarged parathyroids. On histopathology there is increase in the proportion of parenchymal cells as compared to stromal cells. Treatment is surgical and usually removal of three and a half glands is recommended. A small part of parathyroid tissue may be sliced and auto transplanted in the forearm, to maintain calcium homeostasis and to allow easy surgical access in cases of recurrence.

Parathyroid carcinoma

Parathyroid carcinoma is one of the rarest known malignancies that may occur sporadically or as a part of a genetic syndromes (MEN). It accounts for approximately 1% of patients with primary HPT. Most parathyroid carcinomas are hormonally functional and hypersecrete PTH and have significantly elevated serum calcium levels. The clinical features of parathyroid carcinoma are caused primarily by the effects of excessive secretion of PTH

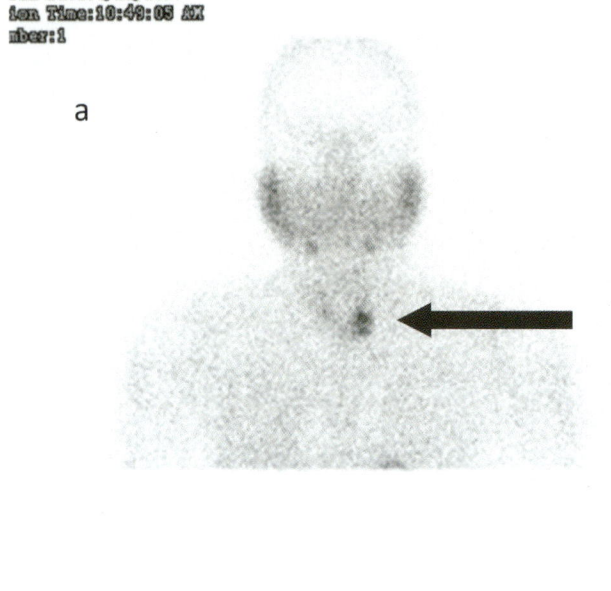
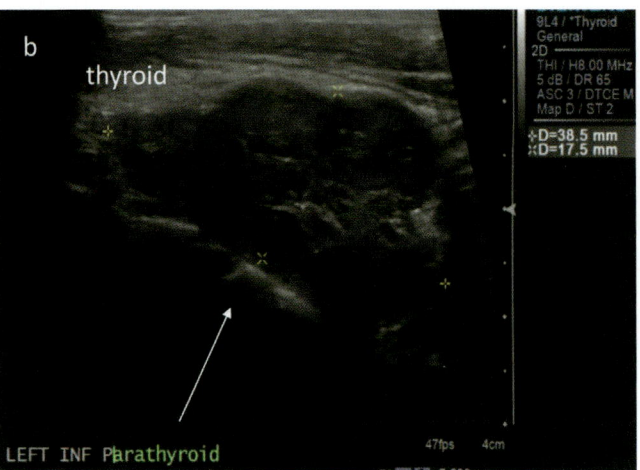
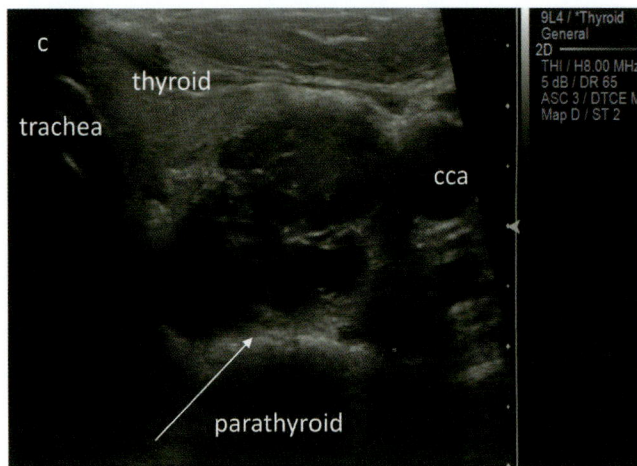
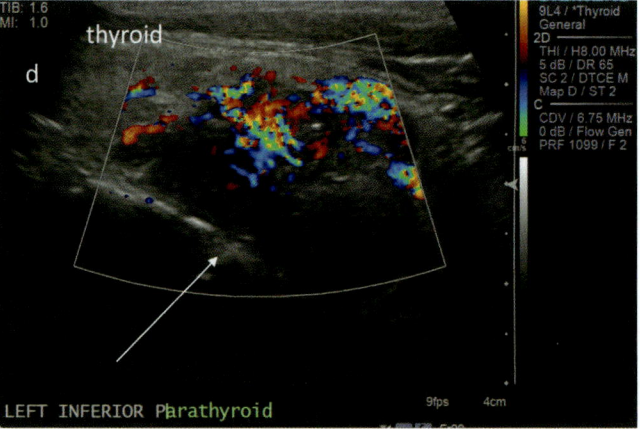

FIGURE 32.31 (a)–(d) Parathyroid carcinoma in a 66-years-old man presenting with PHPT (serum calcium: 10.9 mg/dl, PTH 970 pg/ml). Image (a) MIBI scan showing uptake at the lower pole of left thyroid on delayed scan. Images (b)–(d) ultrasound showing a heterogeneous lobulated hypoechoic mass lesion, measuring 38 × mm 29 mm × 21 mm, located below the lower pole of left thyroid gland, with no distinct margins from the adjacent thyroid. Color Doppler showing heterogenous vascularity. Histopathology showing nuclear polymorphism, with large nucleus and prominent nucleoli. Capsular and vascular is seen. On IHC: Ki67:2%.

by the tumor rather than by the infiltration of vital organs by tumor cells. Serum PTH levels may be three to ten times above the upper limit of normal for the assay employed. Parathyroid carcinoma should be suspected in cases with hypercalcemia of more than 14 mg/dl and with concomitant renal and skeletal disease. Ultrasound features suggestive of parathyroid carcinoma include heterogenous appearance of the nodule with imperceptible margins from the adjacent tissues (Figures 32.31, 32.32 and 32.33). On color Doppler heterogenous vascularity may be seen in the lesion. Recognition of the diagnosis preoperatively helps in appropriate management planning and preoperative patient counseling [35–37].

Parathyroid cyst

Parathyroid cysts are rare and pose a diagnostic challenge on preoperative ultrasound and are often missed [38]. Most cases are initially diagnosed as thyroid cysts and final diagnosis is confirmed at postsurgery histopathology or often discovered only at autopsy. The majority of parathyroid cysts are nonfunctional; however, functioning cysts may lead to HPT. Functioning parathyroid cysts probably originate from cystic degeneration of a parathyroid adenoma. Other theories of origin include persistent embryologic remnant of pharyngeal pouches or enlargement of preexisting microcysts. MIBI scan is often negative in

Localization Studies in Parathyroid Diseases

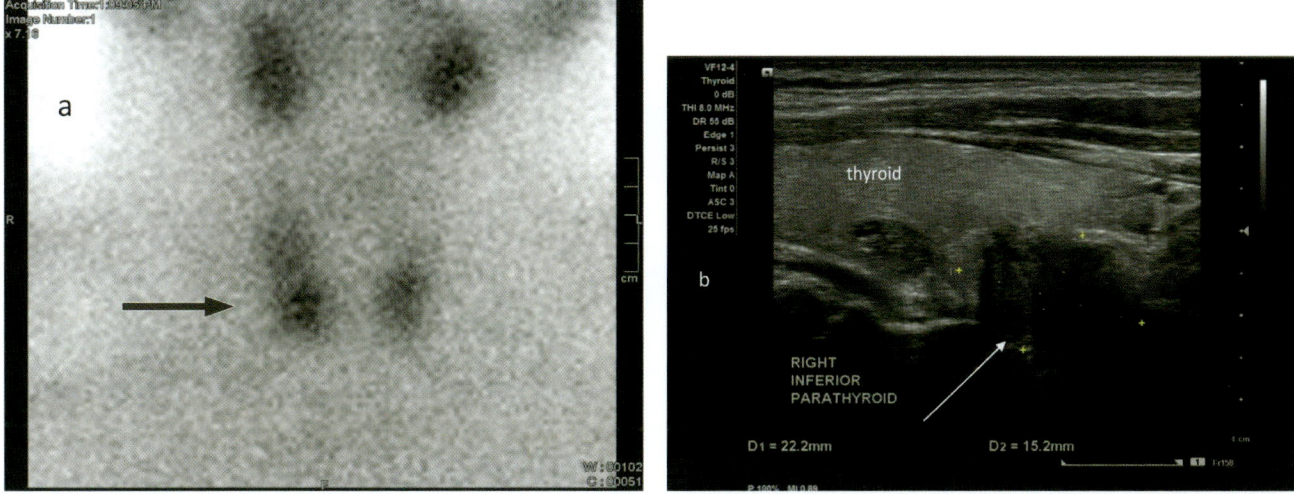

FIGURE 32.32 (a) and (b) Tc 99m sestambi scan and ultrasound longitudinal scan right lobe thyroid Tc 99m sestambi scan on delayed image showing retention of tracer at the lower pole of right thyroid. Ultrasound neck showing n heterogenous right inferior parathyroid with its margins merging with the adjacent thyroid. Postsurgery histopathology showed parathyroid carcinoma.

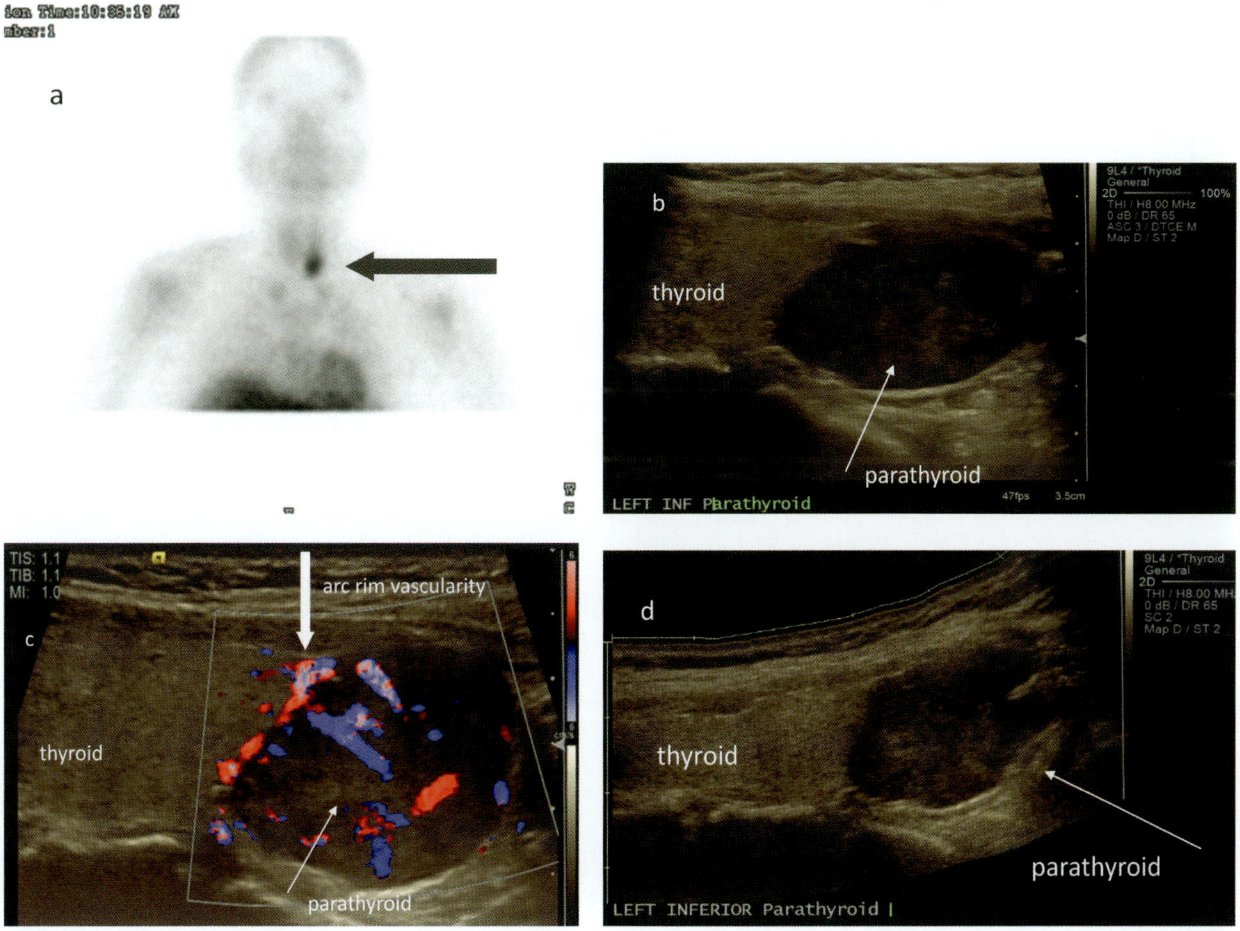

FIGURE 32.33 (a)–(d) PHPT in a 43-year-old woman with serum calcium 13.8 mg/dl and serum PTH 4098 pg/ml. Image (a) Tc 99m sestamibi showing left inferior parathyroid. Images (b)–(d) ultrasound neck showing a corresponding large left inferior parathyroid lesion, slightly heterogenous in echotexture with no clear visualization of the echogenic capsule between the thyroid and parathyroid. Histopathology was reported as suspicious for parathyroid carcinoma.

these cases as there is only minimally compressed parathyroid tissue at the periphery. Adjunct imaging such as ultrasound (Figure 32.34(a)–(f)) or CT can help in establishing a preoperative diagnosis. Needle aspiration of the cyst fluid shows clear watery fluid with elevated serum PTH values.

Parathyroid cysts must be thought of in the differential diagnosis of cystic neck masses and at times may be large and lead to compressive symptoms in the neck region.

Pregnancy with PHPT

Primary HPT is twice more common in women than men. Most patients are older than 45 years; however, about 25% cases are seen in women of child bearing age. Pregnant women have the same incidence of HPT as non-pregnant women; however, the diagnosis is often delayed or unrecognized due to physiological changes in pregnancy [39]. The serum calcium levels are lower in

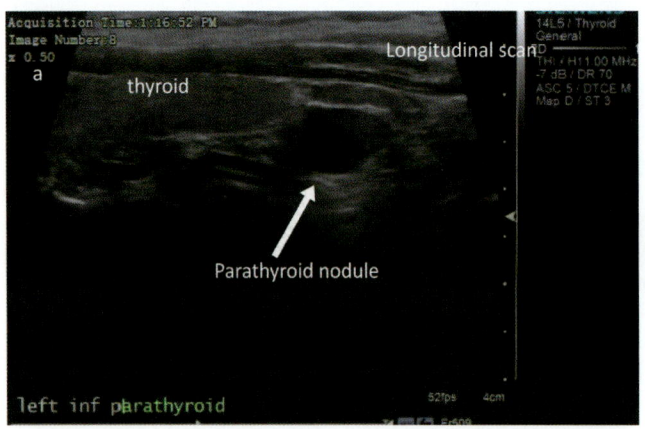
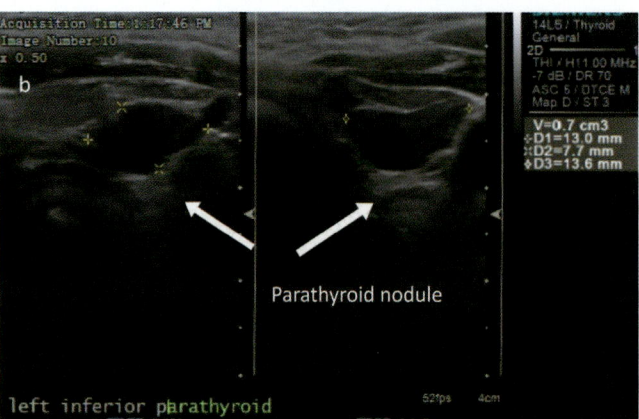
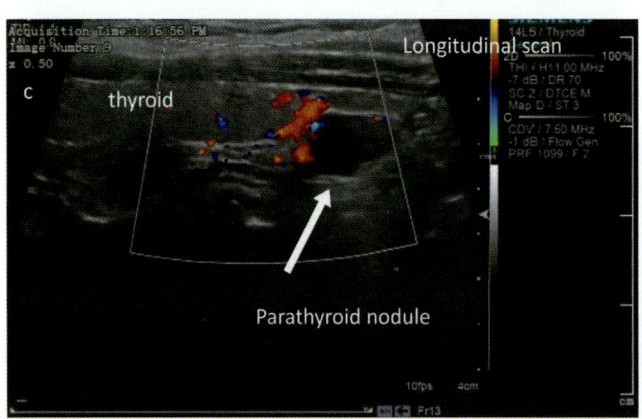
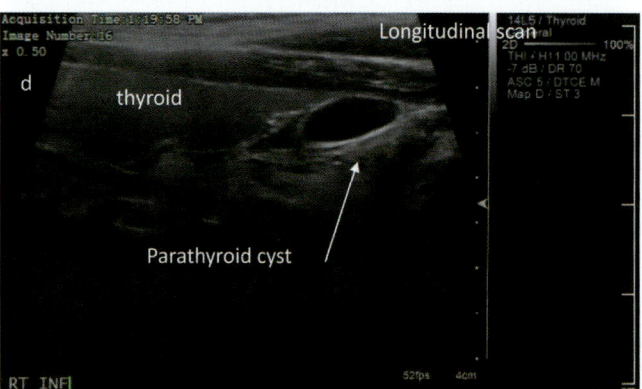
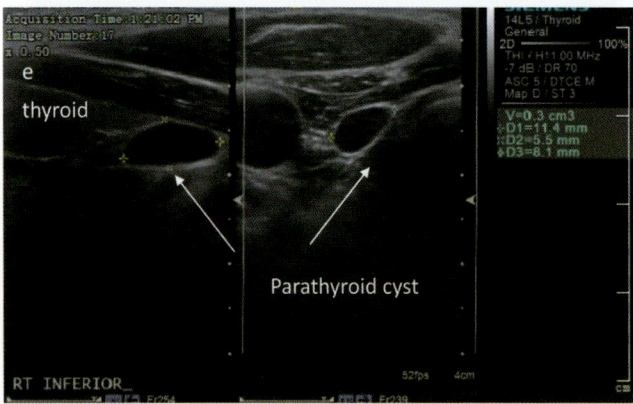
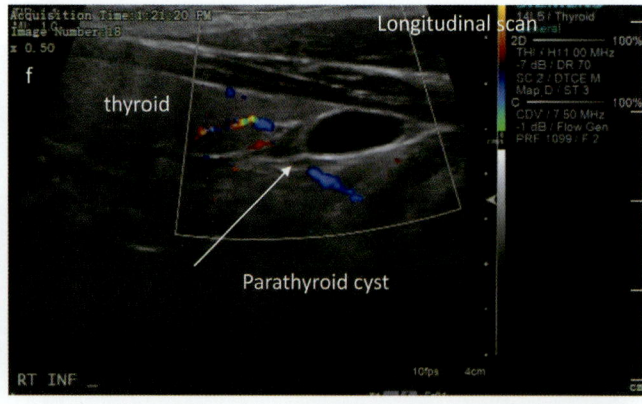

FIGURE 32.34 (a)–(f) A 60-year-old man with PHPT (serum calcium 10.4 mg/dl and serum PTH 140 pg/ml) with concomitant left inferior parathyroid adenoma and right inferior parathyroid cyst. Images (a) and (b) showing the typical hypoechoic tear drop shaped left inferior parathyroid adenoma. Images (c) and (d) of the same patient showing a well-defined clear anechoic cyst with thin echogenic capsular rim, suggestive of cyst. Note the lesion is clearly extrathyroidal (arrows). Postoperative histopathology confirmed the findings.

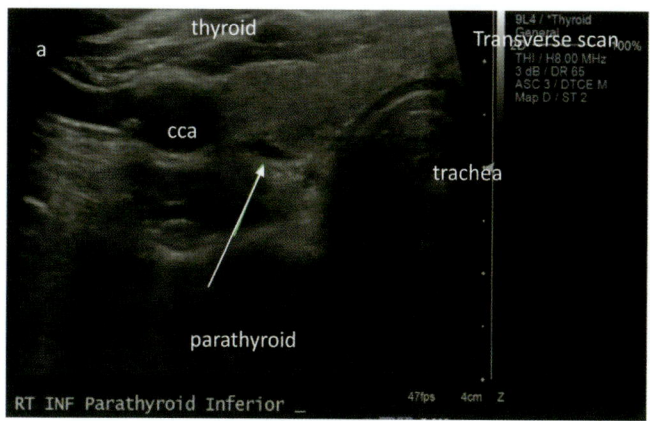
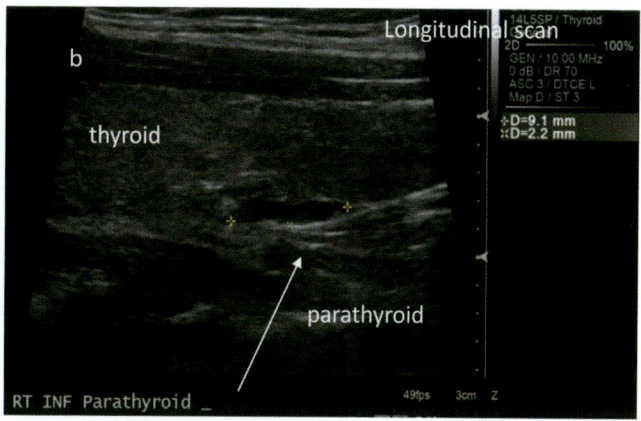
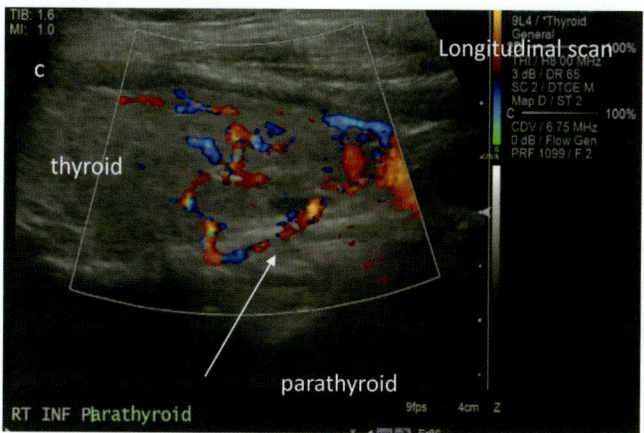

FIGURE 32.35 (a)–(c) A 34-year-old woman G2P1 presented with loss of fetal movements at 27 weeks and subsequently diagnosed as PHPT with pregnancy. Serum calcium 10.9 mg/dl and serum PTH 165 pg/ml. Ultrasound showed a tiny flattened hypoechoic right inferior parathyroid adenoma measuring 9 mm × 2 mm. Patient was taken up for surgery and the corresponding adenoma removed and confirmed at histopathology.

cases of pregnancy with HPT due to the pregnancy pathophysiology. Presenting symptoms and maternal and fetal complications depend on the level of hypercalcemia. Non-specific symptoms of fatigue, nausea and anorexia overlap with pregnancy symptoms. Incidence of preclampsia is reported to be as high as 25% in cases of pregnancy with HPT. Fetal complications include spontaneous abortions, intrauterine growth restriction, low birth weight, preterm delivery, intrauterine fetal demise and neonatal death. Early diagnosis and appropriate timely management is needed to prevent the complications. Since Technetium 99m sestamibi scan is contraindicated in pregnancy, importance of ultrasound in the localization of abnormal parathyroids cannot be overemphasized in this case (Figure 32.35(a)–(c)).

Parathyroid autotransplantation

In cases of MEN1 and 2, refractory HPT and renal failure patients with secondary and THPT, three and a half parathyroidectomy is done and remaining part of the parathyroid is cut into thin 10–20 thin slices or cubes (1-mm thickness), which are inserted into individual muscle pockets and marked with clips for ease of identification for future follow-up [40,41]. The common sites for reimplantation are mid part of sternocleidomastoid, brachioradialis and even subcutaneous tissue of forearm. Implantation into sternocleidomastoid is done to salvage a normal parathyroid removed inadvertently at thyroidectomy. Implantation into brachioradialis muscle or subcutaneous tissues of forearm is chosen for cases of refractory and THPT which can be followed up by venous sampling and ultrasound and reoperated if required, avoiding the complications of cervical re exploration. Imaging follow up of parathyroid autotransplantation is done with MIBI Scintigraphy or ultrasound. In cases of recurrence ultrasound may show enlargement of the implanted parathyroids as an ill-defined hypoechoic area at the site, with or without increased vascularity on color Doppler.

Conclusion

Surgical removal of all the abnormal parathyroid glands is the only definitive management of primary HPT and is also employed in the management of secondary and THPT. The success of surgery is largely dependent on accurate preoperative localization of all the abnormal parathyroid nodules. Minimally invasive surgery has emerged as the preferred surgical technique due to the decrease in possible complications when compared with bilateral neck exploration for the removal of hyperfunctioning parathyroid glands. Preoperative localization has become of utmost importance for performing minimally invasive surgery.

References

1. Pradeep PV, Jayashree B, Mishra Anjali, Mishra SK. Systematic review of primary hyperparathyroidism in India: The past, present, and the future trends. Int J Endocrinol. 2011;2011:921814.
2. Kollars J, Zarroug AE, van Heerden J, Lteif A, Stavlo P, Suarez L, Moir C, Ishitani M, Rodeberg D. Primary hyperparathyroidism in pediatric patients. Pediatrics. 2005 Apr;115(4):974–980.
3. Roizen J, Levine MA. Primary hyperparathyroidism in children and adolescents. J Chin Med Assoc. 2012;75(9):425–434.
4. Goldstein DA. Serum calcium. In: HK Walker, WD Hall and JW Hurst, eds. Clinical Methods: The History, Physical, and Laboratory Examinations. 3rd ed. Boston, MA: Butterworths; 1990. Chapter 143. Available from: https://www.ncbi.nlm.nih.gov/books/NBK250/.
5. Thier M, Daudi S, Bergenfelz A, Almquist M. Predictors of multiglandular disease in primary hyperparathyroidism. Langenbecks Arch Surg. 2018;403(1):103–109.
6. Policeni BA, Smoker WR, Reede DL. Anatomy and embryology of the thyroid and parathyroid glands. Semin Ultrasound CT MR. 2012 Apr;33(2):104–114.
7. Sadowski SM, Vidal Fortuny J, Triponez F. A reappraisal of vascular anatomy of the parathyroid gland based on fluorescence techniques. Gland Surg. 2017;6(Suppl 1):S30–S37.
8. Phitayakorn R, McHenry CR. Incidence and location of ectopic abnormal parathyroid glands. Am J Surg. 2006 Mar;191(3):418–423.
9. Singhal AA, Baijal SS, Sarin D, Arora SK, Mithal A, Khuchay SM. Ectopic undescended left parathyroid adenoma: Diagnosed on ultrasound. J Head Neck Physicians Surg. 2017;5:44–47.
10. Mazeh H, Kouniavsky G, Schneider DF, Makris KI, Sippel RS, Dackiw AP, Chen H, Zeiger MA. Intrathyroidal parathyroid glands: Small, but mighty (a Napoleon phenomenon). Surgery. 2012 Dec;152(6):1193–1200.
11. Singhal AA, Baijal SS, Sarin D, Arora SK, Mithal A, Gautam D, Sharma N. Intrathyroidal parathyroid adenoma in primary hyperparathyroidism: Are we overdiagnosing? Case series and learning outcomes. J Head Neck Physicians Surg. 2018;6:48–53.
12. d'Alessandro AF, Montenegro FL, Brandão LG, Lourenço DM Jr, Toledo Sde A, Cordeiro AC. Supernumerary parathyroid glands in hyperparathyroidism associated with multiple endocrine neoplasia type 1. Rev Assoc Med Bras (1992). 2012 May-Jun;58(3):323–327.
13. Mohebati A, Shaha AR. Imaging techniques in parathyroid surgery for primary hyperparathyroidism. Am J Otolaryngol. 2012;33(4):457–468.
14. Hindié E, Ugur O, Fuster D, et al. 2009 EANM parathyroid guidelines. Eur J Nucl Med Mol Imaging. 2009;36:1201–1216.
15. Nguyen BD. Parathyroid imaging with Tc-99m sestamibi planar and SPECT scintigraphy. RadioGraphics. 1999;19:601–614.
16. McHenry CR, Lee K, Saadey J, Neumann DR, Esselstyn CB Jr. Parathyroid localization with technetium-99m-sestamibi: A prospective evaluation. J Am Coll Surg. 1996;183:25–30.
17. Sun SS, Shiau YC, Lin CC, Kao A, Lee CC. Correlation between P-glycoprotein (P-gp) expression in parathyroid and Tc-99m MIBI parathyroid image findings. Nucl Med Biol. 2001;28:929–933.
18. Tublin ME, Pryma DA, Yim JH, et al. Localization of parathyroid adenomas by sonography and technetium Tc 99m sestamibi single-photon emission computed tomography before minimally invasive parathyroidectomy: Are both studies really needed? J Ultrasound Med. 2009;28:183–190.
19. Shi Lam and Brian Hung-Hin Lang (May 21st 2014). A Review of the Pathogenesis and Management of Multinodular Goiter, Thyroid Disorders – Focus on Hyperthyroidism, Gonzalo Diaz Soto, IntechOpen, DOI: 10.5772/57547.
20. Wolf RJ, Cronan JJ, Monchik JM. Color Doppler sonography: An adjunctive technique in assessment of parathyroid adenomas. J Ultrasound Med. 1994;13(4):303–308.
21. Mohammadi A, Moloudi F, Ghasemi-Rad M. Preoperative localization of parathyroid lesion: Diagnostic usefulness of color Doppler ultrasonography. Int J Clin Exp Med. 2012;5(1):80–86.
22. Varsamidis K, Varsamidou E, Mavropoulos G. Color Doppler sonography in the detection of parathyroid adenomas. Head Neck. 1999;21(7):648–651.
23. Okabe M, Graham A. The origin of the parathyroid gland. Proc Natl Acad Sci USA. 2004;101(51):17716–17719.
24. Gilmour JR. The embryology of the parathyroid glands, the thymus and certain associated rudiments. J Pathol Bacteriol. 1937;45:507–522.
25. Roy M, Mazeh H, Chen H, Sippel RS. Incidence and localization of ectopic parathyroid adenomas in previously unexplored patients. World J Surg. 2013;37(1):102–106.
26. Noussios G, Anagnostis P, Natsis K. Ectopic parathyroid glands and their anatomical, clinical, and surgical implications. Exp Clin Endocrinol Diabetes. 2012;120:604–610.
27. Hu J, Ngiam K, Parameswaran R. Mediastinal parathyroid adenomas and their surgical implications. Ann R Coll Surg Engl. 2015;97(4):259–261.
28. Elhelf IAS, Kademian JC, Moritani T, Capizzano AE, Policeni B, Maley J. Ectopic mediastinal parathyroid adenoma localized with four-dimensional CT: A case report. Radiol Case Rep. 2017;12(2):247–250.
29. Pattou FN, et al. Supernumerary parathyroid glands: Frequency and surgical significance in treatment of renal hyperparathyroidism. World J Surg. 2000;24:1330–1334.
30. Bann DV, Zacharia T, Goldenberg D, Goyal N. Parathyroid localization using 4D-computed tomography. Ear Nose Throat J. 2015;94(4–5):E55–E57.
31. Chazen JL, Gupta A, Dunning A, Phillips CD. Diagnostic accuracy of 4D-CT for parathyroid adenomas and hyperplasia. Am J Neuroradiol. 2012 Mar;33(3):429–433.
32. Barczyński M, Bränström R, Dionigi G, Mihai R. Sporadic multiple parathyroid gland disease – a consensus report of the European Society of Endocrine Surgeons (ESES). Langenbecks Arch Surg. 2015 Dec;400(8):887–905.
33. Bergenfelz A, Almquist M. Predictors of multiglandular disease in primary hyperparathyroidism. Langenbecks Arch Surg. 2018;403(1):103–109.
34. Repplinger D, Schaefer S, Chen H, Sippel RS. Neurocognitive dysfunction: A predictor of parathyroid hyperplasia. Surgery. 2009;146(6):1138–1143.
35. Kwon JH, Kim EK, Lee HS, Moon HJ, Kwak JY. Neck ultrasonography as preoperative localization of primary hyperparathyroidism with an additional role of detecting thyroid malignancy. Eur J Radiol. 2013;82(1):e17–e21.
36. Shane Elizabeth. Parathyroid carcinoma. J Clin Endocrinol Metab. 2001 Feb;86(2):485–493.
37. Sharretts JM, Kebebew E, Simonds WF. Parathyroid cancer. Semin Oncol. 2010;37(6):580–590.
38. Guner A, Karyagar S, Ozkan O, Kece C, Reis E. Parathyroid cyst: The forgotten diagnosis of a neck mass. J Surg Case Rep. 2011;2011(8):4.
39. Som M, Stroup JS. Primary hyperparathyroidism and pregnancy. Proc (Bayl Univ Med Cent). 2011;24(3):220–223.
40. Hicks G, George R, Sywak M. Short and long-term impact of parathyroid autotransplantation on parathyroid function after total thyroidectomy. Gland Surg. 2017;6(Suppl 1):S75–S85.
41. Wells SA Jr, Gunnells JC, Shelburne JD, Schneider AB, Sherwood LM. Transplantation of the parathyroid glands in man: Clinical indications and results. Surgery. 1975 Jul;78(1):34–44.

33

FAMILIAL HYPERPARATHYROIDISM

S. Dhalapathy and Smitha Rao

Introduction

Primary hyperparathyroidism (PHPT) is a commonly identified cause of hypercalcemia. They could be sporadic or familial. Familial causes can account for 5%–50% of cases: FHH, multiple endocrine neoplasia (MEN-1, MEN-2A, MEN-4), autosomal dominant moderate hyperparathyroidism (ADMH) or familial isolated hyperparathyroidism (FIHP), hyperparathyroidism jaw-tumor (HPT-JT) syndrome, neonatal severe hyperparathyroidism (NSHPT). Various germline mutations like MEN1, RET, CaSR, GNA11, CDKIs, CDC73/HRPT2, AP2S1 have been identified to be pathogenic in the recent times. Hereditary hyperparathyroidism generally presents with multiglandular parathyroid disease in contrast to a solitary parathyroid adenoma in sporadic disease. Severity of each familial condition has wide variation due to variable penetrance mandating distinct prognosis and treatment strategies. Genetic subtyping plays an integral role in treatment decision-making with the advent of molecular genetics.

Goldman and Smyth in 1936 were the first ones to report a brother and a sister with non-MEN familial HPT (NMFH). Subsequently, many cases have been reported. Hillman et al. described NSHPT in two siblings in 1964. Similar to the classification of medullary thyroid cancer, HPT can be classified into four types: (1) familial HPT with MEN 1 and 2; (2) NMFH or familial isolated HPT (FIHP); (3) NMFH associated with jaw tumor (HPT-JT) syndrome; and (4) sporadic HPT. As NMFH is relatively uncommon, these patients are included in the series of patients with familial HPT with MEN or benign familial hypocalciuric hypercalcemia (BFHH). The differences between sporadic and hereditary PHPT are given in Table 33.1.

Familial hyperparathyroidism (FHPT) is believed to be due to various genetic mutations, but, overall, they represent a minority in incidence.

Two germline mutations including in the tumor suppressor genes *MEN1* (menin) with loss of heterozygosity and *CDC73* (formerly *HRPT2*) with another second somatic cell mutation have increased possibility of having parathyroid tumors. Sporadic adenomas and carcinomas are caused due to the somatic mutations in the same genes. Familial parathyroid adenomas have an autosomal dominant inheritance and most commonly caused by *MEN1* mutation. Autosomal dominant FHPT tumor-jaw syndrome (HPT-JT), parathyroid carcinomas and familial isolated hyperparathyroidism are due to *CDC73* gene germline mutations. HPT-JT with autosomal dominant inheritance consists of parathyroid adenomas with PHPT (or carcinomas), maxillary or mandibular fibro osseous tumors and renal tumors. MEN2A (associated with parathyroid adenomas) and various other endocrine syndromes are caused due to RET mutations in the proto-oncogene. Although *CDKN1B* mutations are responsible for rare cases of MEN4, Murk Jansen metaphyseal chondrodysplasias, a variety of skeletal dysplasia, are caused by mutations in the parathyroid hormone receptor *PTH1R*. (1, 2)

Multiple endocrine neoplasia type 1

Clinical features

Hereditary hyperparathyroidism is most commonly caused by MEN 1 mutation. PHPT is the first manifestation of MEN1 in 90% patients and is also the most common manifestation in MEN1 (95%). Mild hypercalcemia is seen usually irrespective of gender predilection with an average age of onset of 20 years in familial cases. Hence, they have to undergo timely investigation and follow-up as a routine to pick up the onset of symptoms and avoid complications in MEN1. Timely intervention involves total parathyroidectomy (TPTX) whenever needed. Most common associated tumors include pancreatic islet cell tumors including recurrent peptic ulceration of the Zollinger-Ellison syndrome and gastrinomas. These gastrinomas account for one of the major causes of morbidity and mortality in MEN1. Other frequent associations could be insulinomas and asymptomatic pancreatic polypeptidomas; rarely there could be VIPomas and glucagonomas. Most commonly associated pituitary tumors include seen in one-third of MEN1 cases. Corticotropinomas, somatotropinomas and nonfunctioning pituitary tumors are other associations including adrenocortical carcinoma, thyroid follicular carcinoma, carcinoids, collagenomas, lipomas and facial angiofibromas.

Genetics

MEN1-associated tumors are implicated to be due to loss of heterozygosity in *MEN1 gene. It is* located by analysis on the chromosome 11q13 in various diagnosed families. Tumor initiation in *MEN1 is* postulated to be due to Knudson two-hit model in this tumor suppressor gene. Positional cloning modality in linkage analysis has identified *MEN1* gene and various somatic and germline mutations. Parathyroid adenoma, anterior pituitary tumors, gastrinoma, insulinoma and lung carcinoid are known to occur due to these somatic mutations. Tumor is due to loss of alleles in menin gene. New mutations not involving the coding region is seen in 25% of MEN1 patients and de novo mutations occur in 10% of the *MEN1* cases. (3, 4)

Sporadic parathyroid adenomas are frequently reported to have LOH and somatic *MEN1* mutations in 40% of cases. There are a few cases known to have germline *MEN1* mutations as causes of sporadic parathyroid adenomas. FIHP is also seen with *MEN1* mutations in some cases. Parathyroid carcinomas are rarely part of MEN1 but have been reported.

TPTX with removal of all four glands and autologous parathyroid tissue graft or subtotal parathyroidectomy (SPTX) with removal of at least three or three-and-half glands plus transcervical thymectomy is considered the treatment of choice in MEN1-related PHPT. The choice of surgery in these cases is debatable

TABLE 33.1: Differences Between Sporadic and Hereditary PHPT

	Sporadic	Hereditary PHPT
Age	Any	Young (<45 years)
Sex	Postmenopausal women	Equal M:F
Family history	–	+
Glandular involvement	Single gland	Multiglandular
Mutation	–	+/Denovo
Nature	Homogenous	Heterogenous
Preoperative localization	+by ultrasound, SESTAMIBI	–
Treatment	Focused approach/ (MIS) Minimally invasive surgery	4 gland exploration
Recurrence/Persistence	–	Very high
Carcinoma incidence	<1%	15% with CDC73/ HRPT2 mutation
Prognosis	Good	Slightly worse
Monitoring	Not required	Lifelong, genetic counseling

and various among various surgeons. Calcimimetics constitute the medical management recurrent PHPT and/or in those cases with surgical contraindications. (5, 6)

Menin

Menin gene contains 610 amino acids and has nuclear location. Menin gene loss by various genetic mechanisms like TGF Beta signaling pathway loss and epigenetic mechanisms have been traced to be the source of tumorigenesis but not well understood. It acts as an oncogene in the pathogenesis of leukemias in MLL fusion proteins as along with being a tumor suppressor gene. The crystal structures for menin have been identified in human being as well as the sea anemone (*Nematostella vectensis*). The tumorigenic pathway and its association with menin seem to be beyond just endocrine control. (7)

Multiple endocrine neoplasia Type 2A

Clinical features
MEN2A is type of MEN2 which is most commonly seen. MEN2A consists of medullary thyroid carcinoma as the most common manifestation accounting for 95% of patients, while pheochromocytoma and hyperparathyroidism are seen in 50% and 20% patients. respectively. Multiple parathyroid adenomas or parathyroid hyperplasia could be responsible for PHPT. The reasons for the presence of parathyroid disease in most cases are known to be multiglandular disease seen during surgery in MEN2A cases and calcium infusion test showing incomplete response of suppression of PTH. MEN 2A has milder hypocalcemia as compared to MEN 1 cases, and hence, a less aggressive approach in surgery is advisable.

Genetics
Rearranged during transfection (*RET*) proto-oncogene is responsible for *MEN2*. This tyrosine kinase receptor containing MEN2 gene is mapped to chromosome 10q11.2. This receptor contains two domains – cysteine-rich, cadherin-like extracellular and an intracellular tyrosine kinase domain.

All variants of MEN2 show RET point mutations. Any one of these five codons (609, 611, 618, 620 in exon 10 and 634 in exon 11) containing cysteine show missense mutations of recurring type, which cause variable receptor function responsible for MEN2A. Majority (85%) of MEN2A consists of the *RET* mutation in codon 634 (p.Cys634Arg). (8, 9)

Nonfamilial hyperparathyroidism shows the involvement of RET gene. M918T mutation is the chief RET mutation predominantly seen in MEN2B – are known to be causative of pheochromocytomas and some sporadic medullary thyroid carcinomas. Sporadic parathyroid tumors surprisingly fail to show these mutations. Glial cell–derived neurotrophic factor mutations which is a ligand in the RET receptor have no role in parathyroid adenomas or MEN2 neoplasms.

PHPT in the form of adenoma/hyperplasia may be rarely diagnosed during thyroidectomy but mostly diagnosed much later after thyroid surgery in MEN2A (~15 years) patients. SPTX or TPTX with parathyroid forearm autograft could be offered as treatment for all the enlarged parathyroid glands (single/multiglandular). Those patients who undergo SPTX without auto transplant are scheduled for a routine annual screening with calcium and parathormone levels. Patients with limited survival, with contraindications to surgery or recurrent/persistent PHPT after 1 or more prior surgeries should be offered medical treatment to reduced morbidity due to high calcium levels.

Multiple endocrine neoplasia type 4

Few (10%) MEN1 patients might have other mutations in contrary to presence of MEN1 gene mutations. This category is designated as MEN 4 encoding *CDNK1B* gene which has 196 amino acids. Various other families have also been identified with other CDKI mutations of p15, p18, 021 and p27 as well. In mutation-negative MEN1 cases, such mutations are uncommon (~2%). MEN4 has to be differentiated MEN1, MEN2A and MEN2B (older MEN3) as to MEN1 with the classical CDKN1B mutation. MEN4 compulsorily has parathyroid involvement but other presentations can be variable. Sporadic hyperparathyroidism as *CDKN1B* mutations including germline mutations in a few cases. This is evidence enough that *CDKN1B* gene is susceptible to various mutations. Parathyroid adenomas and carcinomas show a moderate and significant reduction in p 27 levels, respectively. (10)

Hyperparathyroidism-jaw tumor syndrome

Clinical spectrum
Recurrent parathyroid tumors, fibrous ossifying maxillary and mandibular tumors, uterine, renal and other tumors are characteristic of HPT-JT syndrome with early parathyroid involvement. It is a familial endocrine disorder with multisystem involvement and is inherited in an autosomal dominant fashion. It has been found to have variable penetrance with severe hypercalcemia in childhood and adolescence, few cases with metabolic bone disease of severe degree and few with risk of hypercalcemic crisis. Bone disease could lead to pathological fractures and even death. Unlike other inherited diseases with multiglandular disease, this syndrome has a characteristic involvement of a single gland which is enlarged and cystic. Though the calcium levels normalize after surgery, patients could present with recurrences due to double adenomas. HPT-JT is known to have much higher number (>15%) of parathyroid carcinoma as compared to MEN or sporadic PHPT. X-rays give a classic cystic appearance of fibro osseous jaw tumors. These are maxillary and mandibular tumors with an independent natural history not

associated with hyperparathyroidism. Untreated PHPT show the presence of brown tumors on histopathology, consisting of osteoclasts which are different in HPT-JT. Brown tumors here comprise of woven trabecular bone with no aberrant cell type but with a background of stroma. Renal tumor associations like mentioned earlier may comprise of Wilms' tumor, polycystic kidneys, hamartomas and uterine tumors like leiomyomas, benign fibromas and adenosarcoma have been identified.

Risk of questionable reproductive fitness necessitates sound gynecologic assessment due to high incidence of uterine leiomyomas. Families with jaw tumors have frequent associations with renal and uterine anomalies.

Surgical therapy includes parathyroid adenomectomy in uniglandular disease, while SPTX or TPTX with forearm parathyroid auto transplant (TPX + AT) with thymectomy is performed when multiglandular involvement is suspected.

Genetics

Parafibromin/CDC73 is a transcription factor which is encoded by *CDC73/HRPT2*, mapped to 1q21–31 based on analysis of wide variety of mutations in affected families. The Knudson two-hit hypothesis was tested positive in *CDC73* gene just like in MEN and its' association has been tested in parathyroid carcinomas and eventually postulated in sporadic and familial type of carcinomas. This is another autosomal dominant pattern of inheritance just like other familial types with variable incomplete penetrance according to age. Those families sharing a common mutation with a similar genetic background will have reduced phenotype variability within families but with limited knowledge on genotype-phenotype correlations. Familial isolated hyperparathyroidism (FIHP or HRPT1) is a unique entity where there are a few families with hyperparathyroidism as the only feature with no other features of MEN 1 which contributes to the heterogenous genetic nature of this variety. (11)

Parafibromin/CDC73

Parafibromin is a protein comprising of 531 amino acids coded by *CDC73/HRPT2* gene as mentioned on chromosome 1 consisting of 17 exons with a transcript measuring 2.7 kb. The carboxy terminal of the protein is very homologous with the cell division cycle (cdc73) of the yeast which is the reason for the designation conferred on the gene (CDC73/HRPT2). It is ubiquitous in expression and has a nuclear location. Parafibromin is involved in the elongation of mRNA transcript by interacting with the enzyme RNA polymerase II, since it is a part of the polymerase-associated factor 1 (PAF1) complex. Like menin, parafibromin can behave as an oncogene/tumor suppressor depending on the context. There are lot of mutations reported including germline and somatic (2/3, 1/3) accounting for more than 110 in number till date. They include premature stop codons and truncation types. Only 50% of kindreds with HPT-JT have these mutations even if there is significant family history identifying the gene mapped to chromosome 1. Along with parental mosaicism, de novo mutations have also been reported in this disease.

Parafibromin/CDC73 in parathyroid carcinoma

Sporadic hyperparathyroidism usually does not show somatic mutations in CDC73. Parathyroid carcinomas associated with HPT-JT have been shown to have tumor suppressive activity by parafibromin due to the proposed LOH as referred to earlier in the chapter. HPT-JT-associated parathyroid carcinomas have shown to house LOH in the carriers and somatic mutations in sporadic parathyroid carcinomas in various studies. Occasionally germline mutations have also been known to occur in sporadic carcinomas. Carcinoma of parathyroid localized to the gland is potentially curable, but metastasis poses significant risk of cure. A detailed family history and *CDC73* mutation screening should be the standard management of all patients with a fresh diagnosis of parathyroid carcinoma according to recommendations. At risk families should be screened with parafibromin immunostaining and may be offered a genetic testing for germline mutation in CDC73 based on these results. Asymptomatic carriers may be kept on serial monitoring as recommended by proposed guidelines. Histopathologic criteria may not suffice to differentiate parathyroid adenoma from carcinoma. Parenchymal mitoses, thick fibrous bands trabeculated parenchyma, capsular and vascular invasion are the features which may be common to both atypical adenomas and parathyroid carcinomas. The classical feature on histopathology pointing toward carcinoma and metastatic behavior would be capsular breach with lymphovascular invasion. Immunohistochemical tumor markers have emerged as an important modality in diagnosis. The most classical, highly sensitive and specific immunomarker in the recent times is the loss of expression of parafibromin in association with other markers or alone. It is still regarded as a useful marker of malignancy. Galectin-3 overexpression and loss of RB1 are other markers in addition to loss of parafibromin. Those patients with parathyroid carcinoma may have a combination of calcium-sensing receptor (CASR) downregulation with loss of parafibromin, which marks a high malignant potential of these tumors with possible aggressive and metastatic behavior. (12, 13)

Familial hypocalciuric hypercalcemia

Familial heterozygous benign hypercalcemia (FBH) syndrome or familial hypocalciuric hypercalcemia (FHH) is characterized by autosomal dominant pattern of inheritance. It is usually asymptomatic with mild type of hypercalcemia which may persist throughout the patient's life with incidentally detected higher calcium levels. It mimics any other mild variety of PHPT but with a pathology associated with renal handling of calcium which is malfunctioning. Foley first described it in 1972. Serum parathormone levels can be misleading as they are exceedingly normal. Due to the mild variety of hypercalcemia in FHH, those patients posing a confusion as to having normal/upper limit of normal PTH levels will require a calcium creatinine ratio to differentiate between FHH and PHPT in 10% of patients, where the value lies less than 0.01. The consensus is to avoid surgery in FHH patients since those who undergo parathyroidectomy remain hypercalcemic postoperatively. Surgery may prove futile in these cases of FHH, suggesting that the underlying pathology is a continued increased calcium absorption by the renal tubules which is not controlled by PTH. Calcium set point abnormality that dictates secretion of PTH cannot be corrected with TPX, but SPTX in symptomatic PHPT can be beneficial, though it can lead to a possibility of persistent postoperative hypercalcemia.

Neonatal severe hyperparathyroidism

PHPT is a rare occurrence in infancy and childhood, usually fatal. It usually presents as 'failure to thrive' syndrome. The various presentations of PHPT in infancy are (1) autosomal recessive familial parathyroid hyperplasia; (2) an inactivating heterozygous mutation of the calcium sensing receptor (CaSR) gene causing autosomal dominant familial hypocalciuric hypercalcemia (FHH); (3) *de novo* heterozygous CaSR mutations producing sporadic neonatal hyperparathyroidism; and (4) homozygous or double heterozygous mutations of CaSR gene causing NSHPT in children. There are very few reported cases and a handful of small series on PHPT in children with no large prospective studies in literature due to its rarity. Long-term medical treatment could lead to 70%–87% mortality, whereas mortality rate due to surgery could be reduced to 25%.

Multiglandular involvement is a feature of NSHPT and very rarely single adenomas. Severe hypercalcemia which is grossly symptomatic and is refractory to routine management in these patients with florid rickets and other bony changes of the chest cavity and other bones due to hyperparathyroidism. Causes of infantile hypercalcemia like (1) hyperparathyroidism with maternal hypoparathyroidism, (2) idiopathic infantile hypercalcemia, (3) blue diaper syndrome and (4) subcutaneous fat necrosis have to be ruled out before arriving at a diagnosis of neonatal severe PHPT (NSPHPT). Death or a severely morbid neurodevelopmental disorder can be an eventuality if the treatment is delayed. Some types of neonatal hyperparathyroidism will present with a milder form of hypercalcemia which may be transient or less symptomatic.

Surgery is restricted to high volume endocrine surgeons with sufficient expertise in anatomy in these cases of NSPHPT. TPTX with transcervical thymectomy, with practical removal of all functioning parathyroid, should be the treatment of choice in the initial months of life whenever feasible to prevent fatality. The author's experience, due to be published in Indian Journal of Endocrinology and Metabolism, would provide a good insight to management of these cases. (14, 15)

(1) Reproducible hypercalcemia (two or more high values) and (2) a normocalcemic interval (at least one normal calcium level more than three months after surgery prior to diagnosis of postoperative hypercalcemia are the two required criteria to diagnose postoperative recurrent hypercalcemia. Likewise persistent hypercalcemia is diagnosed by the following criteria – (1) reproducible hypercalcemia and (2) absence of normocalcemic interval after surgery (as defined in criteria for recurrence). The calcium levels normalize gradually over a period of 2 weeks in these cases, which is why postoperative calcium levels may not be a good marker of disease cure. Postoperative parathormone levels less than 10 pg/ml or negligible levels would be the most accurate marker of cure in addition to a histopathology evidence of atleast four parathyroids with thymic tissue.

Genetics

Several hypotheses have been offered to explain the familial coincidence of FHH and NSPHPT: (1) NSHPT may represent an extreme phenotype that occurs within the spectrum of clinical severity in FHH; (2) mutated FHH gene product may interact with an unidentifiable protein to cause NSHPT; (3) it is reported in the offspring of unaffected mothers and fathers with FHH, NSHPT may represent in utero development of severe secondary hyperparathyroidism in an FHH child in response to normocalcemia in the mother; and (4) it was also seen in several off springs of consanguineous marriages between those with FHH, which is considered to be homozygous type of FHH.

FHH has complete penetrance with an autosomal dominant manner of inheritance. The infrequency of recognition rather than rarity is the probable reason for poorly defined prevalence in the population. *CASR* gene mutation mapped to chromosome 3q13–21 has been documented in most FHH kindreds while the trait was mapped to 19p13 in one of the families.

Thus, FHH could be genetically heterogeneous with atypical features (age-related rise in PTH and osteomalacia) reported in some kindreds.

Calcium-sensing receptor

The *CASR* gene in humans consists of 1078 amino acids in its protein and has been associated with chromosome 3q13.3–21. This chromosome has eight exons, out of which CASR protein is coded by exons 2–7. Cell signaling is initiated by the CASR gene which functions as a dimer with calcium and others binding to clefts. Varying Ca2+ concentrations guide the allosteric modulators, which bind within the transmembrane region of CASR and desensitize or sensitize the CASR categorized as calcilytics/calcimimetics. NSPHPT, severe hypercalcemia in parathyroid carcinoma patients with chronic kidney disease on dialysis have been treated with calcimimetics. These drugs do not majorly affect the bone mineral density and bone turnover and also reduce serum calcium and PTH levels, increasing serum phosphate levels. Majority of the CASR mutations which have been identified are inactivating (2/3), responsible for FHH/NSHPT, while the others (1/3) are activating, causing autosomal dominant–type hypocalcemia. Most commonly missense mutations, followed by insertion, deletion, truncation, splice and frame-shift mutations are the myriad inactivating type of mutations noted. Significant symptomatic impairment may be seen due to any single critical mutation in any one of the complex functional components.

FHH syndrome does not present with overt hyperparathyroidism. The major histological difference seen in NSPHPT is markedly hypercellular multiglandular disease while FHH would have a few hyperplastic areas rarely. Increased PTH levels with identified adenomas may be seen in a few FIHP kindreds with *CASR* mutations and FFH families. In such cases, parathyroidectomy might an effective cure. Heterozygous CASR mutations in particular have a negative effect on the proliferation of parathyroid cells while somatic CASR mutations will produce tumors. This was evidenced by analysis of parathyroid and calcium sensing and signaling pathways. Sporadic parathyroid adenomas are usually not cause by somatic mutations according to recent evidence. Reduced expression of CASR is seen in most of the cases of PHPT. Increased serum calcium and parathyroid levels and enlargement of parathyroid gland in these cases occur due to the shift of the calcium set point to the right. Also, the pathophysiology of neoplasm in the parathyroid tissue is said to be due to inhibition of CASR expression by the regulator of G protein signaling 5 (RGS5). PHPT has been predominantly associated with vitamin D insufficiency and a progressive disease with severity is usually noted in vitamin D deficiency. The proliferation of parathyroid cells including the expression of PTH and CASR genes is known to be due to 1,25(OH)2D, an active metabolite of vitamin D. Increased PTH levels with significant parathyroid hyperplasia, falsely mimicking PHPT, is known to be the manifestation of homozygous inactivation of the VDR or its ligand. Though there is an under expression

Familial Hyperparathyroidism

of VDR in PHPT, somatic mutation of the same will not cause parathyroid tumors like the *CASR*. VDR under expression may lead to reduced expression of *CASR* expression. FHH affected individuals may in fact present with clinically symptomatic hypercalcemia when associated with Vitamin D deficiency. Such a condition can be treated with supplementation of vitamin D, resulting in mild hypercalcemia with normalized PTH levels in FHH, thus averting misdiagnosis. (1, 2)

Familial isolated hyperparathyroidism

Another hereditary type of PHPT associated with MEN 1 with no other related tumors is familial isolated hyperparathyroidism (FIHP or HRPT1). These cases are monogenic variants of the diseases like FHH, MEN1 or HPT-JT with no specific genes mapped to this disease. Subtotal or TPTX is the treatment of choice resulting in reduction of calcium levels.

Patients with NMFH are diagnosed by means of (1) a thorough personal family history concerning the clinical manifestations of MEN and (2) laboratory tests that should include pituitary hormone, gastrin, chromogranin, pancreatic peptide, calcitonin, CEA and urinary calcium-to-creatinine clearance ratio (Cca/Ccr) to rule out BFHH and MEN-associated parathyroid disease. Recently, progressive genetic tests have proved useful in clarifying more about the genetic picture of NMFH.

Pathogenesis of FHPT: The pathogenesis has been compared with the sporadic ones and detailed in the table. (Figure 33.1)

Cyclin D1 oncogene and FIPH parathyroid neoplasia

CCND1 encoding cyclin D1 earlier known as parathyroid adenomatosis 1(PRAD 1) is the only oncogene known to be associated with parathyroid neoplasia. The CCND 1 gene is controlled by the PTH gene in the 5′ regulatory region due to the centromeric mutation, resulting in overexpression of cyclin D1. Expression of PTH in such tumors is caused by the single intact copy of the *PTH* gene, cyclin D1 overexpression (40%) is seen in both sporadic adenomas and parathyroid carcinomas.

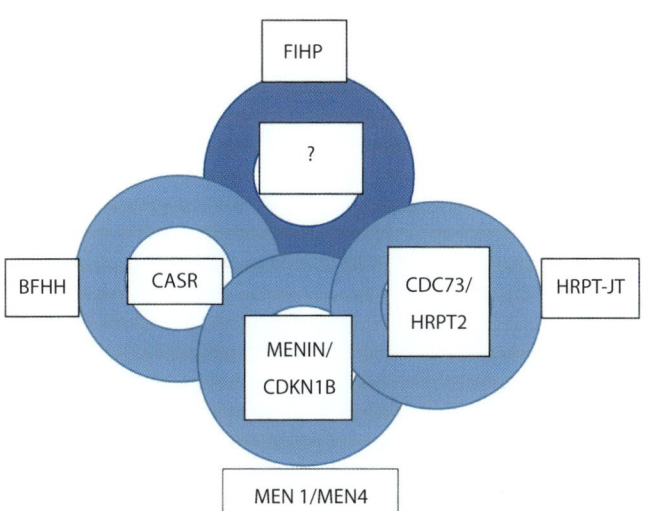

FIGURE 33.1 Pathogenesis of FHPT.

Extensive studies are being conducted on overexpression of genes. It may be more of a regulatory disturbance than clonal mutation of an allele.

Regulation of G1-S phase transition in the normal cell cycle and progression of cycle is controlled by cyclin. There are different types of cyclins described in literature, each one responsible for activating cyclin-dependent kinases (CDKs) by both transcriptional and posttranscriptional mechanisms.

Parathyroid gland calcium set point may vary, acting as a stimulus for cell proliferation. 'Set point' genes may not necessarily initiate the disease. (6)

Other aspects of parathyroid tumorigenesis

Alternate mutations responsible for parathyroid tumorigenesis like truncation have been reported. There may be presentations with undetectable circulating intact PTH but they still exhibit skeletal changes of PHPT and hypercalcemia. Heterozygous leukocyte DNA mutation with deletion of the wild-type *PTH* allele would be noted in the tumor. This mutated PTH will be secreted by the gland, being biologically active in the tissues. Another important cause of PHPT which is increasingly seen is neck irradiation. may contribute to the tumorigenesis. Genes like *p53, RB, H-ras, K-ras, N-ras,* Beta-catenin (Wnt pathway target) with *CTNNB1* gene and epigenetic modifications, few repair and recombinant genes are responsible for various tumors.

HIC1 plays an important regulatory part in the growth of parathyroid tumor. Under expression or nil expression in adenomas and hypermethylation in carcinomas would be characteristic.

MicroRNAs (miRs) are negative regulators of gene expression and are non-coding. They cause mRNA degradation, translation inhibition or a gene silencing. They may act as oncogenes or tumor suppressor genes causing growth or tumor suppression. They can have a differential expression in parathyroid carcinomas. 2D electrophoresis and mass spectrometry with a proteomic approach classified different functional categories of 20 different proteins identified.

Sporadic parathyroid adenomas were analyzed with whole genome sequencing too recently, consisting of examining selective genes in a large panel.

Rare mutations like histone methyltransferase *EZH2* gene and frequent (35%) mutations like MEN1 were reported. The various forms of FHPT and their characteristics are given in Table 33.2.

South Asian perspective: Though the western world has documented more of asymptomatic presentation (85%–90%) in PHPT in the recent time owing to better biochemical testing methods, symptomatic hypercalcemia remains a significant presentation in most of South East Asia. Vitamin D deficiency and its' association with PHPT has been studied extensively off late. The correction of vitamin D has unmasked most of these cases. Increased awareness with regard to PHPT, particularly FHPT has increased the diagnosis of hypercalcemia from infants to adults. There have been reports of successful detection and surgical treatment of FHPT in children including NSPHPT. The incidence of FHH still remains low as compared to general literature due to the milder nature of the disease with lack of availability of investigations resulting in underdiagnosis. MEN 1 remains the most common cause of FHPT by and large, while HPT-JT and FIHP remain the least common in the list.

TABLE 33.2: Description of Various FHPT and Its' Characteristics

	MEN 1	MEN2A	MEN4	FIHP	FHH	NSHPT	HPT-JT
Genetic locus	11q13	10q11.2	12q13.1	2p130.3-14	3q13.3-21	3q13.3-21	1q31.2
Mode of inheritance	AD	AD	AD	AD	AD	AR	AD
Mutation	MEN 1	RET	CDKN1B	–	CASR	CASR	CDC73/HRPT2
Genetic product	MENIN	RET	P27 (Kip1)	–	CASR	CASR	Parafibromin/CDC73
Sporadic parathyroid tumor defects	Inactivation in 25%–35% benign tumors, rare in carcinoma	Mutation not found in benign tumors	Mutation found in a few sporadic tumors	–	Mutation very rare in benign tumors	–	Inactivation in 70% carcinomas, rare in benign tumors
Associated tumors	Pancreatic islet cell tumors, pituitary tumors, other nonendocrine tumors	Medullary thyroid carcinoma and pheochromocytoma	Pituitary tumors, carcinoids and lipomas	–	Chondrocalcinosis and pancreatitis	–	Jaw fibromas, renal and uterine tumors

Abbreviations: AD, autosomal dominant; AR, autosomal recessive.

Conclusion

- The knowledge of various causes of FHPT will help distinguish symptomatic, atypical presentations from the sever hypercalcemia.
- Timely biochemical diagnosis in few patients and the requirement of necessary imaging in others should be clearly defined.
- The procedure of total parathyroidectomy with thymectomy, technique of thymectomy and bilateral exploration of the neck to identify the parathyroids should be known to the operating surgeon.
- Futile surgeries can translate into significant patient morbidity and add to the difficulties of a second surgery.
- Follow-up of symptomatic cases biochemically is another point of emphasis in many of these cases.
- Genetic testing in the patient and screening among kindreds would prevent unnecessary delay in diagnosis.
- Future research in this direction will definitely identify many more genes associated with this condition and various other treatment modalities, particularly the persistent/recurrent hypercalcemia.

References

1. Duan K, Mete O. Familial hyperparathyroidism syndromes. Diagn Histopathol. 2016;22:1–9.
2. Hendy GN, Cole DEC. Genetic defects associated with familial and sporadic hyperparathyroidism. In: C.A. Stratakis, ed., Endocrine Tumor Syndromes and Their Genetics. Front Horm Res. Basel: Karger; 2013. vol. 41, pp. 149–165.
3. Giusti F et al. Hereditary hyperparathyroidism syndromes. J Clin Densitom. 2013;16(1):69–74.
4. Clark OH. Familial hyperparathyroidism. In: Textbook of Endocrine Surgery. 3rd ed. New Delhi: Jaypee Brothers Medical Publishers; 2016. pp. 831–843.
5. Bilezikian JP. Primary hyperparathyroidism. J Clin Endocrinol Metab. 2018;103(11):3993–4004.
6. Pollak et al. FHH and NSHPT: effects of mutant gene dosage on phenotype. J Clin Invest. 1994; 93:1108–1112.
7. Law et al. Autosomal recessive inheritance of familial hyperparathyroidism. NEJM 1983;309(11):650–653.
8. Matsuo et al. Neonatal hyperparathyroidism. Am J Dis Child. 1982;136:728–732.
9. Naseri et al. Hypercalcemia due to PHPT. Int J Clin Pediatr. 2014;3(3):94–96.
10. Shiva S et al. Neonatal hypercalcemia due to primary hyperparathyroidism. Iran J Pediatr. 2008;18(3):277–280.
11. Rizzoli et al. Parathyroidectomy in familial endocrine neoplasia type I. Am J Med. 1985;78:467–474.
12. Ross et al. Primary hyperparathyroidism in infancy. J Pediatr Surg. 1986;21(6):493–499.
13. Spiegel et al. Neonatal primary hyperparathyroidism with autosomal dominant inheritance. J Pediatr. 1977;90(2):269–272.
14. Heath H III: Familial benign hypercalcemia—from clinical description to molecular genetics. West J Med. 1994;160:554–561.
15. Sacharan D, et al. Neonatal severe primary hyperparathyroidism: a series of four cases and their long-term management in India. Indian J Endocr Metab. 2020;24:196–201.

34

SECONDARY AND TERTIARY HYPERPARATHYROIDISM

Lee Kai Yin and Rajeev Parameswaran

Introduction

Secondary hyperparathyroidism (SHPT) and tertiary hyperparathyroidism (THPT) are conditions that are closely associated with end-stage renal disease and renal transplantation. The development of hyperparathyroidism occurs early in chronic kidney disease and progresses as renal function worsens, and majority of patients would have developed SHPT by the time they require dialysis. This results in biochemical abnormalities of phosphate, calcium and parathyroid hormone (PTH) levels, which eventually results in various mineral and bone disorders. In THPT, persistent hypercalcemia or PTH levels may affect allograft survival. Persistent HPT also results in higher mortality.

In this chapter, we will discuss definitions and pathogenesis of SHPT and THPT, as well as their clinical presentations. Diagnostic evaluations and current medical treatment and surgical techniques and adjuncts will be discussed. We will also discuss the prevalence of diabetic end-stage renal disease (ESRD) and SHPT and THPT in Asia, with our suggestions on feasible and cost-effective treatment of SHPT and THPT.

Definitions of secondary and tertiary HPT

Secondary hyperparathyroidism (SHPT) is defined by elevated PTH levels caused by conditions outside of the parathyroid glands. The most common cause is chronic kidney disease (CKD), and this develops early in CKD and worsens in severity as the glomerular filtration rates decrease and renal function worsens (1). It is estimated that more than 90% of all patients develop SHPT by the time of dialysis initiation (2–5). Less common causes include conditions related to Vitamin D deficiency (osteomalacia, rickets) and malabsorption conditions (chronic pancreatitis, malabsorption-dependent bariatric surgery), as well as long-term use of lithium (6).

Tertiary hyperparathyroidism (THPT) refers to the development of autonomous parathyroid function after a prolonged period of hyperparathyroidism. This is usually discussed in the context of patients with SHPT that have persistent or recurrent elevated PTH levels after a renal transplant (7). This may occur in 30% of patients after renal transplant. However, autonomous function of parathyroid glands may also be seen in prolonged hypocalcemia such as those with chronic malabsorptive diseases or those with long dialysis vintage. Serum calcium levels may become normal or even elevated.

Physiology of parathyroid hormone

PTH is a single-chain hormone produced by chief cells in parathyroid glands. It plays a major role in calcium hemostasis and bone remodeling. It acts mainly on bone and kidneys and, to a lesser extent, on blood vessels. The synthesis and secretion of PTH are regulated by extracellular calcium (8). Calcium-sensing receptors (CaR) are located on the surface of chief cells in the parathyroid glands and detect changes to extracellular calcium levels (9). Hypercalcemia reduces overall PTH secretion and favors release of PTH fragments, while hypocalcemia favors PTH secretion and active PTH release.

Parathyroid hormone-related protein (PTHrP) is protein member of the PTH hormone family (10). While commonly associated with tumor cells causing paraneoplastic syndromes, they are also found in normal body function. It a major regulator of bone formation and to a smaller extent is associated with controlling vascular tone.

The main signaling receptor for both PTH and PTHrP is PTH/PTHrP receptor, which is a G protein–coupled transmembrane receptor. It is highly expressed in bone and kidney and at lower levels in blood vessels. PTH and PTHrP bind to PTH/PTHrP receptor and exert various actions at different target organs. Termination of its signaling is occurs with negative feedback of PTH secretion but may also be achieved with desensitization-internalization process with chronic activation of the receptor (11).

Effect of PTH on target organs

The three primary target organs for PTH activity are the kidneys, intestines and bones. PTH causes increased renal excretion of phosphate, increased renal tubular reabsorption of calcium, increases the formation of 1,25-dihydroxycholecalciferol and this increases intestinal absorption of calcium. In the bone, PTH acts directly on osteoblasts and osteocytes and indirectly on osteoclasts. Intermittent increases in PTH levels promote osteoblastic activity and increased number of osteoblasts and, hence, bone formation (12). However, continuous exposure to high PTH levels results in higher osteoclastic activity and inhibition of proliferation of osteoblasts and overall bone resorption (13, 14).

In the kidney, PTH acts primarily on the distal convoluted tubules to increase calcium reabsorption and decrease calcium excretion (13). It also increases phosphate urinary excretion at the proximal convoluted tubules. It also indirectly promotes calcium and phosphate reabsorption in the intestines by increasing 1,23-dihydroxy-vitamin D_3 production in the kidney (15). PTH and PTHrP both have vasodilatory actions on vascular smooth muscle cells (16). They also reduce oxidative stress as well as procalcification and pro-fibrotic signals that drive atherosclerosis in vessels (17).

Pathogenesis of secondary HPT

In chronic kidney disease, there is loss of phosphate and calcium homeostasis, resulting in electrolyte derangements, secondary hyperparathyroidism and bone disorders (18). These are termed collectively as chronic kidney disease-mineral bone disorder (CKD-MBD) in KDIGO guidelines (19). PTH levels have been shown to be closely related to glomerular filtration rate (11). As renal function worsens, increased PTH synthesis and secretion with parathyroid hyperplasia drive rising PTH levels.

Impaired excretion of phosphate in the renal tubes result in hyperphosphatemia and consequently decreased extracellular calcium concentrations. Hyperphosphatemia also drives also increased fibroblast growth factor 23 (FGF23) levels but decreased expression of FGF receptors (20). Vitamin D levels are low due to impaired conversion of 25-hydroxycholecalciferol to 1,25-dihydroxycholecalciferol (calcitriol) and also from increased FGF23 concentrations. Vitamin D receptors (VDRs), calcium-sensing receptors (CaRs) are downregulated (20).

The combination of hyperphosphatemia and decreased vitamin D production results in decreased levels of serum calcium. Hypocalcemia is detected by CaR receptors in parathyroid chief cells and results in increased PTH secretion. CKD also decreases CaR expression and drives PTH production and parathyroid cell proliferation (20). Elevated phosphate levels stimulate PTH synthesis and parathyroid chief cell proliferation (21). CKD also results in resistance of PTH on skeletal cells, driving persistently elevated PTH levels (20).

Calcitriol inhibits parathyroid cell proliferation and suppresses PTH secretion, and decreased circulating calcitriol levels with decreased expression of VDRs results in a loss of inhibition of PTH and also drives progression of parathyroid chief cell diffuse hyperplasia toward nodular hyperplasia (22, 23). Tominaga et al. studied expression of VDR in parathyroid glands and found that there was significantly less expression of VDR in areas of nodular hyperplasia compared to diffuse hyperplasia (24, 25).

FGF23 plays an important role in phosphate homeostasis and acts on the renal proximal convoluted tubules by binding to FGF receptors to reduce phosphate reabsorption and increase phosphate urinary excretion. It also inhibits expression of 1-α-hydroxylase and, hence, decreases synthesis of calcitriol in the renal tubules (26). In chronic kidney disease, FGF23 levels are elevated, but actions are limited due to decreased expression of FGF receptors (27, 28). FGF23 is also associated with increased risk of cardiovascular disease (29) and, hence, mortality in patients with CKD (30).

Parathyroid cellular proliferation most commonly forms diffuse hyperplasia. However, there is asymmetric enlargement, and nodular hyperplasia may occur with chronic hypocalcemia driving elevated PTH levels (31, 32). It is observed that the chief cells first follow a hyperplastic patter and then progressed to diffuse hyperplasia, nodular hyperplasia and finally a single nodule (21, 32).

Pathogenesis of tertiary hyperparathyroidism

THPT occurs commonly after renal transplant, where patients with SHPT continue to have elevated PTH levels after transplant (33, 34). Possible factors may be chronic SHPT drives development of autonomous nodular parathyroid adenomas. These nodules are transformed monoclonally and proliferate aggressively and do not undergo involution. The exact mechanisms are not well understood but are speculated to stem from genetic abnormality (34). VDR density has also been noted to be reduced in areas of nodular formation (25).

Prevalence of 2°/3° HPT in Asia

There is a high burden of chronic kidney disease in the Asian population, with a large majority of patients developing chronic kidney disease and ESRD as a result of diabetes (35-37). The exact incidence is unknown, but several studies across Pakistan (38), Bangladesh (39), Sri Lanka (40), Singapore (41), Thailand (42), Malaysia (43), Indonesia (44) and India (45) show prevalence of CKD ranging from 6.3% to 26%. Population studies revealed prevalence of CKD in China as 11.6% (46) and 12.9% in the United States (47). In Singapore, the prevalence of CKD was reported to be 15.6% (48); it is estimated that the incidence of chronic kidney disease will triple that of the incidence in 2007 (41).

The prevalence of both CKD and ESRD is expected to increase in Asia. The two main factors responsible for the increasing incidence of CKD are diabetes and hypertension. The prevalence of diabetes and hypertension in Singapore in 2010 was around 11% and 24%, respectively (49). There was an increase of more than 50% in the incidence of diabetes and 7% in the incidence of hypertension when compared to 2004. It is estimated that the incidence of diabetes in Singapore will further increase to about 20% (50). Adding to this, the increasing life span will pose a big challenge to the nation on both economic and health front (51).

Although there are many patients with ESRD in Southeast Asia, there remains a large gap in access to treatment. A significant part of Southeast Asia are still developing nations, with majority of patients from low income families. There is limited access to health care and hemodialysis facilities due to both cost and location. The average cost of two to three dialysis sessions of four hours duration per week ranged from 5,869 to 8,804 USD (52), and this places a significant financial burden for patients in the long term. In Pakistan, it is estimated that only 10% of patients with ESRD undergo renal replacement therapy, and <5% undergo kidney transplant (53). However, many governments in Asia have taken steps to develop stronger health economic policies and fundings to improve the accessibility and financial support for renal replacement therapy. This will hopefully increase the number of patients with ESRD who are able to receive RRT.

The exact incidence of secondary hyperparathyroidism in Asia is unknown, but with our understanding on the onset of SHPT and CKD, it is estimated that almost all patients with ESRD will develop SHPT. A population study in India estimated that the number of patients with iPTH >300 pg/mL was 27.9%, while it was 11.5% in a Japanese study (54). SHPT is especially prevalent in Asia, as the access to renal transplant is limited. With a high burden of ESRD, the demand for kidney transplantation far outweighs the number of donors available (55). Only a small proportion of patients with ESRD are able to receive hemodialysis, and even fewer are aware about the options of transplantation. In addition, many developing nations do not have a national transplantation program, and illegal organ trade remains a difficult issue to resolve. In Singapore, cadaveric donors still account for majority of kidney transplantations, due to social and ethnic barriers surrounding living related kidney donors. The average waiting time for a kidney transplant is 9 years, and majority of patients develop worsening SHPT that may eventually require surgery.

Clinical presentation

Majority of patients with SHPT and THPT are asymptomatic. SHPT is well recognized as a disease that begins early on in CKD, and most renal units worldwide check serum PTH levels routinely and start treatment early. Patients who undergo kidney transplant also undergo regular surveillance including blood tests such as serum PTH, phosphate and calcium levels.

Bone

Changes in bone turnover begin early in CKD and continue to progress in ESRF and dialysis (56, 57). Studies have shown the incidence of osteitis fibrosa cystica to be about 30% in patients with CKD and adynamic bone disease in 40% (58). With better control of SHPT without over treatment, bone disorders have decreased in prevalence.

There are several subsets of bone disorders related to hyperparathyroidism (59) and CKDMBD:

1. *Osteitis fibrosa cystica* – High bone turnover due to SHPT
2. *Adynamic bone disorder* – Low bone turnover due to excessive suppression of parathyroid glands
3. *Osteomalacia* – Low bone turnover due to delayed bone mineralization. This was associated with the use of aluminum-containing antacids as phosphate binders, resulting in aluminum deposition in bone
4. *Mixed uremic osteodystrophy* – May be either high or low bone turnover due to abnormal bone mineralization
5. *Bone cysts* – Amyloid deposits presenting as bone cysts in patients on long-term dialysis

Patients may present with bone pain as a results of osteitis fibrosa cystica. Radiological features such as salt and pepper appearance of the skull and subperiosteal bone resorption of the middle phalanges and brown tumors for long bones are classical for osteitis fibrosa cystica. Pathological fractures may occur due to osteoporosis. Decreased bone mineral density as a result of overall osteoclastic activity and vitamin D deficiency results in thinning of the cortical bone with preserved trabecular bone. Patients are more predisposed to osteoporotic fractures in areas such as forearm, hip and spine.

Calciphylaxis

Calciphylaxis is a rare but serious complication of persistent hyperparathyroidism resulting in calcium deposition of dermis and subcutaneous adipose tissues, resulting in painful skin ischemia and necrosis. Patients present with painful, violaceous plaque-like subcutaneous nodules and later progress to ischemic ulcers and eschars (60, 61).

Tertiary hyperparathyroidism

Patients with tertiary hyperparathyroidism do not usually present with symptoms, but symptoms are associated with hypercalcemia. The mnemonic "bones, moans, stones and groans" is often used to describe symptoms of hypercalcemia. Patients may present with vague neuromuscular symptoms, such as weakness and fatigue. They may also present with psychiatric symptoms such as lethargy, depression, psychosis or cognitive impairment. As a result of elevated PTH levels, they may also develop bone pain and pathological fractures. As serum calcium levels are persistently elevated, they may develop vascular and soft tissue calcifications, resulting in worsening atherosclerosis. They also may develop nephrolithiasis and may present with ureteric colic.

Diagnosis and investigations

Diagnosis of SHPT and THPT is a combination of history, clinical findings and laboratory investigations. A clear clinical history is taken to establish the chronicity and progression of CKD, dialysis vintage, renal transplantation if any and its complications. One should also look for complications such as history of fractures, bone pain, lethargy as well as new onset psychiatric symptoms.

Laboratory markers

Serum PTH, phosphate and calcium are most commonly used for diagnosis and monitoring of SHPT and THPT. The biochemical derangements are summarized in Table 34.1.

Preoperative serum ALP levels reflect the state of bone turnover and, therefore, the degree of osteoclast activity and bone resorption. ALP levels are, thus, a good surrogate marker of the degree and duration of hypocalcemia (62).

Imaging

The routine use of imaging is not performed in the diagnosis of SHPT and THPT. Imaging is usually considered for preoperative planning for localization of parathyroid glands in the context of parathyroidectomy or reoperative surgery for SHPT or THPT. This will be discussed later in the chapter. An ultrasound of the thyroid may be considered to guide preoperative planning; however, not all parathyroid glands may be visualized on the ultrasound. However, abnormalities of the thyroid gland may be picked up which may necessitate concomitant surgical resection of the thyroid.

Treatment strategies

Medical treatment

Medical treatment remains the first line for SHPT. Majority of patients are managed with medical therapy and do not require surgery. The goals of treatment are to correct hyperphosphatemia, hypocalcemia, vitamin D deficiency and finally PTH itself. KDIGO 2017 guidelines suggest maintaining iPTH levels in the range of two to nine times the upper limits (63).

Treatment of hyperphosphatemia

KDOQI guidelines recommend maintenance of normal ranges of serum phosphate, although no specific threshold was given for treatment. In general, most renal physicians recommend that dietary phosphate should be restricted in patients with CKD and treatment with serum phosphate levels of >1.78 mmol/L. Phosphate binders may be calcium containing (calcium acetate, calcium carbonate) or non–calcium containing (sevelamer, lanthanum, ferric citrate). KDIGO guidelines recommend restricting the dosage of calcium-containing phosphate binders, and some

TABLE 34.1: Biochemical Findings for SHPT and THPT

	Corrected Calcium	Phosphate	PTH
SHPT	↓ or normal	↑	↑↑↑
THPT	↑	normal	↑↑

guidelines have recommended that calcium-containing binders should be avoided (63), due to concerns of vascular calcification with calcium-containing phosphate binders in the absence of hypocalcemia. However, non–calcium containing binders are more expensive than binders that contain calcium (63) and may be an unrealistic option for patients in developing nations. The use of calcium-containing binders is still safe but should be restricted to elemental calcium doses of less than 1,500 mg a day, and regular checks on serum calcium should be performed (63).

Maintenance of normocalcemia
Hypocalcemia is associated with increased mortality and drives persistent hyperparathyroidism. However, there are also concerns for vascular calcification with oral calcium administration, especially when given concurrently with Vitamin D and calcium-containing phosphate binders. Mild hypocalcemia is not generally treated if patients are otherwise asymptomatic and not on dialysis.

Treatment of vitamin D deficiency
Vitamin D deficiency is common in patients with CKD. In patients with persistent SHPT, patients should be started on vitamin D analogs such as calcitriol, rather than ergocalciferol or cholecalciferol. However, calcitriol should not be given if patients are hyperphosphatemic or hypercalcemic. It is also commonly used in conjunction with calcimimetics for treatment of progressive SHPT.

Calcimimetics
Calcimimetics were first introduced in the United States in 2014 and are allosteric activators of calcium-sensing receptor (CaSR) (64). They bind to CaSR on parathyroid glands, allowing for activation at lower calcium levels and, hence, lowering plasma PTH levels by inhibiting PTH release, decreasing PTH gene expression and also increasing VDR expression in parathyroid glands (65). Currently, combination therapy with both calcimimetics and vitamin D analogs have been superior to monotherapy for treatment of decreasing PTH levels to target levels (66, 67) and may potentially avoid parathyroidectomy.

Longer term data for cinacalcet use, however, has not shown to be consistently superior in maintaining low PTH levels. A study by Brunaud et al. comparing ESRD patients who received cinacalcet to those who did not and found that at 2 years, the use of cinacalcet did not significantly reduce PTH levels compared to those who did not receive cinacalcet (68). In the EVOLVE trial (EVOLVE), the authors did not find significant reduction in mortality and cardiovascular outcomes in patients who received cinacalcet compared to those on conventional therapy (69). Cinacalcet is expensive and, hence, not routinely used in Asia.

Role of medical treatment in THPT
THPT is the most common cause for hypercalcemia in renal transplanted patients, affecting up to 25% of patients at 1 year after renal transplant (Finnerty). Cinacalcet has been shown to be effective in reducing PTH and calcium levels in the short term (70). There were initial concerns that PTX may cause hypoparathyroidism and, hence, graft dysfunction and graft loss (71). Chudzinski et al. showed that graft dysfunction with decreased eGFR occurs early on postoperative days 2 and 3, with subsequent recovery of function by days 4 and 5 (71). Finnerty et al. compared patients with THP to treatment with cinacalcet vs PTX and found that PTX group was associated with lower rates of allograft failure (9% vs 33%, P = 0.07) and had significantly lower median levels of PTH and serum calcium compared to cinacalcet group (72). However, further studies will be needed to compare the treatment modalities.

TABLE 34.2: Indications for Parathyroidectomy in Secondary and Tertiary Hyperparathyroidism

Indications for parathyroidectomy in SHPT
Calciphylaxis
Osteoporosis or fragility fracture
Symptomatic – pruritus, bone pain
Failure of medical therapy
• Hyperphosphatemia
• Hypercalcemia
• PTH levels >nine times upper limit, or >800 pg/mL
Indications for parathyroidectomy in THPT
Hypercalcemia-related complications
• Severe hypercalcemia
• Persistent hypercalcemia >1 year after renal transplant
• Symptomatic hypercalcemia including bone pain, neuropsychiatric symptoms, pruritus, nephrolithiasis, peptic ulcer disease
Severe osteopenia

Parathyroidectomy
Indications of parathyroidectomy
Parathyroidectomy is indicated in patients with SHPT or THPT that are symptomatic or in patients with progressive severe hyperparathyroidism that is not responding to medical therapy (63). The various indications for parathyroidectomy are summarized below in Table 34.2. While SHPT is more commonly treated with medical therapy, THPT is more likely to be treated with surgery. Hypercalcemia, hypophosphatemia and elevated PTH levels are associated with decreased allograft survival, bone loss and overall survival (72).

Types of parathyroidectomy
Currently, several types of parathyroidectomy are performed for the treatment of SHPT and THPT. Subtotal parathyroidectomy and total parathyroidectomy with or without autotransplantation are all acceptable surgical options. All parathyroidectomies start with a neck exploration to identify all four parathyroid glands. The middle thyroid vein may sometimes be ligated to allow for full exposure of the neck thyroid bed to identify the glands. In up to 40% of patients, the parathyroid glands may be in an ectopic location (73). The paraesophageal, retroesophageal, retropharyngeal, paralaryngeal, superior mediastinal spaces may be explored. The carotid sheath should be opened and explored, and the thymus or thyroid lobectomy may be performed. Once all four parathyroid glands are confidently identified, various parathyroidectomies may then be performed.

Role of ioPTH
The use of intraoperative PTH (ioPTH) levels is not used routinely in parathyroidectomy for SHPT and THPT. It may not be available in all centers, especially in Asia. However, its use may be useful in cases where parathyroid glands are not confidently identified, and a persistently elevated ioPTH level may suggest an ectopic location of parathyroid gland. It may also be useful in reoperative neck surgery for persistent or recurrent hyperparathyroidism. While cutoffs are clearly defined and accepted in SHPT, it is less

so in SHPT and THPT. In SHPT, the goal is >50% drop in ioPTH 10–30 minutes after parathyroidectomy (74). However, reduced PTH clearance may affect ioPTH readings, making interpretation difficult. In THPT, various cutoffs have been used, from 65 to 200 pg/mL (75–78).

Thymectomy with parathyroidectomy

Concurrent thymectomy with parathyroidectomy remains controversial. The thymus is the most common site of an ectopic or supernumerary parathyroid and occurs in up to 15% of patients (79). A study by Soares et al. found intrathymic parathyroids in 7.5% and did not significantly increase surgical time with no increased complications (79). However, evidence on thymectomy in SHPT in limited and is not routine in many surgical practices (4).

Cryopreservation of parathyroid tissue

Cryopreservation of parathyroid tissue is a new advancement in parathyroid surgery, which involves preserving excised parathyroid tissue and reimplanting them should patients develop hypoparathyroidism after surgery. The success rates remain variable, and cryopreserved tissue beyond 2 years were found to be nonfunctional (4, 80). However, few surgeons particularly in Asia have access to cryopreservation facilities and, hence, rarely used.

Subtotal parathyroidectomy (SPTX)

This involves resection of three and a half parathyroid glands. The smallest, most normal gland is chosen and the nonvascular pole is excised, leaving approximately 40 mg of parathyroid tissue. It is important to ensure that its vascularity is preserved. The main benefit for SPTX is minimal risk of permanent hypoparathyroidism postoperatively and is important for patients who are likely to undergo renal transplant in the future. Hypoparathyroidism is associated with allograft dysfunction and increased allograft loss.

Total parathyroidectomy (TPTX) with or without autotransplantation (AT)

In TPTX, all four glands are resected. However, autotransplantation involves selecting the most normal looking gland with the least nodularity and obtaining a small portion (40 mg) of the gland, dicing it up and transplanted into either the nondominant forearm or deltoid muscle via open cutdown or intramuscular injection. Other sites of autotransplantation include the chest or neck. The main argument for TPTX + AT allows for easy surgical management SHPT recurrence by excising the parathyroid tissue in a superficial space with local anesthesia and, hence, avoiding the risks related to reoperative neck surgery.

SPTX vs TPTX +/– AT

Both SPTX and TPTX + AT have been considered acceptable options for treatment of SHPT. A metanalysis comparing SPTX vs TPTX + AT showed no significant difference in recurrence and postoperative reduction in biochemical markers including serum calcium, PTH, phosphate and ALP (81, 82). In countries where access to renal transplant is limited and patients are likely to be on long-term dialysis, the risk of recurrent SHPT in higher. TPTX + AT may be advantageous as it allows for easy access to autotransplanted parathyroid tissue. A study in our institution also found that long-term recurrence rates were lower in TPTX + AT compared to SPTX (10.5% vs 20.8%), although not statistically significant (83).

TPTX vs TPTX + AT

TPTX without autotransplantation is relatively new and is associated with lower recurrence of SHPT compared to patients who received TPTX + AT (84). This may be useful in patients who are at highest risk for recurrent HPT, such as patients who have calciphylaxis, or are not candidates for renal transplant. A metanalysis comparing TPTX vs TPTX + AT found that TPTX was superior to TPTX + AT for recurrence (OR = 0.20; 95% CI, 0.11–0.38; $P < 0.01$), as well as operating time and and reoperation rates (85). However, TPTX is associated with increased risk for hypoparathyroidism (OR = 2.97; 95% CI, 1.09–8.08; $P = 0.01$), although no patients reported adynamic bone disease of permanent hypocalcemia. However, the studies were limited to cohort studies and 1 RCT, and there is concern for permanent hypoparathyroidism (85). A prospective RCT (TOPAR-PILOT) comparing TPTX + AT to TPTX was performed from 2007 to 2013 and currently awaiting results (86). However, preliminary results show no statistical differences in recurrence or postoperative hypoparathyroidism (87).

Parathyroidectomy for THPT

In patients in THPT, SPTX is considered to be the surgery of choice. SPTX is associated with the lowest risk of permanent hypoparathyroidism. Normal PTH levels and normocalcemia are important for kidney graft survival, and hypoparathyroidism is associated with decreased graft survival. A retrospective study compared PTX to cinacalcet therapy for patients with THPT and showed that PTH group had higher normalization of PTH compared to cinacalcet (67% vs 15%, $P < 0.01$) and also had fewer allograft failure (9% vs 33%, $P = 0.07$) (72).

Role of ethanol and vitamin D chemical ablation

Chemical ablation of parathyroid glands guided by ultrasound is a possible treatment modality for patients indicated for parathyroidectomy but are not fit for surgery. This procedure can be performed at the bedside with local anesthetic, and either ethanol or calcitriol is injected directly into hyperplastic parathyroid glands. Although the procedure may have to be repeated to achieve ablation of the parathyroid glands, it has shown promising efficacy in controlling SHPT (88, 89).

Complications of parathyroidectomy

Complications related to parathyroidectomy may be divided into intraoperative and postoperative complications. Parathyroidectomies are usually safe and technical complications are rare.

Intraoperative complications include:

- Bleeding and hematoma. Patients are often on antiplatelets and may be complicated by uremic coagulopathy, placing them at higher risks of developing a postoperative hematoma. Rarely, a cervical neck hematoma causes life threatening airway compromise, requiring urgent intubation, release of neck hematoma and surgical reexploration and hemostasis.
- Infection
- Injury to recurrent laryngeal nerve
- Failure to identify all four parathyroid glands

Postoperative complications may be early or late. Compared to patients with primary HPT, the patient population with SHPT and THPT are frail and are more likely to develop complications including hypocalcemia and hypoparathyroidism. Hypocalcemia is the most common complication after PTX, and while majority are mild and transient, some patients may develop symptomatic or refractory hypocalcemia, which may be life threatening. Hypocalcemia after parathyroidectomy has been reported in more than 80% of patients, with median length of stay 4.7–10.2 days (90, 91). Postoperative hypocalcemia is an important cause of prolonged hospital stay, readmissions and increased morbidity for patients.

Hungry bone syndrome (HBS) occurs in an estimated 20%–30% of patients with SHPT after PTX (92). It is a result of rapid bone remodeling following the acute withdrawal of high PTH levels. The rate of bone mineralization exceeds that of bone resorption, resulting in severe hypocalcemia. This is most commonly seen in patients with preexisting fibrosa osteitis cystica, although other risk factors include age >60 years old, serum ALP >3 times upper limit, preoperative PTH levels >1,000 pg/mL (92–94). HBS occurs in an estimated 20%–30% of patients with SHPT after PTX. There is no clear clinical criteria for HBS, but clinical parameters of sever hypocalcemia <2.1 mmol/L, despite infusional calcium replacement lasting beyond a few days should suggest ongoing HBS. Some patients may have hypophosphatemia with hyperkalemia. Calcium loading pre- and postoperatively in both oral and intravenous form prevents symptomatic hypocalcemia.

Routine titrated calcium replacement protocol

Studies have shown that a titrated calcium replacement protocol has been shown to be effective in managing postoperative hypocalcemia (95, 96). Preoperative loading of calcium and vitamin D has also shown to reduce requirements of postoperative intravenous calcium and, hence, reducing length of stay (90).

Our institution developed a multidisciplinary protocol for patients undergoing parathyroidectomy for SHPT and THPT. This involves preoperative loading with oral calcium and vitamin D, as well as intravenous calcium replacement following a protocol that commences immediately after all four parathyroid glands are removed. The recommended intravenous calcium dose is based on preoperative ALP levels. Postoperatively, patients are also started on oral calcium and vitamin D replacement, which is titrated based on regular checks on serum calcium levels with the aim of reducing intravenous calcium requirements. After introduction of the protocol, fewer patients developed symptomatic hypocalcemia (33.6% vs 8.9%).

Recurrence of SHPT and THPT

SHPT and THPT may be persistent or recurrent after initial PTX. Persistent HPT refers to failure of PTH to fall below three times of normal upper limit, and recurrent HPT is assumed when PTH levels increases more than three times above the normal upper limit beyond 6 months of initial parathyroidectomy. The reported rates of persistent or recurrent SHPT are variable, ranging from 5% to 25% (87), with no consistent evidence showing superiority of the surgical techniques. In THPT, recurrence rates range from 0% to 8% (4, 83).

The most common cause for recurrence is supernumerary parathyroid glands or ectopic locations (4, 87). Supernumerary glands are estimated to occur in 13%–14% of the population (36), while ectopic glands have a report incidence of 2%–22% (97, 98). In patients who continue to have high PTH levels or persistent symptoms, reoperative neck surgery may be considered.

Preoperative imaging modalities

In reoperative neck surgery for recurrent SHPT and THPT, preoperative localization of the ectopic or supernumerary gland increases success rates to 95% (99). At present, the best imaging or combination has not been determined. 99mTc-sestamibi has been showed to identify the location of the parathyroid remnant in 85% of patients with persistent of recurrent SHPT (4). The combination 99mTc-sestamibi with single-photon-emission CT may improve accuracy (87). In patients with THPT, ultrasound of neck, 99mTc-sestamibi scans and MRI were all successful in identifying the parathyroid gland (4, 100). In addition, adjuncts such as radioguided surgery (101–103) and ioPTH (as discussed earlier in the chapter) may also be useful for reoperative parathyroid surgery.

Conclusion

The development of hyperparathyroidism occurs early in chronic kidney disease and progresses as renal function worsens. Majority of patients of SHPT are managed with medical treatment. The goals of treatment are to correct hyperphosphatemia, hypocalcemia, vitamin D deficiency and finally PTH itself. Parathyroidectomy is indicated in patients with SHPT or THPT that are symptomatic or in patients with progressive severe hyperparathyroidism that is not responding to medical therapy. Intraoperative PTH is not used routinely in parathyroidectomy for SHPT and THPT. The most common cause for recurrence is supernumerary parathyroid glands or ectopic locations and patients who continue to have high PTH levels or persistent symptoms, reoperative neck surgery may be considered.

References

1. Rosen CJ, Bouillon R, Compston JE, Rosen V. Primer on the Metabolic Bone Diseases and Disorders of Mineral Metabolism. 8th ed. Hoboken (NJ): Wiley; 2013.
2. Messa P, Alfieri CM. Secondary and tertiary hyperparathyroidism. Front Horm Res. 2019;51:91–108.
3. Klempa I. [Treatment of secondary and tertiary hyperparathyroidism–surgical viewpoints]. Chirurg. 1999;70(10):1089–1101.
4. Pitt SC, Sippel RS, Chen H. Secondary and tertiary hyperparathyroidism, state of the art surgical management. Surg Clin North Am. 2009;89(5):1227–1239.
5. van der Plas WY, Noltes ME, van Ginhoven TM, Kruijff S. Secondary and tertiary hyperparathyroidism: a narrative review. Scand J Surg. 2020;109(4):271–278.
6. Chandran M, Wong J. Secondary and tertiary hyperparathyroidism in chronic kidney disease: An endocrine and renal perspective. Indian J Endocrinol Metab. 2019;23(4):391–399.
7. Dulfer RR, Franssen GJH, Hesselink DA, Hoorn EJ, van Eijck CHJ, van Ginhoven TM. Systematic review of surgical and medical treatment for tertiary hyperparathyroidism. Br J Surg. 2017;104(7):804–813.
8. Truszkowski R, Blauth-Opieńska J, Iwanowska J. Parathyroid hormone. Biochem J. 1939;33(6):1005–1011.
9. Gensure RC, Gardella TJ, Juppner H. Parathyroid hormone and parathyroid hormone-related peptide, and their receptors. Biochem Biophys Res Commun. 2005;328(3):666–678.
10. Wysolmerski JJ. Parathyroid hormone-related protein: an update. J Clin Endocrinol Metab. 2012;97(9):2947–2956.
11. Evenepoel P, Bover J, Urena Torres P. Parathyroid hormone metabolism and signaling in health and chronic kidney disease. Kidney Int. 2016;90(6):1184–1190.
12. Silva BC, Bilezikian JP. Parathyroid hormone: anabolic and catabolic actions on the skeleton. Curr Opin Pharmacol. 2015;22:41–50.
13. Goltzman D. Physiology of parathyroid hormone. Endocrinol Metab Clin North Am. 2018;47(4):743–758.
14. Kazama JJ, Wakasugi M. Parathyroid hormone and bone in dialysis patients. Ther Apher Dial. 2018;22(3):229–235.
15. Kritmetapak K, Pongchaiyakul C. Parathyroid hormone measurement in chronic kidney disease: from basics to clinical implications. Int J Nephrol. 2019;2019:5496710.
16. Rambausek M, Ritz E, Rascher W, Kreusser W, Mann JF, Kreye VA, et al. Vascular effects of parathyroid hormone (PTH). Adv Exp Med Biol. 1982;151:619–632.
17. Shan J, Pang PK, Lin HC, Yang MC. Cardiovascular effects of human parathyroid hormone and parathyroid hormone-related peptide. J Cardiovasc Pharmacol. 1994;23 Suppl 2:S38–S41.

18. Cunningham J, Locatelli F, Rodriguez M. Secondary hyperparathyroidism: pathogenesis, disease progression, and therapeutic options. Clin J Am Soc Nephrol. 2011;6(4):913–921.
19. Waziri B, Duarte R, Naicker S. Chronic kidney disease-mineral and bone disorder (CKD-MBD): current perspectives. Int J Nephrol Renovasc Dis. 2019;12:263–276.
20. Silver J, Kilav R, Naveh-Many T. Mechanisms of secondary hyperparathyroidism. Am J Physiol – Renal Physiol. 2002;283(3):367–376.
21. Tominaga Y. Mechanism of parathyroid tumourigenesis in uraemia. Nephrol Dial Transplant. 1999;14 Suppl 1(90001):63–65.
22. Tokumoto M, Taniguchi M, Matsuo D, Tsuruya K, Hirakata H, Iida M. Parathyroid cell growth in patients with advanced secondary hyperparathyroidism: vitamin D receptor, calcium sensing receptor, and cell cycle regulating factors. Ther Apher Dial. 2005;9 Suppl 1:S27–S34.
23. Chen CL, Chen NC, Liang HL, Hsu CY, Chou KJ, Fang HC, et al. Effects of denosumab and calcitriol on severe secondary hyperparathyroidism in dialysis patients with low bone mass. J Clin Endocrinol Metab. 2015;100(7):2784–2792.
24. Arcidiacono MV, Sato T, Alvarez-Hernandez D, Yang J, Tokumoto M, Gonzalez-Suarez I, et al. EGFR activation increases parathyroid hyperplasia and calcitriol resistance in kidney disease. J Am Soc Nephrol: JASN. 2008;19(2):310–320.
25. Fukuda N, Tanaka H, Tominaga Y, Fukagawa M, Kurokawa K, Seino Y. Decreased 1,25-dihydroxyvitamin D3 receptor density is associated with a more severe form of parathyroid hyperplasia in chronic uremic patients. J Clin Invest. 1993;92(3):1436–1443.
26. Komaba H, Fukagawa M. FGF23–parathyroid interaction: implications in chronic kidney disease. Kidney Int. 2010;77(4):292–298.
27. Wetmore JB, Santos PW, Mahnken JD, Krebill R, Menard R, Gutta H, et al. Elevated FGF23 levels are associated with impaired calcium-mediated suppression of PTH in ESRD. J Clin Endocrinol Metabol. 2011;96(1):E57–E64.
28. Quarles LD. Role of FGF23 in vitamin D and phosphate metabolism: Implications in chronic kidney disease. Exp Cell Res. 2012;318(9):1040–1048.
29. Faul C, Amaral AP, Oskouei B, Hu M-C, Sloan A, Isakova T, et al. FGF23 induces left ventricular hypertrophy. J Clin Invest. 2011;121(11):4393–4408.
30. Isakova T, Cai X, Lee J, Xie D, Wang X, Mehta R, et al. Longitudinal FGF23 Trajectories and Mortality in Patients with CKD. J Am Soc Nephrol: JASN. 2018;29(2):579–590.
31. Dusso AS, Sato T, Arcidiacono MV, Alvarez-Hernandez D, Yang J, Gonzalez-Suarez I, et al. Pathogenic mechanisms for parathyroid hyperplasia. Kidney Int. 2006;70(S102):S8–S11.
32. Tominaga Y, Kohara S, Namii Y, Nagasaka T, Haba T, Uchida K, et al. Clonal analysis of nodular parathyroid hyperplasia in renal hyperparathyroidism. World J Surg. 1996;20(7):744–752.
33. Gioviale MC, Bellavia M, Damiano G, Lo Monte AI. Post-transplantation tertiary hyperparathyroidism. Ann Transplant. 2012;17(3):111–119.
34. Massari PU. Disorders of bone and mineral metabolism after renal transplantation. Kidney Int. 1997;52(5):1412–1421.
35. Singh AK, Farag YMK, Mittal BV, Subramanian KK, Reddy SRK, Acharya VN, et al. Epidemiology and risk factors of chronic kidney disease in India – results from the SEEK (Screening and Early Evaluation of Kidney Disease) study. BMC Nephrol. 2013;14(1):114.
36. Li PKT, Chow KM, Matsuo S, Yang CW, Jha V, Becker G, et al. Asian chronic kidney disease best practice recommendations: positional statements for early detection of chronic kidney disease from Asian Forum for Chronic Kidney Disease Initiatives (AFCKDI). Nephrology. 2011;16(7):633–641.
37. Ene-Iordache BD, Perico NMD, Bikbov BMD, Carminati SIT, Remuzzi AE, Perna AM, et al. Chronic kidney disease and cardiovascular risk in six regions of the world (ISN-KDDC): a cross-sectional study. Lancet Global Health. 2016;4(5):e307–e319.
38. Imtiaz S, Salman B, Qureshi R, Drohlia MF, Ahmad A. A review of the epidemiology of chronic kidney disease in Pakistan: A global and regional perspective. Saudi J Kidney Dis Transpl. 2018;29(6):1441–1451.
39. Das SK, Afsana SM, Elahi SB, Chisti MJ, Das J, Mamun AA, et al. Renal insufficiency among urban populations in Bangladesh: A decade of laboratory-based observations. PLOS ONE. 2019;14(4):e0214568.
40. Wimalawansa SJ. Escalating chronic kidney diseases of multi-factorial origin in Sri Lanka: causes, solutions, and recommendations. Environ Health Prev Med. 2014;19(6):375–394.
41. Wong LY, Liew AST, Weng WT, Lim CK, Vathsala A, Toh MPHS. Projecting the burden of chronic kidney disease in a developed country and its implications on public health. Int J Nephrol. 2018;2018:5196285–5196289.
42. Ingsathit A, Thakkinstian A, Chaiprasert A, Sangthawan P, Gojaseni P, Kiattisunthorn K, et al. Prevalence and risk factors of chronic kidney disease in the Thai adult population: Thai SEEK study. Nephrol Dial Transplant. 2010;25(5):1567–1575.
43. Ismail H, Abdul Manaf MR, Abdul Gafor AH, Mohamad Zaher ZM, Ibrahim AIN. Economic burden of ESRD to the Malaysian health care system. Kidney Int Rep. 2019;4(9):1261–1270.
44. Prodjosudjadi W, Suhardjono, Suwitra K, Pranawa, Widiana IGR, Loekman JS, et al. Detection and prevention of chronic kidney disease in Indonesia: initial community screening. Nephrology. 2009;14(7):669–674.
45. Rajapurkar MM, John GT, Kirpalani AL, Abraham G, Agarwal SK, Almeida AF, et al. What do we know about chronic kidney disease in India: first report of the Indian CKD registry. BMC Nephrol. 2012;13(1):10.
46. Yang C, Wang H, Zhao X, Matsushita K, Coresh J, Zhang L, et al. CKD in China: evolving spectrum and public health implications. Am J Kidney Dis. 2019; vol. 76/no. 2, (2020;2019;), pp. 258–264.
47. Myers OB, Pankratz VS, Norris KC, Vassalotti JA, Unruh ML, Argyropoulos C. Surveillance of CKD epidemiology in the US–a joint analysis of NHANES and KEEP. Sci Rep. 2018;8(1):15900–15909.
48. Sabanayagam C, Lim SC, Wong TY, Lee J, Shankar A, Tai ES. Ethnic disparities in prevalence and impact of risk factors of chronic kidney disease. Nephrol Dial Transplant. 2010;25(8):2564–2570.
49. Singapore. Ministry of Health E, Disease Control D. National Health Survey 2010, Singapore. Singapore: Ministry of Health; 2011.
50. Wong LY, Toh MPHS, Tham LWC. Projection of prediabetes and diabetes population size in Singapore using a dynamic Markov model. J Diabetes. 2017;9(1):65–75.
51. Reisman D, NetLibrary I. Social Policy in an Ageing Society: Age and Health in Singapore. Northampton, MA: Edward Elgar; 2009.
52. Mushi L, Marschall P, Fleßa S. The cost of dialysis in low and middle-income countries: a systematic review. BMC Health Serv Res. 2015;15:506.
53. Rizvi SA, Naqvi SA, Zafar MN, Hussain Z, Hashmi A, Hussain M, et al. A renal transplantation model for developing countries. Am J Transplant. 2011;11(11):2302–2307.
54. Hedgeman E, Lipworth L, Lowe K, Saran R, Do T, Fryzek J. International burden of chronic kidney disease and secondary hyperparathyroidism: a systematic review of the literature and available data. Int J Nephrol. 2015;2015:184321–15.
55. Schmidt VH, Lim CH. Organ transplantation in Singapore: history, problems, and policies. Soc Sci Med. 2004;59(10):2173–2182.
56. Chiang C. The use of bone turnover markers in chronic kidney disease-mineral and bone disorders: Detection and evaluation of CKD-MBD. Nephrology. 2017;22:11–13.
57. Ott SM. Bone disease in CKD. Curr Opin Nephrol Hypertens. 2012;21(4):376–381.
58. Drüeke TB, Massy ZA. Changing bone patterns with progression of chronic kidney disease. Kidney Int. 2016;89(2):289–302.
59. Spaulding C, Young G. Osteitis fibrosa cystica and chronic renal failure. J Am Podiatric Med Assoc. 1997;87(5):238–240.
60. Nigwekar SU, Thadhani R, Brandenburg VM. Calciphylaxis. N Engl J Med. 2018;378(18):1704–1714.
61. Sandra Tan NKY, Lim DGZ, Parameswaran R. Calciphylaxis in renal hyperparathyroidism: a case-based review. World J Endocrine Surg. 2016 May–Aug;8(2):156–159.
62. Ho L-Y, Wong P-N, Sin H-K, Wong Y-Y, Lo K-C, Chan S-F, et al. Risk factors and clinical course of hungry bone syndrome after total parathyroidectomy in dialysis patients with secondary hyperparathyroidism. BMC Nephrol. 2017;18(1):12.
63. Kidney Disease: Improving Global Outcomes CKDMBDUWG. KDIGO. 2017 Clinical practice guideline update for the diagnosis, evaluation, prevention, and treatment of chronic kidney disease–mineral and bone disorder (CKD-MBD). Kidney Int Suppl. 2017;7(1):1–59.
64. Ballinger AE, Palmer SC, Nistor I, Craig JC, Strippoli GFM. Calcimimetics for secondary hyperparathyroidism in chronic kidney disease patients. Cochrane Database Syst Rev. 2014(12):CD006254.
65. Harrington P, Fotsch C. Calcium sensing receptor activators: calcimimetics. Curr Med Chem. 2007;14(28):3027–3034.
66. Fukagawa M, Kurokawa K. Pathogenesis and medical treatment of secondary hyperparathyroidism. Semin Surg Oncol. 1997;13(2):73–77.
67. Vestergaard P, Susanna vid Streym T. Medical treatment of primary, secondary, and tertiary hyperparathyroidism. Curr Drug Saf. 2011;6(2):108–113.
68. Brunaud LMDP, Ngueyon Sime WMD, Filipozzi PMD, Nomine-Criqui CMD, Aronova AMD, Zarnegar RMD, et al. Minimal impact of calcimimetics on the management of hyperparathyroidism in chronic dialysis. Surgery. 2016;159(1):183–192.
69. Parfrey PS, Chertow GM, Block GA, Correa-Rotter R, Drüeke TB, Floege J, et al. The clinical course of treated hyperparathyroidism among patients receiving hemodialysis and the effect of cinacalcet: the EVOLVE trial. J Clin Endocrinol Metabol. 2013;98(12):4834–4844.
70. Bergua C, Torregrosa JV, Cofán F, Oppenheimer F. Cinacalcet for the treatment of hypercalcemia in renal transplanted patients with secondary hyperparathyroidism. Transplant Proc. 2007;39(7):2254–2255.
71. Chudzinski W, Wyrzykowska M, Nazarewski S, Durlik M, Galazka Z. Does the parathyroidectomy endanger the transplanted kidney? Transplant Proc. 2016;48(5):1633–1636.
72. Finnerty BM, Chan TW, Jones G, Khader T, Moore M, Gray KD, et al. Parathyroidectomy versus cinacalcet in the management of tertiary hyperparathyroidism: surgery improves renal transplant allograft survival. Surgery. 2019;165(1):129–134.
73. Schneider R, Waldmann J, Ramaswamy A, Fernandez ED, Bartsch DK, Schlosser K. Frequency of ectopic and supernumerary intrathymic parathyroid glands in patients with renal hyperparathyroidism: analysis of 461 patients undergoing initial parathyroidectomy with bilateral cervical thymectomy. World J Surg. 2011;35(6):1260–1265.
74. Pitt SC, Panneerselvan R, Chen H, Sippel RS. Secondary and tertiary hyperparathyroidism: the utility of ioPTH monitoring. World J Surg. 2010;34(6):1343–1349.
75. Ohe MN, Santos RO, Kunii IS, Carvalho AB, Abrahao M, Neves MC, et al. Intraoperative PTH cutoff definition to predict successful parathyroidectomy in secondary and tertiary hyperparathyroidism. Braz J Otorhinolaryngol. 2013;79(4):494–499.
76. Cheung CK, England RJ, Bhandari S. The utility of intraoperative PTH measurement in surgical parathyroidectomy after renal transplantation. Clin Nephrol. 2011;76(2):104–109.
77. El-Husseini A, Wang K, Edon A, Saxon D, Lima F, Sloan D, et al. Value of intraoperative parathyroid hormone assay during parathyroidectomy in dialysis and renal transplant patients with secondary and tertiary hyperparathyroidism. Nephron. 2018;138(2):119–128.
78. Weber KJ, Misra S, Lee JK, Wilhelm SW, DeCresce R, Prinz RA. Intraoperative PTH monitoring in parathyroid hyperplasia requires stricter criteria for success. Surgery. 2004;136(6):1154–1159.
79. Soares MR, Cavalcanti GV, Iwakura R, Lucca LJ, Romao EA, Conti de Freitas LC. Analysis of the role of thyroidectomy and thymectomy in the surgical treatment of secondary hyperparathyroidism. Am J Otolaryngol. 2019;40(1):67–69.
80. Shepet K, Alhefdhi A, Usedom R, Sippel R, Chen H. Parathyroid cryopreservation after parathyroidectomy: a worthwhile practice? Ann Surg Oncol. 2013;20(7):2256–2260.
81. Yuan Q, Liao Y, Zhou R, Liu J, Tang J, Wu G. Subtotal parathyroidectomy versus total parathyroidectomy with autotransplantation for secondary hyperparathyroidism: an updated systematic review and meta-analysis. Langenbecks Arch Surg. 2019;404(6):669–679.

82. Chen J, Jia X, Kong X, Wang Z, Cui M, Xu D. Total parathyroidectomy with autotransplantation versus subtotal parathyroidectomy for renal hyperparathyroidism: a systematic review and meta-analysis. Nephrology (Carlton). 2017;22(5):388–396.
83. Rajeev P, Lee KY, Tang XJ, Goo TT, Tan WB, Ngiam KY. Outcomes of parathyroidectomy in renal hyperparathyroidism in patients with No access to renal transplantation in Singapore. Int J Surg. 2016;25:64–68.
84. Li C, Lv L, Wang H, Wang X, Yu B, Xu Y, et al. Total parathyroidectomy versus total parathyroidectomy with autotransplantation for secondary hyperparathyroidism: systematic review and meta-analysis. Ren Fail. 2017;39(1):678–687.
85. Liu ME, Qiu NC, Zha SL, Du ZP, Wang YF, Wang Q, et al. To assess the effects of parathyroidectomy (TPTX versus TPTX+AT) for secondary hyperparathyroidism in chronic renal failure: a systematic review and meta-analysis. Int J Surg. 2017;44:353–362.
86. Schlosser K, Veit JA, Witte S, Fernandez ED, Victor N, Knaebel HP, et al. Comparison of total parathyroidectomy without autotransplantation and without thymectomy versus total parathyroidectomy with autotransplantation and with thymectomy for secondary hyperparathyroidism: TOPAR PILOT-Trial. Trials. 2007;8:22.
87. Rodriguez-Ortiz ME, Pendon-Ruiz de Mier MV, Rodriguez M. Parathyroidectomy in dialysis patients: indications, methods, and consequences. Semin Dial. 2019;32(5):444–451.
88. Schamp S, Dunser E, Schuster H, Kramer-Deimer J, Kettenbach J, Funovics M, et al. Ultrasound-guided percutaneous ethanol ablation of parathyroid hyperplasia: preliminary experience in patients on chronic dialysis. Ultraschall Med. 2004;25(2):131–6.
89. Fletcher S, Kanagasundaram NS, Rayner HC, Irving HC, Fowler RC, Brownjohn AM, et al. Assessment of ultrasound guided percutaneous ethanol injection and parathyroidectomy in patients with tertiary hyperparathyroidism. Nephrol Dial Transplant. 1998;13(12):3111–3117.
90. Alsafran S, Sherman SK, Dahdaleh FS, Ruhle B, Mercier F, Kaplan EL, et al. Preoperative calcitriol reduces postoperative intravenous calcium requirements and length of stay in parathyroidectomy for renal-origin hyperparathyroidism. Surgery. 2019;165(1):151–157.
91. Mittendorf EA, Merlino JI, McHenry CR. Post-parathyroidectomy hypocalcemia: incidence, risk factors, and management. Am Surg. 2004;70(2):114–119; discussion 9-20.
92. Jain N, Reilly RF. Hungry bone syndrome. Curr Opin Nephrol Hypertens. 2017;26(4):250–255.
93. Goldfarb M, Gondek SS, Lim SM, Farra JC, Nose V, Lew JI. Postoperative hungry bone syndrome in patients with secondary hyperparathyroidism of renal origin. World J Surg. 2012;36(6):1314–1319.
94. Ge Y, Yang G, Wang N, Zha X, Yu X, Mao H, et al. Bone metabolism markers and hungry bone syndrome after parathyroidectomy in dialysis patients with secondary hyperparathyroidism. Int Urol Nephrol. 2019;51(8):1443–1449.
95. Loke SC, Kanesvaran R, Yahya R, Fisal L, Wong TW, Loong YY. Efficacy of an intravenous calcium gluconate infusion in controlling serum calcium after parathyroidectomy for secondary hyperparathyroidism. Ann Acad Med Singapore. 2009;38(12):1074–1080.
96. Tan JH, Tan HCL, Loke SC, Arulanantham SAP. Novel calcium infusion regimen after parathyroidectomy for renal hyperparathyroidism. Nephrology (Carlton, Vic). 2017;22(4):308–315.
97. Taterra D, Wong LM, Vikse J, Sanna B, Pękala P, Walocha J, et al. The prevalence and anatomy of parathyroid glands: a meta-analysis with implications for parathyroid surgery. Langenbeck's Arch Surg. 2019;404(1):63–70.
98. Uslu A, Okut G, Tercan IC, Erkul Z, Aykas A, Karatas M, et al. Anatomical distribution and number of parathyroid glands, and parathyroid function, after total parathyroidectomy and bilateral cervical thymectomy. Medicine. 2019;98(23):e15926–e15926.
99. Hiramitsu T, Tomosugi T, Okada M, Futamura K, Tsujita M, Goto N, et al. Pre-operative localisation of the parathyroid glands in secondary hyperparathyroidism: a retrospective cohort study. Sci Rep. 2019;9(1):14634.
100. Taïeb D, Ureña-Torres P, Zanotti-Fregonara P, Rubello D, Ferretti A, Henter I, et al. Parathyroid scintigraphy in renal hyperparathyroidism: the added diagnostic value of SPECT and SPECT/CT. Clin Nucl Med. 2013;38(8):630–635.
101. Ardito G, Revelli L, Giustozzi E, Giordano A. Radioguided parathyroidectomy in forearm graft for recurrent hyperparathyroidism. Br J Radiol. 2012;85(1009):e1–e3.
102. Pitt SC, Panneerselvan R, Sippel RS, Chen H. Radioguided parathyroidectomy for hyperparathyroidism in the reoperative neck. Surgery. 2009;146(4):592–599.
103. Somnay YR, Weinlander E, Alfhefdi A, Schneider D, Sippel RS, Chen H. Radioguided parathyroidectomy for tertiary hyperparathyroidism. J Surg Res. 2015;195(2):406–411.

35

NORMOCALCEMIC HYPERPARATHYROIDISM

Mayur Agrawal and Subhash Yadav

Introduction

Primary hyperparathyroidism (PHPT) is a common endocrinological disorder and frequently encounter this in clinical practice. The classical symptoms are described by stones, bones, groans, moans and overtones, i.e., renal stones, bony pain, fractures and osteitis fibrosa cystica; abdominal pain, gall stone disorder, acid peptic disease, pancreatitis; psychiatric moans, mood disorder, irritability and fatigue overtones, myalgia or myopathy. Besides that this classical pentad of severe symptomatic and sometimes life-threatening hypercalcemia is now less often seen than previously as more and more biochemical testing is done routinely, and people present to clinic with asymptomatic hypercalcemia (1–3).

A newer clinical presentation of PHPT is normocalcemic hyperparathyroidism (NPHPT) characterized by normal total and ionized serum calcium levels and consistently elevated parathyroid hormone (PTH) levels provided that more common cause for secondary elevations of PTH, such as renal disease and vitamin D deficiency, are ruled out. This was firstly recognized in 2008 by the panel of experts of the Third International Workshop on Asymptomatic Primary Hyperparathyroidism (4).

Definition

NPHPT is defined as persistent normal fasting total and ionized serum calcium levels and consistently elevated PTH levels after ruling out secondary caused of hyperparathyroidism.

Many times, in abnormal calcium states, total calcium frequently disagrees with ionized calcium (iCa) in classifying calcium status. So measurement of iCa is required to accurately assess calcium status and improve diagnostic accuracy (5). NPHPT has been increasingly detected in patients who are evaluated for low BMD (6).

It is also important to note that many patients with PHPT may have intermittent hypercalcemia or may have only raised ionized calcium and more clinical setting is that of a patient of PHPT after parathyroidectomy may have elevated PTH with normal calcium level. One should also pay attention to history of drugs or treatment, such as bisphosphonates and denosumab, causing serum calcium to normalize in PHPT (5, 7).

Other causes of hyperparathyroidism due to a normal physiological stimulus to increased PTH levels that is secondary hyperparathyroidism states should be excluded. Secondary causes of an elevated PTH level includes renal disease, vitamin D deficiency, hypercalciuria, gastrointestinal disorders associated with calcium malabsorption and drugs like loop diuretics and lithium use (8). The diagnosis of parathyroid gland autonomy in the setting of chronic kidney disease is more challenging. Defining vitamin D optimal level is also controversial, and the recommended threshold value of the Institute of Medicine (IOM) for 25(OH)D is 20 ng/mL (50 nmol/L) and that of Endocrine Society is 30 ng/mL (75 nmol/L) (9, 10).

Prevalence

There are very few epidemiological studies to estimate the prevalence of NPHPT and also difficult to determine the epidemiology of NPHPT as a very few number of studies have examined the prevalence in the general population, and the existing studies have been inconsistent in their disease definition. A study is done by Natalie E. Cusano et al. to find out prevalence of NPHPT in nonselected, nonreferral populations (The Osteoporotic Fractures in Men [MrOS] study and Dallas Heart Study [DHS]). In the Osteoporotic Fractures in Men, the prevalence of normocalcemic hyperparathyroidism was 0.4%. Similarly, the Dallas Heart Study of men and women aged 18–65 years determined prevalence of normocalcemic hyperparathyroidism of 3.1% (11). In a prospective study conducted in Spain, a cohort of 100 healthy postmenopausal women is studied. Six patients (prevalence 6%) had high PTH with 25-OH vitamin D >30 ng/mL and were classified as normocalcemic hyperparathyroidism (12). In a population-based survey of 5202 postmenopausal women in Sweden in 1991–1992 between the ages of 55 and 75 showed that 0.5% had elevated PTH levels with normal serum calcium values (13). Comparing prevalence within and between countries is problematical owing to varying levels of screening availability and sources of information.

Pathophysiology

There are various hypotheses proposed for NPHPT, and it may be early or mild form of hypercalcemic hyperparathyroidism that is like a subclinical stage (14). This hypothesis went on to state that the second phase of the evolution of PHPT would be the clinical stage when hypercalcemia became overtly present. Another hypothesis postulated by Maruani et al. is that in NPHPT, there is resistance to target tissues. They have showed that after an oral calcium load, normocalcemic subjects showed inadequate suppression of PTH when matched with a cohort of subjects with hypercalcemic PHPT (15). Other authors have suggested that it is a response to persistent hypocalcemic stimuli, and this happened because of persistent leak of calcium from kidney (16).

Data on the specific genetic background of the parathyroid tumors associated with NPHPT are lacking. Genes involved in regulating the cell cycle are thought to be implicated in sporadic parathyroid adenomas. Studies have revealed gene involved like CCND1, MEN1, CDC73, CTNNB1, CDKN1B and AIP (17).

In a prospective study in Spain, 61 consecutive normocalcemic and asymptomatic hyperparathyroidism patients were followed up for 1 year. A986S polymorphism of calcium sensing receptor (CaSR) was an independent predictor of PTH level in normocalcemic hyperparathyroidism patients but not in asymptomatic hyperparathyroidism. Therefore, PTH levels in NPHPT may be partially regulated by the A986S polymorphism, acting as a resistance factor due to a relative loss of CASR function (18).

Natural course

Data are limited regarding the natural history of the NPHPT. It is believed that manifestations of PHPT develop chronologically; initially it has normal levels of calcium with increased PTH, that is, normocalcemic hyperparathyroidism is subclinical phase of PHPT, and later classical hyperparathyroidism develops where hypercalcemia occurs with increased levels of PTH and clinical manifestation appears (19). But the rate and duration of this conversion is not clear as different studies have defined normocalcemic hyperparathyroidism differently, and many studies have not even ruled out secondary causes of hyperparathyroidism (20). It is also seen that for a long time, calcium remains within normal range with elevated PTH (21).

In a longitudinal cohort study by Lowe et al., 37 patients of normocalcemic hyperparathyroidism were followed for median of 3 years (1–8 years). Seventeen patients (19%) became frankly hypercalcemic (seven hypercalcemia; one kidney stone; one fracture; two marked hypercalciuria; six had >10% bone mineral density [BMD] loss at one or more sites) within 3 years, suggesting that at least in certain patients, the condition progresses from the preclinical to the clinically evident stage (20).

In another study by Tordjman et al., 32 patients with normocalcemic hyperparathyroidism were evaluated. A total of 12 patients underwent parathyroid surgery, and remaining 20 patients were followed for a mean of 4.1 ± 3.2 years (1–13 years). None of these patients developed hypercalcemia in follow-up, also there was no significant change in mean urinary calcium excretion or PTH levels (22).

Clinical presentations

PHPT can present with hypercalcemia crisis or features of hypercalcemia and target organ involvements. Normocalcemic means normal calcium but does not imply that the patient is without clinical manifestations. Normocalcemic hyperparathyroidism can present without any symptoms or with target organ involvement, although usually in milder forms. As stated previously, most cases of NPHPT are found during evaluation of low BMD or nephrolithiasis (20).

Although the clinical manifestations of NPHPT should be milder than those of overt disease, most studies have high rates of bone disease and nephrolithiasis. However, this could be just a selection bias as most cases of normocalcemic hyperparathyroidism are diagnosed during the evaluation of a skeletal or a renal disease (20).

In PHPT, dual-energy X-ray absorptiometry (DEXA) and histomorphometry suggest low BMD, especially in distal third of radius, i.e., cortical sites, with a relative preservation of the trabecular bone. Newer methods of imaging such as high-resolution peripheral quantitative computed tomography and trabecular bone score revealed altered bone microarchitecture and increased risk of fractures at both cortical and trabecular sites (23). In two studies, one by Amaral et al. and the other by Lowe et al., it was revealed that BMD in the distal radius was more preserved in the normocalcemic patients than in hypercalcemic hyperparathyroidism (20, 24).

In a retrospective study of 307 patients, prevalence of low BMD and kidney stones was similar between NPHPT and hypercalcemic hyperparathyroidism (25). Similarly, retrospective study of 70 patients of PHPT showed previous history of fractures in 15% of normocalcemic patients and 10.8% of hypercalcemic patients, although it was statistically nonsignificant. It also revealed nephrolithiasis in 18.2% normocalcemic hyperparathyroidism and 18.9% in the hypercalcemic PHPT (24).

Symptomatic renal stones have been seen in about 10% of patients with PHPT, and occult renal stones have been reported in about 20–50%. Whereas there was no difference in the incidence of vertebral fracture and osteoporosis between symptomatic and asymptomatic patients, more stones were detected in symptomatic (78%) than asymptomatic (35.5%) in a prospective study on 140 patients by Cipriani et al. (26).

While hypercalcemic hyperparathyroidism has been linked to adverse cardiovascular outcomes, effects of NPHPT on various metabolic outcomes have been addressed in a few small cohorts. In a retrospective study, 11 normocalcemic hyperparathyroidism were compared to 296 normal PTH individuals, and no significant differences were found in terms of age, sex, body mass index, serum calcium, 25-hydroxyvitamin D, serum creatinine, fasting plasma glucose, triglycerides, total cholesterol, high-density lipoprotein and low-density lipoprotein. Normocalcemic hyperparathyroidism had higher risk of high blood pressure. The proposed mechanisms are: (1) PTH receptors are expressed in the vessel and myocardium and may be involved in vascular stiffness and left ventricular hypertrophy, (2) endothelial dysfunction and (3) PTH-induced hypertension includes activation of the renin-aldosterone system, secretion of cortisol from the adrenal cortex and sympathetic activity (27).

In a metanalysis of 12 studies, PTH excess indicated an increased risk for total CVD events: pooled HR (95% CI), 1.45 (1.24–1.71) and the results for fatal CVD events and nonfatal CVD events were: HR 1.50 (1.18–1.91) and HR 1.48 (1.14–1.92) respectively. The metanalysis indicates that higher PTH concentrations are associated with increased risk of CVD event (28).

In a prospective study, 25 patients with normocalcemic hyperparathyroidism, 24 with hypercalcemic hyperparathyroidism and 30 age-gender matched controls were compared. Normocalcemic hyperparathyroidism patients had significantly higher prevalence of glucose intolerance and hypertension, whereas similar prevalence of metabolic syndrome, glucose intolerance and previous history of hypertension/antihypertensive medications was found between normocalcemic and hypercalcemic hyperparathyroidism (29). Current data do not support a cardiovascular evaluation or surgery for the purpose of improving cardiovascular markers (30).

Diagnosis and evaluation

The expert panel from the Fourth International Workshop on the Management of asymptomatic PHPT recommended that the PTH level remains above the normal range on at least two subsequent measurements during a 3–6 months period to confirm hyperparathyroidism (31). Laboratory evaluation should include measurements of serum calcium, phosphate, albumin, alkaline phosphatase, ionic calcium, intact PTH (iPTH) levels, renal function tests and serum 25-hydroxyvitamin D levels. USG abdomen and 24-hour urinary calcium level (>400 mg/day) should also be measured to rule out nephrolithiasis and hypercalciuria, respectively, and a BMD to look for osteoporosis. A urinary calcium clearance/creatinine clearance ratio should be calculated to rule out familial hypocalciuric hypercalcemia, and ratio of <0.01 suggests, but does not prove, FHH (31).

Management

Though the optimal management strategy for the NPHPT has not been established, the guidelines are available from the Fourth International Workshop on the Management of Asymptomatic PHPT based on expert recommendation (31). Presently in absence of evidence, all the recommendations advised for asymptomatic hyperparathyroidism may not be applicable as it is to normocalcemic hyperparathyroidism, so treatment can be individualized. Surgery is main treatment for patients with hypercalcemic hyperparathyroidism for all symptomatic as well as asymptomatic patients with target organ damage, i.e., significant kidney and bone disease. In patients without complications at the time of presentation, monitoring should include annual clinical assessment, measurement of biochemical parameters, including total/ionized calcium and PTH annually, and bone density measurement every 1–2 years (32). There are limited data for management of patients with NPHPT.

It was also found that it was difficult to locate adenoma in patient with NPHPT. A study by Cunha-Bezerra et al. found the sensitivity of all imaging procedures was lower for the normocalcemic individuals compared to the hypercalcemic cohort, with four-dimensional computed tomography performing best for normocalcemic patients: ultrasound 22 vs. 58%, scintigraphy 11 vs. 75% and four-dimensional computed tomography 56 vs. 75% (33). While another study by Traini et al. found insignificant differences in the accuracy of preoperative sestamibi or ultrasound imaging between normocalcemic and hypercalcemic patients (34). In some series, it has noted higher percentage of normocalcemic patients with multiglandular disease (35, 36).

When patients with NPHPT have parathyroid surgery, though there are limited data but it indicate similar improvement in bone density as for patients with hypercalcemic disease. In a study by Traini et al., it was documented that 42% had improvement in bone density postoperatively with 50% showing stability without further progression. In the same cohort, they showed patients with nephrolithiasis, and there was improvement in 40% of patients and stability in 60% (34). BMD after parathyroidectomy in patients with normocalcemic hyperparathyroidism showed that 46% of patients who had surgery were followed for 1 year and had gains at the spine and hip BMD. Alkaline phosphatase levels above median were identified as an independent predictor of individual BMD gain (37).

As an algorithm for the management of NPHPT patients, the panel of experts suggested, based on the monitoring of serum calcium and PTH annually and bone density by DEXA every 1–2 years, to consider surgery in the following conditions (31):

1. Progression to hypercalcemic hyperparathyroidism: indication to parathyroidectomy according to the guidelines.
2. Progression of the disease, that means worsening of BMD or fracture and/or kidney stones or nephrocalcinosis.

There is paucity of data available about the impact of medical therapy on patients with NPHPT. It is not recommended to limit calcium intake in patients with PHPT who do not undergo surgery. Patients with low serum 25-hydroxyvitamin D should be replete. Supplemental doses of 600–1000 IU cholecalciferol were considered than large doses. The goal of cautiously administered repletion regimens should be to increase the serum 25(OH)D levels to >50 and up to 75 nmol/L (20–30 ng/mL) (32).

Alendronate has shown benefit in BMD with NPHPT at 1 year. This prospective study also revealed significant decrease in bone turnover markers at 3 and 6 months in normocalcemic hyperparathyroidism receiving alendronate vs. vitamin D alone(38).

A pilot study by Brardi et al. demonstrated that of cinacalcet normalized PTH concentrations significantly and reduced the number and diameter of kidney stones in both hypercalcemic and normocalcemic patients over 10 months of therapy (39).

South Asian perspective

In developing countries of South Asia, particularly India, PHPT is still an uncommonly diagnosed. This may be because screening of the healthy population for hypercalcemia is not a routine practice, and there is limited access to medical treatment, especially in the rural areas. PHPT in South Asia is a severe issue with symptomatic involvement of skeletal, muscle and kidney at a young age. The mean calcium, PTH and alkaline phosphate levels are high with low Vit D levels as compare to Western population (40, 41). Prevalence of NPHPT is quite low in South Asian countries, and many times cofounding factor of vitamin D is present.

Conclusion

Normocalcemic hyperparathyroidism is newer clinical entity, and physician should be well versed with it, especially keeping in mind to rule out secondary causes of hyperparathyroidism. Presently NPHPT becomes more evident as countries adopt biochemical screening methods. Though it has normal serum total calcium and ionic calcium, it has many of features pertaining to hypercalcemic hyperparathyroidism. It may also evolve into hypercalcemic hyperparathyroidism, so patients must be followed carefully. The available data suggest that patients with NPHPT develop complications, including nephrolithiasis and osteoporosis, at similar or higher rates to patients with traditional hypercalcemic disease, so treatment modalities should be discussed with patient and mutual decision should be taken. Further studies are warranted for better understanding of natural course of the disease.

References

1. Yadav SK, Mishra SK, Mishra A, Mayilvagnan S, Chand G, Agarwal G, et al. Changing profile of primary hyperparathyroidism over two and half decades: a study in tertiary referral center of North India. World J Surg [Internet]. 2018 Sep 1 [cited 2020 Jul 17];42(9):2732–2737.
2. Mithal A, Kaur P, Singh VP, Sarin D, Rao DS. Asymptomatic primary hyperparathyroidism exists in North India: retrospective data from 2 tertiary care centers. Endocr Pract [Internet]. 2015 Jun 1 [cited 2020 Jul 17];21(6):581–585.
3. Cusano NE, Silverberg SJ, Bilezikian JP. Normocalcemic primary hyperparathyroidism. J Clin Densitom. 2013 Jan;16(1):33–39.
4. Eastell R, Arnold A, Brandi ML, Brown EM, D'Amour P, Hanley DA, et al. Diagnosis of asymptomatic primary hyperparathyroidism: proceedings of the third international workshop. J Clin Endocrinol Metab. 2009;94(2):340–350.
5. Ong GSY, Walsh JP, Stuckey BGA, Brown SJ, Rossi E, Ng JL, et al. The importance of measuring ionized calcium in characterizing calcium status and diagnosing primary hyperparathyroidism. J Clin Endocrinol Metab [Internet]. 2012 Sep [cited 2020 Jul 17];97(9):3138–3145.
6. Eastell R, Brandi ML, Costa AG, D'Amour P, Shoback DM, Thakker RV. Diagnosis of asymptomatic primary hyperparathyroidism: Proceedings of the fourth international workshop. J Clin Endocrinol Metabol [Internet]. 2014 [cited 2020 Jul 17];99(10):3570–3579.
7. Schini M, Jacques RM, Oakes E, Peel NFA, Walsh JS, Eastell R. Normocalcemic hyperparathyroidism: study of its prevalence and natural history. J Clin Endocrinol Metab. 2020;105(4):e1171–e1186.
8. Bilezikian JP, Cusano NE, Khan AA, Liu JM, Marcocci C, Bandeira F. Primary hyperparathyroidism. Nat Rev Dis Prim. 2016 May;2:1–16.
9. Ross AC, Manson JAE, Abrams SA, Aloia JF, Brannon PM, Clinton SK, et al. The 2011 report on dietary reference intakes for calcium and vitamin D from the Institute of Medicine: what clinicians need to know. J Clin Endocrinol Metabol. 2011;96(1):53–58.

10. Holick MF, Binkley NC, Bischoff-Ferrari HA, Gordon CM, Hanley DA, Heaney RP, et al. Evaluation, treatment, and prevention of vitamin D deficiency: an endocrine society clinical practice guideline. J Clin Endocrinol Metab. 2011;96(7):1911–1930.

11. Cusano NE, Maalouf NM, Wang PY, Zhang C, Cremers SC, Haney EM, et al. Normocalcemic hyperparathyroidism and hypoparathyroidism in two community-based nonreferral populations. J Clin Endocrinol Metab [Internet]. 2013 Jul [cited 2020 Jul 17];98(7):2734–2741.

12. García-Martín A, Reyes-García R, Muñoz-Torres M. Normocalcemic primary hyperparathyroidism: one-year follow-up in one hundred postmenopausal women [Internet]. Endocrine; 2012 [cited 2020 Jul 17]; 42:764–766.

13. Lundgren E, Hagström EG, Lundin J, Winnerbäck K, Roos J, Ljunghall S, et al. Primary hyperparathyroidism revisited in menopausal women with serum calcium in the upper normal range at population-based screening 8 years ago. World J Surg [Internet]. 2002 [cited 2020 Jul 17];6(8):931–936.

14. Rao DS, Wilson RJ, Kleerekoper M, Parfitt AM. Lack of biochemical progression or continuation of accelerated bone loss in mild asymptomatic primary hyperparathyroidism: evidence for biphasic disease course. J Clin Endocrinol Metab [Internet]. 1988 [cited 2020 Jul 20];67(6):1294–1298.

15. Maruani G, Hertig A, Paillard M, Houillier P. Normocalcemic primary hyperparathyroidism: evidence for a generalized target-tissue resistance to parathyroid hormone. J Clin Endocrinol Metab. 2003;88(10):4641–4648.

16. Palmieri S, Eller-Vainicher C, Cairoli E, Morelli V, Zhukouskaya VV, Verga U, et al. Hypercalciuria may persist after successful parathyroid surgery and it is associated with parathyroid hyperplasia. J Clin Endocrinol Metab [Internet]. 2015 Jul 1 [cited 2020 Jul 20];100(7):2734–2742.

17. Brewer K, Costa-Guda J, Arnold A. Molecular genetic insights into sporadic primary hyperparathyroidism [Internet]. Vol. 26, Endocrine-Related Cancer. BioScientifica Ltd.; 2019 [cited 2020 Jul 20]. p. R53–72.

18. Díaz-Soto G, Romero E, Castrillón JLP, Jauregui OI, De Luis Román D. Clinical expression of calcium sensing receptor polymorphism (A986S) in normocalcemic and asymptomatic hyperparathyroidism. Horm Metab Res [Internet]. 2016 Mar [cited 2020 Jul 20];48(3):163–168.

19. Bilezikian JP, Silverberg SJ. Hiperparatiroidismo normocalcêmico primário [Internet]. Vol. 54, Arquivos Brasileiros de Endocrinologia e Metabologia. Sociedade Brasileira de Endocrinologia e Metabologia; 2010 [cited 2020 Jul 20]. p. 106–109. Available from: https://pubmed.ncbi.nlm.nih.gov/20485897/

20. Lowe H, McMahon DJ, Rubin MR, Bilezikian JP, Silverberg SJ. Normocalcemic primary hyperparathyroidism: Further characterization of a new clinical phenotype. J Clin Endocrinol Metab [Internet]. 2007 [cited 2020 Jul 19];92(8):3001–3005.

21. Maruani G, Hertig A, Paillard M, Houillier P. Normocalcemic primary hyperparathyroidism: evidence for a generalized target-tissue resistance to parathyroid hormone. J Clin Endocrinol Metab [Internet]. 2003 Oct [cited 2020 Jul 19];88(10):4641–4648.

22. Tordjman KM, Greenman Y, Osher E, Shenkerman G, Stern N. Characterization of normocalcemic primary hyperparathyroidism. Am J Med [Internet]. 2004 Dec [cited 2020 Jul 19];117(11):861–863.

23. Makras P, Anastasilakis AD. Bone disease in primary hyperparathyroidism. Metabolism. Metabolism. 2018 Mar;80:57–65.

24. Amaral LM, Queiroz DC, Marques TF, Mendes M, Bandeira F. Normocalcemic versus hypercalcemic primary hyperparathyroidism: more stone than bone? J Osteoporos. 2012; 2012:128352.

25. Tuna MM, Çalışkan M, Ünal M, Demirci T, Doğan BA, Küçükler K, et al. Normocalcemic hyperparathyroidism is associated with complications similar to those of hypercalcemic hyperparathyroidism. J Bone Miner Metab. 2016 May;34(3):331–335.

26. Cipriani C, Biamonte F, Costa AG, Zhang C, Biondi P, Diacinti D, et al. Prevalence of kidney stones and vertebral fractures in primary hyperparathyroidism using imaging technology. J Clin Endocrinol Metab [Internet]. 2015 Apr [cited 2020 Jul 19];100(4):1309–1315.

27. Chen G, Xue Y, Zhang Q, Xue T, Yao J, Huang H, et al. Is normocalcemic primary hyperparathyroidism harmful or harmless? J Clin Endocrinol Metab [Internet]. 2015 Jun [cited 2020 Jul 19];100(6):2420–2424.

28. Van Ballegooijen AJ, Reinders I, Visser M, Brouwer IA. Parathyroid hormone and cardiovascular disease events: a systematic review and meta-analysis of prospective studies [Internet]. Am Heart J. 2013 [cited 2020 Jul 19];165:655–664.

29. Ozturk FY, Erol S, Canat MM, Karatas S, Kuzu I, Cakir SD, et al. Patients with normocalcemic primary hyperparathyroidism may have similar metabolic profile as hypercalcemic patients. Endocr J [Internet]. 2016 Feb [cited 2020 Jul 19];63(2):111–118.

30. Silverberg SJ, Clarke BL, Peacock M, Bandeira F, Boutroy S, Cusano NE, et al. Current issues in the presentation of asymptomatic primary hyperparathyroidism: Proceedings of the fourth International Workshop. J Clin Endocrinol Metab. 2014;99(10):3580–3594.

31. Bilezikian JP, Brandi ML, Eastell R, Silverberg SJ, Udelsman R, Marcocci C, et al. Guidelines for the management of asymptomatic primary hyperparathyroidism: summary statement from the fourth international workshop. J Clin Endocrinol Metab. 2014;99(10):3561–3569.

32. Cusano NE, Cipriani C, Bilezikian JP. Management of normocalcemic primary hyperparathyroidism [Internet]. Vol. 32, Best Practice and Research: Clinical Endocrinology and Metabolism. Bailliere Tindall Ltd; 2018 [cited 2020 Jul 19]. p. 837–845. Available from: https://pubmed.ncbi.nlm.nih.gov/30665550/

33. Cunha-Bezerra P, Vieira R, Amaral F, Cartaxo H, Lima T, Montarroyos U, et al. Better performance of four-dimension computed tomography as a localization procedure in normocalcemic primary hyperparathyroidism. J Med Imaging Radiat Oncol [Internet]. 2018 Aug [cited 2020 Jul 20];62(4):493–498.

34. Traini E, Bellantone R, Tempera SE, Russo S, De Crea C, Lombardi CP, et al. Is parathyroidectomy safe and effective in patients with normocalcemic primary hyperparathyroidism? Langenbeck's Arch Surg [Internet]. 2018 May [cited 2020 Jul 20];403(3):317–323.

35. Lim JY, Herman MC, Bubis L, Epelboym I, Allendorf JD, Chabot JA, et al. Differences in single gland and multigland disease are seen in low biochemical profile primary hyperparathyroidism. In: Surgery (United States) [Internet]. Mosby Inc.; 2017 [cited 2020 Jul 20]. p. 70–77. Available from: https://pubmed.ncbi.nlm.nih.gov/27847113/

36. Kiriakopoulos A, Petralias A, Linos D. Classic primary hyperparathyroidism versus normocalcemic and normohormonal variants: do they really differ? World J Surg [Internet]. 2018 Apr [cited 2020 Jul 20];42(4):992–997.

37. Koumakis E, Souberbielle JC, Payet J, Sarfati E, Borderie D, Kahan A, et al. Individual site-specific bone mineral density gain in normocalcemic primary hyperparathyroidism. Osteoporos Int [Internet]. 2014 [cited 2020 Jul 20];25(7):1963–1968.

38. Cesareo R, Di Stasio E, Vescini F, Campagna G, Cianni R, Pasqualini V, et al. Effects of alendronate and vitamin D in patients with normocalcemic primary hyperparathyroidism. Osteoporos Int [Internet]. 2015 Apr [cited 2020 Jul 17];26(4):1295–1302.

39. Brardi S, Cevenini G, Verdacchi T, Romano G, Ponchietti R. Use of cinacalcet in nephrolithiasis associated with normocalcemic or hypercalcemic primary hyperparathyroidism: results of a prospective randomized pilot study. Arch Ital Urol Androl [Internet]. 2015 Mar [cited 2020 Jul 19];87(1):66–71.

40. Pradeep P V, Jayashree B, Mishra A, Mishra SK. Systematic review of primary hyperparathyroidism in India: the past, present, and the future trends. Int J Endocrinol [Internet]. 2011;2011:921814.

41. Mishra SK, Agarwal G, Kar DK, Gupta SK, Mithal A, Rastad J. Unique clinical characteristics of primary hyperparathyroidism in India. Br J Surg [Internet]. 2001 May [cited 2020 Jul 24];88(5):708–714.

36

SURGICAL APPROACHES IN PARATHYROID DISEASES

Dhritiman Maitra, Chitresh Kumar and Anurag Srivastava

Introduction

The first parathyroidectomy was performed in Vienna, Austria by Felix Mandl in 1925 in a patient with florid symptoms of hyperparathyroidism, classically described as painful bones, abdominal groans, psychic moans, urinary stones and fatigue overtones (1). With the advances in radiology and nuclear medicine, precise preoperative localization of the parathyroids has become a reality, and there has been gradual emergence of minimally invasive parathyroidectomy (MIVAP) targeting only a specific pathological gland in suitable cases.

With the discovery of multichannel serum analyzer around 1970, entities like asymptomatic hyperparathyroidism and normocalcemic hyperparathyroidism have been diagnosed ever more frequently. This has led to an evolution of the actual indications of surgery (2). Familial and hereditary conditions with multigland disease have been described and management protocols for them have been devised. The patients of chronic renal failure, having secondary or tertiary hyperparathyroidism, have started having a longer life expectancy, thanks to a wide availability of hemodialysis and renal transplant services. Hence, more of such patients are becoming candidates for parathyroid surgery.

Development and relevant surgical anatomy

The parathyroid glands develop from the endoderm of the pharyngeal pouches. The superior parathyroids develop from the fourth pharyngeal pouch along with the lateral parts of the thyroid lobes and have a short course of descent in the neck. The inferior parathyroid and the thymus develop from the third pharyngeal pouch, have a long trajectory of descent and may be found anywhere from the base of the skull to the aortopulmonary window along their course of descent (3). In most of the patients (85%), there are four parathyroid glands (4). But there could be a supernumerary or absent gland in approximately 13% and 5% patients, respectively (4).

In 85% patients, parathyroid glands are found within 1 cm of the intersection of inferior thyroid artery and recurrent laryngeal nerve (RLN). The superior parathyroid is located superior to this intersection and generally posterior to the RLN. The inferior parathyroid is typically located in a plane anterior to the RLN (4, 5).

The blood supply to the parathyroid is endarterial, through branches of the inferior thyroid artery. Sometimes (15%), the superior glands may have blood supply from superior thyroid artery or a dual supply from both the inferior and superior thyroid arteries (6). Venous drainage is through superior, middle into the internal jugular vein or inferior thyroid vein into the subclavian or innominate vein. Some inferior glands also drain through the thymic veins.

Ectopic positions may be due undescended or overdescended parathyroids in course of embryonic development. It may also be because of gravity on enlarged glands which may then fall to ectopic sites (7). The details of the sites to look for ectopic glands will be described with the operative steps.

Preoperative localization of glands

As the famous saying of John Dappman goes, "The only localization that a patient needs who has primary hyperparathyroidism (PHPT) is the localization of an experienced surgeon" (8); however, there is no denying that a precise preoperative localization helps in the diagnosis of adenoma vis-à-vis hyperplasia and also gives an idea of variant anatomy with respect to ectopic and supernumerary parathyroids. This aids in planning the operative approach; as in case of a well-localized adenoma, targeted (focused) parathyroidectomy to remove only the criminal gland would suffice. For the initial surgery, most surgeons would first do an ultrasonography of neck along with a Technetium 99m sestamibi planar imaging or sestamibi SPECT fused with or without CT to localize the gland(s). Sometimes I-123 subtraction along with Tc sestamibi is also done. Negative findings of imaging do not, however, rule out hyperparathyroidism in the presence of biochemical diagnosis then bilateral neck exploration (BNE) has to be done to identify all the parathyroid glands and to look for all the ectopic sites in the neck (9–13). Occasionally if a hyperfunctioning ectopic gland is identified in the mediastinum, a suitable approach is planned.

The minimum localization tools are USG neck and sestamibi. If the images are concordant, they have a sensitivity of identifying the single diseased gland in 96% of the cases (11). However, if the images are negative or discordant 4D CT, 4D MRI, 18F Fluorocholine or 13C Methionine PET scans are advised depending on availability. Despite resorting to all these imaging modalities, if a single diseased gland cannot be localized with surety, USG neck may be performed during the surgery just prior to or even after making an incision to localize a gland in real time, even if a minimally invasive approach has already been planned based on preoperative imaging. USG is not helpful in locating parathyroid in the chest or in the paratracheal, paraesophageal or retroesophageal locations (11–13).

Surgery in primary hyperparathyroidism

Indications:

1. Significant bone, renal, abdominal, neurophsychiatric, muscular symptoms typical of PHPT
2. Current indications of surgery in asymptomatic PHPT
   a. Age <50 years
   b. Serum calcium >1 mg/dl or > 0.25 mmol/l of the upper limit of the reference interval for total calcium and >0.12 mmol/l for ionized calcium.

    c. Bone mineral density (BMD) T-score ≤ –2.5 at the lumbar spine, femoral neck, the total hip or the one-third radius for postmenopausal women or males >50 years. Z-scores should be used instead of T-scores for BMD in premenopausal women and men younger than 50 years as per international society for clinical densitometry.

    d. A prevalent low-energy fracture in the spine is also considered an indication for surgery, which can be seen on a routine X-ray of the thoracic and lumbar spine or vertebral fracture assessment by DXA or CT, MRI

    e. A glomerular filtration rate of <60 ml/min. All asymptomatic patients should be evaluated with renal imaging (X-ray, CT or ultrasound) to detect silent kidney stones or nephrocalcinosis. A complete urinary stone risk profile should be performed in those individuals whose urinary calcium excretion is > 400 mg/day. If stone(s), nephrocalcinosis, or high stone risk is determined, surgery is indicated.

    f. Surgery is also indicated in patients for whom medical surveillance is neither desired nor possible or patients opting for surgery, as long as there are no medical contraindications.

3. Parathyroid carcinoma

Anesthesia and position

BNEs and endoscopic parathyroidectomy are preferably done under general anesthesia as swallowing movements in an awake person may make this procedure difficult. Minimally invasive focused parathyroidectomy (FP) is mostly done under locoregional anesthesia (superficial cervical plexus or deep cervical plexus block) because of less postoperative pain and speedy recovery.

The patient is generally placed in semi-Fowler sniffing position with neck extended with a sandbag underneath the shoulder blade, roll behind the neck and arms tucked by the side.

Bilateral neck exploration for primary hyperparathyroidism

2BNE in PHPT was the procedure of choice before the era of localizing tools. It is primarily indicated when there are discordant or equivocal findings on preoperative localization studies (12–21), evidence of multigland disease in preoperative localization, MEN 1 associated PHPT (22–24) and coexisting thyroid pathology. It may also be considered in radiation-induced PHPT and MEN 2A-associated PHPT, though nowadays removal of a pre-localized single adenoma has been shown to suffice for MEN 2A patients. In them, multigland disease is rarely encountered, and following FP, recurrence rate within a lifetime is also low due to indolent nature of the disease. Unavailability of preoperative imaging facilities and ioPTH sometimes drives a surgeon to perform BNE (25, 26). An FP is converted to a BNE when the pre-localized gland is not successfully detected during surgery if there is detection of more than one pathological gland on one side and if there is unsatisfactory or no drop of ioPTH (27–29).

BNE ensures a thorough search for all the glands including common sites of ectopia; finally, all abnormal glands are removed (30). However, if all four glands are enlarged total parathyroidectomy (removal of all glands) and autotransplantation or, subtotal parathyroidectomy (removal of 3.5 glands) is done.

The neck is accessed through a symmetrical 4-cm cervical collar incision in a neck skin crease about two fingerbreadths above the suprasternal notch. Incision is deepened to reach the avascular sub-platysmal plane in which flaps are raised superiorly to the tip of the thyroid cartilage and inferiorly to the suprasternal notch. The median raphe of the investing layer of deep cervical fascia is incised in the midline and strap muscles are separated and retracted off the midline with gentle and often blunt dissection in an avascular plane. This is called the conventional or "front-door" technique. There is an alternate "back–door" technique or the lateral approach, in which instead of separating the strap muscles in the midline, dissection is begun laterally in between the medial border of the sternocleidomastoid and the lateral border of the strap muscles. The strap muscles are retracted medially and the sternocleidomastoid laterally. If possible, dissection is started on the side of the suspected abnormal gland(s).

In both approaches, finally the space between the lateral surface of the thyroid lobe and the carotid sheath is exposed. The middle thyroid vein is divided, and the thyroid lobe is retracted anteromedially over the trachea. The carotid sheath is gently retracted laterally. The intersection of the RLN and the inferior thyroid artery is identified. The superior glands are generally superior and posterior to this point. The inferior gland is generally anterior to the nerve. Abnormal parathyroid tissue is generally larger than normal, firmer and has a characteristic color (orange tan or brown). They are not distinctly palpable but ballotable within the enveloping fat. Benign adenomas are generally not adherent to surrounding structures. Adhesions, if present, indicate the possibility of malignancy. The dissection is carried out along the capsule of the tumor trying not to grasp the parathyroid to avert rupture and spillage, leading to subsequent parathyromatosis. The surrounding tissue is dissected off the parathyroid rather than dissecting the parathyroid off the surrounding tissues. The vascular pedicle of the parathyroid is controlled with ligaclips, ligature or energy device. Special care is exercised to keep the RLN out of harm's way. If any gland is apparently normal, one should avoid injuring or devascularizing in course of the surgery. The absence of brisk bleeding on pricking any gland with a needle may point toward devascularization. If a normal gland is inadvertently damaged, it should be minced into 10–15 pieces of 1–2 mm each and immediately autotransplanted in a vascularized tissue bed like the sternocleidomastoid muscle by creating small pockets within the muscle.

The initial primary survey for all the glands to identify the pathology and a final decision-making, prior to removing any of the glands even if single-gland disease is suspected, is a prudent way of doing the surgery. In case of single-gland disease when no other gland is found to be pathological, drop in ioPTH acts as an important adjunct to predict biochemical cure and to assist the surgeon to decide whether to further look for any more pathological glands.

In case of double adenoma, most surgeons remove the pathological glands and confirm with a satisfactory drop in ioPTH levels before terminating the procedure. However, some advocate total or subtotal parathyroidectomy for even double adenoma as they believe it to be a variant of hyperplasia where two glands have disproportionately enlarged over the other glands which are also hyperplastic but enlarged only to a lesser extent.

When multigland disease is detected or suspected, especially in patients with syndromes like MEN 1, cervical thymectomy is also done to remove any potential ectopic inferior parathyroid which may be embedded in it. It also takes care of any thymic carcinoid which is commonly present in patients with MEN 1 syndrome.

If a total parathyroidectomy is planned, all the glands are removed and half of the most normal appearing gland, amounting up to about 50 mg of tissue should be autotransplanted in pockets of the sternocleidomastoid muscle to prevent postoperative hypoparathyroidism. Simultaneously some parathyroid tissue is sent for cryopreservation, so that it can be used in future lest the autotransplanted tissue is not functional.

However, before autotransplantation, frozen section is advisable to make sure that some lymph node or other non-parathyroid tissue is not being used for autotransplantation. Frozen section also helps to make sure that all tissues removed as suspected parathyroids are indeed parathyroid glands. In cases, where chances of hyperfunctioning of the autotransplanted parathyroid is high, especially in syndromes like MEN 1, the parathyroid tissue may be placed in pockets of the brachioradialis muscle of the non-dominant forearm. In that case, in the event of any recurrence in the autotransplanted parathyroid, neck exploration would not be necessary.

If a subtotal parathyroidectomy is planned, half of the most normal appearing gland, amounting up to about 50 mg of tissue, should be left in situ with intact blood supply, followed by excision of rest three and a half glands. First, a part of the most normal gland is sent for frozen section to confirm that it is indeed a parathyroid gland. It is only after this confirmation that the blood supply of the other glands is severed and the glands taken out. If on frozen section the tissue is identified as something else, the next normal looking gland is sent for frozen section and so on. Some surgeons advocate to preferably preserving one of the inferior glands if it is not grossly involved for ease of reoperation if needed in future due to the location of the gland anterior to the RLN.

In course of surgery, if any of the glands is not detectable around its normal position, some special maneuvers must be performed. For a missing superior gland, sometimes mobilization and inferomedial rotation of the superior pole of thyroid does the trick, and the missing gland is found around it in 80% cases. Other locations to look for it are deep to the organ of Zuckerkandl, tracheoesophageal groove, paralaryngeal, paratracheal, paraesophageal and retroesophageal areas. Sometimes it may be intrathyroidal or lying within the carotid sheath near the clavicular head. Rarely, it may migrate along the retroesophageal plane to the posterior mediastinum and hence not found in course of a neck exploration.

For a missing inferior gland, the thyrothymic ligament, the cephalad 6–7 cm of the thymus after delivering it into the neck by superior traction, carotid sheath from skull base to its bifurcation must be explored. Sometimes an undescended gland may be located around the hyoid or submandibular area. Occasionally an inferior gland may be fully or partially intrathyroidal near its inferior pole or located deep down in the anterior mediastinum or around the aortopulmonary window.

Any thyroid pathology must be addressed at the same time, if detected during surgery. In case of intrathyroidal glands, thyroid lobectomy may be required.

Suspicion of parathyroid carcinoma arises if there is a palpable and grossly enlarged gland with gross adhesions, loss of plane with the thyroid, RLN involvement and palpable lymph nodes. In such a case, following BNE, en bloc excision of the pathological gland along with ipsilateral lobe of the thyroid is done with central compartment lymph node dissection for enlarged nodes. Lateral neck dissection is done if lateral compartment is also involved. Sometimes the RLN cannot be preserved and has to be sacrificed.

Some surgeons take the aid of serial ioPTH values in case of double adenoma and also multigland disease, after excising each of the glands to make sure that biochemical cure has been achieved. However, 50% drop criteria may not be adequate to predict end point of such procedures. If all potential sites have been looked for and yet the value of ioPTH remains persistently raised, procedure should be abandoned, and further localization studies done to rule out presence of hyperfunctioning glands in the mediastinum or skull base.

Unilateral neck exploration for primary hyperparathyroidism

Unilateral neck exploration (UNE) was first proposed in 1970, this approach gained acceptability over the years owing to advances in technology for precise preoperative and intraoperative localization of glands as well as advantages in operative time, pain, cosmesis and reduced incidence of postoperative hypoparathyroidism (16, 30–33).

It is a subset of minimally invasive procedures for parathyroid; the difference from FP is that in FP, only one pre-localized pathological gland is removed, whereas in UNE, one side of the neck is explored. This could be achieved by a 2–2.5 collar incision in the neck on the side intended to be explored.

The indications of UNE are unilateral double adenoma or concomitant ipsilateral thyroid pathology where a BNE is not necessarily required. Intraoperative frozen section biopsy and ioPTH monitoring are extremely helpful in determining the adequacy of the procedure against the decision to convert into a BNE.

Minimally invasive parathyroidectomy for primary hyperparathyroidism

1. *Minimally invasive open parathyroidectomy* Unless otherwise specified, it refers to FP, also called concise parathyroidectomy (Worsey, 1998). It significantly relies on preoperative imaging and intraoperative adjuncts like ioPTH monitoring. The procedure is done through a small incision 1–1.5 cm just overlying the expected location of the diseased gland, and excision is accomplished with minimal dissection so that cervical reexploration, if indicated in future, does not become cumbersome. It has the definite advantages of better cosmesis, lesser operative time, pain, hematoma, RLN injury and ensures an early discharge (34–42). Moreover, FP has been found to attain same cure rates as BNE in suitably selected cases.

    Classically indicated in sporadic single-gland disease, it has also been seen to be effective in MEN 2A patients in whom, following removal of single pathological gland, most patients achieve permanent cure without a recurrence in the other glands. However, intraoperative findings like more than one enlarged gland or no abnormal gland on the side of surgery and failure of ioPTH levels to drop may prompt a surgeon to convert the procedure to UNE/BNE.

    Like BNE, FP may also be done either through a midline or a lateral approach. Sometimes, exposure is restrictive, but the gland should never be grasped to avoid capsular rupture and subsequent parathyromatosis. Surrounding tissue should be dissected off it. The RLN is identified and preserved. The RLN is anterior to superior parathyroid adenoma and posterior to inferior parathyroid adenoma.

Intraoperative use of ultrasound is of paramount importance for accurate placement of incision and as a guide to the area of interest. Sometimes, Tc-99m sestamibi is also injected intravenously, and a handheld gamma probe is used to detect the area of highest radioactivity to place the incision accordingly. It is known as radioguided parathyroidectomy. It has poor sensitivity to detect multigland disease and is also taken up by the thyroid leading to high background noise (43, 44). However, due to absence of any background uptake in the chest, it is particularly helpful for adenomas located in the mediastinum. The standard for ioPTH monitoring is the Miami criteria which states that a fall of 50% or more in the values of ioPTH in the 5, 10, 15–20 minutes post-excision venous sample compared to the pre-incision or pre-excision samples (whichever is higher) indicates successful removal of the diseased gland with no residual adenoma.

2. *Minimally invasive video-assisted parathyroidectomy*
MIVAP comprises of procedures done through a mini-incision as described above or a mini-access as done in MIVAP. Miccoli performed the first MIVAP in 1998 (46). The advantage of this procedure is not only a cosmetic smaller scar but the utilization of magnification of the operative field using a video endoscope. However, this procedure has a long and steep learning curve and needs dedicated specialized instruments. It is classically indicated in patients of sporadic PHPT with a single adenoma less than 3 cm localized by preoperative imaging. (47, 48)

With the gradual increase in experience, the indications are expanding to even cover cases with concomitant goiter, in intrathymic and retrosternal adenoma, and even in multigland disease with a provision to convert to BNE if needed. However, patients with previous neck surgery or undergoing reoperative parathyroid surgery are generally not considered for this procedure albeit, some surgeons are currently practicing MIVAP in these circumstances also (47–50).

The procedure is done by a 1-cm incision in the midline of the neck, midway between the cricoid cartilage and the suprasternal notch. Previously it was used to be done following insufflation with CO_2 gas, but now it is being done as a gasless procedure. Retractors are used to create and maintain space. Through this incision, a 5-mm 30° telescope is inserted along with any two small 2-mm working hand instruments. In video-assisted technique, trocars are not used. This helps to keep the endoscope more flexible. This enables to move the endoscope in all directions, thereby making it easy to have access to all possible locations of the parathyroid glands. The dissection and subsequent steps are like open procedures. Lorenz modified the procedure by adding a separate 5-mm incision inferior to the first, in the midline and using it to introduce the endoscope through a 5-mm trocar (49, 51). The midline incision is versatile and can be extended if it is required to convert the procedure to BNE or if any incidentally detected thyroid pathology needs to be addressed. If single-gland removal is being contemplated, ioPTH monitoring is performed as in conventional procedures.

Conversion rates vary from 0.9% to 43% in different studies. Initially operative times are higher than conventional FP but gradually decrease with experience (48, 52, 53). Miccoli et al. reported a cure rate of 98.2% at 35.1 months with acceptable complication rates, better cosmesis and early discharge (48).

Endoscopic parathyroidectomy for primary hyperparathyroidism

The first endoscopic parathyroidectomy was done to remove a mediastinal parathyroid. Gagner performed the first fully endoscopic parathyroid surgery in the neck in 1996 (55). A video-assisted approach merely uses the endoscope for some steps, whereas an endoscopic parathyroidectomy involves conventional trocar placement and all the steps are done endoscopically. Gagner had initially described a midline approach which over time has evolved; now it is done by a lateral approach (EPLA). It can be done robotically as well. The various accesses to perform thyroidectomy like transoral vestibular, trans-axillary, axillo-breast, postauricular may all be used for parathyroidectomy also. In all these procedures, though the incision for access is small, the actual dissection done to reach the parathyroid from the site of remote access is more extensive, and hence, it may not be correct to call this procedure a minimally invasive one.

In the most done endoscopic approach through lateral access, first a 12-mm ipsilateral circum-areolar incision is made. Subcutaneous tunnel heading toward the adenoma made with blunt dissector. Another 10-mm trocar is placed at opposite areola or in ipsilateral midclavicular line. A 5-mm trochar is placed at ipsilateral anterior axillary line in axillary fold. A 30° 10-mm endoscope is introduced. CO_2 insufflation is done. Subplatysmal flaps are raised with scissors and monopolar hook. The thyroid lobe is retracted medially. The adenoma is identified and resected following similar principles as in FP. The endoscopic approaches have the advantage of magnification and illumination of the field.

The indications are like that of MIVAP. However, indications are expanding with gain of experience. It is preferred over open technique for posteriorly located adenomas by some surgeons due to better visualization. Parathyroid carcinoma still seems to remain an absolute contraindication and so is an adenoma more than 3 cm as there is greater chance of rupture of such a big adenoma leading to seeding of the field and future occurrence of parathyromatosis.

Cure rates with EPLA are more than 95%, but the reason for such good outcomes may also be the carefully selected patient cohorts in which it is performed (56, 57). It is superior to BNE in cosmetic outcomes, pain and hospital stay and comparable with the other minimally invasive procedures. Video-assisted thoracoscopic surgery has also been employed for deep mediastinal parathyroids.

Surgery for secondary and tertiary hyperparathyroidism

The current indications of parathyroidectomy in secondary hyperparathyroidism are

a. Calcium × phosphate product > 70
b. Serum calcium level > 11.5 mg/dl
c. Progressive renal osteodystrophy, osteitis fibrosa cystica, symptoms of bone pain and pruritus
d. Calciphylaxis
e. Calcification of soft tissues and tumor calcinosis in spite of maximal medical therapy with cinacalcet for over 2 years.

Some groups also advocate removal of glands more than 1 cm in dimension (500-cm^3 volume) (58, 59). Parathormone levels above 800 pg/ml or >10 times the normal value is also considered as an indication of surgery.

In posttransplant patients (tertiary hyperparathyroidism), the indications of surgery are severe subacute hypercalcemia (12.5 mg/dl), sustained hypercalcemia (>12 mg/dl for >1 year after transplant), symptomatic hypercalcemia including acute pancreatitis and asymptomatic hypercalcemia with impaired renal function (60–64).

Most of these patients present with multigland disease in the form of hyperplasia. In some cases, a single enlarged gland may be identified which may be treated by FP. However, most patients require a formal BNE with total parathyroidectomy with autotransplantation or subtotal parathyroidectomy (removal of three and half glands leaving behind about 50 mg or half of the most normal looking gland or that of one of the inferior glands on a vascular pedicle). A cervical thymectomy may be done to remove any ectopic glands. These patients are generally sick and merit a quick in quick out straight forward procedure. So, an open approach is preferred. Regarding the autotransplantation, using sternocleidomastoid pockets may be a matter of concern in view of future recurrence and need of a cervical reexploration. Using the brachioradialis of nondominant arm for transplantation is also not advisable as these patients often have arteriovenous fistulae. So, pectoralis major muscle may be accessed through an infraclavicular incision and transplantation done creating 15–20 pockets within the muscle. Some patients who are not candidates for renal transplant may also do with a total parathyroidectomy without autotransplantation. Cryopreservation with delayed autotransplantation is also an option though not as efficacious as immediate autotransplantation (success rate 60% versus 95%) (65–67). The postoperative period in these patients may be stormy due to hungry bone syndrome leading to hypocalcemia. Permanent hyocalcemia also occurs and so does recurrent hyperparathyroidism (in autotransplanted parathyroid, remnant parathyroid after subtotal parathyroidectomy or an ectopic missed gland) (68, 69). There is no consensus as to which procedure is better between total parathyroidectomy with auto transplantation and subtotal parathyroidectomy with respect to permanent hypoparathyroidism and recurrence.

ioPTH monitoring may be resorted to, but one has to keep in mind that patients of chronic renal failure have prolongation of $t_{1/2}$ of parathormone. Hence, delayed samples up to 30 minutes post excision may have to be tested to confirm a significant drop in PTH.

Reoperative surgery

Hyperparathyroidism following initial surgery indicated by hypercalcemia within 6 months of surgery is called persistent and that after 6 months is called recurrent hyperparathyroidism. The cure rates in this setting are 10%–15% lower and complication rates are much higher due to obliteration of operative field by postoperative adhesions.

First, the diagnosis should be reviewed and familial hypocalciuric hypercalcemia and non-parathyroid dependent causes of hypercalcemia must be ruled out. The previous operative note must be scanned to find out the nature of procedure done, access, number, site and side of gland(s) removed, spillage if any, suspicion of carcinoma and whether auto transplantation was done or not. Histopathology reports are reviewed to confirm that parathyroid gland(s) had indeed been removed.

In this setting, about 37% patients present with multigland disease (70). These patients could be those with MEN 1 syndrome with no family history or no involvement of other glands in the patient leading to a missed initial diagnosis. Recurrence could also be due to a missed supernumerary or ectopic gland, excessive tissue left behind after subtotal parathyroidectomy, a missed double adenoma or due to hyperfunctioning of autotransplanted tissue or parathyromatosis.

In this setting, if a patient is asymptomatic with only a biochemical recurrence, risk versus benefit between observation and reoperation have to be considered as second surgeries are fraught with both higher failure and complication rates.

After diagnosis of recurrence has been made and reexploration is being planned, suitable imaging for parathyroid localization must be done. In a patient who had primarily undergone a thorough BNE, a mediastinal recurrence is possible apart from a neck recurrence as well. A patient who had undergone FP may have recurrences in the neck itself. USG, Tc-99m sestamibi scan with or without SPECT/SPECT-CT, 4D CT, 4D MRI, fluorocholine PET may be serially used for a comprehensive localization of disease. In remedial settings, selective venous sampling to detect the side and site of recurrence more precisely could be of help. FNA-PTH under image guidance is also helpful to characterize a suspicious lesion. Parathyroid angiography with or without embolization may help in both localization and treatment. Ablation of suspicious glands with alcohol under image guidance is also currently under investigation.

In reoperative circumstances, the objective is to locate the abnormal gland and remove it without disturbing or devascularizing the other normal glands. Hence, a limited focal cervical exploration is ideal. However, it is possible only in the presence of an accurate preoperative localization and ioPTH monitoring.

In absence of localization and ioPTH monitoring facility, a blind extensive reexploration may have to be done. However, such exploration should be undertaken only if a patient merits the surgery due to severe symptoms.

The RLN must be carefully preserved even as all sites of possible missed glands are explored. The nerve monitor should be used in reoperative cases if available. The esophagus is also identified and preserved. Insertion of a nasogastric tube may effectively aid in identifying the esophagus. Sometimes, the inferior gland may be found superior to the superior gland and vice versa. Intraoperative frozen section, FNA with rapid PTH testing for suspicious and intrathyroidal glands, intraoperative selective venous sampling is all considered as extremely useful tools. Radioguided surgery, as described earlier, may also be helpful in this scenario. Hemithyroidectomy may have to be done for suspicious intrathyroidal parathyroids.

Most of the mediastinal parathyroids can be removed via a cervical approach during neck exploration located above arch of aorta. However, video-assisted thoracoscopic surgery and mediastinoscopy are often required for glands which are deep down and posteriorly located in the mediastinum.

Sometimes removal of an autotransplanted tissue from its intramuscular pockets is enough. However, complete removal may be impossible as they develop in-growths into the muscle to become functional and stay viable.

Autotransplantation following BNE and total parathyroidectomy or cryopreservation for delayed transplantation are seriously considered after extensive reexplorations for the concern of permanent hypoparathyroidism.

South Asian perspective

Majority of patients with PHPT have associated vitamin D deficiency or insufficiency in South Asia. Associated vitamin D deficiency aggravates the PHPT and patients have more severe bone disease. These patients have higher PTH **levels**, calcium and alkaline phosphatase; lower plasma phosphate levels, greater adenoma weight, lower BMD particularly at cortical sites, higher bone turnover and increased fracture risk and a greater risk of hungry bone syndrome after parathyroid surgery. As previously thought, PTH-stimulated conversion of 25OHD to $1,25(OH)_2D$ is not responsible for decreased levels of serum 25OHD in PHPT and probably elevated $1,25(OH)_2D$ levels stimulate 24-hydroxylase gene expression and enhanced conversion of 25OHD to 1,24-dihydroxy vitamin D (71, 72).

The minimally invasive video-assisted and endoscopic procedures for thyroid and parathyroid surgery originated in Asia. There are training programs in institutes in India, South Korea, China and Vietnam for these procedures. State of the art institutes equipped with the entire range of investigations for preoperative localization and facility for ioPTH are available in this region. However, a lot of hospitals still to have rely only on USG for localization at most with a planar sestamibi scan. As a result, BNE remains the most commonly done procedure with excellent cure rates. In our institute, however, FP is the preferred procedure (after thorough preoperative localization), which is mostly done under locoregional anesthesia as a day-care procedure.

Conclusion

The definitive cure of PHPT is from surgery, and all symptomatic patients of PHPT and with defined criteria in asymptomatic patients should be managed with surgery. BNE is gold standard operation, but in todays' era, single-gland excision by open or endoscopic technique is the most preferred operation.

References

1. Clark OH. Captain Charles Martell. America's first parathyroid patient. In: M.A. Zeiger, W.T. Shen and E.A. Felger, eds., The Supreme Triumph of the Surgeon's Art: A Narrative History of Endocrine Surgery. Berkeley, CA: The University of California Medical Humanities Press; 2013. pp. 86–97.
2. Heath H, 3rd, Hodgson SF, Kennedy MA. Primary hyperparathyroidism: Incidence, morbidity, and potential economic impact in a community. N Engl J Med. 1980;302(4):189–193.
3. Gauger P, Doherty G, eds. Parathyroid gland. In: Sabiston Textbook of Surgery. 17th ed. Philadelphia, PA: Elsevier and Saunders; 2004. pp. 985–999.
4. Akerstrom G, Malmaeus J, Bergstrom R. Surgical anatomy of human parathyroid glands. Surgery. 1984;95(1):14–21.
5. Pyrtek L, Painter RL. An anatomic study of the relationship of the parathyroid glands to the recurrent laryngeal nerve. Surg Gynecol Obstet. 1964;119:509–512.
6. Flament JB, Delattre JF, Pluot M. Arterial blood supply to the parathyroid glands: Implications for thyroid surgery. Surg Radiol Anat. 1982;3:279.
7. Simeone DM, Sandelin K, Thompson NW. Undescended superior parathyroid gland: A potential cause of failed cervical exploration for hyperparathyroidism. Surgery. 1995;118(6):949–956.
8. Brennan MF. Lessons learned. Ann Surg Oncol. 2006;13(10):1322–1328.
9. Udelsman R, Pasieka JL, Sturgeon C, et al. Surgery for asymptomatic primary hyperparathyroidism: Proceedings of the third international workshop. J Clin Endocrinol Metab. 2009;94(2):366–372.
10. Chen H, Mack E, Starling JR. A comprehensive evaluation of perioperative adjuncts during minimally invasive parathyroidectomy: Which is most reliable? Ann Surg. 2005;242(3):375–380; discussion 380-83.
11. Arici C, Cheah WK, Ituarte PH, et al. Can localization studies be used to direct focused parathyroid operations? Surgery. 2001;129(6):720–729.
12. Siperstein A, Berber E, Barbosa GF, et al. Predicting the success of limited exploration for primary hyperparathyroidism using ultrasound, sestamibi, and intraoperative parathyroid hormone: Analysis of 1158 cases. Ann Surg. 2008;248(3):420–428.
13. Siperstein A, Berber E, Mackey R, et al. Prospective evaluation of sestamibi scan, ultrasonography, and rapid PTH to predict the success of limited exploration for sporadic primary hyperparathyroidism. Surgery. 2004;136(4):872–880.
14. Aarum S, Nordenstrom J, Reihner E, et al. Operation for primary hyperparathyroidism: The new versus the old order. A randomised controlled trial of preoperative localisation. Scand J Surg. 2007;96(1):26–30.
15. Bergenfelz A, Kanngiesser V, Zielke A, et al. Conventional bilateral cervical exploration versus open minimally invasive parathyroidectomy under local anaesthesia for primary hyperparathyroidism. Br J Surg. 2005;92(2):190–197.
16. Bergenfelz A, Lindblom P, Tibblin S, et al. Unilateral versus bilateral neck exploration for primary hyperparathyroidism: A prospective randomized controlled trial. Ann Surg. 2002;236(5):543–551.
17. Miccoli P, Barellini L, Monchik JM, et al. Randomized clinical trial comparing regional and general anaesthesia in minimally invasive video-assisted parathyroidectomy. Br J Surg. 2005;92(7):814–818.
18. Miccoli P, Berti P, Materazzi G, et al. Endoscopic bilateral neck exploration versus quick intraoperative parathormone assay (qPTHa) during endoscopic parathyroidectomy: A prospective randomized trial. Surg Endosc. 2008;22(2):398–400.
19. Slepavicius A, Beisa V, Janusonis V, et al. Focused versus conventional parathyroidectomy for primary hyper parathyroidism: A prospective, randomized, blinded trial. Langenbecks Arch Surg. 2008;393(5):659–666.
20. Sozio A, Schietroma M, Franchi L, et al. Parathyroidectomy: Bilateral exploration of the neck vs minimally invasive radioguided treatment. Minerva Chir. 2005;60(2):83–89.
21. Westerdahl J, Bergenfelz A. Unilateral versus bilateral neck exploration for primary hyperparathyroidism: Five year follow-up of a randomized controlled trial. Ann Surg. 2007;246(6):976–980; discussion 980-71.
22. Carling T, Udelsman R. Parathyroid surgery in familial hyperparathyroid disorders. J Intern Med. 2005;257(1):27–37.
23. Rubin MR, Bilezikian JP, McMahon DJ, et al. The natural history of primary hyperparathyroidism with or without parathyroid surgery after 15 years. J Clin Endocrinol Metab. 2008;93(9):3462–3470.
24. Silverberg SJ, Shane E, Jacobs TP, et al. A 10-year prospective study of primary hyperparathyroidism with or without parathyroid surgery. N Engl J Med. 1999;341(17):1249–1255.
25. Carneiro-Pla DM, Solorzano CC, Irvin GL, 3rd. Consequences of targeted parathyroidectomy guided by localization studies without intraoperative parathyroid hormone monitoring. J Am Coll Surg. 2006;202(5):715–722.
26. Mazeh H, Chen H, Leverson G, et al. Creation of a "Wisconsin index" nomogram to predict the likelihood of additional hyperfunctioning parathyroid glands during parathyroidectomy. Ann Surg. 2013;257(1):138–141.
27. Irvin GL, 3rd, Solorzano CC, Carneiro DM. Quick intraoperative parathyroid hormone assay: Surgical adjunct to allow limited parathyroidectomy, improve success rate, and predict outcome. World J Surg. 2004;28(12):1287–1292.
28. Lew JI, Rivera M, Irvin GL, 3rd, et al. Operative failure in the era of focused parathyroidectomy: A contemporary series of 845 patients. Arch Surg. 2010;145(7):628–633.
29. Lee S, Ryu H, Morris LF, et al. Operative failure in minimally invasive parathyroidectomy utilizing an intraoperative parathyroid hormone assay. Ann Surg Oncol. 2014;21(6):1878–1883.
30. Wang CA. Surgical management of primary hyperparathyroidism. Curr Probl Surg. 1985;22(11):1–50.
31. Worsey MJ, Carty SE, Watson CG. Success of unilateral neck exploration for sporadic primary hyperparathyroidism. Surgery. 1993;114(6):1024–1029, discussion 1029-30.
32. Irvin GL, Sfakianakis G, Yeung L, et al. Ambulatory parathyroidectomy for primary hyperparathyroidism. Arch Surg. 1996;131(10):1074–1078.
33. Sosa JA, Udelsman R. Minimally invasive parathyroidectomy. Surg Oncol. 2003;12(2):125–134.
34. Miccoli P, Berti P, Conte M, et al. Minimally invasive video assisted parathyroidectomy: Lesson learned from 137 cases. J Am Coll Surg. 2000;191:613–618.
35. Norman, J, Chheda H, Farrell C. Minimally invasive parathyroidectomy for primary hyperparathyroidism: Decreasing operative time and potential complications while improving cosmetic results. Am Surg. 1998;64:391–395.
36. Miccoli P, Bendinelli C, Berti P, et al. Video-assisted versus conventional parathyroidectomy in primary hyperparathyroidism: A prospective randomized study. Surgery. 1999;126:1117–1122.
37. Henry JF, Raffaelli M, Iacobone M, et al. Video-assisted parathyroidectomy via the lateral approach vs conventional surgery in the treatment of sporadic primary hyperparathyroidism: The results of a case-control study. Surg Endosc. 2001;15:1116–1119.
38. Lombardi CP, Raffaelli M, Traini E, et al. Video-assisted minimally invasive parathyroidectomy: Benefits and long term results. World J Surg. 2009;33:2266–2281.
39. Melck AL, Armstrong MJ, Yip L, et al. Case-controlled comparison of video-assisted and conventional minimally invasive parathyroidectomy. Am Surg. 2012;78:125–132.
40. Kunstman JW, Udelsman R. Superiority of minimally invasive parathyroidectomy. Adv Surg. 2012;46:171–189.
41. Beyer, TD, Solorzano CC, Starr F, et al. Parathyroidectomy outcomes according to operative approach. Am J Surg. 2007;193:368–373.
42. Miccoli P, Bendinelli C, Vignali E, et al. Endoscopic parathyroidectomy: Report of an initial experience. Surgery. 1998;124:1077–1080.
43. Chen H, Mack E, Starling JR. Radioguided parathyroidectomy is equally effective for both adenomatous and hyperplastic glands. Ann Surg. 2003;238:332–338.
44. Norman J, Lopez J, Politz D. Abandoning unilateral parathyroidectomy: Why we reversed our position after 15,000 parathyroid operations. J Am Coll Surg. 2012;214:260–269.
45. Stavrakis AI, Ituarte PHG, Ko CY, et al. Surgeon volume as a predictor of outcomes in inpatient and outpatient endocrine surgery. Surgery. 2007;142:887–899.
46. Miccoli P, Pinchera A, Cecchini G, et al. Minimally invasive, video-assisted parathyroid surgery for primary hyperparathyroidism. J Endocrinol Invest. 1997;20:429–430.
47. Berti P, Materazzi G, Picone A, et al. Limits and drawbacks of video-assisted parathyroidectomy. Br J Surg. 2003;90:743–747.

48. Miccoli P, Berti P, Materazzi G, et al. Results of video assisted parathyroidectomy: Single institution's six-year experience. World J Surg. 2004;28:1216–1218.
49. Alesina PF, Hinrichs J, Heuer M, et al. Feasibility of video assisted bilateral neck exploration for patients with primary hyperparathyroidism and failed or discordant localization studies. Langenbecks Arch Surg. 2013;398:107–111.
50. Garimella V, Yeluri S, Alabi A, et al. Minimally invasive video-assisted parathyroidectomy is a safe procedure to treat primary hyperparathyroidism. Surgeon. 2012;10:202–205.
51. Lombardi CP, Raffaelli M, Traini E, et al. Advantages of a video-assisted approach to parathyroidectomy. ORL J Otorhinolaryngol Relat Spec. 2008;70:313–318.
52. Dralle H, Lorenz K, Nguyen-Thanh P. Minimally invasive video-assisted parathyroidectomy—Selective approach to localize single gland adenoma. Langenbecks Arch Surg. 1999;384:556–562.
53. Hessman O, Westerdahl J, Al-Suliman N, et al. Randomized clinical trial comparing open with video-assisted minimally invasive parathyroid surgery for primary hyperparathyroidism. Brit J Surg. 2010;97:177–184.
54. Barczyński M, Cichoń S, Konturek A, et al. Minimally invasive video-assisted parathyroidectomy versus open minimally invasive parathyroidectomy for a solitary parathyroid adenoma: A prospective, randomized, blinded trial. World J Surg. 2006;30:721–731.
55. Gagner M. Endoscopic parathyroidectomy. Br J Surg. 1996;83:875.
56. Henry JF, Sebag F, Cherenko M, et al. Endoscopic parathyroidectomy: Why and when? World J Surg. 2008;32:2509–2515.
57. Bergenfelz A, Hellman P, Harrison B, et al. Positional statement of the European Society of Endocrine Surgeons (ESES) on modern techniques in pHPT surgery. Langenbecks Arch Surg. 2009;394:761–764.
58. Tezelman S, Siperstein AED, Duh QY, et al. Tumoral calcinosis: Controversies in the etiology and alternatives in the treatment. Arch Surg. 1993;128:737.
59. Dug QY, Lim RC, Clark OH. Calciphylaxis in secondary hyperparathyroidism: Diagnosis and parathyroidectomy. Arch Surg. 1991;126:1213.
60. D'Alessandro AM, Melzer JS, Pirsch JD, et al. Tertiary hyperparathyroidism after renal transplantation: Operative indications. Surgery. 1989;106(6):1049–1055.
61. Chatterjee SN, Friedler RM, Berne TV, et al. Persistent hypercalcemia after successful renal transplantation. Nephron. 1976;17(1):1–7.
62. Chatterjee SN, Massry SG, Friedler RM, et al. The high incidence of persistent secondary hyperparathyroidism after renal homotransplantation. Surg Gynecol Obstet. 1976;143(3):440–442.
63. Christensen MS, Nielsen HE. The clinical significance of hyperparathyroidism after renal transplantation. Scand J Urol Nephrol Suppl. 1977;(42):130–133.
64. Pieper R, Alveryd A, Lundgren G, et al. Secondary hyperparathyroidism and its sequelae in renal transplant recipients. Long term findings in a series of conservatively managed patients. Scand J Urol Nephrol. 1977;(42):144–148.
65. Wagner PK, Seesko HG, Rothmund M. Replantation of cryopreserved human parathyroid tissue. World J Surg. 1991;15:751.
66. Brennan MF, brown EM, Spiegel AM, et al. Autotransplantation of cryopreserved parathyroid tissue in man. Ann Surg. 1979;189:139.
67. Alveryd A, El-Zawahry Md, Herlitz P, et al. Primary hyperplasia of the parathyroid. Acta Chir Scand. 1975;141:24.
68. Lundgren G, Asaba M, Magnusson G, et al. The role of parathyroidectomy in the treatment of secondary hyperparathyroidism before and after renal transplantation. Scand J Urol Nephrol Suppl. 1977;42:149.
69. Prinz RA, Gamrros OI, Sellu D, et al. Subtotal parathyroidectomy for chief cell hyperplasia of the multiple endocrine neoplasia type I syndrome. Ann Surg. 1981;193:26.
70. Clark O, Siperstein AE. The hypercalcemic syndrome: Hyperparathyroidism. In: S.R. Friesen and N.W. Thompson, ed., Surgical Endocrinology Clinical Syndromes. Philadelphia, PA: J.B. Lippincott Co.; 1990. p. 311.
71. Shah VN, Shah CS, Bhadada SK, Rao DS. Effect of 25(OH)D replacements in patients with primary hyperparathyroidism (PHPT) and coexistent vitamin D deficiency on serum 25(OH)D, calcium and PTH levels: A meta-analysis and review of literature. Clin Endocrinol (Oxf) 2014;80:797–803.
72. Rolighed L, Rejnmark L, Sikjaer T, et al. Vitamin D treatment in primary hyperparathyroidism: A randomized placebo controlled trial. J Clin Endocrinol Metab. 2014;99:1072–1080.

# REMOTE ACCESS THYROID AND PARATHYROID SURGERY

Hyeong Won Yu and June Young Choi

Introduction

Although thyroid and parathyroid surgery through cervical incisions is a safe operation with relatively few complications, esthetic complications have led to patient demands for small or invisible scars. The development of endoscopic subtotal parathyroidectomy led to the development of endoscopic total thyroidectomy (1–3). These endoscopic methods have reduced the sizes of cervical incisions and hence scarring. Moreover, the introduction of robotic equipment led to the development of robotic thyroidectomy, first reported in 2009 (4,5).

Thyroid and parathyroid surgery that does not leave a scar on the neck is classified as remote access surgery. Types of remote access thyroid and parathyroid surgery include cervical approach (2, 3), minimally invasive video-assisted thyroidectomy (MIVAT) (6, 7), an anterior chest approach (8), an axillary approach (8, 9), a gasless trans-axillary approach (TAA) (10), an anterior breast approach (11), an axillo-bilateral breast approach (ABBA) (12), a bilateral axillo-breast approach (BABA) (13), a postauricular and axillary (PAA) approach (14), a sublingual transoral approach (15), and a transoral endoscopic thyroidectomy vestibular approach (TOETVA) (16). Remote access surgery is being increasingly used throughout Asia because of the cultural stigma of neck wounds.

Classification of remote access surgery by access level

Remote access surgery can be classified into five levels based on the location accessed. These five levels include the head, cervical, anterior chest, axillar, and breast and axillar levels (Figure 37.1).

The cervical level is the level at which open thyroidectomy and parathyroidectomy are traditionally performed, leaving a cervical scar. This scarring may be reduced by a cervical approach and MIVAT surgery. The head level is above the cervical level, with the anterior chest, axillar, and breast and axillar levels located below the cervical level. Surgery at the head level includes facelifts, the sublingual transoral approach, and TOETVA. The anterior chest approach is performed at the anterior chest level; the axillary approach and TAA at the axillary level; and the anterior breast approach, ABBA, and BABA at the breast and axillar level.

Endoscopic surgery

Marked advances in remote access surgery have occurred since endoscopy was first reported able to remove the parathyroid gland in 1996 (1). Several surgical approaches and methods have become standardized and verified in many studies. Figure 37.2 shows the history of the development of endoscopic remote access surgery over time.

Cervical approach and MIVAT

Because the cervical approach and MIVAT leave cervical scars, they are more accurately described as minimally invasive surgery (MIS) rather than remote access surgery. However, these two methods have had a great impact on the development of remote access surgery. The cervical approach is a method of performing surgery through three or four endoscopic ports on the cervical or lateral neck above the sternal notch and with the assistance of CO_2 insufflation (2, 3). MIVAT, which consists of operations using small incisions on the cervix (17), has been reported to improve patient satisfaction and reduce postoperative pain, length of hospital stay, and rates of surgical complications (7).

The anterior chest approach

Surgery on the thyroid gland can also be performed by maintaining CO_2 insufflation with an anterior chest approach (8, 18). This surgical method uses one 12-mm port and two 5-mm ports. Subsequent modifications resulted in a surgical method using a 4 cm incision on the chest and a 5-mm port on the neck, with a wire attached to the skin (19).

Axillary approach (CO_2 insufflation)

An axillary approach to thyroidectomy was first shown to be feasible, safe, and without complications in 2000 (9,20). This approach involves raising an arm on the operation side to expose the axilla (20). After inserting a 12-mm trocar through a 3 cm incision in the axillar, the area is insufflated with 4 mmHg CO_2 to secure an adequate working space. Afterward, two 5-mm trocars are inserted downward to perform surgery, and the surgical wounds are covered in the natural resting position. This approach is used to treat adenomatous goiters and follicular nodules <6 cm in size, as well as nodules identified as benign on fine needle aspiration (FNA) (21). Hemithyroidectomy can also be performed to remove low-risk papillary microcarcinomas without lymph node metastases and treat patients with Graves' disease <100 ml. A comparison of 20 patients who underwent surgery using the axillary approach and 20 who underwent MIVAT found that postoperative pain was significantly lower in the MIVAT group, whereas cosmetic satisfaction scores were higher in the group that underwent surgery using the axillary approach (21), suggesting that the latter may be preferred in patients who selectively value cosmetic results. The axillary approach also has advantages in preserving the ipsilateral recurrent laryngeal nerve (RLN) and the parathyroid gland (22), but it has a longer operation time due to poor visual field when operating on the contralateral lobe (21).

Gasless trans-axillary approach

The gasless TAA is a modification of the axillar approach that does not use CO_2 insufflation (10). In this method, an incision of about 5–6 cm is made in the axilla, the flap is secured to the clavicle, and the surgical field of view is secured with a specially designed external elevating retractor (10). A single-arm study of the TAA in 581 patients resulted in a low rate of complications,

Remote Access Thyroid and Parathyroid Surgery

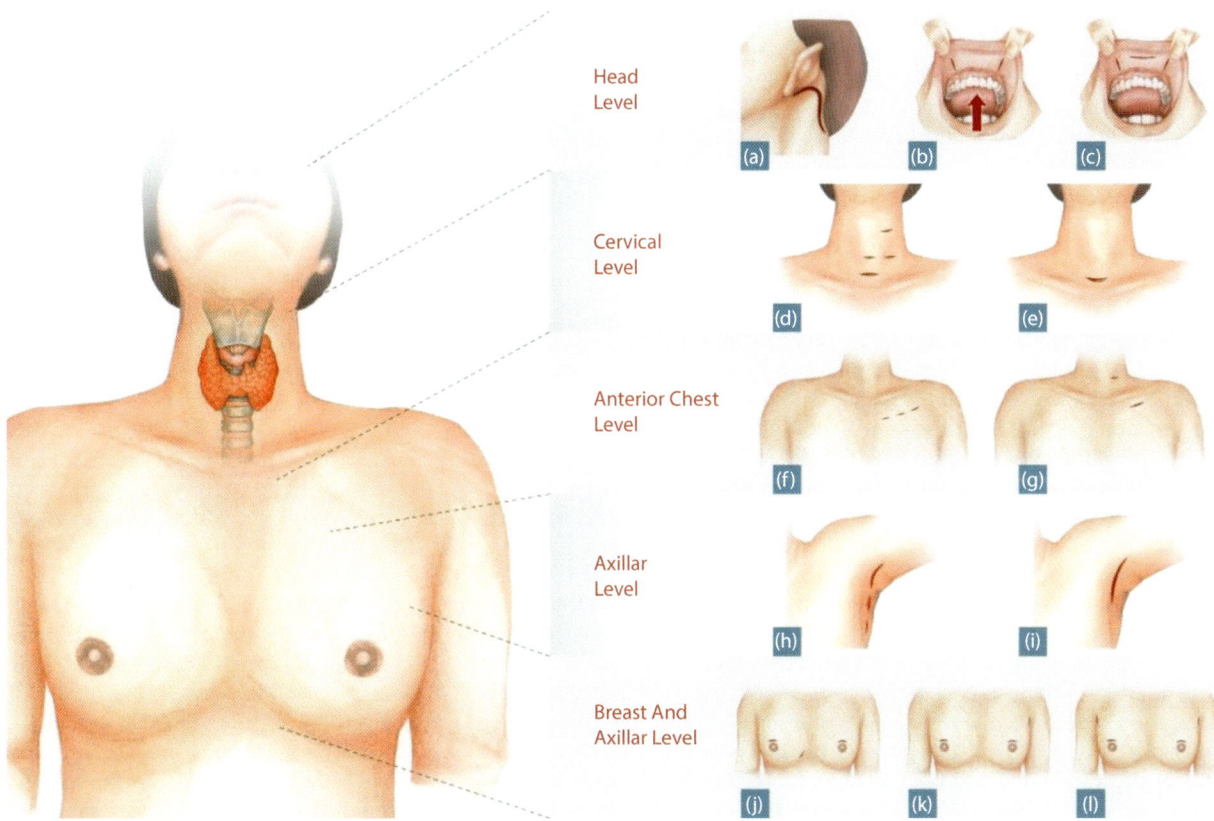

FIGURE 37.1 Classification of types of remote access thyroid and parathyroid surgery. (a) Postauricular and axillary approach, (b) the sublingual transoral approach, (c) transoral endoscopic thyroidectomy vestibular approach (TOETVA), (d) cervical approach, (e) minimally invasive video-assisted thyroidectomy (MIVAT), (f) the anterior chest approach, (g) modification of the anterior chest approach, (h) axillary approach (CO_2 insufflation), (i) gasless trans-axillary approach, (j) anterior breast approach, (k) axillo-bilateral breast approach (ABBA), (l) bilateral axillo-breast approach (BABA).

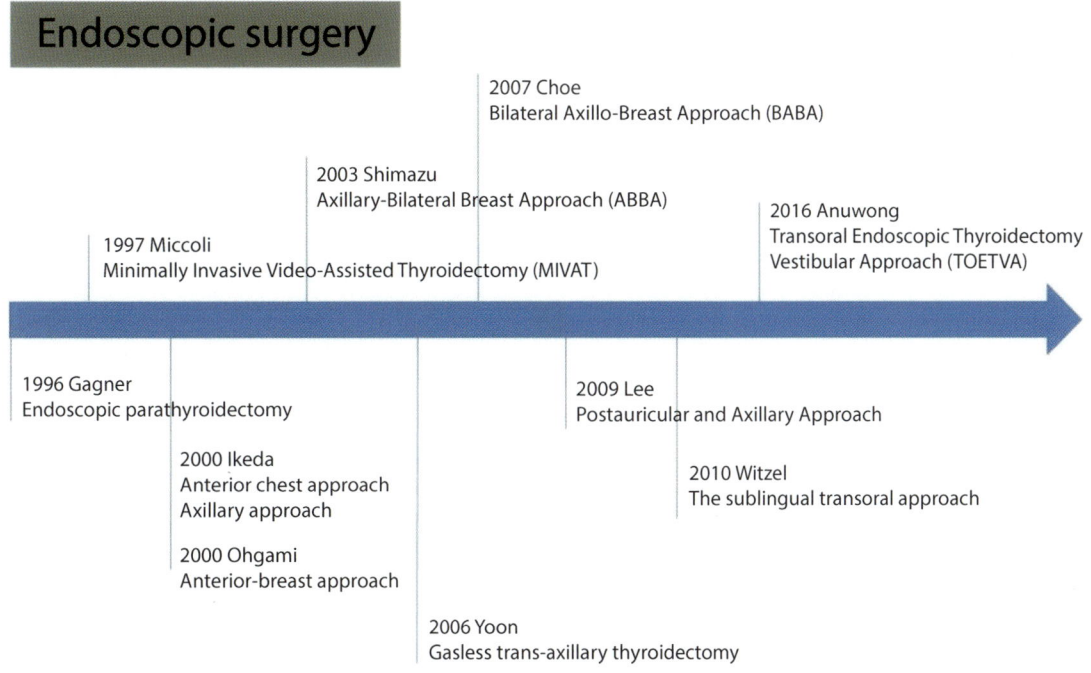

FIGURE 37.2 History of remote access surgery using endoscopy.

with 19 patients experiencing transient hypocalcemia, 13 experiencing transient hoarseness, and 2 having permanent vocal cord palsy (23). Of the 410 malignant tumors, 366 (89.2%) were stage I. In a study comparing gasless endoscopic trans-axillary thyroidectomy in 275 patients with conventional open thyroidectomy in 224 patients, transient hypocalcemia, transient RLN palsy, tracheal injury, and esophageal injury were observed in the endoscopic surgery group (24). Of these patients in the endoscopic surgery group, 12% underwent total thyroidectomy. These findings suggested that gasless endoscopic trans-axillary thyroidectomy may be effective in selected patients. A subsequent study comparing total thyroidectomy using the TAA in 200 patients and conventional open surgery in 538 patients found no differences in the rates of permanent hypocalcemia, permanent RLN palsy, seroma, and hematoma (25). The scope of surgery using the gasless endoscopic TAA encompasses both thyroid glands. However, one possible drawback of this surgical method is the requirement for skilled operators to remove the contralateral lobe.

Anterior breast approach

Endoscopic thyroidectomy can also be performed through an anterior breast approach (11). In this method, a 15-mm transverse skin incision is made at the parasternal border of the breast and a trocar is inserted into the circumareolar areas of both breasts. Thereafter, a working space is created by maintaining a low CO_2 gas insufflation of 5–6 mmHg. This surgical method is mainly indicated for benign thyroid nodules <5 cm and follicular neoplasm confirmed by FNA biopsy (26, 27). Moreover, this approach can be utilized for well-differentiated thyroid carcinomas and Graves' disease <100 g (28, 29). However, it is difficult to apply this surgical method to patients who had previously undergone open neck surgery and those with thyroiditis, a history of breast malignancy, and substernal goiter. In the initial study of five patients who underwent hemithyroidectomy using this approach, none required conversion to open surgery or experienced surgery-related complications (11). The mean operation time was 226 min (range: 177–281 min), and all patients' scars were covered by their clothes. In a study of 92 patients in their 30s, the mean cosmetic satisfaction score was 9.3 (on a scale from 0 to 10) (30). A drawback to this surgical method is that the parasternal scar is likely to become a hypertrophy wound.

Axillo-bilateral breast approach (ABBA)

The axillary-bilateral breast approach (ABBA), using both breasts and one axilla (12), is similar to the anterior breast approach but transfers the parasternal incision of the latter to the axilla. A 10-mm trocar is inserted into both circumareolar incisions and axillae, with low CO_2 insufflation of 4–6 mmHg maintained during the operation to secure the field of view. Although similar to the anterior breast approach, this method has the advantage of an improved visual field through the use of the axillar port. This procedure is indicated for low-risk papillary thyroid microcarcinomas (PTMCs) without lymph node metastases, follicular neoplasms <3 cm, and benign thyroid nodules. A study comparing 12 patients who underwent ABBA and 4 treated with an anterior breast approach found that ABBA was not only cosmetically superior but also provided a wider surgical field of view and free movement of surgical instruments (12).

Bilateral axillo-breast approach (BABA)

The BABA, using both breasts and axillae, was found to overcome the drawbacks of ABBA, enabling its use in total thyroidectomy (13). BABA endoscopic thyroidectomy is performed using 12-mm trocars on both breasts and 5- or 8-mm trocars on both axillae, with insufflation of 5–6 mmHg CO_2 to provide an adequate working space. BABA surgery has the advantage of providing a comfortable environment for the operator because it provides a surgical field of view similar to that of traditional open cervical thyroidectomy. Because there are no restrictions on operations on both the left and right sides and very few collisions between surgical instruments, the scope of surgery is wide (31). A comparison of 102 patients who underwent BABA surgery and 25 who underwent ABBA surgery found that none of the former developed hypertrophic scars (13). In addition, 76.5% of the patients who underwent BABA surgery reported that their cosmetic outcomes were excellent. A study analyzing 512 patients who underwent BABA surgery, including 397 with malignant and 115 with benign lesions, reported that the rates of transient and permanent RLN palsy were 20.1% and 1.7%, respectively, the rate of transient hypercalcemia was 31.1%, and the rate of permanent hypocalcemia was 4.2% (31). A propensity score–matched analysis of 95 patients who underwent BABA ET and 262 patients who underwent open thyroidectomy for lesions that were benign or indeterminate by FNA found no difference in complication rates between the two groups (32). A recent retrospective propensity score analysis of 41 patients who underwent BABA ET and 52 who underwent open thyroidectomy for nonmalignant lesions found that the rates of postoperative symptoms (p = 0.03), tiredness (p = 0.03), impaired social life (p = 0.03), cosmetic complaints (p = <0.001), and the overall QoL (p = <0.001) were significantly lower in the BABA group (33).

Postauricular and axillary approach

The PAA approach, which was developed to avoid breast incision, entails the use of two axillary and two postauricular ports (14). In this method, one 12-mm trocar is inserted into one axilla, 5-mm trocars are inserted into the other three sites, and CO_2 insufflation is maintained at 5–6 mmHg. Indications for PAA surgery are benign thyroid nodules <4 cm, low-risk PTMCs, and follicular neoplasms <3 cm (14). A study of ten patients who underwent PAA, including seven who underwent total thyroidectomy, found that none required conversion to open surgery. The mean operation time was 210.0 ± 43.7 min, and three patients had transient RLN injuries. Similar to BABA, the PAA approach maintains a good surgical field of view on both sides, although there is a risk of facial nerve injury.

The sublingual transoral approach

Sublingual transoral thyroid surgery has two major advantages, the absence of a scar on the skin and the short distance from the incision to the thyroid gland (15). In this method, a 5-mm trocar is inserted through the midline sublingual incision, followed by insufflations of 6 mmHg CO_2 and insertion of the second and third trocars through the vestibular mucosa (34). Although the first study of this method found no complications, a follow-up study of eight patients reported permanent RLN palsy in one and mental nerve palsy in six, with three patients requiring conversion to open surgery (35).

Transoral endoscopic thyroidectomy vestibular approach (TOETVA)

The transoral vestibular approach, first tested in cadavers, involves placing all transoral incisions in the vestibular mucosa (36). Although this method showed good surgical results (37, 38), its major drawback was the potential for mental nerve injury (39). This shortcoming was overcome (16), with transoral endoscopic thyroidectomy via the vestibular approach showing good results in 425 patients (40). Mean operation time was 100.8 min and surgical prognosis was good, with rates of transient and permanent hypoparathyroidism of 10.9% and 0%, respectively, and rates of transient and permanent RLN palsy of 5.9% and 0%, respectively (40). Only three patients (0.7%) experienced mental nerve injury, a major improvement over previous methods (40). This surgical method is receiving considerable attention because it is scarless and requires minimal dissection. By contrast, its craniocaudal approach is difficult for some surgeons because of the unfamiliar surgical field of view. Although oral infection was thought to be a problem, its safety was confirmed through many studies (35, 38, 40). Despite studies showing that this approach is stable and feasible, with a low rate of postoperative complications, the surgical area is relatively limited and there are no reports of long-term results, making it necessary to accumulate additional evidence prior to its being recommended.

Robotic surgery

The robotic system most frequently used is the da Vinci system (Intuitive Surgical, USA). This instrument supports a three-dimensional view of the operating field, a 15-times magnified view, and a greater degree of movement from its use of "wristed" instruments (41, 42). In addition, its tremor elimination function enhances the safety and precision of the procedure (43). Since robotic trans-axillary thyroidectomy was first reported in 2009 (4), BABA, retroauricular ("facelift"), and transoral approaches have been mainly implemented (Figure 37.3).

Gasless trans-axillary approach

Outcomes of 100 patients who underwent robotic thyroidectomy via a TAA were first reported in 2009 (4). At the beginning of the study, axillary incisions were made and an additional chest port was inserted. Subsequently, the approach was improved to use only the axillary port. The da Vinci robot can provide a three-dimensional view of the surgical field, and use of the free endo-wrist does not restrict the movements of surgical instruments (41, 44). In addition, the TAA can preserve the RLN and parathyroid well and enable both lobectomy and total thyroidectomy (4). A study comparing robotic trans-axillary surgery with conventional open thyroidectomy revealed no differences in rates of complications, including blood loss, hypocalcemia, and RLN injury (45). Potential risks of this surgery include anterior chest paresthesia, brachial plexus injury, tracheal injury, and esophageal injury (46–50). A large meta-analysis compared robotic trans-axillary thyroidectomy, endoscopic trans-axillary thyroidectomy, and conventional open surgery in 2881 patients (51). Operation times did not differ in patients who underwent robotic and endoscopic trans-axillary thyroidectomy, but both were longer than the operation time in patients who underwent conventional open surgery. Postoperative complication rates did not differ in these three groups, but cosmetic satisfaction was superior in patients who underwent robotic and endoscopic trans-axillary thyroidectomy compared with those who underwent conventional open thyroidectomy. A retrospective analysis of 5000 patients who underwent gasless trans-axillary robotic thyroidectomy, including 4804 with cancer (4102 with stage I tumors), found that the mean operation time was 134.0 ± 122.0 min and the mean tumor size was 8.0 ± 6.0 mm (52). This study found that 24.1% of patients experienced more than one complication, whereas recurrences were observed in 0.5% (n=26). In addition, a recent study reported the results of trans-axillary hemithyroidectomy in ten patients with 3-cm incisions using the da Vinci SP system (53). TAA has the advantage of not using CO_2, making it one of the most frequent operations performed worldwide. Drawbacks of this approach include the possibility of brachial plexus injury associated with arm extension and the need for skilled operators to perform surgery on the contralateral lobe.

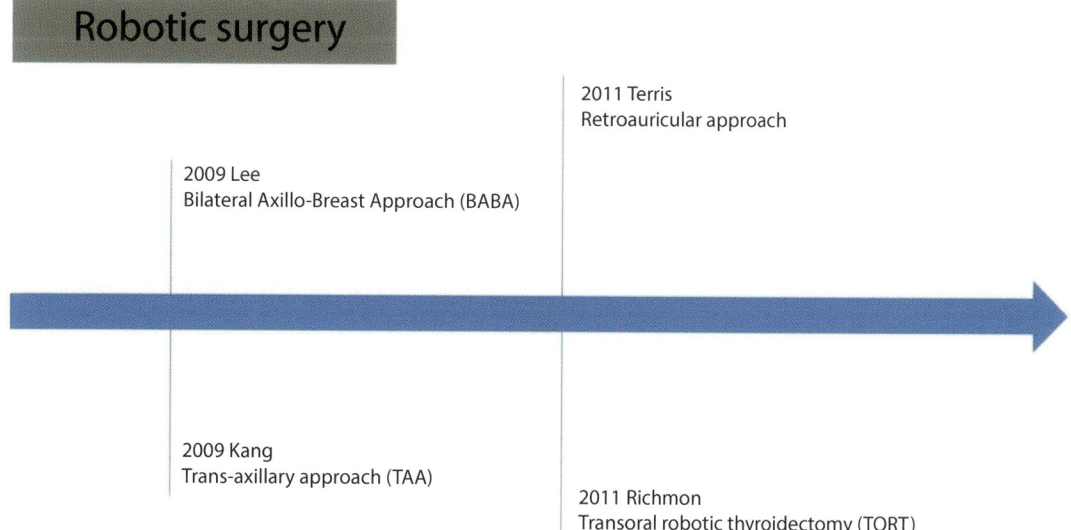

FIGURE 37.3 The history of remote access surgery using robots.

Bilateral axillo-breast approach (BABA)

BABA robotic thyroidectomy consists of the application of the da Vinci robot to the previously described BABA endoscopic thyroidectomy (54). The initial large-scale study of BABA robotic thyroidectomy analyzed 1026 patients (42). An analysis of 872 patients who underwent total thyroidectomy showed that the rates of transient and permanent hypoparathyroidism were 39.1% and 1.5%, respectively, and that the rates of transient and permanent vocal cord palsy were 14.2% and 0.2%, respectively (42). Although BABA robotic thyroid surgery was initially performed in South Korea and developed mainly in Asia, it has become one of the most common types of surgery performed worldwide (55–57). The advantages of BABA robotic thyroidectomy include its provision of a symmetrical field of view, providing the surgeon with a comfortable surgical field and enabling surgery on both thyroid glands (58). In addition, the lack of collision between surgical instruments enables the robotic arm to be used freely and the performance of surgery in a wide surgical field. The robot's camera, which magnifies the field of view of 15 folds, offers advantages in finding and preserving RLNs and parathyroid gland. Initially, the surgical indications for BABA robotic surgery were limited to benign thyroid nodules and low-risk PTMCs, but its indications expanded as experience accumulated (59). In addition, this method has been reported effective even in patients with papillary thyroid carcinoma (PTC) with metastasis and those with unilateral and bilateral modified radical neck dissection (MRND) without limiting the surgical range (60–62). This method also has the advantage of preserving the parathyroid gland. The use of a subcapsular saline injection (SCASI) in patients undergoing BABA RT has been found to drastically reduce transient hypoparathyroidism (63). A study comparing BABA robotic and endoscopic thyroidectomy found no differences in hospital stay and the rates of postoperative complications such as RLN injury, hypoparathyroidism, and bleeding (64, 65). However, operation time was about 1.5 times longer with robotic than endoscopic thyroid surgery, and the number of acquired lymph nodes was greater with BABA robotic than BABA endoscopic thyroidectomy (64, 65). A study comparing BABA robotic thyroidectomy in 2003 patients and BABA endoscopic thyroidectomy in 1029 patients found no difference in the rate of transient hypoparathyroidism (66), whereas the rates of permanent hypoparathyroidism (2.3% vs. 5.2%, p = 0.05) and transient VC palsy (9.1% vs. 14.4%, p = 0.006) were significantly lower in the robotic than in the endoscopic group (66). Although both methods are good, safe, and effective, BABA robotic thyroidectomy can overcome the lack of experience and skills of inexperienced surgeons.

Robotic retroauricular "facelift" approach

The robotic retroauricular (facelift) approach, first reported in 14 patients in 2011 (67), is a modified version of a previously described endoscopic surgery method (14). A study of 91 patients found that the operation times for hemithyroidectomy and total thyroidectomy were 108 and 118 min, respectively (51). Two patients required conversion to open surgery, but none experienced permanent vocal cord palsy. Retroauricular surgery can be applied more easily than trans-axillary surgery to patients with a higher body mass index (BMI) (67). In addition, this method is safe because there is no risk of brachial plexus injury, a potential complication of trans-axillary surgery (68, 69). By contrast, the disadvantages of this surgical method include the possibility of damage to the great auricular nerve and the limited direction of the operation, requiring two incisions to perform total thyroidectomy (70).

Transoral robotic thyroidectomy (TORT)

The application of endoscopic transoral thyroidectomy to robotic systems was first assessed in cadavers (36). In subsequent application to patients, three of four complained of paresthesia due to mental nerve injury (71). Based on TOETVA, a modified incision was suggested to avoid mental nerve injury and subsequently applied to robots (16). A study of 17 patients found that the average operation time was 254 min, with one patient requiring open conversion (72). Complications included hypoesthesia in three patients, lip weakness in one, and a small lateral lip tear in another. A recent study of transoral robotic thyroidectomy (TORT) in 100 patients found that nine experienced perioperative morbidity, including two each with zygomatic bruising, commissure tearing, and chin dimpling, and one each with transient RLN palsy, postoperative bleeding, and chin flap perforation (73). Despite the possibility of mental nerve injury and complications around the lip, TORT has been widely adopted because of its advantage of reaching the thyroid gland without skin injury. Although it also has the advantage of providing the same surgical field of view on both sides, a certain training period is required to become familiar with the craniocaudal direction.

South Asian perspective of remote access thyroid and parathyroid surgery

Resection of the thyroid and parathyroid glands formerly required incisions in the neck. Technological developments, however, resulted in smaller neck incisions and eventually the displacement of these incisions from the neck. Remote access surgery is defined as surgery on the neck in which the incision has been moved outside the neck. Remote access surgery has been widely studied in Asian patients due to cultural concerns regarding neck scars. Initially, remote access surgery was performed with an endoscope but is now increasingly performed with the da Vinci robot.

Many endoscopic and robotic remote access surgery developed in Asia included axillary approach, the anterior chest approach, gasless TAA, anterior breast approach, ABBA, BABA, PAA approach, and TOETVA. Among these surgeries, there are few methods that are consistently performed in various countries. Endoscopic trans-axillary and BABA surgical approaches were originally developed in South Korea and later extended to robotic surgery. Robotic thyroidectomy was initially limited to patients with benign nodules and small PTCs but gradually expanded to include patients with Graves' disease and larger PTCs. The advantage of TOETVA is that its flap area is relatively small; therefore, many surgeons are practicing it. Currently, the surgical extent is relatively limited, but it will continue to expand. For remote access surgery to become widespread, good teaching methods and educational opportunities will be needed (55, 74, 75).

Conclusion

Remote access thyroid surgery has already become an important option for patients. Remote access thyroid surgery was originally limited to benign nodules and PTCs <1 cm. Increased experience has expanded its indications to large benign nodules and goiters and, in patients with PTC, the dissection of lymph nodes. Robotic remote access surgery has become safe and effective, and its use and importance will likely increase in the future.

References

1. Gagner M. Endoscopic subtotal parathyroidectomy in patients with primary hyperparathyroidism. Br J Surg. 1996;83(6):875.
2. Huscher CS, Chiodini S, Napolitano C, Recher A. Endoscopic right thyroid lobectomy. Surg Endosc. 1997;11(8):877..
3. Gagne M, Inabnet WB. Endoscopic thyroidectomy for solitary thyroid nodules. Thyroid. 2001;11(2):161–163.
4. Kang SW, Jeong JJ, Yun JS, Sung TY, Lee SC, Lee YS, et al. Robot-assisted endoscopic surgery for thyroid cancer: Experience with the first 100 patients. Surg Endosc. 2009;23(11):2399–2406.
5. George EI, Brand TC, LaPorta A, Marescaux J, Satava RM. Origins of robotic surgery: From skepticism to standard of care. JSLS J Soc Laparoendosc Surg. 2018;22(4): e2018.00039.
6. Miccoli P, Bendinelli C, Vignali E, Mazzeo S, Cecchini GM, Pinchera A, et al. Endoscopic parathyroidectomy: Report of an initial experience. Surgery. 1998;124(6):1077–1080.
7. G Scerrino NC, Paladino V, Di Paola G, Morfino A, Inviati E, Amodio G, Gulotta SB. Minimally invasive video-assisted thyroidectomy: Four-year experience of a single team in a General Surgery Unit. Minerva Chir. 2013;68(3):307–314.
8. Ikeda Y, Takami H, Tajima G, Sasaki Y, Takayama J, Kurihara H, et al. Total endoscopic thyroidectomy: Axillary or anterior chest approach. Biomed Pharmacother. 2002;56:72s–78s.
9. Ikeda Y, Takami H, Sasaki Y, Kan S, Niimi M. Endoscopic neck surgery by the axillary approach. J Am Coll Surg. 2000;191(3):336–340.
10. Yoon JH, Park CH, Chung WOY. Gasless endoscopic thyroidectomy via an axillary approach: Experience of 30 cases. Surg Laparosc Endosc Percutan Tech. 2006;16(4):226–231.
11. Ohgami M, Ishii S, Arisawa Y, Ohmori T, Noga K, Furukawa T, Kitajima M. Scarless endoscopic thyroidectomy: Breast approach for better cosmesis. Surg Laparosc EndoSc Percutan Tech. 2000;10(1):1–4.
12. Shimazu K, Shiba E, Tamaki Y, Takiguchi S, Taniguchi E, Ohashi S, et al. Endoscopic thyroid surgery through the axillo-bilateral-breast approach. Surg Laparosc Endosc Percutan Tech. 2003;13(3):196–201.
13. Choe JH, Kim SW, Chung KW, Park KS, Han W, Noh DY, et al. Endoscopic thyroidectomy using a new bilateral axillo-breast approach. World J Surg. 2007;31:601–606.
14. Lee KE, Kim HY, Park WS, Choe JH, Kwon MR, Oh SK, et al. Postauricular and axillary approach endoscopic neck surgery: A new technique. World J Surg. 2009;33:767–772.
15. Witzel K, Von Rahden BHA, Kaminski C, Stein HJ. Transoral access for endoscopic thyroid resection. Surg Endosc Other Interv Tech. 2008;22(8):1871–1875.
16. Anuwong A. Transoral endoscopic thyroidectomy vestibular approach: A series of the first 60 human cases. World J Surg. 2016;40(3):491–497.
17. Miccoli P, Berti P, Conte M, Bendinelli C, Marcocci C. Minimally invasive surgery for thyroid small nodules: Preliminary report. J Endocrinol Invest. 1999;22(11):849–851.
18. Ikeda Y, Takami H. Endoscopic parathyroidectomy. Biomed Pharmacother. 2000;54(Suppl 1):52–56.
19. Shimizu K, Kitagawa W, Akasu H, Hatori N, Hirai K, Tanaka S. Video-assisted endoscopic thyroid and parathyroid surgery using a gasless method of anterior neck skin lifting: A review of 130 cases. Surg Today. 2002;32(10):862–868.
20. Ikeda Y, Takami H, Niimi M, Kan S, Sasaki Y, Takayama J. Endoscopic thyroidectomy by the axillary approach. Surg Endosc. 2001;15(11):1362–1364.
21. Ikeda Y, Takami H, Sasaki Y, Takayama JI, Kurihara H. Are there significant benefits of minimally invasive endoscopic thyroidectomy? World J Surg. 2004;28(11):1075–1078.
22. Ikeda Y, Takami H, Sasaki Y, Takayama J, Niimi M, Kan S. Comparative study of thyroidectomies: Endoscopic surgery vs conventional open surgery. Surg Endosc Other Interv Tech. 2002;16(12):1741–1745.
23. Kang SW, Jeong JJ, Yun JS, Sung TY, Lee SC, Lee YS, et al. Gasless endoscopic thyroidectomy using trans-axillary approach; surgical outcome of 581 patients. Endocr J. 2009;56(3):361–369.
24. Jong JJ, Kang SW, Yun JS, Tae YS, Seung CL, Yong SL, et al. Comparative study of endoscopic thyroidectomy versus conventional open thyroidectomy in papillary thyroid microcarcinoma (PTMC) patients. J Surg Oncol. 2009;100(6):477–480.
25. Kim EY, Lee KH, Park YL, Park CH, Lee CR, Jeong JJ, et al. Single-incision, gasless, endoscopic trans-axillary total thyroidectomy: A feasible and oncologic safe surgery in patients with papillary thyroid carcinoma. J Laparoendosc Adv Surg Tech. 2017;27(11):1158–1164.
26. Park YL, Han WK, Bae WG. 100 Cases of endoscopic thyroidectomy: Breast approach. Surg Laparosc Endosc Percutan Tech. 2003;13(1):20–25.
27. Cho YU, Park IJ, Choi KH, Kim SJ, Choi SK, Hur YS, et al. Gasless endoscopic thyroidectomy via an anterior chest wall approach using a flap-lifting system. Yonsei Med J. 2007;48:480–487.
28. Yamamoto M, Sasaki A, Asahi H, Shimada Y, Sato N, Nakajima J, et al. Endoscopic subtotal thyroidectomy for patients with Graves' disease. Surg Today. 2001;31(1):1–4.
29. Kitagawa W, Shimizu K, Akasu H, Tanaka S. Endoscopic neck surgery with lymph node dissection for papillary carcinoma of the thyroid using a totally gasless anterior neck skin lifting method. J Am Coll Surg. 2003;196(6):990–994.
30. Sasaki A, Nakajima J, Ikeda K, Otsuka K, Koeda K, Wakabayashi G. Endoscopic thyroidectomy by the breast approach: A single institution's 9-year experience. World J Surg. 2008;32(3):381–385.
31. Choi JY, Lee KE, Chung KW, Kim SW, Choe JH, Koo DH, et al. Endoscopic thyroidectomy via bilateral axillo-breast approach (BABA): Review of 512 cases in a single institute. Surg Endosc Other Interv Tech. 2012;26:948–955.
32. Alramadhan M, Choe JH, Lee JH, Kim JH, Kim JS. Propensity score-matched analysis of the endoscopic bilateral axillo-breast approach (BABA) versus conventional open thyroidectomy in patients with benign or intermediate fine-needle aspiration cytology results, a retrospective study. Int J Surg [Internet]. 2017;48:9–15.
33. Johri G, Chand G, Mishra A, Mayilvaganan S, Agarwal G, Agarwal A, et al. Endoscopic versus conventional thyroid surgery: A comparison of quality of life, cosmetic outcomes and overall patient satisfaction with treatment. World J Surg [Internet]. 2020; Available from: https://doi.org/10.1007/s00268-020-05732-7.
34. Wilhelm T, Metzig A. Endoscopic minimally invasive thyroidectomy: First clinical experience. Surg Endosc. 2010;24(7):1757–1758.
35. Wilhelm T, Metzig A. Endoscopic minimally invasive thyroidectomy (eMIT): A prospective proof-of-concept study in humans. World J Surg. 2011;35(3):543–551.
36. Richmon JD, Holsinger FC, Kandil E, Moore MW, Garcia JA, Tufano RP. Transoral robotic-assisted thyroidectomy with central neck dissection: Preclinical cadaver feasibility study and proposed surgical technique. J Robot Surg. 2011;5(4):279–282.
37. Park JO, Kim CS, Song JN, Kim JE, Nam IC, Lee SY, et al. Transoral endoscopic thyroidectomy via the tri-vestibular routes: Results of a preclinical cadaver feasibility study. Eur Arch Otorhinolaryngol. 2014;271(12):3269–3275.
38. Park JO, Sun D Il. Transoral endoscopic thyroidectomy: Our initial experience using a new endoscopic technique. Surg Endosc. 2017;31(12):5436–5443.
39. Anuwong A, Sasanakietkul T, Jitpratoom P, Ketwong K, Kim HY, Dionigi G, et al. Transoral endoscopic thyroidectomy vestibular approach (TOETVA): Indications, techniques and results. Surg Endosc. 2018;32(1):456–465.
40. Anuwong A, Ketwong K, Jitpratoom P, Sasanakietkul T, Duh QY. Safety and outcomes of the transoral endoscopic thyroidectomy vestibular approach. JAMA Surg. 2018;153(1):21–27.
41. Ban EJ, Yoo JY, Kim WW, Son HY, Park S, Lee SH, et al. Surgical complications after robotic thyroidectomy for thyroid carcinoma: A single center experience with 3,000 patients. Surg Endosc. 2014;28(9):2555–2563.
42. Lee KE, Kim E, Koo DH, Choi JY, Kim KH, Youn YK. Robotic thyroidectomy by bilateral axillo-breast approach: Review of 1026 cases and surgical completeness. Surg Endosc Other Interv Tech. 2013;27:2955–2962.
43. Tolley N, Arora A, Palazzo F, Garas G, Dhawan R, Cox J, et al. Robotic-assisted parathyroidectomy: A feasibility study. Otolaryngol Head Neck Surg. 2011;144(6):859–866.
44. Lee J, Chung WY. Robotic thyroidectomy and neck dissection: Past, present, and future. Cancer J (United States). 2013;19(2):151–161.
45. Piccoli M, Mullineris B, Santi D, Gozzo D. Advances in robotic transaxillary thyroidectomy in Europe. Curr Surg Rep. 2017;5(8):1–7.
46. Arora A, Garas G, Sharma S, Muthuswamy K, Budge J, Palazzo F, et al. Comparing transaxillary robotic thyroidectomy with conventional surgery in a UK population: A case control study. Int J Surg [Internet]. 2016;27:110–117.
47. Yuk-Wah Liu S, Hung-Hin Lang B. Revisiting robotic approaches to endocrine neoplasia: Do the data support their continued use? Curr Opin Oncol. 2016;28(1):26–36.
48. Dralle H. Robot-assisted transaxillary thyroid surgery: As safe as conventional-access thyroid surgery? Eur Thyroid J. 2013;2(2):71–75.
49. Rabinovics N, Aidan P. Robotic transaxillary thyroid surgery. Gland Surg. 2015;4(5):397–402.
50. Luginbuhl A, Schwartz DM, Sestokas AK, Cognetti D, Pribitkin E. Detection of evolving injury to the brachial plexus during transaxillary robotic thyroidectomy. Laryngoscope. 2012;122(1):110–115.
51. Jackson NR, Yao L, Tufano RP, Kandil EH. Safety of robotic thyroidectomy approaches: Meta-analysis and systematic review. Head Neck. 2014;36(1):137–143.
52. Kim MJ, Nam KH, Lee SG, Choi JB, Kim TH, Lee CR, et al. Yonsei experience of 5000 gasless transaxillary robotic thyroidectomies. World J Surg. 2018;42(2):393–401.
53. Kim K, Kang SW, Kim JK, Lee CR, Lee J, Jeong JJ, et al. Robotic transaxillary hemithyroidectomy using the da Vinci SP robotic system: Initial experience with 10 consecutive cases. Surg Innov. 2020;27(3):256–264.
54. Lee KE, Rao J, Youn Y-K. Endoscopic thyroidectomy with the da Vinci robot system using the bilateral axillary breast approach (BABA) technique: Our initial experience. Surg Laparosc Endosc Percutan Tech. 2009;19(3):e71–e75.
55. Sun HX, Gao HJ, Ying XY, Chen X, Li QY, Qiu WH, et al. Robotic thyroidectomy via bilateral axillo-breast approach: Experience and learning curve through initial 220 cases. Asian J Surg [Internet]. 2020;43(3):482–487.
56. Liu SYW, Kim JS. Bilateral axillo-breast approach robotic thyroidectomy: Review of evidences. Gland Surg. 2017;6(3):250–257.
57. He Q, Zhu J, Zhuang D, Fan Z. Robotic total parathyroidectomy by the axillo-bilateral-breast approach for secondary hyperparathyroidism: A feasibility study. J Laparoendosc Adv Surg Tech [Internet]. 2015;25(4):311–313. Available from: http://online.liebertpub.com/doi/10.1089/lap.2014.0234
58. Lee KE, Koo DH, Kim SJ, Lee J, Park KS, Oh SK, et al. Outcomes of 109 patients with papillary thyroid carcinoma who underwent robotic total thyroidectomy with central node dissection via the bilateral axillo-breast approach. Surgery [Internet]. 2010;148(6):1207–1213.
59. Chai YJ, Suh H, Woo J-W, Yu HW, Song R-Y, Kwon H, et al. Surgical safety and oncological completeness of robotic thyroidectomy for thyroid carcinoma larger than 2 cm. Surg Endosc [Internet]. 2016; Available from: http://link.springer.com/10.1007/s00464-016-5097-1.
60. Yu HW, Chai YJ, Kim S, Choi JY, Lee KE. Robotic-assisted modified radical neck dissection using a bilateral axillo-breast approach (robotic BABA MRND) for papillary thyroid carcinoma with lateral lymph node metastasis. Surg Endosc [Internet]. 2017;0(0):0. Available from: http://link.springer.com/10.1007/s00464-017-5927-9.
61. Choi JY, Kang KH. Robotic modified radical neck dissection with bilateral axillo-breast approach. Gland Surg. 2017;6(3):243–249.
62. Song RY, Sohn HJ, Paek SH, Kang KH. The first report of robotic bilateral modified radical neck dissection through the bilateral axillo-breast approach for papillary thyroid carcinoma with bilateral lateral neck metastasis. Surg Laparosc Endosc Percutan Tech. 2020;30(3):E18–E22.
63. Yu HW, Bae IE, Yi JW, Lee J-H, Kim S, Chai YJ, et al. The application of subcapsular saline injection during bilateral axillo-breast approach robotic thyroidectomy: A preliminary report. Surg Today [Internet]. 2019;0(0):0. Available from: http://link.springer.com/10.1007/s00595-018-1748-2.

64. Kim WW, Kim JS, Hur SM, Kim SH, Lee SK, Choi JH, et al. Is robotic surgery superior to endoscopic and open surgeries in thyroid cancer? World J Surg. 2011;35:779–784.
65. Kim SK, Woo JW, Park I, Lee JH, Choe JH, Kim JH, et al. Propensity score-matched analysis of robotic versus endoscopic bilateral axillo-breast approach (BABA) thyroidectomy in papillary thyroid carcinoma. Langenbecks Arch Surg. 2017;402(2):243–250.
66. Choi JY, Bae IE, Kim HS, Yoon SG, Yi JW, Yu HW, Kim S-j, Chai YJ, Lee KE, Youn Y-K. Comparative study of bilateral axillo-breast approach (BABA) endoscopic and robotic thyroidectomy: a propensity score matching analysis of large multi-institutional data. Ann Surg Treat Res. 2020;98(6):307–314.
67. Terris DJ, Singer MC, Seybt MW. Robotic facelift thyroidectomy: II. Clinical feasibility and safety. Laryngoscope. 2011;121(8):1636–1641.
68. Terris DJ, Singer MC. Qualitative and quantitative differences between 2 robotic thyroidectomy techniques. Otolaryngol Head Neck Surg (United States). 2012;147(1):20–25.
69. Kuppersmith RB, Holsinger FC. Robotic thyroid surgery: An initial experience with North American patients. Laryngoscope. 2011;121(3):521–526.
70. Alabbas H, Ali DB, Kandil E. Robotic retroauricular thyroid surgery. Gland Surg. 2016;5(6):603–606.
71. Lee HY, You JY, Woo SU, Son GS, Lee JB, Bae JW, et al. Transoral periosteal thyroidectomy: Cadaver to human. Surg Endosc. 2015;29(4):898–904.
72. Richmon JD, Kim HY. Transoral robotic thyroidectomy (TORT): Procedures and outcomes. Gland Surg. 2017;6(3):285–289.
73. Kim HK, Chai YJ, Dionigi G, Berber E, Tufano RP, Kim HY. Transoral robotic thyroidectomy for papillary thyroid carcinoma: Perioperative outcomes of 100 consecutive patients. World J Surg [Internet]. 2019;43(4):1038–1046.
74. Kang SW, Lee SC, Lee SH, Lee KY, Jeong JJ, Lee YS, et al. Robotic thyroid surgery using a gasless, transaxillary approach and the da Vinci S system: The operative outcomes of 338 consecutive patients. Surgery [Internet]. 2009;146(6):1048–1055.
75. Kim WW, Jung JH, Park HY. The learning curve for robotic thyroidectomy using a bilateral axillo-breast approach from the 100 cases. Surg Laparosc Endosc Percutan Tech. 2015;25(5):412–416.

38

INTRAOPERATIVE ADJUNCTS IN THYROID AND PARATHYROID SURGERY

Sunnel Mattoo, Shreyamsa M, Roma Pradhan and Amit Agarwal

Introduction

It is the surgeon's duty to tranquillize the temper, to beget cheerfulness, and to impart confidence of recovery.

– Astley Cooper

The history of thyroid surgery is a fascinating one and indeed exemplifies the evolution from a horrible butchery to a highly sophisticated procedure, from bloody dissection to clean surgical fields, from a death warrant to a safe haven, from clinging limbs to diligent toiling, and from vocal crippling to melodious singing.

The *Atharva Veda* (2000 BC), an ancient Hindu collection of incantations, contains exorcisms for goiter. In 1600 BC, the Chinese used burnt sponge and seaweed for the treatment of goiters. Galen also referred to "*spongiausta*" (burnt sponge) for the treatment of goiter in 150 AD. One of the earliest references to a successful surgical attempt for the treatment of goiter is in the medical writings ("*Al Tasrif*") of the Moorish physician Ali Ibn Abbas. In 952 AD, he recorded his experience with the removal of a large goiter under opium sedation using simple ligatures and hot cautery irons as the patient sat with a bag around his neck to catch the blood. The first successful typical partial thyroidectomy was performed by the French Surgeon, Desault, in 1791. Dupuytren did the first total thyroidectomy in 1808, but the patient died 36 h after the operation. Thyroid surgery in the 19th century carried a frightful mortality of 40% even in most skilled hands, mainly due to infection and hemorrhage. The French and German Academy of Medicine banned thyroid surgery, and across the Atlantic, Samuel Gross also denounced thyroid surgery as "horrid butchery". The efforts of "the magnificent seven" surgeons (Billroth, Kocher, Halsted, Mayo, Crile, Lahey, and Dunhill), however, heralded a new era in history with a drastic reduction in perioperative morbidity and mortality. The present research efforts continue in the same direction with the use of ever-evolving technology to make thyroidectomy even more highly effective, safe, and cosmetically appealing. Table 38.1 has a list of all intraoperative adjuncts used in thyroid surgery.

Hemostasis

Thyroid surgery involves meticulous devascularization of the thyroid gland that has one of the richest blood supplies of all organs. Hemostasis is of paramount importance because of two reasons.

TABLE 38.1: Intraoperative Adjuncts in Thyroid Surgery

Aim	Technology
Better hemostasis	Handheld energy devices, e.g. bipolar and ultrasonic devices
Minimize laryngeal nerve palsy	Intraoperative neuromonitoring (IONM)
Neural prognostication	
Prevent hypocalcemia	Parathyroid fluorescence with indocyanine green (ICG)
Cosmesis	Endoscopic and robotic surgery

One of the major concerns following thyroid surgery is the risk of life-threatening hematoma, the incidence of which is 0.3–3%. Postoperatively drain is often used but the presence or the absence of drain doesn't have any influence on hematoma formation or bleeding [1–3]. The other reason is bleeding during thyroidectomy blurs vision, thus putting the recurrent laryngeal nerve (RLN) and parathyroid glands at increased risk of injury.

Two of the most used techniques for hemostasis are suture ligation and electrocoagulation. The disadvantages of these techniques are the prolonged operating time, thermal damage to vital structures, and possibility of granuloma formation. Furthermore, one of the important causes of post-thyroidectomy bleeding is loosening of the surgical knot. Evolutions in technology have allowed surgeons to achieve a better balance between hemostasis and tissue preservation.

Newer devices include the following:

- Bipolar energy sealing system
- Ultrasonic coagulation

Bipolar energy sealing system

It transfers radiofrequency energy to tissues through a bipolar device creating a coagulum by melting collagen and elastin. It can seal vessels up to 7 mm. This has a unique design that prevents electrical power transmission and heat transfer, thus avoiding thermal damage [4]. A significantly lower operation time for total thyroidectomy was seen in the study by Molnar et al. while using bipolar energy system [4]. In a randomized controlled trial comparing bipolar energy system with conventional thyroidectomy, a decrease in operative time and intraoperative bleeding was found compared to conventional technique [5].

Ultrasonic coagulation

It transfers frictional energy through vibrations at 55,000 Hz to tissues causing protein denaturation by rupture of hydrogen bonds. No electrical energy is transmitted to the patient.

The use of ultrasonic coagulation is useful in shortening the duration of thyroid surgery. This is likely attributable to the fact that tissue can be detached, coagulated, and dissected in a continuous operation without the need to change instruments. Lateral thermal spread is also less compared to monopolar cautery (Table 38.2).

However, the evidence for showing the impact of these energy devices on postoperative complications is unclear. Some studies have reported lower rates of complications, whereas others failed to demonstrate benefits over conventional hemostasis [6–9].

Minimize laryngeal nerve palsy

The relationship of RLN with voice has a fascinating story, which dates back as early as 6th century BC as written in Sushruta Samhita. Thyroid surgery seems to revolve around the preservation of integrity of RLN.

TABLE 38.2: Advantages of Hemostatic Devices

Minimal collateral damage for safe dissection near vital structures [10]
Less smoke formation
No neuromuscular stimulation
No electrical energy passed to or through the patient (ultrasonic)
Cuts, coagulates, grasp, and dissects by the same instrument: minimal instrument exchanges
Reliably seal and divide vessels

Injury to the RLN is the most feared injury in thyroid surgery as compared to external branch of superior laryngeal nerve that supplies only the cricothyroid muscle; hence, the damage of the nerve has varied effect on voice and is less troublesome except in singers and teachers.

Before the modern thyroid surgery developed, general surgeons never exposed the RLN for fear of damaging the RLN. However, modern thyroid surgery involved exposure and visualization of the entire course of RLN and this brought down the RLN damage rate to as low as 1–5%. But general and occasional thyroid surgeons continued to avoid exposure of the RLN perhaps because of the lack of adequate training. Furthermore, even for expert surgeons, certain challenging situations make exposure and identification of RLN exceedingly difficult.

Intraoperative neuromonitoring (IONM)

IONM is considered a safe procedure to complement the traditional method of visualizing the nerve, which is considered the gold standard. It can also be used to prognosticate the postoperative nerve function, hence used as an adjunct tool for thyroid surgery. Neuromonitoring can be intermittent or continuous. The intermittent neuromonitoring in thyroid surgery for recognition of RLN was first done in Sweden way back in the late 1960s [11]. All the 15 nerves investigated could be easily identified by it. Though its popularity and use are increasing, it is still considered an adjunct in thyroid surgery and not a necessity. Visual identification of the nerve remains the gold standard. The guidelines and literature suggest its importance in difficult cases like retrosternal goiter, toxic goiter, recurrent goiter, or recurrent thyroid cancer; however, its use regularly in all cases is debatable (Table 38.3).

Current neuromonitoring equipment can be divided into audio-only system or audio and visual waveform system. Audio-only system is inferior as it provides less information regarding waveform.

TABLE 38.3: Advantages of IONM

Prevent bilateral RLN injury by allowing staged surgery when there is LOS on one side, thus avoiding the need for tracheostomy
Prognosticate postoperative function that is difficult to detect by visual identification as most injured nerves appear intact
Detect anatomical variation and abnormal courses of nerves, which are at higher risk of injury if not detected
Beneficial in higher risk patients, e.g. locally advanced thyroid cancer, patients with prior surgery and scarring, and patients with large goiters
Prevent potential nerve injury by detecting signal changes indicating an adverse condition like suture compressing the nerve
Gauge trauma to nerve and increase surgeon's confidence
C-IONM is also able to detect the most proximal injuries that may be missed by intermittent monitoring
Several investigators have suggested that low-volume thyroid surgeons may benefit from IONM

Electromyography response to RLN stimulation cannot be quantified. Recording electrodes can be either needle based or endotracheal tube (ETT) based. Use of needle electrodes may lead to trauma, including vocal cord or laryngeal hematoma, infection, cuff deflation, or accidental needle dislodgment. Endotracheal-based systems record EMG data from vocal cord and do not require any additional equipment beyond ETTs. Endotracheal-based electrodes can be of two types – those embedded into the tubes and the other ones being the stick-on types.

Anesthesia prerequisites

IONM is based on sensitivity of nerves to mechanical stimulation and subsequent response recording in the form of EMG. Muscle relaxants reduce amplitude of EMG and significantly reduce the sensitivity of neuromonitoring to impending nerve injury. Therefore, it is absolutely essential to have full muscular activity soon after intubation. Patient is induced with a short acting intravenous neuroblocking agent like succinylcholine (2–2.5 mg/kg) or a small dose of a nondepolarizing muscle relaxant (e.g. 0.5 mg/kg of atracurium/rocuronium) may be used at intubation, as they allow early return of spontaneous respiration and resumption of normal muscle twitch activity. Inhalational agents used in induction do not interfere with EMG amplitude. The depth of anesthesia from inhalational agents must be sufficient enough to inhibit spontaneous vocal cord activity. A lighter plane of anesthesia may result in high baseline EMG activity and prevent differentiation between spontaneous and stimulated activity. Anticholinergic agents like glycopyrrolate can be used to prevent pooling of saliva at vocal cord level, as it may result in altered signal transmission.

A larger size ETT is preferred as it snugly fits for good contact with vocal cords for better EMG signals. Baseline amplitude of 30–70 mV indicates proper positioning of the ETT. The placement of ETT is the important step.

After patient positioning is complete, monitor settings should be checked. Then this monitor should be checked for an appropriate event threshold at 100 mV, and a stimulator probe should be set on a value of 1–2 mA (Figure 38.1).

To make sure proper functioning of the circuit, vagus stimulation should be done before dissection. The stimulator probe sends signals at 4 per second; hence, the probe should be dragged over the tissue rather than just point touch. Monitor settings should

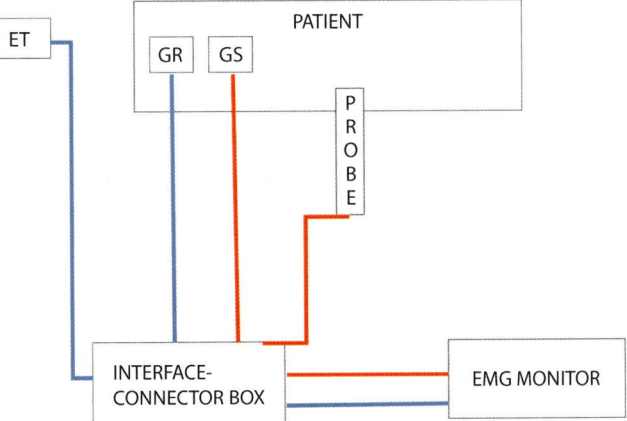

FIGURE 38.1 IONM set-up. Blue = recording side, red = stimulation side. ET – endotracheal tube, GR – ground electrode recording, GS – ground electrode stimulation.

Intraoperative Adjuncts in Thyroid and Parathyroid Surgery

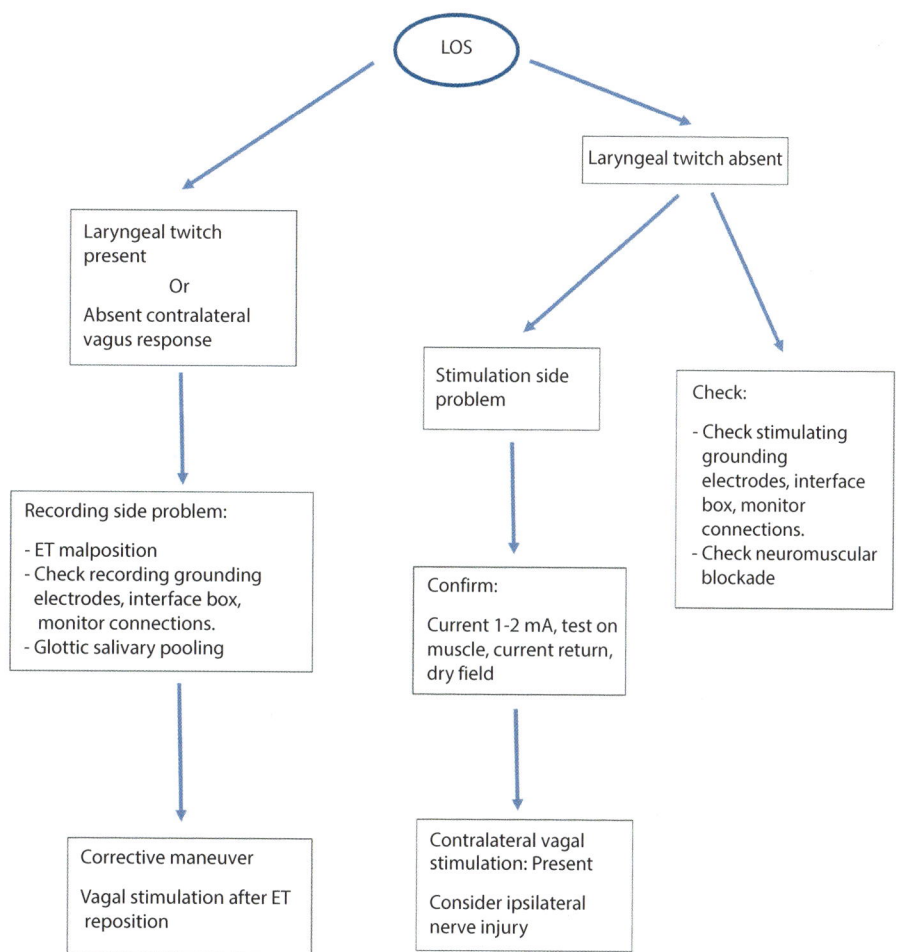

FIGURE 38.2 LOS evaluation algorithm.

include impedance values (<5 kohm), event threshold at 100 mV, and stimulator probe at 1–2 mA value.

Loss of signals (LOS) is defined by EMG change from previous satisfactory EMG, very low or no response (<100 μV) with stimulation. LOS can be due to loss of nerve function or malfunctioning. Once the LOS occurs, the first thing to do is to see and feel the laryngeal twitch. If present, it is likely to be a recording side problem (ETT malposition, ground electrodes detachment, interface box problems, or monitor/connections problems) (Figure 38.2–38.4).

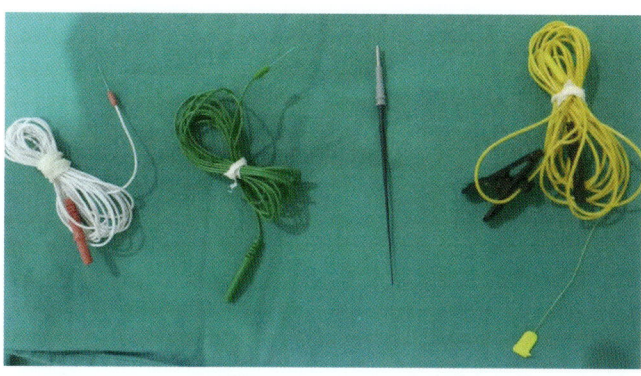

FIGURE 38.3 Equipment used in neuromonitoring.

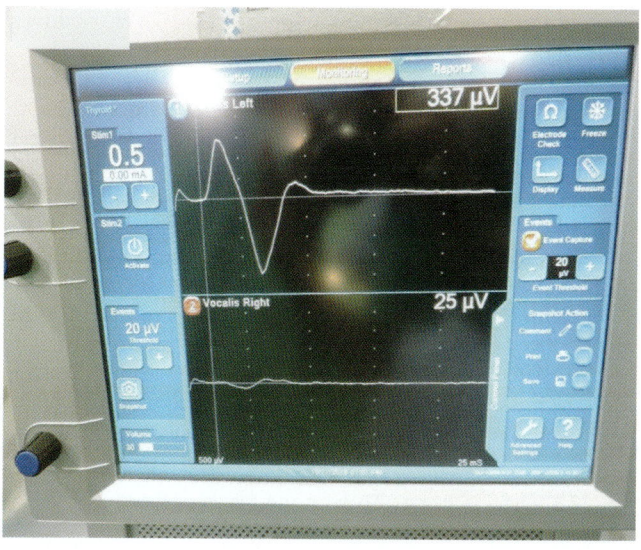

FIGURE 38.4 Good response (positive signal). The evoked waveform shows latency time, has a biphasic curve, and has good amplitude (>100 mV).

If with LOS we have absent laryngeal twitch as well as absent strap muscle twitch, the problem is from stimulating side (current problems, stimulator probe problems, or neuromuscular blockade). If strap muscle twitch is present and signal is obtained after stimulating contralateral vagus nerve, it indicates ipsilateral RLN injury.

Continuous neuromonitoring

Continuous neuromonitoring is a step forward from intermittent neuromonitoring and helps us to react even before the injury happens. It provides real-time status of the nerve function and gives the opportunity to reverse the surgical maneuver, which caused the EMG changes.

In continuous neuromonitoring, the ETT needs to be placed in the same way as in intermittent monitoring. The addition in this is the automatic periodic stimulation (APS) electrode also called the vagal electrode that needs to be placed on the ipsilateral vagal nerve. This involves opening of the carotid sheath, and this has been one of the reasons for criticism of continuous neuromonitoring. This step in continuous neuromonitoring requires precision and experience.

The initial stimulation is with 1 mA and 1 Hz and system calibration is done with the highest amplitude, preferably be more than ≥500 µV, to guarantee a stable and reliable EMG signal. Once the baseline is achieved, changes in it (amplitude and latency) are displayed on a timeline. It is possible to set an audible and visual alert when threshold values are exceeded, to help the surgeon identify risky manipulations.

All events are recorded and classified as baseline amplitude reduction below 75%, 50%, 25%, or LOS, as well as latency increase of 10%. Events with amplitudes less than 100 µV are counted as LOS regardless of the baseline amplitude. After confirmation of LOS, a 20-min wait period allows the surgeon to know if the affected nerve will recover fully or not and whether a *staged surgery* should be considered after the completion of the first side.

The most common cause of RLN injury is due to the traction of nerve especially at the area of ligament of Berry as suggested by Schneider [12] and other authors subsequently in their study [13–15].

Dionigi et al. studied 281 injured nerves associated with temporary or permanent postoperative vocal cord palsy and identified intraoperatively by LOS, found that only 14% of such injuries were visually evident intraoperatively, emphasizing the importance of neural signal loss information and the lack of sensitivity of visual neural inspection [16].

The most important controversy that hovers around neuromonitoring is its cost-effectiveness. The literature is varied with the results of IONM use. Some meta-analysis have demonstrated IONM to reduce the overall and transient vocal cord palsy rates [17], whereas many others have failed to demonstrate it [18, 19]. Cost-effectiveness of IONM was mentioned in few studies [20,21,22]. In a study by Rocke et al. [19], visual RLN identification was more cost-effective than using IONM. Moreover, IONM is cost-effective only if a surgeon can reduce palsy rate by 50.4% or more using IONM, which is impossible to achieve. In fact, it is difficult to analyze the cost associated with IONM since it should also take into consideration the indirect costs associated with RLN palsy like rehabilitation cost and economic compensations for legal claims.

IONM in remote access thyroidectomy

Remote access thyroidectomy is a fast-developing technique, which aimed at a better cosmetic outcome post surgery. IONM has been shown to be feasible in remote access procedures and is considered safe as well as useful in preventing neural injury. The stimulation probes are inserted either percutaneously, directly into the operating field, or via the endoscopic port using long probes. Studies have shown that IONM in remote access procedures helps identify the RLN better and aid in better maneuvering of thyroid without causing tractional injury. The disadvantages are the lack of space and routine exposure of vagus for continuous IONM, which makes the procedure more tedious and is associated with a high failure rate. Hence, it has not been widely adopted in remote access procedures yet.

Although there is no consensus that IONM decreases RLN injury when compared to visual identification, it has many advantages as follows.

Prevention of postoperative hypocalcemia

The reported incidence of transient and permanent hypocalcemia ranges from 3 to 52% and 0.4 to 13%, respectively [23, 24].

Various methods for diagnosing and managing postoperative hypocalcemia have been used. It is known that postoperative hypoparathyroidism leading to hypocalcemia is one of the most common complications after a total thyroidectomy. There are three methods of managing hypocalcemia. The most common approach used by surgeons is *supplementing* the calcium only if the patient develops signs and symptoms of hypocalcemia by monitoring the serum calcium but thus increasing the days of hospitalization. This reactive method of managing hypocalcemia is still being used by many institutions worldwide because the nadir of hypocalcemia typically occurs within 48 h after surgery. The *prophylactic or routine* use of postoperative oral calcium and/or vitamin D supplementation has been advocated by some surgeons to minimize the incidence of hypocalcemia and shorten hospital stay. More recently, with the aim of finding an earlier predictor for hypocalcemia, the short half-life of the parathyroid hormone (PTH) has led to increased interest in early postoperative serum *intact PTH (iPTH)* as an early marker of hypocalcemia [25]. Various studies, including a review [26], have evaluated the utility of postoperative serum iPTH measurement to predict post-thyroidectomy hypocalcemia. Several researches have relied on the utility of iPTH to foresee hypocalcemia after total thyroidectomy using hemithyroidectomy procedure as control group [27–29] but none could characterize an absolute iPTH serum level or percentage hormone decline with 100% sensitivity and specificity values. Some studies concluded that low perioperative PTH levels significantly correlate with the presence of postoperative hypocalcemia but cannot be used to predict it [30].

Therefore, iPTH done early in the postoperative period has the potential to allow early discharge from the hospital without the need of the patient undergoing serial calcium monitoring.

Among the newer techniques, intraoperative parathyroid gland angiography during thyroidectomy can also be used to evaluate parathyroid gland perfusion and function [31–33].

Intraoperative detection of parathyroid gland

Parathyroid detection presents the greatest difficulty in cases such as total thyroidectomy, completion thyroidectomy, central neck lymph node dissection, and re-operative thyroid surgery. The incidence of inadvertent parathyroidectomy during thyroidectomy ranges from 8 to 19%. There remains a clinical need for an intraoperative technique to detect the parathyroid gland instantly with high accuracy. There is, however, no objective intraoperative tool to determine if an ISPG (in situ parathyroid glands) is well perfused or not. Laser Doppler flowmetry was previously used for assessing parathyroid perfusion but has not been widely practiced. Therefore, surgeons often must rely on either visual inspection alone (i.e., by looking at the color changes in the ISPGs) or the "knife" test as ways of estimating parathyroid perfusion and viability. Indocyanine green (ICG) is an inert, water-soluble, nonradioactive, and nontoxic contrast agent that has been approved by the US Food and Drug Administration since 1959. After intravenous injection, ICG is distributed throughout the intravascular space and rapidly bound to plasma proteins. When illuminated at 806 nm with a low-energy laser, these plasma-bound ICG molecules become fluorescent and this fluorescence is recorded by a charge-coupled device camera. Because the fluorescence intensity (FI) in a focused area is directly proportional to the perfusion in that area, the FI value of the ISPGs measured on the ICG fluorescence angiography (ICGA) may provide information regarding the perfusion and the extent of viability of the ISPGs. This technology is not novel and has been used in various clinical areas, including assessing perfusion of skin flaps, bowel anastomosis, and lower limbs. Although this technique has been used for assessing parathyroid remnant in subtotal parathyroidectomy, to our knowledge, its use in assessing parathyroid perfusion during thyroid operations is being increased as reported. It is hypothesized that the FI in the ISPGs may reflect not only the perfusion of the ISPGs but also the residual parathyroid function and the subsequent risk of hypocalcemia. Given that parathyroid perfusion plays a vital role in normalizing early parathyroid function, perhaps patients with a greater FI value in their ISPGs (i.e., good parathyroid perfusion) have a lower chance of postoperative hypocalcemia than those with a lower FI value.

In a recent RCT [34] of 196 patients, a well-vascularized parathyroid gland could be identified in 146 patients (74.5%) and none of the subsequently randomized patients presented with hypocalcaemia. Therefore, serum calcium and/or iPTH measurements may no longer be necessary in patients with at least one well-perfused parathyroid gland, as demonstrated by ICG angiography after thyroidectomy.

A difficulty with ICG angiography is identification of parathyroid glands. Even an experienced thyroid surgeon might misinterpret other anatomical structures for a parathyroid gland. In experienced hands, however, the rate of correct identification of a structure as a parathyroid gland should exceed 95% [31] and hence a systematic biopsy is not necessary to confirm that the structure identified is indeed a parathyroid gland. In less experienced hands, a tool may be needed to help detect and identify parathyroid glands. New reports on parathyroid gland autofluorescence [35, 36] make use of a combination of autofluorescence first to identify the parathyroid glands, followed by ICG angiography to confirm about their vascularization.

Intraoperative parathormone monitoring in parathyroid surgery

Primary hyperparathyroidism (PHPT) is not an uncommon disorder. The commonest cause of PHPT is a single gland adenoma present in 80–85% of patients, followed by hyperplasia in 15–20% and carcinoma in less than 1%. The management also evolved with the first parathyroidectomy performed by Mandl in 1926 [37] with visualization of all the four glands and excising the enlarged gland. As the clinical spectrum of disease evolved from severe symptomatic to asymptomatic disease, the surgical approach also evolved from bilateral neck exploration to a focused approach with the evolution of various preoperative investigations along with adjuncts.

For focused parathyroidectomy, it is essential to get preoperative imaging, i.e., one anatomic and one functional. The goal of preoperative imaging for hyperparathyroidism is to identify the location of abnormal parathyroid tissue as precisely as possible in order to perform focused parathyroidectomy.

Technetium (99mTc) SestaMIBI scan is the imaging of choice with sensitivity ranging from 54 to 88% [38–41] The high-resolution ultrasound has sensitivity ranging from 59 to 89% [38, 39] The sensitivity of combined imaging is more than individual test.

Intraoperative PTH (IOPTH) is the most commonly used adjunct with focused parathyroidectomy. Numerous large studies have documented excellent cure rates after IOPTH-guided parathyroidectomy.

Protocol for blood sampling

A peripheral line access with a 16 ga needle or arterial line for sampling is used. The line is kept patent with saline infusion. It is necessary to instruct anesthetist to discard 10 ml of blood with saline to avoid dilution of sample. A total of 3–5 cm^3 of blood is collected in EDTA vial at a specific time of surgery (Figure 38.5).

Criteria for IOPTH [42–48]

1. *Miami criteria*: More than 50% drop from the highest either pre-incision or pre-excision levels 10 min after the excision of all abnormal parathyroid gland(s) (Figure 38.6).
2. *Vienna criteria*: More than 50% drop from pre-incision level only (disregarding pre-excision level) 10 min after parathyroid gland excision.
3. *Criteria 3*: More than 50% drop from the highest either pre-incision or pre-excision level 10 min after parathyroid excision with the requirement that IOPTH returns to a normal range.
4. *Criteria 4*: More than 50% drop from the highest pre-incision or pre-excision values 10 min after excision and falling below the pre-incision IOPTH level.
5. *Criteria 5*: More than 50% drop from the highest either pre-incision or pre-excision values 5 min after tumor excision.
6. *Criteria 6*: More than 50% drop from pre-excision level only 10 min after gland removal.
7. *Halle criteria*: IOPTH decays into the low normal range (35 ng/l) within 15 min after removal of the hyperfunctioning parathyroid tissue predicts cure.
8. *Residual criteria by Libutti et al.*: Residual criterion is calculated as the residual PTH concentration divided by baseline IOPTH (pre-excision) and expressed as a percentage.

Outcome after IOPTH

Numerous large studies have confirmed excellent outcomes or cures after IOPTH-guided parathyroidectomy. In the series by Chen et al. [49], they divided patients into two groups, one without IOPTH and the other with IOPTH monitoring. In the group without IOPTH, 10% were still hypercalcaemic postoperatively owing to additional unidentified hyperfunctioning parathyroid glands. In contrast, in group with IOPTH, 10% did not have an adequate reduction of IOPTH levels and underwent bilateral

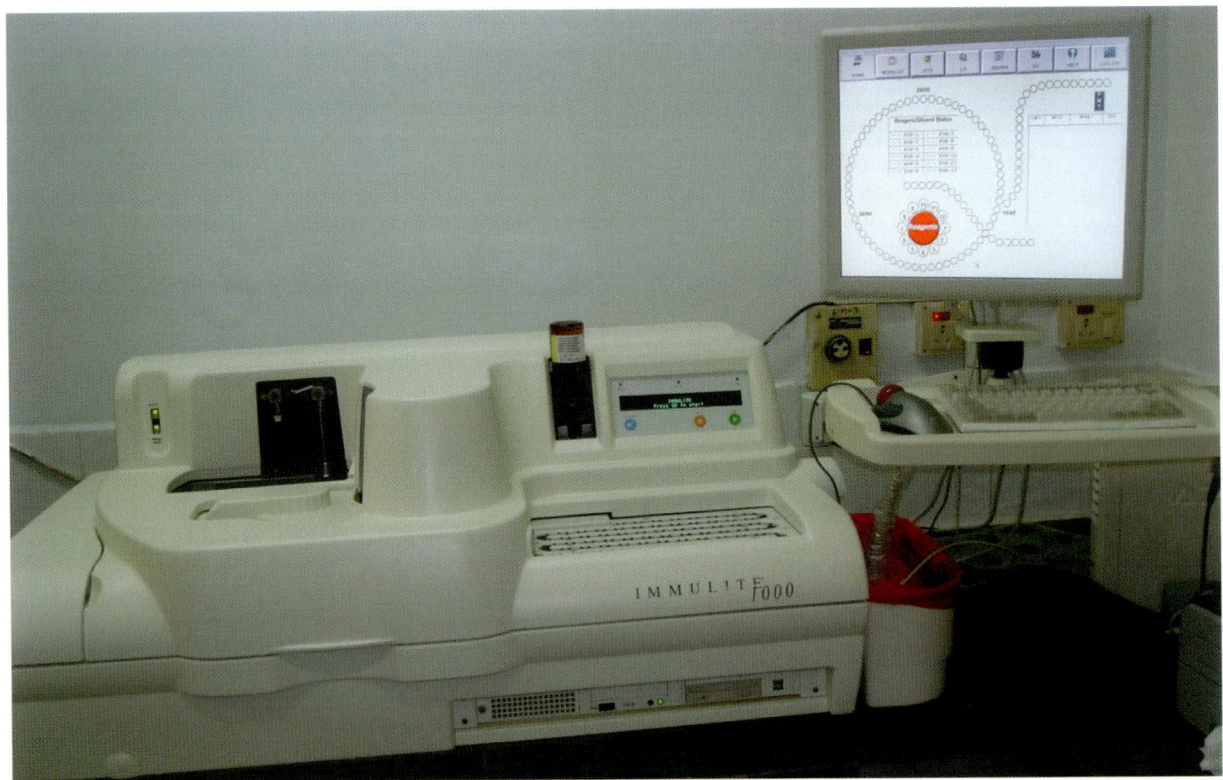

FIGURE 38.5 Immunochemiluminescent machine in central laboratory being utilized for IOPTH.

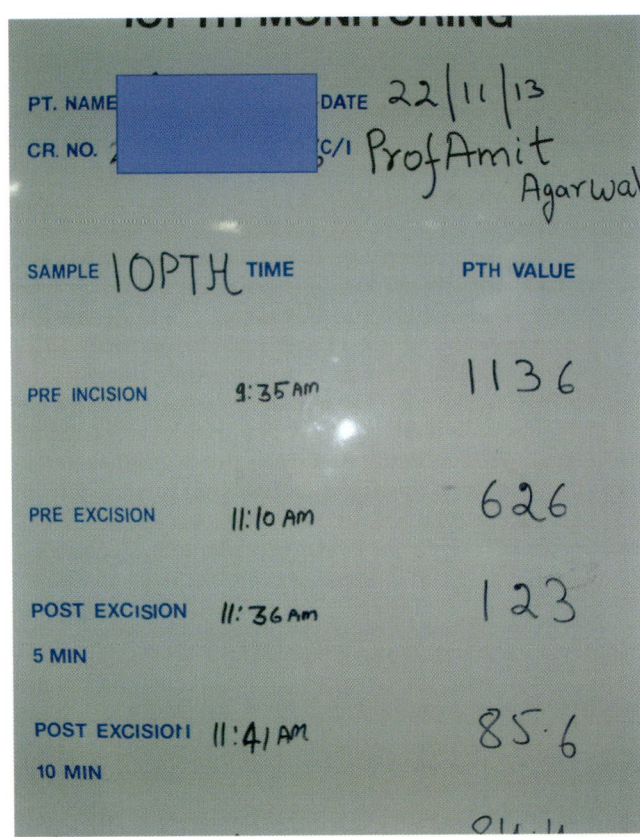

FIGURE 38.6 Miami criteria being followed for defining cure in IOPTH.

exploration with resection of additional parathyroid. Of these 18 patients, 9 had double adenomas, and 9 had 3 or 4 gland hyperplasia. All patients in IOPTH group were subsequently cured. The authors concluded that IOPTH testing allowed intraoperative recognition and resection of additional hyperfunctioning parathyroids missed by preoperative imaging.

Another advantage of using IOPTH is its utility in suggesting the presence of double adenomas even when the preoperative imaging detected a single adenoma. In the study by Haciyanli et al. [50], the combined accuracy of USG, MIBI, and IOPTH assay in predicting a double adenoma was 80%. However, there are numerous criteria to define a cure when IOPTH is used. A number of other criteria are mentioned in literature like the Vienna criteria, 5 min criteria, Halle criteria, and the residual criteria by Libutti. Most commonly followed criteria for defining cure is using a decline of ≥50% within 10 min after excision of the gland during surgery for PHPT (Miami criteria). Because of cost constraints in India where IOPTH is used only in selected centers as a routine adjunct, therefore, a method to reduce time and financial burden was suggested in our study [51].

Two modifications can help in bringing down the cost of IOPTH. One way could be to reduce the number of samples needed to define a cure. The second modification that could be made is the use of central laboratory for quick results.

Various published criteria for IOPTH monitoring, including iteration analysis of IOPTH kinetic data, reported variable success rates in predicting cure. The study from SGPGI [52] itself showed the Miami criteria to be most sensitive. Halle criteria had the highest specificity and positive predictive value.

South Asia perspective

These modern technological tools, even though useful, have a flip side as far as the cost to the patient is concerned. However, despite this disadvantage, the modern thyroid and parathyroid surgeon should be trained in the use of these adjuncts so that he/she can use these judiciously should the need arise or if the patient can afford these. Most of the dedicated units in South Asia used these modern adjuncts for patient care and resident training.

Conclusions

Use of surgical adjuncts is desirable to have a better outcome following thyroidectomy and parathyroidectomy. It's imperative that the trainees of endocrine/thyroid surgery are exposed to the newer tools but nonetheless are also taught to use these wisely and selectively for our patient while keeping cost-effectiveness in mind before using these tools.

References

1. Samraj K, Gurusamy KS. Wound drains following thyroid surgery. Cochrane Wounds Group, editor. Cochrane Database Syst Rev [Internet]. 2007 Oct [cited 2020 Sep 17]; Available from: http://doi.wiley.com/10.1002/14651858.CD006099.pub2.
2. Memon Z, Ahmed G, Khan S, Khalid M, Sultan N. Postoperative use of drain in thyroid lobectomy – A randomized clinical trial conducted at Civil Hospital, Karachi, Pakistan. Thyroid Res. 2012;5(1):9.
3. Khanna J, Mohil R, Chintamani, Bhatnagar D, Mittal M, Sahoo M, et al. Is the routine drainage after surgery for thyroid necessary?—A prospective randomized clinical study [ISRCTN63623153]. BMC Surg. 2005 Dec;5(1):11.
4. Molnar C, Voidazan S, Rad CC, Neagoe VI, Ro C. Total thyroidectomy with LigaSure Small Jaw versus conventional thyroidectomy—A clinical study. Chirurgia (Bucur). 2014 Sep–Oct;109(5):608–612.
5. Ramouz A, Rasihashemi SZ, Safaeiyan A, Hosseini M. Comparing postoperative complication of LigaSure Small Jaw instrument with clamp and tie method in thyroidectomy patients: A randomized controlled trial [IRCT2014010516077N1]. World J Surg Oncol. 2018 Dec;16(1):154.
6. Lombardi CP, Raffaelli M, Cicchetti A, Marchetti M, De Crea C, Di Bidino R, et al. The use of "harmonic scalpel" versus "knot tying" for conventional "open" thyroidectomy: Results of a prospective randomized study. Langenbecks Arch Surg. 2008 Sep;393(5):627–631.
7. Hallgrimsson P, Lovén L, Westerdahl J, Bergenfelz A. Use of the harmonic scalpel versus conventional haemostatic techniques in patients with Grave disease undergoing total thyroidectomy: A prospective randomised controlled trial. Langenbecks Arch Surg. 2008 Sep;393(5):675–680.
8. Ecker T, Carvalho AL, Choe J-H, Walosek G, Preuss KJ. Hemostasis in thyroid surgery: Harmonic scalpel versus other techniques—A meta-analysis. Otolaryngol Neck Surg. 2010 Jul;143(1):17–25.
9. Miccoli P, Berti P, Dionigi GL, D'Agostino J, Orlandini C, Donatini G. Randomized controlled trial of harmonic scalpel use during thyroidectomy. Arch Otolaryngol Head Neck Surg. 2006;132:6.
10. Sutton PA, Awad S, Perkins AC, Lobo DN. Comparison of lateral thermal spread using monopolar and bipolar diathermy, the Harmonic Scalpel™ and the Ligasure™. Br J Surg. 2010 Mar;97(3):428–433.
11. Flisberg K, Lindholm T. Electrical stimulation of the human recurrent laryngeal nerve during thyroid operation. Acta Otolaryngol (Stockh). 1970 Jan;69(sup 263):63–67.
12. Schneider R, Randolph G, Dionigi G, Barczyński M, Chiang F-Y, Triponez F, et al. Prospective study of vocal fold function after loss of the neuromonitoring signal in thyroid surgery: The International Neural Monitoring Study Group's POLT study: Vocal Fold Function After Persistent LOS. Laryngoscope. 2016 May;126(5):1260–1266.
13. Phelan E, Schneider R, Lorenz K, Dralle H, Kamani D, Potenza A, et al. Continuous vagal IONM prevents recurrent laryngeal nerve paralysis by revealing initial EMG changes of impending neuropraxic injury: A prospective, multicenter study: Continuous Vagal IONM Prevents RLN Paralysis. Laryngoscope. 2014 Jun;124(6):1498–1505.
14. Schneider R, Lamade W, Hermann M, Goretzki P, Timmermann W, Hauss J, et al. Kontinuierliches intraoperatives Neuromonitoring des N. laryngeus recurrens in der Schilddrüsenchirurgie (CIONM)—Wo stehen wir? Ein Update zum Europäischen Symposium Kontinuierliches Neuromonitoring in der Schilddrüsenchirurgie. Zentralblatt Für Chir. 2012 Feb;137(01):88–90.
15. Chiang F-Y, Lu I-C, Kuo W-R, Lee K-W, Chang N-C, Wu C-W. The mechanism of recurrent laryngeal nerve injury during thyroid surgery—The application of intraoperative neuromonitoring. Surgery. 2008 Jun;143(6):743–749.
16. Dionigi G, Wu C-W, Kim HY, Rausei S, Boni L, Chiang F-Y. Severity of recurrent laryngeal nerve injuries in thyroid surgery. World J Surg. 2016 Jun;40(6):1373–1381.
17. Pisanu A, Porceddu G, Podda M, Cois A, Uccheddu A. Systematic review with meta-analysis of studies comparing intraoperative neuromonitoring of recurrent laryngeal nerves versus visualization alone during thyroidectomy. J Surg Res. 2014 May;188(1):152–161.
18. Higgins TS, Gupta R, Ketcham AS, Sataloff RT, Wadsworth JT, Sinacori JT. Recurrent laryngeal nerve monitoring versus identification alone on post-thyroidectomy true vocal fold palsy: A meta-analysis: Ionm vs. ID in thyroidectomy. Laryngoscope. 2011 May;121(5):1009–1017.
19. Rocke DJ, Goldstein DP, de Almeida JR. A cost-utility analysis of recurrent laryngeal nerve monitoring in the setting of total thyroidectomy. JAMA Otolaryngol Neck Surg. 2016 Dec;142(12):1199.
20. Wang LY, Ganly I. Nodal metastases in thyroid cancer: Prognostic implications and management. Future Oncol. 2016 Apr;12(7):981–994.
21. Cabot JC, Lee CR, Brunaud L, Kleiman DA, Chung WY, Fahey TJ, et al. Robotic and endoscopic transaxillary thyroidectomies may be cost prohibitive when compared to standard cervical thyroidectomy: A cost analysis. Surgery. 2012 Dec;152(6):1016–1024.
22. Wang T, Kim HY, Wu C-W, Rausei S, Sun H, Pergolizzi FP, et al. Analyzing cost-effectiveness of neural-monitoring in recurrent laryngeal nerve recovery course in thyroid surgery. Int J Surg. 2017 Dec;48:180–188.
23. Vescan A, Witterick I, Freeman J. Parathyroid hormone as a predictor of hypocalcemia after thyroidectomy. Laryngoscope. 2005 Dec;115(12):2105–2108.
24. Which therapy to prevent post-thyroidectomy hypocalcemia?—PubMed [Internet]. [cited 2020 Sep 17]. Available from: https://pubmed.ncbi.nlm.nih.gov/16371185/.
25. Lombardi CP, Raffaelli M, Princi P, Santini S, Boscherini M, De Crea C, et al. Early prediction of postthyroidectomy hypocalcemia by one single iPTH measurement. Surgery. 2004 Dec;136(6):1236–1241.
26. Noordzij JP, Lee SL, Bernet VJ, Payne RJ, Cohen SM, McLeod IK, et al. Early prediction of hypocalcemia after thyroidectomy using parathyroid hormone: An analysis of pooled individual patient data from nine observational studies. J Am Coll Surg. 2007 Dec;205(6):748–754.
27. Fabio FD, Casella C, Bugari G, Iacobello C, Salerni B. Identification of patients at low risk for thyroidectomy-related hypocalcemia by intraoperative quick PTH. World J Surg. 2006 Aug;30(8):1428–1433.
28. Lo CY, Luk JM, Tam SC. Applicability of intraoperative parathyroid hormone assay during thyroidectomy. Ann Surg. 2002 Nov;236(5):564–569.
29. Alía P, Moreno P, Rigo R, Francos J-M, Navarro M-Á. Postresection parathyroid hormone and parathyroid hormone decline accurately predict hypocalcemia after thyroidectomy. Am J Clin Pathol. 2007 Apr;127(4):592–597.
30. Ghaheri BA, Liebler SL, Andersen PE, Schuff KG, Samuels MH, Klein RF, et al. Perioperative parathyroid hormone levels in thyroid surgery. Laryngoscope. 2006 Apr;116(4):518–521.
31. Lang BH-H, Wong CKH, Hung HT, Wong KP, Mak KL, Au KB. Indocyanine green fluorescence angiography for quantitative evaluation of in situ parathyroid gland perfusion and function after total thyroidectomy. Surgery. 2017 Jan;161(1):87–95.
32. Zaidi N, Bucak E, Yazici P, Soundararajan S, Okoh A, Yigitbas H, et al. The feasibility of indocyanine green fluorescence imaging for identifying and assessing the perfusion of parathyroid glands during total thyroidectomy: Assessment of parathyroids using ICG. J Surg Oncol. 2016 Jun;113(7):775–778.
33. Vidal Fortuny J, Belfontali V, Sadowski SM, Karenovics W, Guigard S, Triponez F. Parathyroid gland angiography with indocyanine green fluorescence to predict parathyroid function after thyroid surgery: Indocyanine green parathyroid angiography in thyroid surgery. Br J Surg. 2016 Apr;103(5):537–543.
34. Vidal Fortuny J, Sadowski SM, Belfontali V, Guigard S, Poncet A, Ris F, et al. Randomized clinical trial of intraoperative parathyroid gland angiography with indocyanine green fluorescence predicting parathyroid function after thyroid surgery: Use of indocyanine green angiography to predict postoperative parathyroid function. Br J Surg. 2018 Mar;105(4):350–357.
35. McWade MA, Sanders ME, Broome JT, Solórzano CC, Mahadevan-Jansen A. Establishing the clinical utility of autofluorescence spectroscopy for parathyroid detection. Surgery. 2016 Jan;159(1):193–203.
36. De Leeuw F, Breuskin I, Abbaci M, Casiraghi O, Mirghani H, Ben Lakhdar A, et al. Intraoperative near-infrared imaging for parathyroid gland identification by autofluorescence: A feasibility study. World J Surg. 2016 Sep;40(9):2131–2138.
37. Mandl F. Therapeutischer versuch bein einem falle von ostitis fibrosa generalisata mittels exstirpation eines epithelk orperchen tumors. Zentralbl Chir. 1926;5:260.
38. Ryan JA Jr, Eisenberg B, Pado KM, Lee F. Efficacy of selective unilateral exploration in hyperparathyroidism based on localization tests. Arch Surg. 1997;132:886–890.
39. Arici C, Cheah WK, Ituarte PH, Morita E, Lynch TC, Siperstein AE, et al. Can localization studies be used to direct focused parathyroid operations? Surgery. 2001;129:720–729.
40. Chapuis Y, Fulla Y, Bonnichon P, Tarla E, Abboud B, Pitre J, et al. Values of ultrasonography, SestaMIBI scintigraphy, and intra operative measurement of 1-84 PTH for unilateral neck exploration of primary hyper parathyroidism. World J Surg. 1996;20:835–839.
41. Irvin GL 3rd, Sfakianakis G, Yeung L, Deriso GT, Fishman LM, Molinari AS, et al. Ambulatory parathyroidectomy for primary hyperparathyroidism. Arch Surg. 1996;131:1074–1078.
42. Carneiro DM, Solorzano CC, Nader MC, Ramirez M, Irvin GL 3rd. Comparison of intraoperative PTH assay (QPTH) criteria in guiding parathyroidectomy: Which criterion is the most accurate? Surgery. 2003;134:973–979; discussion 979–981.
43. Riss P, Kaczirek K, Heinz G, Bieglmayer C, Niederle B. A "defined baseline" in PTH monitoring increases surgical success in patients with multiple gland disease. Surgery. 2007;142:398–404.

44. Yang GP, Levine S, Weigel RJ. A spike in parathyroid hormone during neck exploration may cause a false-negative intra-operative assay result. Arch Surg. 2001; 136:945–949.
45. Irvin GL 3rd, Molinari AS, Figueroa C, Carneiro DM. Improved success rate in reoperative parathyroidectomy with intraoperative PTH assay. Ann Surg. 1999;229:874–878; discussion 878–879.
46. Udelsman R, Donovan PI, Sokoll LJ. One hundred consecutive minimally invasive parathyroid explorations. Ann Surg. 2000;232:331–339.
47. Irvin GL 3rd, Deriso GT 3rd. A new, practical intraoperative parathyroid hormone assay. Am J Surg. 1994;168:466–468.
48. Libutti SK, Alexander HR, Bartlett DL, Sampson ML, Ruddel ME, Skarulis M, et al. Kinetic analysis of the rapid intraoperative parathyroid hormone assay in patients during operation for hyperparathyroidism. Surgery. 1999;126:1145–1150; discussion 1150–1151.
49. Cayo AK, Sippel RS, Schaefer S, Chen H. Utility of intraoperative PTH for primary hyperparathyroidism due to multigland disease. Ann Surg Oncol. 2009 Dec;16(12):3450–3454.
50. Mehmet Haciyanli 1, Geeta Lal, Eugene Morita, Quan-Yang Duh, Electron Kebebew, Orlo H Clark. Accuracy of preoperative localization studies and intraoperative parathyroid hormone assay in patients with primary hyperparathyroidism and double adenoma J Am Coll urg. 2003 Nov;197(5):739–746.
51. Pradhan R, Gupta S, Agarwal A. Focused parathyroidectomy using accurate preoperative imaging and intraoperative PTH: Tertiary care experience. Indian J Endocrinol Metab. 2019 May-Jun;23(3):347–352.
52. Singh DN, Gupta SK, Chand G, Mishra A, Agarwal G, Verma AK, et al. Intra-operative parathyroid hormone kinetics and influencing factors with high baseline PTH: a prospective study. Clin Endocrinol (Oxf). 2013 Jun;78(6):935–941.

39

PARATHYROID CARCINOMA

Pooja Ramakant, Chanchal Rana, Kul Ranjan Singh and Anand Kumar Mishra

Introduction

Parathyroid carcinoma (PC) is a rare malignancy (0.005% of all causes of cancers in the United States) and also a rare cause (<1%) of primary hyperparathyroidism (PHPT) (1, 2). In 1904, Swiss surgeon Fritz de Quervain first described PC and since then less than 1000 cases have been mentioned in the literature (3). Patients with PC have an indolent course. Diagnosis is usually not made preoperatively and is a histological diagnosis post surgery. However, occasionally, clinical and radiological features may help us to preoperatively suspect PC. As the tumor is excised mostly as a presumed parathyroid benign adenoma, if there is either tumor capsule rupture or spillage, it may lead to local recurrence.

In patients with PC, metastases may occur in the lung (40%), liver (10%) or lymph nodes (4).

Etiology

PC can happen either due to somatic or germline mutations. Sporadic causes include previous neck irradiation or end-stage renal disease. It usually happens in the fourth decade of life, and there is no sex predilection (5).

PC and genetics

Familial causes include PHPT-JT (CDC73 gene), MEN 1 syndrome (Menin gene), MEN 2A or FIHP. In patients with PHPT-JT syndrome, 80% of them harbor inactivating mutations in CDC73 gene and 15% of the parathyroid tumors are malignant (5). Genetic syndrome associated with PC includes retinoblastoma with p53 gene mutation (5).

Clinical presentation

Patients with PC usually manifest signs and symptoms of severe hypercalcemia (serum calcium levels more than 14 mg/dl) and end organ damage in the form of renal or skeletal damage. Hypercalcemic crisis is a life-threatening disorder and needs urgent management in the form of stabilizing the calcium levels followed by early surgery (6). Palpable hard neck mass is seen in up to 30–76% of patients with PC (7).

If a patient complains of any voice change due to vocal cord palsy in the preoperative setting, this should raise suspicion of PC. Patients may also present with neurocognitive disorders, pancreatitis, peptic ulcer, anemia or cardiac arrhythmias. Rarely, PCs may be nonfunctional in 10% cases, and patients may present with only mass effect due to hard locally infiltrating tumor in the neck. However, all these features are also seen in patients with PHPT due to benign adenoma or hyperplasia especially in Indian scenario (8). Hence, there are no definitive clinical features that are confirmatory for preoperative diagnosis of PC.

Biochemical markers

Serum calcium is usually on higher side as 3–4 mg above the normal range. Serum PTH is usually 3–10 times above the normal range. High levels of serum alkaline phosphatase suggest skeletal damage. High levels of human chorionic gonadotropin (hCG) are seen in serum or urine of patients with PC (9).

Imaging features of patients with PC

On ultrasonography, large (>3 cm) lobulated heterogeneous mass with irregular borders, thick capsule and infiltration to adjacent structures like thyroid, lymphadenopathy, increased vascularity or calcification may lead to suspicion of PC. MIBI scan is used for localization purpose; however, it may not help us to differentiate between benign and malignant parathyroid tumor mass. CT scan or MRI may help in picking up the malignant lesion by infiltrating tumor characteristics or distant metastases. PET scan has no diagnostic role in early stages of PC. FNAC is also not recommended as it may cause tumor cell spillage and capsule tear.

Role of 18F-choline PET scan in detecting primary and metastatic lesions in patients with PC

Few studies in the literature suggest that parathyroid tumors retain their 18F-choline uptake abilities, even when they undergo malignant transformation to PC (10).

Intraoperative findings in PC

Intraoperatively, firm-to-hard parathyroid mass, infiltration, loss of plane between mass and thyroid lobe, grayish white in color and cervical lymphadenopathy may lead to clinical suspicion of PC.

Pathological features of PC

Grossly, these lesions may be well circumscribed or irregular and may weigh >10 g (11, 12). Histologically, a definitive diagnosis of malignancy should be restricted to tumors displaying evidence of vascular invasion, capsular invasion with growth into adjacent tissues or metastases. Criteria for vascular and capsular invasion are similar to those used in thyroid pathology. Hence, adequate sampling of the specimen is of utmost importance, thereby limiting the role of frozen section for intraoperative diagnosis.

Although thick fibrous bands, mitotic activity, trabecular growth pattern and capsular, vascular and adjacent soft-tissue invasion are considered characteristics of PC, morphological features—such as fibrous bands, mitotic activity and trabecular growth—have been identified in parathyroid adenomas as well. To complicate the morphological diagnosis further, a group of neoplasms referred to as "atypical adenomas" exhibit many of these features, but they lack indisputable evidence of malignancy such as angioinvasion and metastases (13). Figure 39.1 shows a case of PC with infiltration of surrounding thyroid parenchyma after capsular invasion.

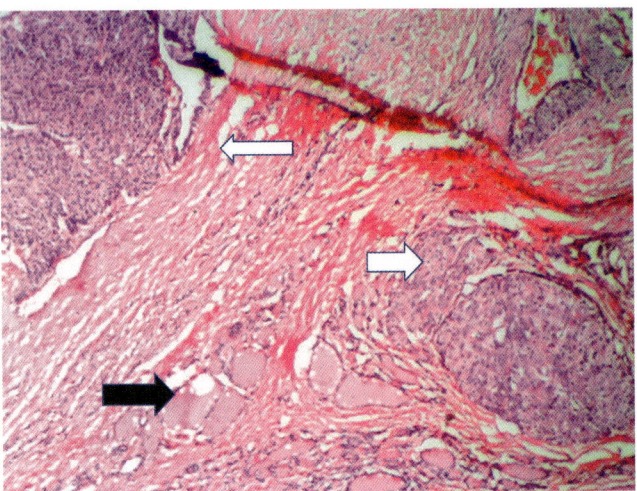

FIGURE 39.1 Photomicrograph displaying infiltration of surrounding thyroid parenchyma by parathyroid carcinoma (hematoxylin and eosin stain; 100× magnifications). White arrow shows tumor component, and black arrow shows normal thyroid parenchyma.

Although the expression of some of the cell-cycle regulatory proteins correlates with the histological type of parathyroid tumors, none is specific for carcinoma. Molecular markers, Ki-67 and p27, may distinguish PC from adenoma. The molecular phenotype, p27(+)Bcl-2(+)Ki-67(−)mdm2(+), appears to be unique to nonmalignant parathyroid tumors, and multimarker phenotypes are more complex in carcinomas (14). Few studies in the past have introduced several immunohistochemical (IHC) biomarkers for PC, including parafibromin, APC, galectin-3, PGP9.5, Ki67 and cyclin D (14, 15). The loss of parafibromin expression due to *CDC73/HRPT2* gene mutation correlates with cell proliferation, transcription and histone modification. However, the usefulness of these IHC markers in PC is unclear. However, a recent meta-analysis has demonstrated that loss of parafibromin expression on immunohistochemistry was significantly higher in PC than in atypical parathyroid adenoma, parathyroid adenoma and parathyroid hyperplasia; therefore, it could be useful for diagnosis and prediction of prognosis of PC in routine practice (16).

PC remains an enigmatic disease, the biological features of which are incompletely defined. Nevertheless, the new techniques of molecular profiling hold potential to further enhance our understanding of this rare tumor.

Prognostic factors in patients with PC in terms of recurrences include the following:

1. Intraoperative tumor rupture.
2. Mitotic figures within tumor parenchyma cells.
3. Schulte differentiated staging classification system Class 3 (17).
4. Nodal involvement.
5. Parafibromin is a protein product of the CDC73/HRPT2 gene. In patients with PC, there is a loss of parafibromin expression due to the gene mutation and associated with a poor prognosis.

Treatment options in PC

Surgery/RT/CT/newer modalities

The best cure rates are achieved by complete resection of the parathyroid tumor mass either itself or if there is no plane with thyroid and en bloc resection with ipsilateral thyroid lobe in the first surgery (18, 19). If a patient presents with hypercalcemic crisis, in preoperative settings, medical management is done to reduce serum calcium levels. Therapeutic lymph node dissection is recommended, and there is no role of prophylactic lymph node dissection. We should avoid capsule tear or tumor spillage by gentle handing of the tumor mass while dissection. If the diagnosis of PC has been made postoperatively on histology, after excision of the tumor mass, we can closely observe the patient, provided all clinical and biochemical parameters are in the normal range.

Postoperative care

Hungry bone syndrome

It is manifested by profound hypocalcemia, hypomagnesaemia and hypophosphatemia, which is exacerbated by low PTH levels post surgery (20). Treatment includes the following:

1. Calcium supplementation in the range of 6–12 g/day
2. Vitamin D (Calcitriol) 2–4 μg/day
3. Correct serum magnesium levels by giving magnesium salts intravenously

Recurrences

Recurrences are common in patients with PC and seen in 33–63% of cases, mostly 2–5 years post surgery (21). Recurrences manifest clinically as well as biochemically. Local recurrences are managed surgically. Lymph node metastases are seen in 15–20% of cases and distant metastases in up to 1% of cases. Common sites of metastases are cervical lymph nodes, lung and liver. Studies have shown that disease biology is the main factor responsible for recurrences, and incomplete surgical extent also plays a significant role in causing multiple recurrences (22). The absence of parafibromin staining also affects recurrences in patients with PC (23).

Radiotherapy (RT)

PC is a radio-resistant tumor. Hence, RT has a limited role. Few studies have shown the use of RT as an adjuvant therapy in high-risk cases or recurrent disease to avoid further disease progression (24).

Chemotherapy has not proved to be effective in PC. In literature, there are anecdotal studies showing that patients with PC with epigenetic silencing of O6-methylguanine DNA methyltransferase gene are more susceptible to Temozolomide (an alkylating agent) (25).

Radiofrequency ablation (RFA) or embolization has been used in some centers for ablating distant metastases in the lung or liver in patients with functioning PC (26). It helps in symptom controls of hypercalcemia in these patients.

Immunotherapy targeting PTH

In literature, some studies have shown the use of immunotherapy-targeting PTH helps in tumor size reduction and reducing the calcium levels in patients with unresectable metastases. In some studies, denosumab, which is a monoclonal antibody having potent anti-resorptive action on bones, has been used to lower serum calcium levels in patients with PC (27).

Tyrosine kinase inhibitors

Sorafenib has been used in metastatic PC patients (28). It has antiangiogenesis effect and delays the disease progression.

Medical management to reduce serum calcium levels in patients with PC

Medical management is especially useful in patients with metastatic or unresectable PC (29). Aim of medical management is to control hypercalcemia.

1. Hydration-forced saline diuresis
2. Bisphosphonates
3. Calcitonin
4. Denosumab
5. Cinacalcet

Controversies in management

The advantage of doing thyroid lobectomy in patients with PC in whom thyroid is not involved is not proven in terms of benefit in local recurrence or survival rates. In one study, patients were stratified in three groups, the first group undergoing parathyroidectomy alone, the second group who had en bloc thyroid lobectomy along with parathyroid mass and the third group who after parathyroidectomy underwent delayed thyroid lobectomy. No statistically significant difference in survival rates or recurrences was seen in all these three groups of patients (30). Prophylactic lymphadenectomy is also debatable with no proven benefits (31).

Follow-up

Patients with PC are followed up lifelong. In the first 5 years, biannually serum calcium and PTH are measured and then annually. USG neck is done annually to look for any local recurrence. Patients who underwent excision of the parathyroid tumor mass and not en bloc resection are closely followed up with 3 monthly serum calcium and PTH for the first 3 years, biannually for the next 2 years, and then annually.

Prognosis

A total of 5-year survival rate is 80–91%, and 10-year survival rate is 49–87% (32). Cause of death is usually related to untreatable hypercalcemia.

South Asian perspective

In South Asia, usually, there is a late presentation of hyperparathyroidism when patients have already developed end organ damage. PC reports are not infrequent from various regions in this area.

Conclusion

PC is a rare malignancy; however, it is associated with an indolent course with multiple recurrences. Surgery is the most effective option.

References

1. Rozhinskaya L, Pigarova E, Sabanova E, Mamedova E, Voronkova I, Krupinova J, Dzeranova L, Tiulpakov A, Gorbunova V, Orel N, Zalian A, Melnichenko G, Dedov I. Diagnosis and treatment challenges of parathyroid carcinoma in a 27-year-old woman with multiple lung metastases. Endocrinol Diabetes Metab Case Rep. 2017 Mar;16–0113.
2. Salcuni AS, Cetani F, Guarnieri V, Nicastro V, Romagnoli E, de Martino D, Scillitani A, Col DEC. Parathyroid carcinoma. Best Pract Res Clin Endocrinol Metab. 2018 Dec;32(6):877–889.
3. Al-Kurd A, Mekel M, Mazeh H. Parathyroid carcinoma. Surg Oncol. 2014 Jun;23(2):107–114.
4. Storvall S, Ryhänen E, Bensch FV, Heiskanen I, Kytölä S, Ebeling T, Mäkelä S, Schalin-Jäntti C. Recurrent metastasized parathyroid carcinoma-long-term remission after combined treatments with surgery, radiotherapy, cinacalcet, zoledronic acid, and temozolomide. JBMR Plus. 2018 Nov;3(4):e10114.
5. Kutahyalioglu M, Nguyen HT, Kwatampora L, Clarke C, Silva A, Ibrahim E, Waguespack SG, Cabanillas ME, Jimenez C, Hu MI, Sherman SI, Kopetz S, Broaddus R, Dadu R, Wanland K, Williams M, Zafereo M, Perrier N, Busaidy NL. Genetic profiling as a clinical tool in advanced parathyroid carcinoma. J Cancer Res Clin Oncol. 2019 Aug;145(8):1977–1986.
6. Rock K, Fattah N, O'Malley D, McDermott E. The management of acute parathyroid crisis secondary to parathyroid carcinoma: A case report. J Med Case Rep. 2010 Jan;4:28.
7. Sadler C, Gow KW, Beierle EA, Doski JJ, Langer M, Nuchtern JG, Vasudevan SA, Goldfarb M. Parathyroid carcinoma in more than 1,000 patients: A population-level analysis. Surgery. 2014 Dec;156(6):1622–1629; discussion 1629-30.
8. Agarwal G, Prasad KK, Kar DK, Krishnani N, Pandey R, Mishra SK. Indian primary hyperparathyroidism patients with parathyroid carcinoma do not differ in clinicoinvestigative characteristics from those with benign parathyroid pathology. World J Surg. 2006 May;30(5):732–742.
9. Rubin MR, Bilezikian JP, Birken S, Silverberg SJ. Human chorionic gonadotropin measurements in parathyroid carcinoma. Eur J Endocrinol. 2008 Oct;159(4):469–474.
10. Deandreis D, Terroir M, AlGhuzlan A, Berdelou A,L acroix L, Bidault F, etal. 18Fluorocholine PET/CT in parathyroid carcinoma: A new tool for disease staging? Eur J Nucl Med Mol Imaging. 2015;42:1941–1942.
11. Kumari N, Mishra D, Pradhan R, Agarwal A, Krishnani N. Utility of fine-needle aspiration cytology in the identification of parathyroid lesions. J Cytol Indian Acad Cytol. 2016;33(1):17–21.
12. Tseng F-Y, Hsiao Y-L, Chang T-C. Ultrasound-guided fine needle aspiration cytology of parathyroid lesions. A review of 72 cases. Acta Cytol. 2002 Dec;46(6):1029–1036.
13. Stojadinovic A, Hoos A, Nissan A, Dudas ME, Cordon-Cardo C, Shaha AR, et al. Parathyroid neoplasms: Clinical, histopathological, and tissue microarray-based molecular analysis. Hum Pathol. 2003 Jan;34(1):54–64.
14. Kumari N, Chaudhary N, Pradhan R, Agarwal A, Krishnani N. Role of histological criteria and immunohistochemical markers in predicting risk of malignancy in parathyroid neoplasms. Endocr Pathol. 2016 Jun;27(2):87–96.
15. Truran PP, Johnson SJ, Bliss RD, Lennard TWJ, Aspinall SR. Parafibromin, galectin-3, PGP9.5, Ki67, and cyclin D1: Using an immunohistochemical panel to aid in the diagnosis of parathyroid cancer. World J Surg. 2014 Nov;38(11):2845–2854.
16. Pyo J-S, Cho WJ. Diagnostic and prognostic implications of parafibromin immunohistochemistry in parathyroid carcinomaT. Biosci Rep. 2019 Apr;39(4).
17. Villar-del-Moral J, Jiménez-García A, Salvador-Egea P, Martos-Martínez JM, Nuño-Vázquez-Garza JM, Serradilla-Martín M, Gómez-Palacios A, Moreno-Llorente P, Ortega-Serrano J, de la Quintana-Basarrate A. Prognostic factors and staging systems in parathyroid cancer: A multicenter cohort study. Surgery. 2014 Nov;156(5):1132–1144.
18. Wilhelm SM, Wang TS, Ruan DT, Lee JA, Asa SL, Duh QY, Doherty GM, Herrera MF, Pasieka JL, Perrier ND, Silverberg SJ, Solórzano CC, Sturgeon C, Tublin ME, Udelsman R, Carty SE. The American Association of Endocrine Surgeons guidelines for definitive management of primary hyperparathyroidism. JAMA Surg. 2016 Oct;151(10):959–968.
19. Wang P, Xue S, Wang S, Lv Z, Meng X, Wang G, Meng W, Liu J, Chen G. Clinical characteristics and treatment outcomes of parathyroid carcinoma: A retrospective review of 234 cases. Oncol Lett. 2017 Dec;14(6):7276–7282.
20. Witteveen JE, van Thiel S, Romijn JA, Hamdy NA. Hungry bone syndrome: Still a challenge in the post-operative management of primary hyperparathyroidism: A systematic review of the literature. Eur J Endocrinol. 2013 Feb;168(3):R45–R53.
21. Thanseer NTK, Parihar AS, Sood A, Bhadada SK, Dahiya D, Singh P, Mittal BR. Evaluation of recurrent parathyroid carcinoma: A new imaging tool in uncommon entity. World J Nucl Med. 2019 Apr-Jun;18(2):198–200.
22. Wei BJ, Shen H, Xing XP, Ji W, Zhao L, Wang J, Xie H, Zhou XH, Yin JS, Jiang T, Chang H, Shi F. [Surgical treatment of recurrent parathyroid carcinoma with invasion of the upper aerodigestive tract]. Zhonghua Er Bi Yan Hou Tou Jing Wai Ke Za Zhi. 2011 Nov;46(11):901–904.

23. Hu Y, Bi Y, Cui M, Zhang X, Su Z, Wang M, Hua S, Liao Q, Zhao Y. The influence of surgical extent and parafibromin staining on the outcome of parathyroid carcinoma: 20-year experience from a single institute. Endocr Pract. 2019 Jul;25(7):634–641.
24. Munson ND, Foote RL, Northcutt RC, Tiegs RD, Fitzpatrick LA, Grant CS, van Heerden JA, Thompson GB, Lloyd RV. Parathyroid carcinoma: is there a role for adjuvant radiation therapy? Cancer. 2003 Dec;98(11):2378–84.
25. Christakis I, Silva AM, Williams MD, Garden A, Grubbs EG, Busaidy NL, Lee JE, Perrier ND, Zafereo M. Postoperative local-regional radiation therapy in the treatment of parathyroid carcinoma: The MD Anderson experience of 35 years. Pract Radiat Oncol. 2017 Nov-Dec;7(6):e463–e470.
26. DasGupta R, Shetty S, Keshava SN, Gupta M, Paul MJ, Thomas N. Metastatic parathyroid carcinoma treated with radiofrequency ablation: A novel therapeutic modality. Australas Med J. 2014 Sep 30;7(9):372–375.
27. Karuppiah D, Thanabalasingham G, Shine B, Wang LM, Sadler GP, Karavitaki N, Grossman AB. Refractory hypercalcaemia secondary to parathyroid carcinoma: Response to high-dose denosumab. Eur J Endocrinol. 2014 Jul;171(1):K1–K5.
28. McClenaghan F, Qureshi YA. Parathyroid cancer. Gland Surg. 2015 Aug;4(4):329–338.
29. Givi B, Shah JP. Parathyroid carcinoma. Clin Oncol (R Coll Radiol). 2010 Aug;22(6):498–507.
30. Medas F, Erdas E, Loi G, Podda F, Pisano G, Nicolosi A, Calò PG. Controversies in the management of parathyroid carcinoma: A case series and review of the literature. Int J Surg. 2016 Apr;28(Suppl 1):S94–S98.
31. Hsu KT, Sippel RS, Chen H, Schneider DF. Is central lymph node dissection necessary for parathyroid carcinoma? Surgery. 2014 Dec;156(6):1336–1341; discussion 1341.
32. Okamoto T, Iihara M, Obara T, Tsukada T. Parathyroid carcinoma: Etiology, diagnosis, and treatment. World J Surg. 2009 Nov;33(11):2343–2354.

40

MANAGEMENT OF RECURRENT PRIMARY HYPERPARATHYROIDISM

Loreno E. Enny, Kul Ranjan Singh and Anand Kumar Mishra

Introduction

Primary hyperparathyroidism (HPT) (PHPT) is a commonly encountered endocrine disease and the most frequently encountered cause of hypercalcemia in the outpatient department, with an estimated incidence of 50.4 cases per 100,000 person-years (1). The underlying pathology in PHPT is a solitary benign adenoma in 80–85%, hyperplasia of multiple glands in 10–15% and carcinoma in less than 1% (2). Surgery is the only curative treatment for symptomatic patients with reported cure rates of >90% and morbidity of <2% (3). However, 2.5–5% of patients may develop recurrent HPT (R-PHPT). Recurrence is established when hypercalcemia is documented after at least 6 months of normocalcemia following initial surgery (4). Adequate preoperative workup, including biochemical and localization studies, is essential before subjecting any patient of HPT to surgery.

Causes for R-PHPT

The most common reported cause for both persistent and recurrent HPT is failed localization of adenoma in ectopic or eutopic position. A missing abnormal gland that was ultimately localized in eutopic and ectopic position in 55.5 and 44.3% patients, respectively, was the cause of R-PHPT. Of the ectopic cases, 50% were in cervical and 50% in mediastinal regions (5).

Other causes of R-PHPT are inadequate resection of multi-gland disease, undiagnosed second adenoma, residual disease in parathyromatosis and malignancy and supernumerary glands (6, 7).

Re-operative parathyroid surgery is challenging due to distorted tissue architecture and the possibility of diseased gland being located in an ectopic position. Re-operative parathyroid surgery is associated with increased morbidity. The reported incidence of permanent recurrent laryngeal nerve (RLN) injury after redo surgery is up to 10 and 35% for hypoparathyroidism (8). PHPT should be confirmed biochemically, and the offending lesion localized or regionalized before redo surgery is contemplated.

Patients with PHPT have an inappropriately raised PTH with respect to serum calcium and vitamin D status with no hypocalciuria. A correct biochemical diagnosis is necessary to avoid unnecessary primary or second surgery as 2–10% of failed operations are attributed to wrong diagnosis (7). Irrespective of the choice of surgical technique, advanced age (>70 years), low volume center (<50 per year), inexperienced surgeon, equivocal sestamibi result has been documented as an underlying factor for R-PHPT (7). Patient-related factors, like obesity, ASA 3 and initial pathology (single adenoma < double adenoma < multi-gland disease), and surgical factors, like inability to identify offending gland or not performing bilateral neck exploration (BNE) when there is inadequate drop in intraoperative PTH (IOPTH), are also associated with a high incidence of R-PHPT (9–11).

Differential diagnosis

Vitamin D deficiency and renal dysfunction lead to a rise in serum parathyroid levels. Benign familial hypocalciuric hypercalcemia (BFHH) is characterized by increased calcium levels with decreased urinary calcium due to a loss of function mutation of the calcium-sensing receptor (CaSR) gene located at the long arm of chromosome 3. Other conditions leading to false increase in PTH are medications, like thiazides and lithium and gastrointestinal abnormalities, including malabsorption syndrome, in patients. Offending medications must be stopped before biochemical evaluation of HPT. Renal calcium leak due to defective calcium reabsorption manifests as hypercalciuria, HPT and the absence of hypercalcemia. This condition can be confirmed by treating the patient with thiazide diuretics, which will lead to a fall in urinary calcium level and normalization of PTH levels.

Establishing the diagnosis

Biochemical workup should include serum calcium (total and ionic), serum PTH, vitamin D, creatinine and 24-hour urinary calcium excretion. Renal creatinine– calcium ratio less than 0.001 should prompt a diagnosis of BFHH. Once the biochemical diagnosis of persistent or R-PHPT is confirmed, a thorough review of all available records, including previous preoperative imaging studies, operative notes and surgical adjuncts used like IOPTH assay and pathological findings, is carried out to zero on the potential causes if failed surgery. Based on this, the treating surgeon is likely to hit upon potential causes of HPT like occult parathyroid adenoma or inadequately treated disease.

A detailed family history is a must to rule out familial cause of HPT (Table 40.1). These familial causes are likely to result in the multi-glandular involvement.

Localization techniques

After the biochemical diagnosis of persistent/recurrent HPT is confirmed, localization studies are mandated for defining the surgical strategy. Although the cure rates of reoperation of parathyroidectomy without localization studies in trained hands have been reported to be as high as 95% (12), localization studies have been advocated for improving the cure rates of repeat surgeries (13). The choice of localization studies can be individualized based on availability, affordability, accuracy and institutional experience. The various localization techniques used include noninvasive imaging, including USG neck, sestamibi scan, four-dimensional (4D) computed tomography (CT) (4D CT), choline positron emission tomography (PET)

TABLE 40.1: Familial Cause of Hyperparathyroidism

Disorder	Gene	Chromosome	Penetrance of PHPT
MEN 1	MEN 1	11q13	Near complete penetrance (approx. 90%)
MEN 2A	RET	10q21	Low penetrance (approx. 20%)
Hyperparathyroidism jaw tumor syndrome (HPT-JT)	HRPT2	1q21	Low
Familial isolated HPT (FIHPT)	HRPT2, MEN 1	1q21, 11q13	Rare
Autosomal dominant moderate HPT (ADMH)	CASR	3q13	Rare
Benign familial hypocalciuric hypercalcemia (BFHH)	CASR	3q13	Rare

and magnetic resonance imaging (MRI), and invasive techniques, like arteriography, selective venous sampling (SVS) and guided aspiration. Coexisting thyroid nodules, lymph nodes and prior surgery affect the performance of localization studies to the various extent and their fallacies should be kept in mind.

Ultrasonography

High-resolution ultrasound using 7.5 or 10 MHz enables proper visualization of thyroid, carotid and jugular areas. It is widely available, easy to perform and well-tolerated modality with no radiation exposure or fear of contrast allergy. It is also used as a first-line imaging modality along with scintigraphy scan by most surgeons. USG has an element of subjectivity, and its efficacy is affected by training/experience of sonologist, size of parathyroid gland, resolution of image and frequency of the transducer (14). It has a reported sensitivity of 76% (70–81%) and positive predictive value of 93% (91–95%). Sensitivity of ultrasound to predict disease is reported to be 26–40% and 30–87% for ectopic gland (15). False-positive results are reported to be as high as 15–20%, which can be caused by the presence of coexisting thyroid nodules (6–15%), lymphadenopathy and esophageal lesion (16–18). The surgeon performing USG has added a new dimension to its role in parathyroidology and also helps plan the incision for focused parathyroidectomy.

Technetium 99m sestamibi scintigraphy

The incorporation of technetium 99m into the cytoplasm and mitochondria of mouse fibroblast in response to certain stimuli was first demonstrated by Chiu et al. in 1990 (19). Parathyroid cells have a large number of mitochondria, and this enables technetium 99m to enter parathyroid cells more intensely. Three different technetium scanning methods have been described.

1. Single-isotope dual-phase scan cervicothoracic planar imaging performed at an interval of 10–15 minutes and 2–3 hours.
2. Dual-isotope subtraction scans where Tc-99m sestamibi is used in conjunction with another radionuclide like iodine-123.
3. Three-dimensional studies.

The overall reported sensitivity of sestamibi scan for R-PHPT, which ranges from 57 to 85% (6, 16, 20), and positive predictive value ranging from 83 to 96%. The sensitivity of sestamibi scan for disease reduces to 30–39% (15). High false-positive result has been reported with the use of sestamibi scan, and this increases with the presence of coexisting thyroid nodules and lymph nodes, and false-negative images are seen in smaller size in the gland (21, 22).

Computed tomography (CT)

CT is a useful localization technique. The sensitivity and specificity of conventional CT range from 40 to 60% and 88 to 89%, respectively (23), with a false-positive rate of up to 50% (24). Nowadays, the use of 4D CT has become popular in many centers, especially in cases of discordant ultrasound and sestamibi scan because of its higher sensitivity and specificity in the localization of abnormal gland. The sensitivity and specificity of 4D CT are 88–93% and 100%, respectively, for localizing abnormal gland in eutopic position, 83 and 92% for localizing ectopic parathyroid glands, including mediastinal (23). However, it has a disadvantage that it cannot be used in patients with renal insufficiency and the total thyroid-specific radiation of MRI is 50 times greater than SPECT. CT imaging has an important and indispensable role in localizing ectopic glands.

Magnetic resonance imaging (MRI)

MRI is more sensitive than CT for localizing abnormal parathyroid gland, and it's preferable as it does not require administration of contrast material and therefore can even be used in patients with renal insufficiency. However, it is expensive and claustrophobic. The abnormal parathyroid gland usually appears hypo-intense on T1-W image and hyper-intense on T2-W image. The reported sensitivity of MRI ranges from 50 to 88% (25, 26). The most common causes of false positive are coexisting thyroid nodule and enlarged lymph nodes, and the most common causes of false negative are adenomas situated close to thyroid goiter and cases of parathyroid hyperplasia (27).

Positron emission tomography

[11]C-methionine has presumed to be involved in pre-pro PTH, a PTH precursor, and reflects amino acid influx into stimulated parathyroid tissue. It accumulates intensively and specifically in enlarged parathyroid glands. The pooled sensitivity and detection rate of 11 C-methionine in patients with suspected parathyroid adenoma are 81% (74–86%) and 70% (62–77%), respectively, which is comparable to that of ultrasound neck and 99mTc sestamibi scan. However, due to its high cost and availability issue, its application in routine is limited (28). Nevertheless, PET imaging has an important role to play in re-operative scenario.

Fluorocholine PET imaging

The clinical utility of 18F-fluorocholine PET/CT (18F-FCH PET/CT) in imaging parathyroid adenoma specifically in multiple or low-sized gland has been demonstrated in various studies.

Cell proliferation in abnormal glands increases choline uptake, which on phosphorylation by choline kinase gets trapped to form a major membrane phospholipid called phosphatidylcholine. Based on this possible mechanism, 18F-FCG is used for the evaluation of parathyroid adenoma (29). A pilot study, involving 24 patients by Lezaic et al., deduced FCH-PET/CT to be an accurate imaging modality for the localization of abnormal parathyroid gland, especially in a setting of hyperplasia or multi-glandular involvement. FCH PET/CT is reported to have a sensitivity and specificity of 92 and 100%, respectively, in contrast to 49 and 100%, 46 and 100%, and 44 and 100% for 99mTc-sestaMIBI SPECT/CT, 99mTc-sestaMIBI/pertechnetate subtraction imaging and 99mTc-sestaMIBI dual-phase imaging, respectively (30). APACH1 study by Quak et al. showed that FCH PET/CT has a better performance in patients with negative or inconclusive conventional imaging. FCH PET/CT helped plan surgery in 88% of patients and avoided bilateral cervical exploration in 75% (31).

Invasive preoperative methods

Invasive methods are usually indicated when combined results of noninvasive test are negative, equivocal or conflicting.

Selective venous sampling (SVS)

SVS is indicated in those with negative/discordant/equivocal/conflicting imaging, unusual neck anatomy and prior neck surgery. It is reserved for remedial cases due to its cost and potential complications. The concept of four parathyroid glands draining into the adjacent superior, middle and inferior thyroid veins, respectively, helps interpret the PTH gradient. A 5 Fr MP catheter is introduced via the femoral vein, and blood samples are obtained from the vena cava, brachiocephalic, internal jugular, thymic, thyroid ima, inferior, middle and superior thyroid veins covering the drainage area of potential eutopic and ectopic parathyroid glands. A twofold gradient between the PTH values obtained at various sites of sampling and peripheral blood regionalizes or localizes the offending gland. The sensitivity of the SVS ranges from 63 to 83% (6, 32–35). Variations in regional venous anatomy of the parathyroids occasionally limit the usefulness of this technique.

Fine needle aspiration

US-guided fine needle aspiration (FNA) combined with the use of the rapid PTH assay is a useful adjunct for patients with equivocal imaging in the setting of prior neck surgery or the confirmation of glands in ectopic locations. FNA enables both PTH assay and cytological examination of the suspected parathyroid gland. The aspirate of FNA specimen is considered positive for a PTH level greater than the normal range (14–72 pg/mL). The sensitivity of FNA combined with the PTH assay ranges from 85 to 94% with specificity ranging up to 100% (36). However, FNA of parathyroid glands should not be performed routinely, as it may increase the difficulty of surgery due to bleeding from the biopsy site, inflammation or even parathyromatosis. McFarlane et al. have also reported the use of PTH assay with favorable outcome with sensitivity of 100% and specificity of 70% (37).

Arteriography

Parathyroid arteriography includes examination of the thyrocervical trunk (to look for parathyroid gland in superior mediastinum, intrathyroidal, tracheesophageal groove or juxtathyroid location), carotids (juxtathyroid or undescended glands), internal mammary arteries (anterior mediastinum and thymus) and sometimes superior thyroid artery. Abnormal parathyroid gland appears highly vascularized and round or oval shaped. The reported sensitivity of arteriography ranges from 60 to 65% (32, 38).

Treatment

Once recurrence or persistence of HPT is biochemically confirmed and offending lesion is localized, the benefits and risks of reoperation should be assessed. Not every patient merit immediate surgery, and many a times mild asymptomatic hypercalcemia is better followed than causing the patient to live with permanent hypocalcaemia and/or RLN palsy. The morbidity associated with redo surgery is high with permanent RLN palsy as high as 6–9% and permanent hypocalcaemia at 10–13%. Preoperative assessment of vocal cord is recommended before any redo thyroid or parathyroid surgery as the risk of RLN injury is higher than primary surgery. Therefore, adjuncts, like intraoperative nerve monitoring, may be of help in improving outcomes of reoperation for R-PHPT (Figure 40.1) (5).

Surgical approach

The surgical approach usually depends on preoperative findings. A classical BNE is recommended in any patient suspected to have a multi-glandular disease. Focused approach remains a valid approach in cases of documented solitary adenoma. Patients with suspected parathyromatosis, carcinoma, intrathyroidal adenoma and graft recurrence should ideally be subjected to en bloc resection. The benefits and risks of subjecting patients with negative localization on multiple imaging studies supplemented with SVS/arteriography to surgery should be kept in mind. The chances of failed intraoperative localization are high in missed adenoma without localization and wait and watch may be a valid option (39). Adjuncts like IOPTH, intraoperative localization techniques and frozen section can help guide the surgeon to adequacy of surgery, and a redo surgery with negative localization is best carried out at specialized centers with such facilities. IOPTH can predict cure or failure in 97–100% and 78% of cases, respectively, in reoperation for R-PHPT.

Minimally invasive parathyroidectomy (MIP)

The most common cause of failed initial surgery is a missed single adenoma. With refinements of imaging modalities and liberal use of intraoperative adjuncts, focused approach can be performed with minimal morbidity. Usually, two concordant imaging modalities are recommended before performing focused approach. There have been several studies that have demonstrated the benefit of focused approach as compared to BNE. The efficacy and safety of focused approach in HPT surgery have been demonstrated by many. Udelsman et al. demonstrated the superiority of minimal invasive surgery based on 1609 patients with PHPT where conventional BNE was performed in 613 patients and MIP in 1037 patients undergoing primary surgery. MIP was associated with a cure rate on 99.4% and

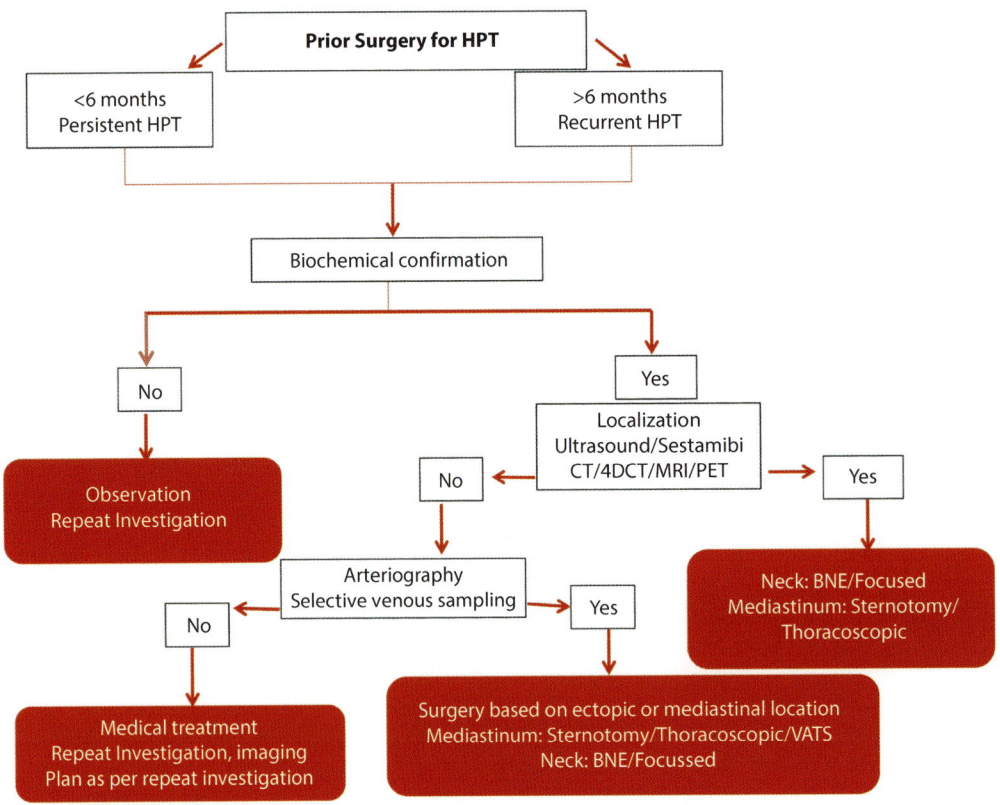

FIGURE 40.1 Management plan in recurrent or persistent HPT.

complication rate of 1.45% compared to BNE with 97.1 and 3.10%, respectively, with added advantage of reduced hospital stay and cost (40). MIP remains a valid option in select group. A cervical lateral approach is usually proposed in the case of missed single adenoma in previous surgery, recurrence due to single adenoma and recurrence of multi glandular disease (MGD) on a parathyroid stump. Thyro-thymic approach is proposed in cases of intra thymic adenoma. Mediastinal approach is usually indicated only in 1–2% of those with R-PHPT (9).

Bilateral neck exploration

The choice of unilateral or bilateral exploration is guided by the possibility of harboring MGD, confidence in imaging outcomes and surgeons preference. A redo parathyroid surgery and BNE demand technical expertise and carry a high risk of RLN damage/permanent hypoparathyroidism. Hence, they are best undertaken at a specialized center. Preoperative localization studies are helpful but may be negative/suboptimal in cases of MGD, a scenario where they are required the most. If the initial approach was a midline ("front-door"), a lateral ("back-door") approach is preferred to minimize the need to dissect through a scarred field. Ideally, all the four parathyroids need to be visualized. When a parathyroid is not found in its normal anatomical confines, a logical and comprehensive exploration is to be carried out for missing parathyroid in ectopic sites, including, retroesophageal space, carotid sheath, thymus and submandibular region, to look for undescended glands. Intraoperative adjuncts like ultrasound, dyes, auto fluorescence and bilateral internal jugular vein sampling can be considered (35). Tissue excised can be confirmed by frozen section. A curative fall on IOPTH helps confirm adequacy of surgical procedure. Partial or complete thyroid lobectomy may occasionally be performed depending on the suspected location of missing gland. The parathyroid can be looked for in the mediastinum if it remains elusive in the neck even after a concerted multi-disciplinary approach.

Operative adjuncts

Intraoperative PTH (IOPTH) assay

The critical importance of IOPTH assay in re-operative surgery has been demonstrated in various studies (2, 41, 42). Various criteria have been used for predicting outcomes of parathyroid surgery. A fall >50% or more from the highest of either preoperative baseline or pre-excision level at 10 minutes after excision (Miami criteria) is the most commonly used parameter for predicting cure. It has a positive predictive value, negative predictive and accuracy rate of 99.6, 70 and 97.3%, respectively (43). IOPTH assay has also various advantages. A curative fall helps confirm that the removed parathyroid gland is the only source of abnormal PTH secretion and also it permits ex-vivo aspiration of excised tissue for the measurement of PTH levels. Raised PTH in tissue aspirate helps differentiate it from similar looking lymph node or thyroid tissue. Irvin L et al. demonstrated the usefulness of IOPTH assay in in 31/33 patients undergoing redo surgery with success rate of 94%, sensitivity, specificity, PPV, NPV and accuracy rate of 100, 93, 97 100, and 98%, respectively (42).

Other invasive treatment modalities besides surgical exploration have also been investigated especially in those patients not willing for surgery, multiple endocrine neoplasia-1 (MEN 1) and patients not fit to undergo surgery. This includes microwave ablation of abnormal parathyroid gland and percutaneous ethanol ablation (PEA) in patients with R-PHPT and MEN 1. Ospina et al. demonstrated the success of PEA for the treatment of R-PHPT in patients with MEN 1. A total of 37 patients underwent 80 PEA resulting in mean calcium level dropping from 10.7 ± 0.57 to 9.6 ± 0.76 mg/dL (p < 0.01). Normocalcemia was achieved in 78%, and hypocalcaemia occurred in 8.1%. Complication rates remained low at 5% (44). The safety and efficacy of microwave ablation in cases with R-PHPT and persistent primary hyperparathyroidism (P-PHPT) were demonstrated by Yu et al.; there was a significant decrease of intact PTH and serum calcium on day 1 after ablation (1570 ± 1765–287 ± 239 pg/mL, p < 0.05 and 2.51 ± 0.23–2.06 ± 0.27 mmol/L, p < 0.001, respectively) with only minor complications (45).

Medical management

Medical options can be offered in those patients who refuse further re-exploration in asymptomatic or mild symptomatic and patients with significant symptoms but unfit to undergo further surgery. For those patients with mild symptoms or asymptomatic, simple observation with the maintenance of adequate hydration may be enough.

Certain drugs have been approved and used with favorable outcomes for the management of HPT. Out of which the most commonly used pharmacological agents include bisphosphonates, estrogen, selective estrogen receptor modulators such as raloxifene and calcimimetic cinacalcet.

Estrogens are usually indicated for postmenopausal osteoporosis prevention. In a patient with PHPT, estrogens are usually indicated in whom surgery is not possible, where skeletal protection is the priority and where other first-line agents for osteoporosis are contraindicated. They reduce bone turnover markers and improve bone mineral density (BMD) but do not significantly lower calcium level. The positive effects of hormone replacement therapy have been shown in various studies (46, 47).

Raloxifene, which is a selective estrogen receptor modulator, has also been used for treatment of PHPT in postmenopausal women. It may produce similar effect as that of estrogen. It decreases bone turnover markers and improves BMD but does not significantly decrease serum calcium level. It has no effect on PTH (48)

Bisphosphonates

This class includes orally administered alendronate, ibandronate and risedronate and intravenous formulation of zoledronic acid and pamidronate. This group of drugs is usually used for the prevention and treatment of postmenopausal osteoporosis. In a patient with PHPT, bisphosphonate especially IV formulation are generally used for severe hypercalcemia in severe PHPT. The choice of bisphosphonates is guided by the drug profile, clinical scenario and affordability. They act by decreasing the bone turnover indices and increase the BMD especially at lumbar spine and femoral neck. They have minimal or no significant effect on serum calcium and PTH level (49)

Calcimimetics

This group of drugs acts by activating the CaSR in parathyroid cells, which mediates the inhibition of PTH secretion and increases calcium renal excretion. The efficacy of cinacalcet in PHPT has been demonstrated in various studies. Its use is generally indicated in patients of PHPT with severe hypercalcemia, parathyroid carcinoma with HPT and secondary HPT on dialysis. It is effective at normalizing the calcium level rapidly and sustainably, has minimal effect on PTH but no effect on BMD and does not reduce bone turnover markers (50)

South Asia perspective

HPT in India is still an uncommon disease, but the incidence seems to be increasing. The age of onset too is earlier with a higher proportion of patients presenting with overt symptoms. Awareness about HPT seems to be lower amongst health care physicians and public alike. Diagnostic modalities for HPT and more so invasive ones are concentrated to select centers, and this is likely to lead to higher rates of recurrence, which is compounded by shortage of specialist endocrine surgeons. However, temporal studies suggest improving parameters. Though there is a paucity of Indian data on persistence and recurrence, available data seems to be in coherence with western data. The reported incidence of persistence and recurrence in India ranges from 0 to 2.7% and 0 to 4.16%, respectively.

Conclusion

Persistent and recurrent HPT is encountered in up to 5% of patients. Biochemical confirmation of diagnosis followed by accurate localization would lay the foundation for optimal outcome. Not all patients merit an immediate surgery, and effective medical management is feasible for variable periods amongst those necessitating treatment but unfit for surgery. Adequate knowledge of parathyroid embryology and anatomy along with certain adjuncts are essential for optimal success of repeat surgery.

References

1. Griebeler ML, Kearns AE, Ryu E, et al. Secular trends in the incidence of primary hyperparathyroidism over five decades (1965–2010). Bone. 2015;73:1–7.
2. Udelsman R, Lin Z, Donovan P. The superiority of minimally invasive parathyroidectomy based on 1650 consecutive patients with primary hyperparathyroidism. Ann Surg. 2011;253:585–591.
3. Uden P, Chan AK, Duh QY, et al. Primary hyperparathyroidism in younger and older patients: Clinical symptoms and outcome of surgery. World J Surg. 1992;16:791.
4. Guerin C, et al. Persistent & recurrent hyperparathyroidism. Updates Surg. 2017 Jun;69(2):161–169.
5. Nawrot I, Chudzin´ski W, Cia̢c´ka T, Barczyn´ski M, Szmidt J. Reoperations for persistent or recurrent primary hyperparathyroidism: Results of a retrospective cohort study at a tertiary referral center. Med Sci Monit. 2014;20:1604–1612.
6. Shen W, Duren M, Morita E, et al. Reoperation for persistent or recurrent primary hyperparathyroidism. Arch Surg. 1996;131(8):861–869.
7. Lappas D, Noussios G, Anagnostis P, Adamidou F, Chatzigeorgiou A, Skandalakis P. Location, number and morphology of parathyroid glands: Results from a large anatomical series. Anat Sci Int. 2012;87(3):160–164.
8. Carty SE, Norton JA. Management of patients with persistent or recurrent primary hyperparathyroidism. World J Surg. 1991;15:716.
9. Henry J-F. Reoperation for primary hyperparathyroidism: Tips and tricks. Langenbecks Arch Surg. 2010;395(2):103–109.
10. Yeh MW, Wiseman JE, Chu SD, et al. Population-level predictors of persistent hyperparathyroidism.Surgery. 2011;150(6):1113–1119.
11. McIntyre CJ, Allen JLY, Constantinides VA, Jackson JE, Tolley NS, Palazzo FF. Patterns of disease in patients at a tertiary referral centre requiring reoperative parathyroidectomy. Ann R Coll Surg Engl. 2015;97(8):598–602.
12. Ippolito G, Palazzo FF, Sebag F, Henry JF. Long-term follow-up after parathyroidectomy for radiation-induced hyperparathyroidism. Surgery. 2007;142(6):819–822.
13. Hessman O, Stålberg P, Sundin A, et al. High success rate of parathyroid reoperation may be achieved with improved localization diagnosis. World J Surg. 2008;32(5):774–781.
14. Gooding GAW. Sonography of the thyroid and parathyroid. Radiol Clin North Am. 1993;31:967.

15. Cheung K, Wang TS, Farrokhyar F, et al. A meta-analysis of preoperative localization techniques for patients with primary hyperparathyroidism. Ann Surg Oncol. 2012;19:577–583.
16. Rodriguez JM, Tezelman S, Siperstein AE, et al. Localization procedures in patients with persistent or recurrent hyperparathyroidism. Arch Surg. 1994;129:870.
17. Miller DL, Doppman JL, Shawker TH, et al. Localization of parathyroid adenomas in patients who have undergone surgery. I. Noninvasive imaging methods. Radiology. 1987;162:133.
18. Levin K, Clark OH. The reasons of failure in parathyroid surgery. Arch Surg. 1989;124:911.
19. Chiu ML, Kronange JF, Piwnica Worms D. Effect of mitochondrial and plasma membrane potentials on accumulation of hexakis (2-methoxyisobutylisonitrile) technetium in cultured mouse fibroblasts. J Nucl Med. 1990;31:1646.
20. Carlson GL, Farndon GL, Clayton B, et al. Thallium isotope scintigraphy and ultrasonography: Comparative studies of localization techniques in primary hyperparathyroidism.Br J Surg. 1990;77:327.
21. Aigner RM, Fueger GF, Wolf G. Parathyroid scintigraphy: First experiences with technetium(III)-99m-Q12. Eur J Nucl Med. 1997;24:326.
22. Sfakianakis GN, Irvin GL III, Foss J, et al. Efficient parathyroidectomy guided by SPECT-MDBI and hormonal measurements. J Nucl Med. 1996;88:798.
23. Rodgers SE, et al. Improved preoperative planning for directed parathyroidectomy with 4-dimensional computed tomography. Surgery. 2006;140(6):932–940.
24. Erdman WA, Breslav NA, Weinreb JC, et al. Noninvasive localization of parathyroid adenomas: A comparison of X-ray, computerized tomography, ultrasound, scintigraphy, and MRI. Magn Reson Imaging. 1989;102:917.
25. Gotway MB, Reddy GP, Webb R, et al. Comparison between MR imaging and 99mTc-MIBI scintigraphy in the evaluation of recurrent or persistent hyperparathyroidism. Radiology. 2001;218:783.
26. Fayet C, Hoeffel C, Fulla Y, et al. Technetium-99m sestamibi scintigraphy, magnetic resonance imaging, and venous sampling in persistent and recurrent hyperparathyroidism. Br J Radiol. 1998;71:108.
27. De Feo ML, Colagrande S, Biagini C, et al. Parathyroid glands: Combination of 99mTc MIBI scintigraphy and US for demonstration of parathyroid glands and nodules. Radiology. 2000;214:393.
28. Caldarella C, et al. Diagnostic performance of positron emission tomography using 11C-methionine in patients with suspected parathyroid adenoma: A meta-analysis. Endocrine. 2013;43(1):78–83.
29. Taywade SK, Damle NA, Behera A, et al. Comparison of 18F-Fluorocholine positron emission tomography/computed tomography and four-dimensional computed tomography in the preoperative localization of parathyroid adenomas-initial results. Indian J Endocr Metab. 2017;21:399–403.
30. Lezaic L, Rep S, Sever MJ, Kocjan T, Hocevar M, Fettich J. 18F-Fluorocholine PET/CT for localization of hyperfunctioning parathyroid tissue in primary hyperparathyroidism: A pilot study. Eur J Nucl Med Mol Imaging. 2014;41:2083–2089.
31. Quak E, Blanchard D, Houdu B, et al. F18-choline PET/CT guided surgery in primary hyperparathyroidism when ultrasound and MIBI SPECT/CT are negative or inconclusive: The APACH1 study. Eur J Nucl Med Mol Imaging. 2018;45:658–666.
32. Jaskowiak N, Norton JA, Alexander HR, et al. A prospective trial evaluating a standard approach to reoperation for missed parathyroid adenoma. Ann Surg. 1996;224:308.
33. Mariette C, Pelliser L, Combemale F, et al. Reoperation for persistent or recurrent primary hyperparathyroidism. Langenbecks Arch Surg. 1998;383:174.
34. Billingsley KG, Fraker DL, Doppman JL, et al. Localization and operative management of undescended parathyroid adenomas in patients with persistent primary hyperparathyroidism. Surgery. 1994;116:982.
35. Ito F, Sippel R, Lederman J, Chen H. The utility of intraoperative bilateral internal jugular venous sampling with rapid parathyroid hormone testing. Ann Surg. 2007 Jun;245(6):959–963.
36. Maser C, Donovan P, Santos F. Sonographically guided fine needle aspiration with rapid parathyroid hormone assay. Ann Surg Oncol. 2006;13:1690–1695.
37. McFarlane MP, Fraker DL, Shawker TH, et al. Use of preoperative fine-needle aspiration in patients undergoing reoperation for primary hyperparathyroidism. Surgery.1994;116:959.
38. Miller DL. Preoperative localization and interventional treatment of parathyroid tumours. When and how? World J Surg. 1991;15:706.
39. Yen TWF, Wang TS, Doffek KM, Krzywda EA, Wilson SD. Reoperative parathyroidectomy: An algorithm for imaging and monitoring of intraoperative parathyroid hormone levels that results in a successful focused approach. Surgery. 2008;144(4):611–621.
40. Udelsman R, Lin Z, Donovan P. The superiority of minimally invasive parathyroidectomy based on 1650 consecutive patients with primary hyperparathyroidism. Ann Surg. 2011;253(3):585–591.
41. Udelsman R, Donovan PI. Remedial parathyroid surgery: Changing trends in 130 consecutive cases. Ann Surg. 2006;244:471–479.
42. Irvin 3rd GL, Molinari AS, Figueroa C, Carneiro DM. Improved success rate in reoperative parathyroidectomy with intraoperative PTH assay. Ann Surg. 1999;229: 874–879.
43. Carneiro DM, Solorzano CC, Nader MC, et al. Comparison of intraoperative iPTH assay (QPTH) criteria in guiding parathyroidectomy: Which criterion is the most accurate? Surgery. 2003;134973–134981.
44. Singh Ospina N, Thompson GB, Lee RA, Reading CC, Young WF. Safety and efficacy of percutaneous parathyroid ethanol ablation in patients with recurrent primary hyperparathyroidism and multiple endocrine neoplasia type 1. J Clin Endocrinol Metab. 2015;100(1):E87–E90.
45. Yu M-A, Yao L, Zhang L, et al. Safety and efficiency of microwave ablation for recurrent and persistent secondary hyperparathyroidism after parathyroidectomy: A retrospective pilot study. Int J Hyperth. 2016;32(2):180–186.
46. Selby PL, Peacock M. Ethinyl estradiol and norethindrone in the treatment of primary hyperparathyroidism in postmenopausal women. N Engl J Med. 1986;314(23): 1481–1485.
47. Grey AB, Stapleton JP, Evans MC, et al. Effect of hormone replacement therapy on bone mineral density in postmenopausal women with mild primary hyperparathyroidism. A randomized, controlled trial. Ann Intern Med. 1996;125(5):360–368.
48. Rubin MR, Lee KH, McMahon DJ, et al. Raloxifene lowers serum calcium and markers of bone turnover in postmenopausal women with primary hyperparathyroidism. J Clin Endocrinol Metab. 2003;88(3):1174–1178.
49. Khan A, Bilezikian JP, Kung AWC, et al. Alendronate in primary hyperparathyroidism: A double-blind, randomized, placebo-controlled trial. J Clin Endocrinol Metab. 2004;89(7):3319–3325.
50. Khan A, Bilezikian JP, Kung AWC, et al. Cinacalcet normalizes serum calcium in a double-blind randomized, placebo-controlled study in patients with primary hyperparathyroidism with contraindications to surgery. Eur J Endocrinol. 2015; 172(5):527–535.

41

ANESTHESIA FOR THYROID AND PARATHYROID SURGERY

Reetu Verma and Yogita Dwivedi

Introduction

Thyroid hormone is a metabolic hormone and its derangement can lead to various intraoperative and postoperative complications, which can lead to delayed recovery of patient from anesthesia. Also, sometimes, the goiter may occur very large in size, creating problem for an anesthetist to maintain airway. Thyroidectomy surgery requires two special considerations before planning anesthetic management. Firstly, assessment of thyroid functions and secondly, proper airway examination and planning, which is the key to successful airway management. The patient should be biochemically and clinically euthyroid before elective surgery to reduce the risk of intraoperative and postoperative complications. A thorough pre-anesthetic checkup should be done for comorbidities, and a detailed drug history regarding the dose, compliance and side effect of antithyroid medications (agranulocytosis, increased aminotransferase) should be documented.

Patients' symptoms, signs and clinical presentation

Symptoms of hyperthyroidism include increased sweating, heat intolerance and sometimes diarrhea. Evaluation of cardiac function required as T3 hormone is directly related to speed of systolic contraction and diastolic relaxation. Hyperthyroidism causes increased systolic blood pressure, decreased diastolic blood pressure, sinus tachycardia and atrial fibrillation. Sinus tachycardia is the most common arrhythmia found in hyperthyroidism. Atrial fibrillation occurs in 2–20% hyperthyroidism patients and its prevalence increases with age [1, 2]. Other features of hyperthyroidism are warm and moist skin, fine tremors and exaggerated tendon reflexes. Signs of ophthalmopathy include staring look, upper eyelid retraction and proptosis. Lid lag phenomenon is common in hyperthyroidism.

In hypothyroidism, patient complains of fatigue, early lethargy, muscle cramps, cold intolerance, decreased sweating, constipation, weight gain and menorrhagia. Cardiac manifestations of hypothyroidism are diastolic hypertension because of increased systemic vascular resistance, sinus bradycardia because of sinus node dysfunction and inability of sinus node to accelerate under various stress conditions like fever and infections. Pericardial effusion and rarely cardiac tamponade may also occur. Pericarditis occurs in approximately 4% of patients with hypothyroidism. Incidence of atherosclerosis also increases with chronic hypothyroidism. ECG may feature sinus bradycardia, low voltage complexes and prolonged QTc with torsades de pointes. Other features associated with hypothyroidism are anemia, coarse and cold skin, dry and brittle hair, brittle nails, periorbital puffiness and delayed ankle reflex.

Clinical examination of swelling

Size, duration and consistency of goiter are important as hard swelling may be malignant. If lower margin of swelling is not palpable, it suggests retrosternal extension. Patient may also complain of dyspnea, cough, stridor, hoarseness of voice and dysphagia. Retrosternal extension of goiter may lead to superior vena cava obstruction, which is assessed by using Pemberton's sign in which patient is asked to raise both hands that result in facial flushing and venous engorgement.

Airway examination and evaluation

A detailed upper airway assessment should be done in patients planned for thyroidectomy focusing on goiter size, its type and extension into surrounding structures. Size of goiter is important for anesthetists as large goiter causing compression or deviation of trachea is a significant predictor of difficult intubation. Tracheal deviation is defined when there is more than 1 cm deviation of trachea from midline. Goiter's type and its extension into surrounding structures should be evaluated as cancerous goiter can infiltrate surrounding tissues and lead to fibrosis that may reduce the mobility of laryngeal structures resulting in difficult laryngoscopy and difficult intubation [3]. Other usual predictive factors that should be considered are advanced age, high BMI, a high Mallampati score, thyromental distance (TMD) <6.5 cm, neck circumference (NC) 40 ≥ cm, NC/TMD ≥5 cm etc. These all are associated with difficult intubation [3–8]. Incidence of difficult intubation in thyroid surgery patients varies from 5.3 to 13.6% [3, 9–11].

Duration of goiter should also be taken into consideration as in long-standing large goiters, tracheomalacia may be present, which may lead to the collapse of trachea after extubation and difficulty in maintaining airway. Tracheomalacia is weakness of tracheal wall, which occurs due to prolonged compression and degeneration of tracheal cartilages. Cuff leak test is done after the completion of surgery to identify any air leak present around the tracheal tube so the patient can be safely extubated. Cuff leak test was originally described for detecting laryngeal edema. In this test, when the spontaneous respiration is regained by patient after the completion of surgery, tracheal tube cuff is deflated and proximal port of tracheal tube is occluded to assess peri tubal leak [12]. It can also be assessed by measuring the difference between inspiratory and expiratory tidal volume before and after deflation of tracheal cuff.

Investigations

Complete blood count, thyroid function test, cervical and chest X-ray AP and lateral view are required in these patients. CT scan of swelling is required in the case of retrosternal goiter to see the extent of goiter, tracheal deviation, compression and stenosis of trachea if present. Indirect laryngoscopy by an ENT specialist to document any preoperative vocal cord dysfunction should also be done before surgery.

Airway management for surgery

In normal goiter patients, endotracheal management is done using direct laryngoscopy technique by central-acting muscle relaxants. But in huge and retrosternal goiter, controlled bag and mask ventilation may be difficult after the administration of muscle relaxants so preservation of spontaneous ventilation is preferred till the intubation is done. Awake fiberoptic intubation may also be considered in huge and retrosternal goiter [13]. Nebulization with local anesthetics and spray-as-you-go technique are recommended for fiberoptic intubation. Inhalational induction with sevoflurane in sitting or semiprone position can also be used. For airway management, reinforced armored tube, North pole Ring Adair Elwyn or neural integrity monitor (NIM) electromyography tube can be used. NIM tube is used for intraoperative monitoring of recurrent laryngeal nerve (RLN) to prevent RLN injury during thyroid and parathyroid surgery. All muscle relaxants reduce the electromyographic amplitude and can interfere with the interpretation of signals and defeat the purpose of using intraoperative nerve monitoring for RLN [14, 15]. Insertion of endotracheal tube requires good relaxation to prevent any airway-related injury so short-acting muscle relaxants like succinylcholine can be used. Succinylcholine at dose of 1 mg/kg results in the return of 90% muscle activity within 9–13 minutes [16]. In patients where we want to avoid succinylcholine, single dose of non-depolarizing muscle relaxants like rocuronium can be used for endotracheal intubation. But the recovery of muscle activity should always be monitored using neuromuscular junction monitor.

Lu IC et al. compared succinylcholine 1 mg/kg, rocuronium .3 mg/kg and rocuronium .6 mg/kg for intraoperative nerve monitoring of RLN in porcine model and observed that with both succinylcholine 1 mg/kg and rocuronium .3 mg/kg, electromyographic signals return to baseline within 30 minutes but with high dose rocuronium electromyographic signals didn't come to baseline until 1 hour after its administration [17].

NIM tube can be placed by direct laryngoscopy, video laryngoscopy or using fiberoptic bronchoscope placing its electrodes exactly between vocal cords [18, 19].

Positioning of patient for surgery

The aim is to provide maximal exposure to the operating surgeon. The patient should be placed in supine position with head up by 15 degrees to reduce chances of bleeding. A shoulder roll is placed at the level of acromion process of scapula to help in the neck extension. Care should be taken to avoid hyperextension of neck and a proper and stable head support is provided. The arms should be gently tucked to either side.

Hyperthyroidism and intraoperative anesthetic management

Hyperthyroidism is characterized by high levels of serum thyroxine and triiodothyronine and low levels of thyroid-stimulating hormone (TSH). Thyrotoxicosis is a clinical syndrome due to the high level of circulating thyroid hormones. It can be primary or secondary. In primary thyrotoxicosis, CNS manifestations such as tremors, increased tendon reflexes and ophthalmopathy dominate. In secondary thyrotoxicosis, cardiovascular symptoms such as tachycardia and arrhythmias predominate. Hyperthyroidism with goiter mainly occurs because of Graves' disease, toxic multinodular goiter or toxic adenoma. Graves' disease is one of the main causes of hyperthyroidism that typically occurs in females in comparison to males (7:1) and between ages from 20 to 40 years. It is an autoimmune disease with antibodies against TSH receptors. Graves' disease features thyrotoxicosis, diffuse goiter, infiltrative orbitopathy and rarely infiltrative dermatopathy and acropathy with thickening of terminal phalanges. Toxic multinodular goiter is another major cause of hyperthyroidism, which usually occurs in long-standing goiter after the age of 50 years and more common in females than males (6:1). Retrosternal extension and obstructive symptoms occur more frequently in toxic nodular goiter than Graves' disease.

Whenever a patient is planned for elective thyroidectomy, patients need to be euthyroid until it is an emergency. In overt hyperthyroidism, drug clearance and distribution of propofol increase so the requirement of propofol may be more [20]. Patients may have exaggerated response to anesthetic drugs with sympathetic stimulation like ketamine, pancuronium, epinephrine, ephedrine and atropine, which are best to be avoided. There may be upregulation of β-adrenergic receptors, so for intraoperative hypotension, directly acting vasopressors like phenylephrine should be used and indirectly acting vasopressors like ephedrine, epinephrine and norepinephrine should be avoided. Antithyroid drugs are given to render the patient euthyroid. In Graves' disease, after achieving a euthyroid state, iodide therapy is started 7–10 days before surgery to decrease the vascularity and hence blood loss during surgery. In the case of emergency surgery, when there is not adequate time to render the patient's euthyroid intravenous β blockers, iodine, glucocorticoids and propylthiouracil (PTU) are used. PTU is given orally via nasogastric tube or rectally. PTU has added advantage that it inhibits conversion of T4 to T3. Dexamethasone is also given in doses of 2 mg every 6 hourly to inhibit conversion of T4 to T3. MAC values of inhalational agents remain unchanged.

Thyroid storm

Thyroid storm is also called accentuated thyrotoxicosis that occurs in association with Graves' disease and sometimes toxic multinodular goiter. Precipitating factors are trauma, infection, surgery, pregnancy, diabetic ketoacidosis and radiation thyroiditis. The clinical presentation is of severe hypermetabolism characterized by fever, profuse sweating, tachycardia, arrhythmias, pulmonary edema and congestive heart failure. Restlessness and tremulousness are present, which may proceed to stupor and delirium.

Treatment aims supportive therapy, management of thyrotoxicosis and precipitating cause. Hyperpyrexia requires vigorous management, and it should be treated with ice packs and cold blankets. Dehydration is treated with glucose-containing intravenous fluids. Thyrotoxicosis treatment involves therapy, which inhibits thyroid hormone synthesis, their release and therapy, which targets peripheral action of thyroid hormone. Antithyroid drugs like PTU or carbimazole are used, but PTU is preferred over others because it also inhibits peripheral conversion of T4 to T3. PTU is given in a loading dose of 500–1000 mg and then 250 mg 4 hourly either orally via nasogastric tube or rectally. Carbimazole is administered at doses of 20–40 mg every

4–6 hours. After 1 hour of initiation of antithyroid drug, Lugols iodine is given 8 drops orally every 6–8 hour to inhibit the release of preformed thyroid hormone from gland. Hydrocortisone 300 mg intravenous loading dose then 100 mg 6 hourly can also be given. It counters the relative adrenal insufficiency, inhibits hormone synthesis and peripheral conversion of T4 to T3. Intravenous β blockers like propranolol should be started immediately unless contraindicated. Propranolol has added advantage of inhibiting peripheral conversion of T4 to T3, but it is contraindicated in asthmatic patient being a nonselective β blocker. Propranolol is given in dosage of 1–2 mg/min every 15 minute till the adequate hemodynamic effect is achieved with maximum dose of 10 mg [21, 22].

For intraoperative thyroid storm Esmolol infusion is given in dosage of .5 mg/kg over 1 minute as loading dose followed by infusion at 50–300 µg/kg/min. Esmolol is a cardio-selective β blocker and has the added advantage of being rapid in onset and also short acting [23].

Hypothyroidism and intraoperative anesthetic management

Hypothyroidism with glandular enlargement occurs in Hashimoto's thyroiditis, which is an autoimmune disease, or endemic goiter, which occurs due to iodine deficiency. Hypothyroidism may be overt or subclinical hypothyroidism. In overt hypothyroidism, fT4 is reduced and TSH is elevated, whereas in subclinical hypothyroidism, fT4 remains low to normal and TSH is elevated. Clinical features can be reversed with the use of thyroxine in overt hypothyroidism patients. So, patients should always be made euthyroid in the case of elective surgery. In the case of emergency surgery, proceeding with deranged values must be weighed against the benefit of surgery. The dose of levothyroxine is 1.6–1.9 µg/kg body weight daily. In obese patients, dose should be adjusted on lean body weight [24].

Hypothyroidism patients are considered potentially full stomach as they have delayed gastric emptying time. Obstructive sleep apnea may also be present so sedative drugs for premedication must be used cautiously. In overt hypothyroidism because of reduced cardiac output and plasma volume, the requirement of inducing agents is decreased with the delayed onset of action so they should be given cautiously to avoid any untoward effects. Clearance of drugs that are excreted through the kidney may be prolonged because of decreased renal blood flow and glomerular filtration rate (GFR), which can lead to delayed recovery from anesthesia. Narcotics and sedatives should be given cautiously because hypoxic and hyperventilatory drives are depressed that may result in respiratory depression in postoperative period [25].

Although MAC values of inhalational anesthetic agents remain unchanged, these should be used cautiously because of baroreceptor reflex dysfunction in hypothyroidism patients, which may result in exaggerated hypotensive response. Hypothyroidism patients are also more prone to develop intraoperative and postoperative hypothermia because of their decreased ability to increased temperature in response to low-temperature stress [2, 26]. Intraoperative bleeding tendencies are increased because of decreased clotting factors VIII and IX and dysfunction of platelets [27, 28].

In subclinical hypothyroidism, whether to proceed with deranged TSH levels in elective surgery is not being studied too much, but in one of the prospective studies, author observed that patients with subclinical hypothyroidism who underwent coronary bypass grafting had higher incidence of postoperative atrial fibrillation in comparison to patients with normal thyroid levels for the same surgery [29]. Also in a study, incidence of postoperative complications was reduced with the supplementation of thyroxine in subclinical hypothyroidism patients undergoing cardiac surgery [30].

Myxedema coma

Myxedema coma is a severe form of hypothyroidism that occurs in long-standing cases of hypothyroidism. Its precipitating factors are exposure to cold, infection, trauma, central nervous depressant drugs and anesthesia. Clinical features are hypothermia, bradycardia, hypotension and delayed relaxation of deep tendon reflexes.

Myxedema coma is a medical emergency with a mortality rate of 20–50%. Intravenous levothyroxine or liothyronine is the treatment of choice. Intravenous levothyroxine 500–800 µg is given as loading dose and 100 µg daily thereafter. Intravenous liothyronine is given at dose of 25 µg 12 hourly. Other supportive measures include intravenous hydration with glucose-containing saline solutions but avoid hypotonic solution because dilution hyponatremia may be present. Temperature management should also be done, but no active warming to be done. Correction of electrolyte imbalances and stabilization of the cardiac and pulmonary systems are necessary. Mechanical ventilation is frequently required. Heart rate, blood pressure and temperature usually improve within 24 hours, and a relative euthyroid state is achieved in 3–5 days. Hydrocortisone 200–400 mg/day IV is also prescribed to treat possible adrenal insufficiency [31].

Postoperative management

Pain
Post thyroidectomy, patient experiences pain through multiple mechanisms due to intraoperative cervical hyperextension, laryngeal discomfort caused by frequent movement of endotracheal tube during manipulations and so on. Multimodal analgesic regime includes opioids, non-steroidal anti-inflammatory drugs, acetaminophen, pregabalin and local infiltration of bupivacaine. Bilateral superficial plexus block of emerging branches of superficial cervical plexus reduces the requirement of analgesics in the first 24 hours postoperative period after thyroid surgery [32].

Nausea and vomiting
Postoperative nausea and vomiting carry the risk of wound dehiscence, hematoma and airway obstruction. Pharmacological interventions include 5-HT3 receptor antagonist. Steroids can also be used to prevent postoperative nausea and vomiting.

Hematoma

Postoperative hematoma may develop even beyond 6 hours of surgery and 24 hours, and its incidence in various studies varies from 0 to 6.5% [33]. The presence of hematoma may result in tracheal compression and respiratory distress, which requires immediate surgical decompression.

Tracheomalacia

Tracheomalacia is defined as weakness of tracheal cartilage because of long-standing goiter that may result in the collapse of trachea after extubation. Tracheostomy of the patient is recommended if trachea is soft and floppy or collapse of trachea occurs following gradual withdrawal of endotracheal tube [34].

Hypocalcemia

It usually occurs between 1 and 7 days after surgery. It occurs because of inadvertent removal or impairment of blood supply to parathyroid glands. Severe hypoparathyroidism is treated with intravenous calcium. In milder cases, oral calcium carbonate and cholecalciferol are recommended.

Recurrent laryngeal nerve injury

Unilateral damage of RLN results in the hoarseness or dysphonia, and bilateral damage of RLN results in acute life-threatening dyspnea.

Anesthetic management for parathyroid surgery

Hyperparathyroidism patients require surgery due to parathyroid hyperplasia that can be primary, secondary and tertiary hyperplasia. Primary hyperparathyroidism is due to oversecretion of parathyroid hormone either due to an adenoma or a tumor. Secondary hyperparathyroidism occurs because of low calcium levels in chronic renal failure. Tertiary hyperparathyroidism is seen after renal transplantation. The main concern for anesthesiologist for parathyroid surgery is levels of calcium and hypercalcemic features. Hypercalcemia may be associated with various nonspecific features involving kidney, neuromuscular, skeletal, gastrointestinal and cardiovascular system. Nephrolithiasis and proximal tubular dysfunction can be present, which may result in the decreased GFR and patient complained of polyuria and polydipsia. Osteitis fibrosa cystica and osteopenia occur in skeletal abnormalities, and patient complains of bone pain. Neuromuscular involvement causes weakness of proximal muscle group and muscle atrophy. Patient may also complain of lethargy and depression. Cardiovascular manifestations are hypertension, which has a prevalence of 40–65% in primary hyperparathyroidism, and ECG features shortened QTc and prolonged PR intervals, which increases the risk of arrhythmias in these patients [35–37]. Peptic ulcer and gastritis are also associated with hypercalcemia because of increased production of peptic acid and gastrin. Preanesthetic evaluation for parathyroid surgery requires evaluation of symptoms associated with increased parathyroid hormone levels and level of calcium. Normalization of calcium levels is recommended before elective surgery. Intraoperative anesthetic concerns are to maintain adequate hydration and urinary output. In postoperative period, calcium level should be checked at 6–24 hours.

Regional anesthesia for thyroid and parathyroid surgery

Thyroidectomy is not routinely performed under regional anesthesia. However, this has been shown to be safe and successful in a selected group of patients, resulting in low morbidity. Local anesthesia infiltration, superficial and deep cervical plexus block with monitored anesthesia care can be used for providing anesthesia in selected patients. Patients who are not cooperative or unable to communicate are poor candidates for regional anesthesia technique [38–41]. Deep cervical plexus block is not routinely used nowadays because of its complications like bradycardia, dysphagia, upper extremity paresthesia, Horner's syndrome, inadvertent intravascular injection and postoperative respiratory failure.

Conclusion

Thyroid disorders are prevalent in South Asian region requiring either medical or surgical treatment. In South Asian region, hypothyroidism is still a high prevalence disease despite the universal iodization program. Endemic goiter that was previously considered prevalent only in iodine-deficient areas has a high occurrence even in iodine-sufficient areas nowadays, maybe because of autoimmune factors and goitrogens etc. Late presentation to hospital when goiter starts causing problems like dysphagia and dyspnea is not a rare entity in this region. In these patients, maintaining airway and extubation is a challenge for anesthesiologist. Preoperative communication between anesthetist and surgeon is very important for proper airway planning, maintaining intraoperative and postoperative airway and avoiding complications.

References

1. Kahaly GJ, Dillmann WH. Thyroid hormone action in the heart. Endocr Rev. 2005;26:704–728.
2. Grais IM and Sowers JR. Thyroid and the heart. Am J Med. 2014;127:691–698.
3. Bouaggad A, Nejmi SE, Bouderka MA, Abbassi O. Prediction of difficult tracheal intubation in thyroid surgery. Anesth Analg. 2004;99:603–606.
4. Kalezić N, Sabljak V, Stevanović K, Miličić B, Marković D, Tošković A, et al. Predictors of difficult airway management in thyroid surgery: A five-year observational single-center prospective study. Acta Clin Croat. 2016;55:9–18.
5. Voyagis GS, Kyriakos PK. The effect of goiter on endotracheal intubation. Anesth Analg. 1997;84:611–612.
6. Tutuncu AC, Erbabacan E, Teksoz S, Ekici B, Koksal G, Altintas F, et al. The assessment of risk factors for difficult intubation in thyroid patients. World J Surg. 2018;42:1748–1753.
7. Meco BC, Alanoglu Z, Yilmaz AA, Basaran C, Alkis N, Demirer S, et al. Does ultrasonographic volume of the thyroid gland correlate with difficult intubation? An observational study. Braz J Anesthesiol. 2015;65:230–234.
8. Mallat J, Robin E, Pironkov A, Lebuffe G, Tavernier B. Goitre and difficulty of tracheal intubation. Ann Fr Anesth Reanim. 2010;29:436–439.
9. Amathieu R, Smail N, Catineau J, Poloujadoff MP, Samii K, Adnet F. Difficult intubation in thyroid surgery: Myth or reality? Anesth Analg. 2006;103:965–968.
10. Olusomi O, Aliyu SZ, Babajide AM, Sulaiman AO, Adegboyega OS, Gbenga HO, Adebisi RG. Goitre-related factors for predicting difficult intubation in patients scheduled for thyroidectomy in a resource-challenged health institution in north central Nigeria. Ethiop J Health Sci. 2018 Mar;28(2):169–176.
11. De Cassai A, Papaccio F, Betteto G, Schiavolin C, Iacobone M, Carron M. Prediction of difficult tracheal intubations in thyroid surgery. Predictive value of neck circumference to thyromental distance ratio. PLOS ONE. 2019 Feb;14(2):e0212976.
12. Fisher MM, Raper RF. The "cuff leak" test for extubation. Anaesthesia. 1992;47:10.
13. Huitink JM, Buitelaar DR, Schutte PF. Awake fibrecapnic intubation: A novel technique for intubation in head and neck cancer patients with a difficult airway. Anaesthesia. 2006 May;61(5):449–452.
14. Marusch F, Hussock J, Haring G, Hachenberg T, Gastinger I. Influence of muscle relaxation on neuromonitoring of the recurrent laryngeal nerve during thyroid surgery. Br J Anaesth. 2005 May;94(5):596–600.
15. Chu KS, Tsai CJ, Lu IC, Tseng KY, Chau SW, Wu CW, et al. Influence of nondepolarizing muscle relaxants on intraoperative neuromonitoring during thyroid surgery. J Otolaryngol Head Neck Surg. 2010 Aug;39(4):397–402.
16. Naguib M, Lien CA, Meistalman C. Pharmacology of neuromuscular blocking drugs. In: RD Miller, ed., Miller's Anesthesia. 8th ed. Philadelphia, PA: Elsevier/Saunders; 2015. p. 1125.
17. Lu IC, Chang PY, Hsu HT, Tseng KY, Wu CW, Lee KW, et al. A comparison between succinylcholine and rocuronium on the recovery profile of the laryngeal muscles during intraoperative neuromonitoring of the recurrent laryngeal nerve: A prospective porcine model. Kaohsiung J Med Sci. 2013 Sep;29(9):484–487.
18. Dralle H, Sekulla C, Lorenz K, Brauckhoff M, Machens A; German IONM Study Group. Intraoperative monitoring of the recurrent laryngeal nerve in thyroid surgery. World J Surg. 2008 Jul;32(7):1358–1366.
19. Lu IC, Chu KS, Tsai CJ, Wu CW, Kuo WR, Chen HY, et al. Optimal depth of NIM EMG endotracheal tube for intraoperative neuromonitoring of the recurrent laryngeal nerve during thyroidectomy. World J Surg. 2008 Sep;32(9):1935–1939.
20. Tsubokawa T, Yamamoto K, Kobayashi T. Propofol clearance and distribution volume increase in patients with hyperthyroidism. Anesth Analg. 1998 Jul;87(1):195–199.

21. Carroll R, Matfin G. Endocrine and metabolic emergencies: Thyroid storm. Ther Adv Endocrinol Metab. 2010 Aug;1(3):139–145.
22. Chiha M, Samarasinghe S, Kabaker AS. Thyroid storm: An updated review. J Intensive Care Med. 2015 Mar;30(3):131–140.
23. Glick DB. The autonomic nervous system. In: RD Miller, ed., Miller's Anesthesia. 8th ed. Philadelphia, PA: Elsevier/Saunders; 2015. pp. 442–443.
24. Santini F, Pinchera A, Marsili A, Ceccarini G, Castagna MG, Valeriano R, et al. Lean body mass is a major determinant of levothyroxine dosage in the treatment of thyroid diseases. J Clin Endocrinol Metab. 2005 Jan;90(1):124–127.
25. Schlenker EH. Effects of hypothyroidism on the respiratory system and control of breathing: Human studies and animal models. Respir Physiol Neurobiol. 2012 Apr;181(2):123–131.
26. Murkin JM. Anesthesia and hypothyroidism: A review of thyroxine physiology, pharmacology, and anesthetic implications. Anesth Analg. 1982 Apr;61(4):371–383.
27. Federici AB. Acquired von Willebrand syndrome associated with hypothyroidism: A mild bleeding disorder to be further investigated. In: Seminars in Thrombosis and Hemostasis (vol. 37, no. 01). Thieme Medical Publishers; 2011. pp. 35–40.
28. Squizzato A, Romualdi E, Buller HR, Gerdes VE. Thyroid dysfunction and effects on coagulation and fibrinolysis: A systematic review. J Clin Endocrinol Metab. 2007 Jul;92(7):2415–2420.
29. Park YJ, Yoon JW, Kim KI, Lee YJ, Kim KW, Choi SH, et al. Subclinical hypothyroidism might increase the risk of transient atrial fibrillation after coronary artery bypass grafting. Ann Thorac Surg. 2009 Jun;87(6):1846–1852.
30. Mahmoud AF, Rehan M, Taha WS, Osman SH, Assad OM, Al Fayoumy OM. Subclinical hypothyroidism affects the intraoperative and postoperative hemodynamics in coronary artery bypass graft surgery: Should we supplement with thyroxine preoperatively. Egypt J Cardiothorac Anesth. 2013 Jul;7(2):43.
31. Wiersinga WM. Myxedema and coma (severe hypothyroidism). In: Endotext [Internet] 2018 Apr 25. MDText. com, Inc.
32. Mayhew D, Sahgal N, Khirwadkar R, Hunter JM, Banerjee A. Analgesic efficacy of bilateral superficial cervical plexus block for thyroid surgery: Meta-analysis and systematic review. Br J Anaesth. 2018;120(2):241–251.
33. Promberger R, Ott J, Kober F, Koppitsch C, Seemann R, Freissmuth M, et al. Risk factors for postoperative bleeding after thyroid surgery. Br J Surg. 2012 Mar;99(3):373–379.
34. Agarwal A, Mishra AK, Gupta SK, Arshad F, Agarwal A, Tripathi M, et al. High incidence of tracheomalacia in longstanding goiters: Experience from an endemic goiter region. World J Surg. 2007:31:832–837.
35. Hedback GM, Oden AS. Cardiovascular disease, hyper-tension and renal function in primary hyperparathyroid-ism. J Intern Med. 2002;251:476–483.
36. Letizia C, Ferrari P, Cotesta D, Caliumi C, Cianci R, Cerci S, et al. Ambulatory monitoring of blood pressure (AMBP) in patients with primary hyperparathyroidism. J Hum Hypertens. 2005 Nov;19(11):901–906.
37. Pepe J, Cipriani C, Sonato C, Raimo O, Biamonte F, Minisola S. Cardiovascular manifestation of primary hyperparathyroidism: A narrative review. Eur J Endocrinol. 2017;177:R297–R308.
38. Snyder SK, Roberson CR, Cummings CC, Rajab MH. Local anesthesia with monitored anesthesia care vs general anesthesia in thyroidectomy: A randomized study. Arch Surg. 2006;141(2):167–173.
39. Saxe AW, Brown E, Hamburger SW. Thyroid and parathyroid surgery performed with patient under regional anesthesia. Surgery. 1988 Apr;103(4):415–420.
40. Spanknebel K, Chabot JA, DiGiorgi M, Cheung K, Lee S, Allendorf J, LoGerfo P. Thyroidectomy using local anesthesia: A report of 1,025 cases over 16 years. J Am Coll Surg. 2005 Sep;201(3):375–385.
41. Kulkarni RS, Braverman LE, Patwardhan NA. Bilateral cervical plexus block for thyroidectomy and parathyroidectomy in healthy and high risk patients. J Endocrinol Invest. 1996 Dec;19(11):714–718.

42

HISTORY OF ADRENAL SURGERY

Asuri Krishna, Mayank Jain, Shardool Vikram Gupta and Subodh Kumar

The text of this chapter is available online at www.routledge.com/9781032136509.

43

ADRENAL GLAND
Embryology and Anatomy

Asuri Krishna and Mayank Jain

Introduction

The adrenal gland consists of two distinct parts that are different histologically and serves different functions owing to difference in their origin, steroid, and catecholamine metabolism. At 5–6 weeks of intrauterine life[1], mesothelium proliferates between the root of the dorsal mesentery and the gonadal ridges (Figure 43.1)[2], which forms the fetal cortex. The cortex forms the outer layer surrounding the inner medulla. At 9 weeks of gestation, the cortex differentiates into distinct zones—the definitive zone and the fetal zone, each zone having different histology[3]. During the period of gestation, these zones play a very important role in the sexual differentiation of the fetus. The fetal cortex produces androgens, and these androgens along with the hormones produced from the gonads effect the sexual differentiation of the fetus.

The fetal adrenal cortex surrounds the developing adrenal medulla (Figure 43.2)[2], and a mesodermal layer that separates the adrenal gland from the adjacent developing gonad and the kidney encapsulates the entire gland. The close approximation of the nascent adrenal cortex to the mesoderm destined to become the kidney and gonads explains both the normal anatomic relationship to the kidney and the occasional finding of ectopic adrenal tissue or adrenal "rests" associated with gonadal vessels and gonads[4]. Up to 50% of newborns have ectopic adrenal tissue, either cortical tissue alone (if it migrated before the invasion of the medullary cells) or a combination of cortical and medullary tissues. This ectopic adrenal tissue atrophies in most children so that adrenal rests are found only in 1% of adults[1].

At 9 weeks of gestation, the fetal adrenal cortex differentiates into histologically distinct zones—the definitive zone and the fetal zone[3]. During gestation, the fetal cortex primarily produces androgens, which along with hormones produced from gonads influence sexual differentiation of the fetus[5]. In the third trimester, a third layer called the transitional zone forms between the definitive and fetal zones. By 6 months of life, the definitive and transitional zones give rise to the zona glomerulosa, the outermost layer of the adrenal cortex, which produces mineralocorticoids, and the zona fasciculata, which produces glucocorticoids. Over the first year of life, the fetal cortex involutes and the zona reticularis, which produces androgens, begins to develop as the innermost layer of the adrenal cortex[6]. The zona reticularis becomes a distinct layer by 3–4 years of age (Figure 43.2)[2].

Chromaffin cells are the functional cells of the adrenal medulla and are derived from the neural crest (Figure 43.1)[2]. Along with chromaffin cells, the neural crest also supplies the chief cells of the paraganglia and the parafollicular C cells of the thyroid to the developing endocrine system[7]. Chromaffin cells in the adrenal produce catecholamines and are the cells of origin of pheochromocytomas and neuroblastomas. Chief cells, found in the varied anatomic locations of the paraganglia, are the cells of origin of extra-adrenal pheochromocytomas and neuroblastomas[7].

The merging of the primitive medullary and cortical cells to create the adrenal gland is accomplished by the migration of medullary cells into the cortex, which begins during the seventh week of gestation. This process continues so that, by the second trimester, the fetal adrenal cortex surrounds the medulla and the entire gland becomes encapsulated by a mesodermal layer separating the adrenal glands from the surrounding retroperitoneal structures[1](Figure 43.2)[2].

Anatomy

Adrenal glands are paired organs in the retroperitoneum, superior and slightly anterior medial to the kidney. The gland lies lateral to the vertebral column, in front of 12th rib on the right and 11th and 12th rib on the left. At birth, weight of both the adrenal glands is about 8 g and is nearly the size of the adult adrenal glands. This size of the adrenal gland reaches up to one-third of the size of the adjacent kidneys[1]. At the age of 1 year, the cortex portion of the fetal adrenal gland involutes and the gland approaches the adult dimensions (approximately $5 \times 3 \times 0.6$ cm) and weight (4–6 g each)[8]. They are enclosed within Gerota fascia and lie on the superomedial aspect of each kidney. This connective tissue plane separating the adrenal gland and the superior pole of the kidney facilitates the dissection of adrenal away from the superior pole of the kidney during adrenalectomy. The adrenal gland has characteristic bright chrome yellow color. The surface has fine granularity, and the gland is firm in consistency. These characteristics are used to differentiate the gland from the

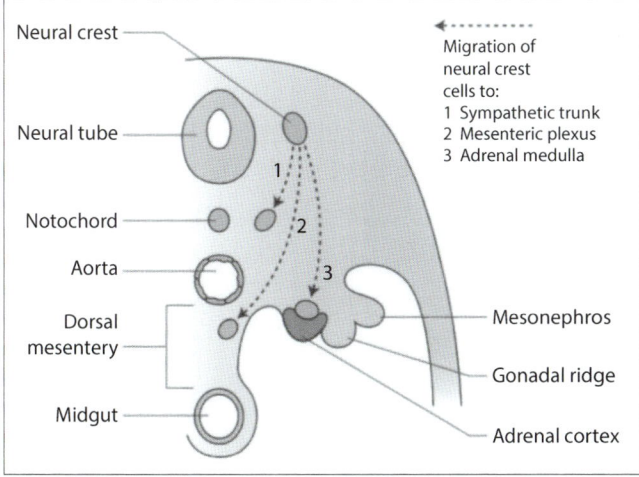

FIGURE 43.1 Embryological migration during development of adrenal glands.

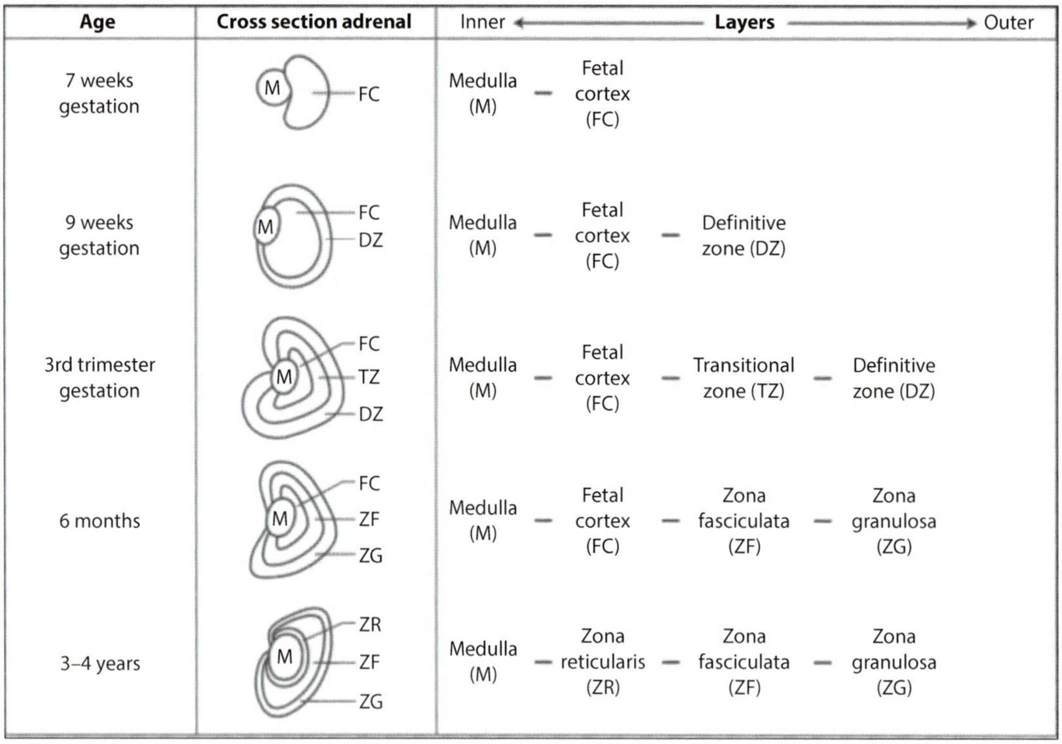

Age
Cross section adrenal
Inner ← Layers → Outer
7 weeks gestation
M
FC
Medulla (M) – Fetal cortex (FC)
9 weeks gestation
M
FC
DZ
Medulla (M) – Fetal cortex (FC) – Definitive zone (DZ)
3rd trimester gestation
M
FC
TZ
DZ
Medulla (M) – Fetal cortex (FC) – Transitional zone (TZ) – Definitive zone (DZ)
6 months
M
FC
ZF
ZG
Medulla (M) – Fetal cortex (FC) – Zona fasciculata (ZF) – Zona granulosa (ZG)
3–4 years
M
ZR
ZF
ZG
Medulla (M) – Zona reticularis (ZR) – Zona fasciculata (ZF) – Zona granulosa (ZG)

FIGURE 43.2 Development of various layers of adrenal gland.

surrounding adipose tissue. This differentiation is more evident in infants and young children than adults due to lesser amount of retroperitoneal fat in the former. This distinct color serves as a useful guide while performing gross total resections of adrenocortical carcinomas, neuroblastomas, and lymph nodes.

Both the glands have different shapes. The right adrenal gland is pyramidal and smaller than the left counterpart (Figure 43.3)[2]. It lies in close proximity to the bare area of the right lobe of the liver anteriorly, the vena cava medially, the duodenum anteromedially, the diaphragm and pleura posteriorly, and the upper pole of the right kidney inferiorly. The right gland lays more cephalad than the left. The position of the right adrenal gland is fixed and does not move down when the kidney is retracted downward. The left adrenal gland is crescentic and bordered by the abdominal

Hepatic veins
Right adrenal vein
Left adrenal vein
1
2
3
3
Arterial blood supply to adrenal:
1 Inferior phrenic arteries
2 Aorta
3 Renal arteries
IVC
Aorta

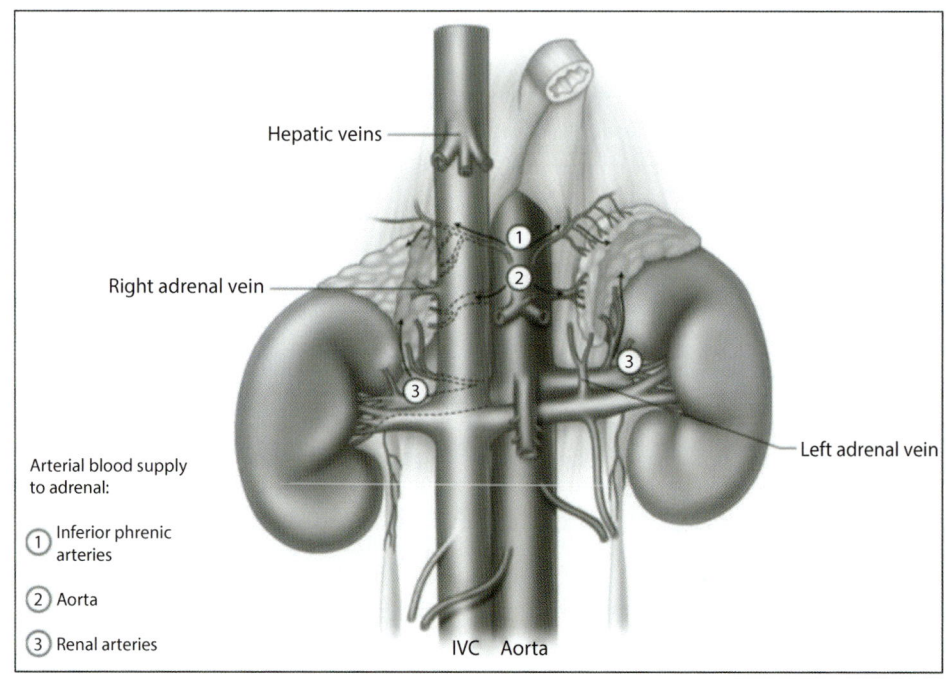

FIGURE 43.3 Anatomical relations of adrenal glands.

Adrenal Gland

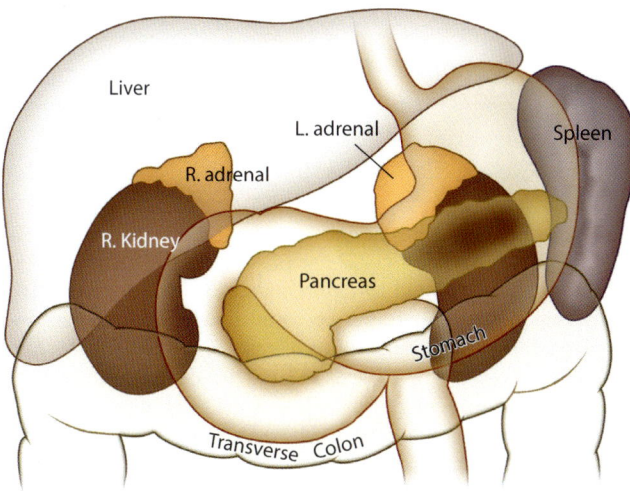

FIGURE 43.4 Anatomical relations of adrenal glands.

aorta medially, the cardiac part of the stomach and the body of the pancreas anteriorly, the spleen superiorly, the kidney inferiorly, and the diaphragm and pleura posteriorly (Figure 43.4). The posterolateral anatomy of both the glands is basically the same.

The right adrenal gland derives its arterial supply through the superior, middle, and inferior adrenal arteries from the inferior phrenic artery, the abdominal aorta, and the renal artery, respectively (Figure 43.3)[2]. Left gland has similar arterial supply as the right gland. The anatomy of the arterial system is unpredictable and variable; sometimes adrenal arteries can also arise from the intercostal or gonadal arteries. These arteries enter the gland along the medial aspect, giving rise to a dense network of vessels supplying the three layers of the adrenal cortex and medulla. The vessels enlarge and engorge in the case of mass lesions within the gland.

Each adrenal has a dominant vein along with some smaller accessory veins adjacent to the adrenal arteries[8]. Various anatomic variants have been reported, the incidence reaches up to 50%[9]. The right adrenal vein takes a short (1 cm) transverse route at an angle of 45 degrees to empty into the posterior segment of the inferior vena cava and is usually not exposed until the adrenal gland is mobilized. Consequently, meticulous dissection of the right adrenal vein is essential to avoid nicking the inferior vena cava. The right inferior phrenic vein and aberrant smaller veins found in 5%–10% of right adrenal glands may drain into the right hepatic or renal vein[10]. These veins should be recognized intraoperatively to avoid accidental ligation of the right renal vein. The left adrenal vein takes a longer course of 2–3 cm, passing downward from the lower medial aspect of the gland, receiving the left inferior phrenic vein before draining into the left renal vein. Occasionally, the left adrenal vein empties into the left inferior phrenic vein before entering the left renal vein or courses over the aorta to enter the inferior vena cava directly. The longer course of the left adrenal vein facilitates venous control during the left adrenalectomy.

The lymphatic drainage also differs for both the glands. On the right, the adrenal lymphatics drain into the paracrural, paraaortic, and paracaval lymph nodes, whereas on the left, the lymphatics from the adrenal drains initially into the paraaortic and left renal hilar lymph nodes. The lymphatics from adrenal may also drain directly into the thoracic duct and the posterior mediastinal nodes[8].

References

1. Barwick TD, Malhotra A, Webb JAW, Savage MO, Reznek RH. Embryology of the adrenal glands and its relevance to diagnostic imaging. Clin Radiol. 2005 Sep;60(9):953–959.
2. Vasudevan S, Brandt ML. Adrenal gland embryology, anatomy, and physiology. In: Ledbetter DJ, Johnson PRV, ed., Endocrine Surgery in Children. Berlin; Heidelberg: Springer; 2018. pp. 77–85.
3. The Developing Human – 10th Edition.
4. Savaş C, Candir O, Bezir M, Cakmak M. Ectopic adrenocortical nodules along the spermatic cord of children. Int Urol Nephrol. 2001;32(4):681–685.
5. Kempná P, Flück CE. Adrenal gland development and defects. Best Pract Res Clin Endocrinol Metab. 2008 Feb;22(1):77–93.
6. O'Leary JP, Tabuenca A, Capote LR. The Physiologic Basis of Surgery. Lippincott Williams & Wilkins; 2008. 778 p.
7. Adams MS, Bronner-Fraser M. Review: The role of neural crest cells in the endocrine system. Endocr Pathol. 2009;20(2):92–100.
8. Avisse C, Marcus C, Patey M, Ladam-Marcus V, Delattre JF, Flament JB. Surgical anatomy and embryology of the adrenal glands. Surg Clin North Am. 2000 Feb;80(1):403–415.
9. Parnaby CN, Galbraith N, O'Dwyer PJ. Experience in identifying the venous drainage of the adrenal gland during laparoscopic adrenalectomy. Clin Anat. 2008 Oct;21(7):660–665.
10. Scholten A, Cisco RM, Vriens MR, Shen WT, Duh Q-Y. Variant adrenal venous anatomy in 546 laparoscopic adrenalectomies. JAMA Surg. 2013 Apr;148(4):378.

44

PHYSIOLOGY OF THE ADRENAL GLAND

Sandeep Bhattacharya

Physiology of adrenal gland

Adrenal gland (also known as suprarenal gland) (ad: near; renal: kidney) are bilateral structures, just above both kidneys, weighing 9–11 g. Adrenal gland is similar to pituitary gland, in the sense that they are derived both from neuronal and epithelial-like tissue.

Around the sixth week of gestation, the outer part, **adrenal cortex**, develops from mesodermal cells near the superior pole of developing kidney. The timing very appropriately coincides with the time of sexual differentiation (seventh to ninth week of gestation). These cells form the endocrine epithelial cells that are steroidogenic. These differentiate into the zona glomerulosa, the zona fasciculata, and the zona reticularis – that produce mineralocorticoids, glucocorticoids, and adrenal androgens, respectively.

The inside core part, **adrenal medulla**, is derived from neural crest cells associated with sympathetic ganglia, called *chromaffin cells*. These form postganglionic sympathetic neuron, synthesizing epinephrine; the preganglionic part is the cholinergic sympathetic neuron.

Adrenal medulla

Adrenal medulla releases catecholamine, epinephrine, into blood, which acts as a hormone. A total of 80% of medullary cells release epinephrine, remaining 20% release norepinephrine. Since adrenal medulla is not the sole source of catecholamine production, this part of the tissue is not essential for life.

Synthesis of epinephrine

Synthesis begins with the transport of amino acid tyrosine into the cytoplasm of chromaffin cells and hydroxylation by tyrosine hydroxylase (rate-limiting step) to dihydroxyphenylalanine (DOPA), which is decarboxylated into dopamine. Dopamine moves inside the granules of chromaffin cells and is hydroxylated by dopamine β-hydroxylase enzymes into norepinephrine that diffuse into the cytoplasm. In the cytoplasm, norepinephrine is methylated by the cytoplasmic enzyme phenylethanolamine-N-methyltransferase (PNMT) to form epinephrine, which is transported back into chromaffin granules.

The primary autonomic centers that initiate sympathetic responses reside in the hypothalamus and brain stem, and they receive input from the cerebral cortex, the limbic system, and other regions of the hypothalamus and brain stem. The increased sympathetic stimulation in response to various stress, including exercise, trauma, pain, shock, and hypoglycemia, increases the release of epinephrine and norepinephrine from the adrenal medulla.

The chemical signal for adrenal medulla to release catecholamine is acetylcholine (Ach), which comes from preganglionic sympathetic neuron to chromaffin cells, where Ach binds to nicotinic receptors on chromaffin cells and increases the activity of rate-limiting enzyme, tyrosine hydroxylase, dopamine β-hydroxylase and increases the release of granules. Increased stimulation causes increased release of catecholamines, so much that the intracellular catecholamine level in the chromaffin cell remains constant even with the increased sympathetic stimulation. Figure 44.1 outlines the major steps in catecholamine synthesis.

Role of arterial structure in adrenal

Cortisol prevents adrenal medulla cells from differentiating into axons and dendrites. Cortisol also increases enzyme PNMT, which is required for the methylation of norepinephrine to epinephrine. All these become possible because medulla remains bathed with a high concentration of cortisol due to special anatomy of its blood supply, a portal venous system, where blood moves centripetally from cortex to medulla. This is the basis of cross talk of adrenal cortex and adrenal medulla. [2]

The outer adrenal capsule is penetrated by three major vessels – superior, middle, and inferior suprarenal arteries. These give rise to two types of branches. Few relatively direct penetrating branches to medulla carry nutrition to chromaffin cells, while numerous others form a network of interconnecting vessels – sinusoids, in the region of adrenal cortex. Cortical cells release their steroid hormones (including cortisol) in these sinusoidal vessels. These vessels continue into the plexus of vessels around adrenal medullary cells, bathing chromaffin cells in cortisol, before joining into suprarenal vein. In this way, cortisol release keeps a control on the release of catecholamines also (by controlling PNMT expression). [3]

Mode of action of catecholamines

Adrenergic receptors are of two major types – alpha and beta. Alpha is further subtyped into α1 and α2 receptors, and the β-adrenergic receptors are divided into β1, β2, and β3 receptors. While both types of receptors are acted upon by both catecholamines, however, epinephrine is more potent than norepinephrine for beta receptors.

Degradation of catecholamines

Both epinephrine and metanephrine are uptaken into the presynaptic terminals and methylated by enzymes catechol-O-methyltransferase (COMT) into metanephrine and normetanephrine, respectively, which is converted into vanillylmandelic acid (VMA) by monoamine oxidase (MAO). Much of the circulating catecholamines are degraded into non-neuronal tissue like the liver and kidney. Urinary VMA and metanephrine are used clinically to assess the level of catecholamine production in a patient. Much of the urinary VMA and metanephrine is derived from neuronal rather than adrenal catecholamines.

Further discussion on sympathetic receptors, their site, and mode of action are beyond the scope of this chapter.

Physiology of the Adrenal Gland

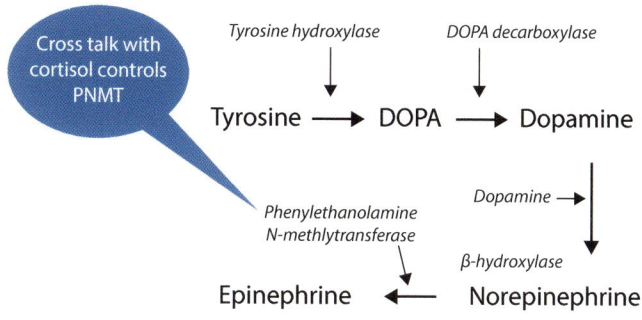

FIGURE 44.1 Biosynthesis of catecholamine. [1]

Adrenal cortex

The adrenal cortex, the outer portion of the adrenal gland, develops from the mesodermal cells, comprises three layers that surround the medulla.

- Outermost layer contains the glomerulosa cells that secrete aldosterone
- Two inner layers of cortex (fasciculata and reticularis) synthesize cortisol and sex steroids

The blood supply enters the cortex in the subcapsular region and flows through anastomotic capillary beds while coursing through both the cortex and the medulla.

Zona fasciculata comprises chords of epithelial cells secreting glucocorticoid hormone, cortisol. These cells take up cholesterol (as LDL or HDL) from blood, storing them as cholesterol esters, which are seen as "foamy cytoplasm," that are nothing but lipid droplets. Stored esters are turned back into cholesterol by enzyme cholesterol ester hydrolase, which is stimulated by ACTH. [4]

Figure 44.2 shows synthetic pathways of all steroid hormones in adrenal cortex [3]

- C21 steroids carry both mineralocorticoids and glucocorticoid activity
- C19 steroids are androgens
- C18 steroid is estradiol

The consequence of deficiency of any of the enzymes can be easily predicted from the above flowchart. The congenital defect leads to increased ACTH secretion, thus causing *syndrome of congenital adrenal hyperplasia*.

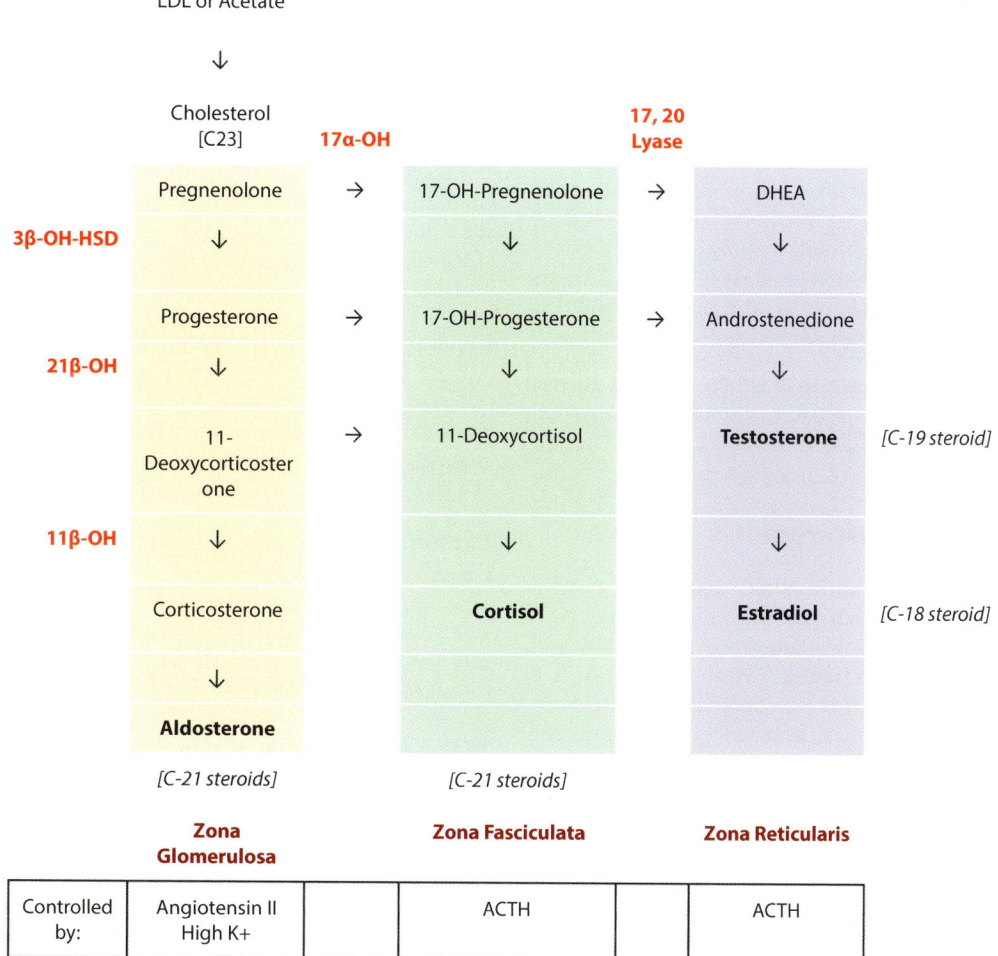

FIGURE 44.2 Synthetic pathways of all steroid hormones in adrenal cortex.

Deficiency of enzymes leading to various congenital syndromes: [3]

Cholesterol desmolase enzyme deficiency is fatal because it prevents the production of Pregnenolone.

3β-Hydroxysteroid dehydrogenase (3β-OH-HSD) deficiency – A lot of DHEA accumulates, while other hormones are not formed. DHEA being a weak steroid causes some masculinization of females but is not able to develop genital organs in genetic males, often presenting as hypospadias.

17α-Hydroxylase (17α-OH) deficiency:

- DHEA, sex hormones are not produced.
- Female external genitals are present.
- Aldosterone pathway remains intact, but cortisol production is decreased.
- High aldosterone leads to mineralocorticoid effect – hypokalemia and hypertension.
- Cortisol activity is partly compensated by glucocorticoid action of corticosterone.

21β-Hydroxylase deficiency is the *most common cause* of congenital adrenal hyperplasia, accounting for almost 90% of cases. 21β-OH Gene is on the short arm of chromosome 6, and its mutation leads to disease spectrum from mild to severe.

- Both cortisol and aldosterone production decreases; thus, intermediary steroids are diverted toward increased androgen production.
- *Females:* High androgen activity leads to virilization causing adrenogenital syndrome in females often presenting later in life.
- *Males:* They are phenotypically normal at birth but develop precocious pseudo-puberty, growth acceleration, premature epiphyseal plate closure, and diminished final height.
- *Low mineralocorticoid:* It often causes salt loss and consequent hypovolemia.
- Neonates may present with salt-wasting crisis.
- Goal of treatment is to inhibit pituitary ACTH by glucocorticoid treatment; this also repairs the glucocorticoid deficiency as well as suppresses adrenal androgen secretion.

11β-Hydroxylase deficiency causes aldosterone and cortisol deficiency with virilization and excess intermediary steroids, which have high mineralocorticoid activity leading to hypertension, salt and water retention.

Aldosterone

Aldosterone determines the extracellular volume by controlling renal Na^+ loss in the principal cells of collecting duct (CD). Sodium being an osmotically active substance retains water with itself and thus the extracellular volume. Extracellular Fluid (ECF) volume is itself a determinant for blood pressure; hence, aldosterone has an important role in the maintenance of blood pressure. The Na^+-conserving action of aldosterone is also seen in salivary ducts, sweat glands, and the distal colon. Aldosterone also causes secretion of H^+ in the intercalated cells and secretion of K^+ in the principal cells of CD. [5]

Thus, primary actions of aldosterone are as follows:

- Na retention (by creating ENac sodium channels)
- K loss in urine (consequential K loss in tubular secretion)
- H^+ loss in urine (activates H^+ pump in distal tubule/CD thus H^+ loss)

Regulation of aldosterone secretion

Unlike zona fasciculata and reticularis, zona glomerulosa secreting aldosterone is less affected by ACTH. Immediately after hypophysectomy, the zona fasciculata and zona reticularis begin to atrophy, whereas the zona glomerulosa is unchanged because of the action of angiotensin II on this zone. The ability to secrete aldosterone and conserve Na^+ is normal for some time after hypophysectomy.

Angiotensin II and plasma K^+ seem to be the major determinant of feedback control for aldosterone. Angiotensin II binds to AT1 receptors in zona glomerulosa causing activation of phospholipase C pathway that activates aldosterone synthase and thus produces aldosterone. Angiotensin II also increases the conversion of cholesterol to pregnenolone.

- Decrease in ECF volume causes → decrease in hydrostatic pressure → decrease in filtration → decrease in Na load delivery to macula densa → renin activates increase in angiotensin II.

Angiotensin II has two primary actions:

a. Vasoconstriction → increase ECF pressure
b. Increase aldosterone → Na reabsorption → water reabsorption → increase ECF volume

Hence, the very cause (decreased ECF volume and pressure) gets corrected.

Compare the action of aldosterone vs vasopressin

Aldosterone is stimulated primarily due to a fall in ECF *volume*, which it corrects by *Na* reabsorption into ECF → correction of ECF volume and pressure. Thus, aldosterone remains a determinant for blood pressure regulation.

Vasopressin is secreted mainly due to ECF *osmolality* (i.e. Na concentration), which it corrects by *water* reabsorption and consequent restoration of osmolality.

Vasopressin does not remain a major determinant for blood pressure regulation.

Mechanism of action of aldosterone

Aldosterone binds to cytoplasmic receptor and moves to nucleus to activate the gene for serum and glucocorticoid regulated kinase (SGK), which causes increased synthesis of epithelial sodium channel (ENaC) that inserts into the epithelium of principal cells of CD. ENaC causes reabsorption of Na^+ from tubular fluid.

Physiological basis of primary hyperaldosteronism: Conn's syndrome [5]

- Etiology is usually an adenoma of the zona glomerulosa, adrenal hyperplasia, and adrenal carcinoma. Bilateral micronodular adrenal hyperplasia is a more common cause (60%) than unilateral.

TABLE 44.1: Conditions that Increase Aldosterone Secretion [5]:

Glucocorticoid secretion also increased:
Surgery, anxiety, physical trauma, hemorrhage
Glucocorticoid secretion unaffected:
High potassium intake, low sodium intake,
Constriction of inferior vena cava in thorax,
Standing
Secondary hyperaldosteronism (congestive heart failure, cirrhosis, and nephrosis)

Physiology of the Adrenal Gland

- Renin secretion is depressed (due to secondary suppression by increased ECF volume).
- Hypokalemia and consequent weakness occur (due to K^+ wasting by aldosterone excess).
- Increased whole-body sodium, fluid, and circulating blood volume occur
- But hypernatremia is infrequent.
- Hypertension occurs due to increased ECF volume and pressure. *Detection of hypertension with hypokalemia is often the initial clue for Conn's syndrome.*
- Edema does *not* occur. This is due to the phenomenon of "aldosterone escape," which is due to increased ANP secretion.
- Metabolic alkalosis occurs due to H^+ loss (aldosterone activates H^+ pump in distal tubule of nephron)

Secondary hyperaldosteronism with hypotension

This occurs due to the collection of blood on the venous side of circulation. Such a condition may be caused by the following:

- Cirrhosis
- Congestive heart failure
- Nephrosis

Thus, leads to decreased arterial blood flow to renal artery and high renin and aldosterone secretion → high ECF volume, high Na and edema.

Edema occurs in secondary hyperaldosteronism since most of the ECF volume is on the venous side, and the escape mechanism does not operate.

Glucocorticoids

Primarily secreted as cortisol, it is mainly bound to corticosteroid-binding protein (CBG) that is secreted in the liver. Protein-bound cortisol and free plasma cortisol remain in dynamic equilibrium, getting unbound from the protein as free cortisol level falls. Free cortisol level gives a negative feedback to pituitary for the release of ACTH.

Metabolic actions of cortisol

Protein metabolism: Cortisol is a catabolic hormone. It promotes the degradation of muscle protein and the activation of gluconeogenesis. Thus, its excess can cause general weakness, muscle loss, and osteoporosis (fractures).

Fat metabolism: Cortisol causes movement of lipid from adipose tissues to FFA, but in high state, it causes deposition of these lipids on the face and trunk, leading to Cushingoid appearance.

The classical triad: Moon-like facies; buffalo like hump; truncal obesity.

Carbohydrate metabolism: Cortisol causes the availability of more glucose for meeting out the stress by its anti-insulin action and by increased gluconeogenesis. Continued high cortisol levels will stimulate insulin resistance to develop and consequently unveil diabetes mellitus.

Other actions of glucocorticoids: High glucocorticoids decrease growth hormone secretion, induce PNMT, and decrease TSH secretion.

In fetal life, glucocorticoids cause the maturation of surfactants. [5]

Regulation of cortisol secretion

Cortisol secretion shows circadian patterns with high cortisol secretion in the morning and low in the evening. A total of 75% of the daily production of cortisol occurs between 4:00 and 10:00 a.m. The bursts are least frequent in the evening. High cortisol levels in the morning coincide with higher glucose levels for an early morning activity.

Cortisol is essentially secreted in response to stress. Free cortisol gives negative feedback stimuli to pituitary and hypothalamus. Hypothalamus secretes corticosteroid regulating hormone (CRH), which stimulates anterior pituitary to secrete ACTH that is released in the blood to stimulate adrenals. ACTH is the primary stimulatory hormone for both cortisol and androgens secretion but to a lesser degree for aldosterone secretion.

Hypercortisolism: It can be primary or secondary.

Primary hypercortisolism: It is ACTH independent, cortisol is increased (ACTH is depressed). Usually, it is due to adrenal adenoma that secretes only cortisol.

Secondary hypercortisolism: It is due to high ACTH that stimulates adrenal to secrete high cortisol and androgens. ACTH can come from either of two sources:

- *Anterior pituitary*: Usually microadenoma in pituitary causing high ACTH.
  Also known as Cushing's disease.
- *Ectopic ACTH*: Usually due to small-cell carcinoma of the lung.

  High ACTH secreting ectopic site is not suppressible with dexamethasone test dose.

Physiological basis of Cushing's syndrome

High cortisol levels due to any cause create characteristic changes in body, which are as follows:

- *Obesity:* Due to movement of lipids and their deposition in central areas like face (moon facies), upper back (buffalo hump), and trunk (truncal obesity).
- Protein depletion due to excessive catabolism, causing muscle breakdown, osteoporosis, and fractures.
- Hyperglycemia due to increased insulin resistance.
- Increased androgens when present in females lead to acne, hirsutism, and amenorrhea.
- Mineralocorticoid effect leads to salt retention, potassium depletion (weakness), and alkalosis.
- Decreased inflammatory response, anxiety, and depression occur due to cortisol. (cf: Cross talk of adrenal medulla and cortex mentioned above)

Hypocortisolism

Addison's disease is primary adrenal insufficiency, with both mineralocorticoids and glucocorticoids usually being deficient. Usual cause of Addison's disease is autoimmune destruction of the adrenal cortex. Different physiological changes that occur are as follows:

1. Decreased cortisol → ACTH secretion increases. → ACTH competes for MC1R in melanocytes and causes an increase in skin pigmentation, especially skin creases, scars, and gums.
2. Decreased mineralocorticoids → contraction of ECF → circulatory hypovolemia and drop in blood pressure.

3. Decreased cortisol → decreases the vasopressive response to catecholamines → peripheral vascular resistance drops → hypotension.
4. Decreased cortisol → prone to hypoglycemia when stressed or fasting, and water intoxication. Also muscle weakness, anemia, decreased GI motility and secretion, reduced iron and vitamin B12 absorption, weight loss, and some psychiatric disorders. [3]

Conclusion

Adrenal gland forms an integral part of metabolic system of body wherein it not only controls various metabolic processes for energy utilization in terms of an emergency situation but also provides permissive effect for most of the other hormones of the body. The cross talk between the two constituents of the gland medulla and cortex helps in the fine tuning of the emergency response, but at the same time in view of increased stressor stimuli at hypothalamus level, it becomes the crux for many of the noncommunicable diseases of this era.

References

1. Bylund DB. Norepinephrine. In: Encyclopedia of the Neurological Sciences; 2003.
2. Trikudanathan S, Williams GH. Primer on the Autonomic Nervous System. 3rd ed., 2012.
3. Koeppen BM, Stanton BA, eds. Berne & Levy Physiology, 6th ed.
4. Walter FB, Boulpaep EL, ed. Medical Physiology: A Cellular and Molecular Approach. 2nd ed.
5. Barrett KE, Barman, SM, Boitano S, Brooks H. Ganong's Review of Medical Physiology. 24th ed. The McGraw-Hill Companies, Inc.
6. Wall RT. Stoelting's Anesthesia and Co-Existing Disease. Chapter 23.

45

BIOCHEMICAL EVALUATION OF AN ADRENAL MASS

Manish Gutch, Sukriti Kumar, Maghvendra Kumar and Manjari Dwivedi

Introduction

Adrenal gland tumors are common diseases in clinical practices. According to the way they manifest themselves, they are classified into functioning (hormone secreting) and nonfunctioning. In terms of biological behavior, they can be divided into benign or malignant tumors [1].

Most adrenocortical tumors are benign, unilateral and nonfunctioning adenomas, presenting less than 4 cm in diameter, perceived during abdominal imaging studies [1].

An adrenal incidentaloma is defined as an adrenal mass, clinically unsuspected, which is found in imaging studies conducted for reasons other than the evaluation of the adrenal glands. In recent years, the prevalence of adrenal adenomas has increased due to the use of abdominal imaging with increasing sensitivity [2]. An adrenal mass is diagnosed in up to 4% of patients imaged for nonadrenal disease [3]. In true incidentalomas, size appears to be predictive of malignancy: Fewer than 2% of incidentalomas smaller than 4 cm but 25% of those larger than 6 cm in diameter are malignant [2].

Functioning tumors with a clear clinical phenotype (pheochromocytomas and those secreting cortisol, aldosterone or sex steroids) and carcinomas account for around 4% of all incidentalomas. Functioning adrenal tumors are usually of the benign adenoma type, which causes Cushing's syndrome, primary aldosteronism (PA) or virilization (less commonly) [4, 5]. Pheochromocytomas, despite being rare, have important implications due to increased risk of associated morbidity and mortality [1].

Epidemiology

In a combined study with different selection and diagnostic criteria, main etiologies of adrenal tumors are described as mentioned in Figure 45.1 [2].

In clinical reports, adrenal incidentalomas show peak incidence in the fifth to seventh decades. The mean age of patients at diagnosis is 55 years, with no significant differences in age between female and male [6].

The prevalence increases with age; the rate is less than 1% for patients under 30 and 7% for patients aged 70 and over [7].

Although most of the adrenal tumors are not functioning, a slightly increased production of certain hormones can be verified in at least 15% of the cases.

Hormonal evaluation

Adenomas or adrenal carcinomas secreting cortisol, pheochromocytomas, aldosteronomas and secretory lesions of androgens are the types of secretory or functioning adrenal masses diagnosed more frequently [4].

Cortisol-producing tumors

These tumors usually produce lesser amounts of cortisol, which, in most cases, are not sufficient to increase the excretion of free cortisol in urine. They are, however, capable of causing the suppression of the hypothalamic-pituitary axis. Usually, there are no manifestations related to Cushing's syndrome in patients. For this reason, this condition is known as subclinical Cushing's syndrome or subclinical hypercortisolism [4]. Subclinical Cushing's syndrome occurs in up to 20–30% of all patients with adrenocortical incidentalomas [3, 8, 9]. The best means to biochemically define this phenomenon is still debatable but serum cortisol after dexamethasone testing has the widest acceptance, although cut-off values vary. The European Society of Endocrinology and European Network for the Study of Adrenal Tumors (ENSAT) have published guidelines for diagnosis and management [10].

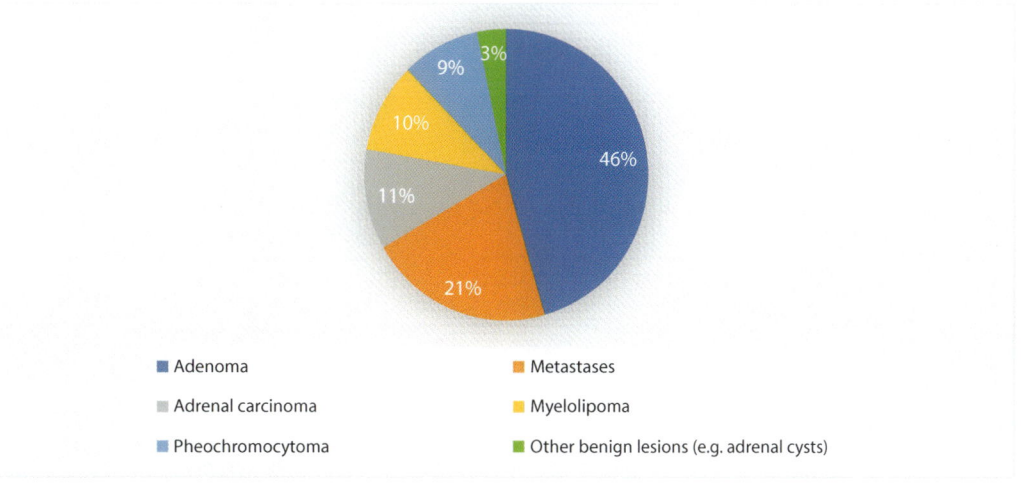

FIGURE 45.1 Etiology of adrenal tumors [2].

It is important to highlight the difference between subclinical Cushing's syndrome, characterized by a clinically non-manifested biochemical abnormality and preclinical Cushing's syndrome, which is the initial stage of the development of the syndrome itself. The subclinical autonomous glucocorticoid hypersecretion (SAGH) is the most current term, proposed to define an autonomous cortisol secretion by an adrenal adenoma in patients without symptoms of Cushing's syndrome [2]. Follow-up of patients with adrenal incidentaloma have shown a very low percentage (<1%) of patients with "autonomous cortisol secretion" actually progress to overt Cushing's syndrome [11].

In adults, the most suggestive signs and symptoms of the presence of hypercortisolism include proximal muscle weakness, facial plethora, loss of fat in limbs with increased fat in the abdomen and face, wide purple striae, hematomas without obvious trauma [11].

However, due to many symptoms of hypercortisolism, among them, hypertension and diabetes are not characteristic, and the degree of their clinical appearance is consistent with the variation in the extent of hormonal overproduction, the precise indication of the prevalence of SAGH, will be subjected to the results obtained by the methods of the tests used and the criteria for the selection of symptomatic patients for the confirmation of the disease [2].

For evaluation of cortisol, excess 1-mg dexamethasone suppression test (DST) should be performed overnight. The day before the collection of serum cortisol that occurs at 8 a.m., the patient takes 1 mg of dexamethasone orally at 11 p.m. [4].

In the case of the diagnosis of subclinical Cushing's syndrome, the most acceptable criterion used is 8 a.m. plasma cortisol >5 μg/dl in the 1-mg DST without any other Cushing's stigmata. 8 a.m. plasma cortisol value following 1 mg DST of <1.8 μg/dl are regarded as normal, whereas the value between 1.8 and 5 μg/dl is defined as "possible autonomous cortisol secretion". The finding of abnormal 1-mg DST need be confirmed with 24-hour urinary free cortisol, ACTH and 8 mg overnight DST.

Testing protocols and cutoffs regarding subclinical Cushing's syndrome are still debatable and the published literature is too limited to make a clear statement on these tests. Thus, it is difficult to reach a consensus for the approach of subclinical Cushing's syndrome, which can be treated clinically or through surgery [5]. For patients with comorbidities that may be related to hypercortisolism, the risk/benefit of adrenalectomy should be considered as a treatment. A large part of the patients undergoing this surgery may develop acute adrenal insufficiency (sometimes fatal), so perioperative coverage with glucocorticoid administration is required.

Figure 45.2 outlines the approach for evaluation and treatment of subclinical Cushing's syndrome.

Catecholamine-producing tumors

Pheochromocytomas are tumors of chromaffin cells of the adrenal medulla that produce, store, metabolized and secrete catecholamines. Paragangliomas (PGLs) are similar tumors, but of extra adrenal origin. Pheochromocytoma/PGL (PPGL) syndrome is a rare disease, with an estimated prevalence between 0.1% and 0.2% of the population of hypertensive individuals [4].

Most catecholamine-secreting tumors are sporadic. However, approximately in 40% the disease, it is familial. In these patients, catecholamine-secreting tumors are more likely to be bilateral adrenal pheochromocytomas or PGLs.

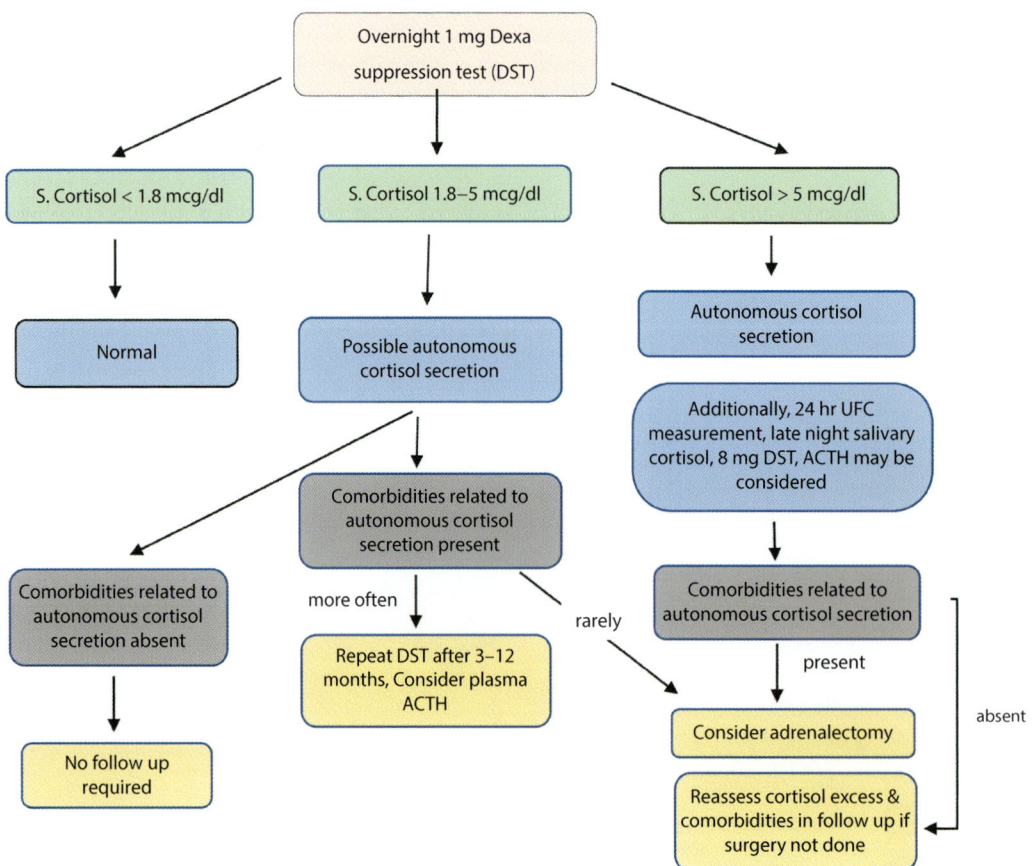

FIGURE 45.2 Algorithm for assessment and management of "autonomous cortisol secretion" in adrenal incidentaloma.

Biochemical Evaluation of an Adrenal Mass

There are several family disorders associated with pheochromocytoma, all with autosomal dominant inheritance:

- Von Hippel-Lindau syndrome (VHL), associated with mutations in the VHL tumor suppressor gene.
- Endocrine multiple neoplasm type 2 (MEN2), associated with mutations in proto-oncogene RET.
- Pheochromocytoma is also observed, although infrequently, of neurofibromatosis type 1 (NF1), due to mutations in the NF1 gene.
- The approximate frequency of pheochromocytoma in these disorders is
  - 10–20% in VHL syndrome,
  - 50% in MEN2 and
  - 3% in NF1 [12].

These tumors are of particular importance because, although rare (as well as the secretory adenomas of aldosterone) give rise to a surgically correctable form of hypertension [13]. Hypertension is often paroxysmal. The classic triad of symptoms in patients with pheochromocytoma consists of episodic headaches, sweating and tachycardia, and a significant number of patients do not present with the three classic symptoms. Besides the patients with the typical clinical manifestations of the disease, the investigation should also be done in individuals with a family history of pheochromocytoma or medullary thyroid carcinoma, in the presence of systemic arterial hypertension in young, systemic arterial hypertension of difficult control or anesthetic induction.

The diagnosis of pheochromocytoma is typically made by measurements of metanephrines and fractionated catecholamines in the urine and plasma, as shown in Figure 45.3 [14].

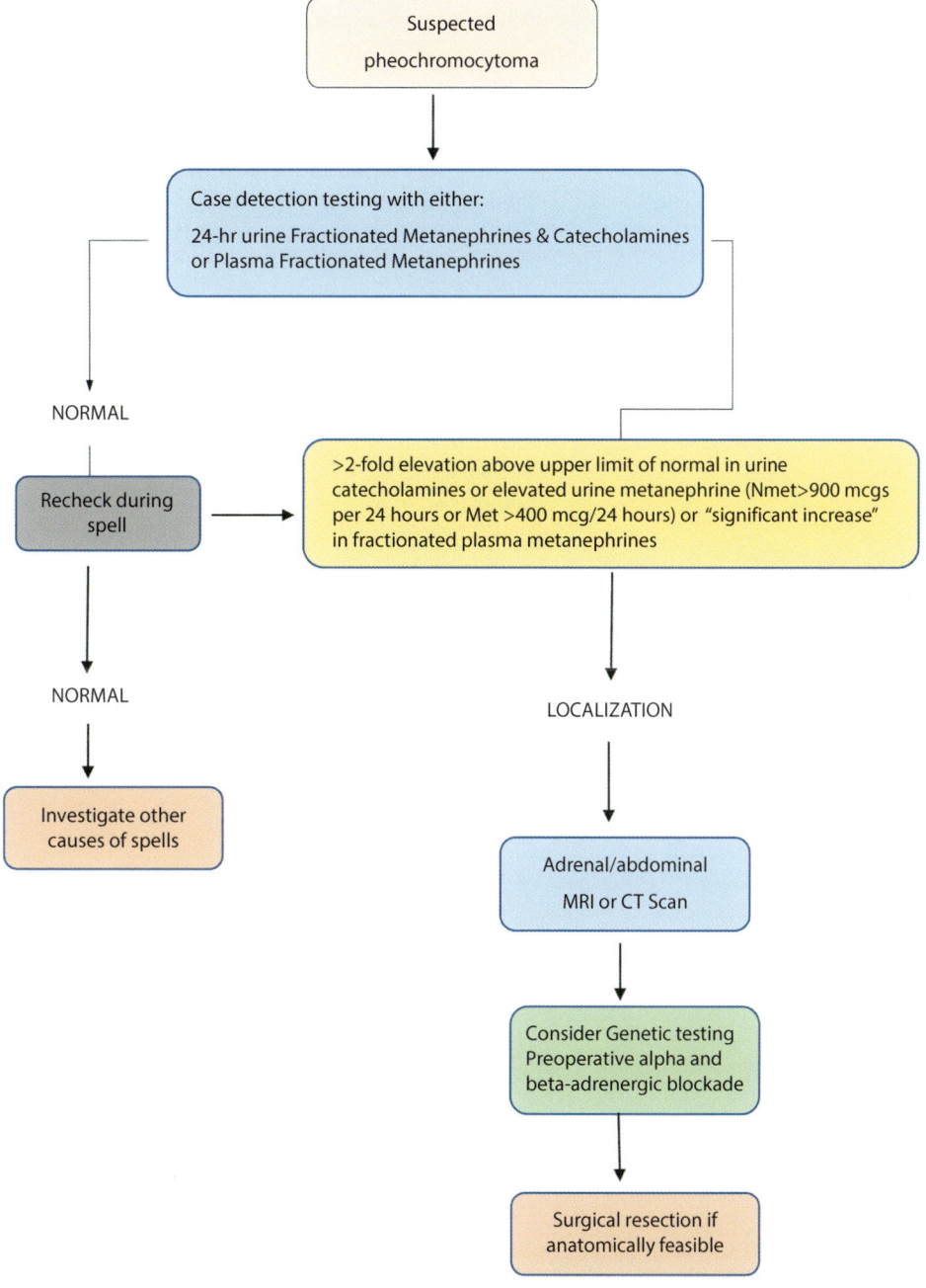

FIGURE 45.3 Algorithm for the investigation of pheochromocytomas in adrenals incidentalomas.

As for the imaging methods, pheochromocytomas have greater attenuation on unenhanced CT (>20 HU), increased vascularization of the mass, delay in contrast medium washing (10 minutes after contrast administration, an absolute contrast medium wash of less than 50%), high signal strength on T2-weighted MRI, cystic and hemorrhagic changes and variable size and can be bilateral.

In contrast, the imaging characteristics that suggest adrenal carcinoma or metastases include: Irregular shape, inhomogeneous density, high unenhanced CT attenuation values (>20 HU), delayed contrast medium washout (e.g., <50% at 10 minutes), diameter >4 cm, and tumor calcification [15].

Aldosterone-producing tumors

Aldosteronomas are uncommon and difficult to detect and are clinically characterized by systemic arterial hypertension associated with hypokalemia. Considering that only a minority of (9–37%) patients with aldosteronomas are hypokalemic [16, 17, 18]. It is recommended that all patients with hypertension associated with adrenal adenoma be evaluated by measuring their plasma aldosterone concentration (PAC) and plasma renin activity (PRA). PA should be suspected if the PRA is suppressed (<1 ng/ml/h) and PAC is increased (e.g., >10 ng/dl). Aldosterone renin ratio (ARR) greater than 30 is highly suggestive of autonomous aldosterone production [4, 18, 19]. A ratio greater than 50 clearly distinguishes PA from other forms of essential hypertension [2, 20–22]. A positive case detection is not diagnostic by itself and must be confirmed by further tests demonstrating inappropriate aldosterone secretion. Oral sodium chloride loading test, intravenous saline infusion and fludrocortisone suppression test are used for confirmation of PA. In patients with spontaneous hypokalemia, plasma renin below detection levels plus plasma aldosterone >20 ng/dl, it is suggested that there is no need for further confirmatory testing [23].

A number of medications may affect the interpretation of ARR as shown in Table 45.1 [5,23].

Adrenal catheterization is the method of evaluation conducive to verifying whether the increase in aldosterone production in patients over 40 years, with confirmed hyperaldosteronism, is actually caused by incidentaloma or adrenal hyperplasia. Figure 45.4 is the investigational algorithm for hyperaldosteronism in adrenal incidentaloma.

TABLE 45.1: Medications Affecting Aldosterone Renin Ratio

False Negative	False Positive
ACE inhibitors	Beta blocker
ARBs	Methyldopa
Mineralocorticoid receptor antagonist	Clonidine
Thiazide diuretic	NSAID
Ca^+ channel blockers (dihydropyridine)	

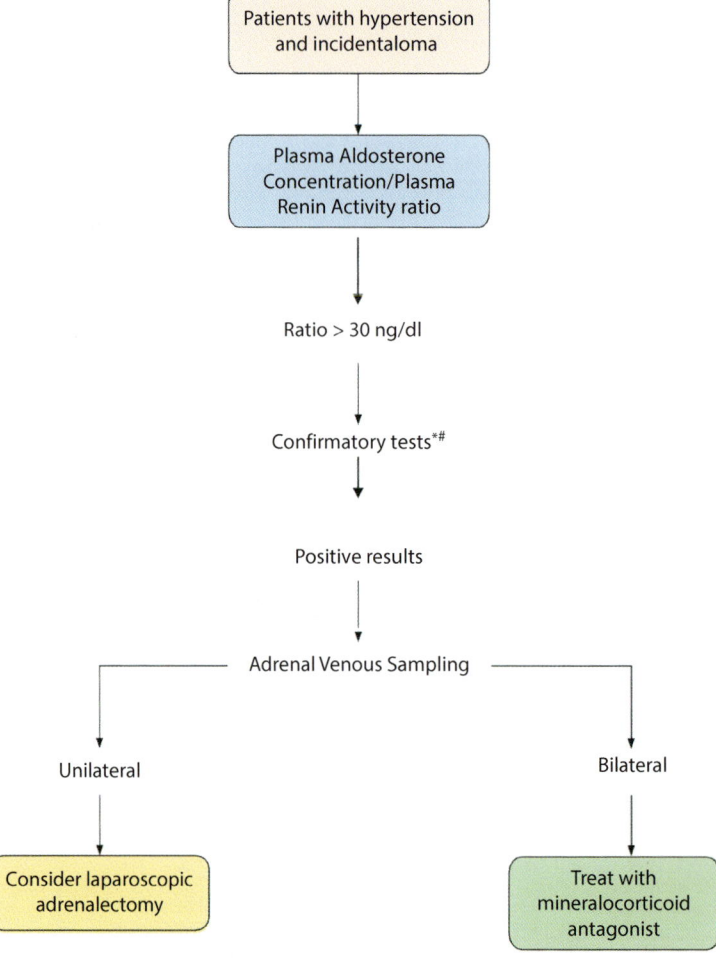

FIGURE 45.4 Algorithm for the investigation of hyperaldosteronism in adrenals incidentalomas. *#Most commonly used confirmatory tests: Oral sodium load test, intravenous saline infusion test.

In such cases, adrenalectomy would not solve hormonal hyperproduction, which should be kept under control with the use of medication, aldosterone antagonists such as spironolactone [5].

Androgen and estrogen producing tumors

In cases of congenital adrenal hyperplasia due to a 21-hydroxylase deficiency, it is common to find adrenal masses, unilateral or bilateral, as a consequence of the chronic excessive stimulation of adrenals by ACTH [4].

The adrenal adenoma that produces sex hormone is very rare. Androgen-producing carcinoma is also uncommon. Cases of androgens or estrogen excesses are rarely described in patients with benign adrenocortical adenomas but in general, they are manifested by symptoms or signs of virilization in women (acne, hirsutism) or feminization in men (gynecomastia). Thus, the need to measure sex hormones and steroid precursors is limited except in cases of adrenal lesions with imaging features suggestive of malignancy, where elevated levels may point to the adrenocortical origin of the tumor and suggesting the presence of an adrenal adenocarcinoma [24]. Adrenalectomy is indicated for the control of hormones in individuals with virilization or high concentrations of androgens [4].

Estrogen-producing tumors are uncommon and, in most cases, malignant. The presence of these tumors in men is usually manifested through feminization with gynecomastia, decreased libido, atrophy of the testicles; in women, it can manifest through breast tenderness and bleeding [19]. In such cases, adrenalectomy may be indicated.

Discussion

In patients presenting with adrenal tumors, a through clinical history and physical examination along with appropriate endocrine tests is required to assess for the evidence of hormone excess. Studies published in medical literature mention several protocols used for hormonal investigation, and the most frequently used are the ones that uses serum cortisol after overnight suppression, with 1-mg dexamethasone (for subclinical hypercortisolism) and plasma metanephrines. The investigation of aldosteronomas, i.e., determination of plasma aldosterone and PRA is only indicated for cases with hypertension and/or hypokalemia. Advancements in the radiological imaging techniques have enabled better differentiation of benign from malignant lesions guiding further management and follow-up. While dealing with adrenal tumors, main concern for general practitioner should be to recognize and evaluate whether the lesion is malignant or functioning, situations in which adrenalectomy is necessary.

Acknowledgments/Conflicts of interest

None of the authors have a conflict of interest.

References

1. Pittella JEH, Coutinho LMB, Hilbig A. Endocrine system. In: F.G. Brazilian, ed., Bogliolo Pathology. 8th ed. Rio de Janeiro: Gen-Guanabara Koogan Group; 2011. p. 1149.
2. Mansmann G, Lau J, Balk E, et al. The clinically inapparent adrenal mass: Update in diagnosis and management. Endocr Rev. 2004;25:309–340.
3. Kloos RT, Gross MD, Francis IR, et al. Incidentally discovered adrenal masses. Endocr Rev. 1995;16:460–484.
4. Vilar L. Handling of adrenals incidentalomas. In: L. Vilar, ed., Endocrinology Clinic. 6th ed. Rio de Janeiro: Koogan Guanabara; 2016. pp. 621–649.
5. Sales P, Santomauro A, Cunha SM, et al. Adrenal incidentaloma. In: P. Sales, A. Halpern and C. Cercato, ed., The Essential in Endocrinology. 1st ed. Rio de Janeiro: Roca; 2016. pp. 121–135.
6. Barzon L, Sonino N, Fallo F, Palu G, Boscaro M. Prevalence and natural history of adrenal incidentalomas. Eur J Endocrinol. 2003;149:273–285.
7. https://emedicine.medscape.com/article/116587-overview#a2.
8. Terzolo M, Bovio S, Reimondo G, et al. Subclinical Cushing's syndrome in adrenal incidentalomas. Endocrinol Metab Clin North Am. 2005;34:423–439, x.
9. Catargi B, Rigalleau V, Poussin A, et al. Occult Cushing's syndrome in type-2 diabetes. J Clin Endocrinol Metab. 2003;88:5808–5813.
10. Fassnacht M, Arlt W, Bancos I, et al. Management of adrenal incidentalomas: European society of endocrinology clinical practice guideline in collaboration with the European Network for the study of adrenal tumors. Eur J Endocrinol. 2016;175(2):G1–G34.
11. Nieman L. Causes and pathophysiology of Cushing's syndrome. In: Basow DS, ed. Waltham UpToDate; 2011.
12. Young WF. Pheochromocytoma in Genetic Disorders. [Internet]. United States: UpToDate; 2018.
13. Kumar V, Abbas A, Fausto N, Mitchell R. Sistema endócrino. In: Robbins Patologia Básica. 9th ed. Philadelphia (PA): Elsevier Health Sciences; 2013. p. 760.
14. Young WF, Lacroix A, Martin KA. Clinical presentation and diagnosis of pheochromocytoma. E-base UpToDate; 2012.
15. Young WF, Kebebew E. TheAdrenal Incidentaloma. E- baser UpToDate; 2018.
16. Mulatero P, Stowasser M, Loh KC, et al. Increased diagnosis of primary aldosteronism, including surgically correctable forms, in centers from five continents. J Clin Endocrinol Metab. 2004;89(3):1045–1050.
17. Piaditis G, Markou A, Papanastasiou L, Androulakis II, Kaltsas G. Progress in aldosteronism: A review of the prevalence of primary aldosteronism in pre-hypertension and hypertension. Eur J Endocrinol. 2015;172(5):R191–R203.
18. Monticone S, Burrello J, Tizzani D, et al. Prevalence and clinical manifestations of primary aldosteronism encountered in primary care practice. J Am Coll Cardiol. 2017;69(14):1811–1820.
19. Stewart PM, Newell-Price JDC. The adrenal cortex. In: S. Melmed, K. Polonsky, P. Reed Larsen, M. Kronenberg and H. Williams, eds., Textbook of Endocrinology. 13th ed. Philadelphia (PA): Elsevier; 2016. pp. 490–555.
20. Young WF Jr, Hogan MJ, Klee GG, Grant CS, Van Heerden JA. Primary aldosteronism: Diagnosis and treatment. Mayo Clin Proc. 1990;65:96–110.
21. McKenna TJ, Sequeira SJ, Heffernan A, Chambers J, Cunningham S. Diagnosis under random conditions of all disorders of the renin-angiotensin-aldosterone axis, including primary hyperaldosteronism. J Clin Endocrinol Metab. 1991;73:952–957.
22. Weinberger MH, Fineberg NS. The diagnosis of primary aldosteronism and separation of two major subtypes. Arch Intern Med. 1993;153:2125–2129.
23. Funder JW, Carey RM, Mantero F, et al. The management of primary aldosternism: Case detection, diagnosis, and treatment: An endocrine society clinical practice guideline. J Clin Endocrinol Metab. 2016;101:1889–1916.
24. https://www.ncbi.nlm.nih.gov/books/NBK279021/.

46

IMAGING OF ADRENAL MASSES

Jyoti Arora, Kulbir Ahlawat and Alka Ashmita Singhal

Introduction

The adrenal glands are routinely visualized on every computed tomography (CT) scan of the abdomen. Although the adrenal gland is involved by a range of diseases, including primary and metastatic malignant tumors, the most common lesion detected is the incidental benign adrenal adenoma.

Adrenal masses can be divided into two physiologic categories based on whether they hypersecrete a hormone or not. Hyperfunctioning adrenal masses produce a hormone that results in a chemical imbalance and include pheochromocytomas, aldosteronomas and cortisol or androgen-producing tumors. Nonfunctioning adrenal masses cause enlargement of the adrenal gland but no significant increased hormone production. Adrenal adenomas and metastases are the most common nonfunctioning adrenal masses.

There are numerous imaging modalities, including CT, magnetic resonance imaging (MRI), ultrasonography and nuclear medicine imaging, which can be used to evaluate the adrenal gland.

CT is the primary modality for both the detection and characterization of adrenal masses. Chemical shift imaging is useful as a problem-solving modality when evaluating the adrenal gland, and T2-weighted imaging may help detect a pheochromocytoma. Nuclear medicine imaging is primarily used for lesions not adequately characterized with CT and MRI. Positron emission tomography (PET) helps in differentiating benign from malignant masses.

Benign adrenal masses

1. Adenoma
2. Myelolipoma
3. Hemorrhage
4. Calcified lesions
5. Adrenal cyst
6. Adrenal cortical hyperplasia
7. Pheochromocytoma

Malignant adrenal masses

1. Adrenal cortical carcinoma
2. Lymphoma
3. Sarcoma
4. Metastasis

Adenoma

Adrenal adenomas are benign neoplasms of the adrenal cortex. Adrenal adenomas are the most common cause of incidentally found adrenal tumors known as "adrenal incidentalomas." Adrenal adenomas can be either hormonally active or inactive, either lipid rich or poor [1].

Typical adenomas (lipid-rich adenomas) are as follows:

- Small (<4 cm).
- Homogenous in attenuation.
- Low density on plain CT scan with HU <10.
- On 15 minutes post-contrast, >60% absolute contrast washout and >40% relative washout.
- *Density evaluation of an adrenal lesion is highly sensitive and specific as 70% of adrenal adenomas contain significant intracellular fat, which are lipid-rich adenomas* (Figure 46.1).

Atypical adenomas (lipid-poor adenomas) can have internal hemorrhage, calcification, necrosis and lack or paucity of fat.

- Larger (>4 cm) in size
- >10 HU on plain CT scan
- On 15 minutes post-contrast, >60% absolute contrast washout and >40% relative washout

Lipid-poor adenomas are more difficult to diagnose as the CT density increases and approaches that of soft tissue density.

- Non-contrast imaging
  - *<0 HU*: Considered 47% sensitive and 100% specific
  - *<10 HU*: Considered 71% sensitive and 98% specific
- Washout imaging
  - 15 minutes post-contrast
  - >60% absolute washout
  - >40% relative washout

MRI: Chemical shift imaging (CSI) is most sensitive for lipid-poor adenomas. It detects minute amounts of intravoxel (i.e. intracellular) fat. It demonstrates signal dropout on opposed-phase images, a drop in signal intensity of >16.5% is considered diagnostic for an adenoma. At T2-weighted MRI, adrenal adenomas tend to be homogeneous and show intermediate-to-low signal intensity compared with skeletal muscle or liver; however, when large, adenomas may undergo cystic degeneration and appear heterogeneous.

Myelolipoma

Myelolipoma is a benign tumor consisting of mature fat interspersed with hematopoietic elements resembling bone marrow [2].

There are four clinicopathological patterns of myelolipoma:

1. Isolated adrenal myelolipoma
2. Adrenal myelolipoma with hemorrhage
3. Extra-adrenal myelolipoma
4. Myelolipoma associated with other adrenal diseases

Imaging of Adrenal Masses

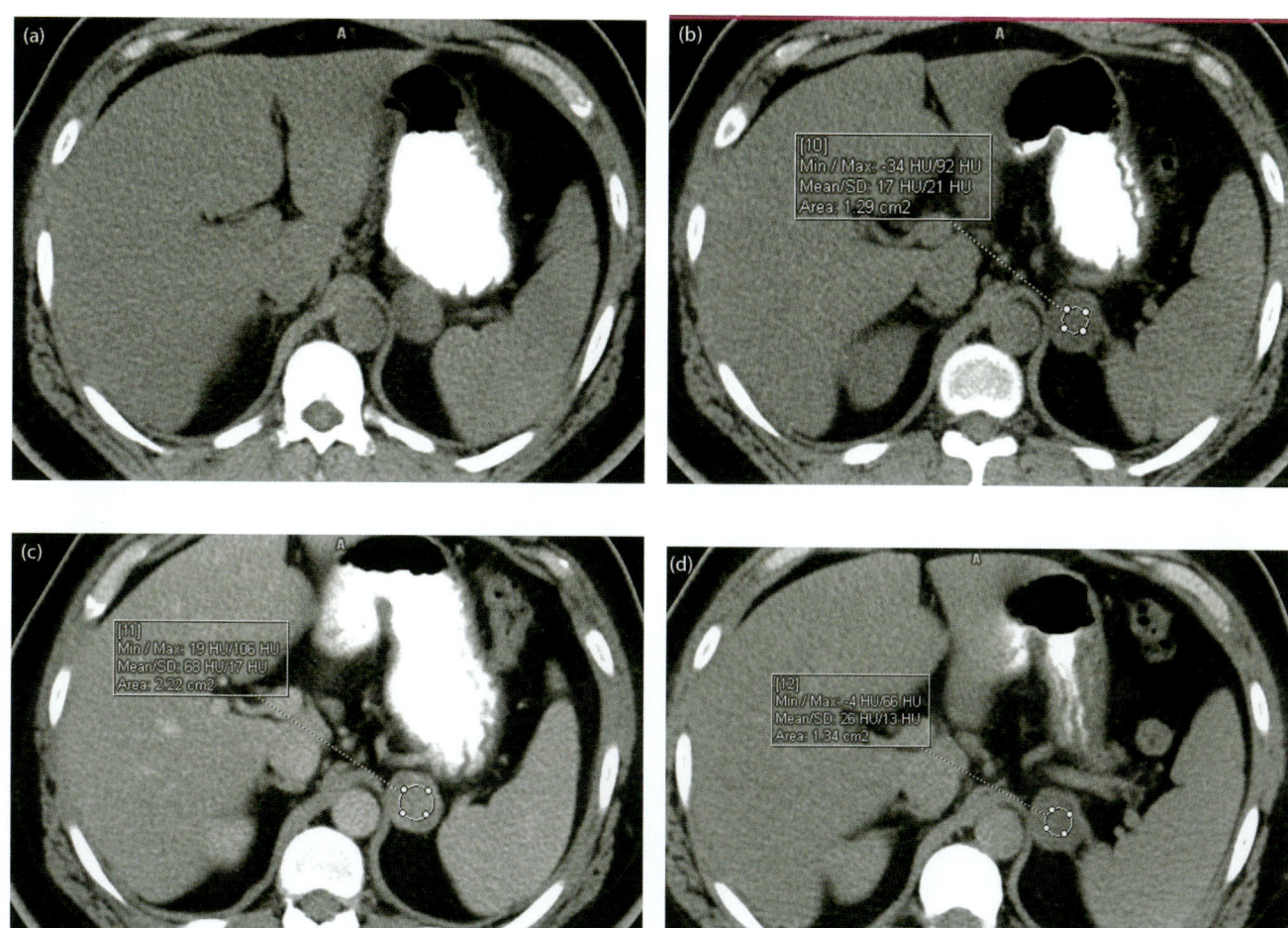

FIGURE 46.1 Adenoma: Axial pre-contrast (a) and (b) and post-contrast (c) and (d). Well-defined round, oval mass lesion with a pre-contrast CT density of 17 HU (b), post-contrast CT density of 68 HU at 1 minute (c) and 26 HU at 15 minutes (d), consistent with adenoma. Absolute washout of 82% (>60% is suggestive of adenoma). Relative washout of 62% (>40% is suggestive of adenoma).

CT:

- Well-circumscribed lucent mass with negative HU if large and shows predominantly fatty component.
- Fatty areas are associated with "smoky" areas of interspersal.
- Higher attenuation tissue that reflects the mixture of fat and marrow elements.
- Internal hemorrhage or calcification can occur, which shows higher attenuation areas.
- Contrast CT shows heterogenous enhancement of the interspersed hematopoietic element (Figure 46.2).

MRI:

- *T1*: Increased signal if fatty component
- *T2WI*: Intermediate to hyperintense signal due to the presence of admixed marrow-like elements
- *Fat-suppressed techniques*: Persistence areas of increased signal if there is a presence of marrow-like elements or hemorrhage
- *Opposed-phase imaging*: Low signal intensity in voxels containing both fat and water tissue
- *T1 C+ gadolinium*: Striking enhancement

Adrenal hemorrhage

Adrenal hemorrhage can be traumatic and nontraumatic. It can be either unilateral or bilateral.

Acute hemorrhage

CT:

- On plain scan, it shows areas of high attenuation (50–90 HU).
- No post-contrast enhancement. Focal preservation of normal adrenal enhancement may be seen and often has a peripheral distribution.
- Periadrenal infiltration.
- Sometimes active extravasation with retroperitoneal bleeding (Figure 46.3).

MRI:

- *Acute stage (<7 days after onset)*: The hematoma typically appears isointense or slightly hypointense on T1-weighted images and markedly hypointense on T2-weighted images.
- *Subacute stage (7 days to 7 weeks after onset)*: The hematoma appears hyperintense on T1- and T2-weighted images

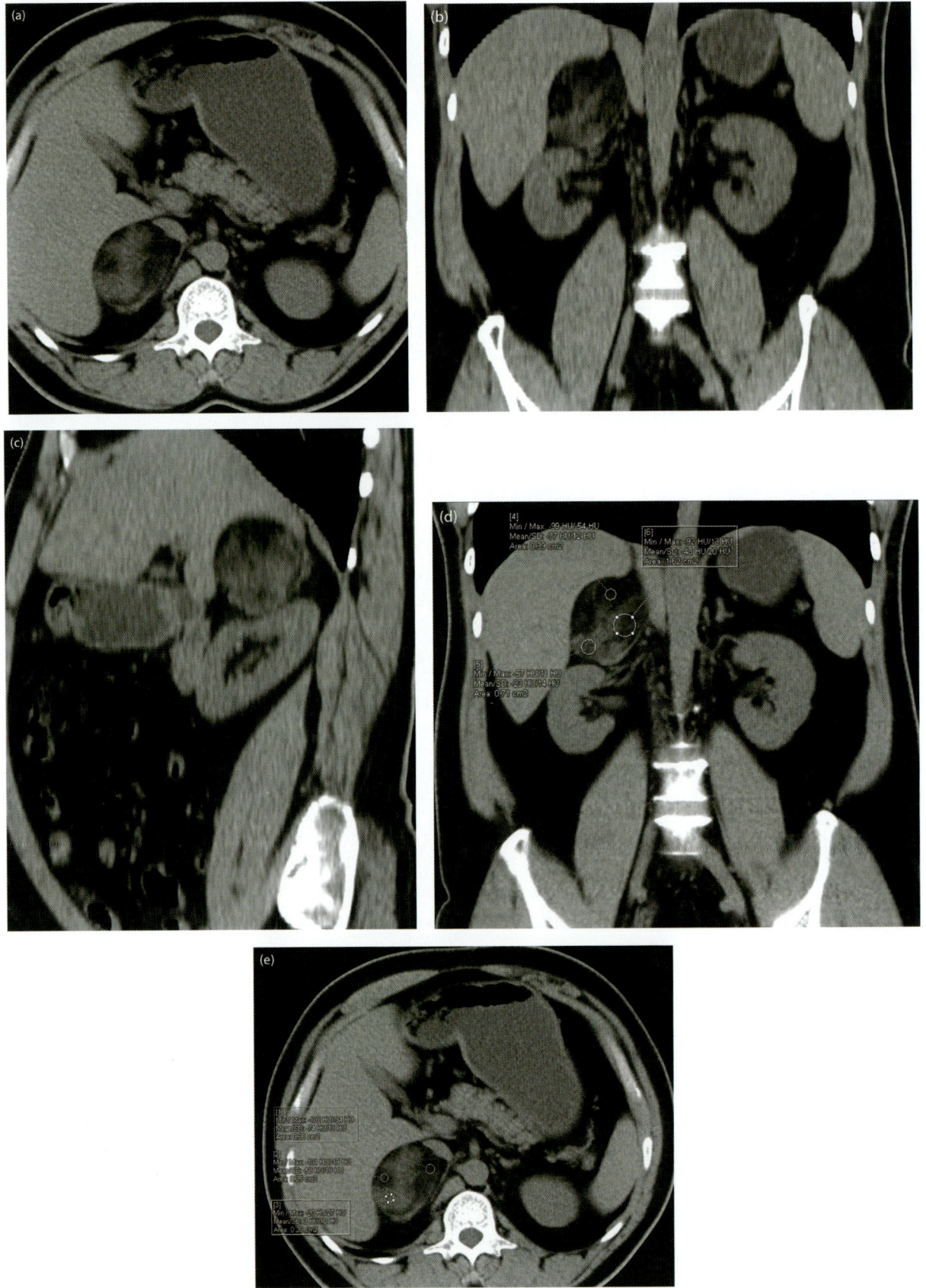

FIGURE 46.2 Myelolipoma: Axial non-contrast (a) and (c), coronal non-contrast (b) and (d) and sagittal non-contrast (e). Well-circumscribed non-infiltrating mass with macroscopic fat and soft tissue component, consistent with myelolipoma. CT density −22 to −77 HU (d).

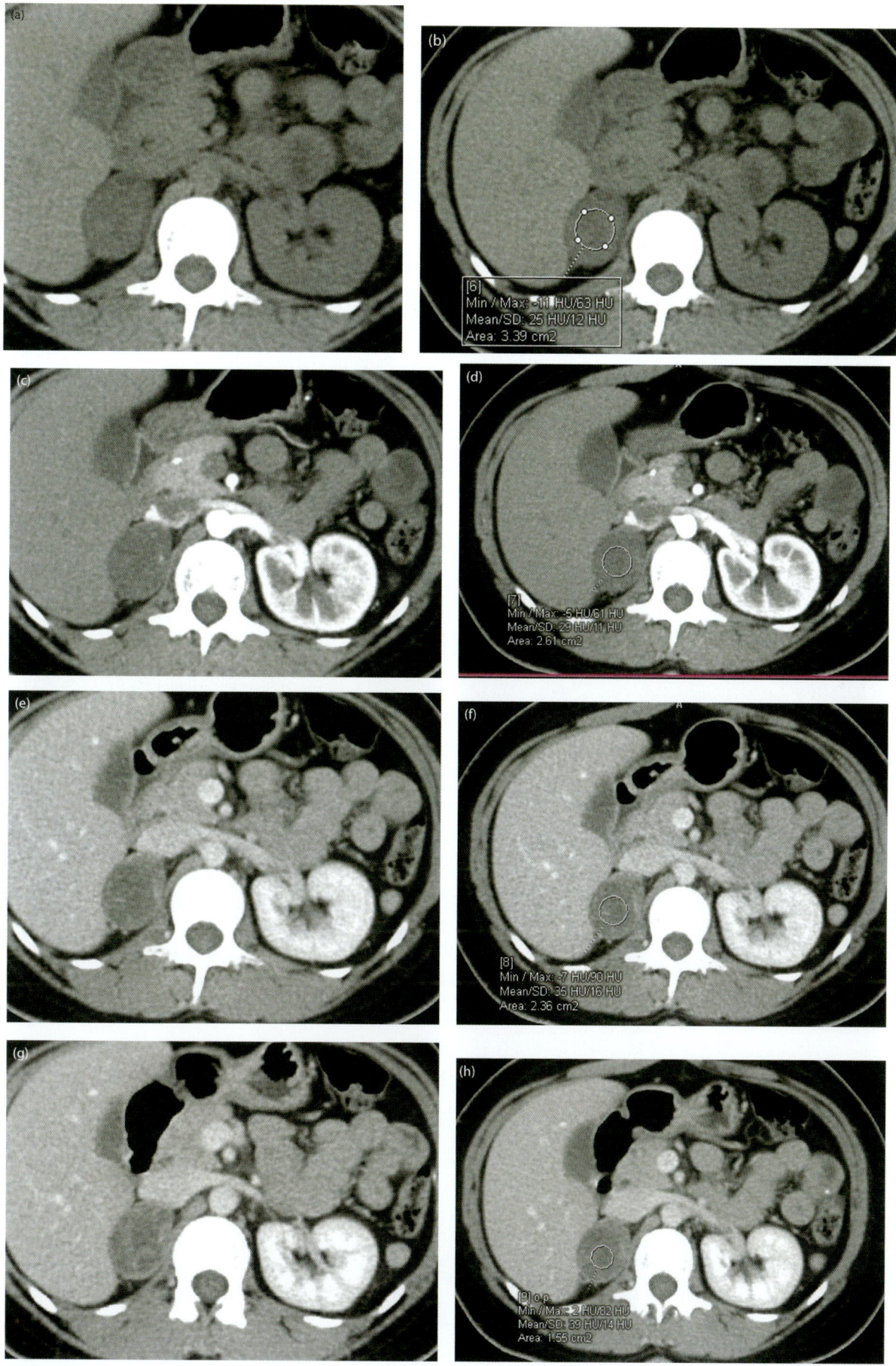

FIGURE 46.3 Adrenal hemorrhage: Axial pre-contrast (a) and (b), axial post-contrast (c)–(h). Well-defined oval mass lesion appearing iso- to hyperdense as compared to kidneys. The pre-contrast CT density is of 25 HU (b). It shows heterogeneous enhancement on post-contrast scan with CT density of 35 HU (f).

Chronic hemorrhage

Adrenal hematomas decrease in size and attenuation over time with simple fluid attenuation, known as adrenal pseudocyst. Organized chronic adrenal hematomas appear as a mass with a hypoattenuating center, with or without calcifications. Chronic hemorrhage may appear as adrenal atrophy.

MRI:

- A total of three-fourths of hypointense signal on both T1- and T2-weighted images with hypointense rim on both T1- and T2-weighted images as the result of hemosiderin deposition and fibrosis

Calcified adrenal lesion

Benign:

1. Hemorrhage
2. *Infection*: Tuberculosis, histoplasmosis (Figure 46.4) and hydatid disease
3. Adrenal cyst
4. Adenoma, myelolipoma, pheochromocytoma and neuroblastoma
5. Addison disease
6. Wolman disease

Malignant:

1. Adrenal cortical cancer
2. Adrenal metastasis
3. Neuroblastoma

Adrenal cyst

- Pseudocyst
- Endothelial cysts
- Epithelial cysts
- Parasitic cysts, usually hydatid
- Cystic lymphangioma

CT:

- A well-circumscribed, thin-walled, non-enhancing, low-density lesion with internal attenuation of less than 20 HU.
- Increased internal attenuation suggests hemorrhage or debris.
- Calcifications may be peripheral, scattered throughout the lesion, or central in location. Peripheral calcification is seen more often with pseudocysts and parasitic cysts, while septal calcification can be present in endothelial cysts (Figure 46.5).

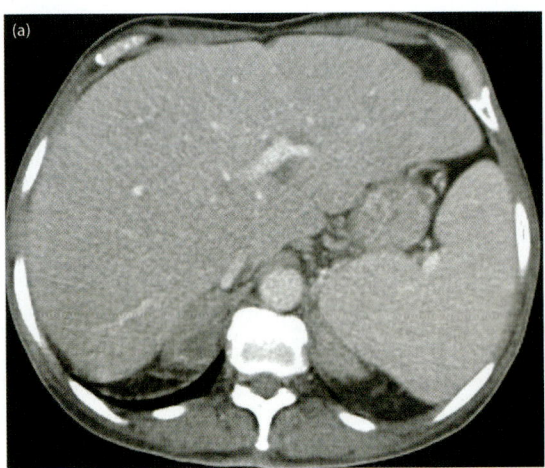
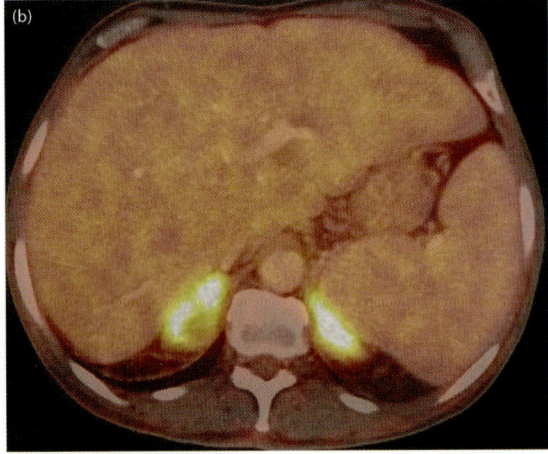
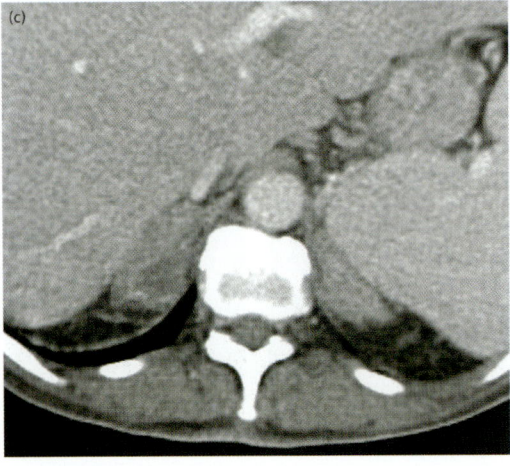

FIGURE 46.4 Histoplasmosis: Axial post-contrast (a) and (b) and FDG PET–CT (c). Bilateral enlarged adrenal glands showing heterogeneous enhancement with hypodense areas and specks of calcification (a) and (b). It shows intense uptake on FDG PET (c). Histopathological examination showed histoplasmosis.

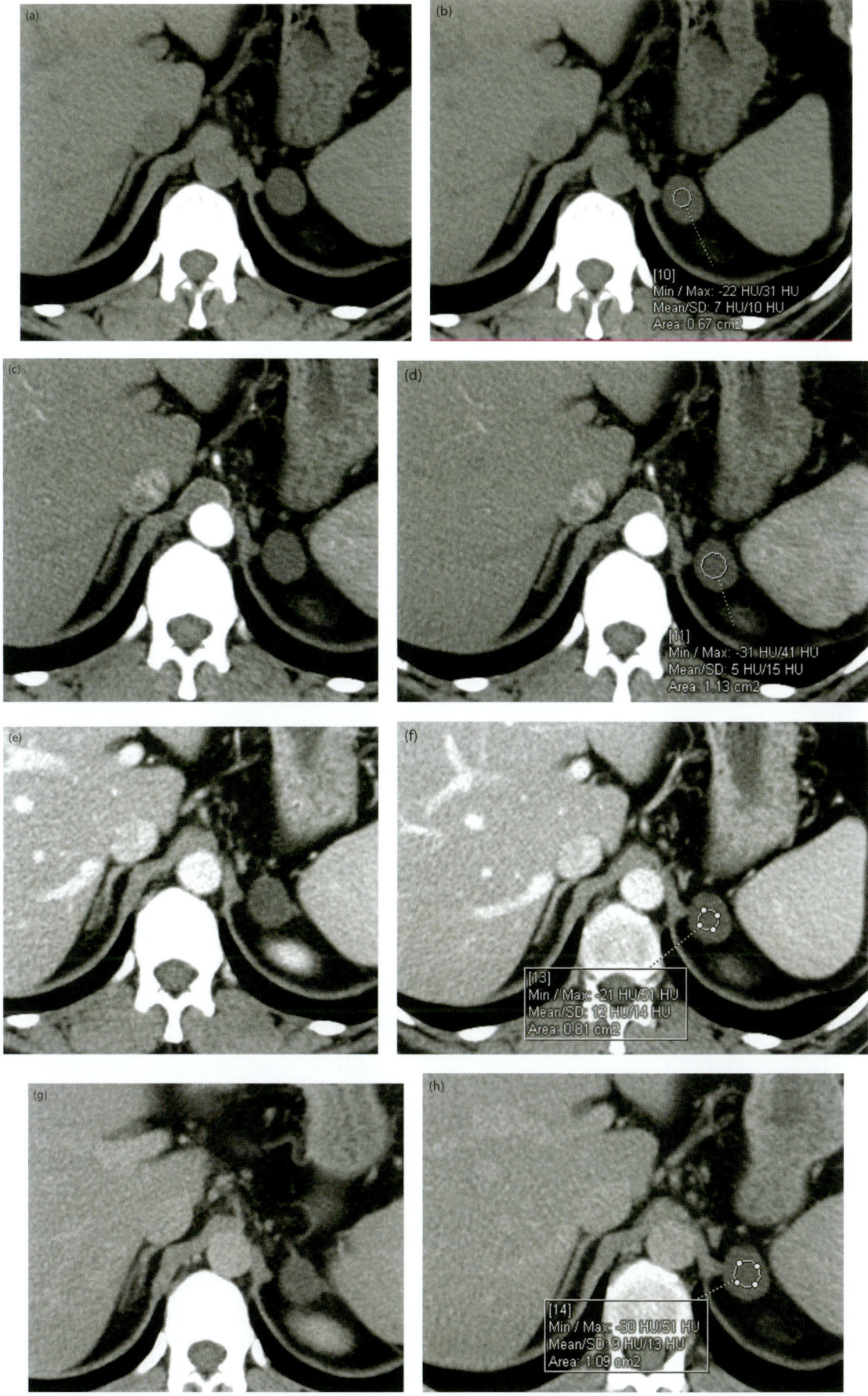

FIGURE 46.5 Adrenal cyst: Axial non-contrast (a) and (b) and axial post-contrast (c)–(h), well-defined non-enhancing hypodense lesion in left adrenal gland with a pre-contrast CT density of 7 HU (b), post-contrast CT density of 5 HU on arterial phase images (d) and 9 HU on hepatic-venous phase images (h).

MRI:

- Hypointensity on T1-weighted images and hyperintensity on T2-weighted images.
- The presence of T1 hyperintense signal is usually secondary to hemorrhage.
- Within the cyst.
- *Hydatid cyst*: Shows findings of a simple cyst, a multilocular lesion with internal septa, focal rounded internal daughter vesicles, the "water lily" sign and septal or mural calcifications [3].

Adrenal cortical hyperplasia

Adrenal hyperplasia is nonmalignant enlargement of the adrenal glands, which is often bilateral. It can be incidental or related to disease process and may be related to benign or malignant etiologies causing biochemical alterations in the hypothalamic–pituitary–adrenal axis. Hyperplasia can manifest as either a diffuse process involving the entire adrenal or nodular hyperplasia. Nodular hyperplasia is usually multifocal and bilateral.

CT:

- Enlarged limbs of one or both adrenal glands >10 mm thick with the maintenance of adrenal morphology
- Nodular or uniform

MRI:
Signal dropout on phase due to high lipid content

Pheochromocytoma

Pheochromocytomas are rare catecholamine-secreting tumors derived from chromaffin cells. More than 90% of pheochromocytomas are located within the adrenal glands, and 98% occur within the abdomen, while 10% are extra-adrenal. Common locations for extra-adrenal pheochromocytomas include the organ of Zuckerkandl, bladder wall, retroperitoneum, heart, mediastinum, carotid and glomus jugulare bodies. Pheochromocytoma follows the rule of "10."

- 10% are extra-adrenal
- 10% are bilateral
- 10% are malignant
- 10% are found in children
- 10% are familial
- 10% are not associated with hypertension
- 10% contain calcification

CT is the most common imaging method used in the diagnosis of pheochromocytomas. CT scans can reveal adrenal pheochromocytomas larger than 5–10 mm with sensitivity >95%.

Attenuation in pheochromocytomas on plain scan is always higher than 10 HU due to the absence of intracytoplasmic lipid, which helps in differentiating from adrenal adenoma [4].

Pheochromocytoma usually displays pronounced enhancement, often more than 130 HU. In smaller solid lesions, the enhancement is relatively homogeneous, while in larger lesions, the character of the enhancement is more or less heterogeneous. Cystic pheochromocytoma shows pronounced enhancement of the peripheral rim of the viable tumor tissue due to central necrosis (Figure 46.6).

MRI is a second-choice imaging tool. The appearance of pheochromocytomas in T1- and T2-weighted images depends on whether the tumor is solid, cystic or hemorrhagic/necrotic. Cystic tumors or those with central necrosis show hyperintensity on T2-weighted images, although classical pattern of a T2 hyperintense pheochromocytoma is relatively uncommon. The signal intensity of the hemorrhage in T1- and T2-weighted images varies and depends on the age of the hematoma. Diffusion-weighted imaging (DWI) and calculation of apparent diffusion coefficient (ADC) maps show significantly higher ADC values in pheochromocytomas compared to adenomas and metastases.

^{123}I-MIBG scintigraphy

Radioactive iodine-labeled ^{123}I-metaiodobenzylguanidine (^{123}I-MIBG) has been used to reveal pheochromocytomas.

Adrenal hemangioma

Adrenal gland cavernous hemangioma is an extremely rare benign vascular tumor composed of angioblastic cells that are mostly discovered incidentally. Adrenal hemangiomas are soft tissue attenuation masses, varying in size from a few centimeters to as large as 25 cm. The larger masses frequently have areas of calcification representing either phleboliths or dystrophic calcification in areas of previous hemorrhage.

On contrast imaging, they enhance similar to hemangiomas elsewhere. It shows mainly peripheral enhancement with gradual filling over time. Central region is often scarred and does not significantly enhance.

Malignant masses

Adrenal cortical carcinoma

This tumor has bimodal age distribution with two peaks: First, in the first decade, and second, in the fourth decade. It is associated with variable presentations, as tumor can be functional or not. Usually, the functional tumors are resulting in opposite adrenal atrophy due to elevated cortisol levels and reduced ACTH.

In children, tumors are usually functional and earlier detected. Presentation is with Cushing's syndrome, feminization, virilization or mixed symptoms.

Hypertension is seen in all functional lesions invariably. Due to size of lesion, abdominal pain and discomfort as well as vomiting can occur.

Imaging pearls

1. *Size >6 cm:* This tumor is larger in size always with mass effect on surrounding structures, pushing the kidneys down, compressing sometimes stomach and reaching up to diaphragm.
2. *Morphology*: Large areas of central necrosis are seen with heterogenous enhancement; sometimes rim enhancement is also seen. Dystrophic microcalcifications are common (Figure 46.7).
3. Relative percentage washout (RPW) on CT scan is less than 40%.
4. *Spread*: Invasion of inferior vena cava (IVC) is a well known complication. It results in significant symptoms due to raised venous pressure. It is also associated with higher incidence of malignancy. However, sometimes IVC invasion can result in the diagnostic dilemma with hepatocellular carcinoma and leiomyosarcoma of retroperitoneal origin that have similar characteristics.
5. *Metastasis*: Liver metastasis is most commonly followed by lung metastasis.

Imaging of Adrenal Masses

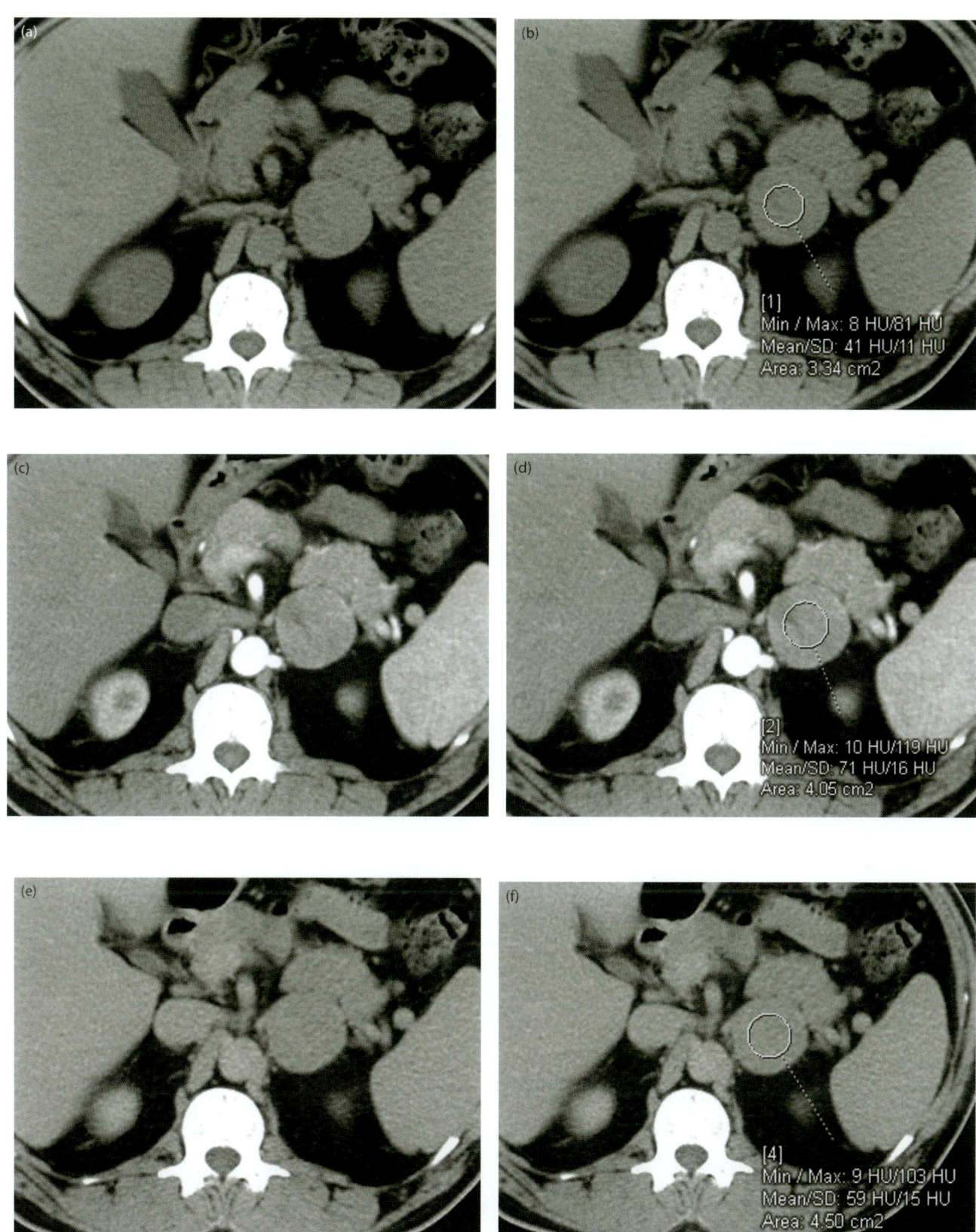

FIGURE 46.6 Pheochromocytoma: Pre-contrast axial (a) and (b), post-contrast arterial phase axial (c) and (d) and post-contrast delayed axial (e) and (f). Well-circumscribed round mass lesion with subtle hypodensity in center shows homogeneous contrast enhancement with pre-contrast CT density of 41 HU (b) and post-contrast CT density of 71 HU at 1 minute (d) and 59 HU at 15 minutes (f) consistent with pheochromocytoma. Absolute washout out is 43% (<60% is indeterminate). Relative washout is 18.3% (<40% is indeterminate).

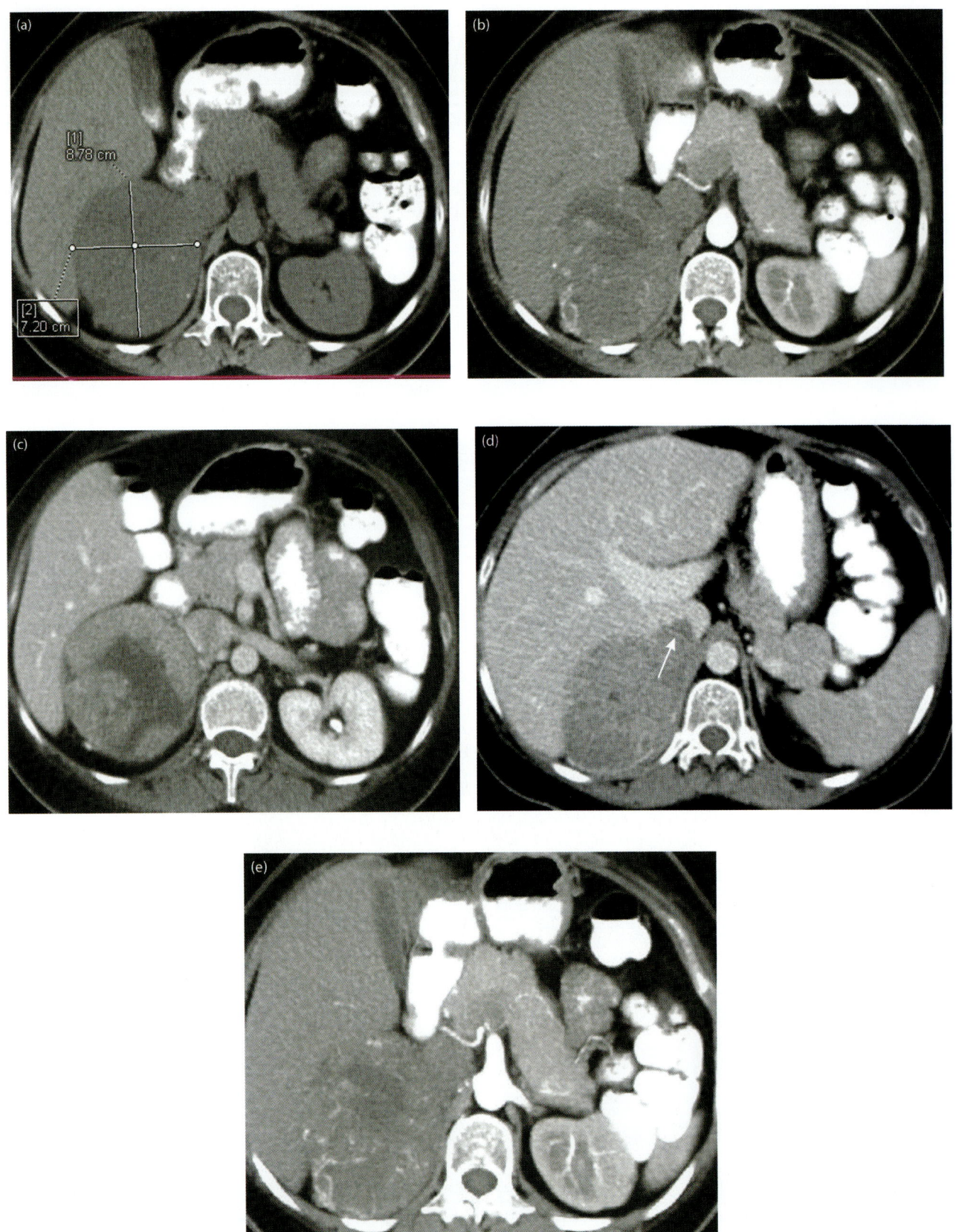

FIGURE 46.7 Adrenal cortical carcinoma: (a)–(e), pre-contrast (a), post-contrast arterial phase (b), portal-venous phase (c), and delayed phase (d) and (e). Large infiltrating mass lesion (8.8 × 7.2 cm) with few specks of calcification shows heterogeneous enhancement on post-contrast study with neovascularity (b) and (e) and central necrosis (d). The mass is infiltrating into the IVC and liver. Findings consistent with adrenal cortical carcinoma.

Lymphoma

Adrenal lymphoma is a well-known entity in older age-groups, around sixth or seventh decade. Constitutional symptoms, like fever, weight loss and pain, occur with few patients showing adrenal insufficiency. Usually, multifocal lymphomatous involvement is seen in the ipsilateral adrenal gland and kidney. Primary lymphoma of adrenal gland is a very rare entity.

Usually, the lesions present with huge size due to late presentation and the presence of larger tumor size, often greater than 10 cm in size. It shows homogenous enhancement with little cystic change or areas of necrosis. It is iso-attenuating to muscles usually. It is having a poor prognosis showing as poor as a 1-year survival rate of patients.

Neuroblastoma

Neuroblastoma is a malignant neoplasm derived from the embryologic neural crest and usually arises within the adrenal medulla but can present anywhere along the sympathetic chain ganglia. It is common in children under 2 years of age. It is a large mass lesion engulfing abdominal vessels and showing dystrophic calcifications. It is also associated with earlier metastasis to the liver and bones. It has a tendency to cross the midline. Wilms tumor is its close differential, which is seen in age-group older than 2 years, usually doesn't cross the midline, displace abdominal vessels and shows no calcification and less commonly shows metastasis [5].

Metastasis

Metastasis to the adrenal gland is the second most common mass after adenoma. Lung and breast tumors have a maximum affinity toward adrenal for metastasis followed by renal, colorectal and thyroid malignancies. Interval change in size, irregular margin and necrotic mass lesion are characteristic features of adrenal metastasis. In case with known primary, FDG-PET is having very high sensitivity to detect adrenal metastasis as normal adrenal gland is not fluorodeoxyglucose (FDG) avid so metastasis is easily picked up. Collision tumors with adenoma being invaded by metastasis are better picked up by PET study (Figure 46.8).

South Asian perspective in adrenal disorders

The imaging features of adrenal masses are similar throughout the globe; however, larger size of the lesions at presentation are common in Southeast Asian region, and this does pose a greater challenge in defining the boundaries and extent of pathology on imaging and planning the consequent management. A slightly higher prevalence of adrenal Cushing's syndrome and tuberculosis is noted in this part of the world.

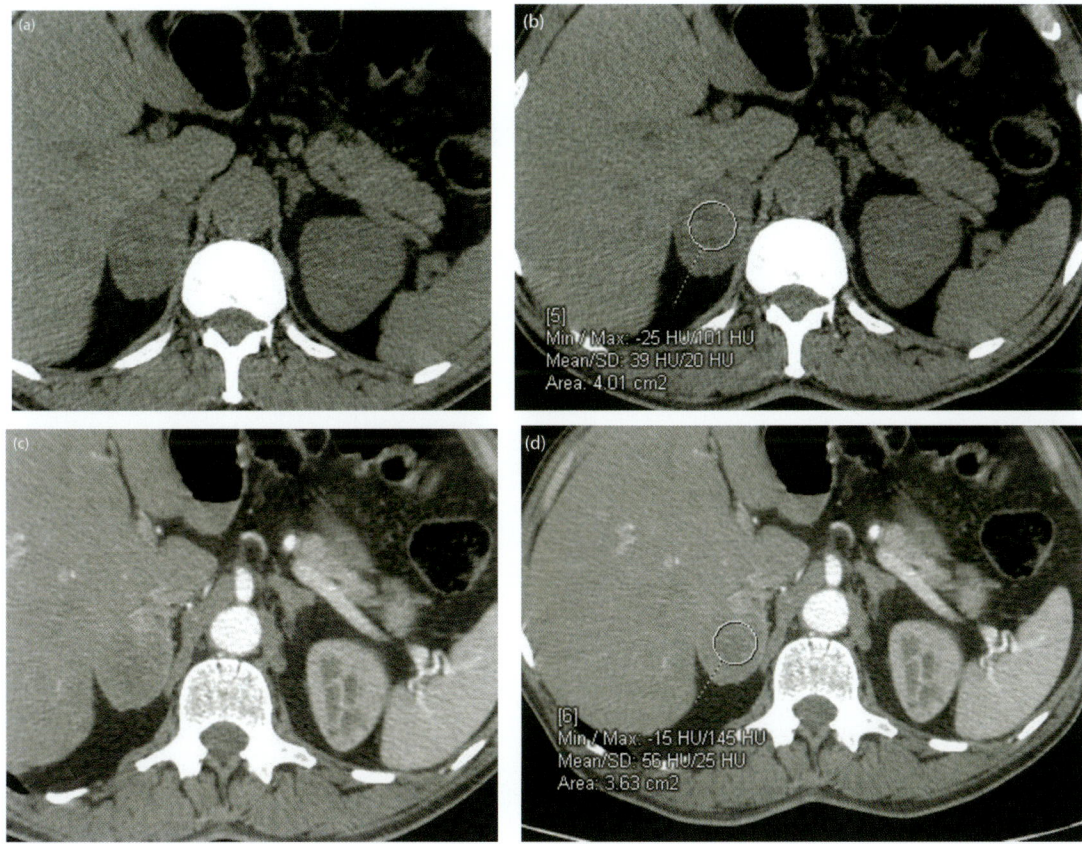

FIGURE 46.8 Metastases: (a)–(h), pre-contrast axial (a) and (b), post-contrast arterial phase (c) and (d), post-contrast delayed (e), (f) and (h) and FDG PET (g). A well-circumscribed heterogeneous hypodense mass lesion with pre-contrast CT density of 39 HU (b) and post-contrast CT density of 56 HU at 1 minute (d) and 58 HU at 12 minutes (f). It shows intense FDG uptake (g). Absolute washout of 11.8% (<60% is indeterminate). Relative washout of 3.6% (<40% is indeterminate). However, in the presence of RCC, this was presumed metastases from RCC, confirmed on subsequent histopathological examination.

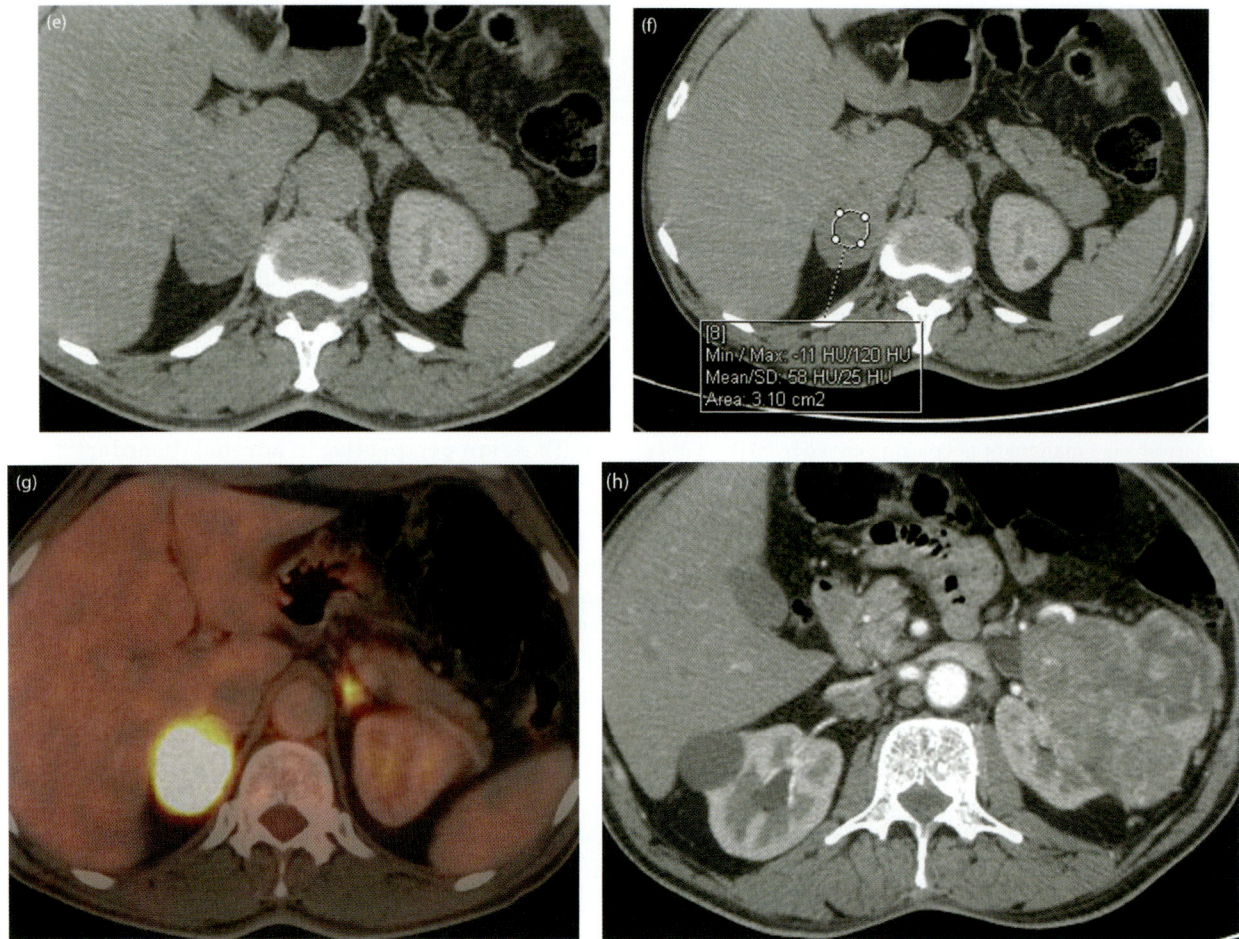

FIGURE 46.8 *(Continued)*

Conclusion

The imaging has dramatically increased the detection of incidental adrenal lesions that are mostly benign and nonfunctioning adenomas. Differentiating a benign adrenal lesion from a malignant one can be challenging and is critical, especially in oncology patients, since it will greatly affect patient management where imaging plays a crucial role.

References

1. Mahmood E, Anastasopoulou C. Adrenal adenoma. [Updated 2020 Jul 6]. In: StatPearls [Internet]. Treasure Island (FL): StatPearls Publishing; 2020 Jan.
2. Albano D, Agnello F, Midiri F, et al. Imaging features of adrenal masses. Insights Imaging. 2019;10:1.
3. Arnold DT, Reed JB, Burt K. Evaluation and management of the incidental adrenal mass. Proc (Bayl Univ Med Cent). 2003;16(1):7–12.
4. Guerrisi A, Marin D, Baski M, Guerrisi P, Capozza F, Catalano C. Adrenal lesions: Spectrum of imaging findings with emphasis on multi-detector computed tomography and magnetic resonance imaging. J Clin Imaging Sci. 2013;3:61.
5. Herr K, Muglia VF, Koff WJ, Westphalen AC. Imaging of the adrenal gland lesions. Radiol Bras. 2014 Jul/Aug;47(4):228–239.

47

PATHOLOGY OF ADRENAL LESIONS

Preeti Agarwal

Pathology of adrenal lesions

Congenital, developmental and infectious lesions

Adrenal gland abnormalities are not very common. (1) Congenital derangements like accessory adrenal, adrenal fusion and aplasia are very rare abnormalities encountered in clinical practice; however, certain storage disorders like Wolman disease and Neimann–Pick disease may show adrenal enlargement with hypofunction. Adrenoleukodystrophy is a rare storage disorder that leads to an atrophic adrenal gland.

Massive hemorrhage, cysts, tuberculosis, malakoplakia and heterotopias are also found to involve adrenal stroma. Adrenal hemorrhage is usually seen in neonates who present with mass, septicemia or adrenal insufficiency (2). True adrenal gland cysts are rare, usually vascular or pseudocysts are seen in adrenal stroma. They may clinically present as mass lesion and mimic neoplasia clinico-radiologically. Heterotropic liver and thyroid tissue have also been reported in adrenal stroma (3) (4).

In South Asian context, adrenal tuberculosis is a known occurrence. Both the glands may be affected. They may or may not be calcified and may present as Addison's disease clinically. On biopsy eosinophilic caseous necrosis, well-formed epithelioid granuloma and/or calcification may be seen. Medical management is recommended in these patients with antitubercular drugs (5) (6).

Disseminated fungal infections involve adrenal gland as well. Histoplasmosis is one of the common etiologic fungal elements. Indian patients usually present with adrenal enlargement; however, infrequently chronic adrenal failure may be presenting clinical sign. Image-guided needle aspiration and biopsy have been proven to provide good diagnostic yield in these cases (7) (8).

Adrenal hyperplasia

Adrenal hyperplasia is considered when an adrenal gland weighs over 6 g provided the adjoining fat has been carefully dissected out. Moreover to histologically interpret the hyperplasia of Adrenal bread loafing of the received adrenal gland and embedding, the cut slices are favored. During gross evaluation, microscopic morphometry is preferred.

Morphological types of hyperplasia are as follows:

1. *Congenital adrenal hyperplasia*
2. *Primary pigmented nodular adrenal cortical hyperplasia*
3. *Acquired hyperplasia*
   a. *ACTH dependent/pituitary dependent*
   b. *ACTH independent/adrenal dependent*
4. *Adrenal medullary hyperplasia*

Congenital adrenal hyperplasia

Commonly called as congenital adrenogenital syndrome is an autosomal recessive disorder leading to masculinization in females, precocious puberty and pseudohermaphroditism in males. Other symptoms include salt wasting and hypertension. The most common deficiency is in $P450_{c21}$, i.e., *21-hydroxylase*, which results in the accumulation of 17OH-progesterone and its catabolite pregnanetriol along with cortisol deficiency, followed by 11β-hydroxylase deficiency which is clinically related to virilization and hypertension (9)–(11). Other rare variants are, namely, P540 oxidoreductase deficiency, 17OH deficiency, lipoid congenital adrenal hyperplasia (STAR mutation), 3 βHSD2 deficiency and P540 cholesterol side chain cleavage enzyme deficiency (10). Morphologically the adrenal is characterized by hyperplasia of cortex especially the reticularis zone. Management consists of hormone replacement therapy and other psychological intervention with rehabilitation.

Primary pigmented nodular adrenal cortical hyperplasia

Isolated forms have been reported along with the above condition being a component of Carney complex (12). It is also referred as micronodular adrenal disease and presents in young individuals as adrenocorticotropic hormone (ACTH)-independent Cushing syndrome. On gross examination, the adrenal gland is either small, normal sized or mildly enlarged. Multiple pigmented (lipofuscin/neuromelanin) cortical nodules are seen with atrophy of intervening cortex (13) (14).

Acquired adrenocortical hyperplasia
ACTH dependent/pituitary dependent

They are usually bilateral with diffuse or nodular enlargement. Commonly diffuse cortical hyperplasias are due to ACTH hyperproduction by either the pituitary gland or an ACTH-producing neoplasm in the lung or some other organ. Thus, they are referred to as ACTH dependent or—in the former instance—pituitary dependent.

ACTH independent/adrenal dependent

It is also known as macronodular cortical hyperplasia that presents clinically with Cushing syndrome (15). The bilateral adrenal glands can become enlarged, mimicking a malignancy, and the cortex between cortical nodules is commonly atrophic. A rare subset of cases presents in children and may be associated with McCune–Albright syndrome (GNAS mutation) (16). Recent studies suggest the presence of germ line or somatic mutations in *ARMC5*, particularly in cortisol-secreting forms of the disease (17) (18).

Adrenal medullary hyperplasia

Hyperplasia of adrenal medulla is at all times is bilateral and both diffuse and nodular involvement may be seen. The clinical symptomatology is similar to pheochromocytoma (19). Proper gross examination and embedding of the specimen plays crucial role in diagnosis. Cases of diffuse hyperplasia show adrenal medullary cells in adrenal tail tissue when embedded properly, making it a characteristic morphological feature for its diagnosis. Morphometry aids diagnosis of early as well as advanced lesions.

Hence, if a clinician is suspecting medullary hyperplasia, a special comment must be added to the requisition form as random embedding of adrenal gland in such cases leads to inadequate diagnosis (20). Medullary hyperplasia has been reported to be component of or associated with multiple syndromes, namely, MEN2A and 2B neurofibromatosis, cystic fibrosis, germ line *SDHB* mutation, *MAX* mutation and Beckwith–Wiedemann syndrome (21)–(25).

Myelolipoma

A variant of lipoma, namely, myelolipoma characterized by presence of marrow elements embedded in lipomatous stroma (Figure 47.1) is seen in adrenal glands in adults. Bilateralism may be seen with or without and Cushing syndrome but is rare (26).

Neoplasms

A. *Adrenocortical neoplasms*
  a. *Adrenocortical adenoma*
  b. *Adrenocortical carcinoma*
B. *Adrenal medulla*
  a. *Neuroblastoma*
  b. *Pheochromocytoma*

Adrenocortical adenoma

Adrenal cortical adenomas are the most frequent principal adrenal lesion. They may be either functional or nonfunctional. On gross examination they are usually well circumscribed encapsulated lesions with tan appearance or central hemorrhage if large.

The tumors are mainly composed of tumor cells disposed in nests or cords separated by thin fibrovascular stroma. The tumor cells may resemble zona fasciculata, the zona glomerulosa or, more commonly, a combination of both. Individual cells are large round with lipid vacuoles clear or mild eosinophilic cytoplasm. Mitosis and necrosis are rare, however, occasional bizarre cells may be seen. Morphological variants include black adenoma (containing neuromelainin or lipofuscin pigment), oncocytoma, myxoid, lipoadenoma and adeoma with areas of myelolipoma (27). Hormone-producing adenomas include primarily cortisone, aldosterone (conn syndrome) or sex hormone–producing adenomas. Morphologically the cells of the adenoma are composite of the cells seen in the entire zone. Distinctively eosinophilic cytoplasmic bodies known as spironolactone bodies may be in cytoplasm of tumor cells of aldosterone-secreting tumors treated with spironolactone (28).

Adrenocortical carcinoma

Carcinoma of adrenal gland is rare occurrence with bimodal age distribution. The peak is seen during the first and fifth decade of life (29). Clinical presentations are varied in form of mass lesion, symptom of excess steroid production, metastatic disease or may be an incidental radiological finding.

On gross examination adrenocortical carcinomas are tan gray with intervening areas of necrosis and hemorrhage. Capsular and vascular invasion may be seen even on gross evaluation. On histology the tumor range from well differentiated from morphologically similar to adenoma or may have sheets of multinucleated bizarre cells (Figure 47.2). Morphological variants recognized are mainly oncocytic, myxoid and sarcomatoid variants. Blood borne metastasis to liver lymph nodes is frequent with loco regional spread to kidney and retroperitoneum. Surgical management is the primary mode; however, in advanced lesions chemotherapy and mitotane therapy are relied on. Radiotherapy is of limited use (30).

Differential diagnosis

Major challenge in diagnosing an adrenal cortical neoplasm is when one has to differentiate it from adenoma or renal cell carcinoma and even adrenomedullary lesions. As far as difference with adenoma is concerned, Weiss criteria are applied. Adenomas have a propensity to be smaller, more homogeneous and lacking hemorrhage and necrosis (31). According to Weiss et al., if a tumor has any three or more of the following microscopic features, it is likely to be malignant rather than benign. The microscopic features recognized by in the *Weiss* criteria laid down are: nuclear grade III or IV, mitotic rate greater than 5 per 50 high-power fields (HPFs), atypical mitoses, less than 25% clear cells, diffuse architecture, necrosis, capsular invasion, venous invasion and sinusoidal invasion. Though the above criteria have been well-utilized for adrenocortical carcinoma, however, it does not help identification of carcinomatous degeneration in oncocytic variant (*Lin–Weiss–Bisceglia criteria*) and myxoid variants (32). Moreover, as far as pediatric lesions are concerned, weight of the tumor is of more importance, and hence, the above criteria are of no use.

Microscopically adrenocortical neoplasm bears a resemblance to renal cell carcinoma, so in cases of metastasis, a differentiation between them becomes a challenge. Immunohistochemistry (IHC) comes to rescue in these circumstances where SF-1, inhibin, Melan-A (Mart-1, A103), calretinin and synaptophysin favors adrenocortical lineage. PAX-8, cytokeratin, EMA and CD10 expression favor renal epithelial cell origin (33) (34). When we have to distinguish adrenocortical from adrenomedullary neoplasms, synaptophysin is of no help instead expression of chromogranin, and GATA 3 should favor adrenomedullary over cortical lesions (35) (36).

Molecular signatures

Mutations frequently associated with aldosterone-secreting adenomas are *KCNJ5* (seen in young females with severe hyperaldosteronism), *ATP 1A1*, *ATP2B3*, *CTNNB1* and *CACNA1D* (37) (38) *PRKACA* mutations are identified in cortisol-producing

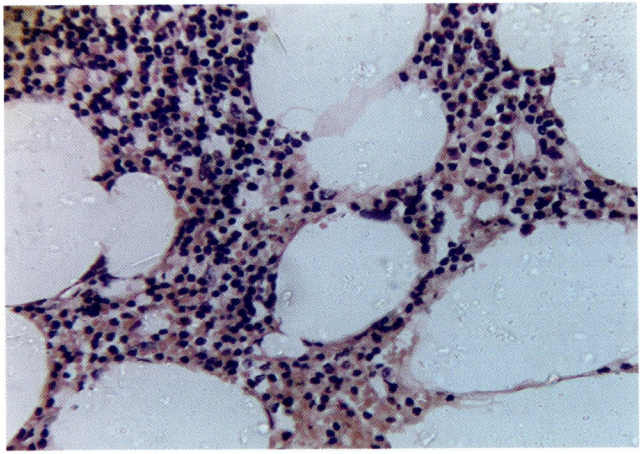

FIGURE 47.1 Myelolipoma: microphotographs displaying a presence of erythroid and myeloid precursors along with megakaryocytes in a lipomatous stroma (hematoxylin and eosin; 400×). (Courtesy of Dr. Chanchal Rana; Orcid Id—000-0002-1783-7689.)

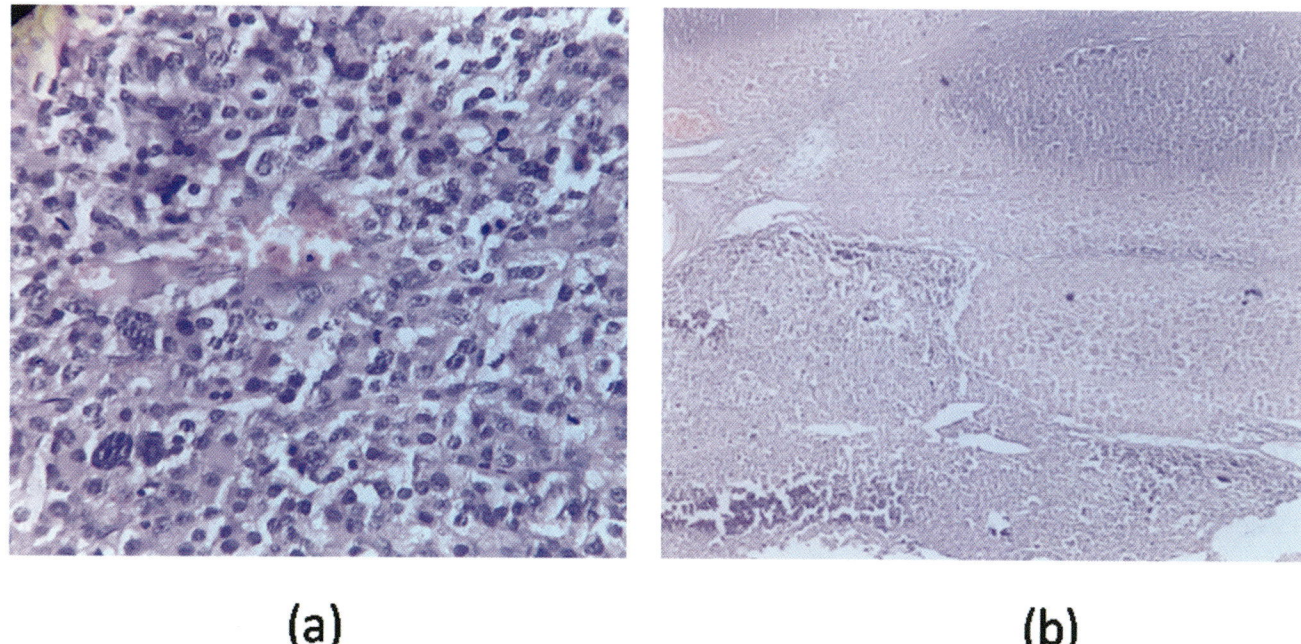

FIGURE 47.2 Adrenocortical carcinoma: (a) Microphotograohs displaying a neoplasm with diffuse architecture, nuclear pleomorphism, hyperchromasia and mitotic figures (Hematoxylin and eosin; 400× magnification) and; (b) Same case with large areas of necrosis (Hematoxylin and eosin; 200× magnification). (Courtesy of Dr. Chanchal Rana; Orcid Id—000-0002-1783-7689.)

adenomas (39). Nonfunctioning adenomas frequently harbor mutations in *CTNNB*, encoding for β-catenin (40). Hereditary syndromes like Carney complex, Li–Fraumeni, MEN type 1, Beckwith–Wiedemann, Familial Adenomatous Polyposis and McCune–Alright syndrome may be associated with adrenocortical adenomas as well as carcinomas. It becomes particularly important when adrenocortical carcinoma is seen in children as germ line p53 mutations must be excluded in them to rule out Li–Fraumeni syndrome. Driver mutations, namely, *p53*, *ZNFR3*, *CTNNB1*, *PRKAR1A*, *CCNE1* and *TERF2* along with frequent IGF2 overexpression, have been seen in adrenocortical carcinomas (41) (42).

Adrenal medulla

Adrenal medulla is primarily involved in epinephrine production and its recreation. Medullary hyperplasia is primarily seen in adults along with pheochromocytoma and rarely ganglioneuroma. In children, neuroblastoma is frequently encountered lesion.

Neuroblastoma

Neuroblastoma, ganglioneuroblastoma and ganglioneuroma are seen involving adrenal medulla usually in children below 4 years with median age of 21 months with no sex predilection. Mass lesion is the most frequent clinical symptom. Child may present watery diarrhea, Cushing syndrome, heterochromia iridis and Horner syndrome (in cervical or mediastinal tumors), opsoclonus/myoclonus (a paraneoplastic autoimmune process) and several other manifestations. They often secrete homovanillic acid (HVA) and vanillylmandelic acid (VMA), both of which may be detected in the urine (43). Sympathetic chain especially of mediastinum or neck can be seen harboring neuroblastoma. I-metaiodobenzylguanidine (MIBG) scintigraphy highlights the primary tumor and foci of metastases.

Morphologic features

On gross examination, the tumor may be large, relatively circumscribed, gray-white with areas of hemorrhage and necrosis. Calcification is often seen but cystic degeneration may also occur. Multifocality may also be seen but in fewer than 10% of the cases (44).

On histology, the tumor is disposed in vaguely nodular or nested pattern with nests of tumor cells separated by thin fibrovascular septa (Figure 47.3). Tumor cells are largely monomorphic

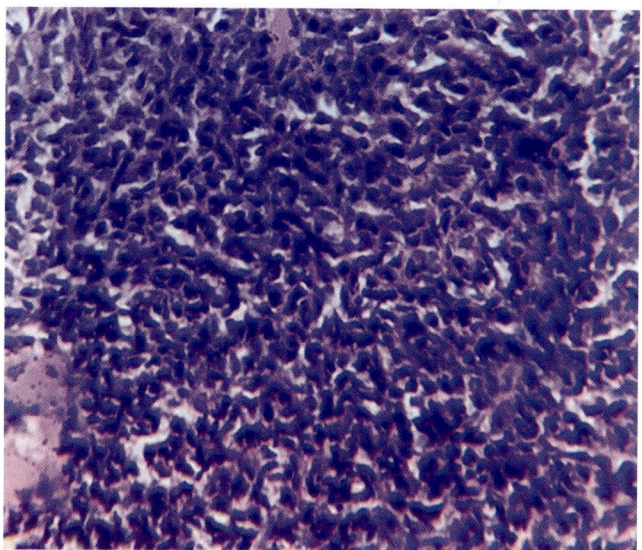

FIGURE 47.3 Neuroblastoma: Composed of small round cell in a neurfibrillary background (Hematoxylin and eosin; 400× magnification). (Courtesy of Dr. Chanchal Rana; Orcid Id—000-0002-1783-7689.)

round with hyperchromatic nuclei and scant cytoplasm. Nucleoli are inconspicuous. Intratumoral hemorrhage leading to cyst-like structure formation with prominent basophilic calcification is frequently seen. Characteristic rosettes which have central eosinophilic fibrillary material-neuropil are seen. These are known as Homer Wright (HW) rosettes. True rosettes with central lumen are not identified in neuroblastoma (45).

International Neuroblastoma Pathology Classification (INPC) is used for classification and mainly depends on relative amount of tumor components. Figure 47.4 provides with a simplified version of classification of neuroblastoma. Postchemotherapy lesions may undergo maturation; hence, they may be just diagnosed as neuroblastoma with chemotherapy effects.

Finally, a rare pleomorphic (anaplastic) form of neuroblastoma characterized by the presence of bizarre giant tumor cells has been described; however, this diagnostic term should not be used in post-therapy specimens where chemotherapy-induced atypia is common (46).

IHC and molecular

Neurites (which form the center of HW rosettes), neurosecretory granules and synaptic endings are seen ultrastructurally (47). Cytoplasmic expression of neuron-specific enolase (NSE), chromogranin, synaptophysin, microtubule-associated proteins and NB-84 is seen in tumor cells (48). PHOXB2 has been identified as most sensitive and specific marker for neuroblastoma (49). IHC plays a very important role in identification of undifferentiated neuroblastoma from its close differentials seen in children, namely, rhabdomyosarcoma, Ewing sarcoma and malignant lymphoma (50). However, it must be emphasized clinical and radiological correlation is of utmost importance in diagnosis of neuroblastoma in children. The commonest alteration seen in neuroblastoma is 17q gain. It confers poor clinical outcome. Oncogenes involved in its development are *MYCN*, *ALK* and paired-like homeobox 2B (*PHBX2B*) genes (51). More than 10 copies MYCN oncogene per diploid genome are regarded as defining criteria of MYC amplification detection by FISH technique. Approximately 25% of cases may show MYCN amplification. MYCN amplification is also regarded as adverse prognostic factor (52). While hyperploidy is considered to confer better prognosis, Germ line *ALK* mutations are associated with familial neuroblastoma.

Spread and metastases

These tumors are locally invasive, intraspinal (dumbbell) extensions (53), or spread into the kidney may also be seen. However, in South Asian context, multiple tumors may be diagnosed late presenting with distant metastases to the lymph nodes, bone marrow, bone, liver, orbit and dura (54). Multiple symmetrical bone metastases may also be seen. Reoccurrence may occur and have been reported within 2 years post excision; however, late reoccurrences are rare (55). INPC and children oncology group (COG) neuroblastoma risk group is a system for risk stratification of neuroblastoma applicable to pretreatment specimens (56)–(58). Simplified form of INPC is summarized in Box 1 with calculation of Mitosis Karyorrhexis index (MKI) in Box 2 and unfavorable molecular signatures in Box 3.

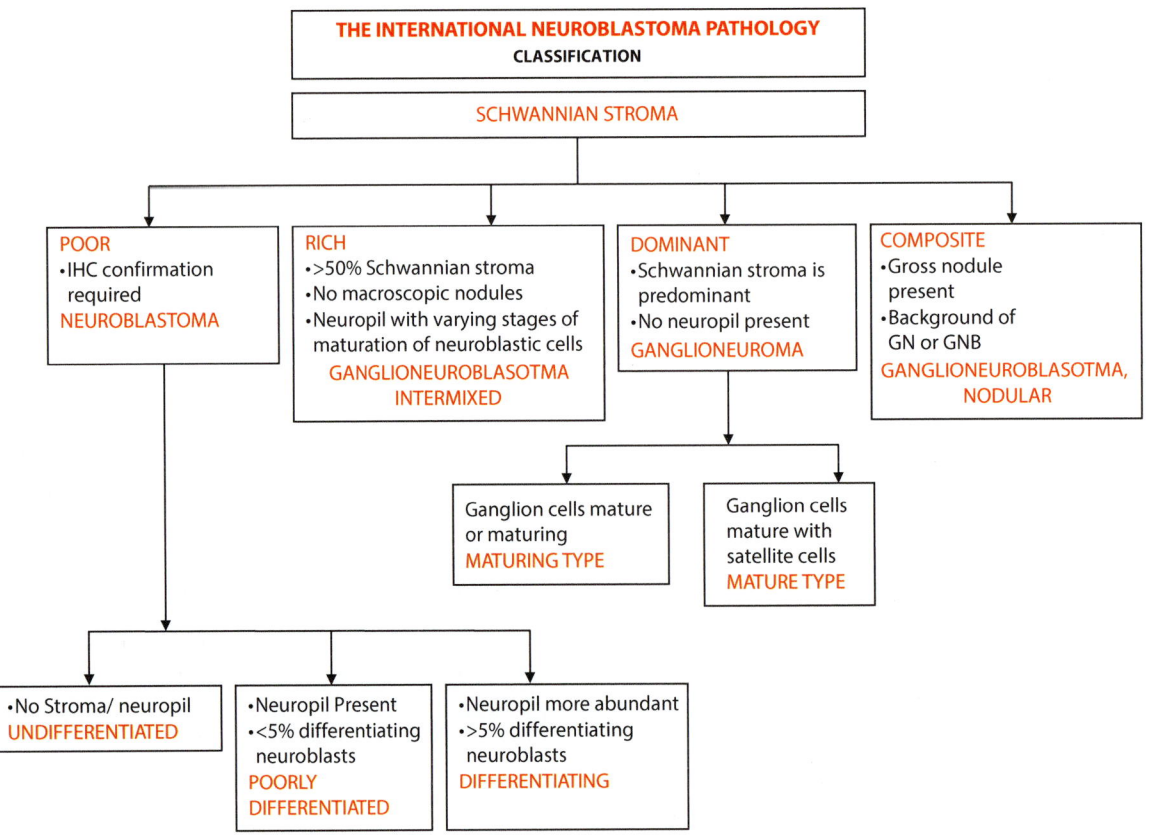

FIGURE 47.4 The flow chart of International Neuroblastoma Pathology classification.

BOX 1

UNFAVORABLE HISTOLOGY

NB undifferentiated
    Neuroblastoma, poorly differentiated
    Neuroblastoma, differentiating, with intermediate MKI — 18 to 60 months of age
    Neuroblastoma, any type—> 60 months of age

FAVORABLE HISTOLOGY

Ganglioneuroblastoma, intermixed either mature or maturing
    Neuroblastoma with intermediate MKI (poorly differentiated or differentiating)—<18 months of age
    Neuroblastoma, differentiating, with low MKI—18–60 months of age

For nodular type of GNB the prognosis is determined by the subtype of NB it is harboring.

BOX 2 MITOSIS AND KARYORRHEXIS INDEX (MKI)

$$MKI = \frac{Mitosis + karyorrhectic\ figures}{5000\ neuroblasts}$$

Low = 2%
Intermediate = 2%–4%
High = >4%

Mitosis: morphologically mitosis must be devoid of nuclear outline displaying condensed chromatin with irregular outline. One may see typical forms like central line or anaphase or atypical forms like multipolar mitosis.

Karyorrhectic figures: these are condensed nuclear remnant with scant eosinophilic cytoplasmic rimming. It should never be assessed in areas of necrosis.

The entire MKI evaluation must be performed under high power (40× magnification).

BOX 3 MOLECULAR UNFAVORABLE SIGNATURES

MYCN amplification
11q deletion and 17q gain
Diploid tumors

Staging

International Neuroblastoma Staging System (INSS) is a surgical staging system that directly relates to surgical pathology evaluation. All lymph nodes attached to the tumor and removed separately must be properly labeled and submitted with the surgical specimen for it reporting. Whereas the International Risk Group Staging System (INRGSS) is a preoperative imaging influenced staging system (59) (60).

International Neuroblastoma Staging System (58)

Stage	Definition
Stage I	Completely excised tumor
	Non-adherent negative lymph nodes (ipsilateral)
	Adherent positive lymph nodes (ipsilateral)
	Microscopic positive margins may be present
Stage IIA	Incompletely excised tumor with gross tumor margins being positive
	Adherent negative lymph nodes (ipsilateral)
Stage IIB	Incompletely excised tumor with gross tumor margins being positive
	Adherent positive lymph nodes (ipsilateral)
	Enlarged negative lymph nodes (contralateral)
Stage III	Unresectable unilateral tumor crossing vertebral column with or without regional nodal involvement
	Completely excised unilateral tumor and contralateral nodal involvement. Unresectable midline tumor having tumor infiltration on both sides or nodal involvement
Stage IV	Tumor with distant metastasis (involvement of distant lymph nodes, bone, bone marrow, liver, skin or other organs)
Stage IVS	Infant younger than 12 months
	Localized primary tumor (stage I, IIA or IIB) with dissemination limited to skin, liver and/or bone marrow
	Bone marrow involvement must have <10% cellularity
	Bone marrow must be metaiodobenzylguanidine scan negative

Pheochromocytoma

These are tumors of the adrenal medullary chromaffin cells which may secrete epinephrine and norepinephrine both. Distinct from their extraadrenal counterparts (paragangliomas pheochromocytomas), they can secrete epinephrine because of presence of adrenal cortex which is essential for its methylation step. Hormonally active tumors may cause intermittent hypertensive episodes, triad of sweating attacks, tachycardia and headaches clinically imply the presence of a pheochromocytoma. Ectopic secretory products leading to Cushing syndrome, diarrhea/achlorhydria/hypokalemia or polycythemia may also be seen (61) (62).

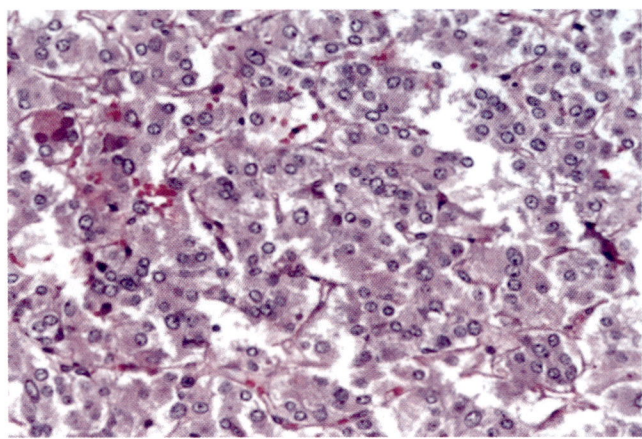

FIGURE 47.5 Pheochromocytoma: A neoplasm displaying a zellballen architecture characterized by tumor cell nests surrounded by delicate fibrovascular septa (Hematoxylin and eosin; 200× magnification). (Courtesy of Dr. Chanchal Rana; Orcid Id—000-0002-1783-7689.)

Morphologic features

On gross well-circumscribed tumor is seen of yellow tan appearance. Necrosis, hemorrhage and cyst formation is usually seen in large tumors. Compressed residual adrenal gland may be identified on careful examination. Histologically characteristic lobular pattern is seen commonly known as 'Zellballen' meaning presence of tumor cells well-defined nests due to presence of thin fibrovascular septa (Figure 47.5) (63). Diffuse, trabercular or sclerotic areas may also be seen. Tumor cells are largely round to oval to polygonal with finely granular basophilic or amphophilic cytoplasm. Nucleolar prominence with intranuclear cytoplasmic inclusions may be seen (64). Subtle cytoplasmic alterations are also known, like clearing due to lipid accumulation, (65) melanin accumulation (66) or oncocytic change (67). Intracytoplasmic hyaline globules are common. Rarely in cases of MEN2A, one may find a true composite tumor with elements both of pheochromocytoma intermixed with ganglioneuroma, ganglioneuroblastoma or neuroblastoma (68).

Molecular and immunohistochemistry

Dense core secretory granules are seen on EM (69). Tumor cells display cytoplasmic expression for synaptophysin, chromogranin which is strong and diffuse along with nuclear expression of GATA 3 in IHC (35). Immunohistochemical loss of SDH has been found to be associated with higher risk of metastatic disease, hence is being now used for predictive screening (70). Infrequently PHOX2B expression may be seen (71). Cytokeratin is variable expression or typically negative; differentiating from paragangliomas of the cauda equina where CK is typically present (72). Surrounding sustentacular cells display S-100 expression (73). Associated genes are, namely, *SDH* family (most common), *NF1*, *VHL*, *RET*, *MAX*, *EPAS1* and *FH*.

Allelic losses at 1p, 3q, 11q, 17p and 22q, are frequent. Alterations in chromosome 11 and losses at 6q and 17p are seen in tumors with malignant potential (74)–(76).

In sporadic tumors somatic mutations of the hereditary genes have been reported, NF1 being the commonest, they may also harbor *HRAS* or *BRAF* mutations (~9% of cases), and *TP53* in 2%–3% (77)–(79).

Spread, metastases, treatment and prognosis

Metastasis is considered as the only features that marks malignancy in pheochromocytoma. No other morphological feature is considered to be directly related to malignant degeneration; however, pheochromocytoma of the Adrenal Gland Scaled Score (PASS) and the Grading System for Adrenal Pheochromocytoma and Paraganglioma (GAPP) have been employed to access the malignant potential with limited role (80) (81).

Pheochromocytoma of the adrenal gland scoring scale (PASS) (82)

Sl. No.	Histomorphological Parameter	Score
1.	Nuclear hyperchromasia	1
2.	Profound nuclear pleomorphism	1
3.	Capsular invasion	1
4.	Vascular invasion	1
5.	Extension into periadrenal adipose tissue	2
6.	Atypical mitotic figures	2
7.	Greater than 3 mitotic figures/10 high-power field	2
8.	Tumor cell spindling	2
9.	Cellular monotony	2
10.	High cellularity	2
11.	Central or confluent tumor necrosis	2
12.	Large nests or diffuse growth (>10% of tumor volume)	2
Total		20

Score of <4 suggests benign tumor and score ≥ 4 suggests malignant lesion.

High proliferative index assessed by Ki67, absence of sustentacular cells which are positive for S-100, increased tenascin or human telomerase reverse transcriptase (hTERT) gene expression have reported as unfavorable prognostic variables (83)–(86). Metastatic tumor deposits have been seen in local lymph nodes, bone, liver and lung. Pheochromocytomas in children are less likely to be malignant, but more likely to be bilateral, or associated with MEN (87).

Other adrenal neoplasms

Mesenchymal lesions with sex cord stromal tumors, sarcomas and lymphomas have been reported in adrenal stroma (88).

Bilateralism is a rule as far as metastatic adrenal tumors are concerned. The most common sites of the primary tumor are lung, breast, gastric, skin (melanoma), pancreas, hepatobiliary and kidney. Renal metastases can be contralateral and may grossly and microscopically simulate the appearance of adrenocortical carcinoma or adenoma (89).

Conclusion

All adrenal specimens to be morphologically evaluated must be supplemented with serological variables and radiological findings. As far as non-neoplastic lesions are concerned in Southeast Asian region, tuberculosis and fungal involvement of adrenal cortex is a known occurrence, so one must keep in mind these entities. Needle biopsy or aspiration cytology may provide with cellular diagnosis in these cases. To avoid erroneous diagnosis, the clinician surgeon must also be very cautious with specimen handling of adrenal excision specimen and avoid making any incision on it during or after surgical delivery.

References

1. Symington T. *Functional Pathology of the Human Adrenal Gland*. Baltimore, MD: Williams & Wilkins; 1969.
2. DeSa DJ, Nicholls S. Haemorrhagic necrosis of the adrenal gland in perinatal infants: a clinico-pathological study. J Pathol. 1972 and 106(3):133–149.
3. Honore LH. Intra-adrenal hepatic heterotopia. J Urol. 1985 and 133(4):652–654.
4. Shiraishi T, Imai H, Fukutome K, et al. Ectopic thyroid in the adrenal gland. Hum Pathol. 1999 and 30(1):105–108.
5. Oelkers W. Adrenal insufficiency. N Engl J Med. 1996 and 335(16):1206–1212.
6. McMurry JF Jr, Long D, McClure R, Kotchen TA. Addison's disease with adrenal enlargement on computed tomographic scanning. Report on two cases of tuberculosis and review of the literature. Am J Med. 1984 and 77(2):365–368.
7. Chakrabarti A, Slavin MA. Endemic fungal infections in the Asia-Pacific region. Med Mycol. 2011 and 49:337–344.
8. Vyas S, Kalra N, Das PJ, et al. Adrenal histoplasmosis: an unusual cause of adrenomegaly. Indian J Nephrol. 2011 and 21(4):283–285.
9. New MI. Congenital adrenal hyperplasia. Pediatr Clin North Am. 1968 and 15(2):395–407.
10. El-Maouche D, Arlt W, Merke DP. Congenital adrenal hyperplasia. Lancet. 2017 and 390:2194–2210
11. Merke DP, Camacho CA. Novel basic and clinical aspects of congenital adrenal hyperplasia. Rev Endocr Metab Disord. 2001 and 2(3):289–296.
12. Stratakis CA. Adrenocortical tumors, primary pigmented adrenocortical disease (PPNAD)/Carney complex, and other bilateral hyperplasias: the NIH studies. Horm Metab Res. 2007 and 39(6):467–473.
13. Iseli BE, Hedinger CE. Histopathology and ultrastructure of primary adrenocortical nodular dysplasia with Cushing's syndrome. Histopathology. 1985 and 9(11):1171–1194.
14. Shenoy BV, Carpenter PC, Carney JA. Bilateral primary pigmented nodular adrenocortical disease. Rare cause of the Cushing syndrome. Am J Surg Pathol. 1984 and 8(5):335–344.
15. Sasano H, Suzuki T, Nagura H. ACTH-independent macronodular adrenocortical hyperplasia: immunohistochemical and in situ hybridization studies of steroidogenic enzymes. Mod Pathol. 1994 and 7(2):215–219.
16. Kirk JM, Brain CE, Carson DJ, et al. Cushing's syndrome caused by nodular adrenal hyperplasia in children with McCune-Albright syndrome. J Pediatr. 1999 and 134:789–792.
17. Albiger NM, Regazzo D, Rubin B, et al. A multicenter experience on the prevalence of ARMC5 mutations in patients with primary bilateral macronodular adrenal hyperplasia: from genetic characterization to clinical phenotype. Endocrine. 2017 and 55:959–968.
18. Bourdeau I, Oble S, Magne F, et al. ARMC5 mutations in a large French-Canadian family with cortisol-secreting β-adrenergic/vasopressin responsive bilateral macronodular adrenal hyperplasia. Eur J Endocrinol. 2016 and 174:85–96.
19. Visser JW, Axt R. Bilateral adrenal medullary hyperplasia: a clinicopathological entity. J Clin Pathol. 1975 and 28(4):298–304.
20. DeLellis RA, Wolfe HJ, Gagel RF, et al. Adrenal medullary hyperplasia. A morphometric analysis in patients with familial medullary thyroid carcinoma. Am J Pathol. 1976 and 83(1):177–196.
21. Romanet P, Guerin C, Pedini P, et al. Pathological and genetic characterization of bilateral adrenomedullary hyperplasia in a patient with Germline MAX mutation. Endocr Pathol. 2016 and 28:302–307.
22. Tischler AS, Semple J. Adrenal medullary nodules in Beckwith-Wiedemann Syndrome resemble extra-adrenal paraganglia. Endocr Pathol. 1996 and 7(4):265–272.
23. Carney JA, Sizemore GW, Sheps SG. Adrenal medullary disease in multiple endocrine neoplasia, type 2: pheochromocytoma and its precursors. Am J Clin Pathol. 1976 and 66(2):279–290.
24. Grogan RH, Pacak K, Pasche L, et al. Bilateral adrenal medullary hyperplasia associated with an SDHB mutation. J Clin Oncol. 2011 and 29:e200–e202.
25. Yoshida A, Hatanaka S, Ohi Y, et al. von Recklinghausen's disease associated with somatostatin-rich duodenal carcinoid (somatostatinoma), medullary thyroid carcinoma and diffuse adrenal medullary hyperplasia. Acta Pathol Jpn. 1991 and 41(11):847–856.
26. Kraimps JL, Marechaud R, Levillain P, et al. Bilateral symptomatic adrenal myelolipoma. Surgery. 1992 and 111(1):114–117.
27. Weissferdt A, Phan A, Suster S, Moran CA. Myxoid adrenocortical carcinoma: a clinicopathologic and immunohistochemical study of 7 cases, including 1 case with lipomatous metaplasia. Am J Clin Pathol 2013 and 139:780–786.
28. Aiba M, Suzuki H, Kageyama K, et al. Spironolactone bodies in aldosteromas and in the attached adrenals. Enzyme histochemical study of 19 cases of primary aldosteronism and a case of aldosteronism due to bilateral diffuse hyperplasia of the zona glomeru.
29. Ayala-Ramirez M, Jasim S, Feng L, et al. Adrenocortical carcinoma: clinical outcomes and prognosis of 330 patients at a tertiary care center. Eur J Endocrinol. 2013 and 169:891–899.
30. McKenney, JK. Adrenal gland and other paraganglia. In: *Rosai and Ackerman's Surgical Pathology*. [eds.] John R, Goldblum MD. Eleventh. s.l.: Elsevier Inc.; 2018. pp. 29, 1190–1221.
31. Weiss LM. Comparative histologic study of 43 metastasizing and nonmetastasizing adrenocortical tumors. Am J Surg Pathol. 1984 and 8:163–169.
32. Bisceglia M, Ludovico O, Di Mattia A, et al. Adrenocortical oncocytic tumors: report of 10 cases and review of the literature. Int J Surg Pathol. 2004 and 12:231–243.
33. Sangoi AR, Fujiwara M, West RB, et al. Immunohistochemical distinction of primary adrenal cortical lesions from metastatic clear cell renal cell carcinoma: a study of 248 cases. Am J Surg Pathol. 2011 and 35:678–686.
34. Gokden N, Gokden M, Phan DC, McKenney JK. The utility of PAX-2 in distinguishing metastatic clear cell renal cell carcinoma from its morphologic mimics: an immunohistochemical study with comparison to renal cell carcinoma marker. Am J Surg Pathol. 2008 and 32(10):1462–1467.
35. Zhang PJ, Genega EM, Tomaszewski JE, et al. The role of calretinin, inhibin, melan-A, BCL-2, and C-kit in differentiating adrenal cortical and medullary tumors: an immunohistochemical study. Mod Pathol. 2003 and 16:591–597.
36. Miettinen M, McCue PA, Sarlomo-Rikala M, et al. GATA3: a multispecific but potentially useful marker in surgical pathology: a systematic analysis of 2500 epithelial and nonepithelial tumors. Am J Surg Pathol. 2014 and 38:13–22.
37. Williams TA, Monticone S, Schack VR, et al. Somatic ATP1A1, ATP2B3, and KCNJ5 mutations in aldosterone-producing adenomas. Hypertension. 2014 and 63:188–195.
38. Akerstrom T, Maharjan R, Sven Willenberg H, et al. Activating mutations in CTNNB1 in aldosterone producing adenomas. Sci Rep. 2016 and 6:19546.
39. Thiel A, Reis AC, Haase M, et al. PRKACA mutations in cortisol-producing adenomas and adrenal hyperplasia: a single-center study of 60 cases. Eur J Endocrinol. 2015 and 172:677–685.
40. Bonnet S, Gaujoux S, Launay P, et al. Wnt/β-catenin pathway activation in adrenocortical adenomas is frequently due to somatic CTNNB1-activating mutations, which are associated with larger and nonsecreting tumors: a study in cortisol-secreting and -nons.
41. Juhlin CC, Goh G, Healy JM, et al. Whole-exome sequencing characterizes the landscape of somatic mutations and copy number alterations in adrenocortical carcinoma. J Clin Endocrinol Metab. 2015 and 100:E493–E502.
42. Wagner J, Portwine C, Rabin K, et al. High frequency of germline p53 mutations in childhood adrenocortical cancer. J Natl Cancer Inst. 1994 and 86:1707–1710.
43. Gambini C, Conte M, Bernini G, et al. Neuroblastic tumors associated with opsoclonus-myoclonus syndrome: histological, immunohistochemical and molecular features of 15 Italian cases. Virchows Arch. 2003 and 442:555–562.
44. Hiyama E, Yokoyama T, Hiyama K, et al. Multifocal neuroblastoma: biologic behavior and surgical aspects. Cancer. 2000 and 88:1955–1963.
45. Joshi VV, Silverman JF. Pathology of neuroblastic tumors. Semin Diagn Pathol. 1994 and 11:107–117.
46. Abramowsky CR, Katzenstein HM, Alvarado CS, Shehata BM. Anaplastic large cell neuroblastoma. Pediatr Dev Pathol. 2009 and 12:1–5.
47. Hachitanda Y, Tsuneyoshi M, Enjoji M. An ultrastructural and immunohistochemical evaluation of cytodifferentiation in neuroblastic tumors. Mod Pathol. 1989 and 2:13–19.
48. Wirnsberger GH, Becker H, Ziervogel K, Hofler H. Diagnostic immunohistochemistry of neuroblastic tumors. Am J Surg Pathol. 1992 and 16:49–57.
49. Hung YP, Lee JP, Bellizzi AM, Hornick JL. PHOX2B reliably distinguishes neuroblastoma among small round blue cell tumors. Histopathology. 2017 and 71(5):786–779.
50. Oppedal BR, Brandtzaeg P, Kemshead JT. Immunohistochemical differentiation of neuroblastomas from other small round cell neoplasms of childhood using a panel of mono- and polyclonal antibodies. Histopathology. 1987 and 11:363–374.
51. Bown N, Cotterill S, Lastowska M, et al. Gain of chromosome arm 17q and adverse outcome in patients with neuroblastoma. N Engl J Med. 1999 and 340:1954–1961.
52. Brodeur GM. Molecular pathology of human neuroblastomas. Semin Diagn Pathol. 1994 and 11:118–125.
53. Holgersen LO, Santulli TV, Schullinger JN, Berdon WE. Neuroblastoma with intraspinal (dumbbell) extension. J Pediatr Surg. 1983 and 18:406–411.
54. Kramer K, Kushner B, Heller G, Cheung NK. Neuroblastoma metastatic to the central nervous system. The Memorial Sloan-kettering Cancer Center experience and a literature review. Cancer. 2001 and 91:1510–1519.
55. Dannecker G, Leidig E, Treuner J, Niethammer D. Late recurrence of neuroblastoma: a reason for prolonged follow-up? Am J Pediatr Hematol Oncol. 1983 and 5:271–274.
56. Shimada H, Ambros IM, Dehner LP, et al. The International Neuroblastoma Pathology Classification (the Shimada system). Cancer. 1999 and 86:364–372.
57. Peuchmaur M, d'Amore ES, Joshi VV, et al. Revision of the International Neuroblastoma Pathology Classification: confirmation of favorable and unfavorable prognostic subsets in ganglioneuroblastoma, nodular. Cancer. 2003 and 15:2274–2281.
58. London WB, Castleberry RP, Matthay KK, et al. Evidence for an age cutoff greater than 365 days for neuroblastoma risk group stratification in the Children's Oncology Group. J Clin Oncol. 2005 and 23:6459–6465.
59. Brodeur GM, Pritchard J, Berthold F, et al. Revisions of the international criteria for neuroblastoma diagnosis, staging, and response to treatment. J Clin Oncol. 1993 and 11:1466–1477.
60. Monclair T, Brodeur GM, Ambros PF, et al. The International Neuroblastoma Risk Group (INRG) staging system: an INRG Task Force report. J Clin Oncol. 2009 and 27:298–303.
61. George DJ, Watermeyer GA, Levin D. Composite adrenal phaeochromocytoma-ganglioneuroma causing watery diarrhoea, hypokalaemia and achlorhydria syndrome. Eur J Gastroenterol Hepatol. 2010 and 22:632–634.
62. Falhammar H, Calissendorff J, Höyberg C. Frequency of Cushing's syndrome due to ACTH-secreting adrenal medullary lesions: a retrospective study over 10 years from a single center. Endocrine. 2017 and 55:296–302.
63. Medeiros LJ, Wolf BC, Balogh K, Federman M. Adrenal pheochromocytoma: a clinicopathologic review of 60 cases. Hum Pathol. 1985 and 16:580–589.
64. DeLellis RA, Suchow E, Wolfe HJ. Ultrastructure of nuclear "inclusions" in pheochromocytoma and paraganglioma. Hum Pathol. 1980 and 11:205–207.
65. Unger PD, Cohen JM, Thung SN, et al. Lipid degeneration in a pheochromocytoma histologically mimicking an adrenal cortical tumor. Arch Pathol Lab Med. 1990 and 114:892–894.
66. Landas SK, Leigh C, Bonsib SM, Layne K. Occurrence of melanin in pheochromocytoma. Mod Pathol. 1993 and 6:175–178.

67. Li M, Wenig BM. Adrenal oncocytic pheochromocytoma. Am J Surg Pathol. 2000 and 24:1552–1557.
68. Brady S, Lechan RM, Schwaitzberg SD, et al. Composite pheochromocytoma/ganglioneuroma of the adrenal gland associated with multiple endocrine neoplasia 2A: case report with immunohistochemical analysis. Am J Surg Pathol. 1997 and 21(1):102–108.
69. Gomez RR, Osborne BM, Ordonez NG, Mackay B. Pheochromocytoma. Ultrastruct Pathol. 1991 and 15:557–562.
70. Assadipour Y, Sadowski SM, Alimchandani M, et al. SDHB mutation status and tumor size but not tumor grade are important predictors of clinical outcome in pheochromocytoma and abdominal paraganglioma. Surgery. 2017 and 161:230–239.
71. Lee JP, Hung YP, O'Dorisio TM, et al. Examination of PHOX2B in adult neuroendocrine neoplasms reveals relatively frequent expression in phaeochromocytomas and paragangliomas. Histopathology. 2017 and 71(4):503–510.
72. Chetty R, Pillay P, Jaichand V, et al. Cytokeratin expression in adrenal phaeochromocytomas and extra-adrenal paragangliomas. J Clin Pathol. 1998 and 51:477–478.
73. Unger P, Hoffman K, Pertsemlidis D, et al. S100 protein-positive sustentacular cells in malignant and locally aggressive adrenal pheochromocytomas. Arch Pathol Lab Med. 1991 and 115:484–487.
74. Edstrom E, Mahlamaki E, Nord B, et al. Comparative genomic hybridization reveals frequent losses of chromosomes 1p and 3q in pheochromocytomas and abdominal paragangliomas, suggesting a common genetic etiology. Am J Pathol. 2000 and 156:651–659.
75. Tanaka N, Nishisho I, Yamamoto M, et al. Loss of heterozygosity on the long arm of chromosome 22 in pheochromocytoma. Genes Chromosomes Cancer. 1992 and 5:399–403.
76. Vargas MP, Zhuang Z, Wang C, et al. Loss of heterozygosity on the short arm of chromosomes 1 and 3 in sporadic pheochromocytoma and extra-adrenal paraganglioma. Hum Pathol. 1997 and 28:411–415.
77. Neumann HP, Berger DP, Sigmund G, et al. Pheochromocytomas, multiple endocrine neoplasia type 2, and von Hippel-Lindau disease. N Engl J Med. 1993 and 329:1531–1538.
78. Irvin GL, Fishman LM, Sher JA. Familial pheochromocytoma. Surgery. 1983 and 94:938–940.
79. Luchetti A, Walsh D, Rodger F, et al. Profiling of somatic mutations in phaeochromocytoma and paraganglioma by targeted next generation sequencing analysis. Int J Endocrinol. 2015 and 2015:138573.
80. Thompson LD. Pheochromocytoma of the Adrenal gland Scaled Score (PASS) to separate benign from malignant neoplasms: a clinicopathologic and immunophenotypic study of 100 cases. Am J Surg Pathol. 2002 and 26:551–566.
81. Kimura N, Watanabe T, Noshiro T, et al. Histological grading of adrenal and extra-adrenal pheochromocytomas and relationship to prognosis: a clinicopathological analysis of 116 adrenal pheochromocytomas and 30 extra-adrenal sympathetic paragangliomas in.
82. Sherwin RP. Histopathology of pheochromocytoma. Cancer. 1959 and 12:861–877.
83. Brown HM, Komorowski RA, Wilson SD, et al. Predicting metastasis of pheochromocytomas using DNA flow cytometry and immunohistochemical markers of cell proliferation: a positive correlation between MIB-1 staining and malignant tumor behavior. Cancer. 1999 and 86(8):1583–1589.
84. Gupta D, Shidham V, Holden J, Layfield L. Prognostic value of immunohistochemical expression of topoisomerase alpha II, MIB-1, p53, E-cadherin, retinoblastoma gene protein product, and HER-2/neu in adrenal and extra-adrenal pheochromocytomas. Appl Immunoh. 2000 and 8(4):267–274.
85. Elder EE, Xu D, Hoog A, et al. KI-67 and hTERT expression can aid in the distinction between malignant and benign pheochromocytoma and paraganglioma. Mod Pathol. 2003 and 16:246–255.
86. Salmenkivi K, Haglund C, Arola J, Heikkila P. Increased expression of tenascin in pheochromocytomas correlates with malignancy. Am J Surg Pathol. 2001 and 25:1419–1423.
87. Caty MG, Coran AG, Geagen M, Thompson NW. Current diagnosis and treatment of pheochromocytoma in children. Experience with 22 consecutive tumors in 14 patients. Arch Surg. 1990 and 125:978–981.
88. Dao AH, Page DL, Reynolds VH, Adkins RB. Primary malignant melanoma of the adrenal gland. A report of two cases and review of the literature. Am Surg. 1990 and 56:199–203.
89. Huisman TK, Sands JP. Renal cell carcinoma with solitary metachronous contralateral adrenal metastasis. Experience with 2 cases and review of the literature. Urology. 1991 and 38:364–368.

48

PHEOCHROMOCYTOMA

M J Paul

Introduction

Pheochromocytoma is a functioning tumor of adrenal medulla, which constitutes about 15% of the normal adrenal gland. The primitive ectodermal cells that migrate down from the neural crest to form the adrenal medulla are known as the sympathogonia. They differentiate to form sympathoblasts and later on differentiate to form ganglion cells or chromaffin cells; the latter secretes catecholamines. Adrenaline, noradrenaline and dopamine are synthesized from tyrosine in the medulla. Adrenaline acts on the alpha receptors producing vasoconstriction, intestinal relaxation and pupillary dilatation. Noradrenaline acts on the beta receptors to increase myocardial contractility and heart rate.

Excessive catecholamine secretion by this tumor classically results in paroxysmal hypertension and a panic syndrome characterized by palpitations, sweating and headache. This clinical feature was first recognized by Felix Frankel in a young girl who expired at Freiburg, Germany, and at autopsy, bilateral adrenal tumors were described in gross and microscopic detail by his pathologist Matt Schottelius in 1886[1]. Later, Takamine extracted the active principle from the adrenal gland and referred to it as Adrenalin in his work published in 1901[2]. The term pheochromocytoma was coined by Ludwig Pick in 1912[3]. It derives its name from the deep yellow-brown color (pheo) acquired on staining with a chromium salt. Cesar Roux in 1926 performed the first surgical excision of a pheochromocytoma.

Clinical presentation

This tumor is found in approximately 0.2% of all hypertensives. It is estimated from autopsy studies that 35–50% of lesions remain undiagnosed during life[4]. Paroxysmal or sustained release of norepinephrine and epinephrine results in multiple physiological effects manifesting in different clinical presentations giving pheochromocytoma the reputation of a 'great mimic'. Hypertension is the most common disorder and is sustained in 50% of patients. Paroxysmal panic attacks may occur spontaneously or may be precipitated by certain foods, alcohol, palpation, defecation, sexual intercourse, diagnostic procedure or general anesthesia. The classic panic attack is a varying mix of adrenergic symptoms like headache, sweating, palpitations, nausea, vomiting, abdominal pain, fainting or a feeling of impending doom. In our series, we found abdominal pain to be a presenting feature in a significant proportion of patients; upper abdominal pain otherwise unexplained in the setting of an adrenal lesion should raise the suspicion of pheochromocytoma. Patients may be noted to have pallor, flushing, tachycardia, very high blood pressure, arrhythmias, cerebrovascular accidents and encephalopathy. Weight loss and glucose intolerance with hyperglycemia is seen in some patients. Pheochromocytoma can rarely be diagnosed during evaluation of an incidentaloma on abdominal imaging done for other reasons, where the clinical features were absent or missed, and has been noted as the diagnosis in 3–10% of incidentalomas in an NIH review[5].

Differential diagnosis

The triad of headaches, palpitations and diaphoresis are common symptoms for a rare disease and, hence, overlap with many other conditions[6]. Labile hypertension, anxiety neurosis and other psychiatric disorders, hyperthyroidism, diabetes mellitus and functional bowel disorder should particularly be considered by primary care providers evaluating patients with panic attacks. Conversely, pheochromocytomas can present in a variety of clinical manifestations mimicking other conditions including cardiomyopathy, cardiac arrhythmias, acute coronary syndrome, heart failure, hypoglycemia syndrome, pyrexia of unknown origin, anxiety disorders and dyspepsia[7].

Pheochromocytoma and paraganglioma

Pheochromocytoma has traditionally been regarded as a '10% tumor', which described the rate of extra-adrenal, bilateral, multiple, familial, pediatric or malignant tumors in early reports. Recent reports have revealed a higher percentage is extra-adrenal, malignant or familial. The majority, 80–90%, arise from the adrenal medulla and the remaining 10–20% from extra-adrenal paraganglia, which extends from the pelvis to the base of the skull. The term functioning paraganglioma (PGL) has replaced the term extra-adrenal pheochromocytoma; together, these catecholamine secreting tumors are termed pheochromocytoma-PGL (PPGL). Most PGL are intra-abdominal arising in the paracaval ganglia at the renal hilum, above the aortic bifurcation (organ of Zukerkandl) or the wall of the urinary bladder. Less than 2% of extra-adrenal lesions occur in the neck, thorax and posterior wall of the atrium. Head and neck PGLs generally arise from the parasympathetic ganglia and do not secrete catecholamines. Thoracoabdominal PGLs tend to secrete catecholamine. Extra-adrenal tumors have a higher malignancy rate. Children have a higher rate of extra-adrenal, multiple and bilateral tumors as chromaffin tissue in these sites regress after puberty.

Screening tests

Plasma studies of fractionated metanephrines are the most sensitive and should be done with the patient resting for 30 minutes with an indwelling catheter. Catecholamines and their major breakdown products via catecholamine-*O*-methyl transferase (COMT), normetanephrines and metanephrines are measured in an acidified 24-hour urine collection. Studies of plasma-fractionated metanephrines have shown them to perform better than plasma or urinary catecholamines as well as the traditional urinary vanillylmandelic acid assay. COMT present in the tumors continuously produce free metanephrines whose assays perform better unlike catecholamine

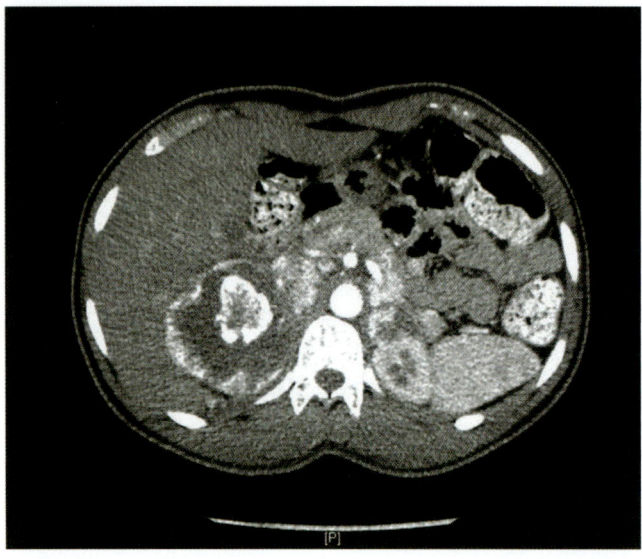

FIGURE 48.1 Contrast-enhanced CT scan of right adrenal pheochromocytoma.

release that may be at low levels or at intermittent bursts leading to lower sensitivity and specificity. Direct comparison studies of plasma versus urine metanephrines using chromatography are not available and urine studies have been independently shown to achieve similar high performance at screening. Plasma tests are expensive and not easily available, so urine studies are generally used most frequently in the South Asian setting.

Imaging

Ultrasound is often the technique that detects an unsuspected adrenal lesion incidentally or on evaluation of abdominal symptoms that may occur in the setting of pheochromocytoma. CT or MRI can be used to locate and characterize a suspected pheochromocytoma with high sensitivity, since most tumors are >3 cm in size. The small tumors are solid, enhancing but larger tumors classically appear inhomogeneous with areas of hemorrhage or necrosis. Figure 48.1 shows contrast-enhanced CT scan of Rt adrenal pheochromocytoma. Figure 48.2 is T1-weighted

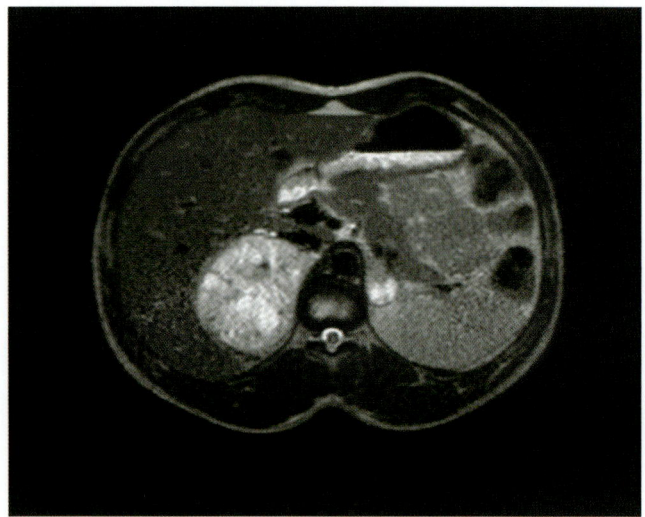

FIGURE 48.2 MRI T1W of same patient in image 1.

MRI image of the same patient. ^{131}I-MIBG isotope scanning has a limited sensitivity of around 70% but is the most widely used when it is indicated in familial disease where multiple/extra-adrenal lesions are suspected and can also detect metastatic lesions of malignant pheochromocytoma. Figure 48.3 shows anterior and posterior planar images of metastatic deposits in ^{131}I–MIBG scan. The newer developments in radionuclide imaging now offer several PET ligands including 18F-FDOPA (fluorodihydroxyphenylalanine), 18F-FDA (fluorodopamine) and 18F-FDG (fluoro-2-deoxy-D-glucose). When available, these are useful in the setting of familial disease, extra-adrenal lesions and suspected malignant metastasis.

Familial disease and genetic testing

Pheochromocytoma is associated with familial syndromes in up to 41% of cases.

1. *Von Hippel Lindau's disease* (CNS ganglioneuroblastomas, retinal angiomas, renal tumors). The most common familial syndrome with pheochromocytoma.
2. *MEN IIA and IIB*, where pheochromocytoma manifests in about 50% of cases.
3. *Von Recklinghausen's disease (multiple neurofibromatosis)* – this is the rarest association.
4. *Familial paraganglioma syndromes* are the most recent to be recognized with multiple tumors arising in extra-adrenal sites. These are caused by mutations in the gene encoding for subunits of the succinate dehydrogenase (SDH) enzyme of the glycolytic pathway. This mutation-causing dysfunction leads to intracellular hypoxia driving hyperplasia and tumor formation responses.

The major advances in the last two decades are the recognition of an increasing role of inherited conditions associated with pheochromocytoma. Genetic screening is now indicated in all cases of pheochromocytoma with inheritable mutations detectable in 30–35% of patients[8].

New genetic mutations have been described apart from the four familial syndromes. Recent research compilation has described three clusters of mutations thought to drive pathophysiology[9]. The clusters 1 and 2 are described below and include germline mutations of the well-known familial syndromes.

1. *Cluster 1: (pseudo-hypoxic signaling)* – hypoxic response from cells via TCA cycle releasing hypoxia-inducible factors and resulting in tumor formation. Germline mutations and intra- or extra-adrenal PCC produce mainly noradrenaline.
   a. *SDH* mutations, *VHL*-related tumors.
2. *Cluster 2: (kinase signaling)* – increased MAP kinase and *P13K-AKT* pathway activity, which increases cell proliferation and catecholamine synthesis. Approximately 20% germline, primarily somatic mutations and intra-adrenal typically produce epinephrine.
   a. *RET, NF1, TMEM-127, MAX, HRAS*
3. *Cluster 3: (Wnt pathway signaling)* – somatic mutations only, intra-adrenal tumors.
   a. *CSDE1, MAML3*

Pheochromocytoma

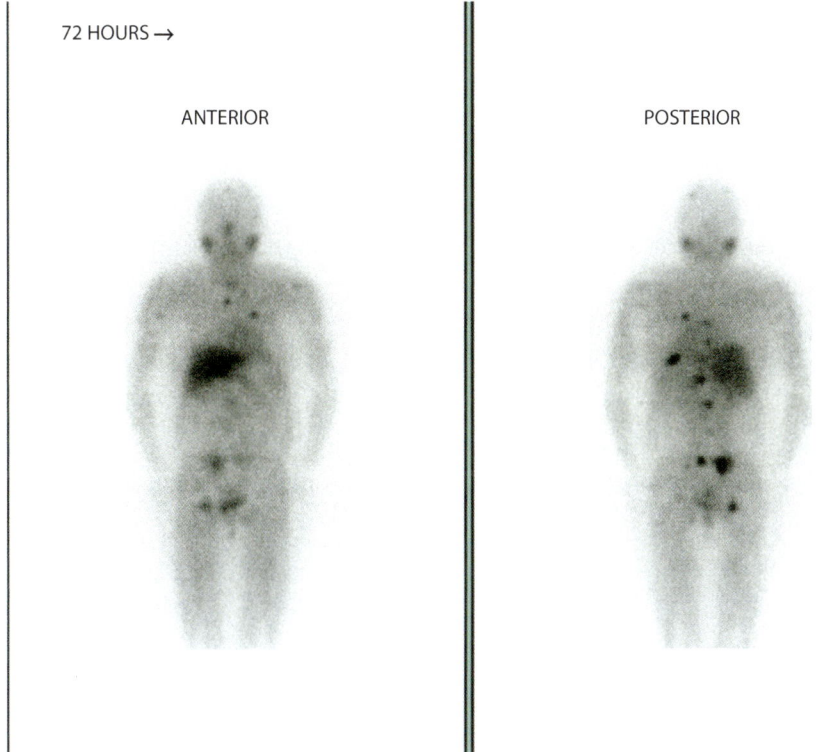

FIGURE 48.3 131I–MIBG therapy scan showing metastasis from malignant PCC.

South Asian perspective on genetic testing

Pheochromocytoma series with genetic data have been reported from three studies in India. The first genetic assay report from **CMC Vellore** analyzed 50 patients with PPGL treated between January 2010 and June 2012; they were screened for mutations in susceptibility genes using an algorithmic approach. Precisely 32% (16/50) of patients were found to be positive for mutations including RET (4), VHL (6), SDHB (3) and SDHD (3) genes. None of these patients were positive for SDHC mutations. A significant association was found between young patients with bilateral tumors and VHL mutations (P = 0.002). NF-1 was not tested in this series[10].

A report from **SGPGI Lucknow** also tested 50 patients, where 10 patients (20%) in all were detected to have a genetic mutation. RET in 6, VHL in 2, SDH in 2 and none with NF1 mutation[11].

In the largest multicenter study, Shah's group based in **KEM Mumbai** analyzed a cohort of one 150 patients in south India; in this study, germline mutations in five susceptibility genes (RET, VHL, SDHB, SDHD and SDHC) were tested by sequencing and NF1 was diagnosed according to phenotype. Of the total population, 49 (32.7%) had germline mutations with commonest being VHL – 23 (15.3%), RET – 13 (8.7%), SDHB – 9 (6%), SDHD – 2 (1.3%) and NF1 – 2 (1.3%). Out of 120 patients with apparently sporadic presentation, 19 (15.8%) had a germline mutation. Mutation carriers were younger (29.9 ± 14.5 vs. 36.8 ± 14.9 years; P = 0.01) and had a higher prevalence of bilateral PCC (26.5 vs 2.9%, P < 0.001) and multifocal tumors (12.2 vs. 0.96%, P = 0.06). Based on syndromic features, metastasis, location and number of tumors, around 96% mutations in this cohort could be detected by appropriately selected single-gene testing[12].

Preoperative preparation

The drug of choice for preoperative preparation is the alpha adrenergic blocking agent phenoxybenzamine, 10 mg twice daily increasing by 10- to 20-mg increments until there is complete elimination of paroxysms of hypertension. A total of 10–14 days of treatment is recommended before surgery; criteria for adequate blockade were given by Roizen et al.[13] which include:

1. No in-hospital blood pressure >160/90 mmHg for 24 hours prior to surgery;
2. No orthostatic hypotension with blood pressure <80/45 mmHg;
3. No ST or T wave changes for 1 week prior to surgery;
4. No more than five premature ventricular contractions per minute.

Side effects of alpha blockade include nasal congestion, postural hypotension, weakness and sedation. In addition, β blockade with a small dose of propranol 40 mg/day is commenced a week prior to surgery. This controls tachycardia and tachyarrhythmias. Beta-blockers are contraindicated in the presence of bronchial asthma and cardiac failure. Prazosin, labetalol, alpha methyl tyrosine and calcium channel blockers have also been tried. Besides alpha blockade, it is also important to see that the intravascular volume deficit, as marked by postural hypotension, is also corrected prior to surgery by increased fluid and salt intake. The hematocrit is known to reduce with fluid status correction and must be rechecked just prior to surgery[14].

Surgery

Surgical excision of pheochromocytoma is the treatment of choice, once diagnosis is made. *Open surgery* via an extended subcostal approach remains the standard technique for larger, invasive adrenal pheochromocytoma. A thoracoabdominal approach has been described for selected cases with large malignant-appearing tumors on the right requiring mobilization or resection of the adjoining liver; alternatively, the liver can be well accessed through the subcostal incision extended in triradiate fashion to the opposite side and to the xiphisternum in the upper midline. The entire tumor should be mobilized carefully taking care not to rupture the capsule. Periadrenal soft tissue should be included in dissecting along the adjacent visceral planes. Adjacent viscera may be invaded by a large malignant PCC and when needed en-bloc resection of kidney, lobe of liver, spleen or distal pancreas may need to be performed to ensure adequate clearance. Formal lymphadenectomy is not required unless significant nodes are visualized on imaging or encountered during dissection. The role of adjuvant postoperative radiation therapy is limited and may be considered in cases of recurrence following second surgery. Figure 48.4 shows the image of operative specimen after adrenalectomy performed for pheochromocytoma in a VHL patient.

Minimally invasive surgery for adrenal tumors began with laparoscopic transperitoneal adrenalectomy[15] (LTA) and is well documented for tumors up to 6–8 cm in size, depending on the surgeon's expertise, and has become the standard of care for smaller noninvasive tumors. Posterior retroperitoneoscopic adrenalectomy (PRA) and robotic adrenalectomy (RA) have also been developed, and there are strong advocates for each method. In a systematic review of the evidence comparing the techniques for all indications, PRA was shown to be more effective than LTA in reducing the operating time, pain scores and hospital stay. RA could not show any superior outcomes and the reducing costs with technical advances will possibly make it more accessible to surgeons in the future. Specifically, for surgery of pheochromocytoma, many studies have shown the suitability of laparoscopic excision and a majority of surgeons prefer the LTA[16,17].

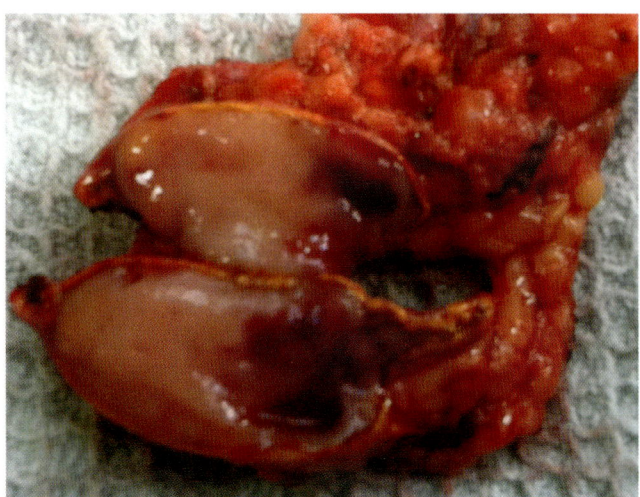

FIGURE 48.4 Operative specimen of pheochromocytoma from a case of VHL.

Cortical sparing surgery – In patients with bilateral disease, such as VHL and MEN II, cortical sparing surgery on the less affected side can be considered. More than 80% of patients will be spared steroid dependence with a small risk (3–8%) of long-term recurrence in the remnant. VHL has been described to have less diffuse disease and is considered most suitable for cortical sparing[18,19].

Anesthesia and perioperative management

Intraoperative surges in blood pressure and heart rate are controlled with intravenous beta-blockers, sodium nitroprusside, glyceryl trinitrate and magnesium infusions. Postoperative fall in blood pressure usually requires transient infusions of noradrenaline for 2–4 hours till stable but may occasionally be prolonged with the need for ICU monitoring. The degree of alpha blockade may impact the duration of postoperative hypotension. Transient fall in blood sugar may occur, which is easily compensated.

Pathological assessment

The histopathologic appearance is characterized by the 'zellballen' pattern with typical nesting of endocrine tumor cells that are large, polygonal with granular cytoplasm. Immunohistochemistry can aid confirmation through positive staining with synaptophysin, chromogranin A, S100 and GATA3.

Malignancy is difficult to diagnose on histopathology as classic features are absent in cytological and architectural detail. According to WHO 2004 criteria, malignancy is reliably diagnosed only by metastasis to tissues where chromaffin tissue is not normally found like lymph nodes, lung, liver and bone[20]. Pathologists have attempted to correlate histopathological features with malignant clinical behavior and formulated two scoring systems to assist clinical management – the PASS and GAPP scores that are widely used, the GAPP score providing a better predictive grouping into three categories with significant difference in metastatic rates and survival:

1. The **PASS** proposed by Thomson et al. scores features of periadrenal adipose invasion, >3 mitoses/10 high-power fields, atypical mitoses, necrosis, cellular spindling, marked nuclear pleomorphism, cellular monotony, large nests or diffuse growth, high cellularity, capsular invasion, vascular invasion; a score of ≥4 predicts malignant behavior[21,22].
2. The **GAPP** score proposed by Kimura from the Japanese study group[22] incorporates histological pattern, cellularity, comedo-type necrosis, capsular/vascular invasion, Ki67 labeling index and catecholamine type. All tumors were scored from 0 to 10 points and were graded as one of the three types: well-differentiated (0–2 points), moderately differentiated (3–6 points) and poorly differentiated (7–10 points); the 5-year survival rate differed significantly at 100%, 66.8% and 22.4%, respectively[23].

Recurrence of PCC has been documented in multiple studies between 6.5% and 16.5% of cases. The recurrence is usually in the adrenal bed; other sites are contralateral adrenal, PGL sites or

Pheochromocytoma

distant metastatic sites in malignant PCC. One study analyzed local recurrence in 13 cases[24] and documented the right retrocaval site is at highest risk due to inadequate dissection of the tumor burrowing posterior to the Inferior Vena Cava size >5 cm is an independent risk factor. Tumor seeding from capsular rupture at surgery or metastatic disease also may cause local recurrence. Close follow-up is required with biochemical screening and routine imaging; CT scanning is more sensitive to pick up early recurrence in up to 25% of cases.

Systemic therapy: Distant metastasis from malignant pheochromocytoma occurs in between 8% and 13% of cases and may be excised when surgically feasible to control disease and hormonal effects. Multiple metastatic sites can also undergo ablative therapy with Radio Frequency Ablation. Residual disease and metastatic disease can be adequately treated with ablative doses of PRRT (peptide receptor radionuclide therapy) – common agents include ^{131}I-MIBG, ^{90}Y-DOTATATE or ^{177}Lu-DOTATATE. Combination chemotherapy with cyclophosphamide, vincristine and dacarbazine can be used to palliate advanced pheochromocytoma. Urinary catecholamines are a good indicator of the response. Though many therapies show tumor response, none have demonstrated significant survival advantage. Tyrosine kinase inhibitors and immunotherapy are in clinical trials and results are eagerly awaited[25]. Figure 48.5 summarizes the management of patient with clinical suspicion of pheochromocytoma.

Special problems in pheochromocytomas

Hypertensive crisis: This is precipitated by drugs, anesthesia or invasive procedures. Here, they must be stabilized with intravenous phentolamine 2.5 mg IV or with sodium nitroprusside 0.5–1.5 µg/kg/min. Surgical excision is often appropriate after adequate medical preparation.

Pheochromocytoma in pregnancy: It is often misdiagnosed as preeclampsia and is potentially life-threatening to mother and child. Emergency cesarean section may be needed with concomitant or delayed excision of the pheochromocytoma. All women with hypertension in the first two trimesters of pregnancy must be screened for pheochromocytoma. Ultrasound and MRI are safe and recommended for adequate assessment for PCC/PGL. When a diagnosis is made in the first/second trimester, the tumor should be excised preferably by laparoscopic surgery after alpha and beta adrenergic blockade during the second trimester before 24-week gestation[26]. In case of bilateral PCC, the larger tumor may be excised followed by cesarean section delivery and planned excision of the second tumor 3 months after delivery. In the third trimester, pharmacological control is obtained and the tumor is excised along with an elective cesarean section. Vaginal delivery should be avoided, which may lead to a fatal outcome.

Conclusions

Pheochromocytoma and PGL have variable clinical behavior and increasingly recognized to occur as inheritable genetic syndromes requiring careful clinical, biochemical and genetic diagnosis. In many locations in South Asia, there is inadequate access to genetic testing, advanced biochemical assays and nuclear imaging. Experience in identifying and managing familial disease is limited outside major centers. Expertise in biochemical assessment, imaging and perioperative anesthesia care is also difficult to accrue on account of the rarity of the disease. The optimal desired care can be provided by endocrinologist, geneticist, surgeon, anesthetist and nuclear physician working in close cooperation as a multidisciplinary team, which is required in larger centers to take care of these complex tumors and associated syndromes. Clinicians interested in providing care can build networks of expertise outside of the larger established hospital systems to promote quality care. It is recommended that cases of PPGL, when diagnosed, are referred to experienced groups with multidisciplinary management to give the patients the appropriate workup and surgical management at the first instance to maximize favorable outcomes.

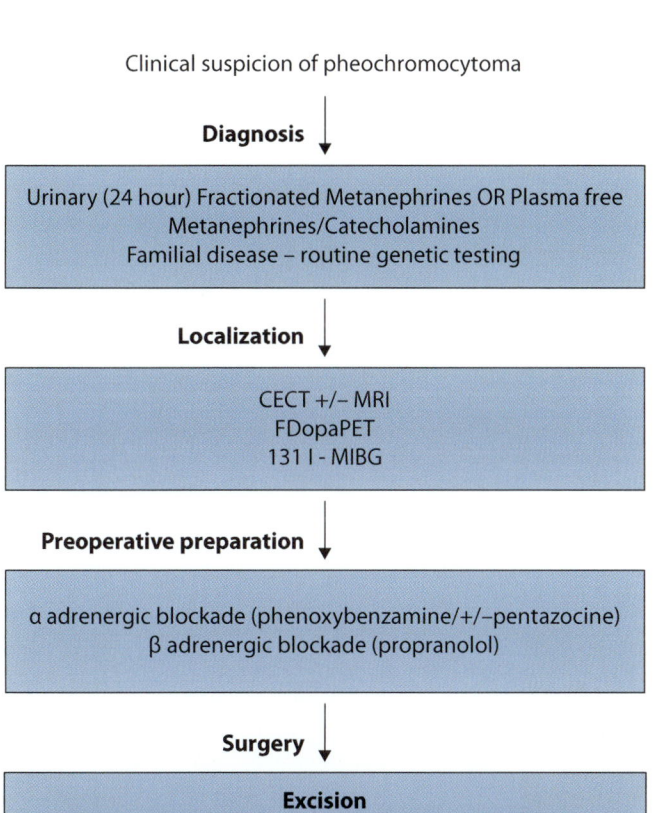

FIGURE 48.5 Management of phaeochromocytoma.

References

1. Birke B, Arthur ST, Kurt W, et al. Pioneer in pheochromocytoma. J Endocr Soc. 2017 Jul;1(7):957–964.
2. Pick L. Das Ganglioma embryonale sympathicum (Sympathoma embryonale), eine typische bösartige Geschwulstform des sympathischen Nervensystems. Berlin Klin Wochenschr. 1912;49:16–22.
3. Takamine J. Adrenalin the active principle of the suprarenal glands and its mode of preparation. Am J Pharm. 1901;73:523–535.
4. Manger WM. An overview of pheochromocytoma: History, current concepts, vagaries, and diagnostic challenges. Ann N Y Acad Sci. 2006;1073:1–20.
5. Grumbach MM, Biller BM, Braunstein GD, et al. Management of the clinically inapparent adrenal mass ("incidentaloma"). Ann Intern Med. 2003;138(5):424.
6. Fogarty J, Engel C, Russo J, et al. Hypertension and pheochromocytoma testing: The association with anxiety disorders. Arch Fam Med. 1994;3:55.
7. Chen H, Sippel RS, O'Dorisio MS, et al. The North American Neuroendocrine Tumour Society (NANETS) consensus guideline for the diagnosis and management of neuroendocrine tumours: Pheochromocytoma, paraganglioma and medullary thyroid cancer. Pancreas. 2010;39:775–783.

8. Fishbein L, Merrill S, Fraker DL, et al. Inherited mutations in pheochromocytoma and paraganglioma: Why all patients should be offered genetic testing. Ann Surg Oncol. 2013;20(5):1444–1450.
9. Dahia PL. Pheochromocytoma and paraganglioma pathogenesis: Learning from genetic heterogeneity. Nat Rev Cancer. 2014;14:108–119.
10. Pai R, Ebenazer A, Paul MJ, et al. Mutations seen among patients with pheochromocytoma and paraganglioma at a referral center from India. Horm Metab Res. 2015 Feb;47(2):133–137.
11. Agarwal G, Rajan S, Valiveru RC, et al. Genetic profile of Indian pheochromocytoma and paraganglioma patients – A single institutional study. Indian J Endocrinol Metab. 2019 Jul-Aug;23(4):486–490.
12. Pandit R, Khadilkar K, Sarathi V, et al. Germline mutations and genotype-phenotype correlation in Asian Indian patients with pheochromocytoma and paraganglioma. Eur J Endocrinol. 2016 Oct;175(4):311–323.
13. Roizen MF, Horrigan RW, Koike M, et al. A prospective randomized trial of four anaesthetic techniques for resection of pheochromocytoma. Anesthesiology. 1982;57:A43.
14. Pacak K. Preoperative management of the pheochromocytoma patient. J Clin Endocrinol Metab. 2007;92:4069–4079.
15. Gagner M, Breton G, Pharand D, Pomp A. Is laparoscopic adrenalectomy indicated for pheochromocytomas? Surgery. 1996 Dec;120(6):1076–1079; discussion 1079-80.
16. Agarwal G, Sadacharan D, Aggarwal V, et al. Surgical management of organ-contained unilateral pheochromocytoma: Comparative outcomes of laparoscopic and conventional open surgical procedures in a large single-institution series. Langenbecks Arch Surg. 2012 Oct;397(7):1109–1116.
17. Chai YJ, Kwon H, Yu HW, et al. Systematic review of surgical approaches for adrenal tumours: Lateral transperitoneal versus posterior retroperitoneal and laparoscopic verus robotic adrenalectomy. Int J Endocrinol. 2014;918346:1–11.
18. Rossitti HM, Söderkvist P, Gimm O. Extent of surgery for phaeochromocytoma in the genomic era. Br J Surg. 2018 Jan;105(2):e84–e98.
19. Neumann HPH, Tsoy U, Bancos I, et al. Comparison of pheochromocytoma-specific morbidity and mortality among adults with bilateral pheochromocytomas undergoing total adrenalectomy vs cortical-sparing adrenalectomy. JAMA Netw Open. 2019 Aug;2(8):e198898.
20. Thompson LD, Young WF, Kawashima A, Komminoth P. Malignant adrenal phaeochromocytoma. In: R.A. DeLellis and R.V. Lloyd, eds., World Health Organization Classification of Tumours Pathology & Genetics Tumours of Endocrine Organs. 3rd ed. Lyon, France: IARC; 2004. pp. 147–150.
21. Thompson LD. Pheochromocytoma of the Adrenal gland Scaled Score (PASS) to separate benign from malignant neoplasms: A clinicopathologic and immunophenotypic study of 100 cases. Am J Surg Pathol. 2002 May;26(5):551–566.
22. Kimura N, Takayanagi R, Takizawa N, et al, Phaeochromocytoma Study Group in Japan. Pathological grading for predicting metastasis in phaeochromocytoma and paraganglioma. Endocr Relat Cancer. 2014 Jun;21(3):405–414.
23. Kimura N, Takekoshi K, Naruse M. Risk stratification on pheochromocytoma and paraganglioma on laboratory and clinical medicine. J Clin Med. 2018 Sep;7(9):242.
24. Sonbare DJ, Abraham DT, Rajaratnam S, et al. Re-operative surgery for pheochromocytoma-paraganglioma: Analysis of 13 cases from a single institution. Indian J Surg. 2018 Apr;80(2):123–127.
25. Ilanchezhian M, Jha A, Pacak K, et al. Emerging treatments for advanced/metastatic pheochromocytoma-paraganglioma. Curr Treat Options Oncol. 2020 Aug;21(11):85.
26. Donatini G, Kraimps JL, Caillard C, et al. Pheochromocytoma diagnosed during pregnancy: Lessons learned from a series of ten patients. Surg Endosc. 2018 Sep;32(9):3890–3900.

49
CUSHING'S SYNDROME
Anand Kumar Mishra

Introduction

Cushing's syndrome (CS) is a symptom complex resulting from chronic exposure to excess glucocorticoids. The most common cause is exogenous intake. Patient can present with varying subclinical, cyclical or mild to rapid-onset severe symptoms, and they have debilitating morbidities and enhanced mortality. Therefore, an early confirmation of hypercortisolism causes identification, and optimum treatment is important in these patients. The diagnosis is sometimes difficult, particularly in mild cases and ectopic sources. Progress in biochemical testing, imaging techniques, endoscopic hypophysectomy, laparoscopic adrenalectomy, and radiotherapy techniques has improved the management of patients. Optimum treatment consists of selective and complete resection of the causative tumor to allow eventual normalization of the hypothalamic-pituitary-adrenal axis and avoidance of tumor recurrence.

Definition

CS is defined as clinical manifestation and metabolic complications of pathologic hypercortisolism. The common clinical manifestations are weight gain with central obesity, facial roundening, skin thinning with easy bruisability, and proximal muscle weakness. Metabolic complications are diabetes mellitus, hypertension, dyslipidemia, and metabolic bone disease.

Epidemiology

CS has incidence of 0.5–2 cases per million per year, prevalence of 39–79 per million in various populations, median age of onset/diagnosis 41.4 years with a female-to-male ratio of 3:1. Hypercortisolism is observed with higher incidence in patients suffering from hypertension (0.5–2%), diabetes (2–3%), early-onset osteoporosis or vertebral fracture (11%). A total of 10% of patients with adrenal masses have hypercortisolism (1–7). Adrenal CS is four times more common in females and is not seen in excess in any ethnicity, race, or region. It mainly affects either the pediatrics age or 20–50 (8–11).

Cushing's disease is seen commonly between 3rd and 5th decade of life; it is rare in children, however one-third cases of childhood CS post puberty are due to pituitary cause. Adrenal tumors have a bimodal age distribution, with small peaks in first decade of life for both adenomas and carcinomas and major peaks at approximately 50 years for adenomas and 40 years for carcinomas. Adrenal carcinoma is responsible for 50% of childhood CS.

Etiology

Exogenous corticosteroid exposure is the most common cause of CS. Endogenous CS can be ACTH (adrenocorticotropic hormone) dependent or independent (Table 49.1). CS caused by pituitary microadenoma, secreting ACTH also known as Cushing's disease is the most common cause of CS among endogenous hypercortisolism. CS caused by adrenal tumors are second in frequency which are ACTH independent and ectopic ACTH secreting tumors are third most common cause of CS (Table 49.2, Figures 49.1–49.4).

Carney complex or syndrome is a rare type of tumor complex which is also responsible for CS (Table 49.3). Adrenal carcinoma usually presents with clinical hypercortisolism alone (45%) or with androgen overproduction (25%). Bilateral adrenal hyperplasias are characterized by nodule diameter greater than 1 cm (macronodular) or less than 1 cm (micronodular). The macronodular is both sporadic and familial with autosomal dominant transmission and also associated with MEN1, familial adenomatous polyposis, and fumarate hydratase gene mutations. The various genetic mutations or abnormal protein expression which are believed to play a part in the pathophysiology are shown in

TABLE 49.1: Causes of Cushing's Syndrome

A. ACTH-dependent (70–80%)
    a. Pituitary corticotroph adenoma or Cushing's disease (60–70%)
    b. Ectopic ACTH syndromes (5–10%)
    c. *Ectopic CRH*: very rare
B. Non-ACTH–dependent (20–30%)
    a. Iatrogenic
    b. Adrenal adenoma (10–22%)
    c. Carcinoma (5–7%)
    d. Primary bilateral macronodular adrenal hyperplasia BMAH (<2%)
    e. Primary pigmented nodular adrenocortical disease (PPNAD) and Carney syndrome
    f. Non-pigmented variant, isolated micronodular adrenocortical disease
    g. Aberrant receptor expression (gastric inhibitory polypeptide, interleukin-1b)
    h. McCune Albright syndrome
C. *Other causes (nonneoplastic)*: alcoholism, depression, obesity, pregnancy

TABLE 49.2: Tumors Causing Ectopic ACTH Syndrome

Tumor	Incidence (%)
Small-cell lung Ca	50
Non-small-cell lung Ca	5
Pancreatic neuroendocrine tumors	10
Thymic neuroendocrine tumors	5
Lung neuroendocrine tumors	10
Others neuroendocrine tumors	2
Medullary carcinoma thyroid	5
Pheochromocytoma and related tumors	3
Rare cancers of prostrate, breast, ovary, gall bladder, colon	10

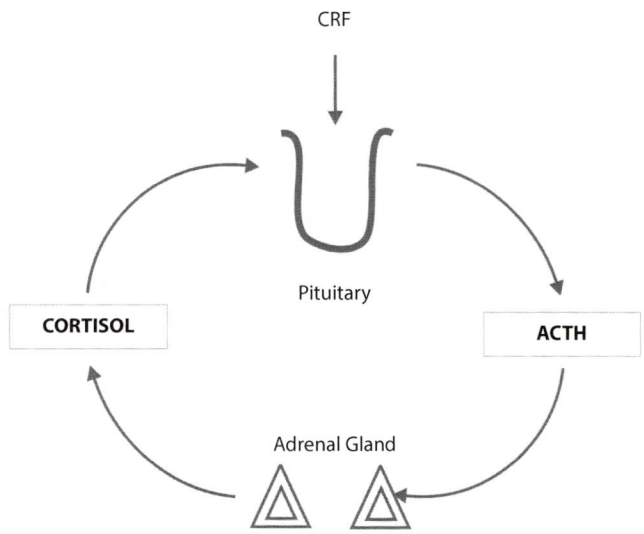

FIGURE 49.1 Normal hypothalamus – pituitary adrenal axis.

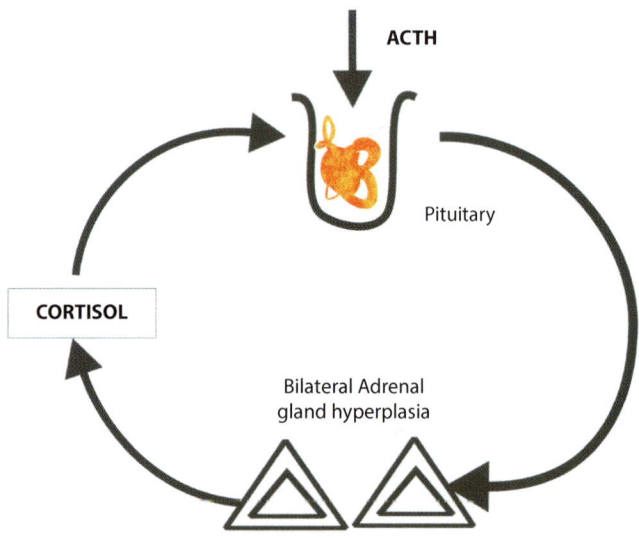

FIGURE 49.2 Cushing's disease.

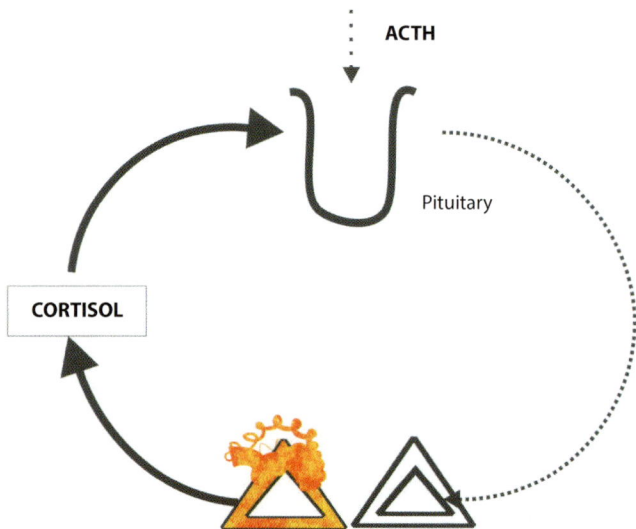

FIGURE 49.3 Adrenal tumor.

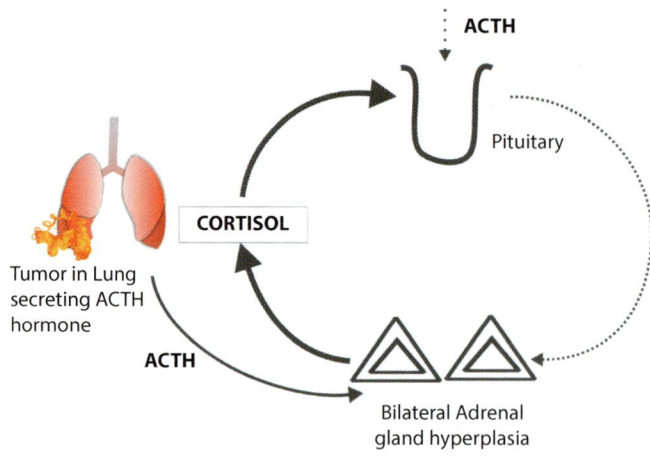

FIGURE 49.4 Ectopic ACTH syndrome.

Table 49.4. The most frequent mechanisms are highlighted in bold characters, and other potential mechanisms are in normal characters while a question mark is shown in bracket in unconfirmed association or genetic predisposition. In bilateral macronodular adrenal hyperplasia (BMAH), the most common mutations observed are in armadillo repeat containing 5 gene (*ARMC5*, chromosome 16p11.2) (8, 9, 12–14).

Pathophysiology

Cortisol is a steroid, catabolic hormone secreted from zona fasciculata of adrenal cortex. In normal physiological conditions, it is secreted by stress. In the circulation, it is 90% bounded by cortisol-binding protein with bioavailability of 60–100%. Excess cortisol causes gluconeogenesis from protein catabolism, glycogenolysis and increases insulin resistance. Due to these three mechanisms, free glucose levels increase. It controls the transcription and translation of enzyme proteins involved in the metabolism of fats, glycogen, proteins synthesis, and Krebs cycle. Prolonged proteins catabolism causes development of purplish striae, osteoporosis, and poor wound healing. High cortisol causes a decrease lymphocytes and increase in neutrophils. Cortisol inhibits the production of IL-2, TNF alpha, IFN alpha, and gamma. Decreased IL-2 levels prevent the proliferation of T-lymphocytes.

TABLE 49.3: Carney Complex: Clinical Features

Clinical Features	Prevalence (%)
Skin lesions: pigmented, blue nevi, cutaneous myxomas	80
Cardiac myxomas	72
Pigmented nodular adrenal hyperplasia	45
Bilateral breast fibroadenomas in females only	45
Testicular tumors in males only	56
Growth hormone secreting pituitary lesions	10
Neural lesions (gastric schwannomas)	Less than 5
Other tumors: thyroid cancers, acoustic neuromas, hepatomas	Rare

Cushing's Syndrome

TABLE 49.4: Frequent Genetic Mutations and Molecular Mechanism in CS

Abnormal protein and gene expression	Cushing's Disease	Mild Hypercortisolism	Overt Hypercortisolism	Ectopic ACTH Secretion
Abnormal protein expression	Brg1, HDAC2, TR4, PTTG, EGFR, others	**GPCR, POMC/ACTH,** PRKAR1A (BMAH)	GPCR, **PRKAR1A**, PRKACA, glucocorticoid receptor	–
Gene mutations	**USP8,** *MEN1, CDKIs, CDKN1B/p27Kip1, AIP, SDHx(?), DICER1,* others	CTNNB1 (16%) **ARMC5** (55% of BMAH) MEN1, FH, GNAS1, PDE11A, PDE8B, MC2R, PRKACA, DOT1L(?)*, HDAC9(?)*, PRUNE2(?)*(BMAH)	PRKACA (35–69%) GNAS (5–17%) **PRKAR1A** (66% of PPNAD)	*RET, MEN1,* others

*(?) – Not established.

Clinical symptoms

Screening of CS is recommended in following situations:

1. Any patient with manifestations consistent with CS
2. Any young adult with hypertension
3. Children with decreasing growth velocity and increasing weight
4. Adrenal incidentaloma
5. Resistant hypertension, progressive osteoporosis, and vertebral compressive fracture
6. Patient having severe proximal muscle weakness features
7. Wide purple voilaceous striae on the abdomen, thigh, or any other area.

The presence and severity of symptoms depends on following factors (8, 9, 12):

- Degree and duration of hypercortisolism
- Presence or absence of androgen excess
- Cause of the hypercortisolism:
  - Hyperpigmentation by high ACTH
  - Androgen excess is seen in women with adrenal Ca or ACTH-stimulated hyperandrogenism as adrenal gland is a major source of androgen production in women but not men)
  - Adenomas generally secrete only glucocorticoids
- Adrenal Ca or ectopic ACTH syndromes have rapid course and small duration of symptoms. Therefore, these patients have more tumor-related symptoms such as weight loss instead of weight gain and less features of hypercortisolism. Ectopic ACTH patients can have electrolyte disturbances with very rapid course.
- Incidentaloma without clinical manifestations of CS usually have mild hypercortisolism (subclinical) on biochemical testing, which is also known as "autonomous cortisol secretion".

In adults, signs and symptoms most suggestive of the presence of CS are proximal muscle weakness, facial plethora, wasting of the extremities with increased fat in the abdomen and face, wide purplish striae, bruising without obvious trauma, and supraclavicular fat pads. The clinical manifestations of CS can be categorized as reproductive, dermatologic, metabolic, cardiovascular, musculoskeletal, neuropsychiatric, and infectious (Table 49.5, Figures 49.5–49.13).

Reproductive
Menstrual irregularities: Oligomenorrhea, amenorrhea, excess, or variable menses

TABLE 49.5: Symptoms and Signs of CS

	Common	Less Common
Symptoms and complications	Especially in young age Hypertension Diabetes mellitus Osteoporosis and vertebral fractures	Fatigue Weight gain Depression, mood and appetite change, Impairment of concentration, memory Back pain Oligomenorrhea Polycystic ovary syndrome Recurrent infections Kidney stones
Signs	Facial plethora Proximal muscle weakness Striae (red-purple, >1 cm wide) Easy bruising In children-weight gain with reduced height	Central obesity Buffalo hump, supraclavicular fullness Facial fullness Acne and hirsutism Skin thinning Poor wound healing Peripheral edema

Signs of adrenal androgen excess: Women suffering from adrenal Ca can have signs of androgen excess as adrenal glands are the major source of androgens in women. These tumors usually secrete large amounts of androgenic precursors, because they are inefficient at converting cholesterol to cortisol. Symptoms are:

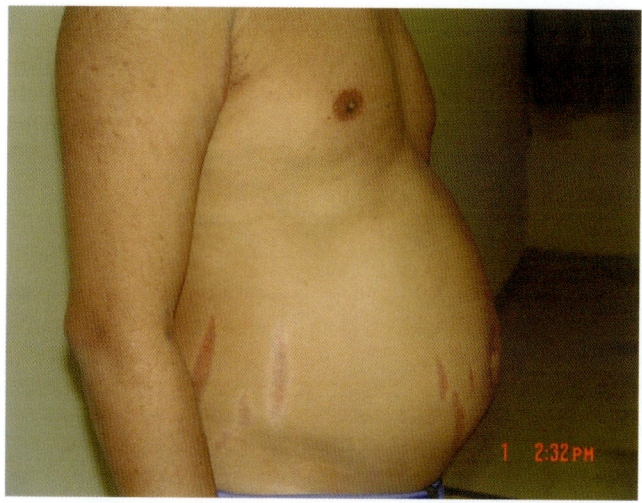

FIGURE 49.5 Centripetal obesity.

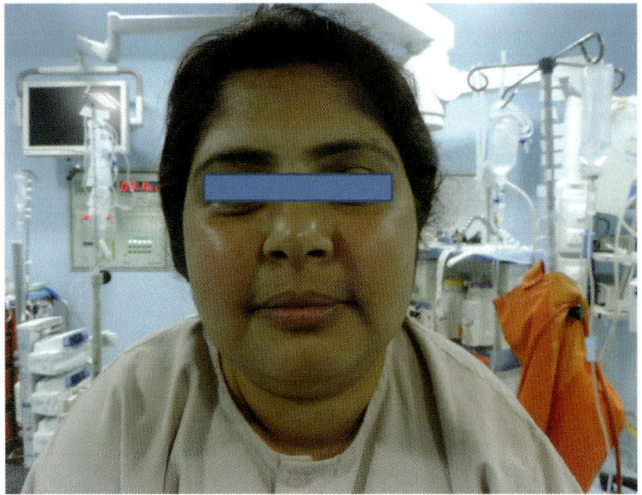

FIGURE 49.6 Moon faces.

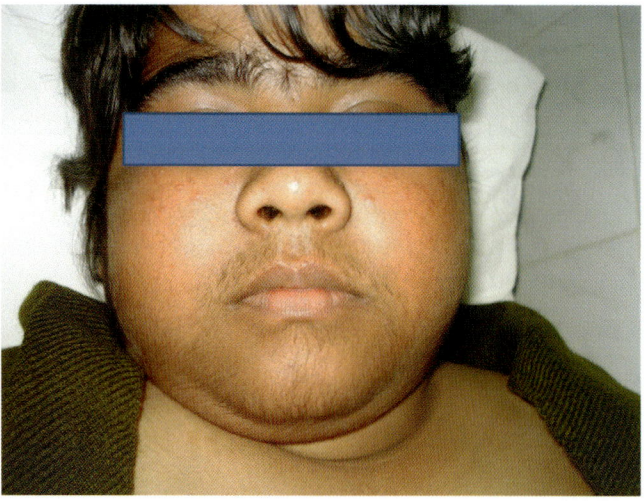

FIGURE 49.7 Hirsutism, moon faces.

1. Hirsutism – mild, limited to face but can be generalized
2. Oily facial skin and acne on the face, neck, or shoulders.
3. Increased libido
4. Temporal balding, deepening voice, male body habitus, male escutcheon, and clitoral hypertrophy, occurs only in girls or women with extremely high serum androgens
5. Premature puberty in prepubertal males

Dermatologic

Catabolic effects of glucocorticoid cause loss of subcutaneous connective tissue and the stratum corneum in skin is thinned. Symptoms are:

1. Easy bruisability after minimal injury
2. Purple wide striae in trunk, breasts, hips, buttocks, shoulders, upper thighs, upper arms, axillae, lower abdomen, and flanks as thin skin does not hide the color of venous blood in the underlying dermis.

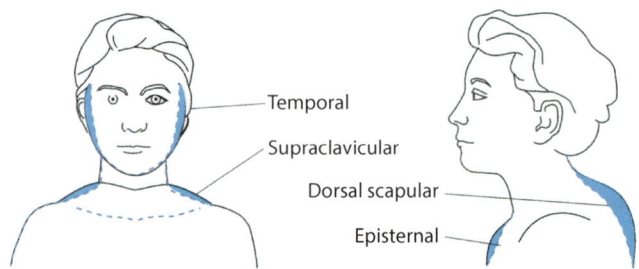

FIGURE 49.8 Distribution of adipose tissue in Cushing's syndrome. Fat deposition in cheeks (moon faces), Fat also may accumulate bilaterally above the clavicles (supraclavicular collar), in front of the sternum (episternal area, or dewlap), and over the back of the neck (dorsal cervical fat pad, or buffalo hump). The dotted line depicts normal contours of patients without Cushing's syndrome.

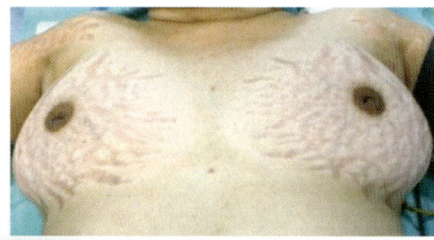

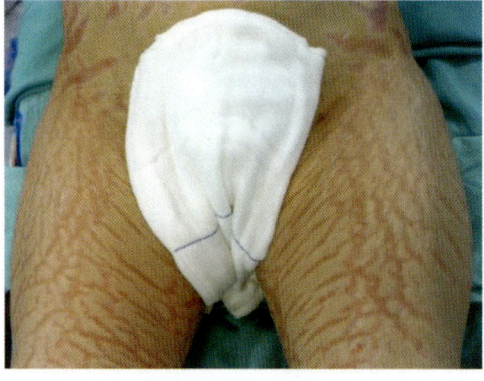

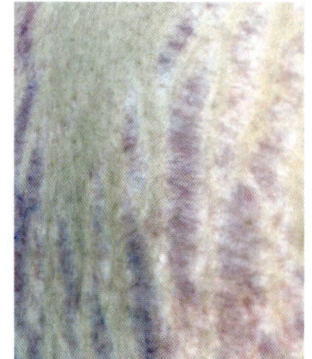

FIGURE 49.9 Large violaceous striae over abdomen, thighs, and chest.

Cushing's Syndrome

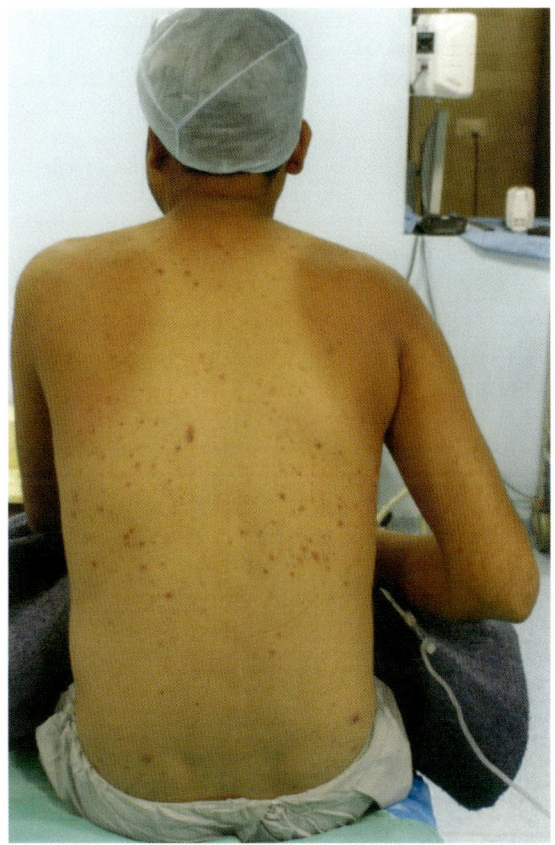

FIGURE 49.10 Hyperpigmentation and petechial hemorrhage.

3. Skin atrophy
4. Cutaneous fungal infections, especially tinea versicolor on trunk, nails
5. Hyperpigmentation: It is induced by high ACTH in ectopic ACTH syndrome and most visible in exposed body parts like face, neck, and back of the hands or body parts vulnerable to trauma, friction, or pressure such as the elbows, knees, spine, knuckles, waist, and shoulders (brassiere straps). Patchy pigmentation may occur on the inner surface of lips and the buccal mucosa along the line of dental occlusion.

Metabolic

- Overt hyperglycemia (10–15%)
- Glucose intolerance
- There is excess fat deposition in the trunk and various places causing progressive central obesity involving face rounding (moon faces), neck (thick short), "buffalo hump", trunk, abdomen, spinal canal, and mediastinum. The extremities are

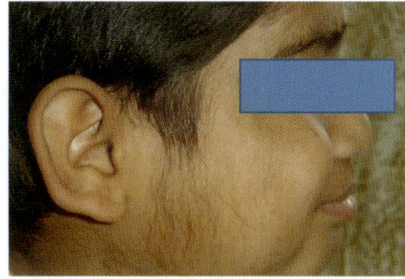

FIGURE 49.11 Excessive facial hairs.

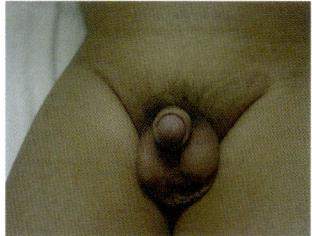

FIGURE 49.12 Early secondary sexual characteristics.

often spared and may be wasted. Children with CS have generalized obesity and growth retardation with age-matched normal children. The suggested cause of central fat distributions is cortisol-induced downregulation of adenosine monophosphate-activated protein kinase (AMPK) that regulates lipid and carbohydrate metabolism, conversion of cortisone to cortisol, and higher serum leptin concentrations.

Cardiovascular

Patients have hypertension, dyslipidemia, heart failure, dilated cardiomyopathy and higher risk of death from myocardial infarction, stroke, and thromboembolism. Angiotensin-converting enzyme (ACE) inhibitors should be considered the first-line treatment of hypertension in CS. Severe hypertension and hypokalemia are more prevalent in patients with ectopic ACTH.

Neuropsychological changes and cognition

In adults, learning, cognition, and memory (especially short-term memory) are impaired by hypercortisolism. Children tend to be overachievers, often ranking near the top of their class.

The common psychological symptoms are:

- Emotional lability
- Depression (37–86% of patients)
- Irritability (86%)
- Anxiety (up to 80%)
- Panic attacks (up to 30%)
- Mild paranoia and mania are less common

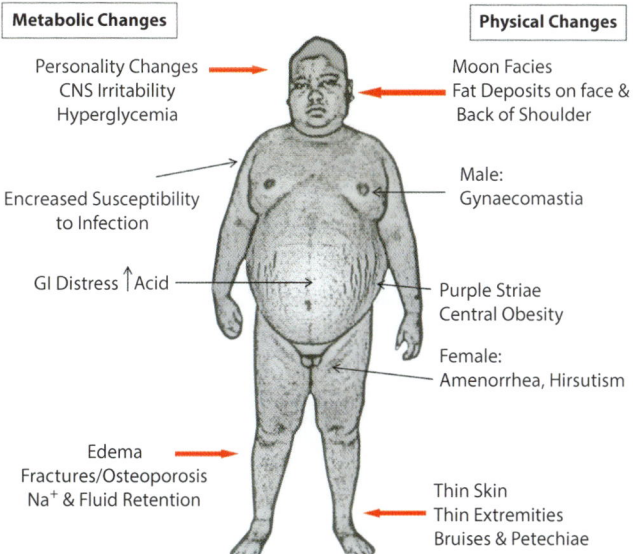

FIGURE 49.13 Cushing's syndrome: Metabolic and physical changes.

Infection and immune function

There is an higher chances of infections caused by inhibition of immune function by glucocorticoids (fall in circulating CD4 cells and decline in natural killer cell activity, inhibit the synthesis of almost all cytokines, inhibition of cytokine release) and thymic atrophy.

Ophthalmologic findings

High intraocular pressure, cataracts, and central serous chorioretinopathy more common with exogenous glucocorticoid administration.

Diagnosis

In a suspected CS, two questions needs to be answered

Q1. Is this patient suffering from CS?
Q2. If yes what is the cause of?

It is essential to confirm endogenous hypercortisolism biochemically and then proceed for radiological investigations to localize the source. Cortisol is secreted in an unbound state but is bound to plasma proteins corticosteroid–binding globulin (CBG or transcortin – 75%) and albumin (15%) in circulation. Only free steroids are biologically active, filtered through kidney, and regulated by ACTH. Plasma free cortisol is about 10% of the circulating cortisol (1 µg/dL). Half-life of plasma cortisol is 60–90 minutes. CBG in plasma has a total cortisol-binding capacity of about 25 µg/dL, and free cortisol increases rapidly if plasma cortisol concentration rises beyond this. 24-hour urinary free cortisol (UFC) is a useful indicator of total cortisol production by the adrenal. Cortisol secretion is tightly matched to ACTH, and both are secreted in a pulsatile fashion. There are normally three mechanisms of control:

1. Circadian rhythm, which is superimposed on episodic secretion
2. Feedback inhibition by glucocorticoids
3. Response to stress (e.g., pain, fright, hypoglycemia) which can override the circadian rhythm *and* feedback inhibition
   Step I: Exclude exogenous glucocorticoids and physiologic hypercortisolism (Table 49.6) by careful history. If wide purplish stria, proximal myopathy, and easy bruising are associated in conditions having physiologic hypercortisolism then only screening tests should be performed.
   Step II: Establish the diagnosis. Diagnosis by three approaches (Table 49.7):

TABLE 49.6: Conditions Associated with Physiologic Hypercortisolism

	Conditions
May have some clinical features of CS	Pregnancy
	Severe obesity (visceral obesity or polycystic ovary syndrome)
	Psychological stress (major depressive disorder)
	Poorly controlled diabetes mellitus
	Chronic alcoholism
	Physical stress (illness, hospitalization/surgery, pain)
	Obstructive sleep apnea
Unlikely to have clinical features of CS	Malnutrition, anorexia nervosa
	Intense chronic exercise
	Hypothalamic amenorrhea
	High corticosteroid-binding globulin
	Glucocorticoid resistance

1. Assessing daily cortisol excretion, by means of 24-hours UFC (at least two samples)
2. Documenting the loss of normal diurnal variation in cortisol secretion, with late-night salivary cortisol (at least two samples)
3. Documenting loss of feedback inhibition of cortisol on the hypothalamic-pituitary-adrenal axis, with 1-mg dexamethasone suppression test or low-dose dexamethasone suppression test (LDDST) (2 mg/day for 48 hours).
   Step III: **Evaluation for the cause (Table 49.7, Figures 49.2–49.4)**

24-hour urinary cortisol excretion: It provides a direct and reliable practical index of cortisol secretion and measure free cortisol. In the given sample, urinary creatinine excretion levels should also be measured simultaneously. The test is interpreted as positive and is a very good "rule in" test for CS when basal urinary cortisol excretion is more than three times the upper limit of normal. False positive results are seen in individuals with high fluid intake.

Late-night salivary cortisol: Cortisol is secreted in saliva and remains stable even at room temperature for several days. Late night salivary cortisol concentration is used to establish the diagnosis. It is noninvasive, can be done by the patient at home and useful in cyclical or intermittent CS but not a good test for patients with erratic sleep schedules or shift work. It is useful to evaluate at least three samples from different days.

Low-dose dexamethasone suppression tests (LDDST): There are two forms of LDDST: the 1 mg "overnight" and the two-day 2 mg test.

1. *Overnight 1-mg test or overnight DST*: Administration of 1 mg of dexamethasone at 11 p.m.–12 a.m. (midnight) and measurement of serum cortisol at 8 AM the next morning. Serum cortisol level should be less than 1.8 µg/dL or 50 nmol/L in normal individual.
2. *Standard two-day 2-mg test or low-dose DST*: Administering 0.5 mg of dexamethasone every 6 hours for 8 doses, and measurement of serum cortisol either 2 or 6 hours after the last dose. Serum cortisol level should be less than 1.8 µ/dL or 50 nmol/L in normal individual. This test has best negative predictive value and overall best sensitivity to rule out hypercortisolism (100%).

For diagnosis, do one of the following first-line tests:

1. Late-night salivary cortisol (two measurements),
2. 24-Hour UFC excretion (two measurements)
3. Overnight 1-mg dexamethasone suppression test (ONDST)
4. Morning ACTH is done after confirmation of endogenous hypercortisolism biochemically. A suppressed level (<10 pg/mL) establishes ACTH independent cause confirming the diagnosis of an adrenal cause.

Pseudo CS: It is characterized by over activity of HPA (hypothalamic-pituitary-adrenal) axis but without features of CS. It is seen in depression, anxiety disorders, alcoholism, poorly controlled diabetes mellitus, and morbid obesity. Two tests can differentiate between CS and Pseudo CS:

1. Midnight single salivary cortisol levels more than 7.5 µm/dL can discriminate with 100% specificity.
2. Combined dexamethasone – CRH test has 100% diagnostic accuracy.

Cushing's Syndrome

TABLE 49.7: Test for Diagnosis and Differential Diagnosis in CS

Name of the Test	Procedure	Result Interpretation and Normal Values	Sensitivity and Specificity	Comments
Overnight dexamethasone suppression test (ONDST)	1-mg dexamethasone (D) between 11 and 12 p.m. and collection of plasma cortisol between 8 and 9 a.m.	Failure to suppress the morning cortisol levels to <1.8 µg/dL or 50 nmol/L	95% sensitivity 80 specificity False +ve in 30% False −ve 2% Preferred test if GFR low or renal failure	**False +ve reasons**: Normal individuals 13% Obese 50% women on estrogens 25% hospitalized and critically ill patients Dexamethasone taken too early Drugs: phenobarbital, phenytoin, estrogens, malabsorption, alcoholism, morbid obesity, pregnancy
24-hour urinary free cortisol (UFC)	Reflection of unbound circulatory cortisol Serum creatinine to be done in all cases UFC decreases when GFR <30 mL/minute Method: HPLC or gas chromatography and mass spectrometry	Normal: 110–138 nmol/24 hours or 40–50 µg/hour If values >normal: positive and >4 times diagnostic	**Best specificity** Preferred test in pregnancy (2nd or 3rd trimester) for values >3 times diagnostic	**10–15% CS will have 1 in 4 samples normal** Milder elevation in pregnancy and pseudo CS False positive in fluid intake >5 L/day
Midnight salivary cortisol	2 methods: Chew cotton pledget for 2–3 minutes, place in plastic tube or passively drool saliva in plastic tube Method: Immunoassay or liquid chromatography–mass spectrometry		Simple, convenient, **Sensitivity 100% Specificity 83%** Positive predictive value: 94% Negative predictive value: 100%	False positive in smokers, tobacco chewers, oral disease Not suitable in patients with less saliva production
Midnight plasma cortisol	After admission IV cannula inserted before 10 PM and when patient is sleeping, midnight blood drawn	7.5 µg/dL or 207 nom/L	**Specific 100%**	
Low-dose dexamethasone (D) suppression test (LDDST)	0.5 mg D × 6 hours × 2 days, start at 9 a.m. and day 2 24 hours UFC collection or S cortisol 9 a.m. day 1 and at 48 hours	Normal UFC <10 mg (27 nmol) per 24 hours in 2nd day or Plasma cortisol <1.8 µm/dL (50 nmol/L)	**Sensitivity 97–100% Sensitivity and specificity >95%**	
High-dose dexamethasone suppression test (HDDST)	2 mg D × 6 hours × two days, start at 9 a.m. and day 2, 24 hours UFC collection or S cortisol 9 AM day 1 and at 48 hours	Suppression of UFC or plasma cortisol >50% diagnostic of CS	Sensitivity and specificity = 60–85% Greater the suppression greater the specificity	Useful for distinguishing between adrenal and ectopic CS
8-mg ONDST	Similar to HDDST 8 a.m. plasma cortisol, 8 mg D at 11 p.m. and 8 a.m. plasma cortisol next morning	Suppression to >5 µg/dL is strongly supportive of CS		
CRH stimulation	Two basal plasma cortisol and ACTH collection 15 minutes apart, 1 µm/kg body weight or single-dose 11 µg of ovine CRH IV, collection of blood sample every 15 minutes for ACTH and plasma cortisol for 2 hours	Normal individuals: ACTH rise: 15%, cortisol rise 20% while in Cushing's disease ACTH rise >50%, cortisol rise >20%		
Plasma ACTH	Differentiates between ACTH dependent and independent cause	Three categories <10 pg/mL: Adrenal disorder >20 pg/mL: Pituitary or ectopic origin 10–20		

Other abnormal laboratory tests may be seen as follows:

1. Total leukocyte count may be normal or raised with relative or absolute lymphopenia (50%).
2. Hypercalciuria (50%), hypokalemia, hypocalcemia, hypochloremia, metabolic alkalosis
3. Elevated fasting blood sugar (15%)
4. Cholesterol and triglycerides are often elevated.
5. Clotting factors V, VIII and prothrombin may be elevated.

Localization of the disease

Imaging tests reveal the size and shape of the pituitary and the adrenal glands and help determine if a tumor is present.

Pituitary imaging: MRI is the best modality for evaluation of the sella and can detect microadenoma in about 50% cases of Cushing's disease.

Adrenal imaging: CECT or MRI of the abdomen is the imaging modality for the adrenals.

Inferior petrosal sinus sampling: In ACTH-dependent CS, if no lesion is identified in pituitary on imaging, inferior petrosal sinus sampling (IPSS) is indicated. Intravenous injection of CRH stimulates ACTH secretion. CRH IV injection is given, and blood samples after cannulation from petrosal sinus and peripheral vein are collected for ACTH. A central to peripheral ACTH gradient of more than 3 is considered suggestive of a pituitary ACTH secreting adenoma.

Differential diagnosis: Exogenous obesity, alcoholism, bulimia, depression

Complications

- Excess hair growth
- Osteoporosis and risk of fractures
- Susceptibility to infections, especially fungal infections
- Delayed wound healing
- Type 2 diabetes
- Peptic ulcer disease
- Hypertension

Treatment

Perioperative management

1. Adequate build up by nutrition
2. Adequate hemoglobin
3. Vigorous chest physiotherapy
4. Prophylaxis for venous thromboembolism
5. Correction of electrolytes
6. Control of blood pressure, blood glucose
7. Control of infections
8. Prophylactic antibiotics and antifungal therapy as and when required
9. Perioperative glucocorticoid coverage and postoperative replacement

The "subclinical" disease is defined as values <1.5 times the upper limit of normal. The risk of death and complications from hypercortisolism is positively correlated to the length of exposure to cortisol excess. Therefore, subclinical disease patients having mild hypercortisolism treatment should be individually tailored making a balance between the benefit and risk of overtreatment (15–17) (Table 49.8).

All overt hypercortisolism patients need treatment, and the curative treatment is surgery. Unilateral adrenalectomy is indicated for unilateral adrenal masses causing CS, and bilateral adrenalectomy is required for bilateral micronodular or macronodular adrenal hyperplasia. Laparoscopic adrenalectomy is the preferred approach as it has less postoperative morbidity, hospital stay. Thromboprophylaxis should be used in patients with CS undergoing surgery as it has hypercoagulable state due to activated coagulation cascade and impaired fibrinolysis. These patients had ten times more risk of developing thromboembolic disease. Figure 49.14 has the flow chart of overall management of CS. The experience of the surgeon is important for the safety of adrenalectomy. Surgeons with lower number of cases had more complications and longer postoperative length of stay when compared to high-volume practitioners (18.2 vs. 11.3%, $p < 0.001$ and 5.5 vs. 3.9 days, $p < 0.001$, respectively) (18).

Treatment of choice for Cushing's disease (ACTH-producing pituitary tumor) is transsphenoidal microadenomectomy for localized pituitary microadenoma. Subtotal or partial hypophysectomy (80–90% resection) is indicated if microadenoma is not localized but pituitary function is unpredictable. The immediate cure rate after successful surgery is 70–80%, but late recurrences reduce the permanent cure rate to approximately 60–70%. Patients of Cushing's disease who are not cured by transsphenoidal surgery or develop recurrence pituitary irradiation are one of the next treatment options. It may also be considered as primary therapy for children under age 18 years.

Optimal treatment for ectopic ACTH syndrome is surgical excision of the tumor. In patients with non-resectable tumors, hypercortisolism can be controlled with adrenal enzyme inhibitors (ketoconazole, metyrapone, and etomidate). Adrenal enzyme

TABLE 49.8: Benefits of Unilateral Adrenalectomy in Patients with Mild Hypercortisolism

	Toniato et al. (16)	Chiodini et al. (17)	Salcuni et al. (18)
Type of study and follow up duration	Randomized control trial with seven year follow-up	Retrospective with 29 month follow-up	Prospective with 40 month follow-up
Patients number having subclinical hypercortisolism	N = 23 vs. 22 controls	Adrenal incidentaloma (N = 108) N = 25 vs. 20 controls	Adrenalectomy on vertebral fractures with unilateral adrenal adenoma N = 32 vs. 23 controls
Reported benefits	DM2 improved in 62% of patients; HTN in 67%; obesity in 50%	Reductions in weight (32%), blood pressure (56%), fasting glucose levels improved (48%)	42.8% lower incidence of vertebral fractures
Reported adverse events	None	None	None

Cushing's Syndrome

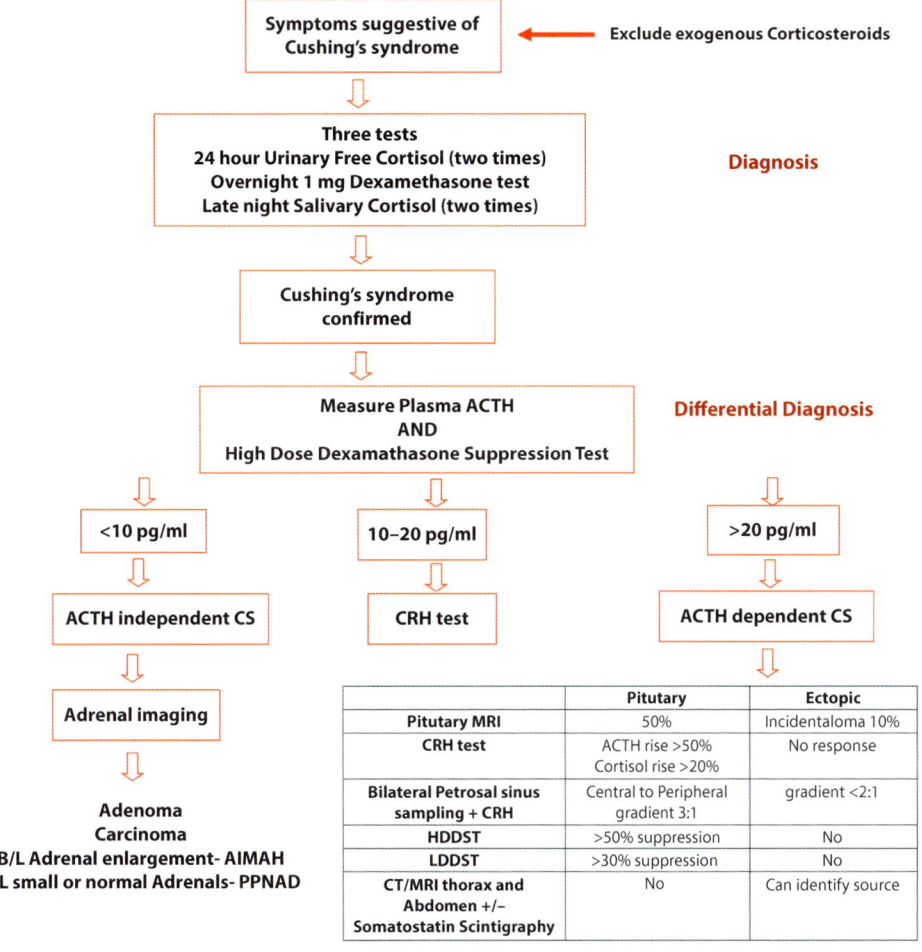

FIGURE 49.14 Flow chart of Cushing's syndrome management.

inhibitor can be continued for a longer period in unlocalized tumors (19). Drugs for medical adrenalectomy are:

- *Adrenocorticolytic drugs*: Mitotane
- *Adrenal enzyme inhibitors*: Aminoglutethimide, ketoconazole, metyrapone
- *Centrally acting drugs*: Bromocriptine, cyproheptadine, valproate.
- Octreotide

A periodical radiological examination by CT or MRI should be continued till the tumor can be located. Bilateral adrenalectomy or long-term treatment with steroidogenesis inhibitors may be used as an alternative to mitotane.

Prognosis

The ultimate prognosis depends on the etiology of CS. Benign adrenal adenomas or benign carcinoids have better prognosis while small-cell lung carcinoma and adrenocortical carcinoma have poor prognosis. Untreated hypercortisolism will always be fatal. The most common cause of death is by cardiovascular events (myocardial infarction, thromboembolic, cerebrovascular and hypertensive complications). The patients have high morbidity and mortality because of low immunity and risk of infections from opportunistic bacterial and fungus. Cushing's disease is a curable variety of CS. Some symptoms and signs of CS resolve after curative therapy between 2 and 12 months, but certain features like associated weight gain, hypertension, and glucose intolerance may never resolve (20–21). Children with CS have improvement in bone density and growth velocity but decline in intelligence quotient and cognitive functional indices persists even after cure.

South East Asia perspective

South East Asian presentation in CS is no different from the Western world; however, CS associated with malignant cause is poor. The average size of the adrenal lesion is higher. The management of CS is limited to most of higher referral centers because of scarcity of the endocrinologist and surgeons.

Conclusion

Clinical presentation of CS is pleomorphic. Cushing's disease or pituitary-dependent CS is the most common cause of endogenous hypercortisolism. Hypercortisolism is associated with 6–9% of incidentally discovered adrenal adenomas. Accurate diagnosis and cause is essential to optimal management in CS. Night salivary cortisol has a sensitivity of 92–100% and specificity of 93–100%. Transsphenoidal surgery is the initial treatment for Cushing's disease. Radiotherapy or bilateral adrenalectomy are second option in surgical failure or relapse in pituitary CS patients. Laparoscopic adrenalectomy is preferably the treatment of choice in adrenal origin CS. In ectopic ACTH syndrome, bilateral adrenalectomy with resection of the source of ACTH, where possible, is the first-choice treatment. CS causes significant impairment in quality of life but improves partially in long term after remission of the disease. Mortality in CS (nonmalignant causes) is two to four times higher because cardiovascular causes are most common.

References

1. Anderson GH Jr, Blankeman N, Streeten DH. The effect of age on prevalence of secondary forms of hypertension in 4429 consecutively referred patients. J Hypertens. 1994;12:609–615.
2. Omura M, Saito J, Yamaguchi K, et al. Prospective study on the prevalence of secondary hypertension among hypertensive patients visiting a general outpatient clinic in Japan. Hypertens Res. 2004;27:193–202.
3. Catargi B, Rigalleau V, Poussin A, et al. Occult Cushing's syndrome in type-2 diabetes. J Clin Endocrinol Metab. 2003;88:5808–5813.
4. Leibowitz G, Tsur A, Chayen SD, et al. Pre-clinical Cushing's syndrome: An unexpected frequent cause of poor glycaemic control in obese diabetic patients. Clin Endocrinol (Oxf). 1996;44:717–722.
5. Reincke M, Nieke J, Krestin GP, et al. Preclinical Cushing's syndrome in adrenal "incidentalomas": Comparison with adrenal Cushing's syndrome. J Clin Endocrinol Metab. 1992;75:826–832.
6. Terzolo M, Pia A, Ali A, et al. Adrenal incidentaloma: A new cause of the metabolic syndrome? J Clin Endocrinol Metab. 2002;87:998–1003.
7. Chiodini I, Mascia ML, Muscarella S, et al. Subclinical hypercortisolism among outpatients referred for osteoporosis. Ann Intern Med. 2007;147:541–548.
8. Lacroix A, Feelders RA, Stratakis CA, et al. Cushing's syndrome. Lancet. 2015;386:913–927.
9. Newell-Price J, Bertagna X, Grossman AB, et al. Cushing's syndrome. Lancet. 2006;367:1605–1617.
10. Ross NS. Epidemiology of Cushing's syndrome and subclinical disease. Endocrinol Metab Clin North Am 1994;23:539.
11. Lindholm J, Juul S, Jørgensen JO, et al. Incidence and late prognosis of Cushing's syndrome: A population-based study. J Clin Endocrinol Metab. 2001;86:117.
12. Loriaux DL. Diagnosis and differential diagnosis of Cushing's syndrome. N Engl J Med. 2017;367(15):1451–1459.
13. Lodish M, Stratakis CA. A genetic and molecular update on adrenocortical causes of Cushing syndrome. Nat Rev Endocrinol. 2016;12:255–262.
14. Nieman LK, Biller BM, Findling JW, et al. Treatment of Cushing's syndrome: An Endocrine Society clinical practice guideline. J Clin Endocrinol Metab. 2015;100:2807–2831.
15. Gadelha MR, Vieira Neto L. Efficacy of medical treatment in Cushing's disease: A systematic review. Clin Endocrinol (Oxf). 2014;80:1–12.
16. Toniato A, Merante-Boschin I, Opocher G, Pelizzo MR, Schiavi F, Ballotta E. Surgical versus conservative management for subclinical Cushing syndrome in adrenal incidentalomas: A prospective randomized study. Ann Surg. 2009 Mar;249(3):388–391.
17. Chiodini I, Morelli V, Salcuni AS, et al. Beneficial metabolic effects of prompt surgical treatment in patients with an adrenal incidentaloma causing biochemical hypercortisolism. J Clin Endocrinol Metab. 2010;95(6):2736–2745.
18. Salcuni AS, Morelli V, Eller Vainicher C, et al. Adrenalectomy reduces the risk of vertebral fractures in patients with monolateral adrenal incidentalomas and subclinical hypercortisolism. Eur J Endocrinol. 2016;174(3):261–269.
19. Park HS, Roman SA, Sosa JA. Outcomes from 3144 adrenalectomies in the United States: Which matters more, surgeon volume or specialty? Arch Surg. 2009;144(11):1060–1067.
20. Mishra AK, Agarwal A, Gupta S, Agarwal G, Verma AK, Misra SK. Outcome of adrenalectomy in Cushing's syndrome: Experience from a tertiary care center. World J Surg. 2007;31:1425–1432.
21. Ritzel K, Beuschlein F, Mickisch A, et al. Clinical review: Outcome of bilateral adrenalectomy in Cushing's syndrome: A systematic review. J Clin Endocrinol Metab. 2013;98:3939–3948.

50

HYPERALDOSTERONISM

Troy H Puar and Meifen Zhang

Introduction

Primary aldosteronism: A common and important cause of secondary hypertension

Primary aldosteronism (PA) is estimated to be the most common cause of secondary and treatable hypertension, affecting 5–10% of all patients with hypertension worldwide (1, 2). Compared to patients with essential hypertension who have similar blood pressure control, patients with primary aldosteronism are at increased risk of cardiovascular events, renal disease, impaired quality of life and death (3–6). This is possibly due to the direct deleterious effects of excess aldosterone hormone (7). Studies have also shown that aldosterone excess in primary aldosteronism directly leads to injury in cardiovascular and renal tissues (inflammation, remodeling, and fibrosis) and induces adverse metabolic effects that are at least partly independent of its effect on blood pressure (7, 8). In addition, patients with primary aldosteronism are more likely to have hypertension that is resistant to the first-line hypertension medications such as calcium channel blockers, ACE inhibitors, angiotensin-receptor blockers, and diuretics (9–11). Hence, identifying and treating this group of patients with hypertension is particularly important and can thus lead to a significant reduction of health-care costs and burden.

Pathophysiology

Primary aldosteronism occurs from excessive and autonomous production of aldosterone from the adrenal cortex. Excess aldosterone causes increased sodium reabsorption via amiloride-sensitive epithelial sodium channels within the distal nephron, leading to hypertension and suppressed renin (12). Urinary loss of potassium and hydrogen ions, exchanged for sodium at the distal nephron, may also result in hypokalemia and metabolic alkalosis (13).

Screening and diagnosis

Screening for primary aldosteronism in patients with hypertension

When first described by Jerome Conn in 1955, hypokalemia was a sine qua non in patients with Conn's disease (unilateral primary aldosteronism) (13). However, improved aldosterone and renin assays, and the adoption of the aldosterone-to-renin ratio (ARR) to screen for patients with primary aldosteronism, have since led to the realization that the majority of patients with primary aldosteronism have normokalemia. Hence, the presence of normokalemia should not preclude the diagnosis of primary aldosteronism. In patients with diuretic-induced hypokalemia, this suggests that they may have a propensity to develop hypokalemia, and they should be actively screened for primary aldosteronism (14).

While primary aldosteronism affects 5–10% of all hypertensive patients, in selected patient groups, the prevalence is even higher. Hence, current guidelines (15, 16) suggest screening patients with:

1. Hypertension and sustained BP > 150/100 mmHg (17)
2. Resistant hypertension (BP > 140/90 mmHg) despite three antihypertensive medications, including a diuretic (9, 18)
3. Controlled hypertension (BP < 140/100 mmHg) on ≥4 antihypertensive medications
4. Hypertension associated with hypokalemia (spontaneous or diuretic-induced)
5. Hypertension associated with obstructive sleep apnea (19, 20), or adrenal incidentaloma

ARR is a useful screening tool

The screening and diagnosis of primary aldosteronism is summarized in Figure 50.1. Patients with primary aldosteronism demonstrate both a high-aldosterone level (due to autonomous aldosterone production) and a suppressed renin level (due to negative feedback), leading to an elevated ARR (21, 22). Hence, ARR is particularly useful as a screening test. It is important to highlight that a suppressed renin is considered a hallmark of primary aldosteronism, and patients with unsuppressed renin should be investigated for causes of secondary hyperaldosteronism. A very low renin (e.g. undetectable renin) can inflate the ratio and lead to false-positive ARR. To avoid this, patients should also demonstrate an elevated aldosterone level, as reflected in Figure 50.1. Instead of using the ARR, an alternative will be to consider patients with both elevated aldosterone and suppressed renin as a positive screening test and offer these patients a confirmatory testing (23).

Medications and their effects on ARR

Several factors are known to alter aldosterone and renin levels and thus may affect the ARR. Hypokalemia can suppress aldosterone secretion and should ideally be corrected with oral potassium supplementation prior to hormonal tests (12). If, however, ARR is assessed and noted to be elevated in the presence of hypokalemia, this is strongly suggestive of PA. Other factors such as increasing age and renal impairment also lead to increased aldosterone and reduced renin levels, which can lead to false-positive results (14). Medications such as ACE inhibitors, angiotensin-receptor blockers, and diuretics can lead to lowering of aldosterone and increased renin, leading to false-negative results, while medications such as beta blockers lead to suppression of renin, leading to false-positive results (24, 25). It has been recommended to discontinue these antihypertensive medications and switch to other medications with minimal effects on aldosterone and renin such as hydralazine, alpha-receptor blockers, and non-dihydropyridine calcium channel blockers (verapamil, diltiazem) (14). However, it is also recognized that many patients with primary aldosteronism have difficult-to-control blood pressure and switching medications for diagnostic tests can be difficult and lead to severe hypertension. This can also

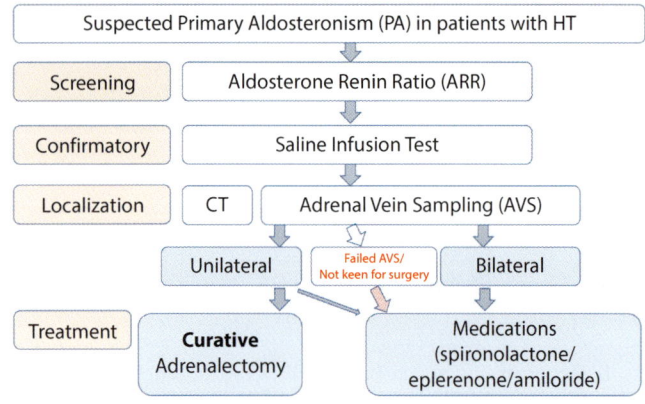

FIGURE 50.1 Overview of the diagnosis and management of patients with primary aldosteronism.

lead to the reluctance of physicians to screen for primary aldosteronism and fewer patients being identified and treated (14). Hence, in our practice, we only stipulate that several medications are discontinued before screening. These include spironolactone, eplerenone, and amiloride that are specific medications used to treat primary aldosteronism, and they should be stopped at least 6–8 weeks prior to testing (Figure 50.1).

Assays of renin and aldosterone and effects on ARR

Different centers may utilize different aldosterone and renin assays, and they may also adopt slightly different ARR threshold cutoffs to define a positive screening result. We have taken a positive screening result to be an ARR > 550 (with aldosterone units measured in pmol/L). Plasma renin activity (PRA) has been widely used by many centers in the past. Over the last decade, there has been a shift toward measuring renin using direct renin concentration (DRC). The advantages of DRC over PRA are that it can be automated on an immunoassay platform, resulting in a shorter turnaround time (few hours) compared to PRA, which was often radioimmunoassay-based, labor-intensive, and required incubations of samples over a day. DRC also has less variability and more reproducibility over different centers (14). DRC generally correlates well with PRA, except when the PRA is <1 ng/mL/h (26). Since low renin is a hallmark of primary aldosteronism, this is particularly important (12). In addition, DRC can be affected by estrogen status and use of oral contraceptive pills in women (27). The scalability of doing more screening tests with DRC may outweigh the cons. Ultimately, the choice of which renin assay is used is often dependent on the laboratory and assay availability.

Confirmatory testing

In patients with spontaneous hypokalemia, suppressed renin, and significantly elevated aldosterone >20 ng/dL (550 pmol/L), this is highly suggestive of primary aldosteronism, and further confirmatory testing may be omitted (14, 28). However, in most patients with a positive ARR test, further confirmatory testing should be done. In the various confirmatory tests, suppression of aldosterone is induced either with salt loading (oral or intravenous), fludrocortisone, or captopril. Failure to adequately suppress aldosterone confirms the diagnosis of primary aldosteronism (12, 14).

The four most commonly used confirmatory tests are listed below (14):

1. Saline infusion test (SIT)
2. Oral sodium loading test
3. Fludrocortisone suppression test (FST)
4. Captopril challenge test (CCT)

None of these confirmatory tests is considered the best, and the choice often depends on each center's experience. One of the most widely used tests is currently the SIT that can be done in the ambulatory setting. The SIT can be done with the patient either in the recumbent or seated position. In a recent comparison between the two, with FST as reference, the seated SIT had a significantly better diagnostic accuracy compared with the recumbent SIT (29). The SIT is usually conducted in the morning, with 2 L of isotonic saline infused over 4 hours. Blood samples for renin, aldosterone, and potassium are drawn before and after infusion. Post-saline infusion aldosterone levels of >10 ng/dL (280 nmol/L) confirms the diagnosis of primary aldosteronism. Cutoff levels vary between different centers, and some centers adopt lower cutoffs ranging between 5 and 10 ng/dL (140–280 pmol/L). In general, post-saline infusion aldosterone levels <5 ng/dL (140 pmol/L) exclude the diagnosis of primary aldosteronism. The SIT should not be performed in patients with severe uncontrolled hypertension, uncontrolled hypokalemia, renal insufficiency, or cardiac arrhythmia (14).

Subtype testing

Primary aldosteronism can be due to unilateral or bilateral adrenal hypersecretion, and subtype tests (computed tomography [CT] imaging and adrenal vein sampling [AVS]) aid to differentiate between the two. Unilateral primary aldosteronism is most commonly due to an aldosterone-producing adenoma (APA), and less commonly due to primary adrenal hyperplasia. Adrenal carcinoma is generally rare in patients with PA. Bilateral disease is often due to bilateral adrenal hyperplasia. The distinction between unilateral and bilateral adrenal disease in primary aldosteronism is important, as treatment options differ. It is generally recommended that patients with unilateral adrenal disease are treated with unilateral adrenalectomy, which is curative for the condition and leads to improvement or cure of hypertension. Patients with bilateral disease are treated with lifelong medications. Bilateral adrenalectomy is not offered for bilateral disease as it will render the patient completely adrenal insufficient, necessitating lifelong steroid replacement, and put the patient at risk of Addisonian crisis. Patients with unilateral disease who are poor surgical candidates or prefer medical treatment may also be treated with lifelong medications. If surgical treatment is not desired, AVS is not required. Figure 50.2 provides an overview of the diagnosis and management of patients with primary aldosteronism.

Predictors of unilateral disease and aldosterone–potassium ratio

About half of the patients with confirmed primary aldosteronism have unilateral adrenal disease and will benefit from subtype tests and surgery. Patients with unilateral disease are more likely to present with a more severe phenotype: uncontrolled hypertension, severe hypokalemia, higher aldosterone levels, and a clear adenoma on CT imaging (30–32). The convenient aldosterone–potassium ratio can be a useful guide for clinicians and patients

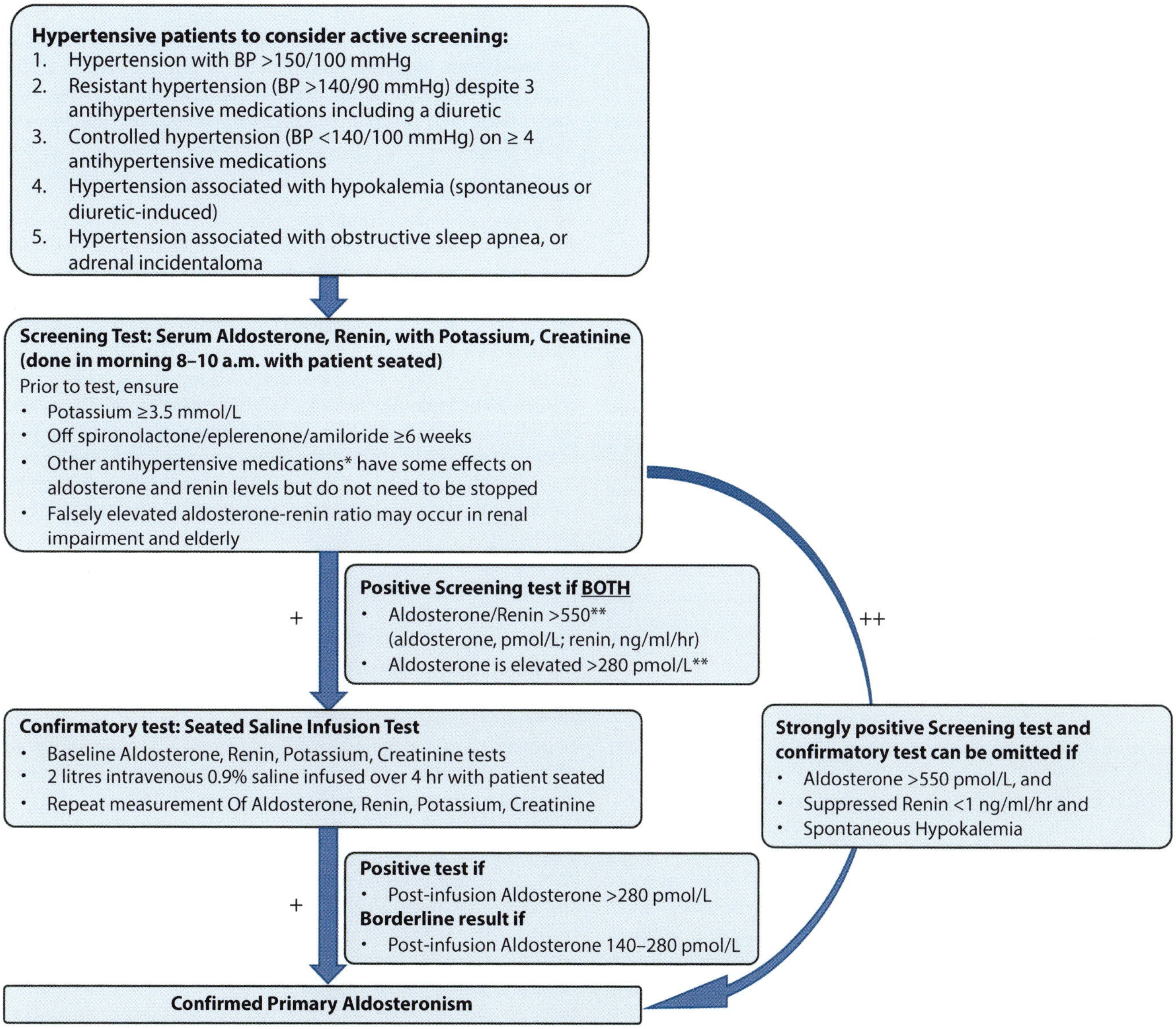

Hyperaldosteronism

Hypertensive patients to consider active screening:
1. Hypertension with BP >150/100 mmHg
2. Resistant hypertension (BP >140/90 mmHg) despite 3 antihypertensive medications including a diuretic
3. Controlled hypertension (BP <140/100 mmHg) on ≥ 4 antihypertensive medications
4. Hypertension associated with hypokalemia (spontaneous or diuretic-induced)
5. Hypertension associated with obstructive sleep apnea, or adrenal incidentaloma

↓

Screening Test: Serum Aldosterone, Renin, with Potassium, Creatinine (done in morning 8–10 a.m. with patient seated)
Prior to test, ensure
- Potassium ≥3.5 mmol/L
- Off spironolactone/eplerenone/amiloride ≥6 weeks
- Other antihypertensive medications* have some effects on aldosterone and renin levels but do not need to be stopped
- Falsely elevated aldosterone-renin ratio may occur in renal impairment and elderly

Positive Screening test if BOTH
- Aldosterone/Renin >550** (aldosterone, pmol/L; renin, ng/ml/hr)
- Aldosterone is elevated >280 pmol/L**

Confirmatory test: Seated Saline Infusion Test
- Baseline Aldosterone, Renin, Potassium, Creatinine tests
- 2 litres intravenous 0.9% saline infused over 4 hr with patient seated
- Repeat measurement Of Aldosterone, Renin, Potassium, Creatinine

Positive test if
- Post-infusion Aldosterone >280 pmol/L

Borderline result if
- Post-infusion Aldosterone 140–280 pmol/L

Strongly positive Screening test and confirmatory test can be omitted if
- Aldosterone >550 pmol/L, and
- Suppressed Renin <1 ng/ml/hr and
- Spontaneous Hypokalemia

Confirmed Primary Aldosteronism

* Medications with minimal interference on aldosterone and renin levels include alpha-blockers, hydralazine, verapamil and diltiazem, and if possible patients can be switched to these antihypertensive medications
** to convert aldosterone to ng/dL, divide value in pmol/L by 27.7

FIGURE 50.2 Diagnostic algorithm for screening and confirming the diagnosis of primary aldosteronism.

on the likelihood of unilateral disease (33) and was developed in an Asian patient cohort and validated in a European patient cohort. This is calculated using the baseline aldosterone level (in ng/dL) divided by the lowest recorded potassium level (mmol/L). Patients with an aldosterone-potassium ratio >10 are likely to have unilateral disease and should be encouraged to pursue subtype tests. Patients with a ratio <5 are more likely to have bilateral disease. However, a low ratio should not completely exclude these patients from pursuing subtype testing, as identifying unilateral disease still offers an important opportunity for cure of disease and reduction of pill burden.

CT

CT of the adrenals is the imaging modality of choice in most centers. While CT imaging can identify the APA responsible for causing unilateral primary aldosteronism, it must be noted that most APA are often less than 2 cm and can be missed on CT, leading to a false-negative result (34). Conversely, nonfunctional adrenal adenomas are also common, in as many as 3–10% of individuals above 40 years old (35), leading to a false-positive result. Hence, the determination of unilateral or bilateral primary aldosteronism should not be based on CT findings alone. In comparing CT or MRI imaging to AVS as the gold standard, CT was inaccurate in 37.8% of patients (359 of 950) (36). Regardless, CT imaging is useful for ruling out any large (>4 cm) or suspicious adrenal tumor (>4 cm) indicated for surgical removal (14). In addition, CT imaging with contrast helps to characterize the adrenal lesion and provides the anatomical location of the adrenal veins, which aids the interventionist during AVS (37).

Adrenal vein sampling (AVS)

AVS is the current reference method for determining unilateral adrenal disease. While cutoffs and AVS protocols vary between centers, the general principle is that unilateral adrenal disease is present when the aldosterone production from one adrenal vein is significantly greater than the contralateral side. AVS involves the insertion of a catheter into the femoral vein under local anesthesia. Under fluoroscopic guidance, the adrenal veins are then cannulated, and blood samples are taken. AVS can be technically challenging, particularly cannulating the right adrenal vein that drains directly into the inferior vena cava. In many centers worldwide, inconclusive results can occur in >50% of patients (38).

Several approaches have been taken to improve AVS rates. Having a dedicated interventionist in each center conducting the procedure can help (37, 39). Use of rapid cortisol assays can improve AVS success (40, 41). After samples are taken, the femoral catheter sheath is kept in situ until cortisol levels are known. If cannulation has failed, the interventionist proceeds with a second AVS attempt. Due to the technical difficulty of cannulating the right adrenal vein, in our center, our interventionist routinely samples the right adrenal vein twice, to improve the likelihood of success. All these measures have led to a high cannulation rate over the last few years. Finally, in centers without adequate experience, consideration could be given to sending the patient to a high-volume center for the AVS (23).

Corticotropin stimulation

AVS protocols differ between centers, and one controversy is whether corticotropin stimulation should be used or not (42). There are several reasons for using corticotropin stimulation. First, it leads to maximal cortisol production from the adrenal glands, leading to higher cortisol levels when the adrenal veins are correctly cannulated. This leads to less procedures being considered inconclusive. Second, this reduces stress-induced fluctuations between the adrenal veins, particularly when sequential cannulation of the adrenal veins is done, as opposed to bilateral simultaneous cannulation. Finally, it has been postulated that APA harbors ACTH receptors, and corticotropin stimulation can increase aldosterone production and better lateralization to the affected side (23). However, this has recently been challenged (43). In centers where corticotropin stimulation is used, samples are usually taken nonsequentially via a single groin catheter. In centers where corticotropin stimulation is not used, two catheters are usually required, with samples from both adrenal veins taken simultaneously. Table 50.1 shows the illustration of AVS of a 59-year-old gentleman with confirmed PA.

Interpretation

To determine if the adrenal veins have been successfully cannulated, the cortisol levels in the adrenal samples should be higher than the peripheral sample (cortisol gradient), and at least >3 (stimulated with corticotrophin), or >2 (unstimulated), and even preferably >5 and >3, respectively (44). Aldosterone levels are also corrected for the cortisol production, giving the aldosterone-to-cortisol (A/C) ratios. This is because left adrenal vein samples are collected at the confluence of the left inferior phrenic vein and the left adrenal vein, leading to the dilution of the adrenal vein sample, whereas the right adrenal vein samples are taken directly from the adrenal vein. A/C ratio in the higher side is divided by the contralateral side to yield the lateralization ratio. In unilateral disease, it is >4 (or >2 if unstimulated AVS). Patients with similar aldosterone-to-cortisol ratios in both adrenals and lateralization ratio <3 are classified as bilateral disease. In addition, there is often suppression of aldosterone production on the contralateral side (ratio <1 in 93% of cases) (34) and calculated by taking the aldosterone-to-cortisol ratio of the contralateral side divided by the peripheral. Contralateral suppression is a prerequisite for confirming unilateral disease in some centers, but not all (45). In general, corticotropin stimulation (compared to unstimulated AVS) is associated with better success rates of cannulation but may lead to decreased lateralization ratios (42, 44).

Importance of AVS

AVS role to differentiate unilateral from bilateral primary aldosteronism has been recently challenged by a randomized controlled clinical trial (46). In the *SPARTACUS* trial, patients with primary aldosteronism were randomized into a CT-only arm, and an AVS arm (with CT), where treatment (adrenalectomy or medications) was directed by the subtype investigations. Interestingly, reduction of blood pressure medications (primary outcome) was similar whether patients underwent

TABLE 50.1: Case Illustration of an Adrenal Vein Sampling (AVS) Procedure in a Patient with Confirmed Primary Aldosteronism

	Adrenal Vein Sampling			
	Right Adrenal Vein #1	Right Adrenal Vein #2	Peripheral (IVC)	Left Adrenal Vein
Aldosterone, pmol/L	40,165	64,264	499	3850
Cortisol, nmol/L	18,883	20,677	666	17,793
Cortisol gradient	28.4	31.0	NA	26.7
A/C ratio	2.13	3.11	0.75	0.22
Potassium, mmol/L			3.8	
Renin, ng/mL/h			<0.6	

Note: Lateralization ratio = 3.11/0.22 = 14.1 (>4 is suggestive of unilateral disease on right). Contralateral suppression = 0.22/0.75 = 0.29 (<1 is suggestive of unilateral disease on right). A 59-year-old gentleman presents with a history of hypertension for 20 years, which was uncontrolled at 180/90 mmHg on four antihypertensive medications (nifedipine 60 mg daily, enalapril 20 mg twice daily, atenolol 50 mg daily, and terazosin 2 mg daily). CT imaging did not reveal any obvious adenoma. AVS achieved bilateral successful cannulation of the adrenal veins (cortisol gradient >5 in the adrenal vein samples). During the procedure, his potassium level was adequately repleted to the normal range, and renin was suppressed, consistent with primary aldosteronism. There was lateralization toward the right (ratio 14.1 that is greater than 4), with appropriate contralateral suppression on the left side (0.29 that is less than 1). He underwent right adrenalectomy. Six months post-surgery, his blood pressure has improved to 130/80 mmHg on only two medications (nifedipine 60 mg daily and enalapril 20 mg twice daily).

adrenalectomy based on CT findings alone, or on AVS results. However, 9 of 46 (19.6%) in the CT arm had biochemical persistence of PA, compared to 5 of 46 (10.9%) in the AVS arm. A criticism of this study was that it was inadequately powered to look at biochemical cure of primary aldosteronism (47), which will be a better assessment of the diagnosis of unilateral disease. While this study has not changed clinical practice, in that AVS is still required to confirm unilateral disease, SPARTACUS brought about a consensus on biochemical cure of primary aldosteronism post surgery (PASO criteria discussed later). In addition, it has now set the standard for future subtype tests (e.g. functional imaging) to be referenced against (48).

Treatment: surgery vs medical

Introduction

Choice of therapy depends on primary aldosteronism subtype, which can be unilateral (~50% of cases), or bilateral (Figure 50.2). It is generally recommended that unilateral primary aldosteronism is treated by laparoscopic adrenalectomy, as it offers an opportunity for cure, and is more cost-effective in the long term (49). Patients either not keen for surgery or unsuitable for surgery may proceed directly to medical treatment without AVS for subtyping (Figure 50.2). Patients with a failed AVS procedure (or indeterminate subtype) are often offered lifelong medications (14). Alternatively, patients may be offered surgery based on CT findings (46) or use of other AVS criteria (50), but there may be a risk of disease persistence post-surgery.

Several studies have shown that patients treated with surgery have better surrogate outcomes than those treated with medications (51), in terms of blood pressure (52), cardiovascular disease (53), and quality of life (54), while others studies have found similar benefits (55–57). Importantly, these patient groups are often different, as patients who undergo surgery have unilateral disease, while those treated medically often have bilateral disease. To address this, a recent retrospective study, which included only patients with unilateral disease, found that surgery was more effective at controlling blood pressure compared to medical treatment (58).

In addition, recent data has provided further evidence in support of surgery with important end points. Hundemer et al. (6) showed that patients with primary aldosteronism treated medically still had increased risk of cardiovascular events and mortality, compared to patients with essential hypertension matched for baseline blood pressure. In addition, these patients on medical treatment also had an increased risk of atrial fibrillation and renal deterioration (59, 60). Conversely, this excess risk was completely ameliorated in patients with primary aldosteronism treated surgically. This suggests that current medical treatment may not completely remove the excess risk. One possible reason is that primary aldosteronism is also associated with mild glucocorticoid excess that has deleterious effects and is not adequately addressed with mineralocorticoid antagonist therapy alone (61).

Surgery

Pre-surgery preparation is mainly aimed at adequate blood pressure control and correction of hypokalemia, which can be managed with conventional antihypertensive medications and potassium supplements. If desired, spironolactone may be started once investigations such as confirmatory tests and AVS have been completed, with close monitoring of potassium levels. Patients with primary aldosteronism are at higher risk of obstructive sleep apnea (62), cardiovascular disease (3), and renal disease (63), and an anesthetist should evaluate the patient prior to surgery.

Laparoscopic adrenalectomy is the treatment of choice in patients with unilateral PA and is associated with shorter hospitalization and fewer complications than open surgery (14). This can be done via the transabdominal or retroperitoneal approach (64). Even in patients with a clear and distinct adenoma, complete adrenalectomy is preferred to nodulectomy, as there is a possibility of other adenomas in the ipsilateral adrenal responsible for aldosterone excess (65). In histological examinations of adrenal tissues, there is often zona glomerulosa hypertrophy of the adrenal tissue adjacent to the nodule (66). Furthermore, AVS only identifies the side of pathology and not the affected segment of the adrenal.

Post-surgery, potassium supplements and spironolactone should be stopped as there may be rebound hyperkalemia. Creatinine levels are also expected to rise post-surgery. This is because hyperaldosteronism causes glomerular hyperfiltration and lowering of creatinine levels, which is reversed after surgery (57). In some cases, mineralocorticoid replacement may be required if hypoaldosteronism is persistent, but this is generally uncommon (67). Importantly, renal function stabilizes thereafter with improved long-term outcomes in terms of albuminuria and renal disease (63). In patients with already established advanced renal disease (chronic kidney disease stage 4 or 5), AVS (due to intravenous contrast load) and adrenalectomy are generally avoided. Antihypertensive medications can be reduced or stopped post-surgery depending on the blood pressure response. While some improvement can be seen in the first week post-surgery, blood pressure may continue to improve over the first few months.

Prediction of cure

Surgery leads to cure of primary aldosteronism, hypokalemia, as well as improvement or cure of hypertension. In about 50% of patients, hypertension is completely cured (14), and clinical scores have been developed to predict complete resolution of hypertension (68). Predictive factors for complete resolution of hypertension post-surgery include younger age, female gender, shorter duration of hypertension, using less medications, absence of left ventricular hypertrophy, and lower BMI (69).

Even if hypertension is not completely cure, it is important to highlight that these patients still experience significant improvement in blood pressure or reduction in pill burden (69), which cannot be otherwise achieved with medical treatment. It is assumed that these patients often have underlying essential hypertension (70), or the long-standing effects of hypertension on vascular remodeling have led to irreversible hypertension. These factors stress the importance of early detection and treatment of patients with PA.

Primary aldosteronism surgical outcome (PASO) criteria

Since many patients with primary aldosteronism currently present with normokalemia, resolution of hypokalemia alone is not a reliable marker of cure of primary aldosteronism post-surgery. A recent expert consensus has decided on several criteria to ascertain for cure post-surgery (69). Complete biochemical remission is defined as resolution of hypokalemia (if present pre-surgery) and normalization of ARR. Patients with a positive ARR post-surgery should proceed with a confirmatory test to establish for persistence of PA. Complete clinical remission requires normalization of blood pressure without antihypertensive medications. Partial clinical remission is defined as either improvement in blood pressure with the same doses of antihypertensive medications or the same blood pressure with lower doses of antihypertensive medications. In this study, spanning 12 centers, patients who underwent surgery after the confirmation of unilateral disease on AVS were prospectively assessed with these new criteria. A total of 94% had complete biochemical resolution, while 37% had complete clinical resolution and 47% had partial clinical improvement in hypertension.

Medication

While medications may be able to control hypertension and hypokalemia in patients with PA, they need to be taken lifelong and may have side effects (71). Mineralocorticoid-receptor antagonists are the first-line medications for the treatment of PA, namely spironolactone and eplerenone. Spironolactone has been used for several decades, is generally inexpensive, effective, and requires only once a day dosing. In some patients, doses of up to 400 mg may be required. However, due to its nonselectivity and antagonistic action on the androgen receptor, it may lead to side effects particularly in males, such as decreased libido, breast tenderness, and gynecomastia (72). These side effects are dose dependent (73). Even in females, it can lead to menstrual irregularities and breast pain. Two separate studies did not find any increased risk of breast cancer with the use of spironolactone (74, 75).

Eplerenone has greater selectivity for the mineralocorticoid receptor, with minimal effects on the androgen and progesterone receptors, resulting in much fewer side effects compared with spironolactone (72). In a head-to-head comparison with spironolactone, it was less efficacious in lowering blood pressure (76). However, this may have been due to a lower equivalent dosage of eplerenone compared to spironolactone. Eplerenone is approved by the FDA for use in essential hypertension up to a dose of 100 mg daily, although higher doses (300 mg daily) were used in trials for primary aldosteronism (76). Notably, eplerenone has about 25–50% potency compared with spironolactone and needs to be dosed twice daily due to its shorter half-life.

Alternatives to mineralocorticoid-receptor antagonists are potassium-sparing diuretics, like amiloride or triamterene. Amiloride acts on the epithelial sodium channels in kidneys and helps to improve hypertension and hypokalemia. It may not have the added benefits of antagonizing the action of aldosterone in other organs such as the heart and brain, but it also does not have the anti-androgen side effects of spironolactone. It may be used in conjunction with spironolactone or eplerenone and thereby reduce their dosage requirements.

The target of medical treatment should be to aim for a high-to-normal potassium level, and possibly nonsuppression of renin levels (6, 23), to ensure blockade of hyperaldosteronism. After initiation or titration of medical treatment, potassium supplementation should be reduced, with close monitoring of potassium and creatinine levels (72).

Histology and genetics

There are several inheritable forms of primary aldosteronism, the most notable of which is familial hyperaldosteronism type 1, or glucocorticoid remediable aldosteronism (77), responsible for about 1% of all cases of PA. This occurs due to a fusion of *CYP11B1* promotor region with *CYP11B2* coding region to form a chimeric gene *CYP11B1/CYP11B2* (78). In this condition, aldosterone production is under control of ACTH. This entity is important to recognize as these patients should be treated with dexamethasone, to suppress aldosterone production, in doses of 0.125–0.25 mg/day (79).

It has been previously thought that patients with unilateral primary aldosteronism have a solitary APA responsible for aldosterone hypersecretion, while patients with bilateral primary aldosteronism have bilateral adrenal hyperplasia. However, in histology specimens of resected adrenals, it has been observed that almost 50% of patients with unilateral primary aldosteronism have hyperplasia, or microscopic nodularity, as opposed to a solitary nodule (66). Furthermore, since 2011, there has been increased discovery of various somatic mutations responsible for the development of APA (80), and currently, almost 50% of adenomas harbor a known somatic mutation. These include mutations in *KCNJ5* (80), *ATP1A1* (81,82), *ATP2B3* (81), and *CACNA1D* (82, 83). These mutations, through various mechanisms, cause membrane depolarization, calcium influx, and increased production of aldosterone (84, 85). *KCNJ5* mutations are currently the most common mutation, and patients with this mutation are more often younger, female gender, with larger adenomas and more severe aldosterone production. The prevalence of *KCNJ5* in Asians appears to be higher (>50%) although it is not currently known why this may be so (86, 87). Patients with ATPase or *CACNA1D* mutations are often older, with a male predominance, and smaller adenomas (88). Adjacent to the adenomas, there are often aldosterone-producing cell clusters (APCCs) seen on histology. Interestingly, recent studies have found similar mutations of ATPase and *CACNA1D* in these APCCs, suggesting that APCCs may be precursors for APA (89).

Future perspectives

11C-metomidate PET–CT imaging

While AVS is considered the current gold-standard test for determining unilateral PA, it is invasive, technically challenging, and may yield inconclusive results (42). 11C-metomidate PET/CT imaging is a promising new modality to identify unilateral PA. This is a noninvasive functional imaging and is not operator dependent (90, 91). In a study by Burton et al. in Cambridge, United Kingdom, in 2010, 35 patients with primary aldosteronism underwent 11C-metomidate PET/CT scan, and they found a specificity of 87% and sensitivity of 76% for identifying unilateral disease (92). Importantly, these findings were using AVS as the reference standard and AVS has also been shown to have its limitations (69). Postoperative cure of primary aldosteronism will be a better standard to assess the accuracy of localization tests, and there are ongoing studies assessing the accuracy of 11C-metomidate PET/CT. 11C-metomidate is able to detect microadenomas (<1 cm) in size. This was a limitation of earlier forms of functional imaging for PA, such as ^{131}I-iodocholesterol scintigraphy, which was not adequately sensitive in detecting adenomas less than 1.5 cm in size (93). This is particularly relevant as a large majority of Conn's adenomas are less than 2 cm in size (23).

Our group in Singapore has recently been the first in Asia to utilize 11C-metomidate PET/CT imaging for subtyping of PA

Hyperaldosteronism

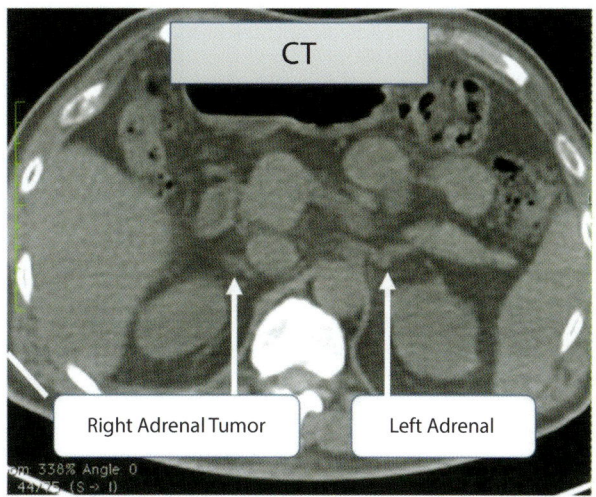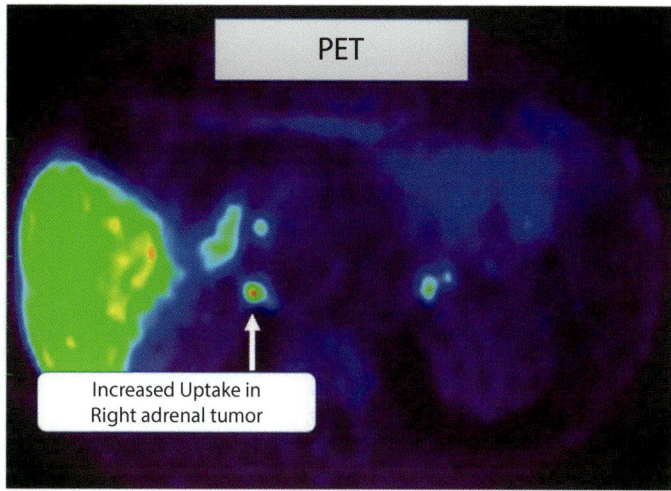

FIGURE 50.3 CECT and PET images of a patient with hyperaldosteronism and right adrenal neoplasm.

and has found it to be effective in detecting both macro- and microadenomas responsible for aldosterone hypersecretion (94) (Figure 50.3). Due to the short half-life of 11-carbon, this radiotracer has to be produced on-site prior to the scan. If shown to be an accurate test, patients may want to travel to centers with these facilities for diagnostic testing and this may also encourage more centers to develop the required capabilities to deliver this.

Ablation

While unilateral adrenalectomy is the choice of treatment for patients with unilateral PA, radiofrequency ablation (RFA) offers a less invasive alternative. Success rates of RFA have been reported to be similar to unilateral adrenalectomy, but these are based on retrospective data, and RFA has been done only in a few centers worldwide (95). The advantages of RFA are that it is less invasive and may be done under sedation instead of general anesthesia, with less morbidity and recovery time (95).

RFA may allow ablation of the nodule while sparing the adjacent adrenal gland. However, similar to partial adrenalectomy, RFA may lead to persistence of disease, as the adjacent adrenal may also be abnormal. In one study, RFA led to 92% of resolution of PA, which is promising data albeit in a single center and a small patient cohort (69, 96). RFA should not be done if there is suspicion of malignancy, e.g. tumor >4 cm. However, most Conn's adenomas are benign. Potential complications of RFA include pneumo- or hemothoraces, bleeding, infection, and potentially hypertensive crisis (95). More long-term prospective data are needed to evaluate the value of RFA in the treatment of PA.

South Asian

Primary aldosteronism is an important problem in South Asians. Prevalence studies in Singapore, with a multiethnic population, found a prevalence of primary aldosteronism of 4.6%, which was comparable to other countries: 10.8% in the United States and 8% in Italy (1). The majority of patients diagnosed in that study had normokalemia, highlighting the importance of screening patients with hypertension for this condition. This should include patients with diuretic-induced hypokalemia, as they likely have a low baseline potassium, which can go into hypokalemia ranges after a diuretic 'challenge' (97).

Patients should be screened with an ARR, which is an effective screening tool to detect patients with primary aldosteronism (15, 16, 98). ARR (aldosterone, pmol/L divided by PRA, ng/mL/h >550) and a concomitant high aldosterone >280 pmol/L are taken to be a positive screening test. These patients should then undergo confirmatory test, such as an intravenous SIT.

Subtype tests include CT imaging and AVS. While AVS remains the gold standard test, it remains a technically challenging procedure to perform, with variable success rates between centers, and there is a need for either improved AVS or an alternative test (48). In our center, we have achieved highly successful bilateral cannulation rates of 100% over the last 5 years in more than 60 patients. This has been possible through various measures, including a dedicated interventional radiologist, use of rapid cortisol results, increase in volume of patients sent for AVS, and a hospital protocol in place. Hence, we believe that these high success rates can be replicated in other centers.

Similar to other endocrine conditions that utilize functional imaging, such as somatostatin-receptor scintigraphy for neuroendocrine tumors (99), 11C-metomidate PET–CT has a promising role in the diagnostic testing for primary aldosteronism. Singapore is currently the first center in Asia to offer 11C-metomidate PET–CT to identify patients with unilateral primary aldosteronism. A multicenter trial (ClinicalTrials.gov: NCT03990701) involving 25 patients with primary aldosteronism will be concluded in 2020. As illustrated below, 11C-metomidate PET–CT is able to detect functional microadenomas in patients with unilateral primary aldosteronism (94). One of the major limitations of 11C-metomidate PET–CT imaging is the short half-life of 11C-isotope, which limits its exportability to other centers. However, if shown to be highly accurate, patients may be willing to travel to a center offering the test, which can be done outpatient, as opposed to an AVS procedure with possibility of an inconclusive result.

The prevalence of KCNJ5 mutations in APA in Asians appears to be higher (>50%) compared to Caucasians (86, 87). Because patients with a KCNJ5 mutation often have a more severe phenotype (hypokalemia and higher aldosterone levels), one possible explanation is patients who are offered surgery in Asia are often those who present with hypokalemia. In our center, many patients referred to endocrinologists have hypokalemia (33), which means that many normalkalemic patients with primary aldosteronism are not being identified. It is currently estimated that fewer than 1% of all patients with primary aldosteronism are being diagnosed and treated, underlining the importance of greater awareness and the need for screening by physicians (100).

Conclusion

Primary aldosteronism is likely the most common treatable cause of secondary hypertension, and these patients are at increased risk of cardiovascular disease and mortality. Unfortunately, many patients remain undiagnosed and increased screening of hypertensive patients with ARR can help to improve case detection. While primary aldosteronism can be treated with aldosterone antagonists, medications need to be taken lifelong and may be associated with side effects. Identifying unilateral primary aldosteronism is important as these patients can be offered curative unilateral adrenalectomy. CT imaging can be inaccurate in many patients, and AVS is required in most patients to accurately identify unilateral adrenal disease. However, vein sampling is invasive, and in inexperienced centers, many patients may have inconclusive results. Functional imaging may potentially help to circumvent this issue and identify more patients who can be offered curative adrenalectomy.

References

1. Mulatero P, Stowasser M, Loh K-C, Fardella CE, Gordon RD, Mosso L, et al. Increased diagnosis of primary aldosteronism, including surgically correctable forms, in centers from five continents. J Clin Endocrinol Metab. 2004;89(3):1045–50.
2. Käyser SC, Dekkers T, Groenewoud HJ, van der Wilt GJ, Carel Bakx J, van der Wel MC, et al. Study heterogeneity and estimation of prevalence of primary aldosteronism: a systematic review and meta-regression analysis. J Clin Endocrinol Metab. 2016;101(7):2826–35.
3. Milliez P, Girerd X, Plouin P-F, Blacher J, Safar ME, Mourad J-J. Evidence for an increased rate of cardiovascular events in patients with primary aldosteronism. J Am Coll Cardiol. 2005;45(8):1243–8.
4. Sukor N, Kogovsek C, Gordon RD, Robson D, Stowasser M. Improved quality of life, blood pressure, and biochemical status following laparoscopic adrenalectomy for unilateral primary aldosteronism. J Clin Endocrinol Metab. 2010;95(3):1360–4.
5. Catena C, Colussi G, Nadalini E, Chiuch A, Baroselli S, Lapenna R, et al. Cardiovascular outcomes in patients with primary aldosteronism after treatment. Arch Intern Med. 2008;168(1):80–5.
6. Hundemer GL, Curhan GC, Yozamp N, Wang M, Vaidya A. Cardiometabolic outcomes and mortality in medically treated primary aldosteronism: a retrospective cohort study. Lancet Diabetes Endocrinol. 2018;6(1):51–9.
7. Funder JW, Zennaro M-C. 30 Years of the mineralocorticoid receptor: the scientific impact of cloning the mineralocorticoid receptor: 30 years on. J Endocrinol. 2017;234(1):E3–6.
8. Fallo F, Sonino N. Metabolic syndrome and primary aldosteronism: time for reappraisal? J Hum Hypertens. 2010;24(10):623–4.
9. Calhoun DA, Nishizaka MK, Zaman MA, Thakkar RB, Weissmann P. Hyperaldosteronism among black and white subjects with resistant hypertension. Hypertension. 2002;40(6):892–6.
10. Douma S, Petidis K, Doumas M, Papaefthimiou P, Triantafyllou A, Kartali N, et al. Prevalence of primary hyperaldosteronism in resistant hypertension: a retrospective observational study. Lancet Lond Engl. 2008;371(9628):1921–6.
11. Williams B, MacDonald TM, Morant SV, Webb DJ, Sever P, McInnes GT, et al. Endocrine and haemodynamic changes in resistant hypertension, and blood pressure responses to spironolactone or amiloride: the PATHWAY-2 mechanisms substudies. Lancet Diabetes Endocrinol. 2018;6(6):464–75.
12. Stowasser M, Gordon RD. Primary aldosteronism: changing definitions and new concepts of physiology and pathophysiology both inside and outside the kidney. Physiol Rev. 2016;96(4):1327–84.
13. Conn JW. Presidential address. I. Painting background. II. Primary aldosteronism, a new clinical syndrome. J Lab Clin Med. 1955;45(1):3–17.
14. Funder JW, Carey RM, Mantero F, Murad MH, Reincke M, Shibata H, et al. The management of primary aldosteronism: case detection, diagnosis, and treatment: an Endocrine Society Clinical Practice Guideline. J Clin Endocrinol Metab. 2016;101(5):1889–916.
15. Gupta V. Mineralocorticoid hypertension. Indian J Endocrinol Metab. 2011;15(Suppl 4):S298–312.
16. Puar THK, Mok Y, Debajyoti R, Khoo J, How CH, Ng AKH. Secondary hypertension in adults. Singapore Med J. 2016;57(5):228–32.
17. Mosso L, Carvajal C, González A, Barraza A, Avila F, Montero J, et al. Primary aldosteronism and hypertensive disease. Hypertension (Dallas, Tex.: 1979). 2003;42(2):161–5.
18. Gallay BJ, Ahmad S, Xu L, Toivola B, Davidson RC. Screening for primary aldosteronism without discontinuing hypertensive medications: plasma aldosterone-renin ratio. Am J Kidney. 2001;37(4):699–705.
19. Dudenbostel T, Calhoun DA. Resistant hypertension, obstructive sleep apnoea and aldosterone. J Hum Hypertens. 2012;26(5):281–7.
20. Di Murro A, Petramala L, Cotesta D, Zinnamosca L, Crescenzi E, Marinelli C, et al. Renin-angiotensin-aldosterone system in patients with sleep apnoea: prevalence of primary aldosteronism. J Renin Angiotensin Aldosterone Syst. 2010;11(3):165–72.
21. Montori VM, Young WF. Use of plasma aldosterone concentration-to-plasma renin activity ratio as a screening test for primary aldosteronism. A systematic review of the literature. Endocrinol Metab Clin North Am. 2002;31(3):619–32, xi.
22. Stowasser M, Gordon RD, Gunasekera TG, Cowley DC, Ward G, Archibald C, et al. High rate of detection of primary aldosteronism, including surgically treatable forms, after "non-selective" screening of hypertensive patients. J Hypertens. 2003;21(11):2149–57.
23. Young WF. Diagnosis and treatment of primary aldosteronism: practical clinical perspectives. J Intern Med. 2019;285(2):126–48.
24. Mulatero P, Rabbia F, Milan A, Paglieri C, Morello F, Chiandussi L, et al. Drug effects on aldosterone/plasma renin activity ratio in primary aldosteronism. Hypertension (Dallas, Tex.: 1979). 2002;40(6):897–902.
25. Browne GA, Griffin TP, O'Shea PM, Dennedy MC. β-Blocker withdrawal is preferable for accurate interpretation of the aldosterone-renin ratio in chronically treated hypertension. Clin Endocrinol (Oxf). 2016;84(3):325–31.
26. Dorrian CA, Toole BJ, Alvarez-Madrazo S, Kelly A, Connell JMC, Wallace AM. A screening procedure for primary aldosteronism based on the Diasorin Liaison automated chemiluminescent immunoassay for direct renin. Ann Clin Biochem. 2010;47(Pt 3):195–9.
27. Ahmed AH, Gordon RD, Ward G, Wolley M, McWhinney BC, Ungerer JP, et al. Effect of combined hormonal replacement therapy on the aldosterone/renin ratio in postmenopausal women. J Clin Endocrinol Metab. 2017;102(7):2329–34.
28. Umakoshi H, Sakamoto R, Matsuda Y, Yokomoto-Umakoshi M, Nagata H, Fukumoto T, et al. Role of aldosterone and potassium levels in sparing confirmatory tests in primary aldosteronism. J Clin Endocrinol Metab. 2019;105(4):1284–89.
29. Stowasser M, Ahmed AH, Cowley D, Wolley M, Guo Z, McWhinney BC, et al. Comparison of seated with recumbent saline suppression testing for the diagnosis of primary aldosteronism. J Clin Endocrinol Metab. 2018;103(11):4113–24.
30. Umakoshi H, Tsuiki M, Takeda Y, Kurihara I, Itoh H, Katabami T, et al. Significance of computed tomography and serum potassium in predicting subtype diagnosis of primary aldosteronism. J Clin Endocrinol Metab. 2018;103(3):900–8.
31. Küpers EM, Amar L, Raynaud A, Plouin P-F, Steichen O. A clinical prediction score to diagnose unilateral primary aldosteronism. J Clin Endocrinol Metab. 2012;97(10):3530–7.
32. Sze WCC, Soh LM, Lau JH, Reznek R, Sahdev A, Matson M, et al. Diagnosing unilateral primary aldosteronism – comparison of a clinical prediction score, computed tomography and adrenal venous sampling. Clin Endocrinol (Oxf). 2014;81(1):25–30.
33. Puar TH, Loh WJ, Lim DS, Loh LM, Zhang M, Foo RS, et al. Aldosterone–potassium ratio predicts primary aldosteronism subtype. J Hypertens. 2019;38(7):1375–83.
34. Young WF, Stanson AW, Thompson GB, Grant CS, Farley DR, van Heerden JA. Role for adrenal venous sampling in primary aldosteronism. Surgery. 2004;136(6):1227–35.
35. Fassnacht M, Arlt W, Bancos I, Dralle H, Newell-Price J, Sahdev A, et al. Management of adrenal incidentalomas: European Society of Endocrinology Clinical Practice Guideline in collaboration with the European Network for the Study of Adrenal Tumors. Eur J Endocrinol. 2016;175(2):G1–34.
36. Kempers MJE, Lenders JWM, van Outheusden L, van der Wilt GJ, Schultze Kool LJ, Hermus ARMM, et al. Systematic review: diagnostic procedures to differentiate unilateral from bilateral adrenal abnormality in primary aldosteronism. Ann Intern Med. 2009;151(5):329–37.
37. Kądziela J, Prejbisz A, Michałowska I, Kołodziejczyk-Kruk S, Schultze Kool L, Kabat M, et al. A single-centre experience of the implementation of adrenal vein sampling procedure: the impact on the diagnostic work-up in primary aldosteronism. Kardiol Pol. 2017;75(1):28–34.
38. Vonend O, Ockenfels N, Gao X, Allolio B, Lang K, Mai K, et al. Adrenal venous sampling: evaluation of the German Conn's registry. Hypertension (Dallas, Tex.: 1979). 2011;57(5):990–5.
39. Young WF, Stanson AW. What are the keys to successful adrenal venous sampling (AVS) in patients with primary aldosteronism? Clin Endocrinol (Oxf). 2009;70(1):14–17.
40. Auchus RJ, Michaelis C, Wians FH Jr, Dolmatch BL, Josephs SC, Trimmer CK, et al. Rapid cortisol assays improve the success rate of adrenal vein sampling for primary aldosteronism. Ann Surg. 2009;249(2):318–21.
41. Blondin D, Quack I, Haase M, Küçükköylü S, Willenberg HS. Indication and technical aspects of adrenal blood sampling. ROFO Fortschr Geb Rontgenstr Nuklearmed. 2015;187(1):19–28.
42. Deinum J, Groenewoud H, Wilt GJVD, Rossi G, Lenzini L. Adrenal venous sampling: cosyntropin stimulation or not? Eur J Endocrinol. 2019;181(3):D15–D26.
43. Rossitto G, Maiolino G, Lenzini L, Bisogni V, Seccia TM, Cesari M, et al. Subtyping of primary aldosteronism with adrenal vein sampling: hormone- and side-specific effects of cosyntropin and metoclopramide. Surgery. 2018;163(4):789–95.
44. Rossi GP, Auchus RJ, Brown M, Lenders JWM, Naruse M, Plouin PF, et al. An expert consensus statement on use of adrenal vein sampling for the subtyping of primary aldosteronism. Hypertension. 2014;63(1):151–60.
45. Kline GA, Chin A, So B, Harvey A, Pasieka JL. Defining contralateral adrenal suppression in primary aldosteronism: implications for diagnosis and outcome. Clin Endocrinol (Oxf). 2015;83(1):20–7.
46. Dekkers T, Prejbisz A, Kool LJS, Groenewoud HJMM, Velema M, Spiering W, et al. Adrenal vein sampling versus CT scan to determine treatment in primary aldosteronism: an outcome-based randomised diagnostic trial. Lancet Diabetes Endocrinol. 2016;16(3):e547–e548.

47. Beuschlein F, Mulatero P, Asbach E, Monticone S, Catena C, Sechi LA, et al. The SPARTACUS Trial: controversies and unresolved issues. Horm Metab Res. 2017;49(12):936–42.
48. Puar TH, Khoo JJ, Ng KS, Kam JW, Wang KW. Adrenal vein sampling versus CT scanning in primary aldosteronism. Lancet Diabetes Endocrinol. 2016;4(11):885–6.
49. Lubitz CC, Economopoulos KP, Sy S, Johanson C, Kunzel HE, Reincke M, et al. Cost-effectiveness of screening for primary aldosteronism and subtype diagnosis in the resistant hypertensive patients. Circ Cardiovasc Qual Outcomes. 2015;8(6):621–30.
50. Strajina V, Al-Hilli Z, Andrews JC, Bancos I, Thompson GB, Farley DR, et al. Primary aldosteronism: making sense of partial data sets from failed adrenal venous sampling-suppression of adrenal aldosterone production can be used in clinical decision making. Surgery. 2017;163(4): 801–6.
51. Muth A, Ragnarsson O, Johannsson G, Wängberg B. Systematic review of surgery and outcomes in patients with primary aldosteronism. Br J Surg. 2015;102(4):307–17.
52. Miyake Y, Tanaka K, Nishikawa T, Naruse M, Takayanagi R, Sasano H, et al. Prognosis of primary aldosteronism in Japan: results from a nationwide epidemiological study. Endocr J. 2014;61(1):35–40.
53. Mulatero P, Monticone S, Bertello C, Viola A, Tizzani D, Iannaccone A, et al. Long-term cardio- and cerebrovascular events in patients with primary aldosteronism. J Clin Endocrinol Metab. 2013;98(12):4826–33.
54. Velema M, Dekkers T, Hermus A, Timmers H, Lenders J, Groenewoud H, et al. Quality of life in primary aldosteronism: a comparative effectiveness study of adrenalectomy and medical treatment. J Clin Endocrinol Metab. 2018;103(1):16–24.
55. Rossi GP, Cesari M, Cuspidi C, Maiolino G, Cicala MV, Bisogni V, et al. Long-term control of arterial hypertension and regression of left ventricular hypertrophy with treatment of primary aldosteronism. Hypertension. 2013;62(1):62–9.
56. Zacharieva S, Orbetzova M, Elenkova A, Stoynev A, Yaneva M, Schigarminova R, et al. Diurnal blood pressure pattern in patients with primary aldosteronism. J Endocrinol Invest. 2006;29(1):26–31.
57. Reincke M, Rump LC, Quinkler M, Hahner S, Diederich S, Lorenz R, et al. Risk factors associated with a low glomerular filtration rate in primary aldosteronism. J Clin Endocrinol Metab. 2009;94(3):869–75.
58. Katabami T, Fukuda H, Tsukiyama H, Tanaka Y, Takeda Y, Kurihara I, et al. Clinical and biochemical outcomes after adrenalectomy and medical treatment in patients with unilateral primary aldosteronism. J Hypertens. 2019;37(7):1513–20.
59. Hundemer GL, Curhan GC, Yozamp N, Wang M, Vaidya A. Incidence of atrial fibrillation and mineralocorticoid receptor activity in patients with medically and surgically treated primary aldosteronism. JAMA Cardiol. 2018;3(8):768–74.
60. Hundemer Gregory L, Curhan Gary C, Yozamp N, Wang M, Vaidya A. Renal outcomes in medically and surgically treated primary aldosteronism. Hypertension. 2018;72(3):658–66.
61. Adolf C, Köhler A, Franke A, Lang K, Riester A, Löw A, et al. Cortisol excess in patients with primary aldosteronism impacts left ventricular hypertrophy. J Clin Endocrinol Metab. 2018;103(12):4543–52.
62. Prejbisz A, Kołodziejczyk-Kruk S, Lenders JWM, Januszewicz A. Primary aldosteronism and obstructive sleep apnea: is this a bidirectional relationship? Horm Metab Res. 2017;49(12):969–76.
63. Sechi LA, Novello M, Lapenna R, Baroselli S, Nadalini E, Colussi GL, et al. Long-term renal outcomes in patients with primary aldosteronism. JAMA. 2006;295(22):2638–45.
64. Chai YJ, Kwon H, Yu HW, Kim S-J, Choi JY, Lee KE, et al. Systematic review of surgical approaches for adrenal tumors: lateral transperitoneal versus posterior retroperitoneal and laparoscopic versus robotic adrenalectomy. Int J Endocrinol. 2014;2014:918346.
65. Ishidoya S, Ito A, Sakai K, Satoh M, Chiba Y, Sato F, et al. Laparoscopic partial versus total adrenalectomy for aldosterone producing adenoma. J Urol. 2005;174(1):40–3.
66. Dekkers T, ter Meer M, Lenders JWM, Hermus ARM, Schultze Kool L, Langenhuijsen JF, et al. Adrenal nodularity and somatic mutations in primary aldosteronism: one node is the culprit? J Clin Endocrinol Metab. 2014;99(7):E1341–51.
67. Fischer E, Hanslik G, Pallauf A, Degenhart C, Linsenmaier U, Beuschlein F, et al. Prolonged zona glomerulosa insufficiency causing hyperkalemia in primary aldosteronism after adrenalectomy. J Clin Endocrinol Metab. 2012;97(11):3965–73.
68. Zarnegar R, Young WF, Lee J, Sweet MP, Kebebew E, Farley DR, et al. The aldosteronoma resolution score: predicting complete resolution of hypertension after adrenalectomy for aldosteronoma. Ann Surg. 2008;247(3):511–8.
69. Williams TA, Lenders JWM, Mulatero P, Burrello J, Rottenkolber M, Adolf C, et al. Outcomes after adrenalectomy for unilateral primary aldosteronism: an international consensus on outcome measures and analysis of remission rates in an international cohort. Lancet Diabetes Endocrinol. 2017;5(9):689–99.
70. Sawka AM, Young WF, Thompson GB, Grant CS, Farley DR, Leibson C, et al. Primary aldosteronism: factors associated with normalization of blood pressure after surgery. Ann Intern Med. 2001;135(4):258–61.
71. Ghose RP, Hall PM, Bravo EL. Medical management of aldosterone-producing adenomas. Ann Intern Med. 1999;131(2):105–8.
72. Deinum J, Riksen NP, Lenders JW. Pharmacological treatment of aldosterone excess. Pharmacol Ther. 2015;154:120–33.
73. Jeunemaitre X, Chatellier G, Kreft-Jais C, Charru A, DeVries C, Plouin PF, et al. Efficacy and tolerance of spironolactone in essential hypertension. Am J Cardiol. 1987;60(10):820–5.
74. Biggar RJ, Andersen EW, Wohlfahrt J, Melbye M. Spironolactone use and the risk of breast and gynecologic cancers. Cancer Epidemiol. 2013;37(6):870–5.
75. Mackenzie IS, Morant SV, Wei L, Thompson AM, MacDonald TM. Spironolactone use and risk of incident cancers: a retrospective, matched cohort study. Br J Clin Pharmacol. 2017;83(3):653–63.
76. Parthasarathy HK, Ménard J, White WB, Young WF, Williams GH, Williams B, et al. A double-blind, randomized study comparing the antihypertensive effect of eplerenone and spironolactone in patients with hypertension and evidence of primary aldosteronism. J Hypertens. 2011;29(5):980–90.
77. Sutherland DJ, Ruse JL, Laidlaw JC. Hypertension, increased aldosterone secretion and low plasma renin activity relieved by dexamethasone. Can Med Assoc J. 1966;95(22):1109–19.
78. Lifton RP, Dluhy RG, Powers M, Rich GM, Cook S, Ulick S, et al. A chimaeric 11 beta-hydroxylase/aldosterone synthase gene causes glucocorticoid-remediable aldosteronism and human hypertension. Nature. 1992;355(6357):262–5.
79. Stowasser M, Bachmann AW, Huggard PR, Rossetti TR, Gordon RD. Treatment of familial hyperaldosteronism type I: only partial suppression of adrenocorticotropin required to correct hypertension. J Clin Endocrinol Metab. 2000;85(9):3313–8.
80. Choi M, Scholl UI, Yue P, Björklund P, Zhao B, Nelson-Williams C, et al. K⁺ channel mutations in adrenal aldosterone-producing adenomas and hereditary hypertension. Science. 2011;331(6018):768–72.
81. Beuschlein F, Boulkroun S, Osswald A, Wieland T, Nielsen HN, Lichtenauer UD, et al. Somatic mutations in ATP1A1 and ATP2B3 lead to aldosterone-producing adenomas and secondary hypertension. Nat Genet. 2013;45(4):440–4, 444e1–2.
82. Azizan EAB, Poulsen H, Tuluc P, Zhou J, Clausen MV, Lieb A, et al. Somatic mutations in ATP1A1 and CACNA1D underlie a common subtype of adrenal hypertension. Nat Genet. 2013;45(9):1055–60.
83. Scholl UI, Goh G, Stölting G, de Oliveira RC, Choi M, Overton JD, et al. Somatic and germline CACNA1D calcium channel mutations in aldosterone-producing adenomas and primary aldosteronism. Nat Genet. 2013;45(9):1050–4.
84. Zennaro M-C, Boulkroun S, Fernandes-Rosa F. Genetic causes of functional adrenocortical adenomas. Endocr Rev. 2017;38(6):516–37.
85. Gomez-Sanchez CE. Channels and pumps in aldosterone-producing adenomas. J Clin Endocrinol Metab. 2014;99(4):1152–6.
86. Warachit W, Atikankul T, Houngngam N, Sunthornyothin S. Prevalence of somatic KCNJ5 mutations in Thai patients with aldosterone-producing adrenal adenomas. J Endocr Soc. 2018;2(10):1137–46.
87. Zheng F-F, Zhu L-M, Nie A-F, Li X-Y, Lin J-R, Zhang K, et al. Clinical characteristics of somatic mutations in Chinese patients with aldosterone-producing adenoma. Hypertension (Dallas, Tex.: 1979). 2015;65(3):622–8.
88. Brown MJ. Primary aldosteronism: the spectre of cure. Clin Endocrinol Oxf. 2015;82(6):785–8.
89. Nishimoto K, Tomlins SA, Kuick R, Cani AK, Giordano TJ, Hovelson DH, et al. Aldosterone-stimulating somatic gene mutations are common in normal adrenal glands. Proc Natl Acad Sci U S A. 2015;112(33):E4591–9.
90. Bergström M, Sörensen J, Kahn TS, Juhlin C, Eriksson B, Sundin A, et al. PET with [11C]-metomidate for the visualization of adrenocortical tumors and discrimination from other lesions. Clin Positron Imaging. 1999;2(6):339.
91. Hennings J, Lindhe O, Bergström M, Långström B, Sundin A, Hellman P. [11C]-metomidate positron emission tomography of adrenocortical tumors in correlation with histopathological findings. J Clin Endocrinol Metab. 2006;91(4):1410–14.
92. Burton TJ, Mackenzie IS, Balan K, Koo B, Bird N, Soloviev DV, et al. Evaluation of the sensitivity and specificity of (11)C-metomidate positron emission tomography (PET)-CT for lateralizing aldosterone secretion by Conn's adenomas. J Clin Endocrinol Metab. 2012;97(1):100–9.
93. Nomura K, Kusakabe K, Maki M, Ito Y, Aiba M, Demura H. Iodomethylnorcholesterol uptake in an aldosteronoma shown by dexamethasone-suppression scintigraphy: relationship to adenoma size and functional activity. J Clin Endocrinol Metab. 1990;71(4):825–30.
94. Puar T, Tan C, Tong A, Zhang M, Khoo CM, Tan A, et al. 11C-metomidate PET/CT identifies unilateral primary aldosteronism in a multi-ethnic cohort. In BioScientifica; 2019 [cited 20 August 2019]. Available from: https://www.endocrine-abstracts.org/ea/0063/ea0063p445.
95. Sacks BA, Sacks AC, Faintuch S. Radiofrequency ablation treatment for aldosterone-producing adenomas. Curr Opin Endocrinol Diabetes Obes. 2017;24(3):169–73.
96. Liu SYW, Chu CCM, Tsui TKC, Wong SKH, Kong APS, Chiu PWY, et al. Aldosterone-producing adenoma in primary aldosteronism: CT-guided radiofrequency ablation-long-term results and recurrence rate. Radiology. 2016;281(2):625–34.
97. Cooray MSA, Bulugahapitiya US, Peiris DN. Rhabdomyolysis: a rare presentation of aldosterone-producing adenoma. Indian J Endocrinol Metab. 2013;17(Suppl 1):S237–9.
98. Nagarajan R, Kuberan K, Senthil Kumar MS, Chandrasekaran M. Is hyperaldosteronism a pathognomonic feature of Conn's syndrome? Indian J Surg. 2010;72(2):146–8.
99. Hope TA, Bergsland EK, Bozkurt MF, Graham M, Heaney AP, Herrmann K, et al. Appropriate use criteria for somatostatin-receptor PET imaging in neuroendocrine tumors. J Nucl Med. 2018;59(1):66–74.
100. Brown MJ. Ins and outs of aldosterone-producing adenomas of the adrenal: from channelopathy to common curable cause of hypertension. Hypertension. 2014;63(1):24–6.

51

ADRENAL MYELOLIPOMA

Himagirish K Rao

Introduction

Myelolipoma is a benign adrenocortical neoplasm that, as the name suggests, comprises of myeloid and adipose tissues. In the World Health Organization classification of adrenal tumors, it is listed under mesenchymal and stromal tumors of the adrenal cortex.[1] The clinical relevance of this invariably benign tumor is that it might cause dilemmas in the diagnosis of adrenal neoplasms. The incidence of myelolipoma has increased in recent times owing to the widespread use of imaging modalities including computed tomography (CT) and magnetic resonance imaging (MRI).

Adrenal myelolipomas are found in one out of 500–1250 autopsies.[2] However, it is difficult to estimate the exact clinical prevalence of the condition since the tumor is benign and invariably asymptomatic. Myelolipoma is the second-most common primary adrenal incidentaloma (6–16% of all adrenal incidentalomas).[3–5] While the vast majority of myelolipomas are adrenocortical in origin, they have been reported in extra-adrenal locations too, including the mediastinum [6], spleen [7], kidney [8], bones [9], thorax [10], the nasal cavity [11], the extradural tissues [12] and even in the eyes.[13] Invariably, myelolipomas are biochemically nonfunctional.

Pathogenesis

Myelolipomas are composed of mature adipocytes with hematopoietic cells interspersed in between. The pathogenesis is obscure. One of the theories suggests metaplasia as the primary event. Stimuli like necrosis, infection and stress might induce metaplastic change within the adrenal cortex [14–16], in the reticuloendothelial cells of the capillaries, in the peri-stromal mesenchymal cells and in the adipose tissue within the stroma. As the adipocytes proliferate, differentiate and mature, they might secrete various inflammatory metabolites that recruit circulating hematopoietic progenitors to settle and differentiate.[17]

Another theory suggests genetic events. One report described the presence of a balanced translocation of (3;21) (q25; p11) in the tumor, but it is not clear how relevant this is pathologically.[18] In another study, the majority of myelolipomas have been found to have nonrandom X-chromosome inactivation, suggesting clonal origin of this tumor.[19]

Hormonal pathways have also been suggested. Many decades ago, Hans Selye performed some experiments in which hypophysectomized rats were treated with methyltestosterone and with lyophilized anterior pituitary extract. The zonae fasciculata and reticularis were transformed into tissue that was very similar to bone marrow.[20] In correlation with these experiments, it has been observed that myelolipomas have developed in some patients with untreated adrenal hyperplasia and very high ACTH levels. Another hormonal theory suggests that myelolipoma could develop as a result of sustained elevations of erythropoietin seen in chronic anemia.[15, 21]

It might be possible that more than one of these factors might work in conjunction to result in the occurrence of myelolipomas.

Myelolipoma and extramedullary hematopoiesis (EMH)

Hematopoiesis occurs within the medulla (bone marrow) as well as in extramedullary locations. In the fetus, the bone marrow isn't fully developed structurally as well as functionally. Hence, hematopoiesis is essentially extramedullary and is seen predominantly in the liver, spleen and other components of the reticuloendothelial system. After birth, as the bone marrow develops function, EMH ceases over time. However, in conditions like hemoglobinopathies and myeloproliferative disorders that involve hemolysis and marrow degeneration, EMH resumes.[22] In rare instances, EMH per se is seen in the adrenal cortex, sometimes causing significant enlargement of the adrenal gland, which can lead to diagnostic dilemma.

EMH and myelolipoma are two different pathological entities but with very similar pathological appearance. In both conditions, the affected tissues include mature adipocytes interspersed with trilinear hematopoietic cells. Both differ from mature bone marrow in that they lack reticular sinusoids. EMH usually occurs in hematological disease, while myelolipoma is associated with healthy marrow tissue with normal function.[23] While myelolipoma is a well-encapsulated tumor with predominance of mature adipose tissue and interspersed hematopoietic cells, EMH is not circumscribed and fat is not an obligatory component.[24]

Pathology

Myelolipomas are round or oval, well-circumscribed and discreet lesions that vary widely in size. The smallest of them are barely a few millimeters across, while the largest reported tumor measured 43 cm.[25] Tumors larger than 10 cm are called giant myelolipomas. In a review of more than 400 cases of myelolipoma by Declan et al., 35% of the tumors were reported to have measured larger than 10 cm. Weight of the specimen correlates poorly with size due to variations in the proportion of adipose and hematopoietic tissue and due to the variable extent of hemorrhage within the tumor.

Common findings on gross examination of the specimen include a capsule or pseudocapsule, yellow and reddish-brown areas on cut surface and hemorrhage in the substance of the tumor (Figure 51.1). The pseudocapsule is the outer layer of compressed adrenal cortex (zonae glomerulosa and fasciculata). The yellow areas on cut surface correspond to the adipose tissue component, while the reddish-brown areas contain the hematopoietic elements. In their review, Decman et al. reported that foci of hemorrhage were seen on cut surface in about a fifth of the cases. [25] On histopathological examination, the adipose and myeloid elements are interspersed with each other within the substance of

Adrenal Myelolipoma

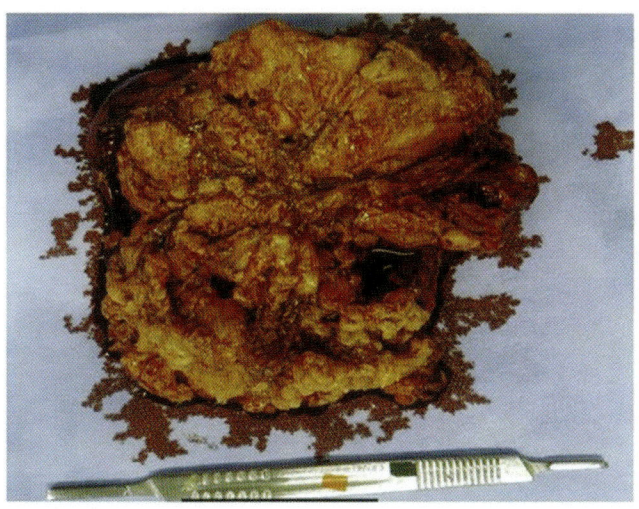

FIGURE 51.1 Myelolipoma gross cut section.

the tumor. The capsule consists of layers of fibrous stroma sometimes, the condensation of normal adrenocortical tissue around the tumor, the pseudocapsule, is evident (Figure 51.2).

Clinical features

Usually, patients are in their 50s and 60s when myelolipoma is diagnosed.[26, 27] However, the youngest patient was 1 year old at diagnosis and the oldest was 83.[28, 29] In a review of 440 case reports, out of which the gender was reported in 438 patients, it was observed that 211 (48.6%) were female and 223 (51.4%) were male.[25] No significant gender preponderance was observed. In another review based on two Chinese studies, female preponderance was reported.[30]

The predominant symptoms were abdominal discomfort, a continuous dull ache in the hypochondrium, lumbar regions, loins or back, dyspepsia, nausea and vomiting and acute abdominal pain [25] Except for giant myelolipomas that produce mass effect, it is difficult to ascribe clinical symptoms exclusively to the tumor.

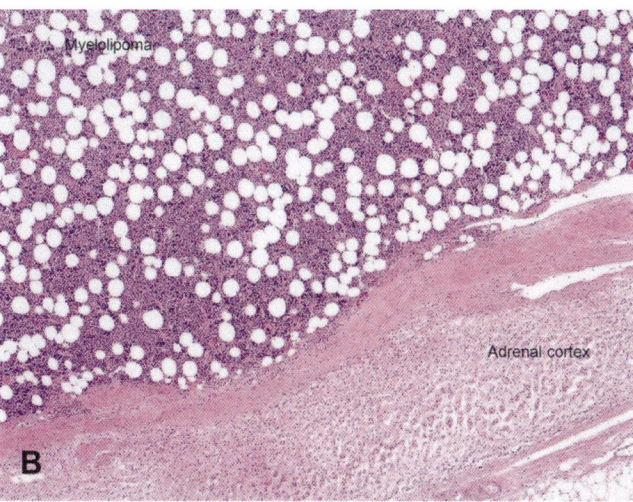

FIGURE 51.2 Myelolipoma HPE.

Generally, myelolipoma occurs more often on the right side when compared to the left.[1, 20, 25, 30] In a systematic review which included various studies with a cumulative total of 438 cases, right-sided tumors were reported in 260 patients (59.3%), left-sided tumors in 111 patients (25.3%) and bilateral myelolipomas in 54 (12.3%). It has been reported that left-sided tumors are slightly larger than right-sided ones, but the difference in size wasn't significant.[25]

The rate of growth of the tumor is an important aspect in the management of adrenal tumors, especially in case of the silent and asymptomatic ones. Myelolipomas are generally slow-growing tumors. Campbell et al., in their study of 69 cases of myelolipomas, found the median growth rate to be 0.16 cm per year (0.08–0.71).[31] Follow-up imaging was performed at a median interval of 3.9 years. In another older study, 12 patients with 13 myelolipomas were studied and the results were more variable, with rate of annual growth ranging between 0.64 and 5.5% per month.[32]

Spontaneous rupture of myelolipomas can result in retroperitoneal hemorrhage. Usually it is chronic, but rarely, it can be acute and torrential, presenting as acute hemorrhagic shock.[33] The median size of ruptured myelolipomas was found to be 12 cm. Most of the bleeding myelolipomas were larger than 10 cm. The smallest myelolipoma with reported rupture and hemorrhage was 6.5 cm.[29] Spontaneous rupture was found in 5% of myelolipomas.[29]

Myelolipomas and associated endocrine disease

Associated endocrine disorders have been found in a significant proportion of patients with myelolipomas (Table 51.1).[34–38] Among the patients with myelolipoma and congenital adrenal hyperplasia (CAH), the commonest disorder was 21-hydroxylase deficiency (35/44). 17-Hydroxylase deficiency was seen in five patients, while only one patient had 11-beta-hydroxylase deficiency. In this subset of patients, nearly half of them (18/44) had

TABLE 51.1: Associated Endocrine Disorders in Patients with Myelolipoma [25]

Disorder	Number of Patients
Hypertension	97
Diabetes mellitus	41
Congenital adrenal hyperplasia	44
Hypercortisolism	23
Primary hyperaldosteronism	9
Primary hyperandrogenism	4
Primary hypogonadism	2
Primary hyperparathyroidism	2
Pheochromocytoma	2
Other conditions	
Carney's complex	
Polycystic ovarian syndrome	
Papillary thyroid carcinoma	
Hyperthyroidism	
Hypothyroidism	
Multiple endocrine neoplasia	
Nelson's syndrome	

TABLE 51.2: Non-endocrine Disorders Associated with Myelolipoma [25]

Hemolytic anemias
Thalassemias
Sickle cell disease
Red cell membrane anomalies
Renal cell carcinoma
Prostatic carcinoma
Atrial fibrillation
Breast cancer
Gastric cancer
Endometrial cancer

bilateral tumors. Left-sided tumors were seen in 12 patients, while right-sided tumors were seen in only 5 patients. This is contrary to the general pattern of laterality. Complaints and symptoms of hypercortisolism, hyperaldosteronism and hyperandrogenism seem to disappear after removal of the tumor. The average size of functioning tumors (68.5 mm) is significantly less that of nonfunctioning tumors (104 mm), which would be explained by earlier presentation in case of functional tumors.

This estimation may not be accurate due to publication bias. The incidence of functioning myelolipomas may be lower than what literature suggests. However, the fact that myelolipomas with associated functional components have been reported might indicate that AML is not a purely mesenchymal tumor with adipose and hematopoietic elements only. It may also include elements of the functional adrenal cortical cells.

Myelolipomas are also associated with non-endocrine disorders like thalassemia and other hemoglobinopathies, renal cell cancer, prostate cancer and atrial fibrillation (Table 51.2). Association with hemoglobinopathies may be significant in that it may hint at common pathways of pathogenesis for the two entities. There have been instances of adrenal gland enlargement due to EMH without the occurrence of a frank myelolipoma.

Imaging and other investigations

Ultrasonography

Often, this is the first imaging investigation that is performed for adrenal lesions. Myelolipoma is generally a well-demarcated, oval or round lesion arising out of the adrenal gland with preserved planes all around the lesion (Figure 51.3). It is seen as a hyperechogenic and heterogenous mass. Calcifications are often observed within the lesion. Ultrasound alone is not adequate to diagnose this lesion, and so, CT and/or MRI are required.[25]

Computed tomography (CT)

On CT scans, myelolipomas are well-circumscribed, round or elliptical lesions with well-preserved fat planes all around the lesion (Figure 51.4). They appear as hypodense lesions due to the significant adipose tissue present and are heterogenous due to the presence of multiple tissue components. Attenuation values of −120 to −90 HU are characteristic of fat and the presence of fat density is pivotal in the diagnosis of an adrenal lesion as myelolipoma. The average attenuation values vary because the proportion of the adipose tissue component within the lesion is variable. If present, features like hemorrhage and calcifications will be appreciable on CT scanning.[15] In these times, positron emission tomography (PET) is widely performed during diagnostic

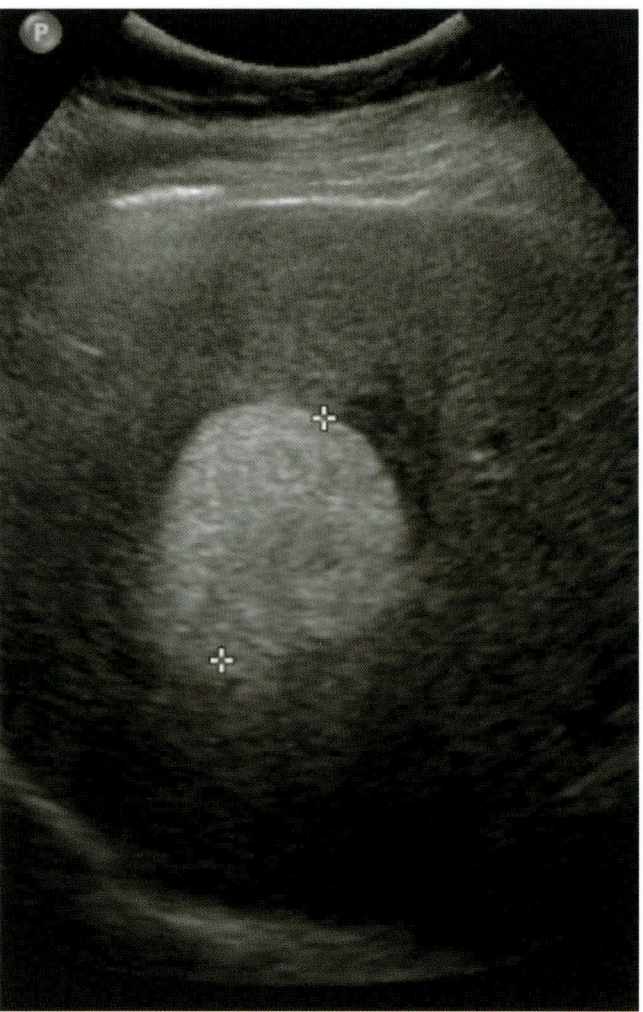

FIGURE 51.3 Myelolipoma USG.

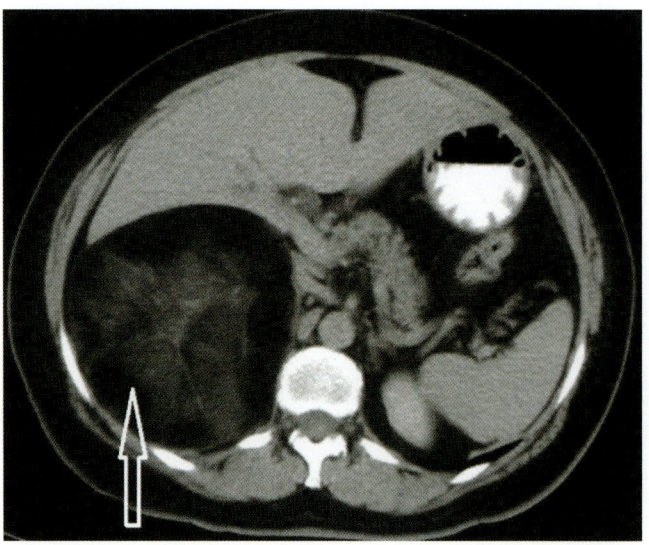

FIGURE 51.4 Myelolipoma CT.

Adrenal Myelolipoma

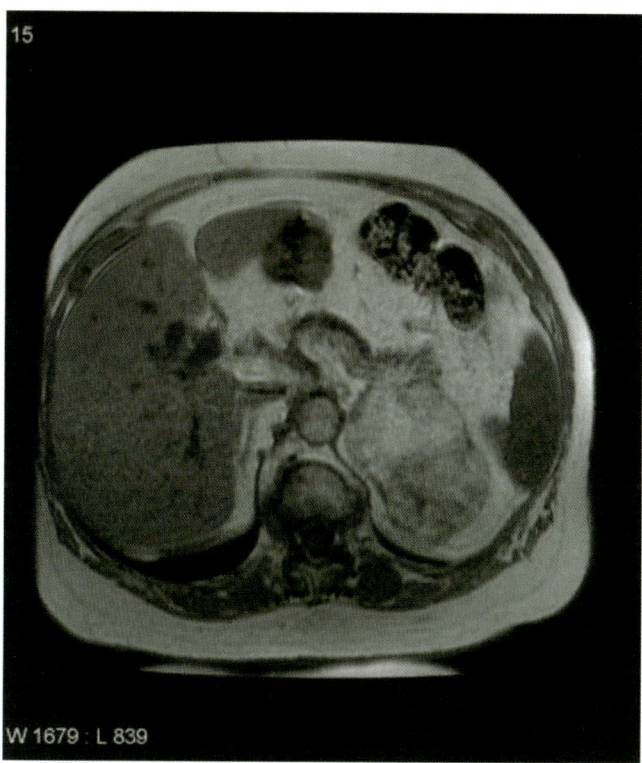

FIGURE 51.5 Myelolipoma MRI.

work-up of adrenal lesions, although PET is not an essential imaging study in this condition. FDG uptake is usually absent in myelolipomas.[39] However, the hematopoietic elements may rarely produce evidence of intense FDG uptake on the scan.[40]

Magnetic resonance imaging (MRI)

Adipose tissue appears hyperintense on T1- and T2-weighted sequences of MRI (Figure 51.5). Hence, the fat component of myelolipoma appears hyperintense and is well-recognizable even without fat suppression. The tumors are well-demarcated and, usually, heterogenous. On the basis of two different and unconnected studies by Boraschi et al. and Musante et al., three different morphologies have been described for myelolipomas: (1) homogenous, hyperintense masses on T1-weighted images with intermediate signals on T2-weighted images, (2) heterogenous masses with at intensity areas and hyperintense areas on T2-weighted images and (3) nodules hypointense to the liver on T1-weighted sequences and after gadolinium administration, hyperintense sequences on T2-weighted images, suggesting myeloid elements in the lesions.[41, 42]

Differential diagnosis

Adrenal myelolipoma can appear similar to other lipid-containing tumors that occur in the region, including adrenocortical adenoma (ACA), adrenocortical carcinoma (ACC), retroperitoneal liposarcoma (RPL), exophytic renal angiomyolipoma and adrenal lipoma.

ACAs can be functioning as well as nonfunctioning tumors. The functional tumors will be diagnosed on biochemical tests of adrenal function. On imaging, ACAs appear as well-defined, homogenous and sharply marginated masses. TO diagnose ACAs in routine clinical practice, an upper threshold of 10 HU is set for lipid-rich ACAs that make up 70% of all ACAs. The attenuation value might be higher (usually 30 HU or less) in the rest of the ACAs. On T1-weighted MRI, ACAs are isointense with respect to the liver and hyperintense with respect to the spleen.[43]

ACCs are often large with multiple lobulations. Fat planes around the lesion might be lost due to extra-adrenal involvement. Cystic spaces and foci of hemorrhage are often seen in the substance of the lesions. The margins are irregular. There might be evidence of invasion into the surrounding structures like kidney, perinephric fat and the inferior vena cava (IVC). Attenuation values on CT are often more than 10 HU. There may be low attenuation at the center of the lesion due to tumor necrosis. Peripheral nodular enhancement on CECT is typical. The tumors give low signal on T1-weighted MRI sequences and heterogeneously high signals on T2-weighted images. On FDG-PET, the uptake will be high.[44–46]

Angiomyolipoma is the most common benign tumor of the kidney. Composed of mature adipose tissue, blood vessels and smooth muscle cells, it is usually a large necrotic tumor. In many cases, it extends through the renal capsule into the perinephric space. On ultrasound, it appears as a heterogeneously echodense mass. On CT, the attenuation values are in the negative range. When a fat-containing solid mass is seen arising from the kidney and extending out into the perinephric space, the suspicion of angiomyolipoma is high. On T1-weighted images, the tumor is hyperintense relative to the renal parenchyma and isointense relative to fat.[47]

RPL grows slowly and infiltrates the surrounding tissues. Distant metastasis is very rare with RPL. The well-differentiated lipogenic type of RPL is the most common subtype and is the one that is mostly similar to myelolipoma on imaging. However, unlike myelolipoma, peri-lesional infiltration is common, fat planes are frequently breached and enhancement with IV contrast is consistent. RPL also takes up FDG avidly when compared with myelolipoma.[48] Adrenal lipoma is devoid of myeloid elements. It is extremely rare (24 documented cases only in history) [49], and differential diagnosis with myelolipoma is not clinically relevant.

Clinical management

There are no specific guidelines as yet for the management of adrenal myelolipoma. Hence, it is wise to individualize management decisions. The majority of myelolipomas are clinically occult and do not trouble the patient – they are the classical incidentalomas. However, since, as per the AACE guidelines on adrenal incidentalomas [50], incidentalomas are generally evaluated for biochemical function before anatomical characterization, most of the patients undergo biochemical work-up by the time a diagnosis is made on the basis of imaging.

That said, the necessity of hormonal evaluation of myelolipomas is debatable. Many authors have not proposed hormonal evaluation for obvious myelolipomas.[50, 51] On the other hand, some authors have found functional myelolipomas to be prevalent enough (20% of all the cases of myelolipoma) to warrant routine biochemical testing for all patients with this tumor.[15] In their review of 440 cases, Decman et al. found that the prevalence of hormonally functional myelolipomas was 18.3%.[25] This included CAH, which was seen in 10% of patients.[25] Considering the evidence of literature so far, it is advisable to consider the clinical picture overall before deciding about functional assessment for patients with myelolipoma.

For cases of asymptomatic myelolipoma, follow-up with serial imaging should be adequate, given that the tumor is benign, slow-growing and inert in nature. There have been isolated reports that have observed the rate of tumor growth in patient cohorts.[49, 50] However, due to lack of sufficient and consistent data, it would be difficult to determine the threshold diameter above which follow-up by serial imaging could be proposed. Follow-up of giant myelolipomas might be warranted, but the frequency of follow-up is yet to be determined. Since myelolipomas are, by and large, larger than ACAs, ultrasound might be accurate enough for follow-up.

Myelolipomas that cause symptoms in patients need to be treated. Surgical resection is the only treatment option available. If and when required, resection can be performed either by minimal access approach or open surgery. Adrenal tumors that are 10 cm or smaller in diameter are amenable to excision by minimal access surgery.

Laparoscopic adrenalectomy is safe and effective and is the standard of care at present for surgical adrenalectomy.[52] The adrenal gland can be approached either transperitoneally (lateral and anterior approaches) or retroperitoneally. There are merits and demerits for each approach, but generally, it is easier to remove the larger tumors through the transperitoneal approach. Tumors that are 6 cm or smaller in size can be removed through the retroperitoneal approach without much difficulty.

The size threshold for laparoscopic adrenalectomy is 10 cm, since the risk of malignancy increases significantly in larger tumors. However, there have been isolated reports where myelolipomas as large as 15 cm have been successfully excised successfully without complications through the transperitoneal approach. Shen et al. have described a retroperitoneal approach for operating large myelolipomas by a technique that includes liposuction.[53]

Rupture of the tumor and the resulting hemorrhage can be a surgical emergency necessitating emergency laparotomy. There have been reports of successful trans-arterial embolization using gelatine sponge in these cases, which has enabled control of bleeding and elective removal of the tumor after optimization.[54, 55]

Conclusion

Adrenal myelolipoma is a benign tumor composed of adipose tissue and elements of extramedullary hematopoietic tissue. It is usually a large tumor, most often diagnosed in the sixth decade of life. Due to its composition, it can sometimes cause severe diagnostic confusion, mostly with adrenocortical cancer. Detailed imaging including CT, MRI and if required, PET, might be helpful. The only feasible modality of treatment is surgery. If the diagnosis is unambiguous and if the lesion causes no symptoms or discomfort to the patient, surgical excision may not be needed at all.

References

1. A.K. Lam, Update on adrenal tumours in 2017 World Health Organization (WHO) of endocrine tumours. Endocr. Pathol. 1–15 (2017). https://doi.org/10.1007/s12022-017-9484-5.
2. C.A. Olsson, R.J. Krane, R.C. Klugo, S.M. Selikowitz, Adrenal myelolipoma. Surgery 73, 665–670 (1973).
3. J.H. Song, F.S. Chaudhry, W.W. Mayo-Smith, The incidental adrenal mass on CT: prevalence of adrenal disease in 1,049 consecutive adrenal masses in patients with no known malignancy. Am. J. Roentgenol. 190, 1163–1168 (2008).
4. X. Bin, Y. Qing, W. Linhui, G. Li, S. Yinghao, Adrenal incidentalomas: experience from a retrospective study in a Chinese population. J. Urol. 29, 270–274 (2011).
5. F. Mantero, A.M. Masini, G. Opocher, M. Giovagnetti, G. Arnaldi, Tumors, on behalf of the N.I.S.G. on A., Adrenal incidentaloma: an overview of hormonal data from the National Italian Study Group. Horm. Res. 47, 284–289 (1997).
6. Y. Minamiya, S. Abo, M. Kitamura, K. Izumi, Mediastinal extraadrenal myelolipoma: report of a case. Surg. Today 27, 971–972 (1997).
7. Y. Zeng, Q. Ma, L. Lin, P. Fu, Y. Shen, Q.-Y. Luo, L.-H. Zhao, J.-H. Mou, H.-L. Xiao, Giant myelolipoma in the spleen: a rare case report and literature review. Int. J. Surg. Pathol. 24, 177–180 (2016).
8. M. Ghaouti, K. Znati, A. Jahid, F. Zouaidia, Z. Bernoussi, N. Mahassini, Renal myelolipoma: a rare extra-adrenal tumor in a rare site: a case report and review of the literature. J. Med. Case Rep. 7, 92 (2013).
9. M. Sundaram, T. Bauer, A. von Hochstetter, H. Ilaslan, M. Joyce, Intraosseous myelolipoma. Skelet. Radiol. 36, 1181–1184 (2007).
10. M. Krismann, G. Reichle, K.M. Müller, [Thoracic bilateral myelolipoma]. Pneumologie 47, 501–503 (1993).
11. S.A. George, M.T. Manipadam, R. Thomas, Primary myelolipoma presenting as a nasal cavity polyp: a case report and review of the literature. J. Med. Case Rep. 6, 127 (2012).
12. S.J. Newman, K. Inzana, W. Chickering, Extradural myelolipoma in a dog. J. Vet. Diagn. Investig. 12, 71–74 (2000).
13. G. Storms, G. Janssens, Intraocular myelolipoma in a dog. Vet. Ophthalmol. 16, 183–187 (2013).
14. R. Sanders, N. Bissada, N. Curry, B. Gordon, Clinical spectrum of adrenal myelolipoma: analysis of eight tumors in seven patients. J. Urol. 153, 1791–1793 (1995).
15. V.G. Shenoy, A. Thota, R. Shankar, M.G. Desai, Adrenal myelolipoma: controversies in its management. Indian. J. Urol. 31, 94–101 (2015).
16. S. De Navasquez, Case of myelolipoma (bone-marrow, heterotopia) of suprarenal gland. Guys. Hosp. Rep. 88, 237–240 (1935).
17. C. Feng, H. Jiang, Q. Ding, H. Wen, Adrenal myelolipoma: a mingle of progenitor cells? Med. Hypotheses 80, 819–822 (2013).
18. K.-C. Chang, P.-I. Chen, Z.-H. Huang, Y.-M. Lin, P.-L. Kuo, Adrenal myelolipoma with translocation (3;21)(q25; p11). Cancer Genet. Cytogenet. 134, 77–80 (2002).
19. E. Bishop, J.N. Eble, L. Cheng, M. Wang, D.R. Chase, A. Orazi, D.P. O'Malley, Adrenal myelolipomas show nonrandom X-chromosome inactivation in hematopoietic elements and fat: support for a clonal origin of myelolipomas. Am. J. Surg. Pathol. 30, 838–843 (2006).
20. H. Selye, H. Stone, Hormonally induced transformation of adrenal into myeloid tissue. Am. J. Pathol. 26, 211–233 (1950).
21. I. Motta, L. Boiocchi, P. Delbini, M. Migone De Amicis, E. Cassinerio, D. Dondossola, G. Rossi, M.D Cappellini, A giant adrenal myelolipoma in a beta-thalassemia major patient: does ineffective erythropoiesis play a role? Am. J. Hematol. 91, 1281–1282 (2016).
22. A. Taher, E. Vichinsky, K. Musallam, M.D. Cappellini, V. Viprakasit, S.D. Weatherall, Guidelines for the Management of Non Transfusion Dependent Thalassaemia (NTDT). Thalassaemia International Federation; 2013. https://www.ncbi.nlm.nih.gov/books/NBK190453/.
23. M.R. Fowler, R.B. Williams, J.M. Alba, C.R. Byrd, Extra-adrenal myelolipomas compared with extramedullary hematopoietic tumors: a case of presacral myelolipoma. Am. J. Surg. Pathol. 6, 363–374 (1982).
24. K.T.K. Chen, E.L. Felix, M.S Flam, Extraadrenal myelolipoma. Am. J. Clin. Pathol. 78, 386–389 (1982).
25. A. Decman, P. Perge, M. Toth, P. Iglas, Adrenal myelolipoma: a comprehensive review. Endocrine 59, 7–15 (2018).
26. G. Low, H. Dhliwayo, D.J. Lomas, Adrenal neoplasms. Clin. Radiol. 67, 988–1000 (2012).
27. K.Y. Lam, C.Y. Lo, Adrenal lipomatous tumours: a 30 year clinico-pathological experience at a single institution. J. Clin. Pathol. 54, 707–712 (2001).
28. I.A. Cardinalli, A.G. de Oliveira-Filho, M.J. Mastellaro, R.C. Ribeiro, S.S. Aguiar, A unique case of synchronous functional adrenocortical adenoma and myelolipoma within the ectopic adrenal cortex in a child with Beckwith–Wiedemann syndrome. Pathol. Res. Pract. 208, 189–194 (2012).
29. M.C. Sebastià, M.O. Pérez-Molina, A. Alvarez-Castells, S. Quiroga, E. Pallisa, CT evaluation of underlying cause in spontaneous subcapsular and perirenal hemorrhage. Eur. Radiol. 7, 686–690 (1997).
30. A.K. Lam, Lipomatous tumours in adrenal gland: WHO updates and clinical implications. Endocr. Relat. Cancer 24, R65–R79 (2017).
31. M.J. Campbell, M. Obasi, B. Wu, M.T. Corwin, G Fananapazir, The radiographically diagnosed adrenal myelolipoma: what do we really know? Endocrine, 1–6 (2017). doi:https://doi.org/10.1007/s12020-017-1410-6.
32. M. Han, A.L. Burnett, E.K. Fishman, F.F. Marshall, The natural history and treatment of adrenal myelolipoma. J. Urol. 157, 1213–1216 (1997).
33. H.-P. Liu, W.-Y. Chang, S.-T. Chien, C.-W. Hsu, Y.-C. Wu, W.C. Kung, C.-M. Su, P.-H. Liu, Intra-abdominal bleeding with hemorrhagic shock: a case of adrenal myelolipoma and review of literature. BMC Surg. 17, 74 (2017).
34. A.A. Reza-Albarran, F.J. Gomez-Perez, J.C. Lopez, M. Herrera, A. Gamboa-Dominguez, C. Keirns, A. Aranda, J.A. Rull, Myelolipoma: a new adrenal finding in Carney's complex? Endocr. Pathol. 10, 251–257 (1999).
35. P. Kalafatis, Bilateral giant adrenal myelolipoma and polycystic ovarian disease. Urol. Int. 63, 139–143 (1999).
36. M. Yoshioka, K. Fujimori, M. Wakasugi, N. Yamazaki, M. Kuroki, T. Tsuchida, H. Seki, M. Sekiya, T. Tamura, Cushing's disease associated with adrenal myelolipoma, adrenal calcification and thyroid cancer. Endocr. J. 41, 461–466 (1994).
37. S. Banik, P.S. Hasleton, R.L. Lyon, An unusual variant of multiple endocrine neoplasia syndrome: a case report. Histopathology 8, 135–144 (1984).
38. I. Maschler, E. Rosenmann, E.N. Ehrenfeld, Ectopic functioning adrenocortico-myelolipoma in longstanding Nelson's syndrome. Clin. Endocrinol. (Oxf.) 10, 493–497 (1979).
39. F. Gemmel, H. Bruinsma, P. Oomen, J. Collins, PET/CT incidental detection of bilateral adrenal myelolipomas in a patient with a huge maxillary sinus carcinoma. Clin. Nucl. Med. 35, 132–133 (2010).

40. V. Ludwig, M.H. Rice, W.H. Martin, M.C. Kelley, D. Delbeke, 2-Deoxy-2-[^{18}F]fluoro-D-glucose positron emission tomography uptake in a giant adrenal myelolipoma. Mol. Imaging Biol. 4, 355–358 (2002).
41. P. Boraschi, G. Braccini, R. Gigoni, F. Cartei, A. Campatelli, A. Di Vito, G. Perri, [Adrenal myelolipomas: their magnetic resonance assessment]. Clin. Ter. 147, 549–557 (1996).
42. F. Musante, L.E. Derchi, M. Bazzocchi, T. Avataneo, G. Gandini, R.S Pozzi Mucelli, MR imaging of adrenal myelolipomas. J. Comput. Assist. Tomogr. 15, 111–114 (1991).
43. D.J. Wale, K.K. Wong, B.L. Viglianti, D. Rubello, M.D. Gross, Contemporary imaging of incidentally discovered adrenal masses. Biomed. Pharmacother. 87, 256–262 (2017).
44. M. Fassnacht, M. Kroiss, B. Allolio, Update in adrenocortical carcinoma. J. Clin. Endocrinol. Metab. 98, 4551–4564 (2013).
45. M.L. Nunes, A. Rault, J. Teynie, N. Valli, M. Guyot, D. Gaye, G. Belleannee, A. Tabarin, 18F-FDG PET for the identification of adrenocortical carcinomas among indeterminate adrenal tumors at computed tomography scanning. World J. Surg. 34, 1506–1510 (2010).
46. M. Fassnacht, W. Arlt, I. Bancos, H. Dralle, J. Newell-Price, A. Sahdev, A. Tabarin, M. Terzolo, S. Tsagarakis, O.M. Dekkers, Management of adrenal incidentalomas: European Society of Endocrinology Clinical Practice Guideline in collaboration with the European Network for the Study of Adrenal Tumors. Eur. J. Endocrinol. 175, G1–G34 (2016).
47. S. Krishna, C.A. Murray, M.D. McInnes, R. Chatelain, M. Siddaiah, O. Al-Dandan, S. Narayanasamy, N. Schieda, CT imaging of solid renal masses: pitfalls and solutions. Clin. Radiol. 72, 708–721 (2017).
48. W.D. Craig, J.C. Fanburg-Smith, L.R. Henry, R. Guerrero, J.H. Barton, Fat-containing lesions of the retroperitoneum: radiologicpathologic correlation. RadioGraphics 29, 261–290 (2009).
49. M. Terzolo, S. Bovio, A. Pia, G. Reimondo, A. Angeli, Management of adrenal incidentaloma. Best. Pract. Res. Clin. Endocrinol. Metab. 23, 233–243 (2009).
50. M. Zeiger, G. Thompson, Q.-Y. Duh, A. Hamrahian, P. Angelos, D. Elaraj, E. Fishman, J. Kharlip, American Association of Clinical Endocrinologists, American Association of Endocrine Surgeons, American Association of Clinical Endocrinologists and American Association of Endocrine Surgeons Medical Guidelines for the Management of Adrenal Incidentalomas: executive summary of recommendations. Endocr. Pract. 15, 450–453 (2009).
51. M. Terzolo, A. Stigliano, I. Chiodini, P. Loli, L. Furlani, G. Arnaldi, G. Reimondo, A. Pia, V. Toscano, M. Zini, G. Borretta, E. Papini, P. Garofalo, B. Allolio, B. Dupas, F. Mantero, A. Tabarin, A.M.E. Position, Statement on adrenal incidentaloma. Eur. J. Endocrinol. 164, 851–870 (2011).
52. S. Yamashita, K. Ito, K. Furushima, J. Fukushima, S. Kameyama, Y. Harihara, Laparoscopic versus open adrenalectomy for adrenal myelolipoma. Ann. Med. Surg. 3, 34–38 (2014).
53. X. Shen, Y. Qiu, Y. Zheng, S. Zhang, Retroperitoneal laparoscopic liposuction for large adrenal myelolipomas: a report of nine cases. J. Laparoendosc. Adv. Surg. Tech. 22, 578–580 (2012).
54. M. Nakajo, S. Onohara, K. Shinmura, F. Fujiyoshi, M. Nakajo, Embolization for spontaneous retroperitoneal hemorrhage from adrenal myelolipoma. Radiat. Med. 21, 214–219 (2003).
55. S.M. Chng, M.B.K. Lin, F.C. Ng, H.C. Chng, T.K. Khoo, Adrenal myelolipoma presenting with spontaneous retroperitoneal haemorrhage demonstrated on computed tomography and angiogram – a case report. Ann. Acad. Med. Singap. 31, 228–230 (2002).

ADRENAL SURGICAL DISEASES IN CHILDREN

Ahmet Çelik and Emre Divarci

Simple anatomy – basic physiology

Adrenal glands are located in the retroperitoneal area and are covered with a perirenal fascia. Each gland is located on the superomedial edge of each kidney like a hat. The glands are located in front of the 11th and 12th ribs on the left and 12th rib on the right. Dorsal and lateral neighborhoods are the same for both glands, but medial and anterior neighborhoods are different (1, 2).

The adrenal glands together weigh 6–8 g at birth and are nearly the size of adult adrenals. Proportionally, they are 10–20 times larger than adult adrenals. By the end of first year of age, it reaches normal dimensions and weight after cortical involution. The mature adrenal gland measures 3–5 cm in length and 4–6 mm in thickness. The right adrenal gland has a triangular, but left adrenal has a larger and more crescentic shape. The surface has a bright yellow-orange color (1, 2).

The anatomy of the arterial system is unpredictable and variable. The aorta, inferior phrenic artery, and renal artery are the main sources of these profuse arterial supplies. Each gland is drained by a single large adrenal vein. The right adrenal vein is draining into the inferior vena cava directly. The left adrenal vein is longer than the right vein and merges with the left inferior phrenic vein prior to draining into the left renal vein (2).

Adrenal glands are divided into two functional parts: cortex and medulla. Adrenal cortex consists of three different cell groups producing different hormones. The zona glomerulosa (outer layer of adrenal and 10% of cortex) is exclusively responsible for the production and secretion of mineralocorticoids (aldosterone regulated by renin-angiotensin axis), the zona fasciculata (middle layer, 80% of adrenal cortex) that produces glucocorticoids (conversion of progesterone to cortisol by 17 alpa-hydroxylase and 11 beta-hydroxylase), and the zona reticularis (10% of adrenal cortex) as the most inner layer of cortex produces androgens (dihydroepiandrosterone: DHEA and DHEA-sulfate). Functional cells of the adrenal medulla are chromaffin cells and derived from neural crest. Chromaffin cells in the adrenal produce catecholamines, which is regulated by the sympathetic nervous system, and there are the cells of the origin of pheochromocytomas and neuroblastomas (NBs).

Adrenal-related surgical problems

Adrenal masses are the most common cause of problems requiring adrenal surgery in childhood. Compared to adults, the majority of masses in children are malignant and 80% are neuroblastic tumors (3, 4). According to our clinical experience and literature, adrenal masses are summarized in Table 52.1 (3).

Evaluation of adrenal masses

The combination of history, physical examination, laboratory tests, and imaging studies, especially modern cross-sectional imaging, in particular, can help in distinguishing this type of masses (5, 6).

Symptoms and sings of adrenal masses

Neuroblastic tumors may present with mass effects or the hormone effects they secrete. An abdominal mass that crosses the midline or unilaterally can be palpated (Figure 52.1). Different types of paralytic problems can be detected with the mass extending into the spinal canal. Paraneoplastic syndromes, such as opsomyoclonus (an immune-mediated paraneoplastic syndrome is characterized by multiple jerking movements), bone pain (Hutchinson syndrome), hepatomegaly (Pepper syndrome), and respiratory distress caused by it, periorbital lesion (raccoon's eyes), and subcutaneous deposits (blueberry muffin), are clinical reflections that may occur as a result of metastases of NBs. Hypertension, palpitations, sweatiness, shakiness, anxiety, and diarrhea can present as a result of catecholamine secretions in both NB and pheochromocytoma.

Adrenocortical tumors (ACTs) secrete hormones causing various clinical symptoms that, depending on the specific hormone, will be present in children. Virilization (the most common presentation, 80% due to secretion of androgens), feminization, Cushing's syndrome (occurs in one-third patients as a result of autogenous corticosteroids), and Conn's syndromes (primary hyperaldosteronism headache, polyuria, tachycardia, hypocalcemia, hypertension, and weakness of proximal muscle groups) are the most common clinical presentations (Table 52.2). These tumors can cause precocious puberty as a result of gonadotropin-independent source of endogen androgens and cortisol, which usually produce pseudoprecocious puberty. Incidentally detected adrenal mass rates are also increasing (3, 6).

Laboratory investigation of adrenal masses

In these cases, history and physical examination also guide the priority of laboratory analysis. The frequency of the probability of tumors becoming malignant requires the investigation of neuroblastic tumor markers first. Investigation includes measuring the adrenal hormone secretions of medulla or cortex. Urine and blood should be collected for homovanilic acid (HVA), vanillylmandelic acid (VMA), and dopamine and norepinephrine levels when medullary tumors are suspected.

Laboratory testing for ACTs includes evaluation of androgens and glucocorticoid levels and its breakdown products in blood and urine samples (urinary 17-ketosteroids are the most important marker for ACT, plasma DEAS-S is the second-most sensitive marker). Briefly, urinary 17-KS, and 17-OH, urinary or plasma cortisol, plasma DHES-S, testosterone, androstenedione, 17-hydroxyprogesterone, aldosterone, and renin activity levels are useful laboratory tests. Serum electrolytes (potassium will be low in Conn's syndrome) and glucose (will be elevated with corticosteroids) levels are also useful (5, 7).

Imaging evaluation of adrenal masses

Mass effect on surrounding organs and calcifications on plain radiographs suggest NBs and/or previous adrenal hemorrhages. Ultrasonography (US) is the first diagnostic method and serves as

Adrenal Surgical Diseases in Children

TABLE 52.1: Childhood Adrenal Masses

Neoplasm	Functional	Adenoma
		Carcinoma
		Pheochromocytoma
		PPNAD
		AIMH/AIMiH
		Oncocytoma
	Nonfunctional	Neuroblastoma
		Adrenal cyst
		Hemangioma/Lipoma
		Teratoma
		Leiomyosarcoma
		Oncocytoma
Metastatic*		Renal cell carcinoma
		Extrarhabdoid tumor
Traumatic		Neonatal hemorrhage
		Child abuse
Infective		
Mimicking adrenal lesions		Extrapulmonary sequestration
		Extramedullary hematopoiesis
		Diaphragmatic lesions

Abbreviations: ACIMAH, ACTH-independent macronodullary/(Mi, micronodullary) adrenal hyperplasia; PPNAD, Primary pigmented nodullary adrenocortical disease; RMS, Rhabdomyosarcoma. *Very rare in children.

TABLE 52.2: Etiology of Cushing Syndrome (CS) in Childhood

ACTH-Dependent Causes *2nd Most Common Cause*
- Cushing disease(CD) (pituitary adenoma – micro or macro)
- *80–85% has surgically identifiable microadenoma in children*
- Ectopic ACTH production=*rare in children*
- Small cell bronchogenic carcinoma
- Carcinoid tumors=*bronchial one is the most frequent cause of ectopic CD in children*
- Pancreatic islet cell carcinoma
- Thymoma/Medullary thyroid carcinoma/Pheochromocytomas

ACTH-Independent Causes (10–15%) (43, 44)
- Adrenal adenoma
- Adrenocortical carcinoma
- Adrenal hyperplasia (macro- or micronodular/pigmented or not)

Iatrogenic=Exogenous (*The Most Common Cause of CS in Adults and Children*) (43, 44)
- Administration of ACTH or glucocorticoids

a good initial study to define the next step of management (5, 6). With US, the location, internal features, neighborhoods, vascularization, and blood supply of the mass can be easily evaluated. Liver metastases can be detected. US with Doppler modality, the extension of the tumor into the renal vein, vena cava, and right atrium can be demonstrated. US feature of ACTs as defined including a wide range in size, a round or ovoid shape, and a thin echogenic capsule-like rim. Unfortunately, no echo pattern has been defined as characteristic enough to allow differentiation of adrenal adenoma from carcinoma. Smaller lesions are more likely to be benign, and larger lesions with areas of necrosis, hemorrhage, and calcification are more likely to be malignant. 'Scar sign' refers to radiating linear echoes that suggest adrenocortical carcinoma (6, 8).

Computerized tomography (CT) provides more accuracy for the definitions of tumor size, location, vascular invasion, lymph nodes, and metastases (Figure 52.2). Magnetic resonance imaging (MRI) is superior to CT and does not expose the patient to radiation, but image quality may deteriorate due to movement artifact in young children (6). Metaiodobenzylguanidine (MIBG) nuclear scan investigations may be used for detection of medullary tumors. MIBG scans particularly useful in localizing such tumors in extra-adrenal sites and metastases (9).

Differential diagnosis of adrenal masses

Adrenal hemorrhage: It is the most common (four times more than NB) adrenal mass in a neonate and differentiating it from NB can be challenging. It can lead to symptoms such as anemia, persistent jaundice, abdominal distension, and abdominal mass. It usually progresses asymptomatically and is detected in imaging performed for other reasons (6, 10, 11). Etiology is not always available; relatively increased size and vascularity of the adrenal gland can explain this predisposition. It can be associated with traumatic birth, hypoxia, shock, septicemia or bleeding diathesis, and sometimes it can develop spontaneously. In severe cases, adrenal insufficiency and shock due to hemorrhage may be observed, especially in the bilateral cases (12). It can be distinguished from a neoplastic adrenal tumor by serial sonograms that demonstrate temporal evaluation of mass through stages of liquefaction, clot retraction, and eventual shrinkage and exhibit cystic transformation over time, eventually resolving completely

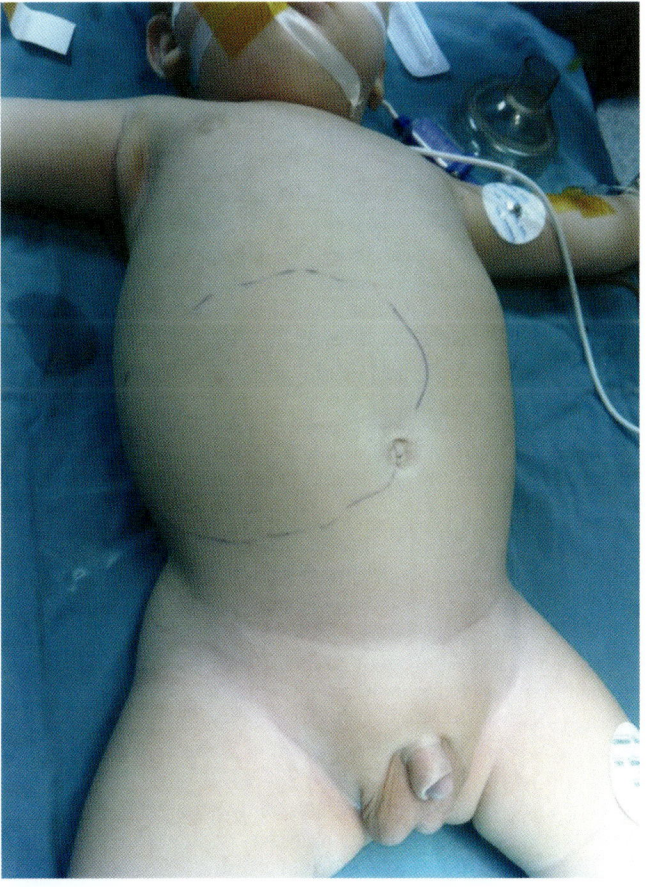

FIGURE 52.1 Child with abdominal (adrenal NB) tumor crossing midline.

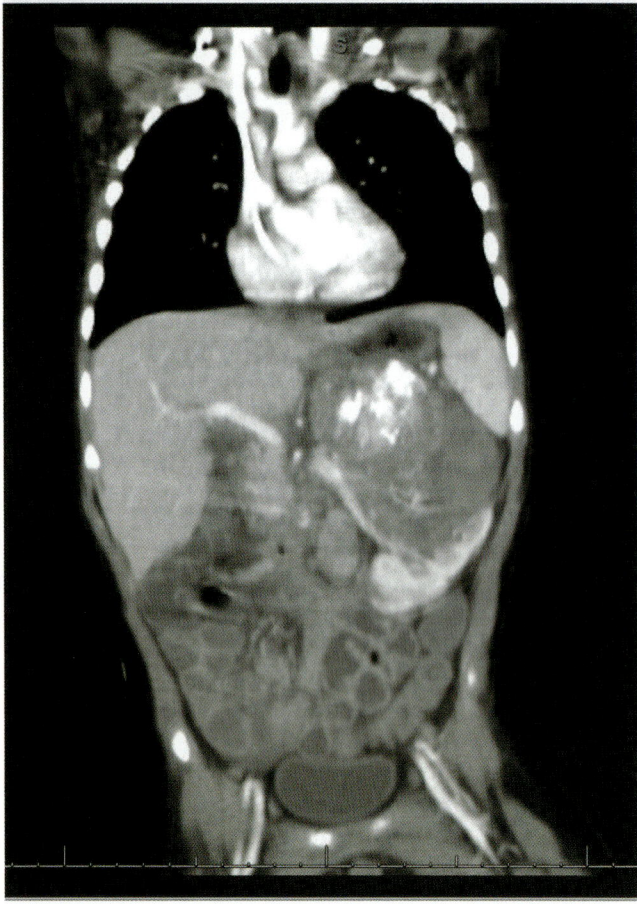

FIGURE 52.2 Left adrenal mass (NB) displacing left kidney.

with or without residual calcifications (5, 11). In benign conditions, this process is expected to be completed in 1–2 weeks. MRI is the most sensitive and specific tool and may also be useful for differentiating NB from a lone hemorrhage (6, 13).

Adrenal abscess: It is a very rare condition. It is thought that adrenal abscess formation mostly develops in neonates following adrenal hemorrhage. In cases not treated early, especially in septic newborns, the complication and mortality risk is high. Optimal therapy is drainage (image-guided percutaneous or surgical) and broad-spectrum antibiotics (14–16).

Extralobar pulmonary sequestrations: It is a form of bronchopulmonary foregut malformation. It mainly occurs in the thorax (90%) but can also occur in other places, such as the abdomen (10%) (6). Dominantly occurring in boys (80%), more than half of cases are associated with other congenital anomalies. The mass of extralobar pulmonary sequestration is often first seen in the second trimester on prenatal US in contrast to congenital NB, which is almost always first detected in the third trimester. CT and MRI can more accurately delineate the lesion and its blood supply than can US. It should be kept in mind in the differential diagnosis of the masses in adrenal localization. Despite some clues, the preoperative exact diagnosis is difficult. Generally, definitive diagnosis can be made after surgery (17–20). Management of extralobar pulmonary sequestration is surgical, with an excellent prognosis.

In our clinical experience, we have two patients with left adrenal mass, explored with initial diagnosis of neuroblastic tumor; definitive diagnosis could only be made by peroperative and postoperative examinations in both (21).

Adrenal cysts: The cystic lesions of adrenal gland are rare but may be recognized at any age. Three major types have been described (22).

(1) *Pure cysts (endothelial-vascular)*: Most frequent type, which has lymphangiomatous or hemangiomatous origin. Second one is a hemorrhagic cyst, also called pseudocyst or hemorrhagic cyst. The rarest subgroup is the epithelial cyst, named true cyst, which is related to a congenital glandular sac and associated liquid retention. (2) *Parasitic cysts:* The adrenals are not a typical site for parasites, yet hydatid cyst formed by the larva of a parasite has been described. (3) *Tumor related cysts:* NB, ganglioneuroma (GN), pheochromocytoma, teratoma, and, exceptionally, adrenocortical carcinoma/adenoma can be shown with a cystic component. Pediatric adrenal cysts vary from simple cysts with a benign behavior to neoplasia-related lesions displaying severe prognosis as seen in cystic NB. A multidisciplinary approach is required for their management. Conservative follow-up or surgical interpretation in selected cases can be required (22).

Adrenal medulla–related masses

NB: NB is a malignant neoplasm that arises from primitive neural crest cells and can be seen in any area where the sympathetic nervous system is located. It is the most common extracranial solid neoplasm in children, accounting for 10% of all pediatric neoplasms; NB accounts for 15% of all childhood mortality from neoplasm (23). It is most frequently located in the abdomen, and the most common location in the abdomen is the adrenal gland (about 45% of NB cases) and typically affects young children (6, 23, 24).

NBs usually secrete catecholamines, their metabolites can be detected in blood and urine (3). High serum levels of neuron-specific enolase (NSE), ferritin, and lactate dehydrogenase (LDH) are associated with advanced disease and poor prognosis. N-myc proto-oncogene, multidrug resistance-associated protein (MRP), CD44, nerve growth factor (NGF), and its associated high-affinity receptor, Trk tyrosine kinase receptor, are several of the crucial molecular markers in NBs. Approximately 30% of primary NBs demonstrate N-myc amplification, which is strongly correlated with advanced-stage tumors and poor prognosis, independent of patient age and staging.

It may be localized, well-shaped, or may be as a retroperitoneal mass that crosses the midline, irregular, encasing vascular structures, and typically showing punctate calcifications on radiologic imaging studies (Figures 52.1 and 52.2) (6, 23). Typically, US is followed by CT or MRI; both modalities can reveal a large heterogeneous mass. I123-MIBG scan is essential for a better evaluation of the primary and metastatic burden of NB (81). As a result of some biochemistrical secretions, these patients may show specific clinical situations named paraneoplastic syndromes and clinical manifestations mentioned earlier.

Stage 4S (age under 1 year, localized tumor, and hepatic, subcutaneous, bone marrow metastasis) is a special stage of NB in which majority of cases may have spontaneous regression; however, in some cases, the tumor is rapidly progressive with poor prognosis and, thus, requires aggressive therapy (25).

NBs are made up of immature neuroblasts of small, uniform cells with dense, hyperchromatic nuclei, and scant cytoplasm. Shimada classification has been widely used to characterize and predict tumor behavior (26). It has been replaced by the more comprehensive International NB Pathological Classification (INPC) system. The new INPC system is based on age at diagnosis, mitosis-karyorrhexis index (MKI), neuroblastic differentiation, and stromal content (27).

The most common sites of metastases include the lymph nodes, bone, bone marrow, liver, and skin. The prognosis for NB varies with age, and cases diagnosed before 18 months of age typically have a much higher 5-year survival rate than those diagnosed at older ages.

NB is treated per protocols dictated by dedicated international study groups (28–31). A combined modality of surgery, chemotherapy, and radiotherapy based on disease stage and patient age at presentation is used for NB. Adrenal-located NB can be a part of low stage or a part of high stage. In localized patients without image-defined risk factor (IDRF), primary surgery is recommended for cure. The goal of surgical intervention is complete resection of tumor. If complete resection is not feasible, the goal is to perform a biopsy and to stage the tumor.

Two main staging systems are used for NB: first, the International NB Staging System (INSS), which is based solely on surgical criteria during excision (30). The second is the newer International Neuroblastoma Risk Group Staging System (INRGSS), published in 2009 to address the need for a unified approach to pretreatment risk assessment (31). The cornerstone of INRGSS system is a group of preset IDRFs used to determine tumor stage and anticipate any surgical complications (4, 31–33). Infiltration of the renal pedicle, encasement of major vessels (inferior vena cava, aorta, superior mesenteric artery, celiac trunk, iliac, and hypogastric vessels), the porta hepatis, dumbbell tumors, muscular infiltration, and compression of kidney or ureter have been identified as IDRFs. Complete resection could be achieved in only 26% of cases presenting with IDRFs in a study of Günther et al. (34). Neoadjuvant chemotherapy is recommended in the presence of IDRF. It is reported that 30% of NB cases, considered unresectable initially, became resectable with this type management (35). For advanced stages (3 and 4 disease) and/or IDRF(+) patients, initial surgical intervention should be limited to open biopsy for tissue diagnosis along with cytogenetic and tumor biomarker analyses. Delaying surgical resection until adjuvant chemotherapy is given has resulted in decreased morbidity and an increased rate of complete resection. Follow-up imaging is required after chemotherapy or surgery to assess response of NB to treatment and detect possible recurrence or metastasis.

Ganglioneuroblastoma (GNB): GNB is an intermediate-grade tumor on the spectrum of neuroblastic tumors (i.e., it arises from neural crest cells) with potentially malignant behavior due to its mixed composition of mature ganglion cells and primitive neuroblasts. GNB tends to be smaller and more well defined than NB and may be predominantly solid or cystic. Differentiation from NB is challenging based on conventional imaging findings alone, and pathologic confirmation is often required.

GN: GN is the most mature or benign form of neural crest tumors that contain mature ganglion cells and nerve fibers but no neuroblasts. They more commonly present in older children as opposed to less mature lesions. The most common locations for GN are the posterior mediastinum (about 40%) and retroperitoneum (about 35%), followed by adrenal glands (about 20%). Most frequently, GN is an incidental finding with no hormonal symptoms (3). Extension into the spinal canal may cause neurologic symptoms due to spinal cord compression.

Pheochromocytoma: The cell origin is neural crest as in NBs, but pheochromocytomas usually occur in older children. Extra-adrenal pheochromocytoma, also termed paraganglioma that originated from cells-migrated extramedullary areas as the paraganglia, can also be seen. The adrenal gland accounts for 85% of all pheochromocytomas in adults. Children have a higher incidence of extra-adrenal pheochromocytoma (30%), multifocal, and familial disease, but a lower incidence of malignancy (10%) compared with adults.

Children typically present with constant or paroxysmal hypertension with resulting headaches. Classical symptom triad (headache, sweating, and palpitation) was reported more often in children (36). Up to 25% of pheochromocytomas are familial, and germline mutations in the following genes have been associated with pheochromocytoma: Pheochromocytomas may occur in patients with neurofibromatosis, von Hippel-Lindau disease, Sturge-Weber syndrome, and multiple endocrine neoplasia (MEN) types IIA and IIB (37–39). In familial patients, tumor bilaterality is common. Less than 10% of pheochromocytomas in children are malignant. On imaging, they tend to be rounded, circumscribed masses (6).

Measurements of plasma and/or urine metanephrines, normetanephrine are the most reliable tests with almost 100% sensitivity. MRI or CT have similar diagnostic sensitivities; I-123 MIBG scintigraphy is a highly specific test for function (6, 39).

Perioperative preparation and handling of patients with dynamic changes are important and should be considered by the surgical and anesthesia team. At operation, it is important to ligate the adrenal vein early and to minimize handling the gland to limit catecholamine surges during the procedure. Laparoscopic transabdominal adrenalectomy has gained significant popularity and been validated for pheochromocytoma resections in children, currently (3, 40). Cortical-sparing adrenalectomies have been proposed for patients with bilateral tumors and those at high risk for developing a metachronous contralateral lesion. In our published series, bilateral pheochromocytoma masses were successfully resected with laparoscopic approach (LA) by adrenal sparing surgery in one case (3, 40).

Adrenal cortex-related diseases

Primary hyperaldosteronism – Conn's syndrome: It is defined as excess production of aldosterone from the adrenal glands with consequent suppression of renin. An adrenal adenoma, or ***Conn's syndrome***, is the most common cause of primary hyperaldosteronism in adults, whereas adrenocortical (nodular)hyperplasia is the most common cause in children (41), but adenoma is also reported (42). Primary hyperaldosteronism is also seen in MEN 1–related adrenal tumors. Signs and symptoms of primary hyperaldosteronism are nonspecific (41, 42). Patients have hypertension, muscle weakness, polydipsia, and polyuria. It is characterized by hypertension and hypokalemic alkalosis. The elevated aldosterone levels suppress renin and angiotensin. The diagnosis should be entertained in any child with hypertension and hypokalemia, even in normokalemia (41, 42). The treatment of a functioning adrenal adenoma is resection, which can be performed laparoscopically. Treatment of patients with bilateral adrenal hyperplasia is with spironolactone.

Cushing syndrome (hypercortisolism): Describes any form of glucocorticoid excess that is caused by endocrine tumors or administration of excess glucocorticoids (most common in children and adults) (Table 52.2). Cushing syndrome (CS) in childhood results mostly from the exogenous administration of glucocorticoids; endogenous CS is a rare disease. The latter is the main reason pediatric patients with CS escape diagnosis for too long (43, 44).

In infants and children younger than 7 years, the most common cause of endogenous CS is an adrenal tumor (ACTH-independent CS). However, in adults and children older than 7 years, adrenal hyperplasia secondary to hypersecretion of pituitary ACTH predominates (45). The classic Cushing appearance may not be seen in children because of its time-consuming development. The most frequent and reliable findings with CS are weight gain and growth failure (43–45). Specifically, any obese child who stops growing should be evaluated for CS (45, 46). Diurnal plasma cortisol levels measurement is the initial tests. The most sensitive screening test is the 24-hour urinary hydroxycorticosteroid or free cortisol value. The overnight dexamethasone suppression test is performed by administering dexamethasone.

Cushing disease: Most pediatric cases (80–85% of those with Cushing disease) are due to pituitary adenomas (mainly microadenomas), which are ACTH-dependent and primarily treated with transsphenoidal surgery (43–45). Adrenalectomy is the preferred treatment when two transsphenoidal procedures fail. Mitotane, an adrenolytic agent, causes a chemical adrenalectomy but has severe side effects, including nausea, anorexia, and vomiting (43–46).

Primary pigmented nodular adrenocortical disease (PPNAD): It is a benign proliferative disorder. PPNAD is characterized by nodules usually less than 4–6 mm in diameter with a brown or black color. The internodular adrenal cortex is atrophic and disorganized, and the adrenal glands are usually of normal weight and size. On imaging studies, the classical beaded appearance has been defined, although not in all cases (47). PPNAD can be single, but it is usually associated with the Carney complex (47). Affected patients often have tumors of two endocrine glands. The problem is usually bilateral and such patients have been treated with bilateral adrenalectomies; however, many patients also benefited from unilateral adrenalectomy (3, 43, 44, 47, 48). In our clinical experience, we had one patient, and its laparoscopic unilateral post-adrenalectomy management was uneventful (3, 48).

ACTH-independent (macronodular/micronodular-nonpigmented) adrenal hyperplasia: AIMAH is an uncommon benign proliferative disorder of the adrenal cortex. Steroid hormone secretion is ACTH independent and associated with both undetectable plasma levels of ACTH and the inability to suppress cortisol secretion with high-dose dexamethasone (43, 44, 49, 50). Histologically, it is composed of nodules with two cell types, lipid rich cells with clear cytoplasm and lipid-poor cells with a compact cytoplasm. Although corticosteroid secretion is independent of ACTH, the cells express the ACTH receptor and patients will respond to exogenous ACTH. Increased hormone secretion is due to increase of adrenocortical mass rather than augmented synthesis within each cell. The primary lesion may be unilateral or bilateral, macroadenoma or hyperplasia, and sporadic or familial (such as part of McCune-Albright syndrome or Carney complex disease). Medical therapy with steroidogenesis inhibitors (such as metyrapone and ketoconazole) can reduce plasma cortisol levels; however, surgical resection of the diseased adrenal is highly and rapidly effective in eliminating the source, and thus, it has been globally accepted as the standard treatment. The problem is usually bilateral and such patients are treated with bilateral (staged or synchronous) adrenalectomy; currently, it can be done laparoscopically (3, 43, 44, 49, 51).

Adrenocortical tumors (ACTs) in children

These tumors are rare in the pediatric population, comprising less than 0.2% of all pediatric neoplasms and 6% of all pediatric adrenal tumors. The incidence of this disease varies depending on geographic location with one region of Brazil having the highest frequency (52). ACT term is currently used to designate both benign and malignant tumors of the adrenal cortex in children. These tumors are less common than NBs but more common than pheochromocytomas (53–55). Tumor weight may range from 2 g to 6 kg (5). There is no laterality predominance, and bilateral tumors occur in about 1% of cases. Typically it is present in the first 5 years of life with median age of presentation between 3 and 4 years of age. There is biphasic age distribution. Second smaller peak is in adolescence. There is a female predominance with 1.5/1 ratio. Ectopic occurrence is not surprising. Most occur in children with no predisposing condition; however, there are some known molecular risk factors for developing ACT, including abnormalities of the p53 tumor suppressor, Ki-67, insulin-like growth factor 2 (IGF-2), and beta-catenin (53, 54). **Adenoma or carcinoma?** In children, clinical findings, tumor size, tumor weight, and histologic features may suggest malignant potential, but no single parameter (except the detection metastases) allows benign tumors to be discriminated from malignant ones (54, 56).

Adrenocortical adenoma: Usually spherical, unilateral, solitary, and well demarcated, but often not truly encapsulated (5). It typically weighs less than 50 g. Adenoma comprises a heterogenous group of benign neoplasms that histologically resemble the appearance of the normal zona fasciculate, the zona glomerulosa, or most often the combination of both (56). In general, adenomas are histologically bland, with low nuclear-to-cytoplasmic ratio. In children, benign tumors are more likely to display marked nuclear atypia, polymorphism, necrosis, and mitotic activity (56). Hormone active functional, and nonfunctional cases have been published (53, 54, 57). We have one case, incidentally defined and nonfunctional adenoma, in our published series (3).

Adrenocortical carcinoma: It represents 1.3% of all carcinomas in children and adolescents in the United States (0.1% of all childhood malignancies) (44, 58). Half of these tumors occur in patients <5 years of age. Tumors equally occur in both sides and are 80–100% hormonally functional. The etiology is unknown, but association with tumor syndromes, Li-Fraumeni, Beckwith-Wiedemann syndrome, Carney complex, MEN 1, and congenital adrenal hyperplasia, has been shown (44, 54).

In contrast to adults, most ACTs are hormonally active, and the clinical presentation is usually associated with steroid overproduction. Virilization, secondary to secretion of adrenal androgens, is the most frequent presenting feature (66%), whereas the remainder of children will be seen with CS symptoms (43, 44, 54). The range of time from symptoms to diagnosis is 6–36 months (59).

Usually weigh over 100 g. Grossly, they have coarse trabeculations, a multinodular contour, and are yellow to brown in color (Figure 52.3). Areas of hemorrhage and necrosis are frequently seen. Cystic changes may be seen in both adenomas and carcinomas, but more common in carcinomas and larger adenomas (56). Carcinoma shows a wide range of differentiation on histologic examination, not only between tumors but also within the same tumor (56).

Prognostic risk factors are age at diagnosis, tumor volume/size, metastatic status, and primary resectability. The presence of two

Adrenal Surgical Diseases in Children

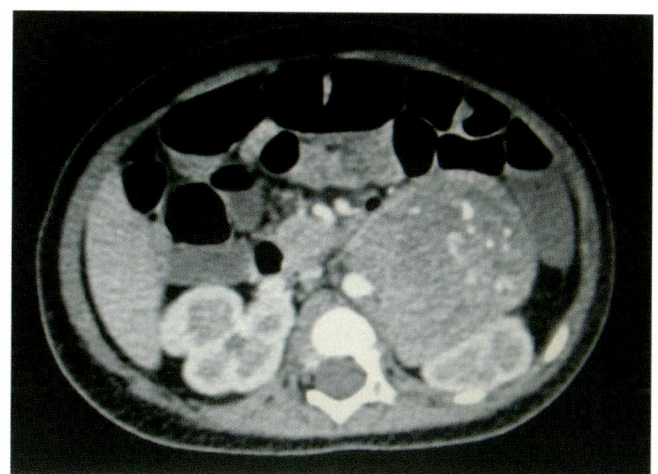
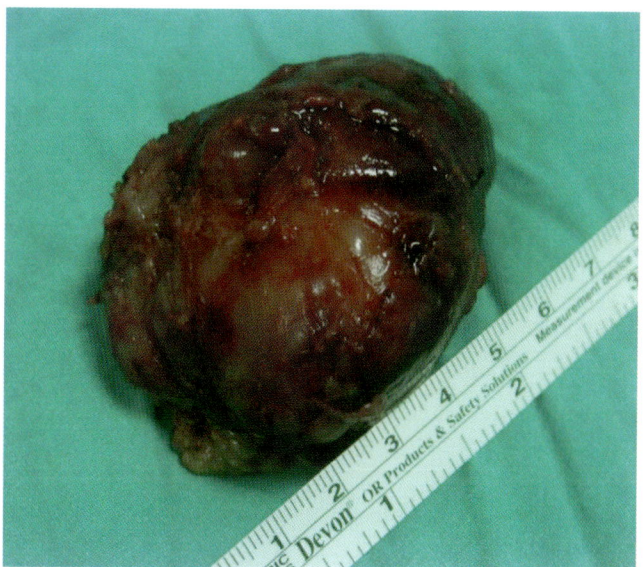
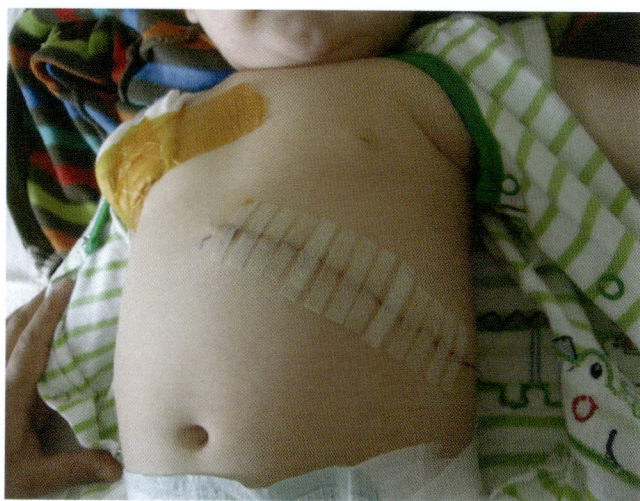

FIGURE 52.3 7-Month-old boy with a left side located neuroblastic tumor, totally resected via open approach: (a) CT image of left adrenal tumor, (b) macroscopic appearances of resected mass, (c) left subcostal incision.

or more factors related to adrenocortical carcinoma (ACC) was associated with an aggressive behavior of disease (60, 61).

As a result of a report of European cooperative study group, distant metastases and large tumor volume (>200 cm³) were the main unfavorable prognostic factors (60). Although tumor size is assessed with different units of measures by different authors (volume, diameter, or weight), the concept that huge ACCs have a worse prognosis is accepted by most (60–66). It has been shown that a tumor volume more than 200 cm³ had a worse impact on pathology free survival (PFS) and overall survival (OS) for localized tumors and on PFS if the whole group is considered (60). The age less than or equal to 4 and more than 10 years at diagnosis showed a significant difference both at OS and PFS (60). In one review of 55 children with adrenal carcinoma, the 2-year survival rates were 82% for children <2 years and 29% for children >2 years (67). It is widely accepted that children have a better outcome than adolescents (60, 61, 67).

Metastatic spread is considered a highly unfavorable prognostic factor, also because the response to medical therapies is normally scarce (60, 68). The International Pediatric Adrenocortical Tumor Registry reported a 20% OS for patients with advanced disease; better results using chemotherapy and mitotane (OS 64.8%) were described recently by the GPOHMET studies (61, 67, 68).

Primary total resectability is also a prognostic factor (61, 67, 69). Survival rates are more than 67% if the tumors were completely excised, but no survivors were found after partial resection (67).

Different criteria have been defined for pathological prognostic evaluation. These are Weiss, Aubert, Wieneke, and Dehner-Hill (63–66). The traditional cutoff of size 5 cm and weight 200 g indicates malignancy, but Wieneke et al. modified the weight and size cutoff to 10.5 cm and 400 g, effectively filtering the more malignant tumors (64). The best clinicopathologic correlation was found with Wieneke and Dehner-Hill pathological (macroscopic and microscopic features) evaluation (62, 64, 65). It is suggested that Wieneke criteria could be applied as gold standard in ACTs' pathologic characterization (62).

These tumors are highly lethal, with nonfunctional tumors and delay in diagnosis leading to worse prognosis. Patients left

TABLE 52.3: Staging Criteria for Pediatric Adrenocortical Tumors

Stage	Description
I	Complete surgical resection
	Tumor <100 g or <200 cm^3//(revised)
	Absence of metastasis
	Normal hormone levels postoperatively
II	Microscopic residual tumor
	Tumor >100 g or >200 cm^3//(revised)
	Tumor spillage during surgery
	Abnormal hormone levels postoperatively
III	Gross residual or inoperable primary tumor
IV	Metastatic disease

untreated with adrenocortical carcinomas have a mean survival of 2.9 months (59).

Staging: Based on preoperative imaging and operative findings. Preoperative imaging defines primary mass, local extent of the tumor, and distant metastases. Direct extension of tumor thrombus into the inferior vena cava represents an important mechanism of nonhematogenous malignant spread and may occur in up to a third of patients (5). The lung is the most common site of distant metastases, followed by the liver. The staging system is based on disease stage and tumor size initially proposed by Sandrini et al. (Table 52.3) (70, 71).

Rare adrenocortical problems

Adrenocortical oncocytomas (AOs): Oncocytomas are tumors predominantly or exclusively composed of oncocytes, cells with granular and eosinophilic cytoplasm filled with mitochondria (72). Although they can occur in every organ, they are rare in adrenal glands, and in pediatric patients, they are even rarer. The development of an AO appears to be a long-term, slow-growing neoplastic process occurring in cells with low proliferative index, which makes this neoplasia extremely rare and unlikely to occur in children (72, 73). Immunohistochemistry to the mitochondrial enzyme succinate dehydrogenase to confirm the oxyphilic nature of AOs is recommended (73). Although, most of these oncocytomas are benign and nonfunctioning, cases with mass that cause clinical manifestations like CS, virilization, precocious puberty had been published, recently (3, 72–76). In children, the treatment of secreting tumors is complete surgical excision, but the management of an incidental nonfunctioning AO is controversial (72). In our published series, we have two patients, nonfunctional, incidentally diagnosed as adrenal mass in left side in both, managed with LA without any complication (3, 76).

Adrenal cytomegaly: In neonatal adrenal, large cells with large and prominent nuclei can sometimes be seen. This phenomenon was first described by Kampmeier and is called adrenal cytomegaly (77, 78). These cytomegalic cells can be found diffusely in the adrenal cortex or in focal areas. It is thought to be not a malign but a degenerative process, because of its very low proliferative activities. In some cases, it may show cystic degenerations, and tissue sampling may be required if it does not regress within a few of follow-up.

Stromal tumors: These tumors are very rare, generally asymptomatic, and may include fibromas, leiomyoma, lipomas, hamartomas, hemangiomas, and sarcomas.

Surgery for adrenal masses

Anatomic basis of surgical approaches to the adrenal

The spectrum of adrenal masses in children varies from benign lesions like adenoma and GN to malignant tumors like adrenocortical carcinoma and NB. Any surgical approach requires careful risk stratification based on oncological and technical criteria. Operations on the adrenal glands can be done using open or minimally invasive techniques (laparoscopic, robotic) from either an anterior or posterior approach (2).

Open technique

Posterior: because the posterolateral anatomy is basically the same for both adrenal glands, the surgical approach through the flank is the same for both glands. Simply, the posterior approach is begun in prone position with an incision along the 12th rib. The latissimus dorsi muscle is divided and the peritoneum is reflected away. The diaphragm and/or the transversalis muscle can be divided and the kidney retracted inferiorly to improve exposure of the glands (1, 2).

Anterior: commonly performed through a subcostal incision in the supine position (Figure 52.3(a)–(c)). A chevron or midline incision can be used for bilateral lesions.

Minimal invasive surgery

Retroperitoneoscopic or the posterior minimally invasive approach is not commonly used in children (3).

- *Retroperitoneoscopic approach:* It begins with a small incision at the tip of 12th rib. A space is created with blunt finger dissection for first port insertion. The space is enlarged using a balloon trocar prior to placing additional trocars (79).
- *LA:* The first LA was performed in an adult patient by Gagner in 1992 (80). The operation can be performed in the supine or lateral position. Although single-incision laparoscopic surgery (SILS), a robot-assisted surgery, has been described, most surgeons continue to prefer a standard anterior LA for adrenal procedures (3, 40, 81, 82). Our approach can be defined as modified Gagner method. The procedure is performed with the patient in a 45° lateral decubitus position, using three to four ports. For right adrenalectomy, need for liver retraction necessitated the use of four ports (Figure 52.4(a)–(c)). For left adrenalectomy, gland exposure is accomplished through mesocolon or with retrocolonic dissection (Figure 52.5(a)–(c)). Specimen-extraction techniques vary according to tumor size. Large tumors require an enlargement of the port incision up to 1–1.5 cm for morcellation, while smaller tumors are removed using endoscopic bag systems through subcostal or umbilical port site. No additional abdominal incisions or drains are required. The children are discharged once their recovery is satisfactory (3, 40). A systematic review of the English literature revealed 22 studies that contained 5 or more laparoscopically managed children with adrenal masses (3). For the period between 2001 and 2017, 416 patients with 437 lesions were identified. Mean operation age was 6.2 years. Gender distribution and laterality were nearly equal. Precisely, 5% of the patients had bilateral adrenal masses. Tumor sizes varied between 1 and 10 cm (mean 4.2 cm) and transperitoneal approach was preferred in the vast majority of the cases. Neuroblastic

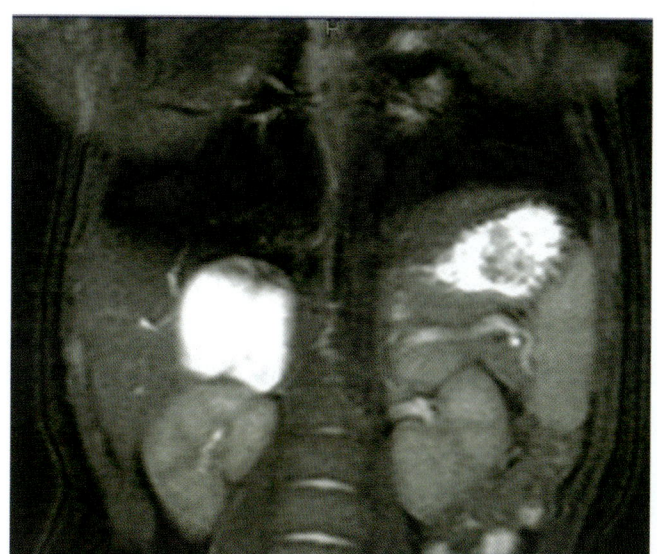
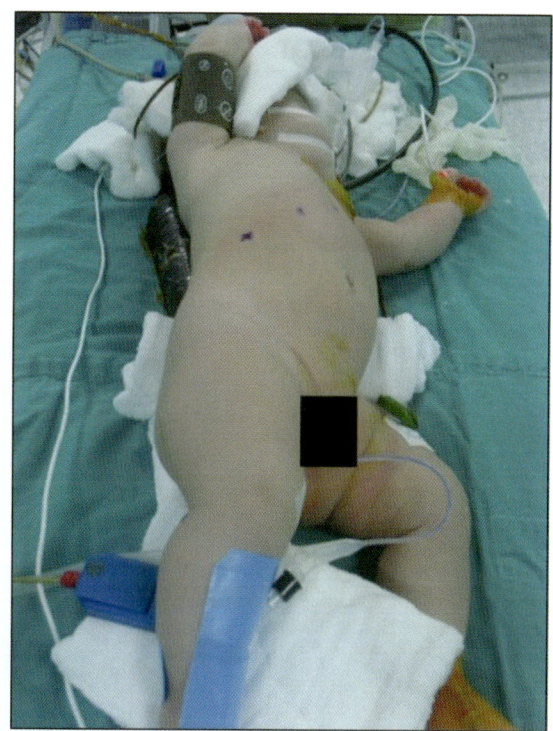
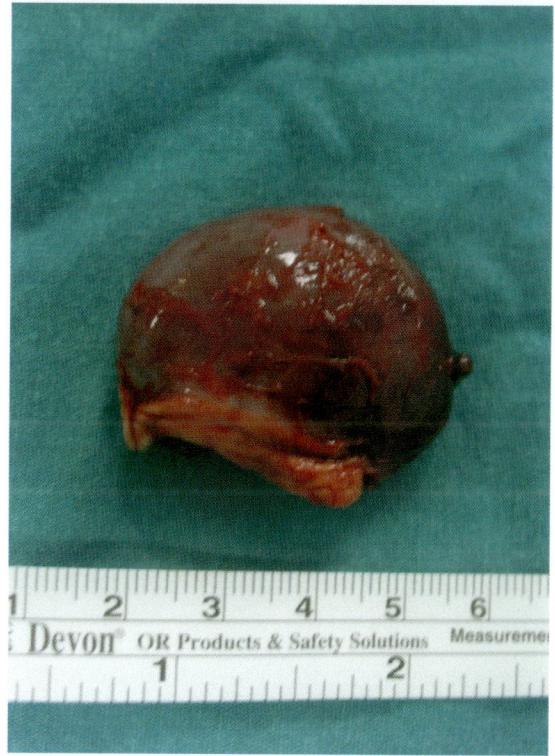

FIGURE 52.4 4-Month-old girl, right adrenal 3.5-cm mass was resected laparoscopically.

tumors (N 50%), pheochromocytomas (12.7%), adenomas (11%), CS (7.4%), and adrenocortical carcinomas (3.9%) were the most common indications. Nonspecified benign cortical tumors (2.9%), cysts (1.2%), hematomas (1.2%), vascular and lymphatic malformations (1%), virilizing tumor (0.7%), lipoma (0.5%), pulmonary sequestration (0.5%), and necrosis (0.2%) were the remaining uncommon benign lesions. There were 31 (7.5%) conversions and 13 (3.1%) intraoperative–postoperative complications (3). LA is safe and effective in selected pediatric patients with benign and malignant adrenal pathologies. Preoperative detailed multidisciplinary evaluation and surgical expertise are the key factors for success (39). The transperitoneal route seems to be the standard approach for pediatric surgeons (3).

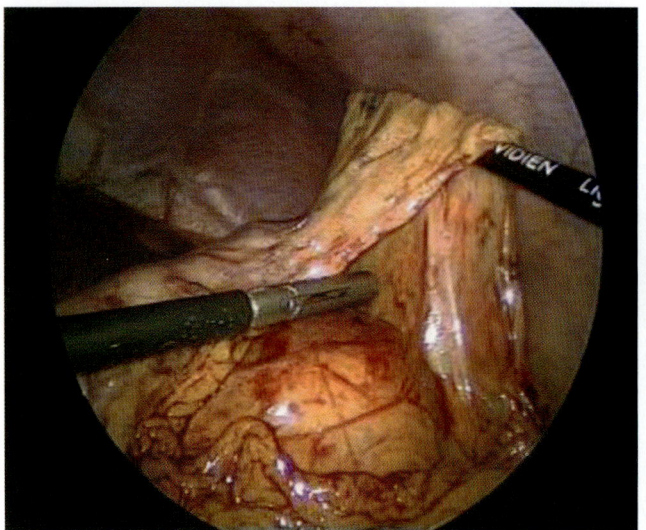
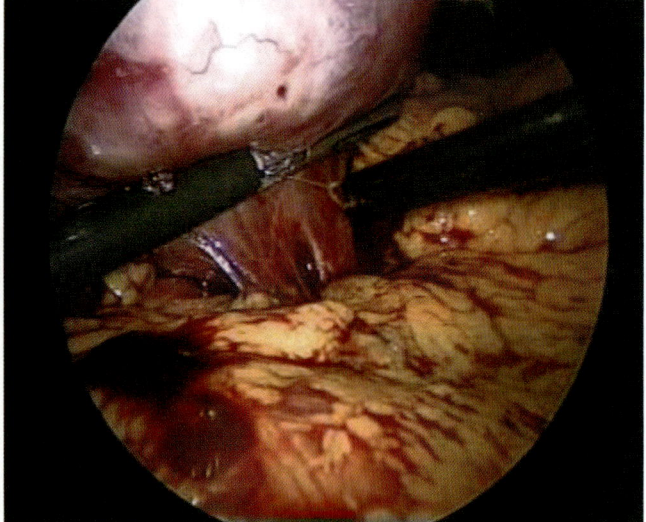
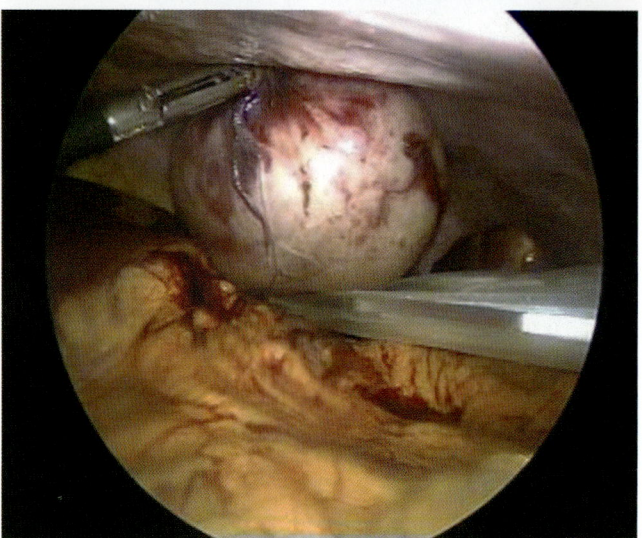

FIGURE 52.5 Left side localized tumor.

Surgery of ACTs: Surgery is the single-most important part of the treatment and requires careful perioperative planning (83, 84). It is important to remember that these patients may be need perioperative steroid coverage, because of contralateral adrenal suppression. Also, special attention to electrolyte balance, blood pressure, wound care, and infection prevention is paramount (5, 83). Generally, open procedures will allow the surgeon the best chance to completely excise the tumor (Figure 52.6(a)–(c)) (2, 5). Total excision should be attempted even if it requires removal of adjacent structures, such as ipsilateral nephrectomy (7). Total resection is essential for cure, and from previous reports, it is clear that incomplete resection has a negative effect on outcome (7, 69, 85). Extreme care must be exercised during surgery as the tumor tends to be friable, and tumor spillage occurs in about 20% of initial operations and in 43% of operations done for tumor recurrence (70, 71). Since tumor spillage worsens prognosis, any maneuver that reduces the risk of spill is advocated (70, 83). Also, infiltration of the vena cava with tumor thrombus may occur in up to 20% of the patients and make complete resection challenging (71). Even in patients with metastatic disease, complete resection is warranted if it is feasible (7, 83).

Retroperitoneal lymph node dissection? The need for lymph node biopsy for staging and for prognosis has not been addressed clearly in the literature. The incidence of lymph node involvement is not known; extensive lymph node biopsy in small ACTs can probably be avoided given the generally good outcome with surgery alone (83). Lymph node sampling is not routinely performed, except if there is obvious lymph node enlargement (5, 83). Patients with large tumors (stage II) also should have an ipsilateral retroperitoneal lymph nodes dissection (5).

Minimally invasive surgery for ACTs in children: It should not be forgotten that the tumor tends to be friable, and tumor spillage occurs in about 20% of initial operations and in 43% of operations done for tumor recurrence (70, 71). International pediatric endosurgery group (IPEG) mentions that there is no absolute contraindication to the LA for ACTs, but notes that principles of cancer surgery must be adhered to (86). In general, the use of open surgeries procedure is recommended for adrenocortical (AC) carcinoma, and a LA for benign, small, localized lesions (3, 7).

Adjuvant therapy: The role of chemotherapy in the management of childhood ACT has not been well established (83).

Adrenal Surgical Diseases in Children

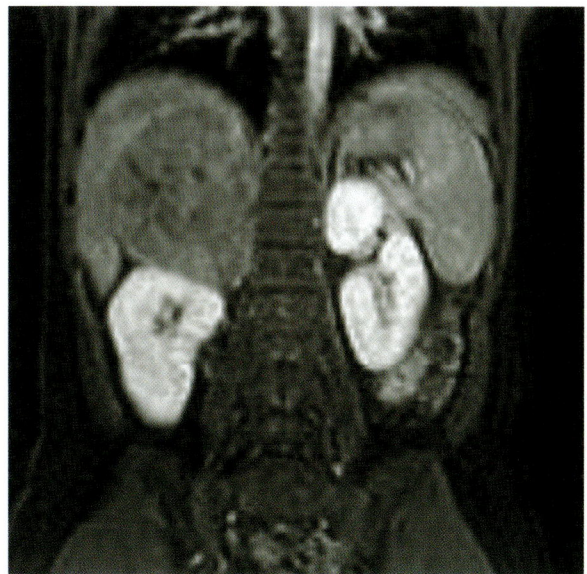
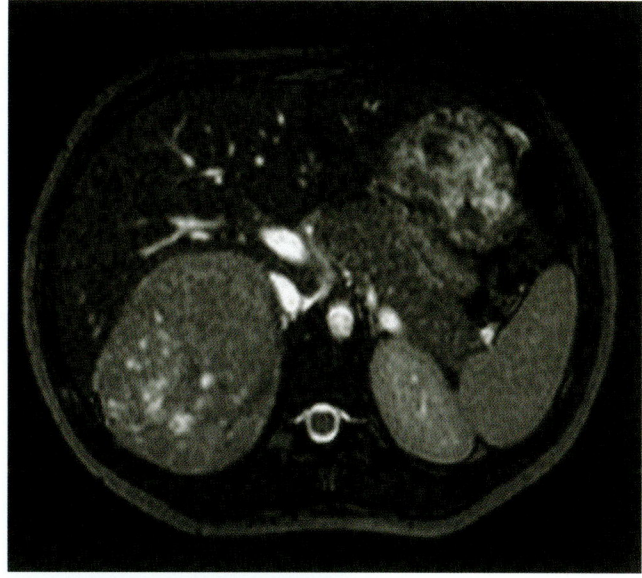
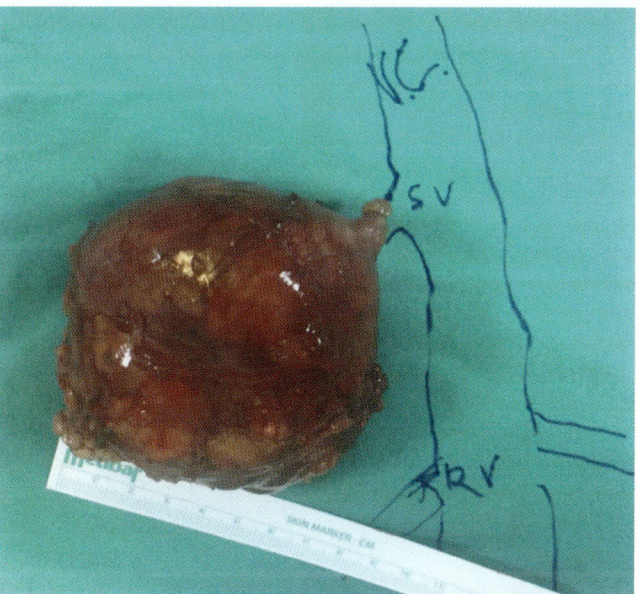

FIGURE 52.6 4-Year-old girl admitted with history of weight gain and virilization for a few months, totally excised with open procedure (note the adrenal vein invasion).

However, for patients with advanced disease or with a high risk of recurrence, the use of systemic therapy with mitotane or chemotherapy (cisplatinum, carboplatinum, etoposide, 5-fluorouracil with leucovorin, and ifosfamide) should be considered even though its impact on the overall outcome is minimal.

Mitotane, the most widely used chemotherapeutic agent, is an insecticide derivative that produces adrenocortical necrosis, and it has been used extensively in adults with ACT. It is used for metastatic disease, for incompletely excised tumors, and for the hormonal effects from the tumors. In the pediatric literature, tumor responses have been reported between 30 and 40%, though the benefit of adjuvant mitotane is controversial.

Radiotherapy: Radiotherapy was shown to have limited success (87), and generally, it is accepted that ACT is radioresistant. Also, because many children with ACT carry p-53 mutations, radiation may increase the incidence of secondary tumors (5).

South Asia perspective

Conclusion

Adrenal masses are the most common cause of problems requiring adrenal surgery in childhood. The majority of masses in children are malignant and 80% are neuroblastic tumors. Neuroblastic tumors may present with mass effects or the hormone effects they secrete. ACTs secrete hormones and cause various clinical symptoms. Virilization is the most common presentation (80%), and Cushing's syndrome is in one-third patients and other presentations are feminization, Conn's syndromes. Imaging is helpful for defining the extent of mass. Surgical planning requires careful risk stratification based on oncological and technical criteria (size, relations with vascular structures). Operations on the adrenal glands can be done using open or minimally invasive techniques (laparoscopic, robotic) from either an anterior or posterior approach. In patients with advanced disease or with a high risk of recurrence, adjuvant systemic therapy with mitotane or chemotherapy (cisplatinum, carboplatinum, etoposide, 5-fluorouracil with leucovorin, and ifosfamide) should be considered even though its impact on the overall outcome is minimal.

References

1. Avisse C, Marcus C, Pattey M, Ladam-Marcus V, Delattre JF, Flament JB. Surgical anatomy and embryology of the adrenal glands. Surg Clin North Am 2000;80(1):403–415.
2. Madani A, Lee JA. Surgical approaches to the adrenal gland. Surg Clin North Am 2019;99(4):773–791.
3. Dökümcü Z, Divarci E, Ertan Y, Çelik A. Laparoscopic adrenalectomy in children: a 25-case series and review of the literature. J Pediatr Surg 2018;53:1800–1805.
4. Emre Ş, Özcan R, Bakır AC, Kuruğoğlu S, Çomunoğlu N, Şen HS, et al. Adrenal masses in children: imaging, surgical treatment and outcome. Asian J Surg 2020;43:207–212.
5. Gow Kenneth W. The evaluation and management of adrenal masses and adrenocortical tumors (Act). In Endocrine Surgery in Children. Eds.: Daniel J. Ledbetter, Paul R.V. Johnson. Springer-Verlag, Germany, 2018. pp. 121–139.
6. Hanafy AK, Mujtaba B, Roman-Colon AM, Elsayes KM, Harrison D, Ramani NS, et al. Imaging features of adrenal gland masses in the pediatric population. Abdom Radiol. 2019. https://doi.org/10.1007/s00261-019-02213-x.
7. Rescorla FJ. Malignant adrenal tumors. Semin Pediatr Surg 2006;15(1):48–56.
8. Hamper UM, Fishman EK, Hartman DS, Roberts JL, Sanders RC. Primary adrenocortical carcinoma: sonographic evaluation with clinical and pathologic correlation in 26 patients. AJR Am J Roentgenol 1987;148(5):915–919.
9. Olecki E, Grant CN. MIBG in neuroblastoma diagnosis and treatment. Semin Pediatr Surg 2019;28:150859.
10. Velaphi SC, Perlman JM. Neonatal adrenal hemorrhage: clinical and abdominal sonographic findings. Clin Pediatr 2001;40:545–548.
11. Bergami G, Malena S, Di Mario M, Fariello G. Sonographic follow up of neonatal adrenal hemorrhage. Fourteen case reports. Radiol Med 1990;79:474–478.
12. Köklü E, Kurtoglu S, Akçakuş M, Köklü S. Adrenal haemorrhage with cholestasis and adrenal crisis in a newborn of a diabetic mother. J Pediatr Endocrinol Metab 2007;20(3):441–444.
13. Eo H, Kim JH, Jang KM, Yoo SY, Lim GY, Kim MJ, Kim OH. Comparison of clinicoradiological features between congenital cystic neuroblastoma and neonatal adrenal hemorrhagic pseudocyst. Korean J Radiol 2011;12(1):52–58.
14. Steffens J, Zaubitzer T, Kirsch W, Humke U. Neonatal adrenal abscesses. Eur Urol 1997;31:347–349.
15. Debnath PR, Tripathi RK, Gupta AK, Chadha R, Choudhury SR. Bilateral adrenal abscess in a neonate. Indian J Pediatr 2005;72:169–171.
16. Blankenship WJ, Bogren H, Stadalnik RC, Vitale DE. Surrenal abscess in the neonate: a case report and review of diagnosis and management. Pediatrics 1975;55:239–243.
17. Chan YF, Oldfield R, Vogel S, Ferguson S. Pulmonary sequestration presenting as a prenatally detected suprarenal lesion in a neonate. J Pediatr Surg 2000;35:1367–1369.
18. Gross E, Chen MK, Lobe TE, Nuchtern JG, Rao BN. Infradiaphragmatic extralobar pulmonary sequestration masquerading as an intra-abdominal, suprarenal mass. Pediatr Surg Int 1997;12:529–531.
19. Singal AK, Agarwala S, Seth T, Gupta AK, Mitra DK. Intra-abdominal extralobar pulmonary sequestration presenting antenatally as a suprarenal mass. Indian J Pediatr 2004;71(12):1137–1139.
20. Agayev A, Yılmaz S, Cekrezi B, Yekeler E. Extralobar pulmonary sequestration mimicking neuroblastoma. J Pediatr Surg 2007;42:1627–1629.
21. Emiroğlu G, Özsan N, Tiryaki S, Çelik A, Ertan Y. A rare case: extralobar pulmonary sequestration mimicking neuroblastoma. Virchows Archiv 2012;461:S99–S100.
22. Carsote M, Ghemigian A, Terzea D, Gheorghisan-Galateanu AA, Valea A. Cystic adrenal lesions: focus on pediatric population (a review). Clujul Medical 2017;90(1):5–12.
23. Rha SE, Byun JY, Jung SE, Chun HJ, Lee HG, Lee JM. Neurogenic tumors in the abdomen: tumor types and imaging characteristics. Radiographics 2003;23(1):29–43.
24. Masiakos PT, Gerstle JT, Cheang T, Viero S, Kim PC, Wales P. Is surgery necessary for incidentally discovered adrenal masses in children? J Pediatr Surg 2004;39:754–758.
25. Mubarak M, Singal AK, Gawdi A. Stage 4S neuroblastoma: a report of two cases presenting with extremes of biological behavior. Gulf J Oncol 2019;1(30):81–84.
26. Schimada H, Chatten J, Newton WA Jr., Sachs N, Hamoudi AB, Chiba T, et al. Histopathologic prognostic factors in neuroblastic tumors: definition of subtypes of ganglioneuroblastoma and an age-linked classification of neuroblastomas. J Natl Cancer Inst 1984;73:405–419.
27. Luo YB, Cui XC, Yang L, Zhang D, Wang JX. Advances in the surgical treatment of neuroblastoma. Chin Med J 2018;131(19):2332–2337.
28. Fisher JP, Tweddle DA. Neonatal neuroblastoma. Semin Fetal Neonatal Med 2012;17:207–215.
29. Cohn SL, Pearson AD, London WB, Monclair T, Ambros PF, Brodeur GM, et al., INRG Task Force. The International Neuroblastoma Risk Group (INRG) classification system: an INRG Task Force report. J Clin Oncol 2009;27:289–297.
30. Brodeur GM, Pritchard J, Berthold F, Carlsen ML, Castel V, Castelberry RP, et al. Revisions of the international criteria for neuroblastoma diagnosis, staging, and response to treatment. J Clin Oncol 1993;11:1466–1477.
31. Cecchetto G, Mosseri V, De Bernardi B, Helardot P, Monclair T, Costa E, et al. Surgical risk factors in primary surgery for localized neuroblastoma: the LNESG1 study of the European International Society of Pediatric Oncology Neuroblastoma Group. J Clin Oncol 2005;23(33):8483–8489.
32. Fischer J, Pohl A, Volland R, Hero B, Dübbers M, Cernaianu G, et al. Complete surgical resection improves outcome in INRG high-risk patients with localized neuroblastoma older than 18 months. BMC Cancer 2017;17(1):520.
33. Monclair T, Mosseri V, Cecchetto G, De Bernardi B, Michon J, Holmes K. Influence of image-defined risk factors on the outcome of patients with localised neuroblastoma. A report from the LNESG1 study of the European International Society of Paediatric Oncology Neuroblastoma Group. Pediatr Blood Cancer 2015;62(9):1536–1542.
34. Günther P, Holland-Cunz S, Schupp CJ, Stockklausner C, Hinz U, Schenk JP. Significance of image-defined risk factors for surgical complications in patients with abdominal neuroblastoma. Eur J Pediatr Surg 2011;21(05):314–317.
35. Avanzini S, Pio L, Erminio G, Granata C, Holmes K, Gambart M et al. Image-defined risk factors in unresectable neuroblastoma: SIOPEN study on incidence, chemotherapy-induced variation, and impact on surgical outcomes. Pediatr Blood Cancer 2017;64(11):e26605.
36. Mishra P, Mehrotra PK, Agarwal G, Agarwal A, Mishra SK. Pediatric and adolescent pheochromocytoma: clinical presentation and outcome of surgery. Indian Pediatr 2014;51(4):299–302.
37. Mittendorf EA, Evans DB, Lee JE, Perrier ND. Pheochromocytoma: advances in genetics, diagnosis, localization, and treatment. Hematol Oncol Clin North Am 2007;21(3):509–525.
38. Bausch B, Wellner U, Bausch D, Schiavi F, Barontini M, Sanso G, et al. Long-term prognosis of patients with pediatric pheochromocytoma. Endocr-Relat Cancer 2014;21(1):17–25.
39. Traynor MD, Jr., Sada A, Thompson GB, Moir CR, Bancos I, Farley DR, et al. Adrenalectomy for non-neuroblastic pathology in children. Pediatr Surg Int 2020;36:129–135.
40. Altıncık A, Özen S, Çelik A, Dökümcü Z, Darcan Ş, Abacı A, Böber E. Pediatric bilateral pheochromocytoma and experience of laparoscopic cortical sparing adrenalectomy. J Pediatr Res 2018;5(4):218–220.
41. Dewez JE, Bachy A. A case of primary aldosteronism in childhood. Arch Pediatr 2009;16(1):37–40.
42. Abdullah N, Khawaja K, Hale J, Barrett AM, Cheetham TD. Primary hyperaldosteronism with normokalaemia secondary to an adrenal adenoma (Conn's syndrome) in a 12 year-old boy. J Pediatr Endocrinol Metab 2005;18(2):215–219.
43. Stratakis CA. An update on Cushing syndrome in pediatrics. Ann Endocrinol (Paris) 2018;79(3):125–131.
44. Lodish MB, Keil MF, Stratakis CA. Cushing's syndrome in pediatrics: an update. Endocrinol Metab Clin North Am 2018;47(2):451–462.
45. Wędrychowicz A, Hull B, Tyrawa K, Kalicka-Kasperczyk A, Zieliński G, Starzyk J. Cushing disease in children and adolescents – assessment of the clinical course, diagnostic process, and effects of the treatment – experience from a single paediatric centre. Pediatr Endocrinol Diabetes Metab 2019;25(3):127–143.
46. Diesen DL, Skinner MA. Endocrine disorders and tumors. In Ashcraft's Pediatric Surgery, 6th ed. Eds.: George W. Holcomb III, Patrick J. Murphy, Daniel J. Ostile. Saunders-Elsevier, Toronto, 2014. pp. 1067–1085.
47. Memon SS, Thakkar K, Patil V, Jadhav S, Lila AR, Fernandes G, et al. Primary pigmented nodular adrenocortical disease (PPNAD): single centre experience. J Pediatr Endocrinol Metab 2019;32(4):391–397.
48. Guanà R, Gesmundo R, Morino M, Matarazzo P, Pucci A, Pasini B, et al. Laparoscopic unilateral adrenalectomy in children for isolated primary pigmented nodular adrenocortical disease (PPNAD): case report and literature review. Eur J Pediatr Surg 2010;20(4):273–275.
49. Simforoosh N, Azar MR, Soltani MH, Nourbakhsh M, Shemshaki H. Staged bilateral laparoscopic adrenalectomy for infantile ACTH-independent Cushing's syndrome (bilateral micronodular non-pigmented adrenal hyperplasia): a case report. Urol J 2017;14(5):5030–5033.
50. Storr HL, Savage MO. Management of endocrine disease: paediatric Cushing's disease. Eur J Endocrinol 2015;173:35–45.
51. Laje P, Mattei PA. Laparoscopic adrenalectomy for adrenal tumors in children: a case series. J Laparoendosc Adv Surg Tech A 2009;19(Suppl 1):27–29.
52. McWhirter WR, Stiller CA, Lennox EL. Carcinomas in childhood. A registry-based study of incidence and survival. Cancer 1989;63:2242–2246.
53. Wu X, Xu J, Wang J, Gu W, Zou C. Childhood adrenocortical tumor: a clinical and immunohistochemical study of 13 cases. Medicine (Baltimore) 2019;98:46.
54. Erickson LA. Challenges in surgical pathology of adrenocortical tumours. Histopathology 2018;72(1):82–96.
55. Lin X, Wu D, Chen C, Zheng N. Clinical characteristics of adrenal tumors in children: a retrospective review of a 15-year single-center experience. Int Urol Nephrol 2017;49(3):381–385.
56. Agrons GA, Lonergan GJ, Dickey GE, Perez-Monte JE. Adrenocortical neoplasms in children: radiologic-pathologic correlation. Radiographics 1999;19(4):989–1008.
57. Ersoy B, Kizilay D, Cayirli H, Temiz P, Gunsar C. Central precocious puberty secondary to adrenocortical adenoma in a female child: case report and review of the literature. J Pediatr Adolesc Gynecol 2017;30(5):591–594.
58. Bernstein L, Gurney JG. Carcinomas and other malignant epithelial neoplasms. In Cancer and Survival among Children and Adolescents: United States SEER Program 1975-1995. Eds.: LAG Ries, MA Smith, JG Gurney, et al. Bethesda, MD, 1999. pp. 139–147.
59. Xu X, Sergi C. Pediatric adrenal cortical carcinomas: histopathological criteria and clinical trials. A systematic review. Contemp Clin Trials 2016;50:37–44.
60. Cecchetto G, Ganarin A, Bien E, Vorwerk P, Bisogno G, Godzinski J, et al. Outcome and prognostic factors in high-risk childhood adrenocortical carcinomas: a report from the European Cooperative Study Group on Pediatric Rare Tumors (EXPeRT). Pediatr Blood Cancer 2017;64:e26368.

61. Gupta N, Riverab M, Novotnyc P, Rodriguezd V, Bancose I, Lteifa A. Adrenocortical carcinoma in children: a clinicopathological analysis of 41 patients at the Mayo Clinic from 1950 to 2017. Horm Res Paediatr 2018;90:8–18.
62. Jehangir S, Nanjundaiah P, Sigamani E, Burad D, Manipadam MT, Lea V, et al. Pathological prognostication of paediatric adrenocortical tumours: is a gold standard emerging? Pediatr Blood Cancer 2019;66:e27567.
63. Weiss L, Medeiros L. Pathologic features of prognostic significance in adrenocortical carcinoma. Am J Surg Pathol 1989;13:202–206.
64. Wieneke J, Thompson L, Heffess C. Adrenal cortical neoplasms in the paediatric population: a clinicopathologic and immunophenotypic analysis of 83 patients. Am J Surg Pathol 2003;27:867–881.
65. Aubert S, Wacrenier A, Leroy X, Devos P, Carnaille B, Proye C, et al. Weiss system revisited: a clinicopathologic and immunohistochemical study of 49 adrenocortical tumours. Am J Surg Pathol 2002;26:1612–1619.
66. Dehner LP, Hill DA. Adrenal cortical neoplasms in children: why so many carcinomas and yet so many survivors. Pediatr Dev Pathol 2009;12:284–291.
67. Sabbaga CC, Avilla SG, Schulz C, Garbers JC, Blucher D. Adrenocortical carcinoma in children: clinical aspects and prognosis. J Pediatr Surg 1993;28:841–843.
68. Klein JD, Turner CG, Gray FL, Yu DC, Kozakewich HP, Perez-Atayde AR, et al. Adrenal cortical tumors in children: factors associated with poor outcome. J Pediatr Surg 2011;46(6):1201–1207.
69. Çiftçi AO, Şenocak ME, Tanyel FC, Büyükpamukçu N. Adrenocortical tumors in children. J Pediatr Surg 2001;36(4):549–554.
70. Sandrini R, Ribeiro RC, DeLacerda L. Extensive personal experience. Childhood adrenocortical tumors. J Clin Endocrinol Metab 1997;82:2027–2031.
71. Michalkiewicz E, Sandrini R, Figueiredo B, Miranda EC, Caran E, Oliveira-Filho AG, et al. Clinical and outcome characteristics of children with adrenocortical tumors: a report from the International Pediatric Adrenocortical Tumor Registry. J Clin Oncol 2004;22(5):838–845.
72. Tahar GT, Nejib KN, Sadok SS, Rachid LM. Adrenocortical oncocytoma: a case report and review of literature. J Pediatr Surg 2008;43(5):E1–E3.
73. Pereira BD, Rios ES, Cabrera RA, Portugal J, Raimundo L. Adrenocortical oncocytoma presenting as Cushing's syndrome: an additional report of a paediatric case. Endocr Pathol 2014;25(4):397–403.
74. Al Badi MK, Al-Alwan I, Al-Dubayee M, Al-Anzi A, Al Turki MS, Aloudah N, Alsaad KO. Testosterone and cortisol secreting oncocytic adrenocortical adenoma in the pediatric age-group. Pediatr Dev Pathol 2018;21(6):568–573.
75. Hong Y, Hao Y, Hu J, Xu B, Shan H, Wang X. Adrenocortical oncocytoma: 11 case reports and review of the literature. Medicine (Baltimore) 2017;96(48):e8750.
76. Ertan Y, Argon A, Özdemir M, Yürekli BPS, Dökümcü Z, Makay Ö. Oncocytic adrenocortical tumors: pathological features of 16 cases and review of the literature. J Environ Pathol Toxicol Oncol 2017;36(3):237–244.
77. Kampmeier OF. Giant epithelial cells of the fetal adrenal. Anat Rec 1927;37:95–102.
78. Noguchi S, Masumoto K, Taguchi T, Takahashi Y, Tsuneyoshi M, Suita S. Adrenal cytomegaly: two cases detected by prenatal diagnosis. Asian J Surg 2003;26(4):234–236.
79. Dickson P, Jiminez C, Chisholm G, Kannamer D, Ng C, Grubbes E, et al. Posterior retroperitoneoscopic adrenalectomy: a contemporary American experience. J Am Coll Surg 2001;212:659–665.
80. Gagner M, Lacroix A, Bolte E. Laparoscopic adrenalectomy in Cushing's syndrome and pheochromocytoma. N Engl J Med 1992;327:1033.
81. Ishida M, Miyajima A, Takeda T, Hasegawa M, Kikuchi E, Oya M. Technical difficulties of transumbilical laparoendoscopic single-site adrenalectomy: comparison with conventional laparoscopic adrenalectomy. World J Urol 2013;31(1):199–201.
82. Fascetti-Leon F, Scotton G, Pio L, Beltrà R, Caione P, Esposito C, et al. Minimally invasive resection of adrenal masses in infants and children: results of a European multicenter survey. Surg Endosc 2017;31:4505–4512.
83. Stewart JN, Flageole H, Kavan P. A surgical approach to adrenocortical tumors in children: the mainstay of treatment. J Pediatr Surg 2004;39(5):759–763.
84. Liou LS, Kay R. Adrenocortical carcinoma in children. Review and recent innovations. Urol Clin North Am 2000;27:403–421.
85. Sawin RS. Functioning adrenal neoplasms. Semin Pediatr Surg 1997;6:156–163.
86. International Pediatric Endosurgery Group. IPEG guidelines for the surgical treatment of adrenal masses in children. J Laparoendosc Adv Surg Tech A 2010;20(2):vii–ix.
87. Lefevre M, Gerard-Marchant R, Gubler JP, Chaussain JN, Lemerle J. Adrenal cortical carcinoma in children: 42 patients treated from 1958 to 1980 at Villejuif. In Adrenal and Endocrine Tumors in Children. Ed.: GB Humphery. Martinus Nijhoff Publishers, Boston, MA, 1983. pp. 265–276.

53
ANESTHETIC MANAGEMENT FOR PHEOCHROMOCYTOMA

Divya Srivastava and Bhavya Naithani

Introduction

Pheochromocytomas are neoplasms of chromaffin tissue that synthesize catecholamines. The 2004 WHO classification of neuroendocrine tumors defines them as intra-adrenal paraganglionomas. They are a catecholamine-producing intra-adrenal tumors arising from the chromaffin cells. Pheochromocytomas produce varying mixtures of norepinephrine, epinephrine and rarely dopamine which in turn lead to myriad clinical manifestations. On the other hand, extra-adrenal paraganglionomas, are tumors of extra-adrenal sympathetic and parasympathetic paraganglia which may or may not secrete catecholamines [1]. They are histologically indistinguishable from pheochromocytomas and therefore may have similar clinical presentations [2]. The anesthetic concerns and challenges regarding these two categories of tumors are therefore the same.

Proper recognition and medical treatment of the condition is necessary before considering any surgery in patients with pheochromocytoma (pheo). It has been estimated that 25–50% of hospital deaths of patients with unmanaged or unknown pheos occur during the induction of anesthesia or operative procedures for other conditions [3]. These patients can present with unexplained severe hypertension, tachycardia, arrhythmias, and cardiovascular collapse after the induction of anesthesia [4] or at any time during the surgery (e.g., after administration of metoclopramide [5]). Unfortunately, the mortality for such patients approaches 80% [6]. Also, since the treatment of most of these tumors is invariably surgical resection, so a lucid understanding of the challenges and complications involved, a careful preoperative assessment, a clear delineation of management goals and preemptive anticipation, and treatment of all complications are imperative in the successful management. This chapter will discuss the preoperative evaluation after the diagnosis has been established, intraoperative management, and postoperative care of patients who will undergo resection of pheochromocytoma.

Goals of anesthetic management

Preoperative alpha-adrenergic blockade may prevent or reduce hypertensive crises during surgery for pheochromocytoma, allow intravascular volume expansion, and improve cardiac function in patients with catecholamine-induced myocarditis and cardiomyopathy. The goals of anesthetic management are as follows:

1. Control of hypertension, including prevention of hypertensive crisis during the surgery (see Figure 53.1).
2. Normalization of intravascular volume: A high-sodium diet is usually incorporated to aid in the expansion of intravascular volume The catecholamines cause intense vasoconstriction through the alpha-1 receptors, and initiation of alpha blockade can lead to severe orthostatic hypotension. To counteract this hypotension, patients are advised to increase fluid and salt intake (2–3 L of fluid orally with 5–10 g of salt to increase the intravascular volume). If oral fluid and salt intake do not improve the orthostatic hypotension while the blood pressure (BP) of the patient still warrants antihypertensive therapy, crystalloids and colloids may be given intravenously. Serial hematocrit measurements give a guide to the effectiveness of volume expansion. Usually, a 5–10% fall in hematocrit is seen in a well-prepared patient. The fall is more a guide to the therapy rather than an end point for adequate volume expansion.
3. Heart rate and arrhythmia control by use of beta blockers and calcium channel blockers.
4. Assessment and optimization of myocardial function–preoperative electrocardiography (E.C.G.) and echocardiography are done.
5. Assessment of end organ damage: These result from excess catecholamine secretion; the system most severely affected is the cardiovascular system. Complications may involve volume depletion, postural hypotension, organ or limb ischemia, aortic dissection, angina, myocardial infarction, acute or chronic cardiomyopathy, congestive heart failure, and arrhythmias [10, 11].
6. Reversal of glucose and electrolyte disturbances – Appropriate therapy for diabetes if required is initiated in the preoperative period with oral hypoglycemic agents and/or insulin.

Preoperative assessment

Patients are assessed at least 7–14 days prior to surgery to allow time for modification of treatment, and titrate therapy to minimize the physiologic impact of catecholamine release. This preoperative medical optimization usually takes 10–14 days.

History and physical examination focuses on the cardiovascular system (like findings of heart failure) and evaluation of vital signs (orthostatic BP). Routine preoperative laboratory testing are performed, including blood glucose, electrolytes, blood urea nitrogen, creatinine, and complete blood count, blood typing, and screening.

Patients with pheochromocytoma and paraganglioma are at risk of catecholamine-induced cardiomyopathy, which is reversed after the removal of the tumor. Preoperative cardiac evaluation includes an electrocardiogram to evaluate for possible ST- and T-wave ischemic changes and rhythm disturbances, all of which usually resolve with preoperative medical preparation prior to surgery, or else surgery is deferred. A Holter monitor is rarely indicated if arrhythmias fail to resolve with medications. A preoperative echocardiogram is performed to assess ventricular function, chamber size, and wall motion and rule out the rare existence of primary cardiac paraganglioma [12, 13].

Anesthetic Management for Pheochromocytoma

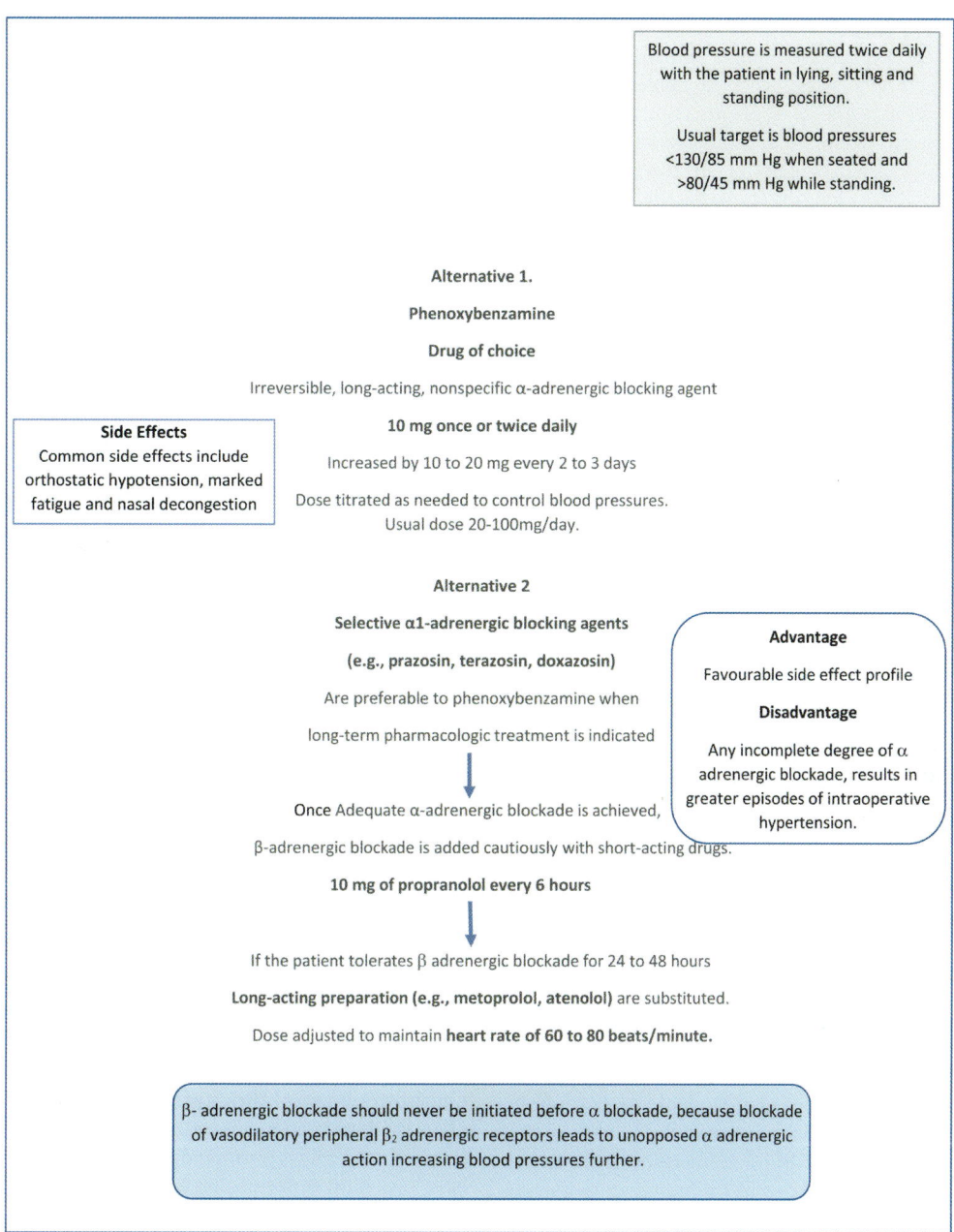

FIGURE 53.1 Preoperative drug therapy in pheochromocytoma [7–9].

Effectiveness of medical preparation is assessed by the following:

1. Twice daily orthostatic BP measurements.
2. A standing systolic BP (SBP) ≥90 mmHg.
3. A heart rate between 60 and 70 beats/minute (bpm) seated and 70–80 bpm standing.
4. No in-hospital arterial BP reading higher than 165/90 mmHg for 48 hours before surgery.
5. Orthostatic hypotension is acceptable as long as arterial BP with the patient standing is not less than 80/45 mmHg.
6. The E.C.G. free of ST–T changes.
7. No more than one premature ventricular contraction (PVC) in 5 minutes [3].

Drug therapy in pheochromocytoma

Alpha-receptor antagonists

Nonselective, irreversible, alpha-receptor antagonists

Phenoxybenzamine is a nonselective, noncompetitive, long-acting alpha blocker. Its mechanism of action is irreversible inactivation of alpha receptors (both alpha 1 and alpha 2) by covalently bonding to the receptor molecule. Phenoxybenzamine is initiated in doses of 10 mg every 6–12 hours and increased to 30–40 mg every 6 hours to a maximum dose of 240 mg/day. Its nonspecific nature also allows presynaptic alpha-2 blockade, which interferes with the norepinephrine negative feedback loop that regulates norepinephrine release. The resulting uninhibited release of norepinephrine from cardiac sympathetic neurones causes a reflex tachycardia via beta-1 stimulation. The drug crosses blood–brain barrier and leads to inactivation of centrally located alpha-1 and alpha-2 receptors and causes side effects such as headache, somnolence, and nasal congestion. The other side effects of phenoxybenzamine such as orthostatic hypotension, tachycardia, dizziness, and syncope are more severe than those seen in patients on selective alpha 1– receptor antagonists. Since it has a long duration of action, postoperative return of adrenergic function is delayed for 24–48 hours, and thus it may lead to postoperative refractory catecholamine-resistant hypotension. A study done by Shao et al. [11] showed that preoperative alpha-1 adrenoceptor antagonist has no benefit in maintaining intraoperative hemodynamic stability in patients with normotensive pheochromocytoma. Kocak et al. [14] and Havlik et al. [15] concluded that preoperative total alpha-adrenergic blockade with phenoxybenzamine offered no advantage over selective blockade with prazosin in terms of perioperative fluid requirements or intraoperative hemodynamic stability. Randle et al. [16] observed that laparoscopic adrenalectomy for pheochromocytoma is safe regardless of the preoperative alpha-blockade strategy employed, but patients blocked selectively may have a higher incidence of transient hypotension during surgery and a greater need for postoperative support. These differences did not result in longer hospital stay or increased complications.

Selective alpha 1–receptor antagonists
The selective alpha 1–receptor antagonist drugs are **prazosin, doxazosin, and terazosin**. Prazosin is the most commonly used drug. The therapy with prazosin is usually initiated at 0.5–1 mg per dose every 4–6 hours and titrated to a maximum of 20–24 mg/day. Many studies and reports have described good preoperative control of symptoms and adequate intraoperative alpha blockade in patients prepared with prazosin preoperatively [10, 17]. Doxazosin is a longer acting drug and thus is usually required as once daily or twice daily dose. Despite being a longer acting drug refractory, hypotension after tumor removal requiring large amounts of intravenous (IV) fluids and vasopressor support is significantly less in patients treated with this drug as compared to patients who receive phenoxybenzamine [18, 19]. Doxazosin is initiated at the dose of 1–2 mg/day and titrated to control BP, up to a maximum dose of 16 mg/day. Terazosin, having a shorter half-life than doxazosin, is also initiated at a dose of 1 mg/day and can be increased up to a maximum of 20 mg/day depending on goals of BP control.

These drugs preferentially act on the alpha-1 receptors and cause vasodilatation but the tachycardia that ensues is of a lesser degree than phenoxybenzamine. Since the alpha-2 receptors are spared, the presynaptic release of NE is not enhanced, and thus severe tachycardia is avoided. The antagonism by this class of drugs is reversible and therefore prolonged hypotension after tumor removal is usually not seen. The common side effects seen are vertigo, dizziness, malaise, mild headache, and gastrointestinal symptoms such as nausea, gastralgia, diarrhea, or vomiting. Postural hypotension can be quite severe especially with the initial doses; hence, the drug is usually started at bedtime and in low doses. Syncope, tachycardia, palpitations, fatigue, drowsiness, rash, and flushes are the rarely encountered side effects [20]. In an observational study of 35 patients with pheochromocytoma or paraganglioma undergoing resection, pretreatment with doxazosin appeared to be as effective as phenoxybenzamine for the control of BP and heart rate before and during surgery [21]. Compared with those receiving phenoxybenzamine, patients treated with doxazosin had less preoperative postural hypotension, required less fluid administration after the effluent vein was clamped (phase II), and recovered to normal BP more rapidly at the end of surgery. **Urapidil** is a selective alpha-adrenergic blocker with a central sympatholytic effect mediated by stimulation of serotonin 5HT receptors and is available in some countries outside the United States [22]. Some studies have described adequate preoperative alpha blockade with three days of IV urapidil [23]. The PRESCRIPT trial compared pretreatment with phenoxybenzamine or doxazosin started 2 to 3 weeks prior to resection of phaeochromocytoma [24]. It concluded that phenoxybenzamin was more effective in preventing intraoperative haemodynamic instability but clinical outcomes were similar in both the groups.

Beta blockers
Beta blockers should never be used before initiation of alpha blockade in patients with functional tumors as they suppress beta 1–mediated cardiac sympathetic drive before adequate arteriolar dilatation, which may precipitate acute cardiac insufficiency and pulmonary edema [25]. Indications of their use are the presence of arrhythmias and features of myocardial ischemia and cardiomyopathy due to excessive catecholamine secretion. Beta blockade is especially important for patients with tumors that secrete large amounts of epinephrine, with resultant tachycardia and arrhythmias. They are started at a low dose using short-acting oral medication (e.g., **metoprolol** 50 mg/day). If the patients tolerate, a longer acting medication or a higher dose is added. Cardioselective beta antagonists are desirable and have less side effects. Labetalol which has both alpha and beta receptor–blocking activity and may be used in place of pure beta antagonists (but never as an alternative to alpha antagonists) [26]. Labetalol reduces the uptake of ^{131}I-MIBG and needs to be stopped two weeks before ^{131}I-MIBG scintigraphy to avoid false-negative test results [27]. It is to be used with caution in patients with asthma or congestive heart failure. Patients with occult catecholamine-induced cardiomyopathy may develop congestive heart failure and pulmonary edema with beta-blocker use.

Calcium channel blockers
They inhibit norepinephrine-induced calcium influx. Although they are not really recommended for monotherapy unless patients have very mild hypertension or develop severe orthostatic hypotension with alpha blockers [28]. Thus, they can be used as an additional drug to patients who are already on alpha blockers. They do not prevent all hemodynamic changes during the surgery. When patients receiving them are anesthetized with potent inhalational agents, hypotension responding to calcium chloride infusion is witnessed. Sustained-release **nicardipine** 30 mg twice daily is a commonly used preparation. **Amlodipine** (5–20 mg/day), **nicardipine** (60–90 mg/day), **nifedipine** (30–90 mg/day), **verapamil** (180–540 mg/day), and **diltiazem** (90–240 mg/day) are other calcium channel blockers used. [26].

Tyrosine Hydroxylase Inhibitor
Metyrosine is a competitive inhibitor of tyrosine hydroxylase, a rate-limiting enzyme, in the formation of catecholamines [29]. Some institutions use a five-day (short term) pre-procedure preparation protocol using metyrosine, while others use metyrosine to supplement preoperative alpha blockade. The most common short-term side effect is hypersomnolence, while side effects of longer term treatment may be disabling. The extrapyramidal effects of haloperidol, if administered during anesthesia, may be potentiated by metyrosine [30].

Intraoperative management

Surgical resection of pheochromocytoma can be divided into two phases based on the ligation of the blood supply to the tumor.

Phase I – Phase I includes dissection and isolation of vascular supply of the tumor, **before clamping of the effluent vein**. This phase is often characterized by periods of severe episodic hypertension and arrhythmias as adrenal manipulation releases catecholamines. Phase I includes the following:

1. Endotracheal intubation – Catecholamine levels rise up till 2000–20,000 pg/mL, with potential for severe hypertension and arrhythmias. Increasing depth of anesthesia keeps it within acceptable limits [31].
2. Peritoneal insufflation – Peritoneal insufflation during laparoscopic resection can lead to hypertension and increased catecholamine levels due to compression of the tumor, change in its blood flow, and sympathetic response to hypercapnia [32].
3. Tumor manipulation – Tumor manipulation during either laparoscopic or open adrenalectomy for pheochromocytoma causes the **greatest release** of catecholamines and increases the BP and heart rate. Catecholamines can remain high even after the ligation of the adrenal vein, which may be related to the hypervascularity of some tumors.

During phase I of the surgery, the aim is to keep the SBP between 100 and 160 mmHg. Titration of vasodilator infusions is mandated. BP elevations are treated with nitroprusside, administered as an infusion of 0.5–4 mcg/kg/minute or a bolus of 20 mcg, supplemented as needed by boluses of phentolamine 1–5 mg IV. Hypotension is treated with phenylephrine, administered as a bolus of 40–160 mcg IV or an infusion of 20–200 mcg/minute IV.

Phase II – Phase II of the surgery begins after the effluent vein is clamped. Precipitous hypotension may result because of the sudden drop in endogenous catecholamine levels, the chronic downregulation of alpha-adrenergic receptors, the presence of alpha-blocking medication, and intravascular volume depletion [25]. Typically, intravascular volume optimization and noradrenaline infusions titrated to effect are utilized to maintain BPs in this phase.

Anesthetic management

Choice of anesthesia: General anesthesia with endotracheal intubation, with or without epidural catheter placement, is used for pheochromocytoma resection.

Monitoring: Apart from the basic standards of monitoring as recommended by the American Society of Anaesthesiologists (BP, E.C.G., oxygen saturation, capnography, and temperature), additional monitoring is required.

Invasive BP (IBP) monitoring is imperative in these patients as hemodynamic instability is invariably encountered even with normotensive individuals. For patients who remain hypertensive preoperatively, arterial catheter is placed prior to induction. For patients with well-controlled preoperative BP, arterial line is placed after sedation but prior to endotracheal intubation.

A central venous access is desirable although not mandatory in these patients. A multi-lumen catheter is placed in a large bore and easily accessible vein such as the internal jugular, axillary, or subclavian vein to provide access to the central vascular compartment for the infusion of vasodilators and vasoconstrictors as and when required.

Measurement of pulmonary capillary wedge pressure using Swan–Ganz catheters or other accurate methods to estimate cardiac filling pressures and function may be needed in patients with catecholamine- or hypertension-induced severe cardiomyopathy [33].

Noninvasive methods for cardiac output estimation and stroke volume variation to diagnose fluid deficit have also been used [34]. Underhydration may lead to severe hypotension. Fluid therapy is a vital and complex component of perioperative management. Assessment of fluid responsiveness may be done either by stroke volume variation or pulse pressure variation methods. Fluid should be given judiciously to avoid pulmonary edema and heart failure as the cardiovascular system of these patients is already compromised.

Depth of anesthesia – Changes in cardiac output due to tumor manipulation can alter blood levels of both inhaled and IV anesthetics [35]. Changing requirements may be reflected in processed electroencephalography monitors (e.g., bispectral analysis monitor [BIS]).

Premedication is done with IV midazolam up to 2 mg in divided doses and small doses of fentanyl (25 mcg IV) titrated to mild sedation.

Induction: Induction of anesthesia should be smooth to avoid the stress response to laryngoscopy and endotracheal intubation. A wide variety of medications can be used except ketamine because of its sympathomimetic properties. Commonly used medications are fentanyl 1–3 mcg/kg IV, lidocaine 1 mg/kg IV, propofol 1–2 mg/kg IV, or etomidate 0.3–0.5 mg/kg. Muscle paralysis with a nondepolarizing neuromuscular blocking agent (NMBA) (e.g., rocuronium 0.5 mg/kg IV) is necessary before attempting endotracheal intubation.

Maintenance of anesthesia: Anesthesia is maintained with either use of inhalational agents or intravenous infusion of propofol. Any inhalation agents can be used except halothane, which is avoided because of its arrhythmogenic potential. Isoflurane, nitrous oxide, enflurane, and total intravenous anesthesia (TIVA) with propofol all have been used safely for pheochromocytoma resection [27].

Medications to avoid – A number of medications commonly used intraoperatively should be avoided or used cautiously in patients with pheochromocytoma (Table 53.1).

TABLE 53.1: Drugs to be Avoided Intraoperatively

Metoclopramide is contraindicated. It inhibits dopaminergic suppression of presynaptic norepinephrine release and stimulates the release of catecholamines directly. It has been reported to induce hypertensive crisis and, in some cases, adrenergic myocarditis with cardiogenic shock in patients with pheochromocytoma

Droperidol (higher amounts) and **haloperidol** cause hypertensive crises

Chlorpromazine and prochlorperazine – have hypotensive effects

Glucagon – releases catecholamines from these tumors and has been associated with hypertensive crisis

Halothane is arrhythmogenic, and it sensitizes the myocardium to catecholamines

Histamine-releasing medications – (e.g., morphine, atracurium) avoided in large doses. However, when given slowly, histamine release can be minimized, and both morphine and atracurium have been used safely in these patients [36]

Ketamine, cocaine-sympathomimetic drugs, may exacerbate preexisting hypertension

Ephedrine – indirect-acting alpha and beta agonists should be avoided until the tumor is excised in order to prevent an exaggerated response via the release of catecholamines from the tumor

Complications

1. **Intraoperative hemodynamic instability**

   Hypertensive crisis occurs invariably, despite adequate preoperative alpha blockade and is independent of preoperative catecholamine levels. Haemodynamic instability presents as hypertension, initially, before tumor removal and hypotension after tumor isolation. Factors influencing it are anesthetic drugs, tumor size and site, associated genetic syndrome, plasma catecholamine levels, and type of surgical approach [36]. In a single-center retrospective review of 258 patients who underwent resection of pheochromocytoma or paraganglioma with preoperative pharmacologic preparation, intraoperative changes in BP and heart rate were greater in patients with increased preoperative catecholamine levels, but substantial variability occurred even in patients with normal hormone levels [3]. In another retrospective single-center study involving 123 patients who underwent laparoscopic resection of pheochromocytoma with preoperative pharmacologic preparation, prolonged hypotension (i.e., requiring continuous catecholamine support for >30 minutes to maintain mean arterial pressure ≥60 mmHg) occurred in 44% of patients following tumor removal [33]. These patients were seen to have higher preoperative levels of epinephrine and dopamine.

   Norepinephrine secretion on tumor manipulation leads to intense hypertension with either bradycardia (more common) or tachycardia. Epinephrine secretion usually causes severe tachycardia but lesser degree of hypertension. Sodium nitroprusside and nitroglycerine are the two drugs, which are commonly used for intraoperative control of hypertension and have established safety profiles. Table 53.2 summarizes the drugs used in the management of intraoperative hypertensive crisis.

   Management of a hypertensive episode involves intimating the surgeon, temporarily ceasing the surgery, anticipatory preparation of easily titratable drugs with rapid onset and quick offset.

   Hypotensive crisis: Hypotension is treated sequentially as follows:

   1. IV fluid boluses of small aliquots of 250 mL crystalloids titrated to affect.
   2. Phenylephrine is a pure alpha agonist with a short half-life that may be given as bolus (40–160 mcg IV) or as infusion (wide range of dosing; 10–200 mcg/minute IV), titrated to effect.
   3. Ephedrine is an indirect-acting alpha and beta agonists. It is given as 5–25 mg bolus IV; repeated if necessary. However, ephedrine should not be used in paraganglioma resection or if incomplete pheochromocytoma resection is suspected to avoid precipitous hypertension due to the release of catecholamines.

TABLE 53.2: Drugs Used for Management of Intraoperative Hypertensive Crisis

Name	Class	Dose	Special Considerations
Nitroprusside Drug of choice for intraoperative hypertensive crisis	An ultrashort-acting vasodilator	Infusion at 0.5–5 mcg/kg/minute and adjusted every few minutes for target BP response	May cause thiocyanate toxicity Infusion should not exceed 3 mcg/kg/minute Reflex tachycardia is often treated with infusion of a short-acting beta blocker
Phentolamine	Nonselective alpha blocker	Initial test dose of 1 mg, followed by a 5-mg bolus and/or continuous infusion (0.5–1 mg/minute IV)	
Nicardipine	Calcium channel blocker	Started at 5 mg/hour and increased by 2.5 mg every 15 minutes to desired effect, not exceeding 15 mg/hour	
Clevidipine	Ultrashort-acting third-generation dihydropyridine calcium channel blocker	Starting dose is 1–2 mg/hour intravenously, usually maintained at a rate of 4–6 mg/hour, doubled every 90 seconds with a maximal dose up to 32 mg/hour, for a maximum duration of 72 hours	It decreases peripheral vascular resistance via direct arteriolar dilatation
Labetalol	Combined alpha and beta blockers	5–20 mg IV	
Esmolol	Ultrashort-acting selective beta-adrenergic blocker	Administered by bolus (10–50 mg IV) or by infusion (25–250 µg/kg/minute)	
Magnesium It is a first-line antihypertensive agent in the intraoperative management of pregnant patients undergoing pheochromocytoma resection	Vasodilator that inhibits catecholamine release from the adrenal medulla and antagonizes alpha-adrenergic receptors, calcium antagonist. Antiarrhythmic with cardiac membrane-stabilizing effects	Administered with a bolus of 2–4 g IV over 20 minutes after induction and endotracheal intubation, followed by infusion at 1–2 g/hour IV, with the infusion adjusted based on blood levels. The infusion is discontinued once the venous drainage from the tumor is ligated or the tumor is removed	Used in patients with arrhythmias who are intolerant of beta blockers Where BP is difficult to control Magnesium potentiates the effects of neuromuscular blocking agents (NMBAs); dosing and reversal of NMBAs should be guided by a neuromuscular monitoring.

4. Norepinephrine is primarily beta adrenergic stimulator with minimal alpha adrenergic agonistic action. It is given as infusion 2–20 mcg/minute IV.
5. Vasopressin (initial dose 0.01–0.03 unit/minute; maintenance dose 0.03–0.04 unit/minute) has been used in cases of refractory hypotension after tumor removal, commonly after significant blood loss or in patients with extremely high preoperative levels of catecholamines [35].

2. **Arrhythmias**

    Different types of arrhythmias ranging from supraventricular tachycardia to ventricular ectopics may be seen. Drugs commonly used are IV lidocaine, beta blockade with esmolol, or amiodarone infusion (in patients with impaired cardiac pump function).

3. **Alterations in blood glucose levels**

    A total of 36% of patients with pheochromocytoma develop diabetes due to catecholamine-induced insulin resistance or suppression. Therefore, blood glucose should be monitored intraoperatively and controlled with an insulin infusion [37].

4. **Blood loss**

    Bleeding occurs during resection of paraganglionomas situated in the intra-aortocaval groove; therefore, blood products should be readily available for transfusion.

Postoperative concerns

Hemodynamic instability – It rears its ominous head throughout the postoperative period; therefore, vigilant hemodynamic monitoring in the PACU is required. Fifty percent of patients remain hypertensive for one to three days post resection, BPs normalize in 75% of patients by the tenth day [38]. Postoperative hypotension is common due to downregulation of alpha-adrenergic receptors, residual effects of long-acting antihypertensive medications, or hypovolemia and should be managed.

Hypoglycemia – Once the tumor is removed, the catecholamine inhibition of insulin secretion is eliminated. Hypoglycemia can occur intraoperatively or postoperatively because of a rebound increase in insulin secretion [39]. It may manifest as delayed emergence, or postoperative weakness or lethargy. Blood glucose should be measured every 6 hours postoperatively and more frequently if hypoglycemia develops.

Adrenal insufficiency – Patients who undergo bilateral adrenalectomy require lifelong steroid supplementation. They are at risk of acute postoperative adrenal insufficiency and therefore require glucocorticoid replacement as given below:

- Hydrocortisone 100 mg IV at induction of anesthesia
- Hydrocortisone 100 mg IV every 8 hours for 24 hours
- Hydrocortisone is tapered over three days to maintenance dose (hydrocortisone 25 mg IV, or prednisone 10 mg PO daily)

Renal failure – Massive catecholamine release causes increased renin activity and hypertensive crisis, causing renal hypoperfusion resulting in acute kidney injury and ischemia. Renal failure may also occur due to rhabdomyolysis caused by skeletal muscle ischemia [39]. Adequate hydration and blood pressures should be maintained throughout the postoperative period to overcome this.

Conclusion

During surgery, there is a risk of massive release of catecholamines, which can cause hemodynamic instability, hypertensive crises, and cardiac arrhythmias. Intra-operative problems and issues can be better managed when patient is adequately prepared preoperatively. Roizen et al. in 1982 [40] proposed criteria for evaluation of preoperative preparation:

1. BP should be less than 160/90 mmHg for 24 hours prior to surgery.
2. Patient should not have orthostatic hypotension with BP reading less than 80/45 mmHg.
3. Electrocardiogram should be free of ST- or T-wave changes for one week prior to surgery.
4. PVCs if any should be less than one per 5 minutes.

A successful perioperative management in cases of pheochromocytoma lies in the adequate preoperative optimization, vigilant intraoperative monitoring, and prompt response to any hemodynamic instability. This vigilance is continued in the postoperative period.

References

1. Pacak K, Eisenhofer G, Ahlman H, et al. Pheochromocytoma: recommendations for clinical practice from the first international symposium. October 2005. Nat Clin Pract Endocrinol Metab 2007;3:92–102.
2. Neumann HPH, Young WF Jr, Eng C. Pheochromocytoma and paraganglioma. N Engl J Med 2019;381:552.
3. Fleisher L, Mythen M. Anesthetic implications of concurrent diseases. In: Miller's Anesthesia, 8th ed., Miller RD, Cohen NH, Eriksson LI, et al. (Eds.), Elsevier, Philadelphia, PA, 2015. p. 1170.
4. Myklejord DJ. Undiagnosed pheochromocytoma: the anesthesiologist nightmare. Clin Med Res 2004;2:59.
5. Sheinberg R, Gao WD, Wand G, et al. Case 1–2012. A perfect storm: fatality resulting from metoclopramide unmasking a pheochromocytoma and its management. J Cardiothorac Vasc Anesth 2012;26:161.
6. O'Riordan JA. Pheochromocytomas and anesthesia. Int Anesthesiol Clin 1997;35:99.
7. Kakoki K, Miyata Y, Shida Y, et al. Pheochromocytoma multisystem crisis treated with emergency surgery: a case report and literature review. BMC Res Notes 2015;8:758.
8. Sauneuf B, Chudeau N, Champigneulle B, et al. Pheochromocytoma crisis in the ICU: a French Multicenter Cohort Study with emphasis on rescue extracorporeal membrane oxygenation. Crit Care Med 2017;45:e657.
9. Subramaniam R. Pheochromocytoma – current concepts in diagnosis and management. Trends Anaesth Crit Care 2011;1:104.
10. Weingarten TN, Cata JP, O'Hara JF, et al. Comparison of two preoperative medical management strategies for laparoscopic resection of pheochromocytoma. Urology 2010;76:508.e6–e11.
11. Shao Y, Chen R, Shen ZJ, et al. Preoperative alpha blockade for normotensive pheochromocytoma: is it necessary? J Hypertens 2011;29:2429–32.
12. Agarwal V, Kant G, Hans N, Messerli FH. Takotsubo-like cardiomyopathy in pheochromocytoma. Int J Cardiol 2011;153:241.
13. Lord MS, Augoustides JG. Perioperative management of pheochromocytoma: focus on magnesium, clevidipine, and vasopressin. J Cardiothorac Vasc Anesth 2012;26:526, 7.
14. Kocak S, Aydintug S, Canakci N. Alpha blockade in preoperative preparation of patients with pheochromocytomas. Int Surg 2002;87:191–4.
15. Havlik RJ, Cahow CE, Kinder BK. Advances in the diagnosis and treatment of pheochromocytoma. Arch Surg 1988;123:626–30.
16. Randle R, Balentine CJ, Pitt S, et al, Selective versus non-selective alpha-blockade prior to laparoscopic adrenalectomy for pheochromocytoma. Ann Surg Oncol 2017;24(1):244–50.
17. Agrawal R, Mishra SK, Bhatia E, et al. Prospective study to compare peri-operative hemodynamic alterations following preparation for pheochromocytoma surgery by phenoxybenzamine or prazosin. World J Surg 2014;38:716–23.
18. Prys-Roberts C, Farndon JR. Efficacy and safety of doxazosin for perioperative management of patients with pheochromocytoma. World J Surg 2002;26:1037–42.
19. Miura Y, Yoshinaga K. Doxazosin: a newly developed, selective alpha 1-inhibitor in the management of patients with pheochromocytoma. Am Heart J 1988;116(6 Pt 2):1785–9.
20. Desiniotis A, Kyprianou N. Advances in the design and synthesis of prazosin derivatives over the last ten years. Expert Opin Ther Targets 2011;15:1405–18.
21. Buch J. Urapidil, a dual-acting antihypertensive agent: current usage considerations. Adv Ther 2010;27:426.
22. Habbe N, Ruger F, Bojunga J, et al. Urapidil in the preoperative treatment of pheochromocytomas: a safe and cost-effective method. World J Surg 2013;37:1141.

23. Gosse P, Tauzin-Fin P, Sesay MB, et al. Preparation for surgery of phaeochromocytoma by blockade of alpha-adrenergic receptors with urapidil: what dose? J Hum Hypertens 2009;23:605.
24. Buitenwerf E, Osinga TE, Timmers HJLM, Lenders JWM, Feelders RA, Eekhoff EMW et al, Efficacy of α-Blockers on Hemodynamic Control during Pheochromocytoma Resection: A Randomized Controlled Trial. J Clin Endocrinol Metab. 2020;105: 2381–91.
25. Prys-Roberts C. Phaeochromocytoma – recent progress in its management. Br J Anaesth 2000;85:44–57.
26. Pacak K. Preoperative management of the pheochromocytoma patient. J Clin Endocrinol Metab 2007;92:4069–79.
27. Solanki KK, Bomanji J, Moyes J, Mather SJ, Trainer PJ, Britton KE. A pharmacological guide to medicines which interfere with the biodistribution of radiolabelled meta-iodobenzylguanidine (MIBG). Nucl Med Commun 1992;13:513–21.
28. Lenders JW, Duh QY, Eisenhofer G, et al. Pheochromocytoma and paraganglioma: an endocrine society clinical practice guideline. J Clin Endocrinol Metab 2014;99: 1915–42.
29. Westfall TC, Westfall DP. Adrenergic agonists and antagonists. In: Goodman and Gilman's The Pharmacological Basis of Therapeutics, 12th ed., Brunton LL, Chabner BA, Knollmann CB (Eds.), McGraw Hill, New York, NY, 2011. p. 309.
30. Young WF, Jr. Endocrine hypertension. In: William's Textbook of Endocrinology, 12th ed., Melmed S, Polonsky KS, Larsen PR, Kronenberg HM (Eds.), Elsevier, Philadelphia, PA, 2011. p. 547.
31. Marty J, Desmonts JM, Chalaux G, et al. Hypertensive responses during operation for phaeochromocytoma: a study of plasma catecholamine and haemodynamic changes. Eur J Anaesthesiol 1985;2:257.
32. de La Chapelle A, Deghmani M, Dureuil B. Peritoneal insufflation can be a critical moment in the laparoscopic surgery of pheochromocytoma. Ann Fr Anesth Reanim 1998;17:1184.
33. Wu S, Chen W, Shen L, et al. Risk factors for prolonged hypotension in patients with pheochromocytoma undergoing laparoscopic adrenalectomy: a single-center retrospective study. Sci Rep 2017;7:5897.
34. Gregory SH, Yalamuri SM, McCartney SL, et al. Perioperative management of adrenalectomy and inferior vena cava reconstruction in a patient with a large, malignant pheochromocytoma with vena caval extension. J Cardiothorac Vasc Anesth 2017;31(1):365.
35. Tan SG, Koay CK, Chan ST. The use of vasopressin to treat catecholamine-resistant hypotension after phaeochromocytoma removal. Anaesth Intensive Care 2002;30:477.
36. Siddiqi HK, Yang HY, Laird AM, et al. Utility of oral nicardipine and magnesium sulfate infusion during preparation and resection of pheochromocytomas. Surgery 2012;152:1027.
37. La Batide-Alanore A, Chatellier G, Plouin PF. Diabetes as a marker of pheochromocytoma in hypertensive patients. J Hypertens 2003;21:1703.
38. Schwartz JJ, Akhtar S, Rosenbaum SH. Endocrine function. In: Clinical Anesthesia. Barash PG, Cullen BF, Stoelting RK, et al. (Eds.), Wolters Kluwer, Philadelphia, PA, 2013. p. 1326. 43. Akiba M, Kodama T, Ito Y, et al. Hypoglycemia induced by excessive rebound secretion of insulin after removal of pheochromocytoma. World J Surg 1990;14:317.
39. Celik H, Celik O, Guldiken S, et al. Pheochromocytoma presenting with rhabdomyolysis and acute renal failure: a case report. Ren Fail 2014;36:104.
40. Roizen MF, Horrigan RW, Koike M, et al. A prospective randomized trial of four anesthetic techniques for resection of pheochromocytoma. Anesthesiology 1982;57:A43.

54

OPERATIVE APPROACH TO THE ADRENAL GLAND PATHOLOGY

Sendhil Rajan and Bharadhwaj Ravindhran

Relevant surgical anatomy and relations

The adrenal glands are located in the perirenal compartment of the retroperitoneum, which also contains the kidney, perirenal/periadrenal fat, and upper ureter. This space is bound by Gerota's fascia anteriorly and posteriorly by the posterior (Zuckerkandl's) renal fascia, quadratus lumborum muscle, paraspinous muscle, transversus abdominis muscle, and thoracolumbar fascia (1).

There is a pervasive arcade of small arteries around the inferior, medial, and superior borders of the adrenal gland, but the venous drainage tends to be solitary. The left adrenal vein drains into the left renal vein after converging with the inferior phrenic vein. In contrast, the right adrenal vein is short, slender, and comes off at a near 90-degree angle from the inferior vena cava (IVC). This makes the cannulation of the right adrenal vein during adrenal venous sampling (AVS) more difficult than the left side (2) and adrenal surgery generally more challenging on the right side. Preoperative cross-sectional imaging should be obtained to determine the position of the tumor within the gland and the relationship of the adrenal/tumor to the renal hilum, kidney, and major vasculature (3).

Pathological considerations

The adrenal gland comprises two distinct tissue zones with special functions. The adrenal medulla, derived from neuroectodermal cells, which produces catecholamines. The adrenal cortex, derived from mesenchymal cells, is formed by three concentric zones: the granulosa that secretes aldosterone, the fasciculata that secretes cortisol, and the inner reticularis that secretes androgens. The most frequent clinical presentations of adrenal disease are related to the hypersecretion of these adrenal hormones.

Partial/cortical-sparing adrenalectomy is useful in benign adenomas and pheochromocytomas and is invaluable in cases of bilateral tumors to preserve endogenous steroid production and prevention of Addisonian crisis. However, this should not be at the expense of leaving behind pathological disease in the remnant.

Hypercortisolism

High levels of circulating plasma glucocorticoids or hypercortisolism result in symptoms and clinical features associated with Cushing's syndrome. Adrenalectomy is indicated in secretory adrenal (Cushing's) adenoma, adrenocortical carcinoma(ACC), and hyperplasia. Hypercortisolism can be associated with significant fat deposition in the subcutaneous tissue, retroperitoneal, and intraperitoneal spaces. Increased subcutaneous tissue may sometimes necessitate the use of longer ports and instruments, as used in bariatric surgery. Deeper fat can make dissection challenging, especially in cases of bilateral hyperplasia – where the ratio of fat:gland tissue is very high, and the gland cannot be easily differentiated from retroperitoneal fat. Occasionally, a "boundary dissection" technique can be employed to clear all fat (and glandular tissue) superior to the kidney. Perioperative care is of utmost importance as these patients are severely immune-compromised, have thinned-out skin, and poor respiratory function (4).

Primary hyperaldosteronism

The most common type of primary hyperaldosteronism is caused by aldosterone-producing adenomas, and less frequently, bilateral adrenal hyperplasia. Solitary adrenal adenomas associated with primary hyperaldosteronism are usually <2 cm in size.

For a unilateral aldosterone-producing adenoma (localized by imaging), surgical resection should be performed, whereas medical treatment is preferred for patients with bilateral hyperplasia.

Typical unilateral Conn adenomas are more easily removed surgically – they are well circumscribed small tumors that rarely grow beyond 2 cm in size. However, a concrete preoperative diagnosis and side localization is crucial. Infrequently, patients may exhibit bilateral tumors on imaging, only one of which is functional – the side must be localized using techniques such as AVS.

Pheochromocytoma

Pheochromocytomas are tumors arising from the chromaffin cells, and their clinical presentation is associated with excess catecholamine production. Minimally invasive adrenalectomy (e.g., laparoscopic transperitoneal approach) is the initial surgical treatment of choice for benign pheochromocytomas. Adequate medical preparation before surgical resection is essential for operative success.

Pheochromocytomas are known to be highly vascular tumors, typically with multiple arterial feeding branches and large caliber adrenal veins. Adequate medical preparation with blockade before surgical resection is essential for operative success. Close liaison with anesthetist should be maintained pre-, intra-, and postoperatively; some surgeons prefer to have a patient monitor turned toward their side during the procedure. Small manipulations of the tumor during surgery can seldom lead to major elevations in blood pressure. It is always preferable to ligate the adrenal vein as early as possible during the procedure, to reduce the amount of catecholamines released into systemic circulation. However, this may always not be possible due to the size and location of the tumor and other anatomical considerations (5). Early vein ligation has the (greater) advantage of preventing systemic complications but carries the disadvantage of engorging the gland with intact arterial supply.

Incidentalomas

Adrenal incidentalomas are usually "incidental" benign adrenal masses (≥1 cm) discovered on imaging studies conducted for other reasons not related to the adrenal glands. Prevalence of incidentalomas now reaches 8% in autopsy series and 4–6% in imaging studies (6, 7).

Surgical indication for nonfunctional adrenal incidentalomas is principally guided by tumor size. Surgical excision is recommended for adrenal tumors >4 cm since most of the adrenocortical carcinomas are usually large (8). Strict adherence to oncological principles is crucial while operating such patients.

Adrenal malignancy

Primary adrenal malignancies are rare and encompass adrenocortical carcinoma and malignant pheochromocytoma. ACC comprises 0.2% of all cancers, and these tumors can secrete excess cortisol, aldosterone, and androgens (9, 10). The incidence of malignant pheochromocytoma ranges from 5 to 26% (11). The preoperative diagnosis of malignant pheochromocytoma by imaging is based on local invasion and distal metastasis.

Assessment for adrenal malignancy is based on the size on imaging studies. Larger adrenal masses are associated with increased risk for malignancy. More specifically, incidental, nonfunctioning adrenal masses that measure ≥4 cm have an increased rate of malignancy and should be surgically removed. Non-contrast CT attenuation coefficient in Hounsfield units (HU) of an adrenal mass revealing densitometry <10 HU demonstrates high fat composition and increases the likelihood of a benign adenoma. CT sensitivity and specificity are 71 and 98%, respectively. However, several adrenal adenomas (30%) are lipid poor, and unenhanced CT is not indicative (12, 13).

The risk of malignancy is very high for larger adrenal tumors with a size threshold of 4 cm having a sensitivity of 96% and specificity of 52% for cancer. An adrenal tumor size threshold of 6 cm has a sensitivity of 90% and specificity of 80% for malignancy (14). The size of an adrenal tumor not only suggests malignancy risk but also a criterion of reference for the choice of surgical approach. Adrenal malignancy is also suggested by morphologic characteristics by imaging studies including irregular border, local invasion, large necrotic areas, and infiltration of the tumor into the periadrenal fat.

Other malignant adrenal lesions are metastases from lung, breast, and other nonadrenal cancers. Removal of such adrenal masses as the only site of metastatic disease is an infrequent indication for adrenalectomy (15).

Indications for adrenalectomy

Most adrenal lesions, within the realm of surgical treatment, are unilateral, presumed benign tumors including functional adrenocortical adenomas, pheochromocytomas, and adrenal incidentalomas. Other less common surgical indications include adrenocortical cancer, adrenal cysts, ganglioneuromas, myelolipomas, androgen-secreting tumors, and bilateral lesions such as macronodular adrenal hyperplasia (16).

Size threshold for laparoscopy

The size threshold of benign and functional adrenal tumors for laparoscopic adrenalectomy has traditionally ranged from 8 to 9 cm. Nevertheless, the size limit of adrenal masses for laparoscopic resection has incrementally increased following the improvement in surgical skills and technologies. Some limitation criteria for laparoscopic removal such as size >9 cm, and preoperative radiologic evidence of intraoperative local infiltration of periadrenal tissue may be useful in patient selection for minimally invasive surgery (17, 18).

Laparoscopy for malignancy

A remaining controversial issue is the laparoscopic resection of highly suspicious or malignant adrenal masses. In the opinion of the authors, well-defined local invasiveness is essential for determining the suitability for laparoscopic adrenalectomy (18–22). Recent data confirm that laparoscopic adrenalectomy can replicate open surgical oncologic resection of ACC, showing comparable survival and recurrence rates. The most important contraindication for the minimally invasive adrenalectomy is local infiltration of periadrenal tissue determined by preoperative imaging and intraoperative inspection (17, 22).

Adrenal metastases may come from primary tumors of lung, breast, stomach, and kidney. Detection of metastasis has increased with the widespread use of imaging studies for cancer surveillance. If solitary metastatic lesions are limited within the capsule of the adrenal gland, adrenalectomy can be performed (23). Laparoscopic adrenalectomy can also be performed for high-risk lesions for malignancy, but general experience is limited, and oncologic effectiveness of minimally invasive approaches remains uncertain in this setting (18, 24–28).

When malignant adrenal tumors, primary or metastatic, are removed laparoscopically, surgical oncologic principles must be followed: low likelihood for conversion, complete removal with the slightest manipulation, and without fragmentation of periadrenal tissues. If required, the conversion to an open procedure must be performed very early, before the advanced dissection of the operative site and possible fragmentation of periadrenal fat or tumor capsule.

Data exit to suggest that laparoscopic adrenalectomy is safe and effective for malignant adrenal tumors. In some studies, outcome results with regard to peritoneal carcinomatosis, positive resection margins, and time to recurrence showed no statistically significant differences between open and laparoscopic approaches (17, 28–32).

Surgical approaches

The surgical approach to the adrenal glands has evolved considerably from the description of the first laparoscopic adrenalectomy (33). This minimally invasive surgical approach has established itself as the "gold standard" for the surgical treatment of most adrenal lesions.

The advantages in performing laparoscopic adrenalectomy include reduced hospital stay, fewer complications, and better aesthetic results. Traditional open adrenalectomy is still reserved for malignant or larger adrenal tumors (16, 34). Regardless of approach, the key to successful adrenalectomy remains the same: proper patient selection for surgery, solid understanding of adrenal pathophysiology, and a thorough knowledge of adrenal anatomy. Over the last two decades, many minimally invasive techniques have been introduced including the lateral transabdominal (LT), posterior retroperitoneal, and robotic approaches. The most frequently performed laparoscopic approach is LT, followed by PRA and anterior transabdominal (AT) access (35). These different laparoscopic approaches are determined by the surgeon's skill set. Laparoscopic LT adrenalectomy was introduced by Gagner in 1992 (35) and is the most popular procedure as it allows for wide exposure of the retroperitoneal space and takes advantage of mobilization of organs due to gravity in both left and right lateral positions: spleen, pancreas, or liver. Adrenalectomy is a unique procedure as there are some differences between right and left adrenalectomy. Open adrenalectomy consists of transabdominal or retroperitoneal approaches that have now been largely adapted to minimally invasive surgery for adrenal resection, except in large tumors and malignant disease (36).

Operative Approach to the Adrenal Gland Pathology

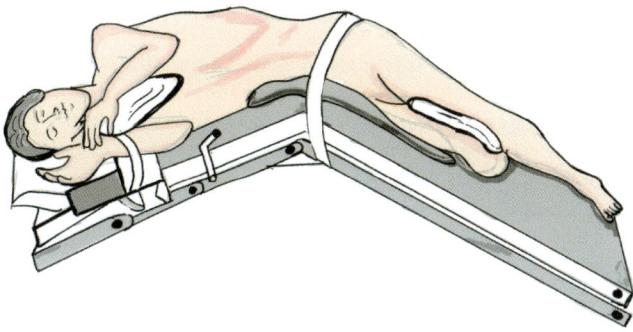

FIGURE 54.1 Patient position for Left Laparoscopic LT Adrenalectomy.

Laparoscopic transabdominal: lateral approach (LT)

Under general anesthesia, the patient is positioned with left lateral side down for right adrenalectomy and the right lateral side down for left adrenalectomy (Figure 54.1). Pneumoperitoneum is induced either through the open method (author's preference), through a Veress needle inserted in the flank or via an optical trocar; with CO_2 pressure regulated at 12–15 mmHg for the whole procedure; a 30-degree laparoscope is introduced through this port. Three other 10-mm ports are inserted for the introduction of atraumatic graspers, hook, retractors, energy devices like ultrasonic shears, clip applicators, and scissors.

Left laparoscopic LT adrenalectomy

Commonly used port positions for left laparoscopic LT adrenalectomy are shown in Figure 54.2. Some surgeons prefer to use the superior-most port for the telescope, and it is often advantageous to not use a fixed port site for the camera during left/right adrenalectomy. Port positions may have to be in a more inferior site than usual in case of larger tumors. The first step of the procedure is the division of phrenicocolic ligament for mobilization of the splenic flexure and left colon – this may not be required in all patients. This is followed by dissection and mobilization of pancreaticosplenic bloc by the division of the splenorenal ligament. The lateral position of the patient allows for better mobilization of the spleen and pancreatic tail. This mobilization allows for the exposure of the left adrenal gland that involves dissection into the retroperitoneal fat above the left kidney. Most important is the careful dissection and ligation of the left adrenal vein, usually by titanium/polymer clips. The left adrenal vein is ligated at least 1 cm above the junction with the renal vein. Identification and ligation of the adrenal vein is recommended early in the procedure, especially in pheochromocytomas. However, this may not always be technically feasible, especially in the obese patient. Laparoscopic ultrasound is useful to identify the adrenal vein, the adrenal gland itself, or the tumor within the gland tissue in difficult cases. The adrenal arteries are smaller in size and are frequently dealt with using vessel-sealing devices like ultrasonic shears, occasionally requiring clips. It is preferred to dissect in a superior-inferior direction in larger lesions – and approach the adrenal vein from above. In smaller lesions, an inferior-superior dissection is feasible with early identification of the adrenal vein. One must be aware of renal vessel anatomical variations – these can often be detected on preoperative CT.

Right laparoscopic LT adrenalectomy

Port positioning for right laparoscopic LT adrenalectomy is shown in Figures 54.3 and 54.4. The epigastric port is used to insert the fan retractor to retract the liver. A grasper might suffice for smaller lesions; alternatively, a Nathanson liver retractor may

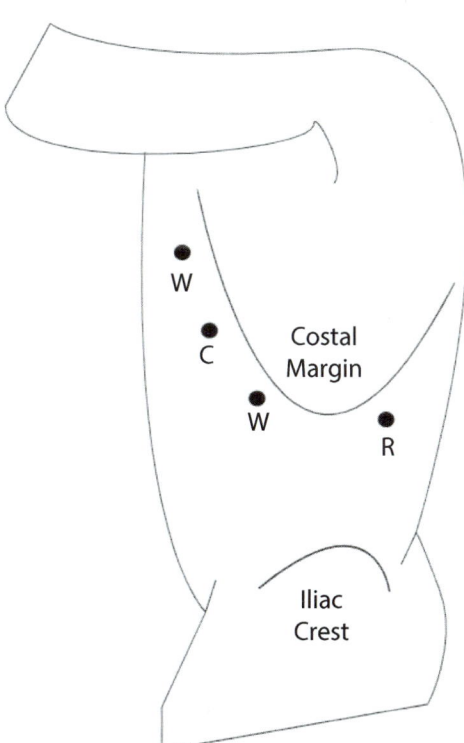

FIGURE 54.2 Port position for left laparoscopic adrenalectomy.

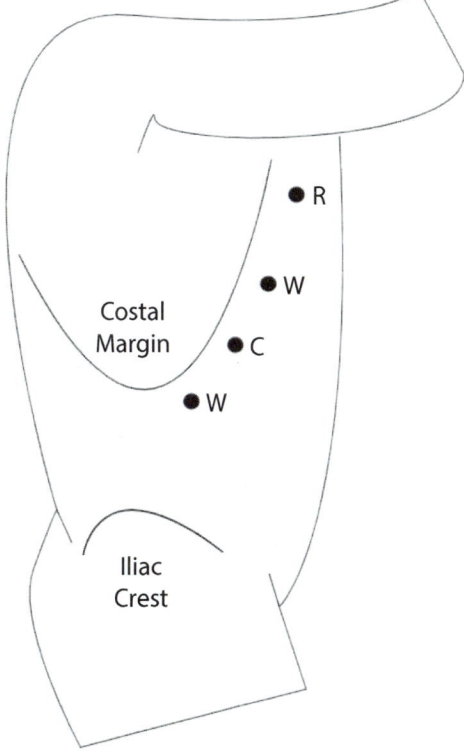

FIGURE 54.3 Port position for right laparoscopic adrenalectomy.

more challenging – especially in cases of hyperplasia, or when the tumor arises from the retrocaval part. The right gland has a very short and broad adrenal vein that runs directly into the IVC. Safe identification and dissection of the vein is of paramount importance during the procedure. A maximum length of the vein should be visualized; it should then be clipped and divided. If it is not possible to get sufficient length of the vein for safe clipping, a vascular stapler may be used. The right adrenal gland can then be dissected free from the retroperitoneal fat; hemostasis is checked, and the adrenal bed is irrigated with saline. The specimen is placed in a plastic bag and extracted through the anterior trocar. A summary of key steps for right laparoscopic LT adrenalectomy done for a 10-cm right adrenal cyst is shown in Figure 54.5.

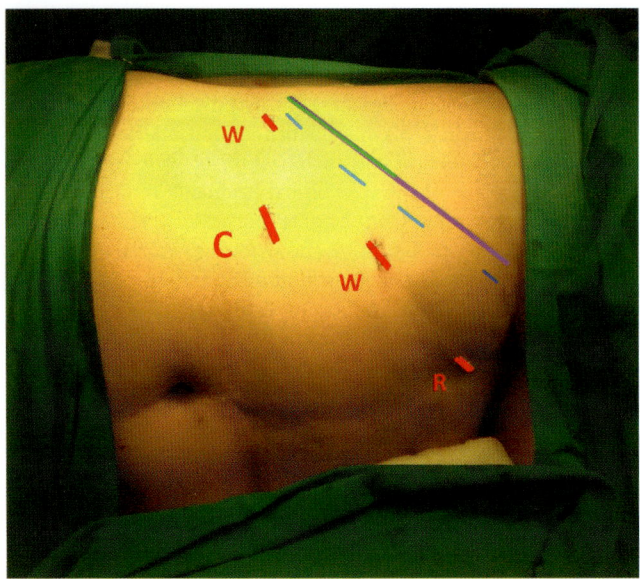

FIGURE 54.4 Patient position for Right Laparoscopic LT Adrenalectomy.

be deployed for effective and atraumatic liver retraction. The retroperitoneum is entered with incision of the right triangular ligament and posterior peritoneum along the inferior surface of the liver. Larger tumors may be adherent to the liver and require considerable dissection. The liver is then retracted superior-medially to expose the surface and superior pole of the right adrenal gland. The next critical step is the identification and exposure of the IVC. The right adrenal gland lies in a partial retrocaval position, and dissection of the segment that lies behind the IVC can be

Anterior approach

The anterior transabdominal approach is a less-preferred initial choice for laparoscopic adrenalectomy (16, 37). Under general anesthesia, the patient is placed in the supine position with containment devices on both sides to allow for table tilting laterally, if required. For left adrenalectomy, four trocars are employed in the following positions: above the umbilicus, in the subxiphoid position, along with the left midclavicular line at the umbilicus level, and in the left flank region along the midaxillary line. The anterior transabdominal approach does not allow for mobilization by the gravity of the spleen and pancreatic tail. Consequently, wide dissection and mobilization of the left colon to the splenic flexure and division of splenocolic and phrenicocolic ligaments is required. The rest of the procedure employs the same steps as that for laparoscopic LT adrenalectomy (38).

Posterior retroperitoneal approach (PRA)

This procedure was popularized by Walz in the early 2000s and has since been gaining popularity worldwide (39). It is ideal for

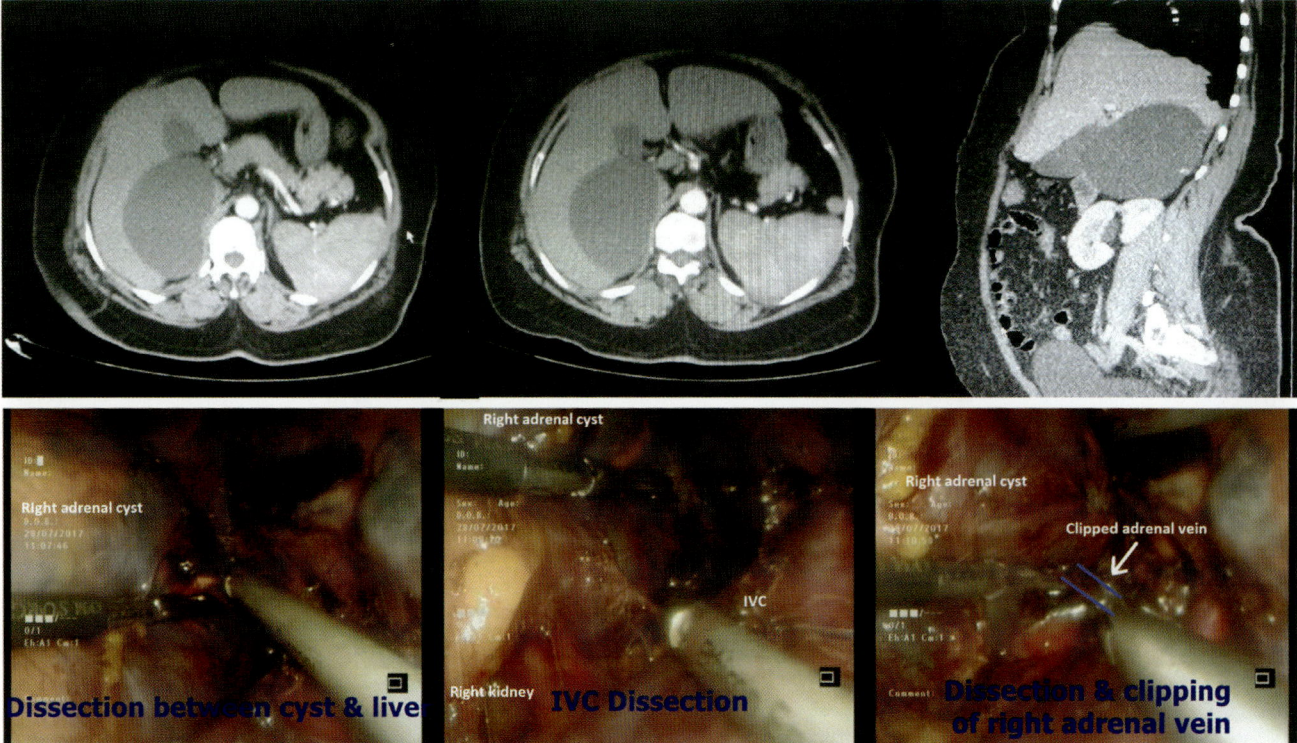

FIGURE 54.5 CT showing Right Adrenal Cyst, key steps of Laparoscopic Right Adrenalectomy.

Operative Approach to the Adrenal Gland Pathology

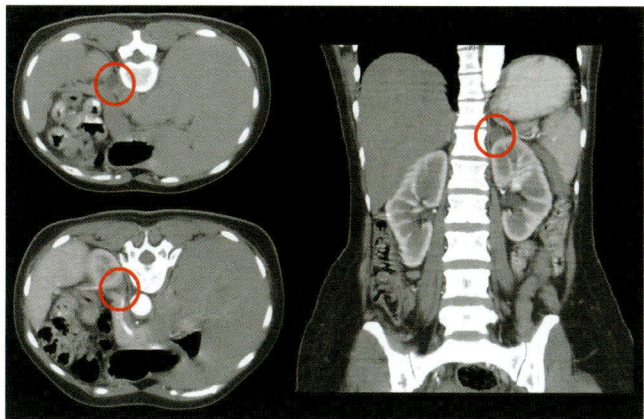

FIGURE 54.6 CT prior to a Left PRA.

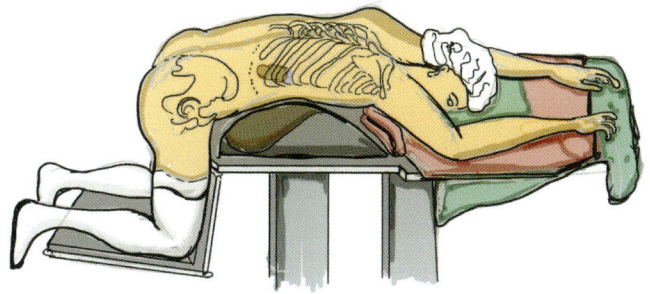

FIGURE 54.7 Patient position for PRA.

smaller tumors and is advantageous in patients with bilateral tumors or prior abdominal surgery. PRA is now the second most common surgical technique utilized for adrenalectomy. It has the advantage of being a more direct route to the adrenal gland without interference from intra-abdominal organs, using the retroperitoneal approach. Shorter operative times, lesser incidence of postoperative ileus, and reduced hospital stay with fewer postoperative fluid collections have been reported with this technique (16, 40–42). The major difficulties associated with the retroperitoneal approach are the learning curve, unfamiliar anatomy to most endocrine surgeons, restricted operative space, and difficult detection of anatomical landmarks that may cause longer operative times and increased carbon dioxide absorption (41, 43, 44). It can be technically challenging in tumors larger than 4–6 cm. Preoperative viewing of the axial CT films with 180-degree rotation helps orient the surgical approach, a left-sided Conn adenoma is depicted in Figure 54.6.

The patient is placed in the prone or jack-knife position, with the hips and knees flexed at 90-degree angles (Figure 54.7).

Access to the retroperitoneum begins with an incision just below the tip of 12th rib (39). A gloved finger is used to create adequate initial working space. Alternatively, a balloon trocar can be inserted and insufflated. Through the incision, a 10-mm trocar is inserted and a laparoscope is guided through to evaluate the retroperitoneal space. CO_2 is injected at 20-mmHg pressure to sustain an adequate retroperitoneal space. Additional trocars are inserted under finger guidance: A lateral 5-mm trocar is inserted under the tip of the 11th rib and another 5 mm/10 mm on 4-cm medial to the first trocar (Figure 54.8). Working space is enlarged by pushing down strands of fibro-fatty tissue anteriorly. Once the posterior surface of the kidney is identified, mobilization of the upper renal pole will allow visualization of the adrenal gland. For proper orientation and safe dissection, the operative field should show the diaphragm cranially, upper pole of kidney caudally, paraspinal muscles medially, and peritoneum laterally, with the muscles of the posterior abdominal wall constituting the roof. It is important to dissect the gland off of the kidney before dividing the superior and medial attachments. The adrenal gland is then mobilized medially and caudally.

On the right side, the vena cava may appear flattened and must be carefully dissected. The adrenal arteries may pass posterior to the vena cava and are ligated by electrocautery/vessel-sealing

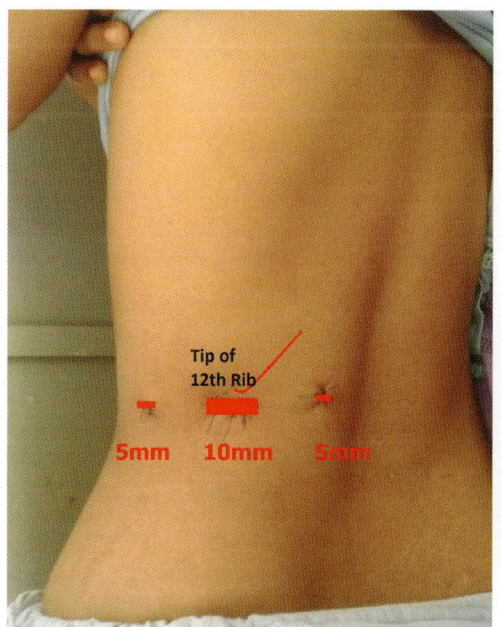
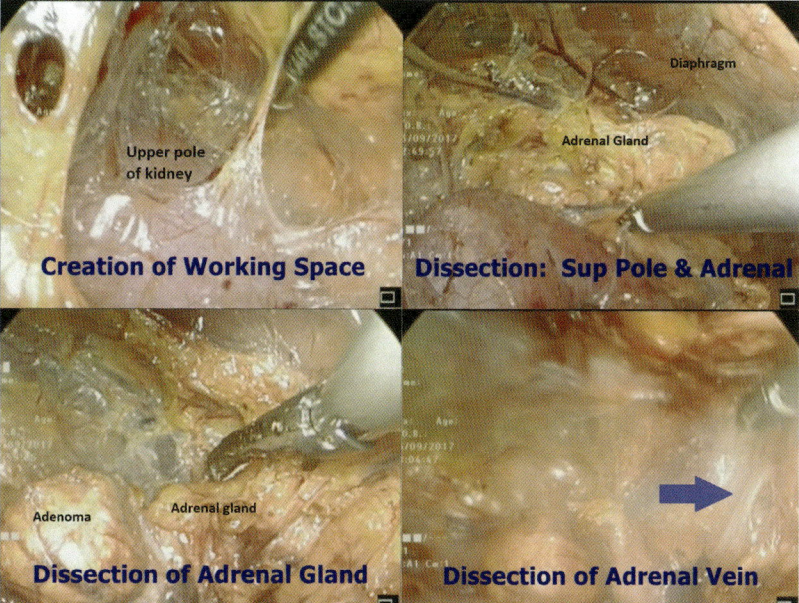

FIGURE 54.8 Port placement and steps of Left PRA.

devices or by clips. The short adrenal vein runs in a posterolateral direction and is skeletonized for at least 1 cm and then clipped and cut. Continued lateral and cranial dissection will completely free the right adrenal gland, which can be extracted in a bag through the central port.

On the left side, the left adrenal vein is isolated in the area between the left adrenal gland and diaphragmatic branch, which is medial to the upper pole of the left kidney. Early ligation of the left adrenal vein will permit traction using the stump to dissect the gland medially, laterally, and then cranially.

Delicate dissection and gentle traction using atraumatic instruments is necessary to avoid damaging of the adrenal capsule during PRA. A drain may be inserted through lateral port, but it is not routine. During surgery, the field may appear bloodless due to the higher insufflations pressure. After extraction of the specimen, pressure is gradually reduced to 8 mmHg to identify bleeding points.

Open adrenalectomy

Open adrenalectomy can be performed by anterior, lateral(flank), and posterior approaches.

It remains preferable to minimally invasive surgery patients with larger tumors and malignancy.

The most common open procedure performed is the *anterior transperitoneal approach* and can be done via different incisions – subcostal, Chevron, Makuuchi, and others. This approach is preferable if open surgery is indicated as it allows maximum visualization of vital structures like the vena cava. Self-retracting systems are invaluable and also free the hands of the assistant. Patient positioning must include placement of a pillow/linen roll below the tumor location.

On the right side, dissection starts with mobilization of the hepatic flexure and division of the triangular ligament with hepatic mobilization. Minimal duodenal kocherization may be required to visualize the vena cava. The parietal peritoneum is then opened to expose the right adrenal gland/tumor. The adrenal vein is carefully identified leaving the gland in a posterolateral direction and entering the IVC. In large tumors, the vena cava may be compressed and will require gentle dissection and retraction to the contralateral side.

On the left side, the splenic flexure and descending colon is first reflected medially by incising the white line of Toldt. The spleen is then mobilized and upper part of left kidney displayed, while protecting the tail of the pancreas. The adrenal gland is then mobilized from medial to lateral, with ligation of the arterial branches when encountered. The left adrenal vein leaves the gland at the inferomedial aspect and drains into the left renal vein. Renal hilar injury can occur in larger tumors and dissection of the hilum may be indicated prior to adrenal vein ligation.

The hand-assisted technique is a hybrid between the open and laparoscopic approach. For some, this technique is useful for large tumor removal with reduced surgical time (45).

The thoracoabdominal approach is made through a midline incision that extends into the chest through the 10th or 11th intercostal space. This approach provides good access, at the cost of increased morbidity. It is generally reserved for larger (>12 cm), invasive malignant tumors.

Robotic adrenalectomy

Although the benefits of laparoscopic adrenalectomy are well known, its drawbacks include the two-dimensional view, unstable camera platform, poor ergonomics, and rigid instrumentation. Subsequently, robotic technology has been recently introduced to join the armamentarium of minimally invasive adrenal surgery with capabilities of three-dimensional view, wristed instrument, and a stable camera platform (46). Since the first fully robotic adrenalectomy (RA) in 2002, many studies have shown the safety and efficacy of RA (47, 48). Transperitoneal and retroperitoneal RA approaches demonstrating the efficacy of both techniques have been described in several reports (49, 50). Current drawbacks, however, associated with RA include its cost, technical difficulty, need of advanced training, and a team with the technical expertise to ensure operative success (51–54). The steps of RA mirror those of laparoscopic/RA. Comparison between laparoscopic and RA outcomes is similar including operative time, postoperative complications, hospital stay, and conversion rate (55).

It is possible that, in the future, RA may assume an increased role in the management of adrenal disease. Research teams are dedicated to the development of robotic systems with greater intelligence and instruments with expanded capabilities, and it is essential that surgeons continue to evaluate these new technologies. The main limitation of robotic surgery has been the cost, availability, and additional learning.

Partial/cortical sparing adrenalectomy

During partial/cortical sparing adrenalectomy, the adrenal vein should be identified, but it is generally not ligated. The arterial supply is dealt with as routine. The gland is then transected at a site well away from the tumor using energy devices like ultrasonic shears, or clips.

Conclusions

Minimally invasive adrenalectomy is favored in the surgical treatment of adrenal tumors and is the standard of care at specialized medical centers worldwide. The choice of laparoscopic transabdominal or retroperitoneal adrenalectomy is strongly influenced by surgeon-related factors such as background, training, and skill. Two limiting issues that exist with minimally invasive approaches are the size of the adrenal mass and margin status in the case of malignant adrenal tumors. Newer techniques, such as robotic surgery, must show robust evidence-based superiority before they can replace conventional minimally invasive approaches.

References

1. Lombardi CP, De Crea C, Raffaelli M, Pennestri F. Surgical anatomy. In Valeri A, Bergamini C, Bellantone RDA, Lombardi CP (Eds.), *Surgery of the Adrenal Gland*. 2013;15–22. https://doi.org/10.1007/978-88-470-2586-8
2. Daunt N. Adrenal vein sampling: How to make it quick, easy, and successful. RadioGraphics 2005 25:suppl_1, S143–S158.
3. Ritchie JE, Balasubramanian S. Anatomy of the pituitary, thyroid, parathyroid and adrenal glands. Surgery. 2011; 29: 403–407.
4. Arnaldi G, Angeli A, Atkinson AB, Bertagna X, Cavagnini F, Chrousos GP, et al. Diagnosis and complications of Cushing's syndrome: A consensus statement. J Clin Endocrinol Metab. 2003;5593–602. Available from: https://pubmed.ncbi.nlm.nih.gov/14671138/.
5. Bravo EL, Tagle R. Pheochromocytoma: State-of-the-art and future prospects. Endocr Rev. 2003;24:539–53.
6. Singh PK, Buch HN. Adrenal incidentaloma: Evaluation and management. J Clin Pathol. 2008;61:1168–73.
7. Bovio S, Cataldi A, Reimondo G, Sperone P, Novello S, Berruti A, et al. Prevalence of adrenal incidentaloma in a contemporary computerized tomography series. J Endocrinol Invest. 2006;29(4):298–302.
8. Kapoor A, Morris T, Rebello R. Guidelines for the management of the incidentally discovered adrenal mass. J Can Urol Assoc. 2011;5(4):241–7.
9. Latronico AC, Chrousos GP. Extensive personal, experience: Adrenocortical tumors. J Clin Endocrinol Metab. 1997;82(5):1317–24.
10. Dackiw APB, Lee JE, Gagel RF, Evans DB. Adrenal cortical carcinoma. World J Surg. 2001;25(7):914–26.

11. Kebebew E, Duh QY. Benign and malignant pheochromocytoma: Diagnosis, treatment, and follow-up. Surg Oncol Clin North Am. 1998;7:765–89.
12. Boland GWL, Blake MA, Hahn PF, Mayo-Smith WW. Incidental adrenal lesions: Principles, techniques, and algorithms for imaging characterization. Radiology. 2008;249:756–75.
13. Hamrahian AH, Ioachimescu AG, Remer EM, Motta-Ramirez G, Bogabathina H, Levin HS, et al. Clinical utility of noncontrast computed tomography attenuation value (Hounsfield units) to differentiate adrenal adenomas/hyperplasias from nonadenomas: Cleveland clinic experience. J Clin Endocrinol Metab. 2005;90(2):871–7.
14. Sturgeon C, Shen WT, Clark OH, Duh QY, Kebebew E. Risk assessment in 457 adrenal cortical carcinomas: How much does tumor size predict the likelihood of malignancy? J Am Coll Surg. 2006;202(3):423–30.
15. Thompson LDR. Pheochromocytoma of the adrenal gland scaled score (PASS) to separate benign from malignant neoplasms: A clinicopathologic and immunophenotypic study of 100 cases. Am J Surg Pathol. 2002;26(5):551–66.
16. Fernández-Cruz L, Saenz A, Taura P, Benarroch G, Astudillo E, Sabater L. Retroperitoneal approach in laparoscopic adrenalectomy: Is it advantageous? Surg Endosc. 1999;13(1):86–90.
17. Machado NO, Al Qadhi H, Al Wahaibi K, Rizvi SG. Laparoscopic adrenalectomy for large adrenocortical carcinoma. J Soc Laparoendosc Surg. 2015;19(3):e2015.00036. https://doi.org/10.4293/JSLS.2015.00036
18. Porpiglia F, Miller BS, Manfredi M, Fiori C, Doherty GM. A debate on laparoscopic versus open adrenalectomy for adrenocortical carcinoma. Horm Cancer. 2011;2(6):372–7.
19. Kebebew E, Siperstein AE, Clark OH, Duh QY. Results of laparoscopic adrenalectomy for suspected and unsuspected malignant adrenal neoplasms. In: Archives of Surgery [Internet]. American Medical Association; 2002 [cited October 31, 2020]. pp. 948–53. Available from: https://pubmed.ncbi.nlm.nih.gov/12146996/.
20. Walz MK, Petersenn S, Koch JA, Mann K, Neumann HPH, Schmid KW. Endoscopic treatment of large primary adrenal tumours. Br J Surg. 2005;719–23. Available from: https://pubmed.ncbi.nlm.nih.gov/15856491/.
21. Palazzo FF, Sebag F, Sierra M, Ippolito G, Souteyrand P, Henry JF. Long-term outcome following laparoscopic adrenalectomy for large solid adrenal cortex tumors. World J Surg. 2006;30(5):893–8.
22. Ramacciato G, Mercantini P, La Torre M, Di Benedetto F, Ercolani G, Ravaioli M, et al. Is laparoscopic adrenalectomy safe and effective for adrenal masses larger than 7 cm? Surg Endosc Other Interv Tech. 2008;22(2):516–21.
23. Kim SH, Brennan MF, Russo P, Burt ME, Coit DG. The role of surgery in the treatment of clinically isolated adrenal metastasis. Cancer. 1998;82(2):389–94.
24. Corcione F, Miranda L, Marzano E, Capasso P, Cuccurullo D, Settembre A, et al. Laparoscopic adrenalectomy for malignant neoplasm: Our experience in 15 cases. Surg Endosc Other Interv Tech. 2005;19(6):841–4.
25. Chuan-Yu S, Yat-Faat H, Wei-Hong D, Yuan-Cheng G, Qing-Feng H, Ke X, et al. Laparoscopic adrenalectomy for adrenal tumors. Int J Endocrinol. 2014;2014:241854. https://doi.org/10.1155/2014/241854
26. Pędziwiatr M, Wierdak M, Natkaniec M, Matłok M, Białas M, Major P, et al. Laparoscopic transperitoneal lateral adrenalectomy for malignant and potentially malignant adrenal tumours. BMC Surg 15, 101 (2015). https://doi.org/10.1186/s12893-015-0088-z
27. Cobb WS, Kercher KW, Sing RF, Heniford BT. Laparoscopic adrenalectomy for malignancy. Am J Surg. 2005;189(4):405–11.
28. Zografos GN, Vasiliadis G, Farfaras AN, Aggeli C, Digalakis M. Laparoscopic surgery for malignant adrenal tumors. J Soc Laparoendosc Surg. 2009;13(2):196–202.
29. Donatini G, Caiazzo R, Do Cao C, Aubert S, Zerrweck C, El-Kathib Z, et al. Long-term survival after adrenalectomy for stage I/II adrenocortical carcinoma (ACC): A retrospective comparative cohort study of laparoscopic versus open approach. Ann Surg Oncol. 2014;21(1):284–91.
30. Porpiglia F, Fiori C, Daffara F, Zaggia B, Bollito E, Volante M, et al. Retrospective evaluation of the outcome of open versus laparoscopic adrenalectomy for stage I and II adrenocortical cancer. Eur Urol. 2010;57(5):873–8.
31. Fosså A, Rosok BI, Kazaryan AM, Holte HJ, Brennhovd B, Westerheim O, et al. Laparoscopic versus open surgery in stage I-III adrenocortical carcinoma-a retrospective comparison of 32 patients. Acta Oncol. 2013;52(8):1771–7.
32. Lombardi CP, Raffaelli M, De Crea C, Boniardi M, De Toma G, Marzano LA, et al. Open versus endoscopic adrenalectomy in the treatment of localized (stage I/II) adrenocortical carcinoma: Results of a multiinstitutional Italian survey. Surgery. 2012;152(6):1158–64.
33. Gagner M, Lacroix A, Bolté E. Laparoscopic adrenalectomy in Cushing's syndrome and pheochromocytoma. N Engl J Med. 1992;327(14):1033.
34. Lee J, El-Tamer M, Schifftner T, Turrentine FE, Henderson WG, Khuri S, et al. Open and laparoscopic adrenalectomy: Analysis of the National Surgical Quality Improvement Program. J Am Coll Surg. 2008;206(5):953–9.
35. Assalia A, Gagner M. Laparoscopic adrenalectomy. Br J Surg. 2004;91:1259–74.
36. Cianci P, Fersini A, Tartaglia N, Ambrosi A, Neri V, Lizzi V, et al. Are there differences between the right and left laparoscopic adrenalectomy? Our experience. Ann Ital Chir. 2016;87(3):242–6.
37. Takeda M. Laparoscopic adrenalectomy: Transperitoneal vs retroperitoneal approaches. Biomed Pharmacother. 2000;54(Suppl. 1):207s–10s.
38. Lezoche E, Guerrieri M, Paganini AM, Feliciotti F, Zenobi P, Antognini F, et al. Laparoscopic adrenalectomy by the anterior transperitoneal approach: Results of 108 operations in unselected cases. Surg Endosc. 2000;14(10):920–5.
39. Walz MK, Alesina PF, Wenger FA, Deligiannis A, Szuczik E, Petersenn S, et al. Posterior retroperitoneoscopic adrenalectomy-results of 560 procedures in 520 patients. Surgery. 2006;140(6):943–50.
40. Fernández-Cruz L, Saenz A, Benarroch G, Astudillo E, Taura P, Sabater L. Laparoscopic unilateral and bilateral adrenalectomy for Cushing's syndrome: Transperitoneal and retroperitoneal approaches. Ann Surg. 1996;224(6):727–36.
41. Chiu AW. Laparoscopic retroperitoneal adrenalectomy: Clinical experience with 120 consecutive cases. Asian J Surg. 2003;26(3):139–44.
42. Bonjer HJ, Sorm V, Berends FJ, Kazemier G, Steyerberg EW, De Herder WW, et al. Endoscopic retroperitoneal adrenalectomy: Lessons learned from 111 consecutive cases. Ann Surg. 2000;232(6):796–803.
43. Fazeli-Matin S, Gill IS, Hsu THS, Sung GT, Novick AC. Laparoscopic renal and adrenal surgery in obese patients: Comparison to open surgery. J Urol. 1999;162(3I):665–9.
44. Wolf JS, Monk TG, McDougall EM, McClennan BL, Clayman RV. The extraperitoneal approach and subcutaneous emphysema are associated with greater absorption of carbon dioxide during laparoscopic renal surgery. J Urol. 1995;154(3):959–63.
45. Bennett IC, Ray M. Hand-assisted laparoscopic adrenalectomy: An alternative minimal invasive surgical technique for the adrenal gland. ANZ J Surg. 2002;72(11):801–5.
46. Horgan S, Vanuno D. Robots in laparoscopic surgery. J Laparoendosc Adv Surg Tech A. 2001;11(6):415–9.
47. Hyams ES, Stifelman MD. The role of robotics for adrenal pathology. Curr Opin Urol. 2009;19(1):89–96.
48. Young JA, Chapman WHH, Kim VB, Albrecht RJ, Ng PC, Nifong LW, et al. Robotic-assisted adrenalectomy for adrenal incidentaloma: Case and review of the technique. Surg Laparosc Endosc Percutan Tech. 2002;12(2):126–30.
49. Desai MM, Gill IS, Kaouk JH, Matin SF, Sung GT, Bravo EL. Robotic-assisted laparoscopic adrenalectomy. Urology. 2002;60(6):1104–7.
50. Berber E, Mitchell J, Milas M, Siperstein A. Robotic posterior retroperitoneal adrenalectomy: Operative technique. Arch Surg. 2010;145(8):781–4.
51. Merseburger AS, Herrmann TRW, Shariat SF, Kyriazis I, Nagele U, Traxer O, et al. EAU guidelines on robotic and single-site surgery in urology. Eur Urol. 2013;64(2):277–91.
52. Brunaud L, Bresler L, Ayav A, Zarnegar R, Raphoz AL, Levan T, et al. Robotic-assisted adrenalectomy: What advantages compared to lateral transperitoneal laparoscopic adrenalectomy? Am J Surg. 2008;195(4):433–8.
53. Winter JM, Talamini MA, Stanfield CL, Chang DC, Hundt JD, Dackiw AP, et al. Thirty robotic adrenalectomies: A single institution's experience. Surg Endosc Other Interv Tech. 2006;20(1):119–24.
54. Taskin HE, Berber E. Robotic adrenalectomy. Cancer J. 2013;19:162–6.
55. Brandao LF, Autorino R, Laydner H, Haber GP, Ouzaid I, De Sio M, et al. Robotic versus laparoscopic adrenalectomy: A systematic review and meta-analysis. Eur Urol. 2014;65:1154–61.

55

PANCREAS
Embryology, Anatomy and Endocrine Physiology

Rahul, Puneet and Sanjeev Kumar

Introduction

Pancreas is a heterocrine organ (endocrine as well as exocrine function). Owing to its retroperitoneal and difficult location, it was labeled as a forbidden structure till the early 20th century. Greeks were the first to acknowledge pancreas as a distinct organ. Eristratos, at around 300 BC, mentioned it in his description of abdominal organs. The name *"Pancreas"* was again given by a great Greek anatomist, Rufus of Ephesus in 100 AD, meaning *"Pan: all"* and *"Kreas: flesh or meat"*. In the 16th century, David Edwards suggested that pancreas served to provide support to lymphovascular channels and Vesalius in his illustrations professed it as an unintelligible organ. It was only in 1642 that its glandular structure could be established by Wirsung. He gave the description of the main pancreatic duct (MPD). This was followed by the discovery of the junction of the pancreatic and bile duct at duodenal papilla. Ampulla was first described by Bidloo in 1685 and later by Vater in 1720. Santorini described the major and minor papilla in 1724 (1,2).

In 1664, de Graff was the first to observe pancreatic juice from a pancreatic fistula in dogs. He cannulated the pancreatic duct in dogs and conducted studies on pancreatic secretion. The specific digestive functions were established later by Eberle (fat emulsification), Purkinje (proteolysis) and Valentin (digestion of starch) in the 19th century. In 1905, Pavlov received Nobel Prize for his work on digestion. The discovery of endocrine function of pancreas was an accident. In 1889, Mering and Minkowski observed that pancreatectomized dogs developed diabetes and blood glucose was under the control of some substance produced in pancreas. This was later found to be produced in the island of cells described as "Islets" by Langerhans. De Meyer, in 1909, named this substance "insulin". In 1923, Canadian scientists Banting, Charles Best and Macleod received Nobel Prize for isolating insulin from the pancreas of dogs. Later in 1958, another Nobel laureate, Sanger described the structure of the hormone. Other hormones secreted by the islets were discovered subsequently (3–5).

Development of pancreas

Pancreas develops from two primordia. On the 26th day of gestation, the dorsal pancreatic bud arises from the dorsal aspect of the foregut endoderm. Ventral bud is an offshoot from the hepatic diverticulum on day 32. In the sixth week, the ventral mesentery of ventral bud disappears. The bud rotates around the duodenum to fuse with the dorsal bud (Figures 55.1 and 55.2). Finally, the duodenum and pancreas take a retroperitoneal position.

With fusion of the two pancreatic buds, both the ducts anastomose. The MPD or duct of Wirsung is formed by the duct of ventral pancreas and the distal portion of the duct of dorsal pancreas. Duct of Santorini (accessory duct) is the proximal duct of the dorsal pancreas. The dorsal pancreas gives rise to the tail, body and superior segment of the pancreatic head, while the ventral pancreatic bud develops into the uncinate process and the inferior portion of the head. The secretory acini and the islet of Langerhans appear by the end of the third month. Critical events in the development of pancreas are rotation and fusion. Malrotation of the ventral bud results in annular pancreas, while the anomalies in fusion may produce different ductal patterns (6, 7).

Congenital anomalies

Annular pancreas

It is a thin band of pancreatic tissue around the second part of duodenum. The band may be free from the duodenum or infiltrating the muscularis. It contains a large duct, which usually opens into the MPD. The incidence is reported as 1 in 1000 on abdominal imaging. The pathogenesis involves genetic factors as it occurs in siblings and offsprings. It is also associated with other congenital anomalies like trisomy 21, malrotation and cardiovascular or genitourinary aberrations (8). The exact mechanism is not known. Some scientists propose early fusion of the tip of ventral pancreatic bud with the dorsal bud, while others propose the division of the ventral bud into two before rotation into opposite directions.

Clinically, half of them present with polyhydramnios on prenatal ultrasound or recurrent non-bilious vomiting and feed intolerance due to duodenal obstruction post delivery. The second peak of presentation is evident in the fourth to seventh decade as pain abdomen, fullness or pancreatitis. At times, the diagnosis is made at laparotomy (9). The treatment of choice as proposed by Gross and Chisolm remains duodenoduodenostomy (10). Annular pancreas carries a high risk for pancreaticobiliary and duodenal neoplasia. Hence, few authors suggest regular screening.

Ectopic and accessory pancreas

Heterotopic pancreas could be detected in 2% of autopsies as stated by Pearson et al. (11). Nearly 6% of Meckel's diverticula contain pancreatic tissue. Common locations include stomach, duodenum and small intestine. They are rarely seen in the colon, gallbladder, omentum and mesentery. Most of them are functional and have an independent blood supply. Islet cells are often present in the ectopic pancreas in the stomach and duodenum (12). Usually asymptomatic, they can present with bleeding, ulcers, intussusception, pancreatitis or malignancy. Incidental detection of ectopic pancreas during exploration does not warrant intervention.

Pancreas divisum (PD)

Failure of fusion of the ventral and dorsal ducts results in pancreas divisum (PD). As a result, the small duct of Santorini drains the head, body and tail through the minor papilla, while the uncinate

Pancreas

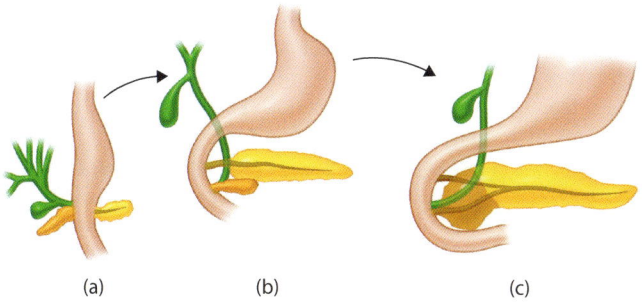

FIGURE 55.1 Embryonic development of pancreas (a) formation of ventral and dorsal pancreatic primordia, (b) rotation of ventral pancreas, (c) fusion of primordia to form an adult pancreas.

drains into the major papilla through the duct of Wirsung. In various autopsy and endoscopic retrograde cholangiopancreatography (ERCP) series, the incidence of PD in asymptomatic patients has been reported to be more than 5% (13). It accounts for 26% of the cases of recurrent pancreatitis (14). Secretin-enhanced magnetic resonance cholangiopancreatography (MRCP) is a useful investigation for the diagnosis. Minor papilla sphincterotomy or ductal stenting is effective in more than three-fourth of the patients with recurrent pancreatitis (15).

Rare pancreatic anomalies

Pancreatic agenesis is very rare and incompatible with life. Congenital short pancreas, wherein the dorsal pancreas fails to develop, has been associated with polysplenia and malrotation (16). Congenital pancreatic cysts are true cysts (epithelial lining), often located in the tail of pancreas. They can be solitary or multiple. They are usually asymptomatic and incidentally detected (17).

Pancreaticobiliary maljunction (PBM)

It is a congenital anomaly, wherein the pancreatic and bile ducts join outside the duodenal wall, forming a long common channel. The average length of the common channel is 4.4 mm (1–12). When pancreaticobiliary junction lies outside the wall, the sphincter function is lost. Reciprocal reflux of bile and pancreatic juice occurs. Hydropressure within the pancreatic duct being higher than the bile duct, the reflux of pancreatic juice into the biliary system is more frequent. This results in premalignant changes (epithelial hyperplasia and k-ras mutation) and higher incidence of malignancy in the bile duct and gallbladder (10%) (18, 19). The pancreaticobiliary maljunction (PBM) has been classified by Komi et al. (20) into three types:

- Type 1 or CP type – common bile duct (CBD) joins the PD at right angle
- Type 2 or PC type – PD joins the CBD at acute angle
- Type 3 – patent accessory duct with or without a complex matrix of ducts

Type 1 and 2 are subclassified into 'a' and 'b' based on dilation or normal caliber of the common channel. Komi et al. documented the prevalence of Type 1, 2 and 3 to be 35%, 22% and 43%, respectively. Similar distribution has been reported in other major series from Japan, while studies from India and other countries have documented low prevalence of Type 3 (~2%) (21).

The CP type is commonly associated with choledochal cysts, while the PC type is associated with gallbladder malignancy and recurrent pancreatitis. PBM may or may not be associated with biliary tract dilatation (choledochal cyst, i.e. CBD > 10 mm). PBM without CBD dilatation is termed "forme fruste" and is closely associated with the development of gall bladder cancer (22).

Pancreatic anatomy

Pancreas is a J-shaped organ that extends transversely from the C-loop of the duodenum to the splenic hilum. It is a retroperitoneal structure at the level of the first and second lumbar vertebrae. It is soft in consistency and pinkish tan in color. The surface appears lobulated to naked eyes. It weighs around 100 g in adult males, 85 g in females and 5 g in a neonate. The length varies from 14 to 18 cm, width from 2 to 9 cm and height from 2 to 3 cm in an adult. The pancreas is composed of 71% water and 13% proteins. The fatty composition varies from 3% to 20%. Specific gravity is 1.04. It is traversed by numerous vascular structures. It lies in close relation to stomach anteriorly, duodenum on the right, spleen and left kidney on the left and major abdominal vessels posteriorly. It is divided into four parts: head and uncinate, neck, body and tail extending from right to left.

Head is the flat portion of pancreas that lies within the duodenal curve. The superior, lateral and inferior margins are lined by the first, second and third parts of duodenum, respectively. The anterior surface is related to the transverse colon and mesocolon, while the posterior surface is in close relation to the inferior

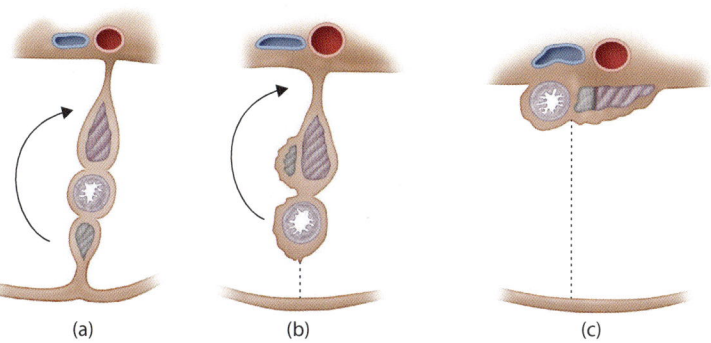

FIGURE 55.2 Rotation of duodenum and pancreas (a) primitive rotation of dorsal and ventral pancreatic primordia, (b) rotation of ventral pancreas, (c) duodenum and pancreas become retroperitoneal organ.

vena cava, right renal vein, right gonadal vessel, right crus and the distal CBD. The CBD may lie on the posterior surface in a groove (15%) or remain embedded (partially/totally) in the parenchyma (85%), inseparable from the pancreas and the duodenum. Osler poetically described this region as the abdominal area of romance, where "the pancreatic head lies folded in arms of duodenum". Any pathology in the head of pancreas requiring its complete excision mandates the removal of duodenum and distal CBD and vice versa. Moreover, lesions in the head tend to involve or compress the bile ducts and result in proximal dilatation of the bile duct as well as the pancreatic duct (5).

The **uncinate process** is a small hook-like projection from the head of pancreas. The word uncinate is derived from the Latin word "uncinatus", which means a hook. It is variable in size, lies between the inferior vena cava (IVC) and aorta and covers the superior mesenteric vessels posteriorly. It may be absent in around 10% cases. When the uncinate process ends near the superior mesenteric vein (SMV), a dense ligament fixes it to the superior mesenteric artery (SMA). A mass in the uncinate process, hence, is often difficult to dissect off the major vessels.

Neck of the pancreas is a narrow segment of 1.5–2 cm between the head and body of pancreas. Anteriorly, it is related to the peritoneal layer of the posterior wall of lesser sac and pylorus. The right border is marked by the origin of the anterosuperior pancreaticoduodenal artery (ASPDA) from the gastroduodenal artery (GDA). The left border is not clearly defined. The posterior surface is related to the SMV and splenic vein (SV) joining to form the portal vein (PV). Behind the neck, the PV receives pancreatic tributaries from the right and left gastric vein and in one-third cases, inferior mesenteric vein (IMV) from the left. In majority, anterior surface of the vein is devoid of pancreatic tributaries. The dissection of the neck over the veins is a critical step in pancreatic head resection and necessitates careful ligation of the tributaries on the right.

The **body** of pancreas extends from the neck toward the left and blends into the tapering tail without a distinct boundary. It is triangular on cross section. The anterior surface is covered by a double layer of peritoneum of the greater omentum that separates it from the stomach. The inferior surface is also covered by the peritoneum that separates it from the duodenojejunal flexure, proximal small intestine and the splenic flexure of colon. The posterior surface is related to the aorta with the origin of SMA, SV, left kidney, adrenal and left renal vessels. Over the anterior surface, a projection of pancreatic tissue is often seen, a little to the neck. This is termed *tuber omentale*. The mid-part of the body overlies the lumbar vertebrae, which makes it most susceptible to injury in blunt abdominal trauma.

The pancreas can be divided into two anatomicosurgical segments. This was described by Busnardo et al. (23) in 1988 based on corrosion casts of pancreas from 30 adult cadavers. An area of paucivascular plane divides the pancreas near the neck and body junction, just to the left of aortomesenteric angle into right (cephalocervical) and left (corporocaudate) segments. The right segment is supplied by the branches from GDA and SMA, while the left segment is supplied by the branches from the splenic artery (SA) (details of arterial supply are described further in arterial supply). The two segments are linked by two arteries (right branch of dorsal pancreatic artery [DPA], a branch of SA and a branch of ASPDA) and a pancreatic duct. Transection of the parenchyma during surgery in this plane after ligation of the two vessels negates the chances of a major bleed. The two segments can be used separately for split pancreatic transplant as well (23).

The **tail** of pancreas lies between the two layers of lienorenal ligament. It is 2–3.5 cm in length and is a relatively mobile structure. It extends up to the splenic hilum and is closely related to the splenic vessels. Careful dissection is imperative during splenectomy to avoid injury to the tail.

Mesopancreas has evolved as a surgical concept rather a true anatomical structure. It was first proposed by Gockel et al. in correlation to the clinical outcomes of total mesorectal excision in rectal cancer (24). Unlike the mesorectum, which is bound by distinct fascia containing the superior rectal artery, nerves and lymphatic tissues, mesopancreas lacks a fascial envelope. There is an absence of a holy plane of dissection around the mesopancreas. Rather, it is an anatomical space bound by the head of pancreas anteriorly, posterior lateral mesopancreas (loose areolar tissue between pancreatic head and IVC) and the mesopancreatic root (relatively denser tissue between pancreas and aorta) posteriorly. The left border is marked by the line joining celiac axis (CA) and SMA. The right border is formed by the second part of duodenum. Superior boundary is formed by the hepatic artery and the inferior by the third part of the duodenum. Mesopancreas contains blood vessels, lymphatics and nerve sheaths. During embryological development, as the pancreatic bud rotates, the inferior pancreaticoduodenal artery (IPDA) from SMA grows along the groove of the duodenum and the pancreas as well as develops a network with GDA. Hence, CA and SMA are considered the intramesopancreatic structures, but full circle dissection of the same during surgery for the head of pancreas malignancy is not routinely warranted (25). Total mesopancreatic resection (TMpE) includes the en bloc excision of the structures within the above defined boundary and dissection of the right semicircumference of SMA and CA. It is safe, increases the R0 resection rate and decreases the blood loss (26).

Ductal anatomy

The MPD begins from the tail of pancreas. It runs through the tail and body halfway between the superior and the inferior borders, but close to the posterior surface. It receives 15–20 tributaries in the body and neck at regular intervals almost at 90°, forming a "herringbone pattern". In the head, the duct turns caudal and posterior, toward the CBD. It joins the CBD in 85% of cases to form a common channel (Type 1). This opens into the second part of duodenum at the major papilla. Papilla is a projection on the posteromedial wall of the duodenum (3–4 in. from the pylorus), where the longitudinal mucosal fold meets a transverse fold to form a **T**. The common pancreaticobiliary channel has a dilatation below the junction called the ampulla of Vater, which is present in 75% of Type 1. Rest has a septum reaching up to the papilla preventing the formation of ampulla. Michels described two other variants: pancreatic and bile ducts opening separately on the major papilla but close to each other (Type 2 – 5%) and the two openings exist at two different points on the duodenum (Type 3 – 9%) (27–29).

Accessory/minor PD (duct of Santorini) is present in 70% of the population. It drains the anterosuperior part of the head into the minor duodenal papilla (2 cm proximal to the major papilla) or the MPD. The accessory duct lies anterior to the CBD. A number of variants of the minor and the major duct have been described (30).

The MPD varies in diameter across the length. It is the widest in the head. The normal diameter described in literature varies from 3.1–4.8 mm in the head to 2–3.5 mm in the body and 0.9–2.4 mm in the tail of pancreas. The upper normal limits in the head and body are 5 and 4 mm, respectively (5, 31).

Pancreas

The ducts follow an oblique course through the duodenal wall. Average diameter of the ducts within the wall gets reduced. Hence, the gallstones usually get lodged in the bile duct rather than the common channel. Only 3.5% of individuals have the dimensions of ampulla of Vater appropriate enough for small stones to slip in. Impaction of stone into the ampulla or passage of stone through the ampulla resulting in bile reflux is one of the explanations for the development of biliary pancreatitis. Additional factors do play a role (32, 33). In normal circumstances, ampulla has mucosal folds that form mucosal valves. They allow passage of fluid into the duodenum but prevent backflow. During passage of a gallstone through the ampulla or the impaction of the same, this mechanism gets compromised. It may allow duodenal contents, capable of activating pancreatic enzymes into the pancreatic duct.

The smooth muscles surrounding the ducts in the duodenal wall form a sphincter complex. This comprises four sphincters well-described by Boyden. The length varies from 6 to 30 mm, and at times, extends beyond the duodenal wall. This includes superior choledochal sphincter and inferior choledochal sphincter around the CBD; sphincter ampullae and the sphincter pancreaticus (Figure 55.3).

Arterial supply

The pancreas, like the duodenum, develops at the junction of foregut and midgut, hence, has a dual supply from the branches of both the major splanchnic vessels – the CA and the SMA. It has a rich blood supply with frequent variations. The head of pancreas and the C-loop of duodenum are perfused by two pancreaticoduodenal arterial arcades. They are invariably present in pairs (anterior and posterior). The superior arteries (anterior or posterior superior pancreaticoduodenal) originate from the branches of celiac trunk (GDA, a branch of common hepatic artery) and the inferior vessels (anterior or posterior inferior pancreaticoduodenal) branch from the SMA. The arcades run close to the medial border of the duodenum. Division of these arcades is imperative in pancreatic head resection, but it leads to duodenal ischemia. Hence, the duodenum is invariably removed with the head. In the case of head coring for chronic pancreatitis, a thin rim of tissue close to the duodenal wall is left intact to preserve the blood supply to the duodenal loop.

The body and tail of the pancreas are supplied by branches from the SA, which runs on the superior border. The DPA arises at the origin of the SA from CA. It gives a right branch that anastomoses with the posterior arcade in the head of pancreas. Branches from the DPA (1, 2) run leftward and supply the body and tail of pancreas. They anastomose with the caudal pancreatic artery that arises from the left gastroepiploic or the distal SA. All the major pancreatic vessels run posterior to the duct (Figure 55.4).

Various arterial anomalies have been described in literature. Anomalous right hepatic artery (accessory or replaced) arises from the SMA in 26% of cases (34). Such an artery courses through the head and neck behind the PV. Anomalous common hepatic artery (CHA) may arise from the SMA in 2%–4% of patients and follow a similar course (35). These aberrations need to be recognized on preoperative imaging and the vessels carefully dissected during head resections in order to avoid postoperative liver failure. Anomalous middle colic artery has also been described in literature arising from the DPA or inferior pancreaticoduodenal, but coursing through the head of pancreas.

A thorough understanding of the arterial network and anomalies is prudent during pancreatic resection. There are three points of arterial control to minimize bleeding. The right gastric, GDA and supraduodenal artery need to be controlled as a first step of pancreaticoduodenal resection. These arteries are the branches of CHA, arising just above and beyond the pylorus. The surgeon should be careful during ligation of GDA as it may be confused

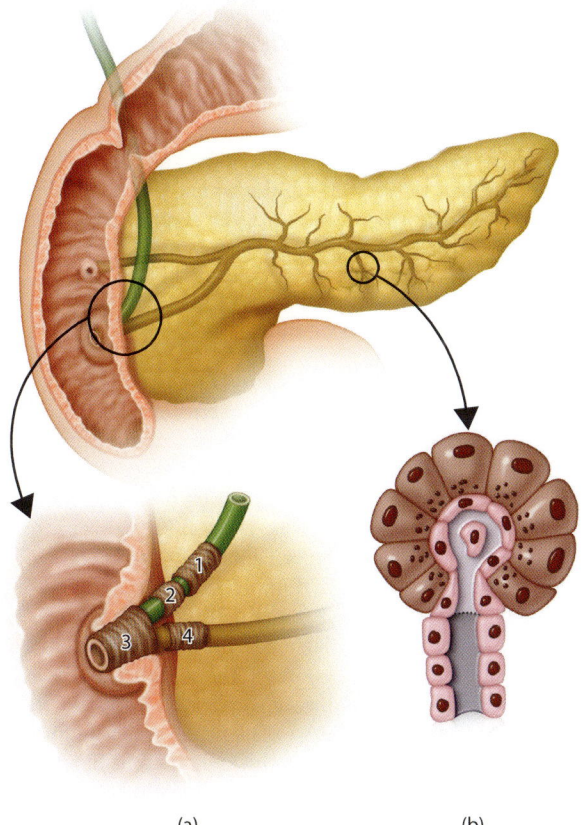

FIGURE 55.3 (a) The four sphincters of Boyden: (1) Superior choledochal, (2) Inferior choledochal, (3) Sphincter ampullae and (4) Sphincter pancreaticus. (b) Functional unit of pancreas – acinus.

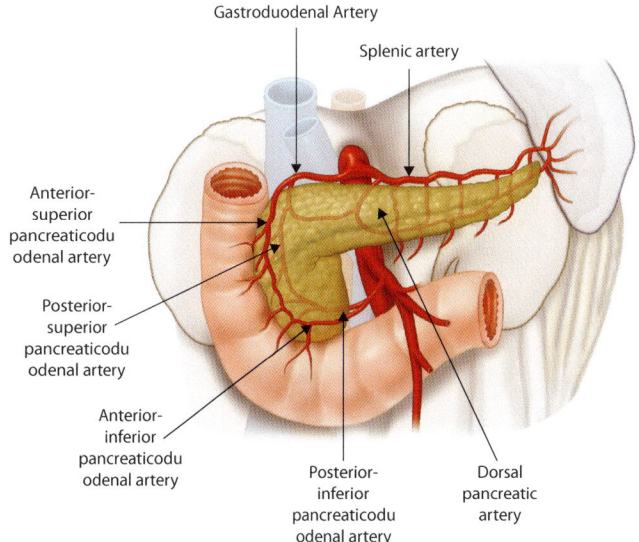

FIGURE 55.4 Arterial supply of the pancreas: (1) gastroduodenal artery, (2) dorsal pancreatic artery, and (3) splenic artery.

with the aberrant hepatic artery. The transverse pancreatic arteries and the DPA can be easily controlled before pancreatic section by simple stitch ligature on the inferior and superior borders of the gland. The third point of control is the inferior pancreaticoduodenal arteries. They leave the SMA to enter the uncinate process behind the SMV. They can be ligated during uncinate mobilization.

Venous drainage

Pancreatic veins run parallel to the corresponding arteries but lie superficial to them. They terminate into the PV, SV, SMV and IMV. In the head and uncinate, the four pancreaticoduodenal veins (PDVs) form arcades similar to the arteries. The anterosuperior PDV vein joins the right gastroepiploic vein. It is joined by the middle colic vein to form the common gastrocolic trunk, which drains into SMV. The posterosuperior PDV drains into the PV on the superior margin. Both the inferior PDVs drain into the SMV. Most of the pancreatic tributaries drain into the SMV or the PV from the right or the left borders. The anterior surface is usually avascular as described in the previous section (36). Venous tributaries from the neck, body and tail of pancreas drain into the SV above and the transverse pancreatic vein below. The latter terminates into the SMV or IMV. Occasionally, it drains into the SV or the gastrocolic vein. The IMV drains into the SV in one-third. In another third, it joins the SMV, and in the rest, it terminates at the junction of the SMV and SV (Figure 55.5).

Pancreatic siphon: Intra-pancreatic venous channels, measuring 1–3 mm, exist in normal individuals. They connect the PV to the SV running through the pancreatic parenchyma. In response to elevated pressure in portosplenic circulation due to PV or SV thrombosis, or due to cirrhosis, they dilate in order to decompress the respective systems. It holds special importance following distal splenorenal shunt (DSRS) for portal hypertension in cirrhotics. These dilated channels develop 1–3 years following DSRS and are responsible for the loss of the selectivity of the shunt. In long term, it leads to progressive worsening of liver functions, especially in alcoholic cirrhotics. The reason stated is decreased hepatopetal flow and hepatotropic factors (insulin, pancreatic hormones) reaching the liver. Ligation of coronary vein and splenopancreatic disconnection reduces the incidence of liver decompensation by maintaining the selectivity of the shunt (37, 38).

Lymphatic drainage

The lymphatics of the pancreas arise from the perilobular region and follow the vessels to drain into five main lymph node (LN) groups described by Cubilla et al. (39): superior, inferior, anterior, posterior and splenic nodes (39) (Figure 55.5). **Superior nodes** receive afferent vessels from the upper half of head and body of pancreas. They include superior head/body nodes along the superior border. Some of the lymphatics from this region may terminate in the hepatic chain (station 8) or gastropancreatic fold nodes. **Inferior nodes** run along the inferior border of the head and body and drain the inferior half of anterior and posterior surfaces of the same area. They may further extend into the superior mesenteric (station 14) and the left lateroaortic group of LNs. **Anterior nodes** includes the infrapyloric (station 6) and anterior pancreaticoduodenal (station 17) LNs. They drain the anterior surface of the head of pancreas and may extend into the superior mesenteric and the root of mesentery group of nodes. **Posterior group** of nodes receive lymphatics from the posterior surface of the head. They comprise the posterior pancreaticoduodenal (station 13), CBD (station 12b) and the right lateroaortic (station 16) LNs. The lymphatics from the tail of the pancreas terminate into the **splenic group** of nodes (splenic hilum, pancreaticolienal ligament, superior and inferior borders of tail of pancreas).

There are various studies on the pattern of lymphatic drainage of pancreas. It is complex and overlapping. No communication prevails between pancreas and the greater or lesser curvature of the stomach. Lymphatics from the head and body never drain into the splenic group or the tail region. In rare circumstances, the tail of pancreas does drain into superior and inferior groups of nodes. The lymphatics from the right of the pancreas terminate onto the right half of the origin of CA and SMA, while those from the left half terminate into the nodes on the left of the two major arteries. They then drain into the abdominal aortic nodes and finally the thoracic duct (39–41).

Innervation

The nerve fibers in the pancreas run close to the blood vessels. The sympathetic supply is from the greater (T5–T9) and the lesser (T9–T10) splanchnic nerves. They contain preganglionic neurons, which pierce the diaphragm and enter the celiac ganglion and plexus, to synapse with the cell bodies of postganglionic efferent fibers to the pancreas. The afferent neurons from the organ cross the midline at the celiac plexus. Their cell bodies are located in the dorsal root ganglion. Here, they may synapse with the somatic sensory fibers. Parasympathetic supply to the pancreas is through the celiac division of the vagus. It contains afferent (preganglionic with cell bodies in the brain) as well as efferent fibers (dendrites of cell bodies in the brain). Both the divisions contain efferent (motor) fibers to the vessel walls, acini and the PD. They also carry pain signals through afferent fibers. During pancreatic inflammation, especially in chronic pancreatitis, the perineurium is damaged allowing biologically active materials to come in contact with endoneurium and stimulate them. In the case of pancreatic tumors, direct invasion of nerve fibers by the tumor produces pain (42, 43).

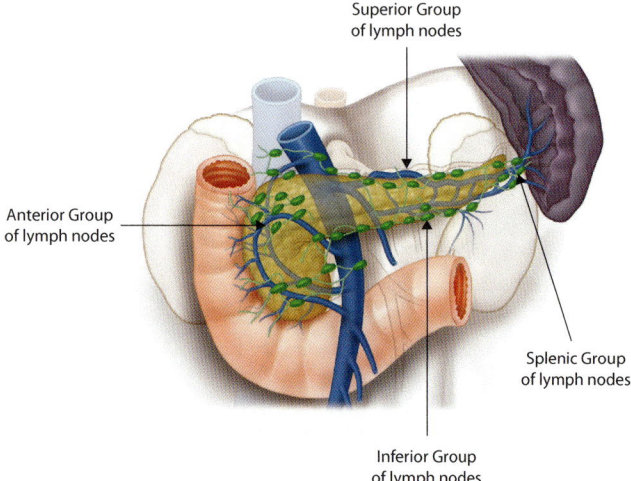

FIGURE 55.5 Venous and lymphatic drainage of pancreas with all the lymph nodes: (1) superior group, (2) inferior group, (3) splenic group, (4) anterior group, and (5) posterior group.

Pancreas

Histology

The pancreas is made up of lobules divided by connective tissue. Each lobule is composed of spherical or tubular group of cells called acinus. It forms the basic functional unit of exocrine pancreas and comprises the major bulk (80%) of the pancreas. Scattered among these acini are specialized cluster of cells called islets of Langerhans, responsible for the endocrine function. Acinus (Latin word for berry) is the functional unit, which synthesizes, stores and secretes digestive enzymes. Each acinus is composed of pyramidal cells arranged in a tubular or spherical fashion with their apex toward the lumen. These cells rest on basolateral membrane that possesses receptors for hormones and transmitters controlling enzyme secretion. Each cell has a big basal nucleus and significant endoplasmic reticulum (ER) for enzyme synthesis. The apical half of the cell contains abundant zymogen granules. These are released into the lumen by exocytosis on stimulation by neurotransmitters, like acetylcholine, and hormones, like secretin and cholecystokinin. The release is regulated by microvilli on the surface of acinar cells. Tight junctions across acinar cells prevent paracellular passage of enzyme molecules (Figure 55.3).

The secretions flow through a tree-like series of ducts: from the intercalated ducts to the intralobular and interlobular ducts, which finally drain into the MPD. The duct epithelium is lined by cuboidal cells. They are rich in small mitochondria that provide energy for active ion transport. The chloride in the pancreatic juice is exchanged for bicarbonate by carbonic anhydrase and cystic fibrosis transmembrane regulator (CFTR) in the duct cells. This neutralizes the acidic pH in duodenum and facilitates digestive action of several enzymes (44, 45).

Islets of Langerhans, the functional endocrine units, have their origin in the neural crest cells. They vary in size from 50 to 250 µm. Small islets remain embedded in between the acini, while the larger ones lie along the MPD or lobular ducts. An adult pancreas contains approximately one million islets. They are pale staining group of polygonal cells, separated from the acini by thin connective tissue. They are scattered throughout the pancreas, with abundance more in the tail than the head and body. They make up 2% of the total volume of pancreas (46). Each islet has a copious blood supply from two to three arterioles branching into a leash of fenestrated capillaries. They drain into numerous venules that pass through the acini. This islet-acinar flow of blood allows local action of islet hormones, especially insulin. Acinar cells around the islets are larger and more abundant in zymogen granules, maybe due to the effect of insulin. The efferent vessels from the islet drain into the interlobular veins and finally terminate into the portal system (unlike other endocrine organs that drain into systemic circulation).

Five major cell types comprise the islets. In the pancreas derived from the dorsal bud, majority of the cells include β cells (75%–80%), followed by α cells (about 15%), δ cells (about 5%) and very few pancreatic polypeptide (PP) cells and epsilon cells. β Cells secrete insulin, while α cells secrete glucagon. α Cells are mostly present at the periphery of the islet and in close contact with vessels. β Cells occupy a more central part, and most of them develop cytoplasmic extension that runs between α cells and reaches the surface of vessels.

The δ cells secrete somatostatin, and the epsilon cells secrete ghrelin. PP cells, also known as F cells, that secrete PP and adrenomedullin, comprise 54%–94% of the pancreas derived from the ventral bud, i.e. the uncinate process (47).

Endocrine physiology

Islets of Langerhans play an important role in homeostasis, especially glucose metabolism. The two hormones, which primarily control the blood glucose level, are insulin and glucagon. β Cells synthesize pre-proinsulin in the ER. It gets cleaved by enzymes to form proinsulin. It contains two chains of insulin connected by a C-peptide. It gets further cleaved to form insulin before secretion. The biologically active insulin is released into the bloodstream along with equimolar C-peptide on stimulation. The insulin is called the "hormone of abundance". Its secretion is regulated by several mechanisms:

Chemical: High levels of blood glucose and amino acids increase secretion. No insulin is secreted when the plasma glucose is below 50 mg/dL. Half of the maximal response occurs at 150 mg/dL, while the maximal insulin response is evident at 300 mg/dL. The secretion is biphasic, with the initial burst of a 5–10-fold increase in secretion for 5–15 minutes following a meal, followed by a sustained gradual release (1 U/hour) till the blood glucose is high. Average daily insulin secreted in an adult is 40 U.

Neural: Activation of parasympathetic nervous system stimulates, while increased sympathetic activity (α-2 adrenergic receptors) inhibits insulin secretion.

Hormonal: The release is regulated by paracrine and endocrine action: inhibitory (glucagon and somatostatin) and stimulatory (gut hormones) effects on insulin secretion.

The half-life of insulin is 5 minutes. It promotes glucose uptake from the blood and energy storage. The uptake is facilitated by glucose transporter (GLUT). GLUT4, which is present on skeletal muscle, cardiac muscle and adipose tissue, is insulin sensitive. The brain, placenta, kidneys and colon possess GLUT1 and GLUT3 receptors that are insulin independent. GLUT2 receptors on the islet, liver and small intestine are insulin independent. Insulin binds to the α subunit of a tetrameric receptor on cells. The β subunit gets autophosphorylated and is responsible for the biological effects. The effects of insulin on various tissues have been listed in Table 55.1. Deficiency of insulin due to decreased secretion (Type 1 diabetes mellitus) or insulin resistance (Type 2 diabetes mellitus) results in persistently high blood glucose, hyperlipidemia and overweight. Long-term uncontrolled hyperglycemia can effect permanent damage to the vessels (atherosclerosis), retina (retinal ischemia), kidneys (proteinuria and glomerulosclerosis), liver (nonalcoholic steatohepatitis) and heart (diastolic dysfunction).

Glucagon is a 29 amino acid peptide secreted by the α cells. It antagonizes the actions of insulin. Its secretion is stimulated by a decrease in blood glucose (exercise and starvation), sympathetic activity through β receptors, protein meal and hormones

TABLE 55.1: Effect of Insulin on Various Organs

Muscle	Promotes glucose uptake, protein synthesis and glycogen synthesis
	Increased potassium uptake
Liver	Stimulates glycogenesis and protein synthesis
	Increased production of lipids (triglycerides and cholesterol)
	Inhibits glycogenolysis, ketogenesis and gluconeogenesis
Adipose tissue	Promotes glucose uptake and triglyceride storage
	Activates lipoprotein lipase
Body cells	Promotes growth of various cells, including nerve cells and axons

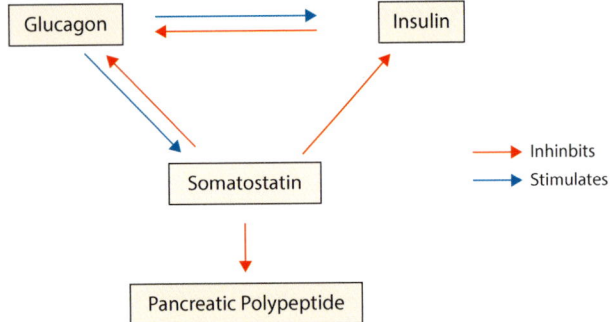

FIGURE 55.6 Paracrine action of islet hormones.

like cholecystokinin (CCK) and gastrin. Secretin and somatostatin inhibit its secretion. It has a half-life of 5 minutes. It acts primarily on the liver. It has a calorigenic action and stimulates glycogenolysis, gluconeogenesis from available amino acids and ketogenesis. The hormone is secreted in an increased amount during starvation and usually reaches a peak on the third day. Glucagon is secreted into the portal system and the majority is deactivated in the liver. The peripheral concentration is very low, but for cirrhosis or acute liver failure. Glucagon does not cause glycogenolysis in muscles. It has a positive inotropic effect on the heart. It also increases the secretion of growth hormone, insulin and somatostatin.

Somatostatin is a universal inhibitor. It has a paracrine action on the islet cells and effect inhibition of insulin, glucagon and PP secretion. It also inhibits CCK secretion and delays gastric emptying. The stimuli that increase insulin secretion (glucose and amino acids) also promote somatostatin secretion.

PP is produced by F cells. The prime function is not known but effects in slowing down the absorption of food. The stimulating factors include protein meal, exercise and parasympathetic activation. It is inhibited by somatostatin and intravenous glucose. The hormones secreted by the islet cells have a paracrine feedback system. The hormones released into the extracellular space diffuse to other islet cells and affect their action. α, β and δ Cells have gap junction that allows passage of small molecules. In synchrony, the various islet cells regulate the utilization of protein and energy. The paracrine effect of various hormones on each other has been depicted in Figure 55.6 (46, 48).

References

1. Fitzgerald PJ. Medical anecdotes concerning some diseases of the pancreas. In: Fitzgerald PJ, Morrison AB, eds. The pancreas. Baltimore, MD: Williams and Wilkins, 1980:1–29.
2. Busnardo AC, DiDio LJA, Tidrick RT, Thomford NR. History of the pancreas. Am J Surg 1983;146(5):539–50.
3. Palade G. Intracellular aspects of the process of protein synthesis. Science 1975;189:867.
4. Garrison FH. An introduction to the history of medicine. Philadelphia, PA: WB Saunders, 1929:554–890.
5. Skandalakis LJ, Rowe JS, Gray SW, Skandalakis JE. Surgical embryology and anatomy of the pancreas. Surg Clin North Am 1993;73(4):661–97.
6. Gittes GK. Developmental biology of the pancreas: A comprehensive review. Dev Biol 2009;326:4–35.
7. Suda K, Mogaki M, Matsumoto Y. Gross dissection and immunohistochemical studies on branch fusion type of ventral and dorsal pancreatic ducts: A case report. Surg Radiol Anat 1991;13:333–7.
8. Jimenez J, Emil S, Podnon Y, Nguyen N. Annular pancreas in children: A recent decade's experience. J Pediatric Surg 2004;39:1654–7.
9. Zyromski N, Sandoval J, Pitt H, et al. Annular pancreas: Dramatic differences between children and adults. J Am Coll Surg 2008;206:1019–25.
10. Gross RE, Chisholm TC. Annular pancreas producing duodenal obstruction. Ann Surg 1944;119:759.
11. Pearson S. Aberrant pancreas. Review of the literature and report of three cases, one of which produced common and pancreatic duct obstruction. Arch Surg 1951;63:168.
12. Curd H. Histological study of Meckel's diverticulum with special reference to heterotopic tissues. Arch Surg 1936;32:506.
13. Smaio T. Proposed nomenclature and classification of the human pancreatic ducts and duodenal papillae: Study based on 200 postmortems. Int Surg 1969;52:125–41.
14. Cotton P. Congenital anomaly of pancreas divisum as cause of obstructive pain and pancreatitis. Gut 1980;21:105–14.
15. Borak GD, Romagnuolo J, Alsolaiman M, et al. Long term clinical outcomes after endoscopic minor papilla therapy in symptomatic patients with pancreas divisum. Pancreas 2009;38:903–6.
16. Kapa S, Gleeson F, Vege S. Dorsal pancreas agenesis and polysplenia/heterotaxy syndrome. A novel association with aortic coarctation and a review of literature. JOP 2007;8:433–7.
17. Auringer S, Ulmer J, Sumner M, Turner C. Congenital cyst of pancreas. J Pediatr Surg 2003;38:1080–2.
18. Shimada K, Yanagisawa J, Nakayama F. Increased lysophosphatidylcholine and pancreatic enzyme content in bile of patients with anomalous pancreaticobiliary ductal junction. Hepatology 1991;13:438–44.
19. Tashiro S, Imaizumi T, Ohkawa H, et al. Pancreaticobiliary maljunction: retrospective and nationwide survey in Japan. J Hepatobiliary Pancreat Surg 2003;10:345–51.
20. Komi N. New classification of anomalous arrangement of the pancreaticobiliary duct (APBD) in the choledochal cyst; a proposal of new Komi's classification of APBD. J Jpn Pancreas Soc 1991;6:234–43.
21. Kimura K, Ohto M, Saiho H, et al. Association of gallbladder carcinoma and anomalous pancreaticobiliary ductal union. Gastroenterology 1985;89:1258–65.
22. Wang HP, Wu MS, Lin CC, Chang LY, Kao AW, Wang HH, Lin JT. Pancreaticobiliary diseases associated with anomalous pancreaticobiliary ductal union. Gastrointest Endosc 1998;48(2):184–9.
23. Busnardo AC, DiDio LJ, Thomford NR. Anatomicosurgical segments of the human pancreas. Surg Radiol Anat 1988;10:77–82.
24. Gockel I, Domeyer M, Wollosheck T, Konerding MA, Junginger T. Resection of the mesopancreas (RMP): a new surgical classification of a known anatomical space. World J Surg Oncol 2007;5:44.
25. Xu J, Tian X, Chen Y, et al. Total mesopancreas excision for the treatment of pancreatic head cancer. J Cancer 2017;8(17):3575–84.
26. Chowdappa R, Challa VR. Mesopancreas in pancreatic cancer: Where do we stand – Review of literature. Indian J Surg Oncol 2015;6: 69–74.
27. Michels NA. Blood supply and anatomy of the upper abdominal organs. Philadelphia, PA, JB Lippincott, 1955.
28. Rienhoff WF Jr, Pickerell KL. Pancreatitis: an anatomic study of pancreatic and extrahepatic biliary systems. Arch Surg 1945;51:205–19.
29. Mishra SP, Gulati P, Thorat VK, et al. Pancreaticobiliary ductal union in biliary diseases. An endoscopic retrograde cholangiopancreatographic study. Gastroenterology 1989;96:907–12.
30. Kleitsch WP. Anatomy of pancreas: A study with special reference to the duct system. AMA Arch Surg 1955;71:795–802.
31. Ladas SD, Tassios PS, Giorgiotis K, et al. Pancreatic duct width: Its significance as a diagnostic criterion for pancreatic disease. Hepatogastroenterology 1993;40:52–5.
32. Mann FC, Giordano AS. The bile factor in pancreatitis. Arch Surg 1923;6:1–30.
33. Opie EL. The etiology of acute hemorrhagic pancreatitis. Bull Johns Hopkins Hosp 1901;12:182–8.
34. Michels NA. The hepatic, cystic, and retroduodenal arteries and their relations to the biliary ducts with samples of the entire celiacal blood supply. Ann Surg 1951;133(4):503–24.
35. Thompson IM. On the arteries and ducts in the hepatic pedicle. A study in statistical human anatomy. Anatomy 1953;1:55.
36. Falconer CWA, Griffiths F. The anatomy of blood vessels in the region of pancreas. Br J Surg 1950;37(147):334–44.
37. Wright AS, Rikkers LF. Current management of portal hypertension. J Gastrointest Surg 2005;9:992–1005.
38. Myburgh JA. Selective shunts: The Johannesburg experience. Am J Surg 1990;160:67–74.
39. Cubilla AL, Fortner J, Fitzgerald PJ. Lymph node involvement in carcinoma of the head of the pancreas area. Cancer 1978;41:880–7.
40. Evans BP, Ochsner A. The gross anatomy of the lymphatics of the human pancreas. Surgery 1954;36:177–91.
41. Skandalakis JE, Gray SW (eds.). Embryology for surgeons. Pancreas. 2nd ed. Baltimore, MD: Williams & Wilkins, 1994:366, 397–9.
42. Bockman DE, Buchler M, Malferthiner P, Beger HG. Analysis of nerves in chronic pancreatitis. Gastroenterology 1988;94:1459–69.
43. Drapiewski JF. Carcinoma of pancreas: a study of neoplastic invasion of nerves and its possible clinical significance. Am J Clin Pathol 1944;14:549–56.
44. Motta PM, Macchiarelli G, Nottola SA, et al. Histology of exocrine pancreas. Microsc Res Tech 1997;37:384–98.
45. Williams JA. Regulation of acinar cell function in the pancreas. Curr Opin Gastroenterol 2010;26:478–83.
46. Barreto SG, Carati CJ, Toouli J, Saccone GT. The islet-acinar axis of the pancreas: More than just insulin. Am J Physiol Gastrointest Liver Physiol 2010;299:G10–22.
47. Stefan Y, Orci L, Malaisse-Lagae F, Perrelet A, Patel Y, Unger R.H. Quantitation of endocrine cell content in the pancreas of nondiabetic and diabetic humans. Diabetes 1982;31(8 Pt 1):694–700.
48. Bonner-Weir S, Orci L. New perspectives on the microvasculature of the islets of Langerhans in the rat. Diabetes 1982;31:883–9.

# 56

INSULINOMA

Anand Kumar Mishra

Introduction

Insulinomas are small, often benign and rare functional neuroendocrine tumors with incidence of four in one million persons. They can occur as sporadic or a part of familial syndromes (multiple endocrine neoplasia type 1 [MEN-1]). Patients present with neuroglycopenic, hypoglycemic or combination of both types of symptoms. The diagnosis is difficult many times and biochemical. The insulinoma is localized preoperatively within the pancreas with a goal of surgical excision as a complete excision will give the patient cure.

Insulinomas are more commonly seen in females (2:1) and usually in fifth or sixth decade while MEN-1 insulinomas are seen in third decade of life.

Historical background

Pancreatic islet cells were first described by a medical student Paul Langerhans in 1869 (1). Insulin, or "isletin," was isolated from a solution extract of a dog's pancreas by Banting and Best in 1922. Harris was the first to suggest a clinical possibility of hyperinsulinism like hypoinsulinism of diabetes in 1923 (2). Wilder and colleagues were the first to describe the association between hyperinsulinism and a functional islet cell tumor in 1926 after they performed an operation on a patient with hypoglycemia and found an islet cell carcinoma with hepatic metastases (3). Graham in 1929 has the credit of the first surgical cure of an insulinoma (2). Whipple described a triad called the "Whipple triad," which became the basis of biochemical diagnosis of insulinoma. The triad consists of hypoglycemia symptoms provoked by fasting with glucose level less than 50 mg/100 mL and relief of symptoms with administration of glucose (2).

Sporadic versus multiple endocrine neoplasia type 1 insulinoma

Insulinoma can occur sporadically, or as part of MEN-1. MEN-1 syndrome is autosomal dominant and caused by MEN-1 tumor suppressor gene "Menin" located on chromosome 11q13, characterized by primary hyperparathyroidism (PHPT), anterior pituitary adenomas and tumors of the endocrine pancreas and duodenum. The most common functioning islet cell tumors in MEN-1 are gastrinomas and insulinomas (4). Insulinoma affects approximately 10–15% of MEN-1 patients. Sporadic insulinomas are solitary, benign, encapsulated lesions while those associated with MEN-1 are multifocal, multiple and more importantly characterized as microscopic small tumors spreading all over the pancreas to large sizes and sometimes malignant tumors in the same patient (5, 6). MEN-1 patients are usually young. Association of PHPT in a patient of insulinoma is virtually diagnostic of MEN-1, and therefore, all patients of insulinoma should have a screening for PHPT by serum calcium determination and parathyroid hormone (PTH). Furthermore, these tumors may produce a variety of hormones. The MEN-1 insulinomas patient may also have gastrinoma. The surgical strategy differs between tumors with MEN-1 and sporadic cases. Total removal of gross disease with adequate prophylactic resection to minimize recurrence without causing endocrine and exocrine pancreatic compromise is the principles of surgery in MEN-1 patient. The best procedure to achieve it is routine distal subtotal pancreatectomy (to the level of portal vein), with enucleation of tumors in the head guided by intraoperative ultrasound (IOUS) for safety.

Pathophysiology

Insulin is synthesized in beta cells through endoplasmic reticulum of the pancreatic islets of Langerhans as preproinsulin. Preproinsulin is converted into proinsulin (which has a 21–amino acid alpha chain, 30–amino acid beta chain and both joined by a 33–amino acid connecting peptide or C-peptide). Proinsulin is stored in secretory granules and transferred to the Golgi apparatus (7). Within these granules, enzyme protease acts on proinsulin, breaks it into C-peptide and the double-stranded insulin molecule. Both these are secreted in equimolar amounts after release (7). Small amount of proinsulin that remains intact in granules is also released and detectable in plasma. Proinsulin represents less than 25% of total immunoreactive plasma insulin in normal subjects, whereas almost more than 90% patients with insulinomas have an elevated proportion of proinsulin relative to total insulin (8).

Clinical approach

Patient presents with hypoglycemic symptoms that are secondary to excessive and uncontrolled secretion of insulin. Symptoms may develop after meals or have no relationship to meals. Typically, they are precipitated by prolonged fasting or exercise and are often nonspecific, episodic, vary among individuals and can differ from time to time in the same individual. Precipitation of symptoms by prolonged fast or avoiding the meals should be kept in mind as in India women keep day-long fasts due to various religious/culture practices. These symptoms can be classified as neuroglycopenic (due to neuronal glucose deprivation in the brain) and neurogenic (due to sympathetic discharge from autonomic nervous system caused by hypoglycemia). Since the symptoms of insulinoma are primarily behavioral, patients are diagnosed as suffering from psychiatric or neurologic disorders and this causes a delay in diagnosis by an average period of 15 months to 3 years. Figure 56.1 outlines the approach to a patient presenting with symptoms consistent with insulinoma.

Presentation: The symptoms can be classified into:

1. **Neuroglycopenic symptoms:** These symptoms are caused by brain glucose deficiency. The spectrum varies from light headedness, visual disturbances, double vision, confusion, amnesia, abnormal behavior, difficulty awakening and

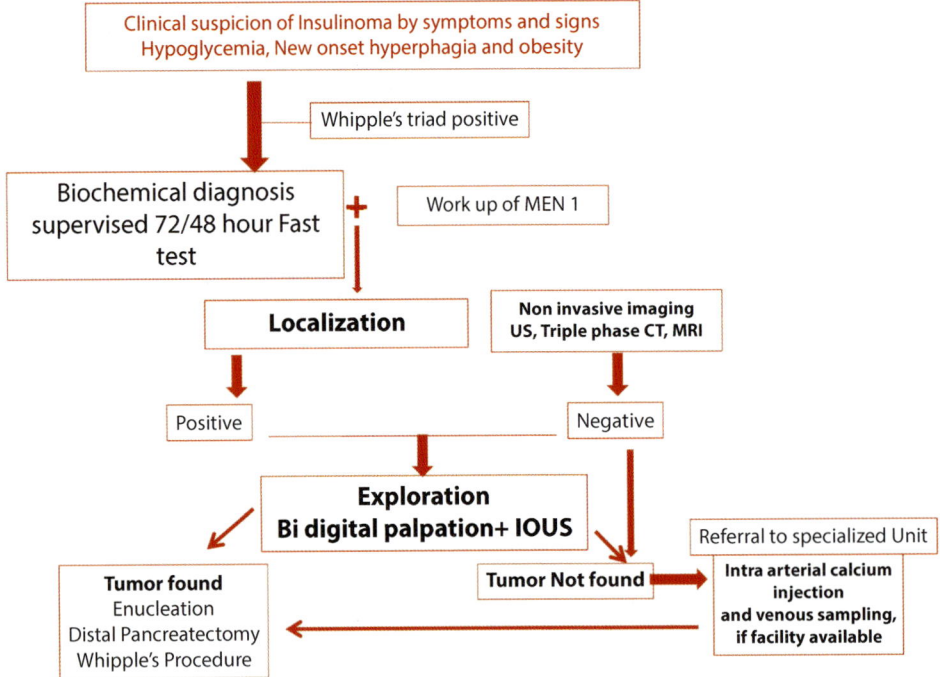

FIGURE 56.1 Flowchart of management in insulinoma.

seizures, which may develop in one third of patients. These symptoms may progress to loss of consciousness.

2. **Neurogenic symptoms:** These symptoms are due to physiological reaction to hypoglycemia. These may be adrenergic or cholinergic (sweating, hunger and paresthesia). Hypoglycemia causes release of catecholamine and patients develop symptoms of weakness, sweating, tremor, nausea, anxiety and palpitations.

Both groups of symptoms can occur in variable combinations in an individual but the symptom complex is individual specific and follows a stereotypic pattern. Patients of insulinoma often learn to avoid the symptoms of hypoglycemia by eating small meals frequently or having snacks, which results in weight gain, and by the time the diagnosis of insulinoma is made, they may be very obese. So, the other two symptoms can be new-onset hyperphagia and new-onset weight gain.

Biochemical diagnosis

Diagnosis of insulinoma is based on demonstrating Whipple's triad during a supervised 72-hour fast. First purpose of the fast is to document hypoglycemia and its relationship to the patient's symptoms, and the second is to demonstrate inappropriate insulin concentrations in relation to hypoglycemia.

1. Classically, the diagnosis of insulinoma is suggested by the presence of "Whipple's triad," which includes three prerequisites. There are symptoms of hypoglycemia (neuroglycopenia ± catecholamine excess) during fasting or exercise, with serum glucose level less than 45 mg/dl and symptoms resolve after oral or intravenous administration of glucose.

2. **Supervised 72-hour fasting test:**

Protocol for 72-hour fast test:

- Discontinue all essential medications and fast is started after admission. An intravenous line is maintained.
- Patient is allowed to have calorie-free drinks and caffeine-free beverages as much as he feels.
- It is ensured that the patient is alert while awake and hemodynamically stable when asleep.
- Plasma glucose, insulin C-peptide and proinsulin is done before the fast and repeated every 6 hours till plasma glucose level is ≤60 mg per deciliter and after this level it is repeated every 1–2 hours.
  - Fast is terminated when plasma glucose level is ≤45 mg per deciliter, and there are symptoms/signs of hypoglycemia.
  - Plasma glucose, insulin, C-peptide, proinsulin, B-hydroxybutyrate and sulfonylurea are done at the end of fast. One-mg intravenous glucagon is injected, and above tests samples are collected immediately and after 10, 20 and 30 minutes. Then patient is allowed for feeding.
  - Plasma cortisol, growth hormone or glucagon can be collected before and after the end of the fast.

Demonstration of inappropriately high level of insulin for the serum glucose during an episode of severe hypoglycemia confirms the diagnosis. The test is terminated if plasma glucose level goes below 40 mg/dl or patient develops symptoms of hypoglycemia. It is observed that approximately 33% of patients become hypoglycemic within 12 hours, 65% within 24 hours, 84% within 36 hours, 93% within 48 hours and 99% within 72 hours (Table 56.1).

Insulinoma

TABLE 56.1: Diagnostic Criteria for Insulinoma after 72-Hour Fast Test

Factor	Concentration
Monitored 72-hour fast or until symptoms develop with blood glucose level less than 50 mg/dl	
Relief of symptoms with oral or intravenous glucose load	
Plasma insulin	≥5–10 micro unit/ml (43 pmol/l)
Plasma C-peptide	≥0.2 nmol/l
Plasma proinsulin	>22 pmol
Plasma or urinary sulphonylurea	Negative
Plasma B-hydroxybutyrate	<2.7 mmol/l
Change in glucose with 1-mg glucagon	≥25 mg/dl at 30 minutes

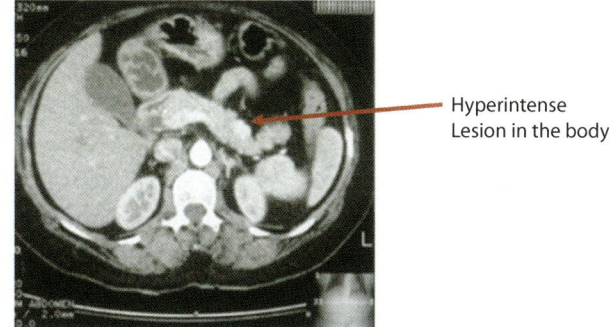

FIGURE 56.2 Spiral CT of a patient with insulinoma in the body of pancreas.

1. Measurement of C-peptide levels: C-peptide secretion is an accurate marker for endogenous insulin secretion as it is secreted in equimolar amounts as insulin by beta cells. Normal C-peptide levels in the setting of elevated blood glucose levels and hyperinsulinemia point toward accidental or surreptitious use of insulin or sulfonylurea.
2. In patients with borderline insulin levels, measurement of proinsulin is useful.
3. C-peptide suppression test: Infusion of exogenous insulin of beef or pork origin is done to suppress endogenous insulin secretion. Hypoglycemia induced by exogenous insulin in healthy subjects will suppress endogenous insulin (measured as C-peptide secretion) by 50–70%. Elevated C-peptide after infusion suggests presence of insulinoma.
4. Measurement of plasma or urinary sulfonylurea: Sulfonylurea causes an elevation of secretion of insulin, C-peptide and proinsulin, similar to insulinoma, and if it is detected in blood sample or urine, should alert the physician of the possibility of exogenous ingestion.

48-Hour supervised fast:

Currently, 48-hour supervised fast with measurement of proinsulin is sufficient for the diagnosis as more than 70–90% patients develop Whipple's triad during this period. The 48-hour fast must be carried out in a supervised setting, and insulin should be determined every 6 hours. Most difficult differential diagnosis for insulinoma is factitious hypoglycemia, especially when oral hypoglycemic medications are used. Insulin and C-peptide levels will be high as in insulinoma. It becomes difficult also as current sulfonylurea assays fail to detect the new generation of non-sulfonylurea hypoglycemic agents.

Localization of the tumor

Tumor localization is required for planning of surgery, and it should be done only after biochemical diagnosis of insulinoma. Although ultrasound, triple-phase contrast CT or MRI have lower sensitivity for localization, but still these imaging studies give essential information about location and the presence of metastases, so they are required in all patients. Despite all efforts for imaging in about 20–50% of patients, the tumor cannot be localized at the time of surgery. And negative preoperative imaging should not deter the planning of surgery if the biochemical diagnosis is certain because the combination of IOUS and bidigital palpation can detect more than 90% of insulinomas during surgery (9, 10).

A wide range of localization methods are available, viz:

Noninvasive imaging

1. Transabdominal ultrasound is operator dependent to a large extent and localization rates vary widely from 13 to 65%.
2. Lower localization rates have been reported for CT scan and MRI. Insulinoma shows up as a hyperintense lesion on contrast enhanced computed tomography. (Figure 56.2).
3. Somatostatin receptor scintigraphy (SRS): This represents a major advance in preoperative tumor imaging. However, only 30% have type 2 somatostatin receptors (11, 12).

Invasive imaging

1. Endoscopic ultrasound (EUS): Results are very good and sensitivity varies with experience of the user and location of the tumor (92.6, 78.9 and 40% in head, body and tail, respectively) and specificity of 100% (11, 12).
2. Selective arterial stimulation and venous sampling (ASVS) is a method when tumor is not localized with other imaging. This is a regionalization modality and utilizes intra-arterial calcium stimulation (selective into branches of the celiac axis and superior mesenteric artery and with hepatic venous sampling). The insulin hormone estimation is done in the hepatic vein sample and by that conclusion is made on the possible region of pancreas likely to harbor the tumor. The principle behind this test is that insulinomas can be stimulated to secrete their hormone when the serum concentration of calcium is raised. In spite of the excellent published result, this technique is technically demanding, invasive, not widely available and carries some risk of complications (13–15).
3. Selective angiography: Historically selective angiography was the method of choice for pancreatic insulinomas. However, because of its cost, invasiveness and potential risk of complications, it is not performed.

Preoperative preparation

All the patients before surgery require a meticulous preoperative preparation to optimize the physiologic condition of the patient so that perioperative period is uneventful. As these patients are obese, vigorous chest physiotherapy is started weeks prior to surgery. Smoking has to be stopped at least 6 weeks prior to surgery in smokers. Previous nights to surgery, light food and liquids are preferred. All these patients require a limited bowel preparation. All patients are started on intravenous infusion of 10% dextrose on the night of surgery to avoid the risk of hypoglycemia as patient is fasting. Octreotide or diazoxide may be given to control severe hypoglycemic episodes in the preoperative period. Both of these are effective in 40–60% of time (16, 17). One disadvantage of perioperative use of octreotide or diazoxide is that intraoperative blood glucose monitoring, which can predict the completeness of excision of insulinoma or biochemical cure cannot be used. Prophylactic antibiotics are given as per institutional protocol. All patients require prophylaxis for deep vein thrombosis. Intraoperative glucose monitoring is required in all cases and intravenous infusion of dextrose should be stopped.

Surgical management: open and laparoscopic resection of insulinoma

Laparoscopic resection of insulinoma

Insulinomas are usually benign tumors (90%) and are solitary, so they are treated with simple enucleation. And because of their benign nature, they can also be excised through the laparoscopic approach. The advantages of minimally invasive procedures are plenty in these patients in terms of hospital stay, postoperative pain and morbidity as these patients are obese. In open surgery, exposure of the pancreas requires a bilateral subcostal incision, which in its self has lot of morbidity. Only disadvantage is that the surgeon should be trained in advanced laparoscopic procedures to perform the resection or distal pancreatectomy (18–23). Laparoscopic intraoperative ultrasound (LIOUS) is used for detection of an insulinoma during laparoscopic procedure. Preoperative tumor location always helps and provides a road map for surgery. In a pre-localized patient, the mobilization and exposure of the pancreas can be limited depending upon the location of the tumor. Open exploration patients have considerable postoperative pain and longer hospital stay.

Open operative technique

Incision: The abdomen is explored through a bilateral subcostal incision. Fixed retractors like Thomson's or Haribhakti is used to elevate the costal margins and provide excellent exposure.

Exploration: The abdomen is initially explored for evidence of metastatic disease on the superior surface of liver, omentum and peritoneum. Wide kocherization of the duodenum is done to mobilize the pancreas head and gland exposure is done by division of gastrocolic ligament, reflecting greater omentum cranially off the transverse colon. The omentum attached to the greater curvature of stomach is retracted superiorly, and congenital adhesions between the posterior wall stomach and pancreas are divided. Uncinate process is mobilized by dividing its small vascular attachments to the superior mesenteric vessels, allowing their full medial retraction. To gain ideal exposure of neck and uncinate process, gastroepiploic artery along the greater curvature of the stomach and the gastroepiploic vein as it joins the gastrocolic venous trunk is sacrificed safely. Adenoma in the uncinate process can be easily missed during palpation if it is not mobilized. Body and tail can be mobilized by incising the peritoneum along the inferior border of the pancreas. Entire body and tail can be rotated around the axis of splenic vessels by gently dissecting beneath the entire posterior surface of the pancreas. While doing this, injury to the underlying adrenal gland should be prevented. If tail of the pancreas is extending deep into the splenic hilum, short gastric vessels can be divided. In this way, spleen becomes free from its peritoneal attachment and it can be lifted along with body and tail. Spleen can be rotated medially to visualize the posterior surface of pancreas.

Selecting the resection procedure

Once pancreas is completely mobilized, bidigital palpation of whole gland is performed systemically along with IOUS to see the relation of tumor to pancreatic duct and portal vein. Palpation by an experienced surgeon and IOUS can detect 98% of insulinomas. Uncommonly, tumor can be identified protruding on the surface as a reddish purple or white mass, but more commonly they can be covered by a variable thickness of normal pancreatic parenchyma. If during exploration, insulinoma is detected early in the course, even then the whole pancreas should be examined to avoid missing multiple tumors. If the tumor is well away from these structures and safe parenchymal margin is available, enucleation is the method of choice. For enucleation, a plane can be developed between the tumor and the softer normal pancreas as insulinoma develops a pseudo capsule around it. It is accomplished by dissecting immediately adjacent to tumor bluntly separating tumor from normal pancreas with fine instruments and sucker. Fine bridging vessels are managed with clips or bipolar cautery. One can put the left hand behind and push forward the tumor and thumb placed anteriorly on tumor can provide countertraction on the tumor. Pancreas can be lifted with one hand and tumor can be pulled in countertraction upwards with a stitch placed through it. After enucleation, the defect is not closed but a drain (preferably a soft silicone drain) is routinely placed as fistula formation is not uncommon. Biological sealants, such as fibrin glue, can be used to limit the occurrence of a pancreatic fistula. If there is suspicion of injury to the duct, intravenous secretin will stimulate secretions and extravasations of pancreatic fluid from the resected area can be seen. An injured duct should be closed by fine sutures or, alternatively, the operation is converted to a resection.

Otherwise, a pancreaticoduodenectomy (Whipple's procedure) can be performed, even for benign disease. In the pancreatic neck or uncinate process, pancreatic duct has oblique course when it meets the confluence, so there are high chances of developing ductal leak. Majority of tumors in the uncinate process of the head, neck or body may be enucleated. In the rare case of a tumor of the mid pancreas, spleen-preserving distal pancreatectomy can be done It has to be kept in mind that extensive resection may result in exocrine pancreatic insufficiency. A technique of central pancreatectomy with distal pancreaticogastrostomy as an alternative to left pancreatectomy has been described to preserve pancreatic function. Tumors of tail may also be enucleated safely. Meticulous technique is the key to safety in pancreatic surgery. Harmonic scalpel if available is particularly useful in resection for its hemostatic effect and limited tissue destruction.

Intraoperative ultrasound (IOUS)

IOUS can be done by operating surgeon or a radiologist. IOUS can detect occult insulinomas as it is superior to bidigital palpation. It can also confirm the abnormality palpated, define relationship of the tumor to pancreatic duct, vessels and can also locate multiple tumors (Figure 56.3).

Intraoperative hormone measurements (IHM)

Intraoperative insulin measurements may be used to confirm the completeness of surgery. Insulin has a very short half-life in the systemic circulation. Serum levels of insulin decrease rapidly

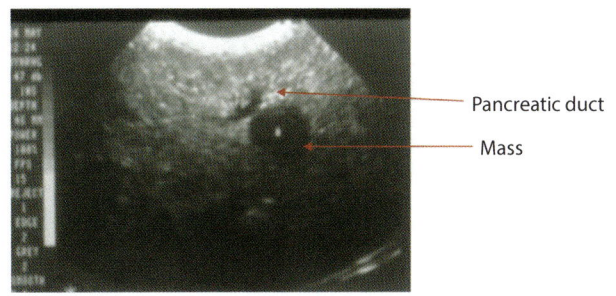

FIGURE 56.3 Intraoperative ultrasound showing the adenoma close to pancreatic duct.

after resection of insulinoma. The overall accuracy of this test is 85%. Intraoperative injection of secretin that stimulates insulin secretion can confirm the excision of tumor tissue. It has been found that secretin stimulates beta-cell insulin secretion in normal tissue but not in tumor cells or in nesidioblastosis. Therefore, insulin rise is observed only after 2 minutes of injection of secretin when complete resection of tumor tissue has been done and inhibition of beta-cell secretion by the autonomous tumor has stopped.

Blood sugar levels also start rising in most patients within 15 minutes of removal of insulinoma, and it predicts the biochemical cure. In very thin patients, hyperglycemic response may be delayed and may take longer in more than 20% of patients.

No tumor identified

Rarely, bidigital palpation and IOUS may fail to reveal a tumor. In these situations, blind distal pancreatectomy, which was recommended in the past, should not be done. Almost 50% of nonpalpable or occult insulinomas are located in head or uncinate process. Pancreatic biopsy in such a situation can be done to exclude adult onset nesidioblastosis.

In case of failed operation, the second exploration should always be performed by an experienced unit. The diagnosis must be reconfirmed in all failed cases and selective venous sampling after intra-arterial calcium injection may redirect subsequent exploration. Surgical reexplorations are always more difficult as dissection is hampered by fibrosis and scarred tissue planes, and pancreas becomes firmer, compromising the surgeon's ability to palpate small tumor.

Complications

The two main complications of pancreatic surgery are

1. Intraperitoneal leak of pancreatic fluid leading to pancreatic ascites
2. Pancreatic fistula and less commonly pseudocysts

With the use of IOUS, fistula rate has decreased tremendously after enucleation. Closed suction drainage should be used to control fistula output in all patients. Pancreatic fluid is rich in amylase, and fluid examination will reveal high amylase concentration. Most of these fistulae resolve spontaneously. In the case of prolonged drainage, drain can be left in place and patient can be orally allowed. Silicone drains are preferred as one may need to keep the drains for a longer duration. Drains should be fixed during operation very cautiously because of the abovementioned reason (24). Octreotide and somatostatin analog have been used prophylactically for prevention of fistula, but evidence shows no obvious benefit.

Special situations

Malignant insulinoma

A total of 5–10% of all insulinomas are malignant. They are generally large and more than 6 cm in size, and commonly, they metastasize to liver and regional lymph nodes. They may be discovered preoperatively or recognized intraoperatively by tumor infiltration, metastases in liver or lymph node or postoperatively by histopathology showing microscopic infiltration (25). Elevated proinsulin or chorionic gonadotropin and its subunits have been correlated with malignancy, but it has poor sensitivity. Patients with malignant insulinomas may have more troublesome hypoglycemic symptoms and rapid course in comparison to patients with benign disease. Intraoperatively, malignant tumor is hard in consistency, may produce puckering of surrounding soft tissue or appear to be infiltrating. A malignant tumor may infiltrate or compress the pancreatic duct and result into distal dilatation of the pancreatic duct.

Management

Treatment of primary: Tumor resection is always indicated to reduce bulk and decrease troublesome hypoglycemia and ultimate outcome. Surgery should not be tried when it is widely spread in peritoneal cavity and involves major vascular structures. Enucleation with a rim of normal pancreatic tissue should be performed in tumors of size more than 2 cm and pseudocapsular margin is unclear. Aggressive resection should be attempted as these tumors are much less virulent than their malignant exocrine counterparts.

Treatment of liver metastases: Metastases are functional and maintain hormonal hypersecretion. Thus, resection should be considered to decrease the bulk and reduce the symptoms. Palliative resection should be planned when at least 90% of the tumor bulk can be excised. The liver metastasis can be treated with nonoperative methods or their combination. The nonsurgical methods are radio frequency ablation, liver hepatic artery embolization and chemotherapy. Cytoreductive hepatic surgery for malignant insulinoma with liver metastases can be performed to provide palliation and probably improve survival (26). Adriamycin and streptozocin chemotherapy have been tried with reports of 70% tumor regression rate and remission of hypoglycemic symptoms up to 18 months. This combination chemotherapy is associated with considerable toxicity (27).

Prognosis: Curative resection results in median disease-free survival of 5 years, but recurrence develops in 63% at a median interval of 2–8 years. Recurrence tumor has median survival of only 19 months. Palliative resection has median survival of 4 years, but biopsy only has survival of 11 months.

Nesidioblastosis: It is characterized by severe recurrent hypoglycemia with hyperinsulinemia, and in neonates, it is the most common cause of severe and persistent hypoglycemia in neonates and children. It is known as persistent hyperinsulinemic hypoglycemia of infancy (PHHI). Rarely, it is also observed in adults. It can be classified into three classes: diffuse (60%), focal and atypical. It is caused by defective genes like ABCC8, KCNJ11, GLUD1,

GCK, HADH, SLC16A1, HNF1A, HNF4A, UCP2, HK1, PGM1, PMM2 and FOXA2 that regulate insulin secretion. Perinatal stress, intrauterine growth retardation, maternal diabetes mellitus, Beckwith-Wiedemann syndrome and Sotos syndrome are seen to be associated with this condition. Nesidioblastosis and insulinoma cannot be distinguished clinically or biochemically. ^{18}F-DOPA-PET scanning is currently the diagnostic imaging tool to accurately localize focal lesions. Management includes dietary, medical and surgical approaches. Near-total pancreatectomy may be required in these patients for a cure. Histologically, there is a proliferation of abnormal beta cells throughout the entire pancreas in diffuse form.

Adult-onset nesidioblastosis

Adult nesidioblastosis is a diagnosis of exclusion where biochemical diagnosis is confirmed but preoperative localization is negative. It may be associated with MEN-1. Also, during exploration, IOUS and bidigital palpation are negative. Intra-arterial calcium angiogram should be performed in these patients and if insulin levels rise after each selective calcium injection, nesidioblastosis is the most likely diagnosis. Various surgical options include distal pancreatectomy and near-total pancreatectomy.

Insulin autoimmune syndrome

Insulin autoimmune syndrome (IAS) presents as hypoglycemic symptoms caused by autoimmune reasons where autoantibodies are produced against insulin (28). This autoimmune-induced hypoglycemia is the third-leading cause of hypoglycemia in Japanese people but rare among other ethnicities.

There are of two types:

1. IAS: This syndrome is characterized by hyperinsulinemic hypoglycemia, elevated autoantibody against insulin (IAA) in the circulation without prior exposure to exogenous insulin and without pathological abnormalities in pancreatic islets. This condition is also known as "Hirata's disease" after Yukimasa Hirata, the author who first described the syndrome in 1970. IAA formation may be triggered by exposure to drugs (containing sulfhydryl groups – antithyroid drugs) or viruses (mumps, rubella, coxsackie B influenza, hepatitis C, chickenpox and measles), dietary supplements containing alpha-lipoic (also called thioctic) acid used to treat diabetic neuropathy or as an antiaging health supplement or spontaneously.
2. Type B insulin resistance syndrome (TBIRS): This syndrome is a rare autoimmune disorder caused by the presence of insulin receptor autoantibodies against the insulin receptor (type B insulin resistance). It results in a very broad array of abnormalities in glucose homeostasis from hypoglycemia to hyperglycemia resistant to high-dose insulin therapy. This condition is also known as Flier's disease. Acanthosis nigricans (areas of skin thickening and hyperpigmentation) is seen associated in up to 88% of patients. These patients have high circulating insulin because of increased insulin secretion from pancreas in an attempt to overcome peripheral insulin resistance in the hypoglycemic phase, which confuses and causes suspicion of insulinoma. High serum insulin levels are accompanied by low proinsulin and C-peptide levels and mimic injectable insulin administration pattern.

South Asia perspective

Insulinoma are rare tumors also in South Asia. There are very few publications from this region. The patients are diagnosed very late as symptoms of insulinoma are primarily behavioral; they are diagnosed as suffering from psychiatric or neurologic disorders and continue to receive treatments. And this causes a delay in diagnosis in most of the patients in this region.

Conclusion

Insulinoma is a rare neuroendocrine tumor arising from beta cells of islets of Langerhans in pancreas. They secrete insulin and cause hypoglycemic symptoms. The tumor is usually benign, well encapsulated and solitary size of less than 2 cm. Biochemical diagnosis of insulinoma is made by a supervised 72-hour fast test with appropriate confirmatory laboratory values. The next step is to localize the tumor in pancreas and evaluate metastases and most commonly a triple-phase CT scan is carried out. If CT is unable to localize the lesion, intra-arterial calcium stimulation and venous sampling is recommended to regionalize the tumor. Surgery will provide the cure and access can be either an open or laparoscopic with IOUS. As most insulinomas are solitary, well encapsulated and benign, enucleation, if feasible, is the procedure of choice. Tumors that are located in close proximity to pancreatic duct or large size and hard will require larger resection (29, 30). Malignant insulinoma metastasizes most commonly to the liver and lymph nodes. As these tumors are functional and secrete insulin hormone, so in patients with metastatic disease, surgical debulking, if possible, provides palliation and improvement in quality of life. When surgical resection is not possible, other noninvasive options like radiofrequency ablation, hepatic artery embolization and chemoembolization may be used along with cytotoxic chemotherapy, molecularly targeted therapy, targeted radiotherapy or other palliative options.

References

1. Langerhans P. Beitragezurmikroskopischen Anatomie der Bauchspeicheldruse. Berlin: Buchdruckerei von Gustav Lange; 1869.
2. Whipple AO, Frautz VK. Adenomas of islet cells with hyperinsulinism: a review. Ann Surg 1935;101:1299–335.
3. Wilder RM, Allan FN, Power MH, et al. Carcinoma of the islets of the pancreas: hyperinsulinism and hypoglycemia. J Am Med Assoc 1927;89:348–55.
4. Rich TA, Perrier ND. Multiple endocrine neoplasia syndromes. Surg Clin North Am 2008;88(4):863–95.
5. Demeure MJ, Klonoff DC, Karam JH, et al. Insulinomas associated with multiple endocrine neoplasia type I: the need for a different surgical approach. Surgery 1991;110:998–1005.
6. O'Riordain DS, Brien T, van Heerden JA, et al. Surgical management of insulinoma associated with multiple endocrine neoplasia type I. World J Surg 1994;18:488–94.
7. Guettier JM, Gorden P. Insulin secretion and insulin-producing tumors. Expert Rev Endocrinol Metab 2010;5:217–27.
8. Thorner MD, Perryman RL, Cronin MJ, et al. Somatotroph hyperplasia. Successful treatment of acromegaly by removal of a pancreatic islet tumor secreting a growth hormone-releasing factor. J Clin Invest 1982;70:965–77.
9. Hashimoto LA, Walsh RM. Preoperative localization of insulinomas is not necessary. Am Coll Surg 1999;189(4):368–73.
10. Lo CY, Lam KY, Kung AW, et al. Pancreatic insulinomas. A 15-year experience. Arch Surg 1997;132(8):926–30.
11. Proye C, Malvaux P, Pattou F, et al. Noninvasive imaging of insulinoma and gastrinomas with endoscopic ultrasonography and somatostatin receptor scintigraphy. Surgery 1998;124:1134–44.
12. Thompson NW, Crako PF, Fritts LL, et al. Role of endoscopic ultrasonography in the localization of insulinomas and gastrinomas. Surgery 1994;116:1131–8.
13. Doppman JL. Pancreatic endocrine tumors; the search goes on. N Engl J Med 1992;326:1770–3.
14. Bottger TC, Junginger T. Is preoperative radiographic localization of islet cell tumors in patients with insulinoma necessary? World J Surg 1993;17:427.

15. Doppman JL, Chang R, Fraker DL, et al. Localization of insulinomas to regions of the pancreas by intra-arterial stimulation with calcium. Ann Intern Med 1995;123:269.
16. Arnold R, Wied M, Behr TH. Somatostatin analogues in the treatment of endocrine tumors of the gastrointestinal tract. Expert Opin Pharmacother 2002;3(6):643–56.
17. Boukhman MP, Karam JH, Shaver J, et al. Insulinoma–experience from 1950 to 1995. West J Med 1998;169(2):98–104.
18. Gagner M, Pomp A, Herrera MF. Early experience with laparoscopic resections of islet cell tumors. Surgery 1996;120:1051–4.
19. Berends FJ, Cuesta MA, Kazemier G, et al. Laparoscopic detection and resection of insulinomas. Surgery 2000;128:386–91.
20. Cogliandolo A, Pidoto RR, Causse X, Kerdraon R, Saint Marc O. Minimally invasive management of insulinomas: a case report. Surg Endosc 2001;15:1042.
21. Jaroszewski DE, Schlinkert RT, Thompson GB, Schlinkert DK. Laparoscopic localization and resection of insulinomas. Arch Surg 2004;139:270–4.
22. Sweet MP, Izumisato Y, Way LW, Clark OH, Masharani U, Duh Q-Y. Laparoscopic enucleation of insulinomas. Arch Surg 2007;142(12):1202–4.
23. Isla A, Arbuckle JD, Kekis PB, Lim A, Jackson JE, Todd JF, Lynn, J. Laparoscopic management of insulinomas. Br J Surg 2009;96:185–90.
24. Ohwada S, Ogawa T, Tanahashi Y, et al. Fibrin glue sandwich prevents pancreatic fistula following distal pancreatectomy. World J Surg 1998;22:494–8.
25. Hirshberg B, Cochran C, Skarulis MC, et al. Malignant insulinoma: spectrum of unusual clinical features. Cancer 2005;104:264–72.
26. Cahin C, et al. Indications and results of liver transplantation in patients with neuroendocrine tumors. Wrold J Surg 2002;26:998–1004.
27. Moertel CG, Mamley JA, Johnson LA. Streptozocin alone compared with streptozocin plus fluorouracil in the treatment of advanced islet cell carcinoma. N Engl J Med 1980;303:1198.
28. Simona C, Caterina M, Corrado B. Insulin autoimmune syndrome: from diagnosis to clinical management. Ann Transl Med 2018;6(17):335–50.
29. Proye CAG. Endocrine tumors of the pancreas: an update. Aust N Z J Surg 1988;68:90–100.
30. Service FHJ, McMahon MM, O'Brien PC, et al. Functioning insulinoma: incidence, recurrence, and long-term survival of patients: a 60-year study. Mayo Clin Proc 1991;66:711.

57

GASTRINOMA

Anand Kumar Mishra

The text of this chapter is available online at www.routledge.com/9781032136509.

58
RARE PANCREATIC ENDOCRINE TUMORS
Anand Kumar Mishra

Introduction

Pancreatic islets of Langerhans arise from the embryonic endodermal cells. The islets have neuroendocrine cells or APUD cells (amine precursor uptake and decarboxylation cells) that possess specialized function of production, storage, and secretion of peptides and biogenic amines (1). In simpler terms, neuroendocrine cells have an ability to receive signals and function, like nerve cells from the brain, and act like an endocrine cell that has capacity to produce hormones. These cells are distributed throughout our body and located in largest number in gastrointestinal tract, lungs, and bronchi and less commonly in thyroid, parathyroid, adrenal, and pituitary. Pancreatic neuroendocrine tumors (PNETs) arise from these specialized cells and are rare tumors. Tumors that produce excess hormones can lead to clinical syndromes and are termed as functional tumors. They include insulinoma, gastrinoma, vasoactive intestinal polypeptide–secreting tumors, glucagonoma, and somatostatinoma. Carcinoid tumors are the most common and can produce carcinoid syndrome by serotonin secreted by the tumor. Other rare PNETs secrete hormones such as adrenocorticotrophic hormone, calcitonin, growth hormone releasing factor, and parathyroid hormone-related peptide and can lead to syndromes also (Table 58.1). A total of 75%–90% of PNETs don't produce any hormone and, thus, do not cause clinical syndrome, and these are called as nonfunctional (NF) (1, 2). Some NF PNETs are associated with high levels of pancreatic polypeptide, neurotensin, or human chorionic gonadotropin but don't produce a clinical syndrome (3). Functional tumors generally have a favorable prognosis than their NF (1), possibly because of earlier detection. NF tumors are more common. In general, PNET that produce ectopic hormones (for example, ACTH) are more aggressive.

Epidemiology

They occur with an estimated incidence of 1–1.5 per lakh population. It accounts for 2%–10% of all detected pancreatic tumors. The peak incidence is seen between 6th and 8th decade of life and have lower 5-year survival in comparison to gastrointestinal NETs. Functional PNET have a prevalence of 1% per lakh while autopsy series report 0.5%–1.5% per lakh. Precisely 95% of PNET are sporadic and only 5% have a family history (4). Familial-inherited conditions that are associated with PNETs include multiple endocrine neoplasia type 1, von Hippel-Lindau syndrome, tuberous sclerosis complex (TSC1 and TSC2), and neurofibromatosis (NF1) (Table 58.2). These tumors are more commonly multifocal and can develop throughout the patient's lifetime, and different tumors may arise in different sites of the body.

Origin and histochemical features

PNET arise from pancreas neuroendocrine cells and are part of the diffuse neuroendocrine cells system scattered throughout the gastrointestinal tract, respiratory tract, and other tissues. Cells of this system have a common embryonic origin from neural crest and endodermal origin shares common cytochemical properties of *a*mine *p*recursor *u*ptake and *d*ecarboxylation. Ultrastructurally, cells have electron-dense granules that contain multiple regulatory hormones and amines, neuron-specific enolase, synaptophysin, and chromogranin. These tumors were previously labeled as APUDoma. APUDomas also included medullary thyroid cancer, pheochromocytoma, and melanoma.

Histologically, there is a homogeneous sheet of small round cells with uniform nuclei and cytoplasm with infrequent mitotic figures (<2 mitoses/high-power field). Necrosis is characteristically uncommon. Malignancy is determined by only metastases or invasion. It is not cellular morphology or ultrastructural studies.

Clinical features

These tumors may present as syndromes caused by excess hormones secreted by the tumor. They may present as asymptomatic, incidentally discovered masses or debilitating hormonal syndromes or diffuse liver metastases (Tables 58.1 and 58.2).

Classification

World Health Organization (WHO) classification proposed in 2010 has classified PNET into three categories on the basis of the anatomic location, mitotic activity, and Ki67 (proliferative index). The three categories are well-differentiated NET with benign or uncertain behavior; well-differentiated carcinoma with malignant characteristics; and poorly differentiated carcinoma (2–5). WHO revised its classification in 2017 as it had considerable confusion in differentiating grade 3 tumors and carcinoma (Table 58.3).

A consensus conference held at the International Agency for Research on Cancer (IARC) in November 2017 and subsequent discussion with experts proposed a classification framework based on the common morphology at different anatomic sites. For PNET, classification is shown in the following Table 58.4.

The 8th edition of the AJCC/UICC staging system uses the same staging system for PNET and exocrine pancreatic adenocarcinomas (12).

T1: Confined to pancreas*, <2 cm
T2: Confined to pancreas, 2–4 cm
T3: Confined to pancreas, >4 cm, or invades duodenum or bile duct
T4: Invasion of adjacent organs or major vessels

TABLE 58.1: Syndromes Associated with Pancreatic Neuroendocrine Tumors (PNETs) (5–8)

Name of PNET	Incidence Per Lakh/Year	Symptoms/Signs	Malignancy (%)/ Hormone Secretion	Primary Location
Insulinoma	1–2	Hypoglycemic symptoms (tremor, palpitations, anxiety, hunger, cognitive impairment, seizure, coma), fasting hypoglycemia, rapid correction with glucose (Whipple's triad)	<10%/Insulin	Pancreas (100%)
Gastrinoma (or Zollinger-Ellison syndrome)	0.5–1.5	Severe, medically refractory peptic ulcer disease, gastroesophageal reflux, diarrhea (Zollinger-Ellison syndrome)	60%–90%/Gastrin	Pancreas (30%), duodenum (60%–70%), other (5%–10%)
VIPoma (Verner-Morrison syndrome, WDHA, pancreatic cholera)	0.05–0.2	Watery diarrhea, hypokalemia, achlorhydria (WDHA syndrome, pancreatic cholera or Verner Morrison syndrome)	>60%/Vasoactive intestinal peptide	Pancreas 85%–95%, other (neural, periganglionic, adrenal) (10%)
Glucagonoma	0.01–0.1	Necrolytic migratory erythema, weight loss, diabetes mellitus, diarrhea, venous thrombosis	50%–80%/Glucagon	Pancreas (100%)
Somatostatinoma	Rare	Diabetes, gallstones, steatorrhea, weight loss	>70%/Somatostatin	Pancreas (50%–60%), duodenal/jejunal (40%–50%)
GRFoma	Unknown	Coarse facial features, enlarged hands and feet, macroglossia, deepening voice, skin thickening, sleep apnea, arthritis, cardiovascular disease, insulin resistance, fatigue, weakness (acromegaly)	>30/Growth hormone–releasing factor	Pancreas (30%), lung (54%), jejunal (75%), other (adrenal, foregut, retroperitoneal) (13%)
ACTHoma	Unknown	Cushing's syndrome features (Ectopic)	>95%/ACTH	4%–25% of all ectopic Cushing syndrome
PNET secreting PTH-rP	Rare	Nephrolithiasis, weakness, bone pain, nausea, constipation, polyuria, depression (hypercalcemia)	85%/PTH-rP (parathyroid hormone related protein)	Pancreas (100%)
Pancreatic carcinoid tumor	<1% of all carcinoids	Flushing, diarrhea, bronchospasm, valvular heart disease (carcinoid syndrome)	77%/Serotonin, tachykinins	Pancreas (100%) (<1% of all carcinoid syndrome)
PNET secreting rennin, erythropoietin, luteinizing hormone, cholecystokinin	Rare	Individual hormones producing their effects like hypertension, polycythemia, masculinization in females, and diarrhea and gallstones	Unknown	Pancreas (100%)
Non-functional PNET	1–5	Asymptomatic, abdominal/back pain, nausea/vomiting, pancreatitis, obstructive jaundice	60%–90%/Pancreatic polypeptide 60%–85%, chromogranin A but without symptoms, neuron-specific enolase, ghrelin, neurotensin, motilin, subunits of human chorionic gonadotropin	Pancreas (100%)

Diagnosis

Functional PNET are suspected on the basis of characteristic clinical features or laboratory values. Nonfunctioning tumors are detected incidentally only. Sometimes there is no clue to diagnosis and imaging features, or histopathology suggests PNET on the basis of the morphology of the lesion. Diagnosis of PNET is confirmed by immunohistochemistry (chromogranin A, synaptophysin, CD56, and neuron-specific enolase, PAX6 [paired box 6], PAX8 [paired box 8], ISL1 – islet 1) and routine hematoxylin and eosin staining is not useful many times in predicting it. Tumor tissue can be obtained by endoscopic ultrasound biopsy or fine needle aspiration of the pancreatic tumor, or percutaneous core needle biopsy of a liver metastasis, or by surgical resection. Before planning definitive surgery, a tissue diagnosis should be tried. However, it has been observed that neuroendocrine carcinomas (NECs) are not always positive for immunochemistry markers. Some PNET may show atypical imaging features, such as cystic change or intraductal growth.

Rare Pancreatic Endocrine Tumors

TABLE 58.2: Hereditary Cancer Syndromes Associated with PNETs

Syndrome	Gene/Inheritance Pattern	Incidence	Component
Multiple endocrine neoplasia type 1 (Wermer syndrome)	MEN1 (11q13; encodes 610 amino acid protein – menin) autosomal dominant	20%–70% symptomatic PNET, nonfunction almost common followed by gastrinoma, nearly 100% develop multiple pancreatic microadenomas	Parathyroid hyperplasia (95%–100%), pituitary tumors (30%–50%), angiofibromas (85%), adrenal adenoma (30%–40%), gastric NETs (10%–35%)
von Hippel-Lindau syndrome	VHL (3p25: encodes 232 amino acid protein) autosomal dominant	10%–20%, all nonfunctional	Retinal and CNS hemangioblastoma (60%–80%), renal cell carcinoma (25%–70%), pheochromocytoma (10%–20%), pancreatic cysts (35%–80%), epididymal cystadenoma (25%–60%)
Neurofibromatosis type 1 (Von Recklinghausen disease)	NF1 (17q11.2: encodes 2485 amino acid protein – neurofibromin) autosomal dominant	0%–10%, characteristically ampullary/duodenal somatostatinomas	Café au lait macules (99%), neurofibromas (99%), skin fold freckling (85%), Lisch nodules (95%), optic pathway glioma (15%), learning problems (60%) skeletal abnormalities, pheochromocytomas, malignant peripheral nerve sheath tumors
Tuberous sclerosis complex (Bourneville disease)	TSC1, TSC2 9q34 (TSC1): encodes 1164 amino acid protein – hamartin; 16p13 (TSC2): encodes 1807 amino acid protein (tuberin) autosomal dominant	Rare, functional or nonfunctional	Variable presentation: hamartomas affecting brain, skin, kidneys, and eyes; classically seizures, developmental delay and angiofibromas
Glucagon cell hyperplasia and neoplasia (Mahvash syndrome)	GCCR autosomal recessive	100%, microglucagonomas and macroglucagonomas	–

TABLE 58.3: WHO Classification: Comparison 2010 and 2017 (10, 11)

WHO 2010	Mitosis (Per 10 High-Power Field) and Ki67	WHO 2017	Mitosis (Per 10 High-Power Field) and Ki67
Well differentiated	Grade 1: <2/<3 Grade 2: 2–20/3–20	Well differentiated	Grade 1: <2/<3 Grade 2: 2–20/3–20 Grade 3: >20/>20
Poorly differentiated	Grade 3: >20/>20	Poorly differentiated	Grade 3: >20/>20 Small-cell type Large-cell type
Mixed adenoma neuroendocrine carcinoma (MANEC)		Mixed endocrine and non-endocrine neoplasm (MiNEN)	

TABLE 58.4: Classification Proposed at Consensus Conference of International Agency for Research on Cancer (IARC) 2017 (9)

	Type of Tumor	Grade	Current Proposed Terminology
Pancreatic neuroendocrine tumor (NET)	Pancreatic neuroendocrine tumor (NET)	G1 G2 G3	PanNET G1 PanNET G2 PanNET G3
Pancreatic neuroendocrine carcinoma (NEC)	Pancreatic NEC, small cell type Pancreatic NEC, large cell type	G3 G3	Small cell NE carcinoma Large cell NE carcinoma

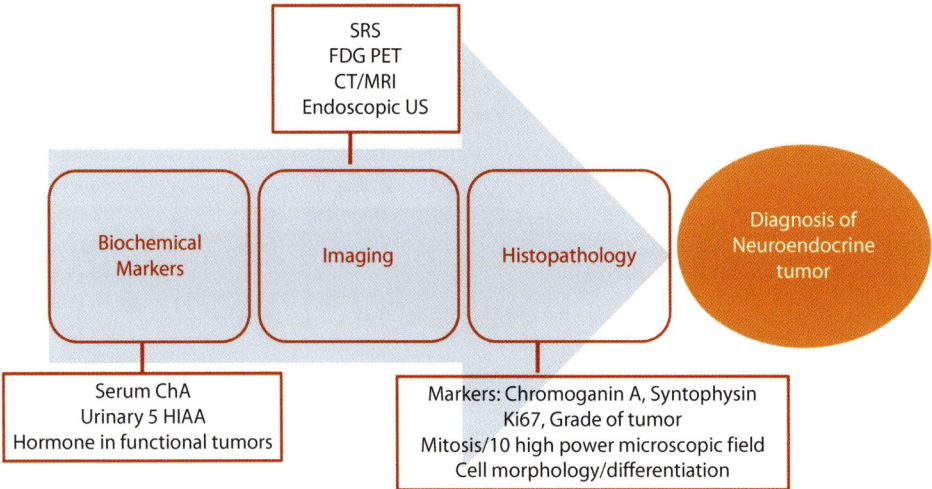

FIGURE 58.1 Diagnostic tool in pancreatic tumors. SRS = somatostatin receptor scintigraphy.

Histopathological examination of biopsy or surgical specimens is, therefore, a must for diagnosis and grading of PNET. Figure 58.1 summarizes the diagnostic algorithm for rare pancreatic tumors.

Imaging

Preoperative imaging and localization are essential for planning of surgical resection. In all patients, a combination of complementary computed tomography (CT), MRI, and nuclear imaging with a novel tracer is required to evaluate local invasion, identification of distant metastasis, and prediction of treatment. It is also required for evaluation of the treatment response. Imaging modalities most commonly used are triple-phase CT scan and MRI with gadolinium contrast. The perfusion techniques like dynamic contrast-enhanced CT and diffusion-weighted imaging MRI are helpful for the evaluation of malignant diseases with regard to both diagnosis and monitoring of treatment. The first imaging of choice is triple-phase CT or pancreatic protocol CT as it has several advantages over other studies. CT is quick, widely available, and provides excellent anatomic delineation of the pancreas, lymph node (LN), or liver metastases. CT also has the advantage of being easier for the surgeon to interpret. It has a mean sensitivity of 82% (13, 14). The other imaging modality is MRI, and it also has a mean sensitivity of 79%. It has an advantage over CT as it is more sensitive for the detection of liver metastases, particularly with hepatocyte-specific contrast agent gadoxetate disodium (Eovist) (14–16). For detection of hepatic metastases, Gadoxetate is superior to conventional contrast agents, but for characterization of the primary and vascular involvement, conventional nonionic contrast is superior. PNET metastases to the liver are typically fed by the hepatic arteries rather than the portal veins and, therefore, are often best seen on the arterial phase. Well-differentiated PNETs are usually smaller than NECs. NETs are hyper-enhancing on both arterial and portal venous phase imaging due to their hypervascular nature. Most NECs show hypoenhancement with the adjacent pancreatic parenchyma, particularly on portal venous phase imaging (17).

Functional imaging is done by PETCT with somatostatin analogues (SSAs). Well-differentiated PNETs are comparatively slow growing and frequently do not show avid glucose uptake. Gallium-68-labeled SSAs (DOTATOC, DOTANOC, and DOTATATE) are more sensitive than CT, MRI, and octreoscan in detecting NETs (100% vs 75%) (18, 19). Somatostatin receptors are expressed by most of the PNETs (80%–100%) except insulinomas (50%–70%) (20). Radiolabeled SSAs using indium-111 somatostatin receptor scintigraphy (111In-SRS, octreoscan) and gallium-68 positron emission tomography (68Ga-PET, Netspot) can provide excellent functional imaging of these tumors. 68Ga-PET is rapidly becoming the functional imaging modality of choice (sensitivity 93%, specificity 91%) (13, 14, 21). Functional somatostatin receptor will often clearly show distant metastases that are not apparent on conventional imaging and is very useful for equivocal lesions on CT or MRI. Functional imaging by PET-CT with a new tracer that uses 18F-dihydroxy-L-phenylalanine, F-DOPA and 11C-5-hydroxy-L-tryptophan, or 11C-5-HTP might have a role in for evaluating the treatment response.

Endoscopic ultrasound examination is the most sensitive test for localizing small PNETs and biopsy via fine needle aspiration can be performed for diagnostic purpose (22–24). It can also provide information regarding multifocality of the tumor but is poor in telling respectability.

Management

The treatment of PNETs is a multidisciplinary effort and includes surgery, radiolabeled SSA, targeted therapy, and cytotoxic chemotherapy. Surgery is the mainstay of treatment for PNETs (25–28). Any patients where resection is possible should be offered and it should be the first in treatment planning. Complete surgical resection provides the only chance for a cure. Any symptomatic patients with unresectable tumor on imaging should also be offered surgical debulking as it may derive significant benefit in terms of both symptom control and survival (29, 30). Various factors that influence the decision regarding type of surgery are size, anatomic location, multifocality, functional status of the tumor and, extent of disease (localized or metastatic), grade, involvement of adjacent structures, and patient comorbidities. The operation can be conservative (enucleation), distal pancreatectomy, or pancreaticoduodenectomy (Whipple procedure) depending upon the size and location of the tumor; however, one should always consider the high morbidity associated with major

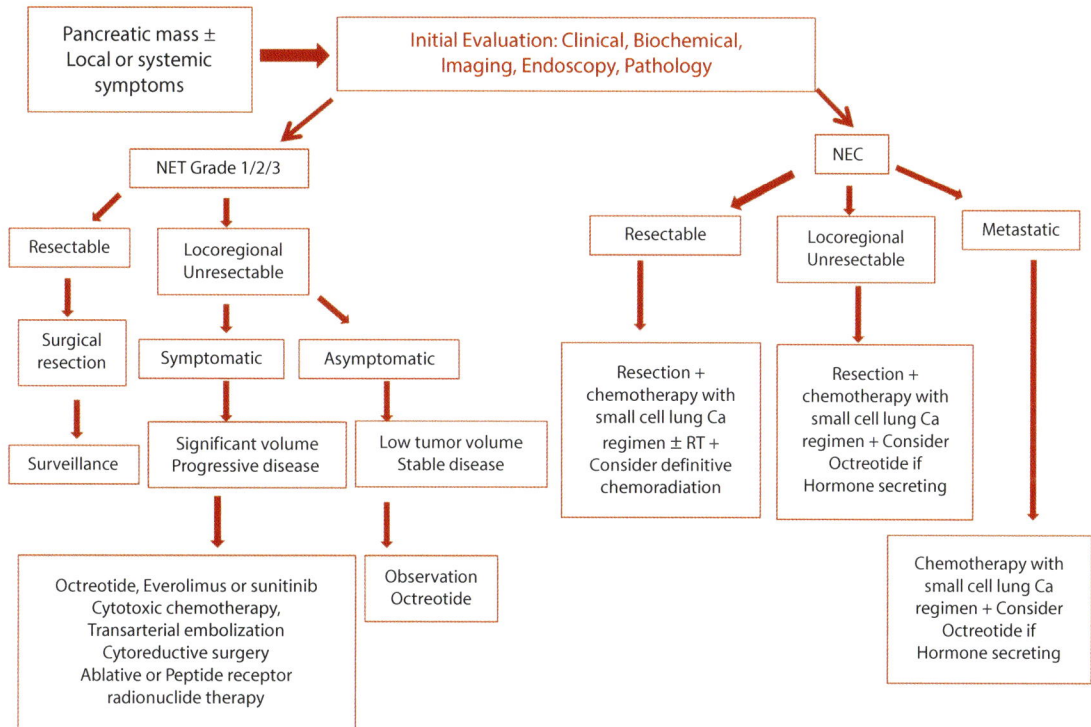

FIGURE 58.2 Stepwise management of pancreatic NET. *Abbreviations:* NEC, neuroendocrine carcinomas; NET, neuroendocrine tumor; RT, radiation therapy.

pancreatic operations and also the indolent growth of well-differentiated PNETs (31, 32). Figure 58.2 outlines the management protocols for PNETs.

For tumors up to 2 cm

Management of asymptomatic PNET between 1 and 2 cm in size should be individualized and these can be managed by either resection or observation depending upon the age and comorbidities, tumor growth over time, estimated risk of symptom development, details of imaging, grade, extent of surgical resection required, patient's wishes, and access to long-term follow-up. In symptomatic patients, the goals of the resection are to control symptoms by removing the source of excess hormone and to improve survival by tumor control. Irrespective of size, all functional tumors biochemically confirmed and localized should be resected. All PNETs have significant malignant potential except insulinoma (33–39). During enucleation, negative margins should be the aim. All major surgical resection should be R0 resection with removal of 11–15 LNs for accurate nodal staging. For smaller PNETs (<2 cm), all suspicious nodes seen on preoperative imaging should be excised and LN sampling may be considered if imaging is negative. Examination of at least 11–15 LNs is required for accurate classification of N stage. In summary, resection is often curative in localized PNETs patients in the absence of recurrence. These patients do not need any further treatment; however, they are kept on clinical or radiological surveillance.

MEN1: All functional PNETs and NF larger than 2 cm should be resected when possible. NF-PNETs size less than 1 cm can be kept under observation depending on factors like development of symptoms, grade of tumor, Ki67, family history, growth rate of tumor, radiographic progression, patient factors, and associated comorbidities. In gastrinomas, medical management by proton pump inhibitors may be considered. Surgical decision-making becomes complex as PNETs are multicentric. Also, surgery is also unlikely to eliminate all disease in the long term. Therefore, excision of the dominant lesion and potentially other easily accessible lesions should be the target as this approach will render a balance between pancreatic function and risk of complications. The aim should be to minimize treatment-related morbidity and mortality. A protocol of watchful surveillance for low-risk tumors, parenchymal-sparing operations to preserve pancreatic endocrine/exocrine functions like enucleation or minimal pancreatic resection for intermediate-risk tumors, and major pancreatic resection for locally invasive, anatomically difficult, or high-risk lesions should be followed. This should be the policy with all familial tumors (40, 41).

VHL: Tumor size, rate of tumor growth, and germline mutation in exon 3 are the three risk factors that correlate with an increased risk of developing or presenting the distant disease. Tumors less than 3 cm in size, with doubling times greater than 500 days and mutations outside of exon 3 can be safely observed with serial imaging every 1–2 years as these patients have less risk of distant disease. Patients with a single high-risk factor (tumor size 3 cm or larger, doubling time less than 500 days, or germline mutations in exon 3) should be considered for surgery vs more frequent imaging at 6- to 12-month intervals depending upon the associated comorbidities and other factors. Any patient who has two or more high-risk factors should be strongly considered for surgical resection (42–46). Spleen-preserving distal pancreatic resection is always preferred. Any patient who is planned for splenectomy should be vaccinated for pneumococcus, meningococcus at least 2 weeks before operation.

Palliative Management

Role of hepatic cytoreductive surgery with liver metastases

Retrospective studies suggest that resection of liver metastases in PNET may lead to improvement in both symptoms (47, 48) and survival (48, 49). However, the studies have been questioned for retrospective data and selection bias (patients with favorable/limited disease treatment by cytoreduction, and with more extensive disease, unfavorable tumor biology, or significant comorbidity of medical therapy or embolotherapy. Extent of liver resection should be individualized and should be based upon number and distribution of metastases, age of the patient, and comorbidities, grade, and rate of progression of tumor. Complete excision of all lesions will surely improve survival; however, resection of more than 70% will definitely improve symptoms and effective survival. Experienced surgeons can perform combined pancreas resection and liver cytoreduction safely with acceptable morbidity and mortality in carefully selected patients. Various factors that influence the decision of cytoreductive surgery in an individual are hepatic tumor burden, tumor grade, previous progression on other therapies, age, the presence of potentially correctable comorbidities, and access to an experienced hepatic surgeon. Indications for debulking or cytoreductive liver surgery are: metastatic PNETs with less than 50% hepatic replacement (preferably <25%) with a surgically amenable distribution (i.e., not miliary) in well-differentiated grade 1 or 2 tumors with normal or near-normal liver function and no evidence of carcinoid heart disease or other major comorbidities. Extrahepatic metastases should not be considered a contraindication to hepatic debulking as peritoneal tumor deposits may be resected concurrently. Liver transplantation seems to be an option in patients with extensive liver involvement with no evidence of extrahepatic disease.

Functional tumors with favorable location (body and tail) may drive benefit in quality of life by resection of primary PNETs with metastatic disease (50). Alternative therapies for oligometastatic and small lesions are radiofrequency ablation (RFA) or microwave ablation or thermal ablation. Embolization of liver metastatic lesion can be done through hepatic artery as metastases lesions predominantly derive their blood supply from the hepatic artery. Various embolization options are bland particle embolization (TAE) producing ischemia, chemoembolization (TACE), and radioembolization (TARE) (51–53).

SSA

SSAs such as octreotide long-acting-repeatable or lanreotide are used for long term in patients with metastatic PNETs. These patients can develop gallstones (incidence 50%), which is significantly higher than in the general population. But the symptomatic biliary disease remains low in these patients, so prophylactic cholecystectomy is not recommended as a separate operation, but it can always be performed in combination with other surgeries.

All metastatic PNETs should undergo routine biochemical and radiographic surveillance at 3–6 months after surgery and then every 6–12 months thereafter. High-grade tumors or patients who have developed progression warrant more frequent surveillance.

Peptide receptor radionucleotide therapy (PRRT)

Various studies have shown PRRT to be an effective treatment with objective response rates up to 70% in primary as well as liver metastases for advanced, unresectable grade 1 and 2 PNETs (54–57). It may be used to decrease tumor burden preoperatively in cytoreductive surgery.

Targeted therapy

Various targeted therapy useful in treatment of PNETs are everolimus (oral MTOR inhibitor), everolimus and octreotide combination, or sunitinib and everolimus combination (58–62).

Role of neoadjuvant therapy

Neoadjuvant therapy can be used to downstage the tumor in patients with advanced or metastatic tumors. It may also be used before cytoreductive surgery. The various options are single agent (oxaliplatin or doxorubicin) (63, 64), or combination of 5-fluorouracil, doxorubicin, and streptozocin (65), or capecitabine and temozolomide (66).

Prognosis

PNETs have heterogenous biologic behavior and prognosis. It varies immensely between indolent limited grade 1 tumors and widely spread grade 3 carcinomas. WHO classifications define different patient subcategories with different prognosis. Median overall survival is reported as 16.2, 8.3, and 0.8 years for grade 1, 2, and 3 tumors, respectively (67). Early recognition, superior therapeutic options, and centralization of care for this rare disease has improved survival over the last decades (68).

South Asia perspective

These tumors present very late and when diagnosed are inoperable. There are publications related to these tumors but essentially the clinical presentation, diagnosis, and management do not differ from the western world.

Conclusion

PNETs are indolent tumors with heterogeneous presentation (asymptomatic, incidentally discovered masses or debilitating hormonal syndromes or diffuse liver metastases) and varying degree of aggressiveness and malignant potential. Patients of neuroendocrine neoplasm should be scrutinized for the presence of a functional hormonal syndrome. The diagnosis is confirmed by histopathology and immunohistochemistry and tumor is graded for classification and treatment purposes. The diagnostic workup includes biochemical testing for NET markers, imaging, which may include CT scans, MRI, endoscopic ultrasound examination, and 68Ga-PET. Imaging by pancreatic protocol CT or contrast-enhanced MRI and functional imaging with gallium-68-labeled SSA and 18F-FDG PET tracers in advanced cases help in deciding extent, staging, resectability, and prognostication. Clinical management requires a multidisciplinary approach. Surgery is the most efficient approach for long-term benefits. Approximately 60% of PNETs at presentation have metastases, most commonly to the liver. The standard treatment for localized PNETs can be observation for small grade 1 NF tumors, enucleation or distal pancreatectomy, or major resections like pancreaticoduodenectomy. The treatment for metastatic PNETs is multimodal and includes primary resection, surgical debulking, liver-directed therapy, and a variety of systemic treatments and targeted therapy (SSAs, everolimus, sunitinib, peptide receptor radionuclide therapy). PNETs have more favorable prognosis when compared with pancreatic adenocarcinoma. High-grade cancers have grave prognosis and palliation can be offered by platinum-based chemotherapy.

References

1. Halfdanarson TR, Rabe KG, Rubin J, et al. Pancreatic neuro endocrine tumors (PNETs): incidence, prognosis and recent trend toward improved survival. Ann Oncol 2008;19:1727–33.
2. Zerbi A, Falconi M, Rindi G, et al. Clinicopathological features of pancreatic endocrine tumors: a prospective multicenter study in Italy of 297 sporadic cases. Am J Gastroenterol 2010;105:1421–29.
3. O'Toole D, Salazar R, Falconi M, et al. Rare functioning pancreatic endocrine tumors. Neuroendocrinology 2006;84:189–95.
4. Kloppel G, Heitz PU. Classification of normal and neoplastic neuroendocrine cells. Ann N Y Acad Sci 1994;733:19–23.
5. Verner JV, Morrison AB. Islet cell tumor and a syndrome of refractory watery diarrhea and hypokalemia. Am J Med 1958;25(3):374–80.
6. Fottner C, Ferrata M, Weber MM. Hormone secreting gastro-entero-pancreatic neuroendocrine neoplasias (GEP-NEN): when to consider, how to diagnose? Rev Endocr Metab Disord 2017;18(4):393–410.
7. Kuo JH, Lee JA, Chabot JA. Nonfunctional pancreatic neuroendocrine tumors. Surg Clin North Am 2014;94(3):689–708.
8. Halfdanarson TR, Rubin J, Farnell MB, et al. Pancreatic endocrine neoplasms: epidemiology and prognosis of pancreatic endocrine tumors. Endocr Relat Cancer 2008;15(2):409–27.
9. Rindi G, Klimstra DS, Abedi-Ardekani B, et al. A common classification framework for neuroendocrine neoplasms: an International Agency for Research on Cancer (IARC) and World Health Organization (WHO) expert consensus proposal. Mod Pathol 2018;31:1770–86.
10. Basturk O, Yang Z, Tang LH, Hruban RH, Adsay V, McCall CM, et al. The high-grade (WHO G3) pancreatic neuroendocrine tumor category is morphologically and biologically heterogenous and includes both well differentiated and poorly differentiated neoplasms. Am J Surg Pathol 2015;39:683–90.
11. Lloyd RV, Osamura RY, Klöppel G, Rosai J. *WHO classification of tumours of endocrine organs*, 4th ed. Lyon: International Agency for Research on Cancer, 2017:209–240.
12. Edge S, Byrd DR, Compton CC, Fritz AG, Greene F, Trotti A. *AJCC cancer staging manual*, 7th ed. New York, NY: Springer, 2010:181–90.
13. Maxwell JE, Howe JR. Imaging in neuroendocrine tumors: an update for the clinician. Int J Endocr Oncol 2015;2(2):159–168.
14. Sundin A, Arnold R, Baudin E, et al. ENETS consensus guidelines for the standards of care in neuroendocrine tumors: radiological, nuclear medicine & hybrid imaging. Neuroendocrinology 2017;105(3):212–44.
15. Dromain C, de Baere T, Lumbroso J, et al. Detection of liver metastases from endocrine tumors: a prospective comparison of somatostatin receptor scintigraphy, computed tomography, and magnetic resonance imaging. J Clin Oncol 2005;23(1):70–8.
16. Tirumani SH, Jagannathan JP, Braschi-Amirfarzan M, et al. Value of hepatocellular phase imaging after intravenous gadoxetate disodium for assessing hepatic metastases from gastro entero pancreatic neuroendocrine tumors: comparison with other MRI pulse sequences and with extracellular agent. Abdom Radiol (NY) 2018;43(9):2329–39.
17. Kim DW, Kim HJ, Kim KW, Byun JH, Song KB, Kim JH, et al. Neuroendocrine neoplasms of the pancreas at dynamic enhanced CT: comparison between grade 3 neuroendocrine carcinoma and grade 1/2 neuroendocrine tumour. Eur Radiol 2015;25:1375–83.
18. Ambrosini V, Campana D, Bodei L, et al. 68Ga-DOTANOC PET/CT clinical impact in patients with neuroendocrine tumors. J Nucl Med 2010;51(5):669–73.
19. Frilling A, Sotiropoulos GC, Radtke A, et al. The impact of 68Ga-DOTATOC positron emission tomography/computed tomography on the multimodal management of patients with neuroendocrine tumors. Ann Surg 2010;252:850–6.
20. Reubi JC. Somatostatin and other peptide receptors as tools for tumor diagnosis and treatment. Neuroendocrinology 2004;80(Suppl 1):51–6.
21. Treglia G, Castaldi P, Rindi G, et al. Diagnostic performance of gallium-68 somatostatin receptor PET and PET/CT in patients with thoracic and gastroenteropancreatic neuroendocrine tumours: a meta-analysis. Endocrine 2012;42(1):80–7.
22. Puli SR, Kalva N, Bechtold ML, et al. Diagnostic accuracy of endoscopic ultrasound in pancreatic neuroendocrine tumors: a systematic review and meta-analysis. World J Gastroenterol 2013;19(23):3678–84.
23. Rosch T, Lightdale CJ, Botet JF, et al. Localization of pancreatic endocrine tumors by endoscopic ultrasonography. N Engl J Med 1992;326(26):1721–6.
24. Zilli A, Arcidiacono PG, Conte D, et al. Clinical impact of endoscopic ultrasonography on the management of neuroendocrine tumors: lights and shadows. Dig Liver Dis 2018;50(1):6–14.
25. Kulke MH, Anthony LB, Bushnell DL, et al. NANETS treatment guidelines: well-differentiated neuroendocrine tumors of the stomach and pancreas. Pancreas 2010;39(6):735–52.
26. Kunz PL, Reidy-Lagunes D, Anthony LB, et al. Consensus guidelines for the management and treatment of neuroendocrine tumors. Pancreas 2013;42(4):557–77.
27. Singh S, Dey C, Kennecke H, et al. Consensus recommendations for the diagnosis and management of pancreatic neuroendocrine tumors: guidelines from a Canadian National Expert Group. Ann Surg Oncol 2015;22(8):2685–99.
28. Falconi M, Bartsch DK, Eriksson B, et al. ENETS consensus guidelines for the management of patients with digestive neuroendocrine neoplasms of the digestive system: well-differentiated pancreatic non-functioning tumors. Neuroendocrinology 2012;95(2):120–34.
29. Morgan RE, Pommier SJ, Pommier RF. Expanded criteria for debulking of liver metastasis also apply to pancreatic neuroendocrine tumors. Surgery 2018;163(1):218–25.
30. Scott AT, Breheny PJ, Keck KJ, et al. Effective cytoreduction can be achieved in patients with numerous neuroendocrine tumor liver metastases (NETLMs). Surgery 2019;165(1):166–75.
31. Finkelstein P, Sharma R, Picado O, et al. Pancreatic neuroendocrine tumors (panNETs): analysis of overall survival of nonsurgical management versus surgical resection. J Gastrointest Surg 2017;21(5):855–66.
32. Howe JR, Merchant NB, Conrad C, Keutgen XM, Hallet J, Drebin JA, Minter RM, et al. Tumors. Pancreas 2020;49(1):1–33.
33. Öberg K. Management of functional neuroendocrine tumors of the pancreas. Gland Surg 2018;7:20–7.
34. Kamp K, Feelders RA, van Adrichem RC, et al. Parathyroid hormone-related peptide (PTHrP) secretion by gastroenteropancreatic neuroendocrine tumors (GEP-NETs): clinical features, diagnosis, management, and follow-up. J Clin Endocrinol Metab 2014;99:3060–9.
35. Mehrabi A, Fischer L, Hafezi M, et al. A systematic review of localization, surgical treatment options, and outcome of insulinoma. Pancreas 2014;43:675–86.
36. Fishbeyn VA, Norton JA, Benya RV, et al. Assessment and prediction of long-term cure in patients with the Zollinger-Ellison syndrome: the best approach. Ann Intern Med 1993;119:199–206.
37. Grant CS. Insulinoma. Best Pract Res Clin Gastroenterol 2005;19:783–98.
38. Norton JA, Fraker DL, Alexander HR, et al. Surgery increases survival in patients with gastrinoma. Ann Surg 2006;244:410–9.
39. Bartsch DK, Waldmann J, Fendrich V, et al. Impact of lymphadenectomy on survival after surgery for sporadic gastrinoma. Br J Surg 2012;99:1234–40.
40. Gonçalves TD, Toledo RA, Sekiya T, et al. Penetrance of functioning and nonfunctioning pancreatic neuroendocrine tumors in multiple endocrine neoplasia type 1 in the second decade of life. J Clin Endocrinol Metab 2014;99: E89–96.
41. Lairmore TC, Chen VY, DeBenedetti MK, et al. Duodenopancreatic resections in patients with multiple endocrine neoplasia type 1. Ann Surg 2000;231:909–18.
42. Keutgen XM, Hammel P, Choyke PL, et al. Evaluation and management of pancreatic lesions in patients with von Hippel–Lindau disease. Nat Rev Clin Oncol 2016;13:537–49.
43. Libutti SK, Choyke PL, Bartlett DL, et al. Pancreatic neuroendocrine tumors associated with von Hippel–Lindau disease: diagnostic and management recommendations. Surgery 1998;124:1153–9.
44. Libutti SK, Choyke PL, Alexander HR, et al. Clinical and genetic analysis of patients with pancreatic neuroendocrine tumors associated with von Hippel–Lindau disease. Surgery 2000;128:1022–7; discussion 1027–8.
45. Marcos HB, Libutti SK, Alexander HR, et al. Neuroendocrine tumors of the pancreas in von Hippel–Lindau disease: spectrum of appearances at CT and MR imaging with histopathologic comparison. Radiology 2002;225:751–8.
46. Blansfield JA, Choyke L, Morita SY, et al. Clinical, genetic and radiographic analysis of 108 patients with von Hippel–Lindau disease (VHL) manifested by pancreatic neuroendocrine neoplasms (PNETs). Surgery 2007;142:814–8.e1–2.
47. Que FG, Nagorney DM, Batts KP, et al. Hepatic resection for metastatic neuroendocrine carcinomas. Am J Surg 1995;169:36–42; discussion 42–3.
48. Mayo SC, de Jong MC, Pulitano C, et al. Surgical management of hepatic neuroendocrine tumor metastasis: results from an international multi-institutional analysis. Ann Surg Oncol 2010;17:3129–36.
49. Sarmiento JM, Heywood G, Rubin J, et al. Surgical treatment of neuroendocrine metastases to the liver: a plea for resection to increase survival. J Am Coll Surg 2003;197:29–37.
50. Bertani E, Fazio N, Radice D, et al. Resection of the primary tumor followed by peptide receptor radionuclide therapy as upfront strategy for the treatment of G1-G2 pancreatic neuroendocrine tumors with unresectable liver metastases. Ann Surg Oncol 2016;23(Suppl 5):981–9.
51. Nazario J, Gupta S. Transarterial liver-directed therapies of neuroendocrine hepatic metastases. Semin Oncol 2010;37(2):118–26. [PubMed: 20494704].
52. Gupta S, Yao JC, Ahrar K, et al. Hepatic artery embolization and chemoembolization for treatment of patients with metastatic carcinoid tumors: the M.D. Anderson experience. Cancer J 2003;9(4):261–7. [PubMed: 12967136].
53. Swärd C, Johanson V, Nieveen van Dijkum E, et al. Prolonged survival after hepatic artery embolization in patients with midgut carcinoid syndrome. Br J Surg 2009;96(5):517–21. [PubMed: 19358175].
54. Partelli S, Bertani E, Bartolomei M, et al. Peptide receptor radionuclide therapy as neoadjuvant therapy for resectable or potentially resectable pancreatic neuroendocrine neoplasms. Surgery 2018;163:761–7.
55. van Vliet EI, van Eijck CH, de Krijger RR, et al. Neoadjuvant treatment of nonfunctioning pancreatic neuroendocrine tumors with [177Lu-DOTA0, Tyr3]Octreotate. J Nucl Med 2015;56:1647–53.
56. Barber TW, Hofman MS, Thomson BN, et al. The potential for induction peptide receptor chemoradionuclide therapy to render inoperable pancreatic and duodenal neuroendocrine tumours resectable. Eur J Surg Oncol 2012;38:64–71.
57. Sowa-Staszczak A, Pach D, Chrzan R, et al. Peptide receptor radionuclide therapy as a potential tool for neoadjuvant therapy in patients with inoperable neuroendocrine tumours (NETs). Eur J Nucl Med Mol Imaging 2011;38:1669–74.
58. Yao JC, Shah MH, Ito T, et al. RAD001 in Advanced Neuroendocrine Tumors, Third Trial (RADIANT-3) Study Group Everolimus for advanced pancreatic neuroendocrine tumors. N Engl J Med 2011;364(6):514–23. [PMCID: PMC4208619] [PubMed: 21306238].
59. Pavel ME, Hainsworth JD, Baudin E, et al. RADIANT-2 Study Group Everolimus plus octreotide long-acting repeatable for the treatment of advanced neuroendocrine tumours associated with carcinoid syndrome (RADIANT-2): a randomised, placebo-controlled, phase 3 study. Lancet 2011;378(9808):2005–12. [PubMed: 22119496].
60. Yao JC, Pavel M, Lombard-Bohas C, et al. Everolimus for the treatment of advanced pancreatic neuroendocrine tumors: overall survival and circulating biomarkers from the randomized, phase III RADIANT-3 study. J Clin Oncol 2016;34(32):3906–13. [PMCID: PMC5791842] [PubMed: 27621394].

61. Pavel M, Unger N, Borbath I, et al. Safety and QOL in patients with advanced NET in a phase 3b expanded access study of everolimus. Target Oncol 2016;11(5):667–75. [PubMed: 27193465].
62. Angelousi A, Kamp K, Kaltsatou M, O'Toole D, Kaltsas G, de Herder W. Sequential everolimus and sunitinib treatment in pancreatic metastatic well-differentiated neuroendocrine tumours resistant to prior treatments. Neuroendocrinology 2017;105(4):394–402. [PubMed: 28122378].
63. Faure M, Niccoli P, Autret A, Cavaglione G, Mineur L, Raoul JL. Systemic chemotherapy with FOLFOX in metastatic grade ½ neuroendocrine cancer. Mol Clin Oncol 2017;6(1):44–8. [PMCID: PMC5245060] [PubMed: 28123727].
64. Sun W, Lipsitz S, Catalano P, Mailliard JA, Haller DG; Eastern Cooperative Oncology Group. Phase II/III study of doxorubicin with fluorouracil compared with streptozocin with fluorouracil or dacarbazine in the treatment of advanced carcinoid tumors: Eastern Cooperative Oncology Group Study E1281. J Clin Oncol 2005;23(22):4897–904. [PubMed: 16051944].
65. Moertel CG, Douglas HO Jr, Hanley J, Carbone PP. Treatment of advanced adenocarcinoma of the pancreas with combinations of streptozotocin plus 5-fluorouracil and streptozotocin plus cyclophosphamide. Cancer 1977;40(2):605–8. [PubMed: 142579].
66. Kunz PL, Catalano PJ, Nimeiri H, et al. A randomized study of temozolomide or temozolomide and capecitabine in patients with advanced pancreatic neuroendocrine tumors: a trial of the ECOG-ACRIN Cancer Research Group (E2211). J Clin Oncol 2018;36(15 Suppl):4004.
67. Dasari A, Shen C, Halperin D, et al. Trends in the incidence, prevalence, and survival outcomes in patients with neuroendocrine tumors in the United States. JAMA Oncol 2017;3(10):1335–42. [PMCID: PMC5824320] [PubMed: 28448665].
68. Hofland J, Kaltsas G, de Herder WW. Advances in the diagnosis and management of well-differentiated neuroendocrine neoplasms. Endocr Rev 2020;41(2):371–403.

59

CARCINOID TUMORS OF THE GASTROINTESTINAL TRACT

Linu Oommen Mathew, Sheeja Sainulabdeen and Rajeev Parameswaran

Introduction

Carcinoid or neuroendocrine tumors (NETs) are rare slow growing neoplasms, which originate in the enterochromaffin cells of the body. *The term neuroendocrine tumor is preferred over carcinoid as tumors are derived from many cell types and include both benign and malignant phenotypes* (1). The first description of carcinoid tumor was given by Theodor Langhans (1839–1915) (2). However, the detailed clinical and histological description was made by Otto Lubarsch (1860–1933) (3). Siegfried Oberndorfer (1876–1944), a pathologist from Munich, coined the term "*karzinoide*" or "carcinoma-like" in 1907. This was a condition whereby the clinical behavior was that of a benign disease; however, it displayed features of a carcinoma on histology (4). It was generally believed that carcinoid tumors were benign, until 140 cases of metastasizing carcinoid tumors were reported in the literature (5, 6). The hormone serotonin was discovered in 1948 (7), and the cell producing this hormone was found to be the Kulchitsky cell (8). Rosenbaum first described "*Carcinoid Syndrome*" (9) following the extraction of serotonin from an ileal carcinoid by Lembeck (10).

Neuroendocrine cells of the gastrointestinal tract form the largest neuroendocrine system in the body. There are two types of neuroendocrine cells in the gastrointestinal tract, "open" and "closed" type, with features shown in Table 59.1. Most cell types are the enterochromaffin cells that originate from Kulchitsky cells widely distributed in the crypts of Lieberkuhn (11). The term "*enterochromaffin*" indicates the ability to stain with chromium salts, a feature of serotonin-secreting cells. Masson suggested the endocrine origin of carcinoid tumors and demonstrated that the tumors had a high affinity for silver stains and hence the term "*argentaffinoma*" (12). Besides the gut, NET can also be seen in the bronchus and pancreas. The most common sites where the tumors are seen are the ileum and appendix, followed by the rectum, lungs, bronchi and stomach (13). A wide range of hormones are actively secreted by the NET, with the most common being the vasoactive peptide serotonin.

Classification

The initial classification of the tumors was based on embryological divisions of the gut, namely the *foregut* tumors arising from lungs, bronchi or stomach, *midgut* tumors from the small intestine, appendix or proximal large bowel, and *hindgut* tumors from the distal colon and rectum (14, 15), as shown in Table 59.2. However, the latest WHO classification is based on the mitotic count and Ki67 proliferative index into "*neuroendocrine tumor*" (Grade 1 or Grade 2), and "*neuroendocrine carcinoma*" (Grade 3, large or small cell type). The European Neuroendocrine Tumour Society (ENETS) has proposed a newer classification and grading system (16). Classification of NETs is also based on the hormone secretions of *functional* or *nonfunctional* types. The hormone-secreting tumors are gastrinoma, somatostatinoma and glucagonoma.

"*Carcinoid syndrome*", which is characterized by severe clinical manifestations, is due to an excess of serotonin (17–20). This entity will be discussed later in the chapter.

Molecular pathogenesis

The mechanisms behind the initiation and progression of NET of the gastrointestinal tract are not well understood unlike other solid tumors. Some improvements in the understanding of the molecular mechanisms have been possible with newer technologies such as next-generation sequencing (NGS), microarray techniques, microRNA (miRNA) and methylation studies (21–23). This led to the detection of various aberrant pathways that play a key role in tumor progression, such as chromatic remodeling, alteration of telomeres and PI3K and MTOR signaling pathways that have paved the way for targeted therapies in the treatment of advanced NET (24, 25). *An important point to understand is that the molecular genetic events are different in tumors from the various sites and also between benign and malignant tumors.* In this section, we will look at the molecular alterations based on the site of origin of the tumors.

Foregut NE tumors

In relation to the pathogenesis of gastric carcinoid genetic mutations, mesenchymal and growth factors and bacterial infections play a role, by affecting multiple cellular pathways. Four studies showed a distinct linkage to MEN1 locus at 11q13 for the loss of heterozygosity in the development of NET in both sporadic and inherited cases (25–28). Aberration of MEN1 gene had no impact on any clinical parameters apart from postoperative tumor recurrence. Another common molecular event reported in many malignancies includes methylation of CpG islands (29, 30). Chan et al. showed p14, p16, MGMT and THBS1 genes were frequently methylated in 16 carcinoid tumors studied (31). Mutations of a few other genes such as TP53, SMAD loci of chromosome 6, KRAS (32), RB1 and ATP_4A (33, 34) have also been reported in poorly differentiated NET or neuroendocrine carcinomas studied.

Midgut NE tumors

Small gut NETs are the most common variety of the gastrointestinal tract. They are classified as *proximal* SI NET involving the duodenum and proximal jejunum and *distal* SI NET involving the distal jejunum and ileum. Most SI NETs are of sporadic type; genetic pattern of the disease seen is only about 1–2% (35, 36). Two genome-wide association studies by Walsh et al. and Ter-Minassian et al. looked at single nucleotide polymorphisms (SNPs) in association with ileal NET (37, 38). Ter-Minassian et al. showed two SNPs, *interleukin 12A*, a gene involved in an inflammatory response, and *DAD1 rs8005354*, a gene that modulates apoptosis to be significantly associated with the development of ileal carcinoids. A study by Walsh did not show any association

TABLE 59.1: Differences between "Open" and "Closed" Neuroendocrine Cell

	Open NET Cell	Closed NET Cell
Definition	Cytoplasm communicates with the lumen of the crypts	Cytoplasm does not communicate with the crypt lumina
Position of cells	Reside at the base of intestinal crypts	Cells lie close to the basement membrane
Physiological response	Do not respond to local, circulating hormones or trophic factors	React to local, circulating hormones or trophic factors
Examples	Gastrin-secreting (G) cells Somatostatin-secreting (D) cells Glucagon-secreting (L) cells	Enterochromaffin-like cells (ECL) Enterochromaffin cells (ECC)

TABLE 59.2: Candidate Genes and Pathways Involved in Pathogenesis of Ileal NETs

Pathways	Genes	Mechanisms
Inflammation	ILI2A	Susceptibility
Apoptosis	DAD1	Susceptibility and amplification
	RYBP	Deletion
	CASP 1,4,5	Deletion
Proliferation	ERBB2/HER2	Amplification
	PRKCA	Amplification
	RET	Upregulation
	APLP1	Upregulation
	RUNX1	Upregulation
Angiogenesis	ECM1	Upregulation
Adhesion	SPOCK1	Upregulation
Unknown	GPR112	Upregulation
	MIRI33A	Downregulation

TABLE 59.3: WHO Grading System for NETs

Grade	Mitotic Count per 10 hpf*	Ki67 Index (%)
G1	<2	≤2
G2	2–20	3–20
G3	>20	>20

Abbreviation: hpf, high-power field.

with the SNPs but showed a small proportion of tumors (6%) carried a copy number variant linked to chromosome 18 (38).

The most frequent genetic alteration seen in ileal NET is loss of heterozygosity (LOH) on chromosome 18, followed by those on chromosomes 9 (*CDKN2A, p16*), 11 (*SDHD*) and 16 (39–41). The molecular events are linked to either *inactivation* of tumor suppressor genes *p16/CDKN2A, WWOX, ZFHX3* (*ATBF1*) and *FOXF1*, *amplification* of ERBB2/HER2 or *activation* of oncogenes such as *OR4A5* (encoding G protein–coupled olfactory receptor) and summarized in Table 59.3 (42–45). LOH on chromosome 18 appears to be an early event in tumor pathogenesis, with additional alterations involving losses and gains on chromosomes associated with disease progression and metastasis. The genomic progression of ileal NET is illustrated in Figure 59.1.

Studies that looked at expression profile in ileal NET have gene expression similar to enterochromaffin cells that are involved in the synthesis of serotonin (46), synaptic vesicles (47, 48), neurotransmitter transport (48), peptide receptors (49–51), adrenoceptors (51) and transcription factors (52, 53). These discoveries aided not only in the diagnosis of SI NET but also develop novel therapies such as somatostatin receptor–mediated therapy (54). The most upregulated genes linked to expression profile include ECM1, LGLAS4, SLC18A1 (VMAT1), HOXC6 and RET (55).

Extracellular matrix protein (ECM1) is known to stimulate angiogenesis. *Ileal NETs that express ECM1 produce abundant stroma that can lead to desmoplastic reaction and small bowel obstruction* (56). Another receptor molecule VMAT1 (*vesicular*

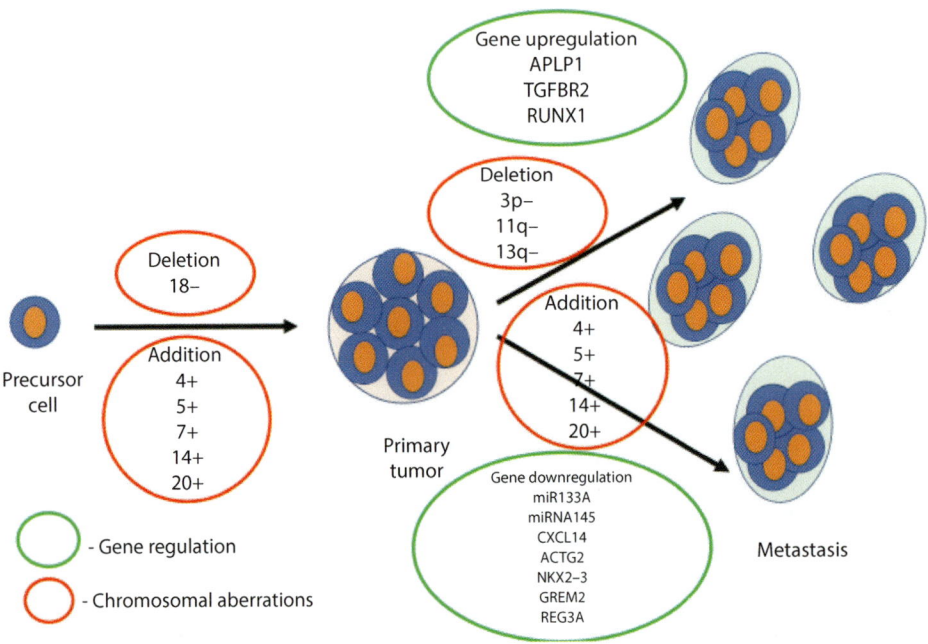

FIGURE 59.1 Chromosomal and genetic aberrations in the progression of NET.

Carcinoid Tumors of the Gastrointestinal Tract

monoamine transporter 1), located in the synaptic vesicular membranes, and chromaffin granules increase the uptake of meta-iodobenzylguanidine (MIBG) and may be an option in the treatment of metastatic ileal NETs using ^{123}I-MIBG in tumors that express VMAT1 (57). Similarly, tumors that express RET may be amenable to targeted kinase therapy (58). The various genes involved with disease progression in ileal NET are shown in Table 59.2.

Hindgut NETs

Molecular aspects of appendicular NET are less well studied, though it is the second commonest site of NET in the bowel. The limited studies that are available are on a subtype of NET called *goblet cell carcinoids* that are not pure carcinoid tumors. A comparative study of 3 cases of appendiceal NET versus 6 goblet cell carcinoid tumors showed no mutation of any of 379 cancer-related genes in appendiceal NET (59).

Colonic NETs are usually very aggressive and have early metastasis. These behave very similar to the poorly differentiated colonic carcinomas but have a poorer prognosis (60–62). The oncogenic mutation profiles those involving *APC*, *KRAS*, *BRAF* and *TP53* genes are similar between colonic neuroendocrine and colorectal carcinomas (33, 63). Other features seen in neuroendocrine carcinomas are decreased *Rb* expression and overexpression of *Bcl-2* and *p16* similar to neuroendocrine carcinomas seen at other sites (33, 63).

In an analysis of rectal NET from 56 patients using miRNA analysis, mutations involving *BRAF, KRAS, NRAS* and *PIK3CA* genes or microsatellite instability (*MSI*) were not detected (64). In another study, epigenetic alterations involving CpG island methylator phenotype (CIMP) were seen in 13% of rectal NET, with *miR-885-5p* being the most common upregulated miRNA, and this correlated with increased lymph nodal spread (64).

Histology

The current classification of NET of the gastrointestinal tract is based on the site, tumor cell type and differentiation (65). For all the sites, there are three main categories of classification and include the following:

1. Well-differentiated endocrine tumors
   a. Tumors with benign behavior
   b. Tumors with indefinite behavior
2. Well-differentiated low-grade endocrine carcinomas
3. Poorly differentiated high-grade endocrine carcinomas

When evaluating and reporting pathology of NET, there is a minimum dataset that is required and includes *histology, tumor cell differentiation, predominant endocrine cell type* and *predictors of malignancy*. As a rule, well-differentiated tumors show structural patterns such as *trabecular, glandular, acinar* or *mixed* type. The cells look uniform with variable cytoplasm, little atypia and low mitotic index (66) (Figure 59.2). Converse is the feature of poorly differentiated carcinoma, where tumors display a solid structure with varying cell sizes, severe atypia, high mitotic index and necrosis (65). A tumor grading and classification system of NET has been proposed by WHO based on the mitotic rate and Ki67 proliferation index (Table 59.3).

Tumor cell differentiation is done by a combination of immunohistochemical neuroendocrine and cell-specific markers (60, 65). Neuroendocrine cells secrete peptides and hormones specific to a tumor cell type and therefore can aid in both diagnosis and prognostication. *Chromogranin A (CgA), synaptophysin* (67–69) and *neuron-specific enolase* (69, 70) are the commonly used hormonal markers and help differentiate the well-differentiated NET from the poorly differentiated type.

Clinical presentation

The majority of the NET are found in the gastrointestinal tract and their clinical presentation depends on site, secretory state and extent of disease. A significant proportion of these tumors are indolent, slow growing and usually asymptomatic. Most NETs

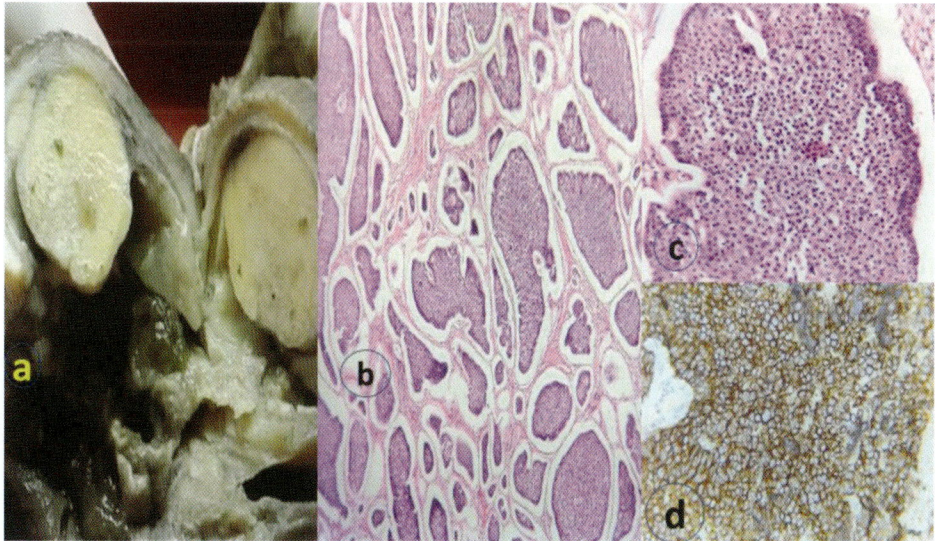

FIGURE 59.2 Histology of ileal NET. (a) Gross ileocaecal region showing a tan yellow mass protruding into the lumen. (b) Neoplastic cells arranged in insular (nesting) and trabecular patterns with peripheral palisading. (c) Monotonous population of small round cells with finely granular cytoplasm and salt and pepper chromatin. (d) Chromogranin and synaptophysin showing diffuse granular cytoplasmic positivity.

TABLE 59.4: Classification of NET Based on Site in the Gastrointestinal Tract

Site	Frequency %	Age Range	% With Metastasis	% With Carcinoid Syndrome
Small intestine	45	60–70	~70	5–7
Rectum	20	50–60	4–18	<5
Appendix	17	40–50	<5	<5
Colon	11	60–70	>60	<5
Stomach	7	60–70	<10	5–10

are found on routine screening endoscopies or imaging investigations. With increased screening, the incidence of gastric and colorectal NET is on the rise. Malignant NET may present with carcinoid syndrome in less than 10% of patients. Over a third of all gastrointestinal NETs arise from the small intestine, appendix and the rectum (Table 59.4).

Gastric NETs are generally of three types: Types I, II and III. Type I gastric NETs are associated with chronic atrophic gastritis type A, type 2 associated with MEN type 1 and Zollinger–Ellison syndrome and type 3 are sporadic. Type I- and II-associated tumors are multicentric and smaller than 2 cm, and metastases are seen in less than 10% of patients (71). Both the lesions are associated with high gastrin levels and produce serotonin, whereas type III lesions do not. Type III gastric NETs are usually large tumors that arise sporadically, generally aggressive and associated with metastasis quite early, with a 5-year survival of less than 75% (71).

The most common site of endocrine gastrointestinal tract NETs is the small intestine and are usually seen in the distal ileum within 60 cm of the ileocecal valve (14, 72). They generally present with small bowel obstruction. The infiltrative nature is due to the dense desmoplastic reaction, which results in kinking, obstruction and ischemia of the small bowel. The tumors are often multicentric, and metastasis to the regional lymph nodes and liver is common (73). A small proportion of patients present with carcinoid syndrome, which has a poor outcome (73, 74). The overall 5-year survival rates are around 65% for locoregional and 35% for distant disease (14).

Appendiceal NETs are the most common tumors seen in the appendix and usually discovered incidentally at surgery or appendectomy. The tumors are commonly situated at the tip or distal part of the appendix and hence do not give rise to many symptoms. Large tumors are usually situated at the base of the appendix, and patients present with clinical features of appendicitis (75). Prognosis is dependent on the size of the tumors and worse when the tumor size is greater than 2 cm (76). Smaller tumors rarely metastasize. The 5-year survival for appendiceal NET is over 90% in local disease, 85% for regional metastasis and 34% when distant metastasis is present (14, 73).

Colorectal NETs are rare and found incidentally in patients when undergoing evaluation for abdominal symptoms such as anorexia, pain and weight loss by colonoscopy (77). The diagnosis is usually made late in the course of the disease. Unlike the colonic NET, rectal tumors usually present with pain or bleeding. There is a difference in the size of the tumors between the colonic and rectal NET. Colonic NET are large with a mean size of 5 cm; metastasis is quite common and the 5-year survival of 25–40% (77, 78). The tumors are smaller in the rectum, but when more than 2 cm is associated with aggressive and malignant potential (14). The 5-year survival for tumors for localized disease is around 90%, with the survival of 49% for nodal metastasis and 26% for distant metastasis (39).

The gastrointestinal tract NETs rarely present with *carcinoid syndrome*.

Diagnosis and imaging

Biochemical diagnosis

Most tumors are asymptomatic at presentation; hence, diagnosing these is a challenge. Diagnosis is made by various tests that include histological examination and immunohistochemistry, biochemical evaluation using serum and urine, and imaging to localize the site of origin and look for distant metastasis. Histological examination and the role of immunohistochemistry were discussed earlier.

Biochemical diagnosis is based on the 24-hour urinary collection for the detection of serotonin metabolites, namely **5-HIAA** (79), and the test has a high specificity but low sensitivity (73, 80). The levels of urinary 5-HIAA are elevated to about 2–50 folds and higher in metastatic disease. It is essential that two 24-hour collections are done. Foods (avocado, banana, chocolate etc.) and drugs (salicylates, L-DOPA, antipsychotics etc.) are to be avoided at the time of collection as they interfere with the measurements (81). *The midgut tumors produce more pronounced elevations in 5-HIAA to foregut and hindgut tumors* (82, 83).

The glycoprotein **CgA** is an important serum marker of disease burden and extent in NET (84). It is particularly useful in conditions where the urinary 5-HIAA is less useful, especially in the diagnosis of foregut and hindgut NET. It is a more sensitive test than urinary 5-HIAA evaluation, but specificity is low (81, 85). *Elevations of CgA are seen more in well-differentiated NE tumors (G1 and G2) in comparison to poorly differentiated types* (86). Conditions such as renal failure, chronic gastritis and the use of proton pump inhibitors can also cause elevations of serum CgA (87). In clinical practice, measurement of both serum CgA and urine 5-HIAA simultaneously offers the best results when evaluating gastrointestinal tract NET.

A few other markers in serum have been evaluated in NET. An enzyme present in the cytoplasm of neuroendocrine cells, neuron-specific enolase (NSE), may be used as a marker for NET. NSE is particularly elevated in patients with poorly differentiated carcinomas (88). Another glycoprotein, human chorionic gonadotropin (HCG), has been shown to be elevated in foregut and hindgut tumors, with little elevation in midgut NET (89, 90). Pancreatic polypeptide, pro-gastrin-releasing peptide (Pro-GRP) and cytokeratin fragments (CKfr) are also expressed in NET (88).

Imaging

A multimodal approach is needed when it comes to imaging the gastrointestinal tract for NET. There are two aspects to imaging: *anatomical* and *functional*. The role of *the anatomical scans is to localize tumors and diagnose metastatic disease*, and commonly, a triple-phase multidetector computed tomography (CT) and magnetic resonance (MR) imaging are used. *Functional imaging*

Carcinoid Tumors of the Gastrointestinal Tract

is done to diagnose, stage and restage following treatment and monitor the status of disease in the body. The most common functional scan used was somatostatin-receptor scintigraphy using indium 111 (^{111}In)–octreotide but now replaced by positron emission tomography (PET).

CT scans can pick up lesions when large. Most gastrointestinal tract NETs are smaller than 2 cm and detection can be quite difficult, with a very low sensitivity (91, 92). The lesions are very vascular and are picked up during the arterial phase of the assessment.

MRI is superior to CT when evaluating soft tissues and best used for focused examination such as the liver for metastasis or where the CT scan results are equivocal (93). MRI is the imaging modality of choice in younger patients due to low risk of irradiation. Imaging findings include a low signal intensity on T1-weighted images and hyperintense lesion on T2-weighted images.

In patients with small bowel NETs who present with obscure gastrointestinal bleeding, CT or MR enterography or enteroclysis is useful with its high sensitivity and specificity (94, 95). CT enterography is sensitive to detect even lesions smaller than 2 cm. The lesions are seen as polyps or circumferential lesions in the duodenum and hyperenhancing polyps or masses or carpet lesions in the ileum (96). Other modalities that have been used to image include endoscopy and barium enema to detect the primary tumor but have less sensitivity.

Functional imaging used in the imaging of gastrointestinal tract NET includes somatostatin-receptor scintigraphy (SRS), PET and iodinated MIBG (^{131}I-MIBG). SRS works on the principle that synthetic somatostatin analogs have a high affinity for tissue expressing somatostatin receptors (SSTR). Of the five subtypes SSTR, type 2 and 5 are expressed in 70–90% of well-differentiated NETs (97, 98) and thus can be used to image these tumors. ^{111}In-DTPA-octreotide is the most common radioligand used for SRS (99, 100). SRS scans are highly sensitive, detects lesions not seen on conventional scans like CT or MRI and identifies a greater load of metastatic disease. Another benefit of SRS scan is that it identifies patients likely to benefit from targeted therapy such as ^{90}Y-DOTA-octreotide or ^{177}Lu-DOTA-octreotate (101–103). Bone metastases are better seen on SRS scans in comparison to technetium bone scan. SRS is not, however, without its limitations: nonspecific uptake in normal glands and inflammatory tissues, and poor spatial resolution (102, 104).

PET is routinely used in clinical oncology for the detection of cancers and assessment of disease progression. A few tracers are used in the assessment of gastrointestinal NET and include gallium 68–tetraazacyclododecane tetraacetic acid–octreotate (^{68}Ga-DOTA-TATE [SSTR-2 analog]), ^{68}Ga-edotreotide (SSTR-2 and SSTR-5 analog) and ^{68}Ga-DOTA-NOC, also known as [^{68}Ga] DOTA-[Nal3]-octreotide (SSTR-2, SSTR-3 and SSTR-5 analog) (104). DOTA imaging is useful in monitoring response to therapy and predicts the more aggressive and poorly differentiated NE cancers. It has a little clinical impact on the evaluation of Grade 1 and Grade 2 NETs (105).

MIBG has been in use for a long time to treat metastatic pheochromocytoma and paragangliomas (106, 107). MIBG is an analog of catecholamine, derived from the drug guanethidine, which gets incorporated into vesicles or secretory granules of a neuroendocrine cell. Both iodine-123 (I^{123}) and iodine-131 (I^{131}) can be tagged with MIBG, but I^{131} is preferentially used due to its beta-ray effect (106). MIBG was used to treat carcinoid tumors in 1986 (108). I^{123} MIBG has a preferential uptake in mid- and hindgut tumors due to the difference in cytochemicals expressed (109).

Studies have shown the sensitivity to be between 36 and 61% (110, 111). In a series of 54 patients with NETs, a comparative study of I^{123} MIBG versus ^{111}In-pentetreotide scintigraphy showed lower sensitivity for MIBG (50 versus 67%) in picking up metastatic lesions. The current indications are therefore for patients requiring targeted therapy with MIBG or those with contraindications to somatostatin analog therapy (112).

Treatment

The most effective treatment for NET of the GI tract is curative surgery. This is, however, not always possible due to a large number of patients presenting with metastasis early in the disease. Surgery is of three types when dealing with NETs:

1. Curative surgery for primary and regional metastasis
2. Cytoreductive surgery of metastasis – regional and distant
3. Palliative surgery for symptom control

Besides surgery, other modalities of treatments include *chemotherapy* with somatostatin analogs, interferons and cytotoxic agents, use of *radiotherapy and radionuclides, ablative therapies with radiofrequency and cryotherapy, chemoembolization* and *palliative symptom control*. The outline of treatment options in NET is shown in Figure 59.3. Each treatment modality is briefly discussed below.

Surgery for primary site disease

The presentation of the disease is in a myriad of ways, based on the site and stage of the disease, and this poses a significant challenge to effective treatment. The main modality of treatment in gastrointestinal tract NET is surgery; however, this is only possible in about a fifth of patients when they present with a small tumor and limited locoregional disease (113). We have also seen earlier that some GI NET presents as emergency either with appendicitis or small bowel obstruction. In this scenario, the diagnosis of NET is only possible after surgical remedy for the acute presentation. Definitive radical surgery should be considered early in such patients. In patients where radical surgery may not be possible, debulking surgery has a role to play, both at the primary and metastatic sites such as the liver.

Small type I and II gastric NETs, less than 1 cm, only require endoscopic surveillance (114). For tumors that are larger in size (more than 1 cm), with polyps less than 6 in number and not involving the muscularis propria on endoscopic ultrasound, endoscopic submucosal surgery is preferred (115, 116). In the presence of six or more polyps, extension into muscularis or positive margins on endoscopic surgery, limited surgery with negative margins in the form of antrectomy is needed (116, 117). In larger tumors (more than 2 cm) or local recurrence following conservative surgery, total gastrectomy is needed (71). In patients with large tumors, gastrectomy with lymph node clearance is required. For poorly differentiated NE carcinomas that usually present with advanced disease, surgical debulking together with chemotherapy is often needed. For lesions in between 1 and 2 cm, the best option of treatment is debatable; both endoscopic surgery and surveillance at 1- to 2-year intervals or surgical management is an option (118–121).

Midgut NET usually presents with obstructing lesions of the small intestine. Typical features of such tumors at laparotomy include a tumor with a lot of nodal metastases and fibrosis (122, 123). Standard treatment includes an en bloc resection of tumor

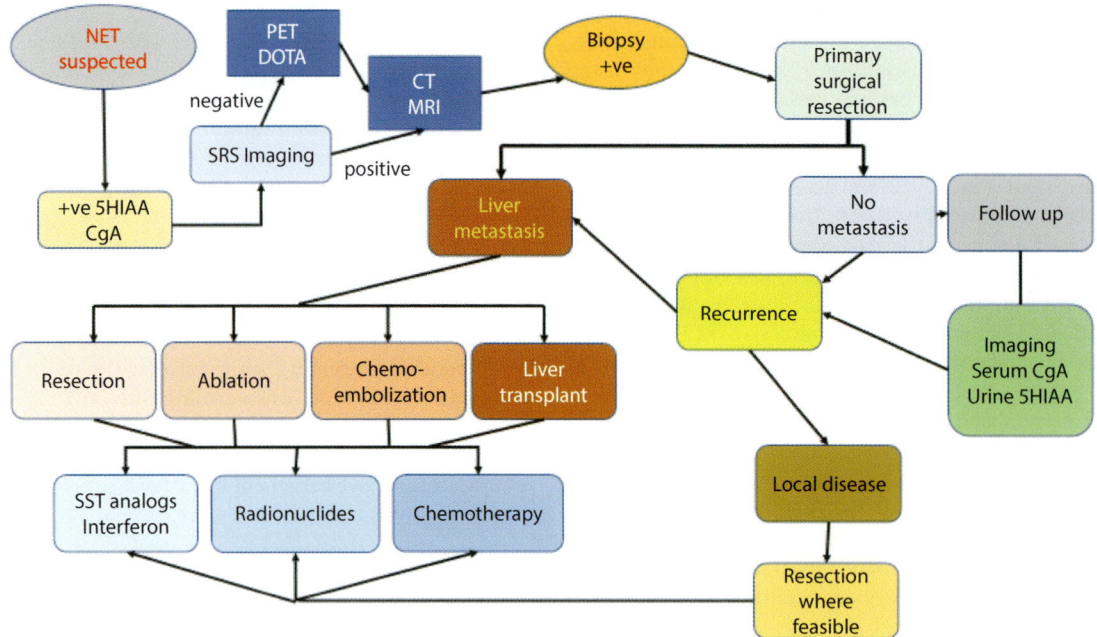

FIGURE 59.3 Treatment algorithm of NETs.

with clear margins, wedge resection of the mesentery and lymphadenectomy. The liver should be examined for any metastases and the whole of the peritoneal cavity should be inspected for any occult disease. Patients do have a tendency for recurrence and require long-term surveillance. Recurrences in the mesentery are not uncommon, and where seen, early surgical intervention is required. Revision surgery can be difficult due to extensive fibrosis that may result in fistulation, devascularization at surgery and short gut syndrome (124).

Appendiceal NETs are commonly during appendicectomy or incidentally at laparotomy. When the NETs are smaller than 1 cm, appendicectomy should suffice. For tumors larger than 2 cm or show features of multicentricity, atypia and invasion should undergo a right hemicolectomy with excision of the mesentery (125).

The treatment of colonic NET is similar to the ileal or midgut disease. Colonic NETs generally have a poorer prognosis and should undergo a radical resection similar to adenocarcinoma whereby the mesentery and the draining lymph nodes are also removed. The smaller rectal NET (less than 1 cm) can be managed by endoscopic or transanal resection (126, 127). Rectal lesions between 1 and 2 cm without lymph nodal disease need a wider excision. The presence of adverse features, such as large tumor size, local invasion and nodal metastases, requires anterior resection with mesorectal excision or abdominoperineal excision if low and near the sphincters (128, 129).

Cytoreductive surgery for metastasis – regional and distant

Peritoneal disease is seen in 10–30% of patients with midgut NET and commonly seen as small nodules at surgery (130, 131). Scoring systems include *Gilly classification* based on nodule size and extent of involvement, and *abdominal gravity. PC scoring system (GPS)*, which combines Gilly classification with lymph nodal involvement and metastases to the liver, was developed to assess the volume of peritoneal disease at surgery (131). Peritonectomy may be considered in fit patients, however is associated with significant morbidity, especially when performing concomitant liver surgery. The evidence of the role of peritonectomy in metastatic NET is lacking at this present time.

Liver metastasis is common in midgut and colonic NETs and has a significant impact on prognosis (132). In patients with well-differentiated NET and liver metastasis, surgical resection should always be considered in the absence of disseminated disease (132). Even in the presence of large metastasis, debulking surgery help control some of the symptoms associated with hormonal excess. A classification has been proposed to guide the feasibility of resection based on the extent of disease in the liver (133):

- Type I: Single or multiple metastases confined to one lobe or adjacent segments
- Type II: One major focus but with contralateral smaller satellites
- Type III: Disseminated spread with both lobes involved

Surgical options for the liver metastases include wedge excisions, enucleation, lobectomy or parenchyma-saving liver resections (134).

Liver transplantation (LT) may be necessary for a small proportion of patients with extensive disease for improved survival and symptom relief. Currently, the two scenarios where LT may be considered in NE cancers are *asymptomatic* unresectable liver secondaries refractory to other modalities of therapy and *symptomatic* unresectable liver secondaries that cannot be treated with other modalities. Retrospective cohort studies have shown the overall 5-year survival rates of 47–97% (135–137) and cure in about 40% (138) following LT. Selection of patients is critical for LT, and to help guide this, the *Milan criteria* were proposed. The patients who would have the highest benefit from LT based on the criteria include the following: (1) *low-grade tumor (WHO G1 or G2)*; (2) *primary tumor drained by the portal system and the absence of extrahepatic disease*; (3) *liver metastasis lesion not exceeding 50% of the liver*; (4) *a stable period of no fewer than 6 months before LT*; and (5) *patient age not exceeding 55 years* (139, 140). There is no role for palliative LT to treat metastatic NET to liver. Currently, there are no studies that have looked at salvage LT after primary liver resection for neuroendocrine metastases to liver (141).

Ablative therapies for NE liver metastases
The ablative therapies used to treat NE liver metastasis include *radiofrequency ablation (RFA), cryosurgical ablation, laser-induced thermal ablation* and *percutaneous ethanol ablation*. RFA induces coagulative necrosis when high frequency alternating current (around 460 kHz) is introduced into the tissues by cause of molecular vibrations and generation of heat. RFA can be delivered through a percutaneous approach or by open and laparoscopic techniques. RFA generally works for smaller tumors (usually less than 3.5 cm), should have normal surrounding liver parenchyma, away from the liver capsule and the hepatic portal veins. The number of metastases that can be ablated is a maximum of seven (142). Published series have shown symptom relief in over 90% of patients over a period of 10–24 months, along with decreased hormonal markers (143–145).

Percutaneous ethanol ablation can also be used in the treatment of metastases from neuroendocrine malignancies (146, 147). A single study involving four patients with liver metastases from NET showed a complete response to ethanol ablation (148). Ethanol ablation can be performed on tumors close to key vital structures such as big vessels and bile ducts (149) and has a much lower collateral damage in comparison to RFA. In general, ablative therapies are not used for tumors situated at the hilum. These procedures are reserved for patients with localized or residual disease and are used as adjuncts to surgery. Complications are generally low for ethanol ablation and commonly include sepsis, bile leak and bleeding.

Transarterial chemoembolization
Transarterial hepatic chemoembolization (TACE) involves occlusion of the hepatic artery to deprive the tumors of their blood supply, so that the tumors get ischemic and undergo necrosis. Chemoembolization can be performed using particles like gel foam, polyvinyl alcohol and microspheres. In chemoembolization, intra-arterial chemotherapy is delivered at high concentrations first and then the artery is embolized to decrease wash out of the chemotherapy (150). Studies have showed that symptomatic relief either partially or completely was seen in 40–100% of tumors over a mean period of 9–24 months (151, 152), associated with a significant reduction in hormonal markers (13–100%) and morphological changes (8–94%) (152). Complications are not uncommon following TACE and include bleeding, infections, transaminitis, carcinoid crisis and *postembolization syndrome* seen in 80–90% of patients (153, 154).

Systemic therapies
Somatostatin functions as an "off switch" due to inhibitory effects on paracrine, exocrine and endocrine glands. The majority of the well-differentiated NETs express the somatostatin receptors 2 and 5. Examples of commonly used SST include lanreotide and octreotide. Besides helping in controlling the symptoms relating to the NET, SST analogs also inhibit the growth of NETs and keep the disease stable (155, 156). The PROMID trial evaluated the effect of octreotide in patients with metastatic well-differentiated NETs (157). *Octreotide therapy is now the standard first-line therapy for midgut metastatic NET not amenable to surgical therapy.* Octreotide is also used in the treatment and prophylaxis of carcinoid crisis. The role of somatostatin analogs in tumors that do not express in foregut and hindgut NET is uncertain. The CLARINET study evaluated lanreotide in nonfunctioning advanced Grade 1 and Grade 2 NETs and showed a progression-free survival of 65% at 24 months of follow-up (158). Side effects are seen with SSR therapy and include nausea, abdominal pain, diarrhea, biliary symptoms, conduction abnormalities and hormonal issues such as hypothyroidism, hyper- and hypoglycemia.

Alpha interferon (INFα) is also used in the treatment of carcinoid syndrome in association with NET. They have significant antiviral and antitumoral properties as a result of immune mediation by inhibition of angiogenesis or arrest of cell growth. INFα has been used as either monotherapy or in combination with SST analogs. Studies have shown a partial radiographic response in 12–20% and urinary 5-HIAA reductions in 39–53% (159, 160). A randomized study of combination therapy of INFα with octreotide in 109 gastrointestinal tract NETs only showed a slight benefit in median survival (161). INFα therapy is associated with significant side effects such as myelosuppression.

Chemotherapy is indicated in patients with NE metastases as a mode of palliative treatment. The common agents that have been used include streptozotocin (STZ), 5-fluorouracil (5-FU), doxorubicin, dacarbazine (DTIC), etoposide and cisplatin as combination therapies. The response to therapies has been disappointing with a response rate of 10–15%, especially for midgut NET, but in contrast pancreatic NET showed a response rate of 33–39% (162). Poorly differentiated Grade 3 NET irrespective of the site of origin showed a response rate of 55–80% to cisplatin and etoposide therapy over duration of 8–11 months (163).

Radionuclide therapy
Radiotherapy is ineffective for gastrointestinal tract NETs as the targets are not stationary and the tumors are not radiosensitive. One way of overcoming this problem is by delivering therapeutic doses of radiation into the cell by linking the radioisotopes to SST analogs, called *radiopeptide targeted therapy* (RPTT). For RPTT to work, the tumors must express the SST receptor, especially type 2, and should demonstrate a high density on SSTR imaging, as outlined by the Rotterdam scale of Grades 2–4 (164). Besides Rotterdam scale, there are few other criteria that need to be met for RPPT therapy and include Karnofsky performance status of more than 60 or ECOF less than 2, G1 or G2 tumors and Ki67 index less than 20 (165,166). The four radioisotopes that can linked to octreotide and currently used in the therapy of NET are ^{90}Y, ^{111}In, ^{131}MIBG and ^{177}Lu. PRRT is recommended for use in patients in unresectable G1 and G2 NETs (167, 168) and has been shown to be highly effective. PRRT studies involving these isotopes showed a tumor response ranging between 8 and 46%, biochemical stability between 52 and 54% and tumor stability between 65 and 92%. PRRT has an excellent safety profile, but carcinoid crisis may occur (169).

Carcinoid syndrome

Carcinoid syndrome is a condition wherein metastatic NET commonly arising from the midgut releases hormones and causes a constellation of signs and symptoms. The most common symptoms include flushing seen in 85% of patients, diarrhea (75–80%), abdominal cramps (75%), bronchospasm and right-sided heart failure (170). The flushing is typically seen in the upper trunk and face and provoked by certain foods or exercise. In terms of right heart disease, tricuspid insufficiency is the commonest abnormality followed by tricuspid stenosis, pulmonary insufficiency, and stenosis.

Diagnosis is made when the patient has a biopsy-proven NET with at least one clinical manifestation and the presence of elevated urinary 5-HIAA. Serum serotonin may be elevated in patients with midgut NET. Similarly, serum CgA may be elevated in well-differentiated NET, and the levels correlate with tumor burden. Imaging of NET was discussed earlier and includes CT, MRI and functional scintigraphy with either octreoscan or PET.

Treatment modalities are surgery and medical therapies as discussed earlier in the chapter. Surgery is the best option, but it may not be possible to resect the tumors, and hence debulking may be necessary. Where metastatic to liver, resections must be done where safe and in the absence of extrahepatic disease. Localized therapies, such as ablative measures with cryotherapy or RFA, or chemoembolization may be needed along with targeted therapies.

SST analogs with and without interferon therapy are possible in tumors that express these receptors especially in G1 and G2 tumors. Evidence suggests that they effectively control the symptoms of carcinoid syndrome and also improve the response of the biological markers. Systemic chemotherapy works for the poorly differentiated NET with limited benefit in well-differentiated disease. Targeted kinase therapies with sunitinib, bevacizumab, sorafenib and everolimus have also been tried in the treatment of the condition with limited efficacy. RPPT therapy with ^{90}Y-DOTA tyr3-octreotide, ^{90}Y-edotreotide, ^{177}Lu-DOTA or Tyr 3-octreotate has shown some beneficial effects in the treatment of carcinoid syndrome in tumors expressing the SST receptor.

Carcinoid crisis is seen in patients where there is a rapid surge of the release of the neuroendocrine hormones and happens usually during tumor handling at surgery or anesthesia or following local ablative therapies (171, 172). The condition is associated with hypotension, confusion, severe dyspnea and flushing, which can be life-threatening. Treatment is supportive with octreotide infusion and drugs to treat diarrhea and bronchospasms (173).

Asian perspective

The incidence of NET has been rising in Asia as well, similar to the trends in the West and United States. The data pertaining to epidemiology and treatment from Asia is limited to studies from a few countries, namely Japan, Taiwan, China, Australia and Singapore (174–181). In an epidemiological study from Japan, the prevalence of NET was 2.23/100,000, and the annual incidence of 1.01/100,000. A similar study from Taiwan showed the incidence to be 1.51 per 100,000 in 2008. Our own study from Singapore showed an incidence that increased from 0.8 to 3 per 100,000 per year over the time period 1993–2014. This is in contrast to the incidence of 0.32 per 100,000 in the United States. The reasons for the high incidence rates in Asia are easier access to imaging modalities such as CT and MRI and improved diagnostic tools during health screening. The epidemiological studies from the five countries are summarized in Table 59.5.

There appears to be a difference in the preferred sites of NETs when comparing the Asian population with published reports from Europe and the United States (84, 174–179). The ileum and colorectal region appear to be the predominant sites of disease in the Western and American population. However, in Asia, the preferred sites of NETs are the colorectum and stomach. Patients commonly present with bowel symptoms in the West, especially with small bowel obstruction, rectal bleeding and dyspepsia. However, in Asia, the presentation is mostly with asymptomatic disease and detected on screening endoscopies or as incidental lesions on imaging. The robust screening programs especially the National Bowel and Gastric Cancer Screening Programs in Japan, Australia and Korea have contributed significantly to the rise of asymptomatic disease. Most centers in Asia show a male preponderance of the disease, and this is like the Western and US studies.

In some Asian countries, patients presenting with metastatic disease ranges from 6 to 36%. This is likely in low-income Asian countries due to the lack of robust National Screening Programmes and access to imaging modalities. Singapore, though a developed nation and with excellent health-care infrastructure, more than a third present with advanced, metastatic disease, and this was due to lack of patient participation for bowel screening. However, this trend is reversing with increased uptake of bowel screening over the last few years. Early detection and treatment have an impact on survival and prognosis as shown in Table 59.5. Clearly one can see that the survival is much improved in countries that have a robust bowel screening program. Diagnosis and treatment of NET are made quite early, and this leads to improved survival.

A study from Canada on 6000 patients with NET showed a difference in survival between patients coming from rural and urban areas (180). This is a possible scenario in the poorer countries of Asia where there is a big gap in the care of patients coming from rural areas due to reasons such as diagnostic delays, lack

TABLE 59.5: Comparison of Studies of NET from Asia (Compiled from References (174–181))

Country of Study	Japan	Taiwan	Singapore	China	South Korea	Australia
Annual incidence per 100,000 population	1.01	1.51	3.0	Increasing trend	Increasing trend	6.3
Gender ratio (M:F)	2:1	2:1	1:1	1.5:1	1.5:1	1:1
Common sites in order of frequency	Colon	Rectum	Rectum	Rectum	Rectum	Appendix
	Rectum	Stomach	Colon	Stomach	Stomach	Ileum
	Stomach	Colon	Stomach	Colon	Colon	Rectum
	Ileum	Ileum	Ileum	Appendix	Ileum	Stomach
	Appendix	Appendix	Appendix	Ileum	Appendix	Colon
Functioning tumors (%)	49%	Not reported	5.5%	4%	Not reported	Not reported
Metastasis at presentation	6%	Not reported	36%	8.3%	Not reported	Not reported
5-year survival	95.8%	50.4%	38.1%	89%	96.7%	68.5–92.6%
Presentation with symptoms	3.4%	Not reported	Not reported	12.4%	Not reported	Not reported

of education and difficulty in access to specialized treatments. Similarly, newer and biological therapies are available in countries with excellent resources but may be difficult to deliver in low-income countries of Asia.

Conclusions

The incidence of GI NET is increasing globally due to early detection and treatment. The disease is usually indolent, but presentation varies with the site of the disease. There is a difference in the site of disease between Asia and the rest of the world, with colorectal and gastric NETs being more common in Asia. Diagnosis is often made late, with distant metastases seen at initial presentation. A small proportion of patients with NETs present with hormonal excess leading to systemic manifestations. The best curative modality is surgery, but other modalities of treatments have emerged for patients with advanced disease due to the better understanding of the molecular mechanisms in these tumors. Prognosis is dependent on factors such as site, size and histology. With improvements in diagnosis, imaging and treatment, disease survival has improved.

References

1. Oberg K, Astrup L, Eriksson B, Falkmer SE, Falkmer UG, Gustafsen J, et al. Guidelines for the management of gastroenteropancreatic neuroendocrine tumours (including bronchopulmonary and thymic neoplasms). Part I – General overview. Acta Oncol. 2004;43(7):617–25.
2. Langhans T. Ueber einen Drüsenpolyp im Ileum. Virchows Arch Pathol Anat. 1867;36:550–60.
3. Lubarsch O. Ueber den primaren Krebs des Ileum, nebst Bemerkungen über das gleichzeitige Vorkommen von Krebs und Tuberkuolose. Virchow Archiv Pathol Anatom Physiol Klin Med. 1867;111:280–317.
4. Oberndorfer S. Karzenoide Tumoren des Dünndarms. Frankf Zschr Pathol. 1907;1:426–30.
5. Pearson C, Fitzgerald PJ. Carcinoid tumors of the rectum-report of three cases, two with metastases. Ann Surg. 1948;128(1):128–43.
6. Pearson CM, Fitzgerald PJ. Carcinoid tumors; a re-emphasis of their malignant nature; review of 140 cases. Cancer. 1949;2(6):1005–26, illust.
7. Rapport MM, Green AA, Page IH. Serum vasoconstrictor, serotonin; isolation and characterization. J Biol Chem. 1948;176(3):1243–51.
8. Erspamer V, Asero B. Identification of enteramine, the specific hormone of the enterochromaffin cell system, as 5-hydroxytryptamine. Nature. 1952;169(4306):800–1.
9. Rosenbaum F, Santer D, Claudon D. Essential telangiectasia, pulmonic and tricuspid stenosis, and neoplastic liver disease-a possible new clinical syndrome. J Lab Clin Med. 1953;42: 941.
10. Lembeck F. 5-Hydroxytryptamine in a carcinoid tumour. Nature. 1953;172(4385):910–1.
11. Gosset A. Tumeurs endocrines de l'appendice. Press Med. 1914;22:37–40.
12. Masson P. Carcinoids (argentaffin-cell tumors) and nerve hyperplasia of the appendicular mucosa. Am J Pathol. 1928;4(3):181.
13. Godwin JD, 2nd. Carcinoid tumors. An analysis of 2,837 cases. Cancer. 1975;36(2):560–9.
14. Modlin IM, Lye KD, Kidd M. A 5-decade analysis of 13,715 carcinoid tumors. Cancer. 2003;97(4):934–59.
15. Williams E. The classification of carcinoid tumours. Lancet. 1963;1:238–9.
16. Rindi G, Klöppel G, Couvelard A, Komminoth P, Körner M, Lopes J, et al. TNM staging of midgut and hindgut (neuro) endocrine tumors: a consensus proposal including a grading system. Virchows Archiv. 2007;451(4):757–62.
17. Lips CJ, Lentjes EG, Hoppener JW. The spectrum of carcinoid tumours and carcinoid syndromes. Ann Clin Biochem. 2003;40(Pt 6):612–27.
18. Grahame-Smith DG, Peart WS, Ferriman DG. Carcinoid syndrome. Proc R Soc Med. 1965;58(9):701–2.
19. Oates JA. The carcinoid syndrome. N Engl J Med. 1986;315(11):702–4.
20. Srirajaskanthan R, Shanmugabavan D, Ramage JK. Carcinoid syndrome. BMJ. 2010;341:c3941.
21. Banck MS, Kanwar R, Kulkarni AA, Boora GK, Metge F, Kipp BR, et al. The genomic landscape of small intestine neuroendocrine tumors. J Clin Invest. 2013;123(6):2502–8.
22. Banck MS, Beutler AS. Advances in small bowel neuroendocrine neoplasia. Curr Opin Gastroenterol. 2014;30(2):163–7.
23. Stalberg P, Westin G, Thirlwell C. Genetics and epigenetics in small intestinal neuroendocrine tumours. J Intern Med. 2016;280(6):584–94.
24. Walenkamp A, Crespo G, Fierro Maya F, Fossmark R, Igaz P, Rinke A, et al. Hallmarks of gastrointestinal neuroendocrine tumours: implications for treatment. Endocr Relat Cancer. 2014;21(6):R445–60.
25. Neychev V, Steinberg SM, Cottle-Delisle C, Merkel R, Nilubol N, Yao J, et al. Mutation-targeted therapy with sunitinib or everolimus in patients with advanced low-grade or intermediate-grade neuroendocrine tumours of the gastrointestinal tract and pancreas with or without cytoreductive surgery: protocol for a phase II clinical trial. BMJ Open. 2015;5(5):e008248.
26. D'Adda T, Pizzi S, Azzoni C, Bottarelli L, Crafa P, Pasquali C, et al. Different patterns of 11q allelic losses in digestive endocrine tumors. Hum Pathol. 2002;33(3):322–9.
27. Zhuang Z, Vortmeyer AO, Pack S, Huang S, Pham TA, Wang C, et al. Somatic mutations of the MEN1 tumor suppressor gene in sporadic gastrinomas and insulinomas. Cancer Res. 1997;57(21):4682–6.
28. Goebel SU, Heppner C, Burns AL, Marx SJ, Spiegel AM, Zhuang Z, et al. Genotype/phenotype correlation of multiple endocrine neoplasia type 1 gene mutations in sporadic gastrinomas. J Clin Endocrinol Metab. 2000;85(1):116–23.
29. Baylin SB, Esteller M, Rountree MR, Bachman KE, Schuebel K, Herman JG. Aberrant patterns of DNA methylation, chromatin formation and gene expression in cancer. Hum Mol Genet. 2001;10(7):687–92.
30. Ahmed AA, Essa MEA. Potential of epigenetic events in human thyroid cancer. Cancer Genet. 2019;239:13–21.
31. Chan AO-O, Kim SG, Bedeir A, Issa J-P, Hamilton SR, Rashid A. CpG island methylation in carcinoid and pancreatic endocrine tumors. Oncogene. 2003;22(6):924–34.
32. Makuuchi R, Terashima M, Kusuhara M, Nakajima T, Serizawa M, Hatakeyama K, et al. Comprehensive analysis of gene mutation and expression profiles in neuroendocrine carcinomas of the stomach. Biomed Res. 2017;38(1):19–27.
33. Sahnane N, Furlan D, Monti M, Romualdi C, Vanoli A, Vicari E, et al. Microsatellite unstable gastrointestinal neuroendocrine carcinomas: a new clinicopathologic entity. Endocr Relat Cancer. 2015;22(1):35–45.
34. Calvete O, Reyes J, Zuniga S, Paumard-Hernandez B, Fernandez V, Bujanda L, et al. Exome sequencing identifies ATP4A gene as responsible of an atypical familial type I gastric neuroendocrine tumour. Hum Mol Genet. 2015;24(10):2914–22.
35. Hiripi E, Bermejo JL, Sundquist J, Hemminki K. Familial gastrointestinal carcinoid tumours and associated cancers. Ann Oncol. 2009;20(5):950–4.
36. Babovic-Vuksanovic D, Constantinou CL, Rubin J, Rowland CM, Schaid DJ, Karnes PS. Familial occurrence of carcinoid tumors and association with other malignant neoplasms. Cancer Epidemiol Biomarkers Prev. 1999;8(8):715–9.
37. Ter-Minassian M, Wang Z, Asomaning K, Wu MC, Liu CY, Paulus JK, et al. Genetic associations with sporadic neuroendocrine tumor risk. Carcinogenesis. 2011;32(8):1216–22.
38. Walsh KM, Choi M, Oberg K, Kulke MH, Yao JC, Wu C, et al. A pilot genome-wide association study shows genomic variants enriched in the non-tumor cells of patients with well-differentiated neuroendocrine tumors of the ileum. Endocr Relat Cancer. 2011;18(1):171–80.
39. Lollgen RM, Hessman O, Szabo E, Westin G, Akerstrom G. Chromosome 18 deletions are common events in classical midgut carcinoid tumors. Int J Cancer. 2001;92(6):812–5.
40. Stancu M, Wu TT, Wallace C, Houlihan PS, Hamilton SR, Rashid A. Genetic alterations in goblet cell carcinoids of the vermiform appendix and comparison with gastrointestinal carcinoid tumors. Mod Pathol. 2003;16(12):1189–98.
41. Wang GG, Yao JC, Worah S, White JA, Luna R, Wu TT, et al. Comparison of genetic alterations in neuroendocrine tumors: frequent loss of chromosome 18 in ileal carcinoid tumors. Mod Pathol. 2005;18(8):1079–87.
42. Cunningham JL, Diaz de Stahl T, Sjoblom T, Westin G, Dumanski JP, Janson ET. Common pathogenetic mechanism involving human chromosome 18 in familial and sporadic ileal carcinoid tumors. Genes Chromosomes Cancer. 2011;50(2):82–94.
43. Kulke MH, Freed E, Chiang DY, Philips J, Zahrieh D, Glickman JN, et al. High-resolution analysis of genetic alterations in small bowel carcinoid tumors reveals areas of recurrent amplification and loss. Genes Chromosomes Cancer. 2008;47(7):591–603.
44. Kim DH, Nagano Y, Choi IS, White JA, Yao JC, Rashid A. Allelic alterations in well-differentiated neuroendocrine tumors (carcinoid tumors) identified by genome-wide single nucleotide polymorphism analysis and comparison with pancreatic endocrine tumors. Genes Chromosomes Cancer. 2008;47(1):84–92.
45. Andersson E, Sward C, Stenman G, Ahlman H, Nilsson O. High-resolution genomic profiling reveals gain of chromosome 14 as a predictor of poor outcome in ileal carcinoids. Endocr Relat Cancer. 2009;16(3):953–66.
46. O'Connor DT, Deftos LJ. Secretion of chromogranin A by peptide-producing endocrine neoplasms. N Engl J Med. 1986;314(18):1145–51.
47. Jakobsen AM, Ahlman H, Wangberg B, Kolby L, Bengtsson M, Nilsson O. Expression of synaptic vesicle protein 2 (SV2) in neuroendocrine tumours of the gastrointestinal tract and pancreas. J Pathol. 2002;196(1):44–50.
48. Jakobsen AM, Andersson P, Saglik G, Andersson E, Kolby L, Erickson JD, et al. Differential expression of vesicular monoamine transporter (VMAT) 1 and 2 in gastrointestinal endocrine tumours. J Pathol. 2001;195(4):463–72.
49. Reubi JC, Kvols LK, Waser B, Nagorney DM, Heitz PU, Charboneau JW, et al. Detection of somatostatin receptors in surgical and percutaneous needle biopsy samples of carcinoids and islet cell carcinomas. Cancer Res. 1990;50(18):5969–77.
50. Nilsson O, Kolby L, Wangberg B, Wigander A, Billig H, William-Olsson L, et al. Comparative studies on the expression of somatostatin receptor subtypes, outcome of octreotide scintigraphy and response to octreotide treatment in patients with carcinoid tumours. Br J Cancer. 1998;77(4):632–7.
51. Modlin IM, Kidd M, Pfragner R, Eick GN, Champaneria MC. The functional characterization of normal and neoplastic human enterochromaffin cells. J Clin Endocrinol Metab. 2006;91(6):2340–8.
52. Wang YC, Zuraek MB, Kosaka Y, Ota Y, German MS, Deneris ES, et al. The ETS oncogene family transcription factor FEV identifies serotonin-producing cells in normal and neoplastic small intestine. Endocr Relat Cancer. 2010;17(1):283–91.
53. Saqi A, Alexis D, Remotti F, Bhagat G. Usefulness of CDX2 and TTF-1 in differentiating gastrointestinal from pulmonary carcinoids. Am J Clin Pathol. 2005;123(3):394–404.
54. Kwekkeboom DJ, de Herder WW, Kam BL, van Eijck CH, van Essen M, Kooij PP, et al. Treatment with the radiolabeled somatostatin analog [177 Lu-DOTA 0,Tyr3] octreotate: toxicity, efficacy, and survival. J Clin Oncol. 2008;26(13):2124–30.
55. Duerr EM, Mizukami Y, Ng A, Xavier RJ, Kikuchi H, Deshpande V, et al. Defining molecular classifications and targets in gastroenteropancreatic neuroendocrine tumors through DNA microarray analysis. Endocr Relat Cancer. 2008;15(1):243–56.

56. Druce M, Rockall A, Grossman AB. Fibrosis and carcinoid syndrome: from causation to future therapy. Nat Rev Endocrinol. 2009;5(5):276–83.
57. Kolby L, Bernhardt P, Levin-Jakobsen AM, Johanson V, Wangberg B, Ahlman H, et al. Uptake of meta-iodobenzylguanidine in neuroendocrine tumours is mediated by vesicular monoamine transporters. Br J Cancer. 2003;89(7):1383–8.
58. Chan JA, Kulke MH. New treatment options for patients with advanced neuroendocrine tumors. Curr Treat Options Oncol. 2011;12(2):136–48.
59. Wen KW, Grenert JP, Joseph NM, Shafizadeh N, Huang A, Hosseini M, et al. Genomic profile of appendiceal goblet cell carcinoid is distinct compared to appendiceal neuroendocrine tumor and conventional adenocarcinoma. Hum Pathol. 2018;77:166–74.
60. Kloppel G. Classification and pathology of gastroenteropancreatic neuroendocrine neoplasms. Endocr Relat Cancer. 2011;18(Suppl 1):S1–16.
61. Brenner B, Tang LH, Shia J, Klimstra DS, Kelsen DP. Small cell carcinomas of the gastrointestinal tract: clinicopathological features and treatment approach. Semin Oncol. 2007;34(1):43–50.
62. Olevian DC, Nikiforova MN, Chiosea S, Sun W, Bahary N, Kuan SF, et al. Colorectal poorly differentiated neuroendocrine carcinomas frequently exhibit BRAF mutations and are associated with poor overall survival. Hum Pathol. 2016;49:124–34.
63. Takizawa N, Ohishi Y, Hirahashi M, Takahashi S, Nakamura K, Tanaka M, et al. Molecular characteristics of colorectal neuroendocrine carcinoma; similarities with adenocarcinoma rather than neuroendocrine tumor. Hum Pathol. 2015;46(12):1890–900.
64. Mitsuhashi K, Yamamoto I, Kurihara H, Kanno S, Ito M, Igarashi H, et al. Analysis of the molecular features of rectal carcinoid tumors to identify new biomarkers that predict biological malignancy. Oncotarget. 2015;6(26):22114.
65. Solcia E, Klöppel G, Sobin LH. Histological typing of endocrine tumours. 2000. Springer Berlin Heidelberg, Berlin, Heidelberg.
66. Soga J, Tazawa K. Pathologic analysis of carcinoids. Histologic reevaluation of 62 cases. Cancer. 1971;28(4):990–8.
67. Janson ET, Holmberg L, Stridsberg M, Eriksson B, Theodorsson E, Wilander E, et al. Carcinoid tumors: analysis of prognostic factors and survival in 301 patients from a referral center. Ann Oncol. 1997;8(7):685–90.
68. Turner GB, Johnston BT, McCance DR, McGinty A, Watson RG, Patterson CC, et al. Circulating markers of prognosis and response to treatment in patients with midgut carcinoid tumours. Gut. 2006;55(11):1586–91.
69. Bajetta E, Procopio G, Buzzoni R, Catena L, Ferrari L, Del Vecchio M. Advances in diagnosis and therapy of neuroendocrine tumors. Expert Rev Anticancer Ther. 2001;1(3):371–81.
70. van Adrichem RCS, Kamp K, Vandamme T, Peeters M, Feelders RA, de Herder WW. Serum neuron-specific enolase level is an independent predictor of overall survival in patients with gastroenteropancreatic neuroendocrine tumors. Ann Oncol. 2016;27(4):746–7.
71. Rindi G, Bordi C, Rappel S, La Rosa S, Stolte M, Solcia E. Gastric carcinoids and neuroendocrine carcinomas: pathogenesis, pathology, and behavior. World J Surg. 1996;20(2):168–72.
72. Kulke MH, Benson AB, 3rd, Bergsland E, Berlin JD, Blaszkowsky LS, Choti MA, et al. Neuroendocrine tumors. J Natl Compr Canc Netw. 2012;10(6):724–64.
73. Sippel RS, Chen H. Carcinoid tumors. Surg Oncol Clin N Am. 2006;15(3):463–78.
74. Yantiss RK, Odze RD, Farraye FA, Rosenberg AE. Solitary versus multiple carcinoid tumors of the ileum: a clinical and pathologic review of 68 cases. Am J Surg Pathol. 2003;27(6):811–7.
75. Roggo A, Wood WC, Ottinger LW. Carcinoid tumors of the appendix. Ann Surg. 1993;217(4):385–90.
76. Moertel CG, Weiland LH, Nagorney DM, Dockerty MB. Carcinoid tumor of the appendix: treatment and prognosis. N Engl J Med. 1987;317(27):1699–701.
77. Rosenberg JM, Welch JP. Carcinoid tumors of the colon. A study of 72 patients. Am J Surg. 1985;149(6):775–9.
78. Spread C, Berkel H, Jewell L, Jenkins H, Yakimets W. Colon carcinoid tumors. A population-based study. Dis Colon Rectum. 1994;37(5):482–91.
79. Feldman JM. Urinary serotonin in the diagnosis of carcinoid tumors. Clin Chem. 1986;32(5):840–4.
80. Feldman JM, O'Dorisio TM. Role of neuropeptides and serotonin in the diagnosis of carcinoid tumors. Am J Med. 1986;81(6B):41–8.
81. O'Toole D, Grossman A, Gross D, Delle Fave G, Barkmanova J, O'Connor J, et al. ENETS consensus guidelines for the standards of care in neuroendocrine tumors: biochemical markers. Neuroendocrinology. 2009;90(2):194–202.
82. Meijer WG, Kema IP, Volmer M, Willemse PH, de Vries EG. Discriminating capacity of indole markers in the diagnosis of carcinoid tumors. Clin Chem. 2000;46(10):1588–96.
83. Baudin E, Bidart JM, Rougier P, Lazar V, Ruffié P, Ropers J, et al. Screening for multiple endocrine neoplasia type 1 and hormonal production in apparently sporadic neuroendocrine tumors. J Clin Endocrinol Metab. 1999;84(1):69–75.
84. Yao JC, Hassan M, Phan A, Dagohoy C, Leary C, Mares JE, et al. One hundred years after "carcinoid": epidemiology of and prognostic factors for neuroendocrine tumors in 35,825 cases in the United States. J Clin Oncol. 2008;26(18):3063–72.
85. Stridsberg M, Oberg K, Li Q, Engstrom U, Lundqvist G. Measurements of chromogranin A, chromogranin B (secretogranin I), chromogranin C (secretogranin II) and pancreastatin in plasma and urine from patients with carcinoid tumours and endocrine pancreatic tumours. J Endocrinol. 1995;144(1):49–59.
86. Baudin E, Bidart JM, Bachelot A, Ducreux M, Elias D, Ruffie P, et al. Impact of chromogranin A measurement in the work-up of neuroendocrine tumors. Ann Oncol. 2001;12(Suppl 2):S79–82.
87. Di Giacinto P, Rota F, Rizza L, Campana D, Isidori A, Lania A, et al. Chromogranin A: from laboratory to clinical aspects of patients with neuroendocrine tumors. Int J Endocrinol. 2018;2018:8126087.
88. Korse CM, Taal BG, Vincent A, van Velthuysen ML, Baas P, Buning-Kager JC, et al. Choice of tumour markers in patients with neuroendocrine tumours is dependent on the histological grade. A marker study of chromogranin A, neuron specific enolase, progastrin-releasing peptide and cytokeratin fragments. Eur J Cancer. 2012;48(5):662–71.
89. Grossmann M, Trautmann ME, Poertl S, Hoermann R, Berger P, Arnold R, et al. Alpha-subunit and human chorionic gonadotropin-beta immunoreactivity in patients with malignant endocrine gastroenteropancreatic tumours. Eur J Clin Invest. 1994;24(2):131–6.
90. Shah T, Srirajaskanthan R, Bhogal M, Toubanakis C, Meyer T, Noonan A, et al. Alpha-fetoprotein and human chorionic gonadotrophin-beta as prognostic markers in neuroendocrine tumour patients. Br J Cancer. 2008;99(1):72–7.
91. Sugimoto E, Lorelius LE, Eriksson B, Oberg K. Midgut carcinoid tumours. CT appearance. Acta Radiol. 1995;36(4):367–71.
92. Woodard PK, Feldman JM, Paine SS, Baker ME. Midgut carcinoid tumors: CT findings and biochemical profiles. J Comput Assist Tomogr. 1995;19(3):400–5.
93. Sundin A, Vullierme MP, Kaltsas G, Plockinger U. ENETS Consensus Guidelines for the Standards of Care in Neuroendocrine Tumors: radiological examinations. Neuroendocrinology. 2009;90(2):167–83.
94. Kamaoui I, De-Luca V, Ficarelli S, Mennesson N, Lombard-Bohas C, Pilleul F. Value of CT enteroclysis in suspected small-bowel carcinoid tumors. Am J Roentgenol. 2010;194(3):629–33.
95. Hakim FA, Alexander JA, Huprich JE, Grover M, Enders FT. CT-enterography may identify small bowel tumors not detected by capsule endoscopy: eight years experience at Mayo Clinic Rochester. Dig Dis Sci. 2011;56(10):2914–9.
96. Paulsen SR, Huprich JE, Fletcher JG, Booya F, Young BM, Fidler JL, et al. CT enterography as a diagnostic tool in evaluating small bowel disorders: review of clinical experience with over 700 cases. Radiographics. 2006;26(3):641–57; discussion 57–62.
97. Reubi J, Kvols L, Krenning E, Lamberts S. Distribution of somatostatin receptors in normal and tumor tissue. Metabolism. 1990;39(9):78–81.
98. Kalkner KM, Janson ET, Nilsson S, Carlsson S, Oberg K, Westlin JE. Somatostatin receptor scintigraphy in patients with carcinoid tumors: comparison between radioligand uptake and tumor markers. Cancer Res. 1995;55(23 Suppl):5801s–4s.
99. Westlin J-E, Janson ET, Arnberg H, Ahlström H, Öberg K, Nilsson S. Somatostatin receptor scintigraphy of carcinoid tumours using the [111In-DTPA-D-Phe1]-octreotide. Acta Oncol. 1993;32(7–8):783–6.
100. Bakker W, Albert R, Bruns C, Breeman W, Hofland L, Marbach P, et al. [111In-DTPA-D-Phe1]-octreotide, a potential radiopharmaceutical for imaging of somatostatin receptor-positive tumors: synthesis, radiolabeling and in vitro validation. Life Sci. 1991;49(22):1583–91.
101. Krenning E, Kwekkeboom DJ, Bakker WH, Breeman W, Kooij P, Oei H, et al. Somatostatin receptor scintigraphy with [111 In-DTPA-D-Phe 1]-and [123 I-Tyr 3]-octreotide: the Rotterdam experience with more than 1000 patients. Eur J Nucl Med. 1993;20(8):716–31.
102. Gibril F, Reynolds JC, Chen CC, Yu F. Specificity of somatostatin receptor scintigraphy: a prospective study and effects of false-positive localizations on management in patients with gastrinomas. J Nucl Med. 1999;40(4):539.
103. Krenning E, Bakker W, Kooij P, Breeman W, Oei H, De Jong M, et al. Somatostatin receptor scintigraphy with indium-111-DTPA-D-Phe-1-octreotide in man: metabolism, dosimetry and comparison with iodine-123-Tyr-3-octreotide. J Nucl Med. 1992;33(5):652–8.
104. Virgolini I, Ambrosini V, Bomanji JB, Baum RP, Fanti S, Gabriel M, et al. Procedure guidelines for PET/CT tumour imaging with 68 Ga-dota-conjugated peptides: 68 Ga-dota-toc, 68 Ga-dota-noc, 68 Ga-dota-tate. Eur J Nucl Med Mol Imaging. 2010;37(10):2004–10.
105. Panagiotidis E, Alshammari A, Michopoulou S, Skoura E, Naik K, Maragkoudakis E, et al. Comparison of the impact of 68Ga-DOTATATE and 18F-FDG PET/CT on clinical management in patients with neuroendocrine tumors. J Nucl Med. 2017;58(1):91–6.
106. Wieland DM, Wu J-I, Brown LE, Mangner TJ, Swanson DP. Radiolabeled adrenergi neuron-blocking agents: adrenomedullary imaging with [131I]iodobenzylguanidine. J Nucl Med. 1980 Apr;21(4):349–53.
107. McEwan AJ, Shapiro B, Sisson JC, Beierwaltes WH, Ackery DM. Radio-iodobenzylguanidine for the scintigraphic location and therapy of adrenergic tumors. Semin Nucl Med. 1985;15(2):132–53.
108. Hoefnagel C, Den FHJ, Van AG, Marcuse H, Taal B. Diagnosis and treatment of a carcinoid tumor using iodine-131 meta-iodobenzylguanidine. Clin Nucl Med. 1986;11(3):150–2.
109. Gopinath G, Buscombe JR, Ratnamm D, Caplin ME, Hilson AJW. Difference in mIBG uptake in foregut, midgut and hindgut carcinoid tumours. Nucl Med Commun. 2004;25(4):416.
110. Feldman JM, Blinder RA, Lucas KJ, Coleman RE. Iodine-131 metaiodobenzylguanidine scintigraphy of carcinoid tumors. J Nucl Med. 1986;27(11):1691–6.
111. Le Rest C, Bomanji J, Costa D, Townsend C, Visvikis D, Ell P. Functional imaging of malignant paragangliomas and carcinoid tumours. Eur J Nucl Med. 2001;28(4):478–82.
112. Grünwald F. & Ezziddin S. "131I-Metaiodobenzylguanidine Therapy of Neuroblastoma and Other Neuroendocrine Tumors", Seminars in nuclear medicine. 2010;40(2):153–163.
113. Plöckinger U, Rindi G, Arnold R, Eriksson B, Krenning EP, de Herder WW, et al. Guidelines for the diagnosis and treatment of neuroendocrine gastrointestinal tumours. A consensus statement on behalf of the European Neuroendocrine Tumour Society (ENETS). Neuroendocrinology. 2004;80(6):394.
114. Merola E, Sbrozzi-Vanni A, Panzuto F, D'Ambra G, Di Giulio E, Pilozzi E, et al. Type I gastric carcinoids: a prospective study on endoscopic management and recurrence rate. Neuroendocrinology. 2012;95(3):207–13.
115. Ichikawa J, Tanabe S, Koizumi W, Kida Y, Imaizumi H, Kida M, et al. Endoscopic mucosal resection in the management of gastric carcinoid tumors. Endoscopy. 2003;35(3):203–6.

116. Zhang L, Ozao J, Warner R, Divino C. Review of the pathogenesis, diagnosis, and management of type I gastric carcinoid tumor. World J Surg. 2011;35(8):1879–86.
117. Gladdy RA, Strong VE, Coit D, Allen PJ, Gerdes H, Shia J, et al. Defining surgical indications for type I gastric carcinoid tumor. Ann Surg Oncol. 2009;16(11):3154.
118. Landry C, Brock G, Scoggins C. A proposed staging system for gastric carcinoid tumors based on an analysis of 1543 patients. Ann Surg Oncol. 2009;16:51–60.
119. Hosokawa O, Kaizaki Y, Hattori M. Long-term follow up of patients with multiple gastric carcinoids associated with type A gastritis. Gastric Cancer. 2005;8:42–6.
120. Soga J. Early-stage carcinoids of the gastrointestinal tract: an analysis of 1914 reported cases. Cancer. 2005;103:1587–95.
121. Guillem P. Gastric carcinoid tumours. Is there a place for antrectomy? Ann Chir. 2005;130:323–6.
122. Öhrvall U, Eriksson B, Juhlin C, Karacagil S, Rastad J, Hellman P, et al. Method for dissection of mesenteric metastases in mid-gut carcinoid tumors. World J Surg. 2000;24(11):1402–8.
123. Makridis C, Öberg K, Juhlin C, Rastad J, Johansson H, Lörelius LE, et al. Surgical treatment of mid-gut carcinoid tumors. World J Surg. 1990;14(3):377–83.
124. Makridis C, Rastad J, Öberg K, Åkerström G. Progression of metastases and symptom improvement from laparotomy in midgut carcinoid tumors. World J Surg. 1996;20(7):900–7.
125. Modlin IM, Lye KD, Kidd M. A 50-year analysis of 562 gastric carcinoids: small tumor or larger problem? Am J Gastroenterol. 2004;99(1):23–32.
126. Okamoto Y, Fujii M, Tateiwa S, Sakai T, Ochi F, Sugano M, et al. Treatment of multiple rectal carcinoids by endoscopic mucosal resection using a device for esophageal variceal ligation. Endoscopy. 2004;36(5):469–70.
127. Higaki S, Nishiaki M, Mitani N, Yanai H, Tada M, Okita K. Effectiveness of local endoscopic resection of rectal carcinoid tumors. Endoscopy. 2008;29(3):171–5.
128. Yangong H, Shi C, Shahbaz M, Zhengchuan N, Wang J, Liang B, et al. Diagnosis and treatment experience of rectal carcinoid (a report of 312 cases). Int J Surg. 2014;12(5):408–11.
129. Koura AN, Giacco GG, Curley SA, Skibber JM, Feig BW, Ellis LM. Carcinoid tumors of the rectum: effect of size, histopathology, and surgical treatment on metastasis free survival. Cancer. 1997;79(7):1294.
130. Norlen O, Stalberg P, Oberg K, Eriksson J, Hedberg J, Hessman O, et al. Long-term results of surgery for small intestinal neuroendocrine tumors at a tertiary referral center. World J Surg. 2012;36(6):1419–31.
131. Kianmanesh R, Ruszniewski P, Rindi G, Kwekkeboom D, Pape UF, Kulke M, et al. ENETS consensus guidelines for the management of peritoneal carcinomatosis from neuroendocrine tumors. Neuroendocrinology. 2010;91(4):333–40.
132. Frilling A, Modlin IM, Kidd M, Russell C, Breitenstein S, Salem R, et al. Recommendations for management of patients with neuroendocrine liver metastases. Lancet Oncol. 2014;15(1):e8–21.
133. Steinmuller T, Kianmanesh R, Falconi M, Scarpa A, Taal B, Kwekkeboom DJ, et al. Consensus guidelines for the management of patients with liver metastases from digestive (neuro)endocrine tumors: foregut, midgut, hindgut, and unknown primary. Neuroendocrinology. 2008;87(1):47–62.
134. Frilling A, Li J, Malamutmann E, Schmid KW, Bockisch A, Broelsch CE. Treatment of liver metastases from neuroendocrine tumours in relation to the extent of hepatic disease. Br J Surg. 2009;96(2):175–84.
135. Le Treut YP, Grégoire E, Belghiti J, Boillot O, Soubrane O, Mantion G, et al. Predictors of long-term survival after liver transplantation for metastatic endocrine tumors: an 85-case French multicentric report. Am J Transplant. 2008;8(06):1205–13.
136. Le Treut YP, Grégoire E, Klempnauer J, Belghiti J, Jouve E, Lerut J, et al. Liver transplantation for neuroendocrine tumors in Europe-results and trends in patient selection: a 213-case European liver transplant registry study. Ann Surg. 2013;257(05):807–15.
137. Mazzaferro V, Sposito C, Coppa J, Miceli R, Bhoori S, Bongini M, et al. The long-term benefit of liver transplantation for hepatic metastases from neuroendocrine tumors. Am J Transplant. 2016;16(10):2892–902.
138. Bagante F, Spolverato G, Merath K, Postlewait LM, Poultsides GA, Mullen MG, et al. Neuroendocrine liver metastasis: the chance to be cured after liver surgery. J Surg Oncol. 2017;115(06):687–95.
139. Mazzaferro V, Pulvirenti A, Coppa J. Neuroendocrine tumors metastatic to the liver: how to select patients for liver transplantation? J Hepatol. 2007;47(4):460–6.
140. Pavel M, Baudin E, Couvelard A, Krenning E, Oberg K, Steinmuller T, et al. ENETS Consensus Guidelines for the management of patients with liver and other distant metastases from neuroendocrine neoplasms of foregut, midgut, hindgut, and unknown primary. Neuroendocrinology. 2012;95(2):157–76.
141. Lim C, Lahat E, Osseis M, Sotirov D, Salloum C, Azoulay D. Liver transplantation for neuroendocrine tumors: what have we learned? Semin Liver Dis. 2018;38(04):351–4.
142. Veenendaal LM, Borel Rinkes IH, van Hillegersberg R. Multipolar radiofrequency ablation of large hepatic metastases of endocrine tumours. Eur J Gastroenterol Hepatol. 2006;18(1):89–92.
143. Berber E, Flesher N, Siperstein AE. Laparoscopic radiofrequency ablation of neuroendocrine liver metastases. World J Surg. 2002;26(8):985–90.
144. Henn AR, Levine EA, McNulty W, Zagoria RJ. Percutaneous radiofrequency ablation of hepatic metastases for symptomatic relief of neuroendocrine syndromes. Am J Roentgenol. 2003;181(4):1005–10.
145. Wessels FJ, Schell SR. Radiofrequency ablation treatment of refractory carcinoid hepatic metastases. J Surg Res. 2001;95(1):8–12.
146. Hellman P, Ladjevardi S, Skogseid B, Åkerström G, Elvin A. Radiofrequency tissue ablation using cooled tip for liver metastases of endocrine tumors. World J Surg. 2002;26(8):1052–6.

147. Giovannini M, Seitz JF. Ultrasound-guided percutaneous alcohol injection of small liver metastases. Results in 40 patients. Cancer. 1994;73(2):294–7.
148. Livraghi T, Vettori C, Lazzaroni S. Liver metastases: results of percutaneous ethanol injection in 14 patients. Radiology. 1991;179(3):709–12.
149. Atwell TD, Charboneau JW, Que FG, Rubin J, Lewis BD, Nagorney DM, et al. Treatment of neuroendocrine cancer metastatic to the liver: the role of ablative techniques. Cardiovasc Intervent Radiol. 2005;28(4):409–21.
150. Ahlman H, Nilsson O, Olausson M. Interventional treatment of the carcinoid syndrome. Neuroendocrinology. 2004;80(Suppl 1):67–73.
151. Granberg D, Eriksson LG, Welin S, Kindmark H, Janson ET, Skogseid B, et al. Liver embolization with trisacryl gelatin microspheres (embosphere) in patients with neuroendocrine tumors. Acta Radiol. 2007;48(2):180–5.
152. Therasse E, Breittmayer F, Roche A, De Baere T, Indushekar S, Ducreux M, et al. Transcatheter chemoembolization of progressive carcinoid liver metastasis. Radiology. 1993;189(2):541–7.
153. Maire F, Lombard-Bohas C, O'Toole D, Vullierme MP, Rebours V, Couvelard A, et al. Hepatic arterial embolization versus chemoembolization in the treatment of liver metastases from well-differentiated midgut endocrine tumors: a prospective randomized study. Neuroendocrinology. 2012;96(4):294–300.
154. Hoffmann RT, Paprottka P, Jakobs TF, Trumm CG, Reiser MF. Arterial therapies of non-colorectal cancer metastases to the liver (from chemoembolization to radioembolization). Abdom Imaging. 2011;36(6):671–6.
155. Aparicio T, Ducreux M, Baudin E, Sabourin JC, De Baere T, Mitry E, et al. Antitumour activity of somatostatin analogues in progressive metastatic neuroendocrine tumours. Eur J Cancer. 2001;37(8):1014–9.
156. Sullivan I, Le Teuff G, Guigay J, Caramella C, Berdelou A, Leboulleux S, et al. Antitumour activity of somatostatin analogues in sporadic, progressive, metastatic pulmonary carcinoids. Eur J Cancer. 2017;75:259–67.
157. Rinke A, Muller HH, Schade-Brittinger C, Klose KJ, Barth P, Wied M, et al. Placebo-controlled, double-blind, prospective, randomized study on the effect of octreotide LAR in the control of tumor growth in patients with metastatic neuroendocrine midgut tumors: a report from the PROMID Study Group. J Clin Oncol. 2009;27(28):4656–63.
158. Caplin ME, Pavel M, Ćwikła JB, Phan AT, Raderer M, Sedláčková E, et al. Anti-tumour effects of lanreotide for pancreatic and intestinal neuroendocrine tumours: the CLARINET open-label extension study. Endocr-Relat Cancer. 2016;23(3):191–9.
159. Oberg K, Norheim I, Lind E, Alm G, Lundqvist G, Wide L, et al. Treatment of malignant carcinoid tumors with human leukocyte interferon: long-term results. Cancer Treat Rep. 1986;70(11):1297–304.
160. Moertel CG, Rubin J, Kvols LK. Therapy of metastatic carcinoid tumor and the malignant carcinoid syndrome with recombinant leukocyte A interferon. J Clin Oncol. 1989;7(7):865–8.
161. Arnold R, Rinke A, Klose KJ, Müller HH, Wied M, Zamzow K, et al. Octreotide versus octreotide plus interferon-alpha in endocrine gastroenteropancreatic tumors: a randomized trial. Clin Gastroenterol Hepatol. 2005;3(8):761–71.
162. Kulke MH, Stuart K, Enzinger PC, Ryan DP, Clark JW, Muzikansky A, et al. Phase II study of temozolomide and thalidomide in patients with metastatic neuroendocrine tumors. J Clin Oncol. 2006;24(3):401–6.
163. Fjällskog MLH, Granberg DP, Welin SL, Eriksson C, Öberg KE, Janson ET, et al. Treatment with cisplatin and etoposide in patients with neuroendocrine tumors. Cancer. 2001;92(5):1101–7.
164. De Jong M, Valkema R, Jamar F, Kvols LK, Kwekkeboom DJ, Breeman WA, et al. Somatostatin receptor-targeted radionuclide therapy of tumors: preclinical and clinical findings. Semin Nucl Med. 2002;32(2):133–40.
165. Bodei L, Ferone D, Grana CM, Cremonesi M, Signore A, Dierckx RA, et al. Peptide receptor therapies in neuroendocrine tumors. J Endocrinol Invest. 2009;32(4):360–9.
166. Kwekkeboom DJ, Krenning EP. Peptide receptor radionuclide therapy in the treatment of neuroendocrine tumors. Hematol Oncol Clin North Am. 2016;30(1):179–91.
167. Hicks RJ, Kwekkeboom DJ, Krenning E, Bodei L, Grozinsky-Glasberg S, Arnold R, et al. ENETS consensus guidelines for the standards of care in neuroendocrine neoplasms: peptide receptor radionuclide therapy with radiolabelled somatostatin analogues. Neuroendocrinology. 2017;105(3):295–309.
168. Hörsch RBD. Erratum to: The joint IAEA, EANM, and SNMMI practical guidance on peptide receptor radionuclide therapy (PRRNT) in neuroendocrine tumours. Eur J Nucl Med Mol Imaging. 2014;41:584.
169. Tapia Rico G, Li M, Pavlakis N, Cehic G, Price T. Prevention and management of carcinoid crises in patients with high-risk neuroendocrine tumours undergoing peptide receptor radionuclide therapy (PRRT): literature review and case series from two Australian tertiary medical institutions. Cancer Treat Rev. 2018;66:1–6.
170. Veenhof C, de Wit R, Taal B, Dirix L, Wagstaff J, Hensen A, et al. A dose-escalation study of recombinant interferon-alpha in patients with a metastatic carcinoid tumour. Eur J Cancer. 1992;28:75–8.
171. Woltering EAMD, Wright AEBSBSN, Stevens MAMPH, Wang Y-ZMD, Boudreaux JPMD, Mamikunian GMS, et al. Development of effective prophylaxis against intraoperative carcinoid crisis. J Clin Anesth. 2016;32:189–93.
172. Marsh HM, Martin JJK, Kvols LK, Gracey DR, Warner MA, Warner ME, et al. Carcinoid crisis during anesthesia: successful treatment with a somatostatin analogue. Anesthesiology. 1987;66(1):89–91.
173. Seymour N, Sawh SC. Mega-dose intravenous octreotide for the treatment of carcinoid crisis: a systematic review. Can J Anesth. 2013;60(5):492–9.
174. Cho M-Y, Kim JM, Sohn JH, Kim M-J, Kim K-M, Kim WH, et al. Current trends of the incidence and pathological diagnosis of gastroenteropancreatic neuroendocrine tumors (GEP-NETs) in Korea 2000-2009: multicenter study. Cancer Res Treat. 2012;44(3):157–65.

175. Fan J-H, Zhang Y-Q, Shi S-S, Chen Y-J, Yuan X-H, Jiang L-M, et al. A nation-wide retrospective epidemiological study of gastroenteropancreatic neuroendocrine neoplasms in China. Oncotarget. 2017;8(42):71699.
176. Ito T, Igarashi H, Nakamura K, Sasano H, Okusaka T, Takano K, et al. Epidemiological trends of pancreatic and gastrointestinal neuroendocrine tumors in Japan: a nationwide survey analysis. J Gastroenterol. 2015;50(1):58–64.
177. Tsai H-J, Wu C-C, Tsai C-R, Lin S-F, Chen L-T, Chang JS. The epidemiology of neuroendocrine tumors in Taiwan: a nation-wide cancer registry-based study. PLOS ONE. 2013;8(4):e62487.
178. Wyld D, Wan MH, Moore J, Dunn N, Youl P. Epidemiological trends of neuroendocrine tumours over three decades in Queensland, Australia. Cancer Epidemiol. 2019;63:101598.
179. Prakash PS, Wijerathne S, Parameswaran R. Rising Incidence of Neuroendocrine Tumors in Singapore: An Epidemiological Study. World J Endoc Surg 2020; 12(1):1-4.
180. Hallet J, Law CH, Karanicolas PJ, Saskin R, Liu N, Singh S. Rural-urban disparities in incidence and outcomes of neuroendocrine tumors: a population-based analysis of 6271 cases. Cancer. 2015;121(13):2214–21.
181. Luke C, Price T, Townsend A, Karapetis C, Kotasek D, Singhal N, et al. Epidemiology of neuroendocrine cancers in an Australian population. Cancer Causes Control. 2010;21(6):931–8.

60
CARCINOID SYNDROME
Anand Kumar Mishra

The text of this chapter is available online at www.routledge.com/9781032136509.

61

GASTROENTEROPANCREATIC NEUROENDOCRINE TUMORS IN CHILDREN

Orkan Ergün

Introduction

Neuroendocrine tumors (NETs) (previously termed "carcinoids") are slow-growing tumors of the neuroendocrine system and are of "small blue cell tumors" family (1). Pediatric NETs are very rare with a reported incidence of 2.8 per million in children. Many of those tumors are diagnosed incidentally; thus, they may remain asymptomatic for a long time or may present with vague symptoms, including abdominal pain, weight loss, fatigue, diarrhea and flushing as well as other symptoms. Early-stage well-differentiated NETs have excellent outcomes with the majority of diseases being cured with surgical resection alone (2). Despite the benign nature of these tumors, there is a definite potential for malignant transformation, and 10–20% of children and young adolescents present with metastatic disease at the time of diagnosis (3, 4).

Depending on the Ki-67 proliferation index, NETs are categorized into Grade I (Ki-67 ≤ 2%), Grade II (Ki-67: 3–20%) and Grade III (Ki-67 ≥ 20%) in which the Grade III tumors are usually poorly differentiated, highly aggressive carcinomas with unfavorable outcomes (5). However, recently Grade III NETs were stratified into well-differentiated and poorly differentiated subgroups; well-differentiated neoplasms are termed "neuroendocrine tumors", while poorly differentiated neoplasms are referred to as "neuroendocrine carcinomas" (6, 7).

Pediatric NETs may involve any organ system, including lungs and tracheobronchial tree, gastrointestinal tract and pancreas (gastroenteropancreatic; GEP-NETs), especially midgut, appendix being the most common site of origin in the gastrointestinal tract (8–13).

Carcinoid symptoms are rare in the pediatric age-group (14). Those NETs displaying systemic symptoms associated with the tumor are referred to as "functioning NETs", while those that remain asymptomatic are called "nonfunctioning NETs". Although rare in pediatric age-group, clinical presentation associated with functioning NETs, especially those arising from the midgut, is termed "carcinoid syndrome" and includes symptoms of colicky abdominal pain, diarrhea, flushing and sometimes wheezing (1).

Most common type of GEP-NET in the pediatric age-group is appendiceal NET, usually presenting as appendicitis. Only 10% of the appendiceal NETs are symptomatic in children; a vast majority of the appendiceal NETs are mainly discovered incidentally at the histopathological examination of the specimen after an appendectomy (1, 15, 16).

Surgical dilemma following an incidentally discovered appendiceal NET is whether to further perform a complimentary surgery such as a right hemicolectomy or consider it surgically cured after appendectomy. Because GEP-NETs are rare in children, most of the information is adopted from adult practice, and the recommendations currently followed in most centers are based on the fact that well-differentiated NETs <2 cm in size are less likely to metastasize (17). However, one should bear in mind that a tumor of a size of 2 cm in a child is proportionately a large tumor compared to that of an adult; therefore, there is always a potential possibility of undertreatment in young children presenting with a relatively large tumor. Completely resected well-differentiated NET with a size that does not exceed 2 cm does not require right hemicolectomy in children. However, tumors that are poorly differentiated or larger than 2 cm in size require a right hemicolectomy. Similarly, NETs breaching serosal surface, invading the mesoappendix by 3 mm, located at the base of the appendix or goblet-cell tumors regardless of the size require a right hemicolectomy (1, 17).

Among the NETs involving the gastrointestinal tract, gastric NETs are very rare in children. They are usually solitary and large tumors, associated with the Zollinger–Ellison (ZE) syndrome and are generally found to have metastasized at the time of presentation (18). The ileum is the most commonly involved site for small bowel NETs in both adults and children and is usually multifocal and aggressive in nature. Carcinoid syndrome is commonly associated with these lesions. Most patients present with local lymphatic spread, and many with distant metastases (10). Colonic NETs are extremely rare in childhood and yet they account for nearly one-third of colorectal tumors in children. In contrast to small bowel NETs in childhood, carcinoid syndrome of colonic and rectal tumors of this origin is very rare; 50% of these lesions are discovered incidentally during an ultrasound study after abdominal pain or weight loss, which are common symptoms for colonic NETs or during endoscopy (1, 19).

Complete surgical resection is the only treatment option and curative for most of the cases. Before planning for the surgical treatment, the possibility of multifocality and thus the presence of local and distant metastatic disease must be taken into consideration and more extensive radical excisional procedures may be required. In the presence of non-resectable or metastatic disease, debulking surgery for reducing the tumor load as well as – depending on the availability – utilizing techniques such as radiofrequency ablation may improve survival (20).

Pancreatic endocrine tumors in children

Pancreatic neoplasms are extremely rare in the pediatric age-group with an estimated incidence of 1–2 patients per 10 million children. Data by Surveillance, Epidemiology, and End Results (SEER) Program released in April 2007 identified 53 new cases in a 31-year period. Nearly 76% of the patients were older than 10 years of age, 51.7% were adolescents and endocrine tumors constituted 32.8% of all pediatric pancreatic neoplasms (21). Brecht et al. analyzing 228 pediatric cases in the SEER database in 2011 have identified 85 patients again constituting 37.3% of all pediatric pancreatic tumors (22). Similarly, evaluation of 109 pediatric pancreatic tumors from the National Database by Picado et al. in 2020 revealed that 27% of all pancreatic malignancies were endocrine tumors, and 94% of those tumors were seen after the age of 10 and accumulated between age intervals of 15 and 17 years (57%) (23).

Pancreatic tumors are classified according to the hormone secreted causing the symptoms. Most common pancreatic endocrine tumors seen in children and adolescents are insulinomas, gastrinomas and VIPomas (tumor of cells secreting vasoactive intestinal polypeptide). Most common of those are insulinomas, still a very rare tumor of the pediatric age-group. Insulinomas are insulin-producing neuroendocrine pancreatic tumors that cause hypoglycemia due to endogenous hyperinsulinism (24). Symptoms include hypoglycemia, low glucose levels at the time of symptoms and improvement of symptoms following carbohydrate administration (*Whipple's triad*) accompanied by inadequately high insulin levels at the time of hypoglycemia (25). Insulinomas are usually isolated benign tumors although some tend to be malignant (26). Ten percent of these tumors are associated with multiple endocrine neoplasia (MEN) type 1 (27). Clinical symptoms may be subtle and sometimes unspecific, including dizziness, drowsiness and behavioral changes, which may be more evident in the mornings due to hypoglycemia after fasting through the night (28), and these symptoms may be initially mistaken for a psychological or neurological disorder (29). Magnetic resonance imaging (MRI), recommended as first-line diagnostic imaging since it does not use radiation, is highly sensitive (30) although the sensitivity of dual-phase computerized tomography is also around 85–100% (31). Definitive diagnosis may be established by endo-ultrasonography guided by fine needle aspiration biopsy in a case with suspected insulinoma following MRI or CT imaging (32).

Gastrinomas, although very rare and hardly diagnosed, are the second most common endocrine tumors of childhood. They usually present at puberty with peptic ulcer disease and diarrhea. The association of gastric hypersecretion, peptic ulcer disease and gastrin-producing tumor, usually at the pancreas, is called ZE syndrome. Although the commoner form of gastrinoma in childhood is a sporadic single tumor, usually located at the pancreas, 20–50% of gastrinomas are associated with MEN 1 syndrome. They present relatively earlier, are usually smaller and multifocal, and often duodenal than pancreatic; 60–90% are malignant and commonly metastasize to the lymph nodes, whereas sporadic forms tend to metastasize to the liver (33). Those associated with ZE have a lower rate of metastatic disease than sporadic gastrinomas at an initial presentation (34). Diagnosis is confirmed by indium-labeled octreotide or pentetreotide scintigraphy. Besides confirming the primary diagnosis of the tumor, scintigraphy also allows for the recognition of possible metastasis (35).

Intraoperative ultrasonography is a valuable tool to exactly locate the tumor(s) for radical resection of all lesions. Proton pump inhibitors and octreotide are first-line medical treatments to control the peptic ulcer disease, and surgical resection of the primary tumor(s), as well as any metastatic lesion remains the key to radical management of gastrinomas. Depending on the site, size and focality of the tumor, surgical options include simple enucleation, nodulectomy, partial pancreatectomy, pancreaticoduodenectomy, partial or total gastrectomy and more extensive resections with an open or laparoscopic approach.

VIPomas are tumors secreting vasoactive intestinal polypeptide resulting in profuse watery diarrhea and severe electrolyte imbalance (hypocalemia and achlorhydria) (36) that may be occasionally fatal. VIPomas are extremely rare and usually extrapancreatic in childhood (37). The incidence in the adult population is estimated to be around 1 in 10 million; the incidence in the pediatric population is unknown (38).

There is no comprehensive series, and most information about childhood VIPomas are based on case reports or series. A recent literature review by Yeh et al., including 45 pediatric cases in 2020, revealed that geographically 80% of cases were from Eurasia where Japanese patients comprised the largest proportion in the Asia-Pacific group. The male-to-female ratio was around 1:2.5, and average age was 3.3 years ranging from 7 months to 15 years. All cases presented with diarrhea; other presentations included flushing, fever, sweating, vomiting, abdominal pain and hypertension. Hypokalemia (84.4%) was the leading abnormal finding followed by achlorhydria in 26.7% and acidosis in 15.6% (39).

Diagnosis is usually delayed; average time to diagnosis from the first onset of symptoms is approximately 3–4 years (38). Elevated plasma VIP levels as well as imaging modalities, including ultrasonography, CT and MRI, are usually diagnostic in locating the tumor(s). The diagnostic performances of FDG PET scan and Ga-DOTATATE for NET are also valuable tools for detecting the tumor; Angelousi et al. reported their sensitivity of 18F-FDG PET scan and 68Ga-DOTATATE as 30 and 79% (38). In the review by Yeh et al., a majority of cases were extrapancreatic; around half of the cases were found in the adrenal and suprarenal regions (46.7%), followed by paravertebral/prevertebral (15.6%) and mediastinum (13.3%). Only 4.4% of cases developed pancreatic lesions (39). Yamaguchi et al. in 1984 reported 38% of metastatic disease in Japanese pediatric cases (40). Surgery seems to be more efficient for the cure when compared to adults; the reviews by Yeh et al. have revealed that at least 90% of cases underwent at least one excisional surgery, and 60% achieved complete resolution of symptoms by surgery alone (39).

Persistent hyperinsulinemic hypoglycemia (PHH)

Persistent hyperinsulinemic hypoglycemia (PHH), formerly named nesidioblastosis, typically occurs in neonates due to dysregulation of insulin secretion in which insulin is continuously secreted to the bloodstream despite low glucose levels. Inappropriate insulin secretion increases glucose consumption as well as inhibits glycogenolysis and gluconeogenesis and thus suppresses endogenous glucose production leading to hypoglycemia. Access insulin also inhibits lipolysis, free fatty acid production and ketogenesis, depriving the brain of ketone bodies, which is an alternative energy substrate (41). Symptoms of hypoglycemia in neonates include lethargy, apnea and seizures. Therefore, it is extremely important to maintain normoglycemia to prevent neurologic impairment due to PHH in neonates.

Pancreatic β cells are responsible for the production and secretion of insulin into the bloodstream to regulate and maintain the blood glucose concentration at physiologic levels. The regulation of insulin secretion in the β cells is controlled by potassium-sensitive ATP (K_{ATP}) channels that play a key role in the electrical excitability of the β-cell membrane and subsequent insulin secretion (42, 43).

PHH is caused by inactivating mutations in β-cell K_{ATP} channels; mutations in *ABCC8* and *KCNJ11* genes result in either lack of channels on the β-cell plasma membrane or channels that are expressed but have impaired function. These channel abnormalities lead to dysregulated insulin secretion, which in a majority of cases are unresponsive to diazoxide, a K_{ATP} channel agonist (44, 45).

PHH may present in diffuse and focal forms; in the "diffuse form", defective mutant β cells are distributed throughout the pancreas showing signs of hyperactivity. In contrast, "focal form" is characterized by a distinct area of β-cell proliferation or adenomatosis (44).

Identification and distinguishing of the two forms are also important; clinical symptoms manifest in the neonatal period right after the birth in the diffuse form; in contrast, focal forms usually present several weeks after the birth with hypoglycemic seizures. However, clinical symptoms are not always enough to differentiate between the two forms.

The aim of the medical treatment in PHH is to maintain serum glucose concentration at stable levels, usually above 60–70 mg/dL to prevent neurologic complications of hypoglycemia. This is usually achieved through parenteral administration of glucose solutions. Enteral feedings are continued, sometimes fortified; however, enteral feeding alone is not sufficient enough to efficiently control serum glucose. First-line medical treatment includes diazoxide that opens the K_{ATP} channels on β cells and inhibits insulin secretion (46). Diazoxide causes fluid retention, which requires a combination with diuretics. Second-line therapy includes octreotide, a somatostatin analogue. However, it should be used with caution in neonates since it has a risk of causing necrotizing enterocolitis in neonates. Glucagon is used to reduce the required dextrose infusion rate in infants waiting for surgery (44).

The two distinct forms as being focal or diffuse also determine the success of management; the resection of the focal lesion is curative. On the other hand, the diffuse form of PHH unresponsive to medical treatment requires near-total pancreatectomy, whereas pancreatectomy in the diffuse form remains palliative with the risk of diabetes mellitus and pancreatic exocrine insufficiency (41). Near-total pancreatectomy may be performed by an open surgery or laparoscopic approach with similar efficiency.

References

1. Johnson PR. Gastroenteropancreatic neuroendocrine (carcinoid) tumors in children. Semin Pediatr Surg. 2014 Apr;23(2):91–95.
2. Farooqui ZA, Chauhan A. Neuroendocrine tumors in pediatrics. Glob Pediatr Health. 2019 Jul;6:2333794X19862712.
3. Parham DM. Neuroectodermal and neuroendocrine tumors principally seen in children. Am J Clin Pathol. 2001 Jun;115(Suppl):S113–S128.
4. Sarvida ME, O'Dorisio MS. Neuroendocrine tumors in children and young adults: Rare or not so rare. Endocrinol Metab Clin North Am. 2011 Mar;40(1):65–80, vii.
5. Bu J, Youn S, Kwon W, et al. Prognostic factors of non-functioning pancreatic neuroendocrine tumor revisited: The value of WHO 2010 classification. Ann Hepatobiliary Pancreat Surg. 2018 Feb;22(1):66–74.
6. Han X, Xu X, Ma H, et al. Clinical relevance of different WHO grade 3 pancreatic neuroendocrine neoplasms based on morphology. Endocr Connect. 2018;7:355–363.
7. Tang LH, Untch BR, Reidy DL, et al. Well-differentiated neuroendocrine tumors with a morphologically apparent high-grade component: A pathway distinct from poorly differentiated neuroendocrine carcinomas. Clin Cancer Res. 2016 Feb;22(4):1011–1017.
8. Howell DL, O'Dorisio MS. Management of neuroendocrine tumors in children, adolescents, and young adults. J Pediatr Hematol Oncol. 2012 May;34(Suppl 2): S64–S68.
9. Khanna G, O'Dorisio SM, Menda Y, et al. Gastroenteropancreatic neuroendocrine tumors in children and young adults. Pediatr Radiol. 2008 Mar;38(3):251–259.
10. Allan B, Davis J, Perez E, et al. Malignant neuroendocrine tumors: Incidence and outcomes in pediatric patients. Eur J Pediatr Surg. 2013;23(5):394–399.
11. Rizzardi G, Marulli G, Calabrese F, et al. Bronchial carcinoid tumors in children: Surgical treatment and outcome in a single institution. Eur J Pediatr Surg. 2009;19(4):228–231.
12. Allan BJ, Thorson CM, Davis JS, et al. An analysis of 73 cases of pediatric malignant tumors of the thymus. J Surg Res. 2013;184(1):397–403.
13. Leake J, Levitt G, Ramani P. Primary carcinoid of the testis in a 10-year-old boy. Histopathology. 1991;19(4):373–375.
14. Wang LT, Wilkins EW Jr, Bode HH. Bronchial carcinoid tumors in pediatric patients. Chest. 1993 May;103(5):1426–1428.
15. Willox SW. Carcinoid tumors of the appendix in childhood. Br J Surg. 1964;51:110–113.
16. Parkes SE, Muir KR, Al Sheyyab M, et al. Carcinoid tumours of the appendix in children 1957-1986: Incidence, treatment and outcome. Br J Surg. 1993;80:502–504.
17. Ramage JK, Ahmed A, Ardill J, et al. Guidelines for the management of gastroenteropancreatic neuroendocrine (including carcinoid) tumors (NETs). Gut. 2012;61:6–32.
18. Zhuge Y, Cheung MC, Yang R, et al. Pediatric intestinal foregut and small bowel solid tumors: A review of 105 cases. J Surg Res. 2009;156(1):95–102.
19. Yang R, Cheung MC, Zhuge Y, et al. Primary solid tumors of the colon and rectum in the pediatric patient: A review of 270 cases. J Surg Res. 2010;161(2):209–216.
20. Maroun J, Koch W, Kvols L, et al. Guidelines for the diagnosis and management of carcinoid tumours. Part 1: The gastrointestinal tract. A statement from a Canadian National Carcinoid Expert Group. Curr Oncol. 2006;13(2):67–76.
21. Perez EA, Gutierrez JC, Koniaris LG, Neville HL, Thompson WR, Sola JE. Malignant pancreatic tumors: Incidence and outcome in 58 pediatric patients. J Pediatr Surg. 2009 Jan;44(1):197–203.
22. Brecht IB, Schneider DT, Klöppel G, et al. Malignant pancreatic tumors in children and young adults: Evaluation of 228 patients identified through the Surveillance, Epidemiology, and End Result (SEER) database. Klin Padiatr. 2011 Nov;223(6):341–345.
23. Picado O, Ferrantella A, Zabalo C, et al. Treatment patterns and outcomes for pancreatic tumors in children: An analysis of the National Cancer Database. Pediatr Surg Int. 2020 Mar;36(3):357–363.
24. Palladino AA, Bennett MJ, Stanley CA. Hyperinsulinism in infancy and childhood: When an insulin level is not always enough. Ann Biol Clin (Paris). 2009 May-Jun;67(3):245–254.
25. Hirshberg B, Livi A, Bartlett DL, et al. Forty-eight-hour fast: The diagnostic test for insulinoma. J Clin Endocrinol Metab. 2000 Sep;85(9):3222–3226.
26. Chaturvedi D, Khadgawat R, Kanakamani J, et al. Management challenges in a child with hyperinsulinemic hypoglycemia. Clin Pediatr Endocrinol. 2008;17(3):61–64.
27. Abu-Zaid A, Alghuneim LA, Metawee MT, Elkabbani RO, Almana H, Amin T, Azzam A. Sporadic insulinoma in a 10-year-old boy: A case report and literature review. JOP. 2014 Jan;15(1):53–57.
28. Mann JR, Rayner PH, Gourevitch A. Insulinoma in childhood. Arch Dis Child. 1969 Aug;44(236):435–442.
29. Kao KT, Simm PJ, Brown J. Childhood insulinoma masquerading as seizure disorder. J Paediatr Child Health. 2014 Apr;50(4):319–322.
30. Padidela R, Fiest M, Arya V, et al. Insulinoma in childhood: Clinical, radiological, molecular and histological aspects of nine patients. Eur J Endocrinol. 2014 May;170(5):741–747.
31. Das CJ, Debnath J, Gupta AK, Das AK. MR imaging appearance of insulinoma in an infant. Pediatr Radiol. 2007 Jun;37(6):581–583.
32. Lee LS. Diagnosis of pancreatic neuroendocrine tumors and the role of endoscopic ultrasound. Gastroenterol Hepatol (N Y). 2010 Aug;6(8):520–522.
33. Gibril F, Jensen RT. Zollinger-Ellison syndrome revisited: Diagnosis, biologic markers, associated inherited disorders, and acid hypersecretion. Curr Gastroenterol Rep. 2004;6:454–463.
34. Quatrini M, Castoldi L, Rossi G, et al. A follow up study of patients with Zollinger-Ellison syndrome in the period 1966–2002: Effects of surgical and medical treatments on long term survival. J Clin Gastroenterol. 2005;39:376–380.
35. Bello Arques P, Hervas Benito I, Mateo Navarro A. Scintigraphy with 111In-octreotide in a case of primary hepatic gastrinoma. Rev Esp Méd Nucl. 2001;20:381–385.
36. Abdullayeva L. VIPoma: Mechanisms, clinical presentation, diagnosis and treatment (Review). World Acad Sci J. 2019;1:229–235.
37. Belei OA, Heredea ER, Boeriu E, et al. Verner-Morrison syndrome. Literature review. Rom J Morphol Embryol. 2017;58(2):371–376.
38. Angelousi A, Koffas A, Grozinsky-Glasberg S, et al. Diagnostic and management challenges in vasoactive intestinal peptide secreting tumors: A series of 15 patients. Pancreas. 2019 Aug;48(7):934–942.
39. Yeh P-J, Chen S-H, Lai J-Y, et al. Rare cases of pediatric vasoactive intestinal peptide secreting tumor with literature review: A challenging etiology of chronic diarrhea. Front Pediatr. 2020;430:1–8.
40. Yamaguchi K, Abe K, Otsubo K, et al. The WDHA syndrome: Clinical and laboratory data on 28 Japanese cases. Peptides. 1984 Mar-Apr;5(2):415–421.
41. Shah P, Demirbilek H, Hussain K. Persistent hyperinsulinaemic hypoglycaemia in infancy. Semin Pediatr Surg. 2014 Apr;23(2):76–82.
42. Hussain K. Congenital hyperinsulinism and neonatal diabetes mellitus. Rev Endocr Metab Disord. 2010;11:155–156.
43. Cook DL, Hales CN. Intracellular ATP directly blocks K1 channels in pancreatic B-cells. Nature. 1984;311:271–273.
44. Lord K, De León DD. Hyperinsulinism in the neonate. Clin Perinatol. 2018 Mar;45(1):61–74.
45. Güemes M, Hussain K. Hyperinsulinemic hypoglycemia. Pediatr Clin North Am. 2015 Aug;62(4):1017–1036.
46. Dayton PG, Pruitt AW, Faraj BA, et al. Metabolism and disposition of diazoxide. A mini-review. Drug Metab Dispos. 1975;3(3):226–229.

62

MULTIPLE ENDOCRINE NEOPLASIA

Anand Kumar Mishra

Introduction

Multiple endocrine neoplasia (MEN) syndromes are autosomal dominant inherited disorders characterized by the occurrence of benign and malignant tumors in two or more endocrine glands in a single patient. They may also occur as sporadic in the absence of family history. MEN syndromes are classified depending on the organs involved. MEN 2 syndrome is characterized by a well-understood genotype–phenotype correlation (1, 2).

Six syndromes are also seen, which are associated with tumors of endocrine and nonendocrine organs. They are hyperparathyroidism (HPT)-jaw tumor syndrome, Von Hippel-Lindau disease, Carney complex, neurofibromatosis type 1, Cowden syndrome, and McCune–Albright syndrome. All of these also inherit as autosomal dominant except McCune–Albright syndrome (3).

Diseases and conditions

Definitions

MEN 1: MEN 1 is defined as the benign or malignant tumors in at least two of the three affected glands (parathyroid, endocrine pancreas, pituitary) in an individual, or at least one gland tumor with one of the first-degree relatives affected by MEN 1.

MEN 2: MEN 2 is characterized by the association of medullary thyroid cancer (MTC) with other benign and nonendocrine diseases. It is of two types A and B. There are four variants of MEN 2 A syndrome: Classic MEN 2 A, MEN 2 A with cutaneous lichen amyloidosis, MEN 2 A with Hirschsprung's disease and familial MTC (FMTC). Hereditary MTC accounts for 80%, 15% and 5% in MEN 2 A, FMTC and MEN 2 B, respectively.

FMTC is arbitrarily defined as MTC in four or more family members across at least two or more generations. In the absence of above criteria, it is necessary to demonstrate the presence of a germline RET mutation without objective evidence of pheochromocytoma and parathyroid disease (1, 2, 4, 5).

Multiple endocrine neoplasia type 1

MEN 1 was first reported by Erdheim in 1903 during the autopsy of a patient with pituitary adenoma and enlarged parathyroid gland (6). Later, it was also named Wermer's syndrome because of the description in 1954 by Dr. Paul Wermer (7, 8). It is an autosomal dominant disorder characterized by parathyroid pituitary and neuroendocrine tumors (NETs) involving duodenum and pancreas. In addition, there may also be tumors of adrenal cortex, carcinoid of thymus and bronchus, and meningioma facial angiofibroma and cutaneous lipomas.

Epidemiology

The prevalence of the syndrome is estimated to be around 1 case per 50,000 to 500,000 of the population. This disorder affects all ages. Male and female are affected equally. MEN 1 affected patients who do not belong to a particular geographical area, and there are no racial or ethnic preferences. No risk factors are known.

Genetic abnormalities (MEN 1)

The MEN 1 gene is called as menin gene and was mapped to human chromosome 11q13 in 1997. The gene encodes for a 610 amino acid nuclear protein termed **menin.** It is a tumor suppressor gene and causes inhibition of proliferation, differentiation, apoptosis, endocrine, metabolic functions and the maintenance of genomic stability by DNA repair (9, 10). More than 13,000 gene mutations have been reported till date. In MEN 1 relatives of the same family sharing the same genetic defects have variable phenotype. Since there is no genotype–phenotype correlation, therefore genetic testing is of no use for the prediction of tumor occurrence, malignant potential and prognosis. But in all patients with clinical diagnosis of index or suspected MEN 1, genetic evaluation of both patient and their first-degree relatives should be performed. All pre-symptomatic individuals with identified positive mutation for MEN 1 should undergo intensive biochemical testing as per schedule in Table 62.1 as biochemical abnormalities can be detected much earlier than their clinical presentation. Pancreaticoduodenal and intrathoracic thymic tumors are potentially malignant and can affect the survival (Table 62.2 and Figure 62.1).

Clinical features

MEN 1 gene has age-related penetrance and approximately 75% of patients will develop one or more tumors by 20 years and 100% by the age of 50 years and unusual in less than 5 years. The clinical features of a patient with clinical diagnosis of MEN 1 depend on hormone hypersecretion and glands involvement. With nonfunctional tumors, patient may have symptoms of mechanical pressure from tumor on the surrounding organs. Approximately 30%–70% of MEN 1 patients die from malignant NETs and thymic carcinoid tumors (11).

Unique features of MEN 1 tumors:

1. They are multiple except in anterior pituitary (multigland disease in parathyroid and multiple submucosal duodenal gastrinomas).
2. The occult metastatic disease is more prevalent in pancreas NETs (50% of MEN 1 insulinomas have metastases, while <10% of non-MEN 1 insulinomas metastasize) (28).
3. MEN 1-tumors may be larger, more aggressive and resistant to treatment observed with anterior pituitary tumors (e.g. macroadenomas at the time of diagnosis 85% vs. 64%, invasion into surrounding tissue 30% vs. 10%, and persistent hormonal oversecretion after appropriate medical, surgical and radiotherapy treatment >45% vs. 10%–40% in MEN 1 and non-MEN 1 patients, respectively (11, 12, 29).

Diagnosis

Diagnosis of MEN 1 in an individual can be established on the basis of one of the following three criteria (12, 13).

1. The presence of two or more primary MEN 1-associated endocrine tumors (parathyroid gland, entero-pancreatic tumor and pituitary adenoma) in an individual.

TABLE 62.1: Characteristics of Multiple Endocrine Neoplasia 1

Chromosome Location/Gene	Tumors (Estimated Penetrance)	Biochemical Imaging Screening Tests	Imaging Screening Tests
Chromosome: 11q13	Parathyroid hyperplasia (95%–100%)	Calcium, PTH annually to start screening at 8 years of age	–
	Gastro-entero-pancreatic tumor (30%–80%): Gastrinoma (20%–60%), nonfunctioning PPoma (20%–55%), glucagonoma (1%–6%), VIPoma (<1%)	Serum gastrin, glucagon, vasoactive intestinal polypeptide, pancreatic polypeptide, chromogranin A at the age of 20 years	MRI, CT, and endoscopic US (annually), gastroscopy with biopsy every 3 years in hypergastrinemia
	insulinoma (10%)	Serum insulin, fasting glucose at the age of 5 years	
	Pituitary adenoma (30%–40%): Prolactinoma (20%), somatotropinoma (10%), corticotropinoma (<5%) nonfunctioning (<5%)	Prolactin, Insulin growth factor 1 annually starts at 5 years of age	MRI (every 3–5 years)
	Associated tumors: Adrenal cortical tumor (20%–40%), pheochromocytoma (<1%)	Biochemical test with tumors <1 cm or with clinical features	CT or MRI (every 3 years)
	Bronchopulmonary NET (2%), thymic NET (2%), gastric NET (10%), lipomas (30%), angiofibromas (85%), collagenomas (70%), meningiomas (8%)	–	CT or MRI (every 1–2 years)

Abbreviation: NET, Neuroendocrine tumor.

2. The presence of one MEN 1-associated tumor in a first-degree relative of a patient with a clinical diagnosis of MEN 1.
3. The presence of a germline MEN 1 mutation in an asymptomatic individual without biochemical or radiological evidence of tumor.

Parathyroid gland

The most common feature of MEN 1 is primary HPT (PHPT) caused by multiglandular parathyroid hyperplasia and usually manifests after 15 years of age. Patient may have only asymptomatic hypercalcemia or symptoms of mild hypercalcemia (e.g. polyuria, polydipsia, constipation or malaise). Patient may present with nephrolithiasis and bony manifestations like brown tumors or peptic ulcers. HPT diagnosis is confirmed by hypercalcemia, with inappropriate high PTH. In summary, MEN 1 HPT is characterized by multiglandular, hyperplastic and asymmetrical parathyroid tumors. Table 62.3 lists the salient differences between sporadic and MEN 1 HPT (14–16).

Endocrine pancreas and duodenum

The second most frequent component of MEN 1 is NETs of the duodenum or pancreas. Tumors can be functioning or nonfunctioning, and pathologic change is typically multifocal, diffuse and potentially malignant. The primary symptoms depend upon the

TABLE 62.2: Characteristic Tumors of Multiple Endocrine Neoplasia 2–4

Phenotype	Chromosome/Genetic Defect and Inheritance Pattern	Features of MTC	Associated Abnormalities
MEN 2 A	10cen-10q11.2/germline missense mutations in extracellular cysteine codons of **RET 634, (Cys-Arg)** autosomal dominant	Multifocal, bilateral (95%)	Pheochromocytoma (50%) Parathyroid adenoma (20%–30%) Cutaneous lichen amyloidosis (10%) Hirschsprung's disease (2%)
MEN 2 B	10cen-10q11.2/germline missense mutation in tyrosine kinase domain of **RET918 (Met-Thr)** autosomal dominant	Multifocal, bilateral (>90%)	Pheochromocytoma (40%–50%) Associated abnormalities (40%–50%) Mucosal neuromas (100%) Marfanoid habitus (70%–100%) Medullated corneal nerve fibers Megacolon (60%)
Familial MTC	Germline missense mutations in extracellular or intracellular cysteine codons of *RET* Autosomal dominant	Multifocal, bilateral (100%)	MTC (100%)
MEN 4	A small subgroup of MEN 1 who don't harbor menin gene mutation but mutation of CDKN1B	–	Parathyroid adenoma Pituitary adenoma Reproductive organ tumors (e.g. testicular cancer and neuroendocrine cervical cancer) ?adrenal + renal tumors*

Abbreviation: MTC, Medullary thyroid cancer.
*(?)- Not established.

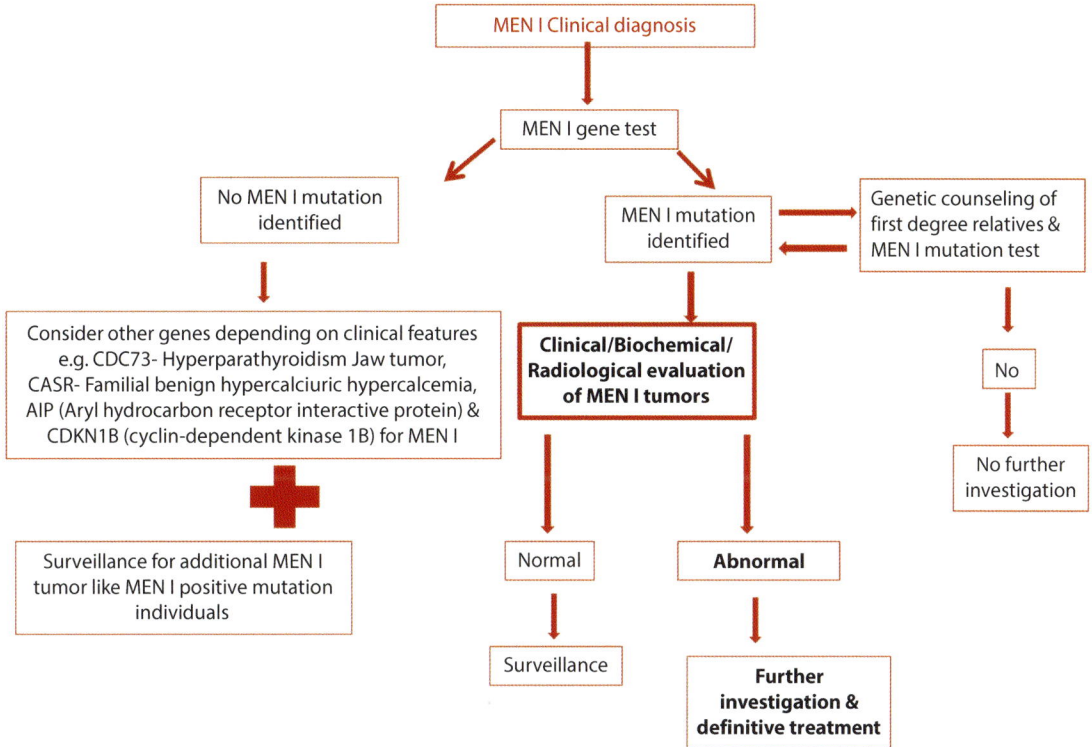

FIGURE 62.1 Approach to genetic testing in MEN 1.

type of hormone oversecretion or symptoms of mass effect especially in nonfunctional tumors (12).

The most common functional NET in MEN 1 is gastrinoma and frequently occurs both within the wall of duodenum and extra-pancreatic sites. Most of gastrinomas are located within the gastrinoma triangle. MEN 1 gastrinomas are usually malignant (≈80%). Patients present with epigastric pain, reflux esophagitis, secretory diarrhea and weight loss as gastrinoma (Zollinger–Ellison syndrome) causes hypersecretion of gastric acid (17). The diagnosis is made by the documentation of hypersecretion of gastric acid (>15 mEq/L in patients without or >5 mEq/L in patients with prior ulcer surgery), with elevated fasting levels of serum gastrin (>100 pg/mL). The diagnosis can be confirmed by an abnormal secretin test result. Primary gastrinoma can develop within lymph nodes; however, there is controversy regarding this. Localized resection is indicated to control tumor burden and prevent subsequent malignant dissemination. Evidence suggests surgery in patients with MEN 1 ZES rarely demonstrate long-term biochemical cure (12, 18–20).

Insulinoma is the second most common pancreatic NETs associated with MEN 1. Insulinoma affects approximately 10%–15% of MEN 1 patients. Insulinomas with MEN 1 are multifocal, multiple and more importantly characterized as microscopic small tumors spreading all over the pancreas to large size and sometimes malignant tumors in the same patient (5, 6). MEN 1 patients are usually young. Association of PHPT in a patient with insulinoma is virtually diagnostic of MEN 1, and therefore all patients of insulinomas should have screening for PHPT by serum calcium determination and PTH. The MEN I insulinoma patients may also have gastrinoma (21–23).

Patients typically present with recurrent symptoms of neuroglycopenia or symptoms of adrenergic sympathetic nervous system activation. Documenting symptomatic hypoglycemia in association with inappropriately elevated plasma levels of insulin and C-peptide during a supervised 72-hour or recently 48-hour fast confirms the diagnosis of insulinoma (23). The preferred treatment is surgical resection of the functioning tumor after accurate localization to correct life-threatening hyperinsulinemia. Preoperative regional localization of the functioning tumor within the pancreas may be provided by selective catheterization of the arteries supplying the pancreas, followed by injection of

TABLE 62.3: Differences From Sporadic Hyperparathyroidism

Features	MEN 1 HPT	Sporadic HPT
Age	20–25 years	50–60 years
Sex	Equal in men and women	Three times more common in women
Gland involvement	Hyperplasia of four glands	Adenoma (80%–85%)
Pathogenesis	Milder hypercalcemia and hyperplasia are caused by multiple cell clones postulated to be caused by a mitogenic factor	Single-cell clones
Neck exploration	Bilateral	Unilateral/focussed/minimal access
Surgery	Subtotal (3.5 glands) or total with autologous forearm tissue graft with transcervical thymectomy	Adenoma excision
Persistent/recurrent hypercalcemia 1,26,27	20%–60% at 10 years	4% at 10 years

an insulin secretagogue (calcium gluconate) and measurement of insulin gradients in the hepatic veins. The surgical strategy differs between tumors with MEN I and sporadic cases. Total removal of gross disease with adequate prophylactic resection to minimize recurrence without causing endocrine and exocrine pancreatic compromise is the principle of surgery in MEN I patient. The best procedure to achieve it is routine distal subtotal pancreatectomy (to the level of portal vein), with enucleation of tumors in the head guided by intraoperative ultrasound for safety.

Pancreatic NETs secreting pancreatic polypeptide are probably the most frequent nonfunctioning NETs in MEN 1. Other functional NETs of the pancreas, such as glucagonoma, somatostatinoma, and tumors secreting vasoactive intestinal peptide or pancreatic polypeptide, occur rarely in association with MEN 1 (24–29).

Pituitary gland
Pituitary microadenomas may present with amenorrhea, galactorrhea (hyperprolactinemia), acromegaly (GH hypersecretion) or Cushing's disease (ACTH hypersecretion). Large tumors present with visual or neurological deficits. Pituitary tumors usually are recognized in the fourth decade of life (30–32).

Treatment
Hyperparathyroidism: The aim of surgical treatment for MEN 1 HPT is to achieve the lowest incidence of recurrent, persistent hypercalcemia with a minimal chance of permanent hypoparathyroidism. Bilateral neck exploration is recommended as MEN 1 patients have multiglandular disease. The two possible operations are subtotal parathyroidectomy (3.5 gland excision) and total parathyroidectomy with intramuscular autotransplantation of parathyroid tissue into the forearm muscle. Transcervical partial thymectomy should always be performed with parathyroid operation to remove ectopic or supernumerary parathyroid gland within the cranial horns of the thymus and to avoid possible development of thymic carcinoid in the future. Postoperative calcium and vitamin D supplementation are given to all patients depending upon the extent of bone disease between 6 and 12 weeks (12).

Pituitary tumors: Surgery is the preferred mode of treatment and depends on size and location of the tumor. It is indicated in patients with large tumors with progressive visual loss. Preferred mode is transsphenoidal surgery. Craniotomy is needed in patients with large suprasellar extensions or cavernous sinus infiltration.

Medical therapy is less effective in growth hormone–secreting adenomas where octreotide gives better response than bromocriptine. Bromocriptine (2.5–20 mg/day) is a drug of choice for prolactinomas. Common side effects include nausea, vomiting, headache and orthostatic hypotension. In patients with incomplete resection, radiotherapy can be used as a postoperative adjunct (12, 31, 32).

Pancreas and duodenum: Controversy exists regarding the optimal timing and most appropriate operation in MEN 1 pancreatic tumors. They are characteristically multifocal, and some of these tumors have a malignant potential, and delays in diagnosis and effective treatment carry the risk of the development of local or distant metastasis. Lack of genotype–phenotype correlation in MEN 1 does not allow genetic stratification of individuals or tumors at higher risk of malignant progression. It is obviously desirable to intervene early to prevent malignant dissemination while minimizing morbidity and mortality from both cancer and surgery. Surgical resection is recommended for all nonfunctioning pancreatic tumors of size more than 1 cm. For tumors less than 1 cm in size, surgical decision is based on tumor doubling time. Resection is planned only after pre- and intraoperative tumor localization (12, 24, 27, 29). Hepatic artery embolization may be used as palliative therapy in patients with advanced, malignant islet cell tumors of pancreas and liver metastasis. Alternative therapies for oligometastatic and small lesions are radiofrequency ablation (RFA), microwave ablation or thermal ablation. Embolization of liver metastatic lesion can be done through hepatic artery as metastatic lesions predominantly derive their blood supply from the hepatic artery. Various embolization options are bland transarterial embolization (TAE)–producing ischemia, chemoembolization (TACE), and radioembolization (TARE). Systemic chemotherapy with drugs such as streptozotocin and 5-fluorouracil may be required in patients in whom surgery is not possible. Tyrosine kinase receptor inhibitors and mTOR inhibitors (everolimus) have been reported as effective in treating pancreatic tumors (33–35).

Screening program in MEN 1 gene carriers
Annual biochemical screening schedule should be planned in MEN 1 carriers, and it should include the following measurements (Table 62.1).

1. *Parathyroid HPT*: Intact PTH and albumin-corrected total serum calcium or ionized serum calcium annually and start at the age of 8 years.
2. *Pituitary tumors*: Serum prolactin and insulin growth factor 1 (IGF-1) by age 5.
3. *Insulinoma*: Serum-fasting glucose and insulin by age 5.
4. *Gastrinoma*: Gastrin, gastric acid output and secretin-stimulated gastrin at the age of 20 years.
5. *Other GEP tumors*: Proinsulin, glucagon, and plasma chromogranin A before the age of 10 years. Biochemical tests for adrenal lesions are recommended in the presence of symptoms or signs of functioning tumors and/or size >10 mm on imaging.

Multiple endocrine neoplasia type 2

The main cancer associated with MEN 2 syndrome is MTC, and it occurs with 100% penetration. This syndrome is of two types A and B, and type A has 4 variants: classic type, associated with cutaneous lichen amyloidosis, associated with Hirschsprung's disease, and FMTC (36) (Table 62.2).

Epidemiology
MEN 2 syndrome is rare with the prevalence of 2–3 patients per 100,000 individuals.

Genetic
The MEN 2 syndrome is caused by activating mutation in RET (**re**arranged during **t**ransfection) proto-oncogene, 21-exon gene, encoding a transmembrane receptor tyrosine kinase, located on chromosome 10q11 and has autosomal dominant pattern of inheritance. The receptor is composed of an extracellular, a transmembrane and an intracellular domain with tyrosine kinase activity. Tyrosine kinase protein is involved in growth, differentiation and migration of developing tissues. The mutations responsible for MTC are missense mutations and cause single amino acid change, which leads to a gain of function (37, 38). The MEN 2 syndromes are characterized by a strong genotype–phenotype correlation. Specific RET mutations are responsible for a particular phenotype with a predictive clinical course of MTC for age

TABLE 62.4: Risk Stratification and Timing of Surgery for Various RET mutations as per ATA

ATA Risk Level for MTC Development	RET Codons	Timing of Thyroid Surgery
A (low)	768, 790, 791, 804, 649, 891	After 5 years
B (medium)	609, 611, 618, 620, 630, 631	Before 5 years of age
C (high)	634	Before 5 years of age
D (highest)	918, 883	As soon as possible in the first year of life

of onset, aggressiveness and the presence or the absence of other endocrine neoplasms (39).

- Most frequent mutations found in typical MEN 2 A families are at codon 634 (exon 11).
- Less common mutations are present at codons 609, 611, 618 and 620.
- Germline RET mutations are found in approximately 95% of families with FMTC (codons 609, 611, 618, 620 and 634).
- Mutation at codon 918 in exon 16 in tyrosine kinase domain of RET gene is responsible for 95% MEN 2 B phenotype, and threonine is substituted for methionine.

Mutation 918 results in the most aggressive forms of MTC seen in MEN 2 B. Mutation 634 is seen in MEN 2 A and has a variable course of MTC, while FMTC patients have the most indolent course. MEN 2 carriers have a 50% risk of genetic transmission to their offspring as RET mutations are inherited in autosomal dominant pattern. Inactivating (loss of function) mutations in RET are associated with Hirschsprung's disease. There is a defect in the migration and development of enteric neurons, which causes megacolon in infancy. Activating (gain of function) germline mutations in RET are associated with the MEN 2 syndromes, while MEN 1, is caused by the loss of function mutations in the predisposition gene that is a tumor suppressor gene (40).

Screening and genetic testing

All patients diagnosed with MTC, with or without familial history, must undergo a germline RET proto-oncogene analysis. If germline mutation is found in the index case, all first-degree relatives should be submitted for RET analysis to identify "gene carriers" from "non-gene carriers." Since RET gene carriers are at very high risk of MTC so diagnostic and therapeutic protocol should be followed with all these carriers. American Thyroid Association (ATA) describes the level of risk of MTC development with codon mutation and age (Table 62.4). Non-gene carriers have a similar risk of development of MTC as general population. Non-carriers should not be submitted to diagnostic protocol (40–43). Tables 62.5 and 62.6 summarizes the differences between genetic mutations between MEN 1 and MEN 2. Pentagastrin-stimulated calcitonin testing is no more used now for screening.

TABLE 62.5: Differences Between MEN 1 and MEN 2 (7, 12, 17, 36–38, 43)

	MEN 1	MEN 2
Synonym	Wermer's syndrome	Sipple's syndrome
Prevalence	2–3 per 100,000	2–3 per 100,000
Definition	MEN 1 tumors, two of three glands (parathyroid, endocrine pancreas, pituitary) or one gland endocrinopathy + one first-degree relative have MEN 1	**MEN 2A:** Two or more specific endocrine tumors-MTC, pheochromocytoma, or parathyroid adenoma/hyperplasia) in a single individual or in close relatives. **FMTC:** Families with 4 or more cases of MTC without pheochromocytoma or parathyroid adenoma/hyperplasia. **MEN 2 B**: Early-onset MTC, mucosal neuromas of lips and tongue + medullated corneal nerve fibers, distinctive facies with enlarged lips + asthenic, marfanoid body habitus.
First endocrine gland involvement	Parathyroid gland Primary HPT: Synchronous or asynchronous benign multiglandular parathyroid hyperplasia (100% penetration 50 years)	Thyroid gland MTC: Bilateral, multicentric and associated with C-cell hyperplasia. Aggressiveness of MTC: MEN 2 B > MEN 2 A > FMTC
Other endocrine glands	Endocrine pancreas, duodenum 70%–80% Commonest: Gastrinoma Second commonest: Insulinoma Pituitary adenoma: 30%–40%	MEN 2 A: Pheochromocytomas: 50% Hyperparathyroidism: 25% and cutaneous lichen amyloidosis: 10% Hirschsprung's disease: 2% MEN 2 B:Pheochromocytomas: 50% Mucosal neuromas: 100% Marfanoid habitus: 100% Ganglioneuromatosis of GIT: 60%
Genetics	Gene menin (tumor suppressor gene) and mutation causes loss of function) located at 11q13, cloned in 1997; >1300 mutations reported; 20%–30% MEN 1 do not have reported mutations	Gene (RET proto-oncogene) located on chromosome 10q11; activating mutation in RET causes II A, II B, FMTC
Prophylactic surgery	**No genotype–phenotype** correlation **No prophylactic surgery** is advised to prevent tumor development	**Strong genotype–phenotype** correlation **Prophylactic surgery** (total thyroidectomy) advocated to prevent MTC development according to codon mutation, which defines risk category.

TABLE 62.6: Difference Between MEN 1 and MEN 2 (RET) gene (9, 10, 12, 37, 38)

Features	MEN 1	MEN 2 (RET)
Gene identification possible	Yes	Yes
Gene location	11q13	10cen
Type of mutation	Inactivate	Activating/transforming
Genotype–phenotype correlation	No	Yes
Can it be used for intervention and prevention	No	Yes
Can it be used to cure cancer	No	Yes

Prophylactic thyroidectomy in RET gene carrier (codon directed surgery)

1. Level D risk individuals or *RET* mutation (918) should have prophylactic total thyroidectomy (TT) as soon as possible within the first year of life.
2. Level B and C mutations individuals should be operated on before 5 years of age.
3. Level A mutation individuals can have delayed TT after 5 years of age or until the calcitonin positivity.

Clinical features: MEN 2

In MEN 2, there is initially C-cell hyperplasia, which progresses to nodular hyperplasia, and later there is malignant transformation (MTC). MTC is usually detected before pheochromocytoma or HPT. Patients present with a neck nodule, and at the time of presentation, 50% have neck or mediastinal lymph node metastases and fewer have lung, liver or bony metastases. These individuals don't have clinical or biochemical thyroid dysfunction. Approximately 30% of patients may have associated diarrhea (unknown etiology, most common systemic manifestation and implies a poor prognosis) or cushingoid features (ectopic ACTH and/or CRH production). Cutaneous lichen amyloidosis is circumscribed, pruritic, lichenoid skin lesion over interscapular region on back. It is seen associated with MEN 2 A. A total of 50% of MEN 2 individuals develop pheochromocytoma. It is usually bilateral, but malignancy is rare. Intermittent headaches, palpitations and sweating with nervousness are usual symptoms but are mild. Predominant epinephrine secretion over norepinephrine is observed in early pheochromocytoma in MEN 2 A.

HPT develops in 10%–25% of MEN 2 A patients but is absent in MEN 2 B. Nephrolithiasis may be the presenting feature in some patients with MEN 2 A.

Ganglioneuromas of lips, tongue, conjunctiva and gastrointestinal tract are observed in 100% of MEN 2 B patients. Intestinal obstruction, flatulence, diarrhea and failure to thrive may occur as a result of gastrointestinal involvement. Mucosal neuromas may affect the ocular tissue and can be picked up on slit lamp examination. Typical facial features of MEN 2 B should alert physician of the possibility of MEN 2. The marfanoid habitus is seen in about two-thirds of MEN 2 B, patients, but does not include cardiac or ocular abnormalities normally associated with Marfan's syndrome. MTC in MEN 2 B develops at an earlier age than MEN 2 A. A total of 25% of all MTC cases are associated with MEN 2, while MTC represents only 5%–10% of all thyroid malignancies. MTC of MEN 2 syndrome is multicentric (90%), bilateral, develops at younger age (even at the age of 1 year) and has a sequence of hyperplasia, nodule and malignancy. Sporadic MTC is solitary (>80%), seen in older population (40–60) years, located in the upper two-thirds of the gland, and there is malignant transformation of C or parafollicular cells (39, 42).

Diagnosis
Biochemical evaluation

1. Plasma calcitonin basal and stimulated collection after 2 and 5 minutes after intravenous calcium administration should be measured. Other calcitonin secretagogues such as pentagastrin can also be used. Plasma calcitonin basal and stimulated equal or above 100 pg/mL is an indication for surgery.
2. Elevated catecholamines and catecholamine metabolites (e.g. norepinephrine, epinephrine, metanephrine, and vanillylmandelic acid [VMA] in plasma or 24-hour urine collections).
3. Elevated serum calcium with elevated or high-normal parathyroid hormone (PTH) suggests PHPT.

Imaging

1. High-resolution ultrasound neck, CT scan with contrast neck and mediastinum in all patients for MTC extent evaluation.
2. Abdominal MRI and/or CT are performed only after biochemical diagnosis pheochromocytoma. MRI is more sensitive than CT in the detection of a pheochromocytoma.
3. 18F-fluorodopamine PET is the best overall imaging modality in the localization of pheochromocytomas. MIBG (123I- or 131I-labeled metaiodobenzylguanidine) scintigraphy should be used for further evaluation if 18FDA PET is unavailable. 68Ga-DOTATATE-PET–CT results correlate best with biochemical parameters of pheochromocytoma.
4. For preoperative adenoma localization, high-resolution ultrasound neck as anatomical imaging and 99mTc-sestamibi scintigraphy with three-dimensional single-photon emission CT (SPECT) as functional imaging combination provide best results.

Differential diagnosis

a. *MTC in individuals with no family history of MTC*: Sporadic MTC tends to be unifocal, has a later age of onset and lacks C-cell hyperplasia. 918 codon variant is the most common.
b. *C-cell hyperplasia (CCH)*: CCH associated with a positive calcitonin stimulation test is seen in about 5% of the general population. Serum calcitonin levels may be elevated in persons with chronic renal failure, sepsis, NETs of the lung or gastrointestinal tract, hypergastrinemia, mastocytosis, autoimmune thyroid disease, and type 1 A pseudohypoparathyroidism.
c. Aging and HPT can cause secondary CCH, but it rarely transforms to MTC and is not related to MEN 2.
d. Up to 25% of individuals with pheochromocytoma without family history of pheochromocytoma have a heterozygous pathogenic variant in one of the genes (*RET, VHL, SDHD* or *SDH*). Approximately 5% of individuals with non-syndromic pheochromocytoma without family history of pheochromocytoma have heterozygous germline *RET mutation*. Biochemically, MEN 2-associated pheochromocytomas do not produce exclusively normetanephrine.

Evaluations following initial diagnosis

After the diagnosis of MEN 2, following evaluations are recommended to establish the extent of disease:

1. Consultation with a clinical geneticist and/or genetic counselor if a facility is available.
2. *Biochemical evaluations*: Serum calcitonin, 24-hour urinary metanephrines, serum calcium and PTH.
3. *Metastatic workup of MTC*: CT with contrast chest and abdomen.
4. MRI of liver in the presence of nodal disease or calcitonin >400 pg/mL.

Treatment

MTC: Treatment of choice in MTC is surgical excision, and all established MTC patients should undergo TT with central neck dissection. The decision to resect lateral nodes depends on the extent of central neck node involvement and the result of preoperative imaging. Lymph node dissection is performed as compartment-oriented dissection. Lateral neck dissection (level II–V nodes) decision depends upon the clinical, radiological, pathological or intraoperative evidence of the presence of lymph node metastases. If unilateral neck lymph node disease is present, bilateral neck dissection should be performed, and if bilateral neck lymph node disease is evident, superior mediastinal lymph node dissection is also indicated along with bilateral neck dissection. With central compartment node dissection, there is a risk of ischemia of parathyroid glands especially lower, so there should be lesser threshold for autotransplantation of devascularized gland. It should be done in sternocleidomastoid muscle in individual muscle pockets in FMTC, MEN 2 B and brachioradialis muscle pockets of non-dominant forearm in MEN 2 A when there is a significant risk of future HPT.

All screen-detected gene carriers who are at risk of developing C-cell disease should undergo TT at an age as per the recommendation of ATA risk classification as described earlier (Table 62.4). Distant metastasis of MTC is treated by resection or radiotherapy. Once TT has been done, the patient will need lifelong thyroid hormone replacement (1.6–2 µg/kg/day). These patients do not require thyroid suppression, and dose is titrated to maintain a normal TSH concentration (43).

Pheochromocytoma: Adrenal surgery for pheochromocytoma should precede thyroid surgery. Pheochromocytomas are not malignant in MEN 2 patients, and they tend to be bilateral. Interval between the development of a pheochromocytoma on one side and the other side is usually more than 10 years. For this reason, unilateral adrenal surgery is recommended for unilateral pheochromocytoma in MEN 2 patients and annual biochemical screening is continued thereafter. Laparoscopic adrenalectomy is the preferred route of surgery.

Patients with bilateral adrenalectomy require lifelong glucocorticoid and mineralocorticoid replacement. Glucocorticoid replacement is done in dose of 0.5–0.6 mg/kg/day of hydrocortisone, or 0.1–0.15 mg/kg/day of prednisolone, and fludrocortisone is the mineralocorticoid of choice.

Hyperparathyroidism: HPT is treated by three and a half gland subtotal parathyroidectomy or total parathyroidectomy with or without autotransplantation. Postoperative hypoparathyroidism is managed with high doses of calcium carbonate and 1,25 dihydroxy vitamin D.

Follow-up

These patients have risk of developing recurrence or new tumors or metastases during follow-up. All patients during follow-up undergo annual serum calcium, plasma calcitonin and urinary catecholamines estimation. In all individuals with *RET* mutations and prophylactic thyroidectomy, annual biochemical screening by serum calcitonin is recommended. Annual screening should begin at 6 months for children with MEN 2 B and 3–5 years for children with MEN 2A or FMTC. Calcitonin results should be interpreted very cautiously in less than 3 years age and especially younger than age 6 months.

South Asia perspective

Both MEN 1 and II have been reported from many referral centers. There is no difference in clinical presentation, genetic mutations from the western world here.

Conclusion

There is no cure for these genetic syndromes. Early suspicion and timely genetic tests help in the diagnosis. With identification of menin and RET gene, better understanding of genotype mutations and phenotype relationship, the subsequent management has changed drastically in the last two decades. MEN 2 has very strong phenotype–genotype relationship. MEN 2 B is the most aggressive form, and early diagnosis increases survival potential. Some patients with MEN 2 A will not exhibit any symptoms at all, and the screening testing for early diagnosis may improve survival.

References

1. Carney JA. Familial multiple endocrine neoplasia syndromes: components, classification, and nomenclature. J Intern Med. 1998;243(6):425–432.
2. Brandi ML, Gagel RF, Angeli A, et al. Consensus: guidelines for diagnosis and therapy of MEN type 1 and type 2. J Clin Endocrinol Metabol. 2001;86(12):5658–5671.
3. Salpea P, Stratakis CA. Carney complex and McCune Albright syndrome: an overview of clinical manifestations and human molecular genetics. Mol Cell Endocrinol. 2014;386:85–91.
4. Thakker RV. Multiple endocrine neoplasia–syndromes of the twentieth century. J Clin Endocrinol Metab. 1998;83:2617–2620.
5. Schernthaner-Reiter MH, Trivellin G, Stratakis CA. MEN1, MEN4, and carney complex: pathology and molecular genetics. Neuroendocrinology. 2016;103:18–31.
6. Erdheim J. Zur normalen und pathologischen Histologie der Glandula thyreoidea, parathyreoidea und Hypophysis. Beitr Pathol Anat. 1903;33:158–263.
7. Wermer P. Genetic aspects of adenomatosis of endocrine glands. Am J Med. 1954;16:363–371.
8. Carney JA. Familial multiple endocrine neoplasia: the first 100 years. Am J Surg Pathol. 2005;29(2):254–274.
9. Agarwal SK, Kester MB, Debelenko LV, et al. Germ line mutations of the MEN1 gene in familial multiple endocrine Neoplasia type 1 and related states. Hum Mol Genet. 1997;6:1169–1175.
10. Lemmens I, Vande Ven WJ, Kas K, et al. Identification of the multiple endocrine neoplasia type 1 (MEN1) gene. The European Consortiumon MEN1. Hum Mol Genet. 1997;6:1177–1183.
11. Goudet P, Dalac A, LeBras M, et al. MEN1 disease occurring before 21 years old: a 160-patient cohort study from the Groupe d'etude des Tumours Endocrines. J Clin Endocrinol Metab. 2015;100:1568–1577.
12. Thakker RV, Newey PJ, Walls GV, et al. Clinical practice guide-lines for multiple endocrine neoplasia type 1 (MEN1). J Clin Endocrinol Metab. 2012;97:2990–3011.
13. Turner JJ, Christie PT, Pearce SH, et al. Diagnostic challenges due to phenocopies: lessons from multiple endocrine neoplasia type1 (MEN1). Hum Mutat. 2010;31:E1089–E1101.
14. Schreinemakers JM, Pieterman CR, Scholten A, Vriens MR, Valk GD, Rinkes IH. The optimal surgical treatment for primary hyperparathyroidism in MEN1 patients: a systematic review. World J Surg. 2011;35:1993–2005.
15. Waldmann J, Lo´pez CL, Langer P, Rothmund M, Bartsch DK. Surgery for multiple endocrine neoplasia type 1-associated primary hyperparathyroidism. Br J Surg. 2010;97:1528–1534.
16. Eller-Vainicher C, Chiodini I, Battista C, et al. Sporadic and MEN1-related primary hyperparathyroidism: differences in clinical expression and severity. J Bone Miner Res. 2009;24:1404–1410.

17. Zollinger RM, Ellison EH. Primary peptic ulcerations of the jejunum associated with islet cell tumors of the pancreas. Ann Surg. 1955;142:709–723; discussion, 724-708.
18. Nell S, Verkooijen HM, Pieterman CR, et al. Management of MEN1 related nonfunctioning pancreatic NETs: a shifting paradigm: results from the Dutch MEN1 Study Group. Ann Surg. 2018;267(6):1155–1160.
19. Yates CJ, Newey PJ, Thakker RV. Challenges and controversies in management of pancreatic neuroendocrine tumours in patients with MEN1. Lancet Diabetes Endocrinol. 2015;3:895–905.
20. Imamura M. Recent standardization of treatment strategy for pancreatic neuroendocrine tumors. World J Gastroenterol. 2010;16:4519–4525.
21. Demeure MJ, Klonoff DC, Karam JH, et al. Insulinomas associated with multiple endocrine neoplasia type I: the need for a different surgical approach. Surgery. 1991;110:998–1005.
22. O'Riordain DS, Brien T, van Heerden JA, et al. Surgical management of insulinoma associated with multiple endocrine neoplasia type I. World J Surg. 1994;18:488–494
23. Ueda K, Kawabe K, Lee L, et al. Diagnostic performance of 48-hour fasting test and insulin surrogates in patients with suspected insulinoma. Pancreas. 2017;46:476–481.
24. Akerström G, Hellman P. Surgery on neuroendocrine tumours. Best Pract Res Clin Endocrinol Metab. 2007;21:87–109.
25. Barbe C, Murat A, Dupas B, et al. Magnetic resonance imaging versus endoscopic ultrasonography for the detection of pancreatic tumors in multiple endocrine neoplasia type 1. Dig Liver Dis. 2012;44: 228–234.
26. Vinik AI, Woltering EA, Warner RR, et al. NANETS consensus guidelines for the diagnosis of neuroendocrine tumor. Pancreas. 2010;39:713–734.
27. O'Toole D, Grossman A, Gross D, et al. ENETS consensus guidelines for the standards of care in neuroendocrine tumors: biochemical markers. Neuroendocrinology. 2009;90:194–202.
28. van Leeuwaarde RS, de Laat JM, Pieterman CRC, et al. The future: medical advances in MEN1 therapeutic approaches and management strategies. Endocr Relat Cancer. 2017;24:T179–T193.
29. Ito T, Igarashi H, Jensen RT. Zollinger-Ellison syndrome: recent advances and controversies. Curr Opin Gastroenterol. 2013;29:650–661.
30. Fernandez A, Karavitaki N, Wass JA. Prevalence of pituitary adenomas: a community-based, cross-sectional study in Banbury (Oxfordshire, UK). Clin Endocrinol (Oxf). 2010;72:377–382.
31. Trouillas J, Labat-Moleur F, Sturm N, et al. Pituitary tumors and hyperplasia in multiple endocrine neoplasia type 1 syndrome (MEN1): a case control study in a series of 77 patients versus 2509 non-MEN1 patients. Am J Surg Pathol. 2008;32:534–543.
32. Verge`s B, Boureille F, Goudet P, et al. Pituitary disease in MEN type 1 (MEN1): data from the France-Belgium MEN1 multicenter study. J Clin Endocrinol Metab. 2002; 87:457–465.
33. Nazario J, Gupta S. Transarterial liver-directed therapies of neuroendocrine hepatic metastases. Semin Oncol. 2010;37(2):118–126.
34. Gupta S, Yao JC, Ahrar K, et al. Hepatic artery embolization and chemoembolization for treatment of patients with metastatic carcinoid tumours: the M.D. Anderson experience. Cancer J. 2003;9(4):261–267.
35. Swärd C, Johanson V, Nieveen van Dijkum E, et al. Prolonged survival after hepatic artery embolization in patients with midgut carcinoid syndrome. Br J Surg. 2009;96(5):517–521.
36. Sipple J. The association of pheochromocytoma with carcinoma of the thyroid gland. Am J Med Sci. 1961;31:163–166.
37. Mole SE, Mulligan LM, Healey CS, Ponder BA, Tunnacliffe A. Localisation of the gene for multiple endocrine neoplasia type 2A to a 480 kb region in chromosome band 10q11.2. Hum Mol Genet. 1993;2:247–252.
38. Machens A, Lorenz K, Sekulla C, et al. Molecular epidemiology of multiple endocrine neoplasia 2: implications for RET screening in the new millenium. Eur J Endocrinol. 2013;168:307–314.
39. Wells SA Jr, Asa SL, Dralle H, et al. Revised American Thyroid Association guidelines for the management of medullary thyroid carcinoma. Thyroid. 2015;25:567–610.
40. Machens A, Dralle H. Therapeutic effectiveness of screening for multiple endocrine neoplasia type 2A. J Clin Endocrinol Metab. 2015;100:2539–2545.
41. Brandi ML, Gagel RF, Angeli A,. Guidelines for diagnosis and therapy of MEN type 1 and type 2. J Clin Endocrinol Metab. 2001;86:5658–5671.
42. Kloos RT, Eng C, Evans DB, Francis GL, Gagel RF, Gharib H, Moley JF, Pacini F, Ringel MD, Schlumberger M, Wells SA Jr. Medullary thyroid cancer: management guidelines of the American Thyroid Association. Thyroid. 2009;19:565–612.
43. Eng C. Multiple Endocrine Neoplasia Type 2. 1999 Sep 27 [Updated 2019 Aug 15]. In: Adam MP, Ardinger HH, Pagon RA, et al., editors. GeneReviews® [Internet]. Seattle (WA): University of Washington, Seattle; 1993-2020.

63

NON-MEN ENDOCRINE SYNDROMES

Kushagra Gaurav, Akshay Agarwal and Kul Ranjan Singh

Introduction

Over the last century, with the huge advancement in the field of molecular diagnostics and discovery of multiple genes, familial endocrine tumors are now being more explicated. Multiple endocrine neoplasia also popularly known as MEN syndrome was described as early as in the early 1900s. The MEN syndromes (MEN 1, MEN 2) are among the more thoroughly studied genetic disorders, which are inherited in autosomal dominant fashion. MEN 1 is characterized by adenomas and/or hyperplasia of the pituitary and parathyroid glands (multiglandular involvement) and neuroendocrine tumors of pancreas, whereas MEN 2 is characterized by the occurrence of unilateral or bilateral adrenal pheochromocytoma and medullary thyroid cancer (MTC) (and parathyroid adenomas in MEN 2A) (1, 2). This chapter deals with newer described entities of non-MEN familial endocrine syndromes. These syndromes are elaborated in the organ-wise format.

Pituitary

Carney complex (CNC)

Carney complex (CNC) is an infrequently encountered entity manifesting with abnormal pigmented lesions of the skin and mucosa, cardiac, cutaneous, and other myxomas, multiple endocrine, and other non-endocrine neoplasms (3, 4). Germline inactivating mutations of PRKAR1A gene, situated at the long arm of chromosome 17 – CNC1 locus, are found in more than one-third and two-thirds of sporadic and familial CNC cases, respectively. It is inherited in an autosomal dominant (AD) fashion having a penetrance of almost 100%. Endocrine neoplasms develop in pituitary, thyroid, adrenal, testis, and ovaries.

Pituitary gland lesions have a wide profile that includes cellular hyperplasia, multiple microadenomas, and invasive macroadenoma. Almost 75% of afflicted individuals have elevated growth hormone (GH) or prolactin levels but only 10% present with clinically apparent acromegaly. On microscopy, there occur multiple areas of somatomammotropic cellular hyperplasia surrounded by non-adenomatous pituitary tissue. A GH-secreting pituitary adenoma manifesting with acromegaly is managed by adrenalectomy, whereas partial or complete hypophysectomy may be required in those with multiple GH-secreting adenoma-associated hyperplasia.

Thyroid gland lesions present with a wide variety of tumors varying from cystic lesions (60–65%) and follicular adenomas (25%) to follicular or papillary carcinoma in approximately 2.5% (5, 6). Long-term clinical and sonographic (USG) surveillance is advised in cases of CNC with suspicious thyroid nodules for the identification of occult thyroid carcinoma. Certain recent studies show the presence of associated hyperthyroidism in about 15% of cases (7).

The commonest endocrine manifestation of CNC is primary pigmented nodular adrenocortical disease (PPNAD). It is detected in 25–60% of patients and more observed in women (3). PPNAD occurs at an earlier age amongst women. Almost half of these patients develop adrenocorticotropic hormone (ACTH)-independent Cushing's syndrome. The manifestations can either be subclinical or overt and occasionally cyclical or atypical. Paradoxical increase of urinary free cortisol by more than 50% may be seen on dexamethasone suppression test. Bilateral sub-centimetric pigmented nodules surrounded by atrophic adrenocortical tissue are seen in adrenal gland(s), which may be of normal size or enlarged. Bilateral adrenalectomy is commonly performed. Rarely ketoconazole or mitotane is used for medical treatment.

Large cell calcifying Sertoli cell tumors (LCCSCTs) are also seen in more than three-quarters of males. LCCSCTs associated with CNC are usually benign, bilateral, and multifocal with the rare occurrence of malignancy and are also associated with decreased sperm counts. These can be distinguished from germ cells and other testicular tumors by their characteristic microcalcifications on USG. Lesions in ovaries are thought to be more frequent in women with CNC. Serous cystadenomas and cystic teratomas, which arise from the surface epithelium, are the most common. However, ovarian carcinomas like mucinous adenocarcinoma or endometrioid carcinoma are rare. Sonographic evaluation and follow-up are advised.

The earliest manifestations of CNC involve the skin, and these are the commonest too. Spectrum of skin lesion varies from lentigines and blue nevi to cutaneous myxomas. Epithelioid blue nevus though not pathognomonic but due to its frequent association with the disease should raise a clinical suspicion of CNC (8). Café-au-lait spots, irregular depigmented areas, and rarely Spitz nevi have also been reported. Cutaneous myxomas are usually asymptomatic sub-centimetric nodules found in the dermis or subcutaneous tissue of eyelids, external auditory canal, breast, and genitalia in about one-third to half unnecessary of all CNC patients.

Cardiac myxomas are the most frequently encountered non-cutaneous lesions in 20–40% of patients. Unlike sporadic myxomas that occur in the left atrium of women predominantly, CNC-associated myxomas can occur anywhere in the heart and do not have any gender predilection. These can cause intracardiac obstruction to blood flow or embolism and are responsible for more than half of the CNC-associated mortality. Early institution of periodic echocardiography has been recommended to improve outcomes.

Other manifestations include – breast myxomas, ductal adenoma, and myxoid fibroadenomas; facial and palpebral lentigines; psammomatous melanotic schwannomas (PMS); osteochondromyxoma; and pancreatic neoplasms (4).

Parathyroid

Hereditary hyperparathyroidism-jaw tumor (HPT-JT) syndrome

Hyperparathyroidism-jaw tumor (HPT-JT) syndrome is a rare AD disorder linked to the HRPT 2 locus located on 1q25-q32 having a high but incomplete penetrance in 70–90% of those involved.

Characteristic features of the disease are familial HPT, ossifying jaw fibromas, and renal abnormalities. Frequently, a single parathyroid gland is involved though multiple glands can also undergo cystic enlargement. There is an associated risk of parathyroid carcinoma in 10–15% of these patients. Hyperparathyroidism-jaw tumor syndrome results from truncating (~80%) or missense variants in the CDC73 gene (also known as HRPT-2). This gene encodes for parafibromin protein. A germline analysis of CDC73 should be considered if there is an absence of nuclear parafibromin staining by immunohistochemistry (IHC) in any parathyroid neoplasm (9, 10). Other manifestations of pathogenic germline CDC73 variants include ossifying fibromas in maxilla and mandible (25–50%), uterine neoplasms (~75% of patients), and renal anomalies (~20%).

Genetic testing is currently the only method used for obtaining a definitive diagnosis of HPT-JT syndrome. HPT-JT syndrome should always be considered when there is

a. Early-onset primary hyperparathyroidism (PHPT) because HPT-JT syndrome commonly occurs in patients of less than 30 years of age, while PHPT typically occurs in much older patients (40–75 years of age)
b. A patient having other family members affected with PHPT (familial HPT to be confirmed by genetic testing)
c. A diagnosis of parathyroid carcinoma.

Surveillance is advised in carriers of CDC73 mutations beginning from age of 5–10 years and the following parameters should be done:

a. Biochemical screening for evidence of HPT: annually
b. Orthopantomograph: at a 5-year interval
c. Renal ultrasonography: at a 5-year interval
d. Uterine ultrasound as clinically indicated for abnormal uterine bleeding (11)

Familial isolated hyperparathyroidism (FIHP)

Familial isolated hyperparathyroidism (FIHP) is an uncommon cause of parathyroid tumors. It is characterized by the absence of a non-parathyroid clinical manifestation of known syndromic primary HPT and is inherited as a dominant trait. Germline mutations in MEN 1, CDC73, and CASR genes have been encountered in patients with FIHP (12, 13), hence for the diagnosis of FIHP, other tumors associated with MEN 1 and HPT-JT should also be screened for. Profound hypercalcemia being the common classical presentation occurs more frequently than in MEN 1. The absence of parafibromin expression is pathognomonic. Usually, a single gland is involved, and limited parathyroidectomy is indicated.

Neonatal severe hyperparathyroidism (NSHPT)

Germline homozygous–inactivating mutations of calcium-sensing receptor (CaSR) gene lead to multiglandular diffuse chief cell hyperplasia (14). Life-threatening hypercalcemia and hypocalciuria occur in the neonatal period. It merits emergent evaluation, and early total parathyroidectomy in the neonatal period improves chances of survival.

Familial hypocalciuric hypercalcemia (FHH)

Familial hypocalciuric hypercalcemia (FHH) is an AD trait, which manifests as mild-to-moderate hypercalcemia and is the most common cause of hereditary hypercalcemia. Symptomatic patients have inappropriate hypocalciuria in the setting of overt hypercalcemia and normal/elevated serum parathyroid hormone (PTH). The majority are clinically symptomatic. In FHH, the normal hypercalciuric response to hypercalcemia is lost due to the derangement in PTH set point due to inactivation of the CaSR-related pathway (15). The parathyroid glands are usually normal in size or only minimally enlarged. Normal phosphate levels and mild hypermagnesemia are often present and may help differentiate FHH from primary HPT. This is important as these patients if not diagnosed may be subjected to unnecessary parathyroidectomy. Calcium tubular resorption is high in FHH, and hypercalcemia will persist post total parathyroidectomy (16).

Thyroid

There is a high degree of preponderance of harboring thyroid tumors (both benign and malignant) among those afflicted by various genetically inherited syndromes. Evaluation of syndromic thyroid nodules aims at ruling out malignancy. Thyroid cancers may derive their origin from follicular cells (~90–95%) and parafollicular cells (C cells) (~5%). Approximately 5% of follicular cell-derived thyroid tumors have a familial disease, which may be 25% in MTC. These familial thyroid syndromes can be classified as familial non-MTC (FNMTC) and familial MTC (FMTC). Under the context of this chapter, we will be focusing on FNMTC syndromes that are further subclassified into two subgroups (17–19):

a. Familial syndromes characterized by a predominance of on-MTC (NMTC) tumors
b. Familial syndromes characterized by a predominance of non-thyroidal tumors

Familial syndromes characterized by a predominance of non-MTC (NMTC) tumors

FNMTC is diagnosed when three or more family members have NMTC tumors and other known syndromes have been excluded. FNMTC is a well-defined clinical entity and represents approximately one-tenth of all follicular cell-derived thyroid carcinomas. Multifocal papillary thyroid cancers (PTC), usually of classical subtype, occurring in FNMTC are usually classic variant PTCs. In these patients, higher rate of multifocality or the presence of multiple benign nodules has been noticed. Frequent locoregional recurrence is reported, thereby decreasing disease-free survival. This entity is further subclassified in the following subgroups (1, 21):

a. **Pure familial PTC with or without oxyphilia:** Multicentric PTC associated with or without oxyphilia characterizes it. Familial PTC with oxyphilia and FNMTC without oxyphilia have been mapped to chromosome 19p13 and 19p13.31, respectively.
b. **Familial PTC with papillary renal cell carcinoma:** This syndrome mapped to Ch 1q21 has no special features, and it presents with classical PTC. It may also manifest as benign thyroid nodules and papillary type of renal cell neoplasm (20).
c. **Familial PTC with multinodular goiter:** Patients usually present with multinodular goiter, but some patients develop PTC. The genetic defect is located on Ch 14q.

Familial syndromes characterized by a predominance of non-thyroidal tumors

There are multiple syndromes that manifest with a predominance of non-thyroidal tumors. Common ones are described below:

a. Familial adenomatous polyposis (FAP)

A germline mutation in the APC gene located on chromosome 5q21 manifests by hundreds to thousands of adenomas throughout the gastrointestinal tract characterizes familial adenomatous polyposis (FAP). It is inherited as a dominant trait. The major clinical consequence of FAP is the occurrence of colorectal carcinoma, but there are certain extra-colonic manifestations as well, which include polyps in the upper GI tract, hepatoblastomas, congenital hamartoma (hypertrophy) of the retinal pigmented epithelium (CHRPE), desmoid tumors, hamartomas, osteomas, thyroid tumors, and epidermal cysts (1, 21, 22). FAP-associated thyroid carcinomas are mostly multifocal and bilateral. Inactivation of the APC tumor suppressor gene has also been seen in FAP-related thyroid tumors. PTC is seen in 10–12% of patients. FAP patients have higher risk of acquiring PTC in their lifetime than other sporadic PTC patients. Cribriform-morular variant (CMV) of PTC was first described with FAP-associated thyroid carcinoma, which is unusual in sporadic PTC (1, 21). Patients with CMV-PTC should further be evaluated for FAP and tested for APC gene mutation as well.

b. PTEN (Phosphatase and TENsin homolog deleted on chromosome 10) hamartoma tumor syndrome (PHTS)

PTEN hamartoma tumor syndrome (PHTS) caused by germline inactivating mutations of the PTEN tumor suppressor gene (10q22-23) is an entity, which includes many syndromes – Cowden syndrome (CS), Bannayan–Riley–Ruvalcaba syndrome (BRRS), Proteus syndrome, and Proteus-like syndrome (23).

Almost two-thirds of individuals with such mutations develop multiple benign as well as malignant neoplasms. CS commonly features with malignancies in thyroid and breast. PHTS is associated with a wide spectrum of thyroid pathologies affecting follicular cells ranging from benign entities such as nodular goiter, adenomatous goiter, and follicular adenoma to pathological ones, which include follicular thyroid carcinoma (FTC) and, occasionally, papillary thyroid carcinoma (PTC) (1, 21). Adenomatous goiter also commonly known as multiple adenomatous nodules (MAN) is classically present in these syndromes, moreover in younger patients. MANs are bilateral, multicentric well-circumscribed nodules, which are yellow-tan on cross section.

Both CS and BRRS are characterized by the presence of FTC. Besides FTC, CS is also associated with multinodular goiter, adenomatous nodules, and follicular adenomas. Though MTC is never seen in this syndrome, anecdotal case reports of C-cell hyperplasia (CCH) are there in the literature (24–26).

c. Pendred syndrome

It is the most common hereditary syndrome associated with bilateral sensory neural deafness and causes early hearing loss in children. Cochlear hypoplasia is an important feature. The syndrome is named after physician Vaughan Pendred. Inherited in autosomal recessive fashion is caused by a gene called SLC26A4 (formerly known as the PDS gene) mapped on chromosome 7q21. Pendrin, the protein encoded by the PDS gene, acts as sodium-independent chloride/iodine transporter in cell membrane. In thyrocytes, pendrin is located in apical membrane and is responsible for iodine transport. Organification step of thyroid hormone synthesis gets impaired upon mutation and thus results in possible hypothyroidism and goiter.

d. Werner syndrome (WS)

First described by Otto Werner in 1904, Werner syndrome (WS/progeria of adults) is a rare autosomal recessive genetic disorder characterized by clinical features suggestive of quickened and premature aging caused due to the mutation in the WRN gene (8p11-12). Patients begin to manifest an aged appearance in the early third decade characterized by a 'pinched' facial appearance, skin atrophy, loss of subcutaneous fat along with graying and loss of hair. Early-onset bilateral cataract is also seen. Those affected commonly develop type 2 diabetes mellitus, hypogonadism, osteoporosis, atherosclerosis, and malignancies (2–60-fold risk) (27). Follicular thyroid cancers followed by malignant melanoma, meningioma, soft tissue sarcomas, primary bone tumors, and leukemia/myelodysplasia are the common malignancies that are associated with WS. Patients with WS usually succumb to cancers or cardiac causes.

Adrenal cortex

Adrenocortical lesions associated with various familial syndromes can be neoplastic or non-neoplastic. Benign adenomas are the most common neoplastic tumors. Adrenocortical carcinomas are rare. Depending on the presence of active hormonal secretions from tumor, they may result in specific syndromes. Nonfunctional lesions may be picked up incidentally or after metastasis.

Characteristic adrenal pathological lesions observed are adrenal cortical adenoma (ACA), adrenal cortical carcinoma (ACC), and nodular hyperplasia (NH) (22).

a. **Beckwith–Wiedemann syndrome (BWS):** BWS results from genetic or epigenetic defects of genomic imprinting on Ch 11p15.5. Patients have multisystem involvement and develop abdominal wall defects, hemihypertrophy, enlarged tongue, abdominal organomegaly, and an increased risk of embryonal neoplasms in childhood. Hepatoblastoma, multifocal Wilms tumor or nephroblastomatosis, and adrenocortical carcinoma are the prominent malignancies that occur in BWS.

b. **Li–Fraumeni syndrome (LFS):** LFS is amongst the most common and aggressive cancer predisposition syndromes arising out of germline mutation in TP53 tumor suppressor gene. Autosomal inherited LFS predisposes the individual to develop various cancers in infancy and early adulthood. Soft tissue sarcoma (STS), osteosarcoma, premenopausal breast cancer, brain tumors, and ACC are commonly associated with LFS and have been designated core cancers. Osteosarcoma (30%) closely followed by ACC (27%), brain tumors (25%), and STS (23%) are the commonest ones in children, whereas breast cancer accounts for four-fifths of all LFS-associated cancers in women (28). Screening for TP53 germline mutation has been advocated in neonatal period in families with documented mutations so that screening may be commenced within the first few months.

c. **MEN 1:** It will be described in detail in a separate chapter on MEN syndrome.

d. **McCune–Albright syndrome (MAS):** Somatic activating mutations in GNAS (Guanine Nucleotide binding protein, Alpha Stimulating activity polypeptide) at 20q13.3 causes MAS. MAS has been characterized by triad of poly/monostotic fibrous dysplasia, café-au-lait spots, and hyperfunctioning endocrinopathies. Acromegaly has been documented in 20% of patients. Precocious puberty and hyperthyroidism are commonly observed. Cushing's syndrome though rare but may happen (29).

e. **Carney complex (CNC):** It has already been described.

f. **Neurofibromatosis 1 (NF1):** Autosomal dominant NF1 affecting 1 out of 2600–3000 was first described by Friedrich von Recklinghausen in 1882. A documented family history is seen only in half of the cases. Germline mutation in the NF1 tumor suppressor gene, mapped on chromosome 17q11.2, results in this syndrome. Neurofibromin, 220 kDa cytoplasmic protein coded by NF1 gene, is a negative regulator of the Ras proto-oncogene. These individuals have a tendency to develop various neoplasms with a propensity of glioma of the optic pathway, glioblastoma, malignant peripheral nerve sheath tumor, gastrointestinal stromal tumor, breast cancer, leukemia, and rhabdomyosarcoma. Endocrine neoplasms like pheochromocytoma, duodenal carcinoid tumor, and ACC have been associated with NF1 (30).

g. **Familial adenomatous polyposis (FAP):** FAP, which has been described earlier, has been commonly associated with adrenal neoplasms. Functions of nonfunctional adenomas arise more frequently in FAP than general population. Aggressive ACC has also been seen in those harboring APC gene mutations.

h. **Hereditary nonpolyposis colorectal cancer (HNPCC): Lynch syndrome (LS):** LS is a familial cancer syndrome having an estimated lifetime risk of colorectal cancers of 80% along with increased incidence of extra-colonic neoplasms of uterus, GI tract, hepatobiliary and urinary tract. LS is inherited in autosomal dominant fashion caused by pathogenic germline mutations in one of the several DNA mismatch repair (MMR) genes (MLH1, MSH2, MSH6, or PMS2). Association of ACC continues to be controversial as it has been seen only rarely in individuals documented with LS (31).

i. **Congenital adrenal hyperplasia (CAH):** It is monogenic autosomal recessive disorders manifested by impaired adrenal steroid hormone synthesis. Various enzymatic deficiencies have been described with 21-hydroxylase deficiency (21OHD) being the commonest (90%). In affected patients, glucocorticoid insufficiency leads to increased ACTH, which further results in adrenal hyperplasia. Long-standing ACTH hypersecretion commonly leads to bilateral adrenal hyperplasia. Tumoral formation is frequent in a hyperplastic adrenal cortex. The high prevalence of 45–82% of these adrenal tumors detected by CT or MRI has been reported in patients with CAH. In CAH cases, adrenal myelolipomas are frequently seen bilaterally. In treatment-resistant cases and tumors progressing despite glucocorticoid treatment, if there are noticeable intra-tumoral heterogeneity, hemorrhage, or other suspicious features, adrenalectomy in CAH is recommended (32, 33).

Adrenal pheochromocytoma and paraganglia

The adrenal medulla and the paraganglia are one of the most studied elements for familial endocrine disorders. Approximately two-thirds to three-fourth of tumors are sporadic and up to one-third to one-fourth of paragangliomas are genetically inherited.

a. **MEN 2 syndrome:** Multiple endocrine neoplasia type 2 (MEN 2), also known as Sipple syndrome, is characterized by the occurrence of three primary types of tumors: MTC, parathyroid tumors, and pheochromocytoma. MEN 2 syndrome is caused due to germline mutations in RET (rearranged during transfection) proto-oncogene mapped at chromosomal location 10q11. Extra-adrenal paragangliomas are rare.

b. **Von Hippel–Lindau (VHL):** Von Hippel–Lindau (VHL) disease results from a heterozygous germline mutation in VHL gene on chromosome 3p25. It is a tumor predisposition syndrome characterized by various neoplasms like central nervous system, retinal hemangioblastomas, clear cell renal cell carcinoma, pheochromocytoma (PC), pancreatic neuroendocrine tumors, endolymphatic sac tumor, epididymal and broad ligament cystadenoma, as well as visceral (renal and pancreatic) cysts. VHL is basically of two types depending on molecular genetics – VHL type 1 arising from truncating variants or exon deletions in the VHL gene confer a low risk of pheochromocytoma. In contrast, VHL type 2 is associated with missense variants that have a high incidence of PC. These patients are at risk of developing bilateral adrenal tumors.

c. **Neurofibromatosis type 1 (NF1):** NF1 patient presenting with the classical triad of headache, sweating, and palpitation should be evaluated for PC as 20–50% of NF1 patients with hypertension, compared to 0.1% of all hypertensive individuals, have secondary hypertension due to pheochromocytoma. However, pheochromocytoma occurs only in 0.1–5.7% of all patients with documented NF1, and the mean age at the diagnosis of pheochromocytoma in patients with NF1 is 42 years (34).

d. **Familial paraglioma syndromes (FPGL):** These are a group of AD disorders (PGL 1–5) arising from the mutation of various subunits of succinate dehydrogenase (SDHx) gene. SDH, located in the mitochondrial membrane, takes part in the mitochondrial respiratory chain and Krebs cycle. The individuals are predisposed to develop PGLs, pheochromocytomas (PCs), renal cell cancers, gastrointestinal stromal tumors, and, rarely, pituitary adenomas. SDH inactivation results in the accumulation of succinate and the increased production of reactive oxygen species, and these have been said to contribute to the buildup of hypoxia-inducible factors within the cell (35). Three different mutations (SDHD, SDHC, and SDHB) are associated with FPGL (PGL 1, PGL 3, and PGL 4, respectively) (1, 36). Other non-SDHx genes associated with hereditary paraganglioma include the MAX gene that co-regulates cellular proliferation and TMEM127 encoding a transmembrane protein that is a negative regulator of mTOR (37–39). PGL 1 (SDHD) and PGL 2 syndromes (SDHAF2) are characterized by a high incidence of multifocal tumors and for parent-of-origin inheritance. Disease usually manifests in subjects inheriting the defective allele from the paternal side. Malignant PGL or PC characterizes PGL 4 syndrome (SDHB). Low-penetrance PGL 3 (SDHC) and PGL 5 syndromes (SDHA) are less common. Diagnosis of these FPGL is largely based on the assessment of multiple factors – comprehensive clinical history, elaborated family history, thorough clinical examination, biochemical workup imaging, and molecular genetic testing (40). Timely detection and prompt removal of tumors help prevent or minimize complications and improve outcomes.

Endocrine pancreas

Pancreatic endocrine tumors originate from the endocrine cells located in the islets and the epithelium of ducts and ductules. Endocrine pancreatic tumors occur as part of inherited familial syndromes, including MEN 1, VHL disease, and NF1. VHL and NF1 here are described below.

a. **Pancreatic endocrine tumors in Von Hippel–Lindau (VHL) syndrome:** VHL is characterized by the occurrence of pancreatic cysts and tumors. Approximately three-fourths of VHL patients develop simple pancreatic cysts that are usually benign and asymptomatic. Symptomatic cysts merit surgical treatment. Approximately 20% of patients with VHL disease develop pancreatic neuroendocrine tumors (NET) (PNET) and approximately 50% of these tumors develop in the head region of pancreas. PNETs in VHL are nonfunctioning so they remain asymptomatic. Almost 50% of VHL-associated PNETs develop metastatic disease. Metastatic potential is higher for primary tumor greater than 3 cm in size or those harboring an exon 3 mutation (41).

b. **Pancreatic endocrine tumors in neurofibromatosis type 1 (NF1):** NETs are reported in about 1% of NF1 with most of them located in the periampullary region. Somatostatinoma (40%) is the most common subtype of NF1-associated PNET. Radiological imaging like endoscopic ultrasound or endoscopy and measurement of 5-hydroxyindolectic acid and chromogranin help clinch the diagnosis. Carcinoid tumors have been reported in about 1% of individuals with NF1 once gain commonly in the periampullary region, presenting with jaundice and nonspecific abdominal pain. Well-differentiated ampullary carcinoids usually >2 cm merit a pancreaticoduodenectomy (42).

South Asian perspective

There is no reported difference in incidence, clinical presentation, diagnosis and management of various Non MEN syndromes.

Conclusion

Non MEN syndromes are rare and require a high degree of clinical suspicion followed by targeted investigations so that early diagnosis and treatment can improve the outcome.

References

1. Nose V, Paner GP, Greenson JK, et al. Diagnostic Pathology: Familial Cancer Syndromes. 1st ed. Manitoba (CA): Amirys Publishing, Inc; 2014.
2. Carney JA. Familial multiple endocrine neoplasia: The first 100 years. Am J Surg Pathol. 2005;29(2):254–274.
3. Kamilaris CDC, Faucz FR, Voutetakis A, Stratakis CA. Carney complex. Exp Clin Endocrinol Diabetes. 2019;127(2–03):156–164.
4. Correa R, Salpea P, Stratakis CA. Carney complex: An update. Eur J Endocrinol. 2015;173(4):M85–M97.
5. Lonser RR, Mehta GU, Kindzelski BA, et al. Surgical management of carney complex-associated pituitary pathology. Neurosurgery. 2017;80:780–786.
6. Stratakis CA, Courcoutsakis NA, Abati A, et al. Thyroid gland abnormalities in patients with the syndrome of spotty skin pigmentation, myxomas, endocrine overactivity, and schwannomas (carney complex). J Clin Endocrinol Metab. 1997;82:2037–2043.
7. Carney JA, Lyssikatos C, Seethala RR, et al. The spectrum of thyroid gland pathology in carney complex: The importance of follicular carcinoma. Am J Surg Pathol. 2018;42:587–594.
8. Mateus C, Palangie A, Franck N, et al. Heterogeneity of skin manifestations in patients with Carney complex. J Am Acad Dermatol. 2008;59:801–810.
9. Gill AJ, Clarkson A, Gimm O, Keil J, Dralle H, Howell VM, et al. Loss of nuclear expression of parafibromin distinguishes parathyroid carcinomas and hyperparathyroidism-jaw tumor (HPT-JT) syndrome-related adenomas from sporadic parathyroid adenomas and hyperplasias. Am J Surg Pathol. 2006;30(9):1140–1149.
10. Cetani F, Ambrogini E, Viacava P, et al. Should parafibromin staining replace HRTP2 gene analysis as an additional tool for histologic diagnosis of parathyroid carcinoma? Eur J Endocrinol. 2007;156(5):547–554.
11. Jackson MA, Rich TA, Hu MI, Perrier ND, Waguespack SG. CDC73-related disorders. In: Pagon RA, Adam MP, Ardinger HH, Wallace SE, Amemiya A, Bean LJH, et al., eds. GeneReviews (R). Seattle (WA); 1993.
12. Simonds WF, James-Newton LA, Agarwal SK, et al. Familial isolated hyperparathyroidism: Clinical and genetic characteristics of 36 kindreds. Medicine (Baltimore). 2002;81(1):1–26.
13. Cetani F, Pardi E, Ambrogini E, et al. Genetic analyses in familial isolated hyperparathyroidism: Implication for clinical assessment and surgical management. Clin Endocrinol (Oxf). 2006;64(2):146–152.
14. Pollak MR, Chou YH, Marx SJ, et al. Familial hypocalciuric hypercalcemia and neonatal severe hyperparathyroidism. Effects of mutant gene dosage on phenotype. J Clin Invest. 1994;93(3):1108–1112.
15. Hannan FM, Nesbit MA, Zhang C, et al. Identification of 70 calcium-sensing receptor mutations in hyper- and hypo-calcaemic patients: Evidence for clustering of extracellular domain mutations at calcium-binding sites. Hum Mol Genet. 2012 Jun;21:2768–2778.
16. Marx SJ, Attie MF, Levine MA, et al: The hypocalciuric or benign variant of familial hypercalcemia: Clinical and biochemical features in fifteen kindreds. Medicine (Baltimore). 1981;60:397–412.
17. Dotto J, Nose V. Familial thyroid carcinoma: A diagnostic algorithm. Adv Anat Pathol. 2008;15(6):332–349.
18. Nose V. Thyroid cancer of follicular cell origin in inherited tumor syndromes. Adv Anat Pathol. 2010;17(6):428–436.
19. Nose V. Familial follicular cell tumors: Classification and morphological characteristics. Endocr Pathol. 2010;21(4):219–226.
20. Malchoff CD, Sarfarazi M, Tendler B, et al. Papillary thyroid carcinoma associated with papillary renal neoplasia: Genetic linkage analysis of a distinct heritable tumor syndrome. J Clin Endocrinol Metab. 2000;85(5):1758–1764.
21. Nose´ V, Erickson LA, Tischler AS, et al. Diagnostic Pathology: Endocrine. 1st ed. Salt Lake City (UT): Amirsys; 2012.
22. Sadow PM, Hartford NM, Nosé V. Familial endocrine syndromes. Surg Pathol Clin. 2014;7(4):577–598.
23. Jelsig AM, Qvist N, Brusgaard K, et al. Hamartomatous polyposis syndromes: A review. Orphanet J Rare Dis. 2014;9(1):101.
24. Laury AR, Bongiovanni M, Tille JC, et al. Thyroid pathology in PTEN-hamartoma tumor syndrome: Characteristic findings of a distinct entity. Thyroid. 2011;21(2):135–144.
25. Nose V. Familial non-medullary thyroid carcinoma: An update. Endocr Pathol. 2008;19(4):226–240.
26. Zambrano E, Holm I, Glickman J, et al. Abnormal distribution and hyperplasia of thyroid C-cells in PTEN-associated tumor syndromes. Endocr Pathol. 2004;15(1):55–64.
27. Ishikawa Y, Sugano H, Matsumoto T, et al. Unusual features of thyroid carcinomas in Japanese patients with Werner syndrome and possible genotype-phenotype relations to cell type and race. Cancer. 1999;85(6):1345–1352.
28. Bougeard G, Renau Petel M, Flaman JM, Charbonnier C, Fermey P, et al. Revisiting Li-Fraumeni syndrome from TP53 mutation carriers. J Clin Oncol. 2015;33:2345–2352.
29. Salenave S, Boyce AM, Collins MT, Chanson P. Acromegaly and McCune-Albright syndrome. J Clin Endocrinol Metab. 2014;99(6):1955–1969.
30. Hirbe AC, Gutmann DH. Neurofibromatosis type 1: A multidisciplinary approach to care. Lancet Neurol. 2014;13(8):834–843.
31. Raymond VM, Everett JN, Furtado LV, et al. Adrenocortical carcinoma is a lynch syndrome-associated cancer. J Clin Oncol. 2013;31:3012–3018.
32. Piskinpasa H, Ciftci Dogansen S, Kusku Cabuk F, et al. Bilateral adrenal and testicular mass in a patient with congenital adrenal hyperplasia. Acta Endocrinol (Buchar). 2019;5(1):113–117.

33. Speiser PW, Arlt W, Auchus RJ, et al. Congenital adrenal hyperplasia due to steroid 21-hydroxylase deficiency: An endocrine society clinical practice guideline. J Clin Endocrinol Metab. 2018;103(11):4043–4088.
34. Walther MM, Herring J, Enquist E, Keiser HR, Linehan WM. Von Recklinghausen's disease and pheochromocytomas. J Urol. 1999;162:1582–1586.
35. Selak MA, Armour SM, MacKenzie ED, et al. Succinate links TCA cycle dysfunction to oncogenesis by inhibiting HIF-α prolyl hydroxylase. Cancer Cell. 2005;7:77–85.
36. Van Nederveen FH, Gaal J, Favier J, et al. An immunohistochemical procedure to detect patients with paraganglioma and pheochromocytoma with germline SDHB, SDHC, or SDHD gene mutations: A retrospective and prospective analysis. Lancet Oncol. 2009;10(8):764–771.
37. Rednam SP, Erez A, Druker H, et al. Von Hippel-Lindau and hereditary pheochromocytoma/paraganglioma syndromes: Clinical features, genetics, and surveillance recommendations in childhood. Clin Cancer Res. 2017;23(12):e68–e75.
38. Comino-Mendez I, Gracia-Aznarez FJ, Schiavi F, et al. Exome sequencing identifies MAX mutations as a cause of hereditary pheochromocytoma. Nat Genet. 2011;43:663–667.
39. Qin Y, Yao L, King EE, et al. Germline mutations in TMEM127 confer susceptibility to pheochromocytoma. Nat Genet. 2010;42:229–233.
40. Benn DE, Robinson BG, Clifton-Bligh RJ. 15 years of paraganglioma: Clinical manifestations of paraganglioma syndromes types 1-5. Endocr Relat Cancer. 2015;22(4):T91–T103.
41. Blansfield JA, Choyke L, Morita SY, et al. Clinical, genetic and radiographic analysis of 108 patients with von Hippel-Lindau disease (VHL) manifested by pancreatic neuroendocrine neoplasms (PNETs). Surgery. 2007;142(6):814–818, discussion 818.e1–818.e2.
42. Relles D, Baek J, Witkiewicz A, Yeo CJ. Periampullary and duodenal neoplasms in neurofibromatosis type 1: Two cases and an updated 20-year review of the literature yielding 76 cases. J Gastrointest Surg. 2010;14:1052–1061.

64

ENDOCRINE EMERGENCIES

VNSSVAMS Mahalakshmi D, Sabaretnam Mayilvaganan, Kul Ranjan Singh and Anand Kumar Mishra

Introduction

Endocrine emergencies, though rare in the general population, comprise important and often encountered entities mostly as complications following surgery and as acute manifestations of a chronic disease process from an endocrine surgeon perspective. Adrenal crisis, myxoedema coma, hypocalcemia with tetany, diabetes is dreaded complications following B/L adrenalectomy, total thyroidectomy, subtotal/total parathyroidectomy, subtotal/total pancreatectomy and constitute emergency visits. Pheochromocytoma crisis, thyrotoxic crisis, hypercalcemic crisis, hypoglycemia, carcinoid crisis may present as manifestations of underlying pheochromocytoma/paraganglioma, Graves' disease, primary hyperparathyroidism (PHPT), insulinoma, neuroendocrine tumors, respectively, necessitating emergency resuscitation with increased risk of mortality and surgery as definitive management of operable cases. Since it is difficult to elaborate on every endocrine emergency, we enlisted them in Table 64.1 and described a few of them in detail.

Hypercalcemic crisis

Hypercalcemic crisis is commonly encountered emergency in hospital setting. However, there is no consensus regarding its diagnostic criteria. Currently, calcium levels >14 mg/dl with symptoms that disappear with lowering of calcium levels is diagnosed as hypercalcemia (1). Incidence of hypercalcemia-induced hypercalcemic crisis (HIHC) ranges in the literature from 1.6% to 6% (2, 3). Hypercalcemic crisis in parathyroid diseases is likely to be because of a carcinoma (3, 4). Patients usually present with fatigue, pancreatitis or altered mental status. The seriousness of clinical manifestations in hypercalcemia differentiates a crisis form noncrisis hypercalcemia (4, 5). In a patient with mild hypercalcemia, hypercalcemic crisis may be precipitated by excessive mobilization or medications like Vit D, diuretics, lithium and calcium-containing antacids (6, 7).

Histopathological specimens of crisis patients is often characterized by a microcystic pattern which is not seen in noncrisis patient leading to an inference that stored parathormone in the vacuoles is released during a partial/total degeneration of the lesion at the time of crisis. Based on this, it's probable that a phase of partial or complete remission may set based on the residual functioning parathyroid tissue. Though rare, PHPT can undergo spontaneous resolution after HIHC (8, 9).

Conventionally, emergency parathyroidectomy has been advocated no later than 72 hours. It has a mortality rate approaching 14% (10, 11). These patients are at risk of cardiac arrhythmias and anesthesia related risks. This along with improvements in pharmacological agents, an emergency surgery is no longer warranted in all patients. Either ways, immediate and adequate hydration along with measures to reduce calcium levels with frequent calcium monitoring should be started.

Hypoglycemia

Classical Whipple's triad that is used to diagnose pancreatic insulinoma is composed of

a. Hypoglycemic symptoms
b. Measured glucose <55 mg/dl
c. Symptom resolution on normalization of glucose levels

There are multiple causes of adult-onset hypoglycemia (Table 64.1) (12). Insulinoma is the most frequently encountered cause of hypoglycemia in endocrine surgery practice. Other causes include infection, trauma, organ failure, hormonal insufficiencies (cortisol, epinephrine and glucagon), medications, various gastric/pancreatic procedures, non-islet cell tumors, antibodies to insulin or insulin receptors, non-insulinoma pancreatogenous hypoglycemia (NIPHS).

Hypoglycemia is characterized by autonomic or neuroglycogenic symptoms (13, 14).

Prolongation of QT interval in ECG is accompanied with episodes of nocturnal hypoglycemia (15, 16). Fatal arrhythmia set off by hypoglycemia in Type 1 DM may cause sudden death during "dead in bed syndrome" (13–17). Traditional nondiabetic hypoglycemia is classified into postabsorptive (fasting) and postprandial (reactive) hypoglycemia. This classification is controversial (18).

Tumor-induced hypoglycemia

Several mechanisms may explain this entity of tumor-induced hypoglycemia. The most common cause, though rare, is insulinoma secreting insulin. Non-islet cell tumor hypoglycemia (NICTH) is also a well-recognized etiology (19). These tumors release insulin-like growth factor 2 (IGF2), high-molecular-weight precursor (big IGF2) etc. Various sarcomas, adrenal cortical carcinoma, pheochromocytomas, hepatocellular carcinomas and gastric cancers may present with hypoglycemia as a neoplastic manifestation (20–28).

Management

Patients with mild-to-moderate symptoms of hypoglycemia can be managed by immediate intake of readily available glucose-rich fluids or food items. An amount of 20 g of glucose would result in symptom alleviation in 15–20 minutes (29). However, this response is usually transient for less than 2 hours in insulin-induced hypoglycemia (30). IV infusion may be required in those unable to take oral glucose. Glucagon (1 mg) can be administered by SC or IM route. This lifesaving drug can cause nausea and vomiting (30).

Insulinomas

Frequent carbohydrate meals along with diazoxide or somatostatin analogues can control symptoms in more than half the patients (31, 32). The only curative treatment is surgery. The surgical procedure would depend on the location of lesion (33).

TABLE 64.1: Endocrine Emergencies

Thyroid gland	Thyroid storm
	Sight – Threatening Graves' ophthalmopathy
	Hyperthyroidism in pregnancy
	Amiodarone-induced thyrotoxicosis
	Severe thyrotoxicosis in the elderly
	Neonatal hyperthyroidism
	Myxedema and coma (severe hypothyroidism)
	Thyroid abscess
	Hashimoto's encephalopathy
	Thyroxine poisoning
	Thyrotoxic periodic paralysis
	CHF, cardiomyopathy in hyperthyroidism
	Sudden hemorrhage into thyroid nodule with respiratory distress
	Anaplastic carcinoma or lymphoma with stridor
	Post-thyroidectomy stridor
	Post-thyroidectomy hypocalcemia
	Post-thyroidectomy hemorrhage
	Post-thyroidectomy bilateral RLN paralysis
Pituitary gland	Pituitary apoplexy, Sheehan's syndrome, diabetes insipidus
Glucose and lipids	Diabetic ketoacidosis
	Hyperglycemia hyperosmolar states
	Emergencies in childhood diabetes
	Hypertriglyceridemic pancreatitis
Mineral disorders	Hypercalcemia
	Hypocalcemia
	Hungry bone syndrome
	Osteoporosis/Vertebral compression fractures
	Kidney stone emergencies
Adrenal gland	Florid Cushing's syndrome
	Adrenal insufficiency
	Pheochromocytoma and paraganglioma emergencies
	Endocrine hypertension
	Congenital adrenal hyperplasia
Neuro endocrine tumors	Carcinoid crisis

TABLE 64.2: Definition of AC by Allolio et al. in a Patient Who is Likely to Develop AC

Major impairment of general health of the patient with at least two of the following signs/symptoms:	Hypotension with [systolic blood pressure (BP) <100 mmHg]
	Nausea and vomiting
	Severe fatigue experienced
	Fever
	Somnolence
	Hyponatremia or hyperkalemia
	Hypoglycemia
Administration of parenteral glucocorticoid (hydrocortisone) results in improvement.	

after best postoperative care, 8.3 AC per 100 patient-years and 0.5 AC-related deaths per 100 patient-years was noted (41–44). Acute AC after bilateral adrenalectomy has been reported in 36.3% ($n = 8/22$) patients by Prajapati et al. from a tertiary referral center from India (45). Of these, single episode occurred in 22.7% patients ($n = 5/22$), whereas 13.6% patients ($n = 3/22$) experienced two or more episodes. In a study from South India of 33 patients, 6 patients (21.4%) experienced at least one AC and were defined by the need for IV glucocorticoid administration (46). In a multicenter consortium-based study, bilateral adrenalectomy for pheochromocytoma resulted in an AC in 18% of patients and 4% of cortical sparing adrenalectomies (47).

Definition and grading of AC

AC is a life-threatening disorder characterized by either low production or action of all steroid hormones (glucocorticoids, mineralocorticoids, adrenal androgens). This condition is classified as primary (diseases affecting the adrenal cortex), secondary (diseases affecting the anterior pituitary gland) or tertiary (diseases affecting the hypothalamus). Diagnosis is biochemical and confirmed by inappropriately low cortisol secretion. Adrenal crisis is defined in a case by Allolio et al. (Table 64.2) (48). Table 64.3 shows the grades the severity of insufficiency.

Several events have been identified that precipitate an AC. Gastroenteritis is the most common cause. Strenuous activities, emotional stress and accidents can trigger a crisis (49–55). Not increasing steroid dose after accidents and perioperative period should be avoided as these are commonly avoidable situations (54–56). Many patients cease to stop steroid replacement and land in AC. AC can be misdiagnosed in pregnancy as hyperemesis gravidarum, and on the other hand, hyperemesis can elicit an AC (57–59).

Pathophysiology

The pathophysiology is not clearly understood. Glucocorticoids influence the stress response by permissive, suppressive, stimulatory and preparative actions. The absence of suppressive action of steroids results in increased TNF α secretion, sensitivity and TNF α-induced glucocorticoid resistance. The lack of supportive action of steroids on adrenergic receptors results in shock (60–63). This is worsened by volume depletion due to lack of

TABLE 64.3: Grade of Adrenal Insufficiency

Grade 1: patient can be managed in outpatient setting
Grade 2: patient needing routine hospital care
Grade 3: patient needing intensive care support
Grade 4: Death attributable to adrenal crisis

Compared to benign insulinomas, which are more common, malignant insulinomas may express somatostatin receptor subtype 2 that can be a therapeutic target for long-acting somatostatin analogues and peptide radionuclide receptor therapy (34–36). Almost half of MEN 1-associated insulinomas are metastatic and malignant insulinomas generally do not respond well to fluorouracil-, doxorubicin- and streptozocin-based regimes (37, 38). Sirolimus and everolimus may stabilize growth and control hypoglycemia (38–40).

Adrenal crisis

Adrenal crisis/insufficiency (AC) is a life-threatening emergency that requires prompt administration of steroids and fluid replacement.

Epidemiology: The incidence of AC ranges between three and six events per 100 patient-years amongst patients of Addison's disease and pituitary dysfunction. This is lower than that after bilateral adrenalectomy 9.3 per 100 patient-years (1–3). Even

mineralocorticoid action along with vomiting and diarrhea (64, 65). Volume depletion is worsened by vomiting and diarrhea.

Clinical features include severe weakness, hypotension, syncope, abdominal tenderness, nausea and vomiting, fever, hyperpigmentation (primary adrenal insufficiency), with laboratory findings of hypercalcemia, hypoglycemia, hyponatremia and hyperkalemia.

Treatment during AC

We should maintain a patent airway and take care of breathing. Samples should be obtained electrolytes, glucose, cortisol, ACTH, bicarbonate and parameters as clinically indicated. Prompt parenteral administration of hydrocortisone in a dose of 100 mg for adults and 50–100 mg/m^2 for children is carried out followed by 200 mg/day (50–100 mg/m^2/day for children divided q6h or via continuous IV therapy for 24–48 hours), and this is tapered to 100 mg/day the next day. If the drug is not available, we can use prednisolone, and dexamethasone is the least preferred. Rapid fluid resuscitation with normal saline or 5% glucose in isotonic saline is necessary, which is guided by volume status and urine output. Mineralocorticoid replacement is not required if the hydrocortisone dose exceeds 50 mg/24 hours. We should treat any infection if present.

Treatment after patient stabilization

Saline infusion is continued and meticulous search for possible life-threatening infections precipitating an adrenal crisis is made and treated. A short synacthen test is performed to confirm the diagnosis. Glucocorticoids are tapered over 3–4 days and equivalent oral maintenance dose started 20 mg on waking and 10 mg at 18:00 hours.

Mineralocorticoid replacement with fludrocortisone (0.1 mg by mouth daily) is done when saline infusion has been stopped.

Dose adjustments

In case of fever 38°C– the dose is doubled until recovery; usual standard dose is resumed after 1–2 days of fever subsiding. The dose is tripled if temp >39°C. Parenteral glucocorticoids should be started in severe gastroenteritis with vomiting or diarrhea.

Patient education is most important in preventing mortality and various prevention strategies include patient education, sick day rules with the administration of stress dose steroids, steroid alerts, steroid emergency pack, etc. Periodical follow-up is essential.

Pheochromocytoma crisis

Pheochromocytoma and paraganglioma (PPGL) crisis is defined as an acute severe manifestation of a catecholamine-induced hemodynamic instability causing end-organ damage or dysfunction (66, 67). It can be divided into types A and B.

Type A represents a limited form of crisis with hemodynamic instability and end-organ dysfunction or damage of one or more organs. It has a mortality of 6%.

Type B crisis a more severe form presenting with sustained hypotension and multiorgan damage of two or more systems and 28% succumb to it (68).

Type A can progress to type B if not managed promptly and adequately.

Catecholamines act primarily on α-adrenergic receptors, causing severe arterial vasoconstriction leading to hypertension and relatively reduced intravascular volume. This results in reduction of end-organ perfusion and failure (69).

Pheochromocytoma crisis can be precipitated by many factors that appear trivial. Some of these triggering factors are normal physiological conditions like advanced pregnancy and peripartum period. Infarction of hemorrhage into tumor or any physical stimulus to the tumor can switch on the cascade. Any surgery or anesthesia without alpha blockade and certain medications like metoclopramide, dopamine antagonists may be responsible for a crisis.

The manifestations are systemic and any major organ dysfunction can occur, most of which are potentially life-threatening. Table 64.4 lists out the various manifestations of PPGL crisis.

TABLE 64.4: Lists of the Various Manifestations of PPGL Crisis

Cardiac	Takotsubo or inverted takotsubo cardiomyopathy, MI, arrhythmias, shock
Respiratory	Pulmonary edema, ARDS, hemoptysis
Neurological	Encephalopathy, stroke, encephalopathy
Kidney	Acute kidney injury
Liver	Acute liver injury
Gastrointestinal	Ileus, ischemia, intestinal perforation
Vascular	Thrombosis, adrenal hemorrhage
Musculoskeletal	Rhabdomyolysis
Metabolic	Lactis acidosis, hypo/hyperglycemia

Management

Pheochromocytoma is usually diagnosed by raised plasma or urine catecholamines. However, cardiogenic shock or hypertensive crisis can also result in catecholamines release, and these patients occasionally receive adrenaline or nor adrenaline infusion. Hence, catecholamines levels during a crisis cannot be diagnostic. In such a scenario, imaging alone will be informative (70).

In case of intraoperative hypertensive crisis in any surgery with or without identifiable mass, a working diagnosis of PPGL crisis should be made and treatment started immediately. Phentolamine, nitroprusside and magnesium sulfate, esmolol, nicardipine and common drugs employed to manage a crisis patient.

Surgery

The ideal timing of surgery for patient having had PPGL crisis remains controversial. Early surgery was thought to be a good strategy as it would remove the source of crisis. However, this was seen to have a higher morbidity or mortality (71, 72). The prognosis is bad, and there is lot of hemodynamic instability during emergency surgery.

Some have argued that these patients with hypertensive crisis may need emergency resection, even without preoperative α-blockade (67, 72–76). However, some showed that optimization of patient with alpha blockade before surgery in a crisis patient improves outcome (77,78,79). In a series by Scholten et al. which reported pheochromocytoma crisis in 18% of 137 patients, all patients were stabilized, and 96% of crisis patients were operated upon laparoscopically with less than 12% conversion after adequate α-blockade prior to surgery. So we advocate stabilization during crisis with planned elective surgery after adequate alpha blockade.

TABLE 64.5: Wartofsky Point Scale for Diagnosis of Thyroid Storm.

		Maximum Score
Fever	5 points per 1°F above 99°F	30
CNS dysfunction	Mild; agitation	10
	Moderate, extreme lethargy, delirium, psychosis	20
	Severe; seizure or coma	30
Heart rate	99–109	5
	100–119	10
	120–129	15
	130–139	20
	>140	25
Atrial fibrillation		10
Cardiac failure	Mild – pedal edema	5
	Moderate – basal crackles	10
	Severe – pulmonary edema	15
Gastrointestinal dysfunction	Moderate	10
	Severe – unexplained jaundice	20
Presence of precipitation factors		10

Note: A total score > 45 is highly suggestive of thyroid storm, score of 25–44 affirms the diagnosis and a score less than 25 rules out the diagnosis (80–85).

Thyroid storm

Though rarely encountered now, thyroid storm is a potentially life-threatening. It's a multisystem disorder having a high mortality rate of 8–25% (80–83). Devised in 1993, Burch-Wartofsky Point Scale (BWPS) is used to arrive at a diagnosis of thyroid storm. A total score >45 is highly suggestive of thyroid storm, score of 25–44 affirms the diagnosis and a score less than 25 rules out the diagnosis (Table 64.5) (80–85). The Japanese Thyroid Association (JTA) scoring system is another diagnostic criterion, but it's less commonly used. Free T3 and T4 should be elevated to make a diagnosis of thyroid storm.

Precipitating factors

Several drugs like iodinated contrast agents, amiodarone and sorafenib can precipitate thyroid storms. Surgery in hyperthyroid patients or any intercurrent infection, illness or sudden stoppage of anti-thyroid medications can also trigger this dreaded clinical situation (80–86).

Management

Management is essentially symptomatic. High-dose corticosteroids (hydrocortisone of dexamethasone) should be administered to avoid relative adrenal insufficiency due to hypermetabolic state in thyroid storm. Corticosteroids inhibit thyroid hormone synthesis and also interfere with its peripheral conversion of T4 to T3. Therapeutic plasma exchange may be considered if thyrotoxic symptoms do not improve within 24–48 hours of initial intensive treatment. Precipitating factor should be treated. Thyroid storm has a high mortality and recurrence should be avoided (80–85).

South Asian perspective

In the developing world, the medical care facilities available may vary and the experience of the doctor in primary setting also varies. In this situation, patient education plays and vital role in the treatment of patients with endocrine emergencies. We should provide emergencies contact numbers and also educate the patient using various tools. Even then there is morbidity and mortality associated with these endocrine emergencies, due to multiple factors. Patient and caregiver education can make a lot of difference in management of these patients. Some of these emergencies require tertiary referral care after initial resuscitation.

Conclusion

Endocrine emergencies are rare and need expertise for appropriate outcomes. Early detection and institution of treatment shall avoid morbidity. Other endocrine emergencies have been covered in appropriate chapters.

References

1. Edelson GW, Kleerekoper M. Hypercalcaemic crisis. Med Clin North Am. 1995;79(1):79–92.
2. Wang C, Guyton SW. Hyper parathyroid crisis. Ann Surg. 1979;190:782–790.
3. Sarfati E, Desportes L, Gossot D, Dubost C. Acute primary hyperparathyroidism: Experience of 59 cases. Br J Surg. 1989;76:979–981.
4. Singh DN, Gupta SK, Kumari N, Krishnani N, Chand G, Mishra A, et al. Primary hyperparathyroidism presenting as hypercalcemic crisis: Twenty-year experience. Indian J Endocrinol Metab. 2015;19(1):100–105.
5. Wei CH, Harari A. Parathyroid carcinoma: Update and guidelines for management. Curr Treat Options Oncol. 2012;13:11–23.
6. Ahmad S, Kuraganti G, Steenkamp D. Hypercalcemic crisis: A clinical review. Am J Med. 2015;128:239–245.
7. Kelly TR, Zarconi J. Primary hyperparathyroidism: Hyperparathyroid crisis. Am J Surg. 1981;142:539–542.
8. Starker LF, Björklund P, Theoharis C, Long WD 3rd, Carling T, Udelsman R. Clinical and histopathological characteristics of hyperparathyroidism-induced hypercalcemic crisis. World J Surg. 2011;35:331–335.
9. Wootten CT, Orzeck EA. Spontaneous remission of primary hyperparathyroidism: A case report and meta-analysis of the literature. Head Neck. 2006;28:81–88.
10. Kovacs KA, Gay JD. Remission of primary hyperparathyroidism due to spontaneous infarction of a parathyroid adenoma. Case report and review of the literature. Medicine (Baltimore). 1998;77:398–402.
11. Baker JR, Wray HL. Early management of hypercalcemic crisis: Case report and literature review. Mil Med. 1982;147:756–760.
12. Lew JI, Solorzano CC, Irvin GL. Long-term results of parathyroidectomy for hypercalcemic crisis. Arch Surg. 2006 Jul;141(7):696–699.
13. Cryer PE, Axelrod L, Grossman AB, Heller SR, Montori VM, Seaquist ER, et al. Evaluation and management of adult hypoglycemic disorders: An Endocrine Society Clinical Practice Guideline. J Clin Endocrinol Metab. 2009;94:709–728.
14. Lee SP, Yeoh L, Harris ND, Davies CM, Robinson RT, Leathard A, et al. Influence of autonomic neuropathy on QTc interval lengthening during hypoglycemia in type 1 diabetes. Diabetes. 2004;53:1535–1542.
15. Robinson RT, Harris ND, Ireland RH, Lee S, Newman C, Heller SR. Mechanisms of abnormal cardiac repolarization during insulin-induced hypoglycemia. Diabetes. 2003;52:1469–1474.
16. Murphy NP, Ford-Adams ME, Ong KK, Harris ND, Keane SM, Davies C, et al. Prolonged cardiac repolarisation during spontaneous nocturnal hypoglycaemia in children and adolescents with type 1 diabetes. Diabetologia. 2004;47:1940–1947.
17. Tattersall RB, Gill GV. Unexplained deaths of type 1 diabetic patients. Diabet Med. 1991;8:49–58.
18. Service FJ. Hypoglycemic disorders. N Engl J Med. 1995;332:1144–1152.
19. de Groot JW, Rikhof B, van Doorn J, Bilo HJ, Alleman MA, Honkoop AH, van der Graaf WT. Non-islet cell tumour-induced hypoglycaemia: A review of the literature including two new cases. Endocr Relat Cancer. 2007;14:979–993.
20. Gorden P, Hendricks CM, Kahn CR, Megyesi K, Roth J. Hypoglycemia associated with non-islet-cell tumor and insulin-like growth factors. N Engl J Med. 1981;305:1452–1455.
21. Daughaday WH, Kapadia M. Significance of abnormal serum binding of insulin-like growth factor II in the development of hypoglycemia in patients with non-islet-cell tumors. PNAS. 1989;86:6778–6782.
22. Shapiro ET, Bell GI, Polonsky KS, Rubenstein AH, Kew MC, Tager HS. Tumor hypoglycemia: Relationship to high molecular weight insulin-like growth factor-II. J Clin Invest. 1990;85:1672–1679.
23. O'Loughlin A, Waldron-Lynch F, Cronin KC, Dinneen S, Lee J, Griffin D, et al. When a nephrectomy cures hypoglycaemia. BMJ Case Rep. 2009;2009:bcr022009161.
24. Ishikura K, Takamura T, Takeshita Y, Nakagawa A, Imaizumi N, Misu H, et al. Cushing's syndrome and big IGF-II associated hypoglycemia in a patient with adrenocortical carcinoma. BMJ Case Rep. 2010;2010:bcr07.2009.2100.
25. Barra WF, Castro G, Hoff AO, Siqueira SA, Hoff PM. Symptomatic hypoglycemia related to inappropriately high IGF-II serum levels in a patient with desmoplastic small round cell tumor. Case Rep Med. 2010;2010:684045.
26. Macfarlane DP, Leese GP. Hypoglycaemia, phaeochromocytoma and features of acromegaly: A unifying diagnosis? QJM. 2011;104:983–986.

27. Ndzengue A, Deribe Z, Rafal RB, Mora M, Desgrottes S, Schmidt F, Becher R, Wright AM, Guillaume J, Jaffe EA. Non-islet cell tumor hypoglycemia associated with uterine leiomyomata. Endocr Pract. 2011;17:e109–e112.
28. Chan JK, Cheuk W, Ho LC, Wen JM. Recurrent meningeal hemangiopericytoma with multiple metastasis and hypoglycemia: A case report. Case Rep Med. 2012;2012:628756.
29. Sugiyama T, Nakanishi M, Hoshimoto K, Uebanso T, Inoue K, Endo H, et al. Severely fluctuating blood glucose levels associated with a somatostatin-producing ovarian neuroendocrine tumor. J Clin Endocrinol Metab. 2012;97:3845–3850.
30. Wiethop BV, Cryer PE. Alanine and terbutaline in treatment of hypoglycemia in IDDM. Diabetes Care. 1993;16:1131–1136.
31. Abboud B, Boujaoude J. Occult sporadic insulinoma: Localization and surgical strategy. World J Gastroenterol. 2008;14657–14665. doi:10.3748/wjg.14.657.
32. Tucker ON, Crotty PL, Conlon KC. The management of insulinoma. Br J Surg. 2006;93:264–275.
33. Levy MJ, Thompson GB, Topazian MD, Callstrom MR, Grant CS, Vella A. US-guided ethanol ablation of insulinomas: A new treatment option. Gastrointest Endosc. 2012;75:200–206.
34. Wild D, Christ E, Caplin ME, Kurzawinski TR, Forrer F, Brandle M, et al. Glucagon-like peptide-1 versus somatostatin receptor targeting reveals 2 distinct forms of malignant insulinomas. J Nucl Med. 2011;521073–521078. doi:10.2967/jnumed.110.085142.
35. Chandra P, Yarandi SS, Khazai N, Jacobs S, Umpierrez GE. Management of intractable hypoglycemia with Yttirum-90 radioembolization in a patient with malignant insulinoma. Am J Med Sci. 2010;340:414–417.
36. Fischbach J, Gut P, Matysiak-Grzes M, Klimowicz A, Gryczynska M, Wasko R, Ruchala M. Combined octreotide and peptide receptor radionuclide therapy ((90)Y-DOTA-TATE) in case of malignant insulinoma. Neuro Endocrinol Lett. 2012;33:273–278.
37. Akerstrom G, Hellman P. Surgery on neuroendocrine tumours. Best Pract Res Clin Endocrinol Metab. 2007;2187–2109. doi:10.1016/j.beem.2006.12.004.
38. Kulke MH, Bergsland EK, Yao JC. Glycemic control in patients with insulinoma treated with everolimus. New Engl J Med. 2009;360:195–197.
39. Bourcier ME, Sherrod A, DiGuardo M, Vinik AI. Successful control of intractable hypoglycemia using rapamycin in an 86-year-old man with a pancreatic insulin-secreting islet cell tumor and metastases. J Clin Endocrinol Metab. 2009;94:3157–3162.
40. Thomas N, Brooke A, Besser G. Long-term maintenance of normoglycaemia using everolimus in a patient with disseminated insulinoma and severe hypoglycaemia. Clin Endocrinol. 2013;78:799–800.
41. Arlt W, Allolio B. Adrenal insufficiency. Lancet. 2003;361:1881–1893.
42. Hahner S, Loeffler M, Bleicken B, Drechsler C, Milovanovic D, Fassnacht M, et al. Epidemiology of adrenal crisis in chronic adrenal insufficiency: The need for new prevention strategies. Eur J Endocrinol. 2010;162:597–602.
43. Ritzel K, Beuschlein F, Mickisch A, Osswald A, Schneider HJ, Schopohl J, Reincke M, Outcome of bilateral adrenalectomy in Cushing's syndrome: A systematic review. J Clin Endocrinol Metab. 2013;98(10):3939–3948.
44. Hahner S, Spinnler C, Fassnacht M, Burger-Stritt S, Lang K, Milovanovic D, et al. High incidence of adrenal crisis in educated patients with chronic adrenal insufficiency: A prospective study. J Clin Endocrinol Metab. 2015;100(2):407Y416.
45. Prajapati OP, Verma AK, Mishra A, Agarwal G, Agarwal A, Mishra SK. Bilateral adrenalectomy for Cushing's syndrome: Pros and cons. Indian J Endocrinol Metab. 2015;19(6):834–840.
46. Nagendra L, Bhavani N, Pavithran PV, Kumar GP, Menon UV, Menon AS, et al. Outcomes of bilateral adrenalectomy in Cushing's syndrome. Indian J Endocrinol Metab. 2019;23(2):193–197.
47. Neumann HPH, Tsoy U, Bancos I, Amodru V, Walz MK, Tirosh A, et al. Comparison of pheochromocytoma-specific morbidity and mortality among adults with bilateral pheochromocytomas undergoing total adrenalectomy vs cortical-sparing adrenalectomy. JAMA Netw Open. 2019;2(8):e198898.
48. Allolio B. Extensive expertise in endocrinology. Adrenal crisis. Eur J Endocrinol. 2015;172: R115–R124.
49. Bornstein SR, Allolio B, Arlt W, Barthel A, Don-Wauchope A, Hammer GD. et al. Diagnosis and treatment of primary adrenal insufficiency: An endocrine society clinical practice guideline. J Clin Endocrinol Metab. 2016;101:364–389.
50. Arlt W; Society for Endocrinology Clinical Committee. Society for endocrinology endocrine emergency guidance: Emergency management of acute adrenal insufficiency (adrenal crisis) in adult patients. Endocr Connect. 2016;5: G1–G3.
51. Hahner S, Loeffler M, Bleicken B, Drechsler C, Milovanovic D, Fassnacht M, et al. Epidemiology of adrenal crisis in chronic adrenal insufficiency: The need for new prevention strategies. Eur J Endocrinol. 2010;162:597–602.
52. Reisch N, Willige M, Kohn D, Schwarz HP, Allolio B, Reincke M, et al. Frequency and causes of adrenal crises over lifetime in patients with 21-hydroxylase deficiency. Eur J Endocrinol. 2012;167:35–42.
53. Ritzel K, Beuschlein F, Mickisch A, Osswald A, Schneider HJ, Schopohl J, Reincke M. Clinical review: Outcome of bilateral adrenalectomy in Cushing's syndrome: A systematic review. J Clin Endocrinol Metab. 2013;98:3939–3948.
54. White K, Arlt W. Adrenal crisis in treated Addison's disease: A predictable but undermanaged event. Eur J Endocrinol. 2010;162:115–120.
55. Omori K, Nomura K, Shimizu S, Omori N, Takano K. Risk factors for adrenal crisis in patients with adrenal insufficiency. Endocr J. 2003;50:745–752.
56. Hahner S, Spinnler C, Fassnacht M, Burger-Stritt S, Lang K, Milovanovic D, et al. High incidence of adrenal crisis in educated patients with chronic adrenal insufficiency: a prospective study. J Clin Endocrinol Metab. 2015 Feb;100(2):407–416.
57. Lewandowski K, Hincz P, Grzesiak M, Cajdler-Łuba A, Salata I, Wilczyński J, Lewiński A. New onset Addison's disease presenting as prolonged hyperemesis in early pregnancy. Ginekol Pol. 2010 Jul;81(7):537–540.
58. George LD, Selvaraju R, Reddy K, Stout TV, Premawardhana LD. Vomiting and hyponatraemia in pregnancy. Br J Obstet Gynaecol. 2000;107:808–809.
59. Gradden C, Lawrence D, Doyle PM, Welch CR. Uses of error: Addison's disease in pregnancy. Lancet. 2011;357:1197.
60. Kalsner S. Mechanism of hydrocortisone potentiation of responses to epinephrine and norepinephrine in rabbit aorta. Circ Res. 1969;24:383–395.
61. Besse JC, Bass AD. Potentiation by hydrocortisone of responses to catecholamines in vascular smooth muscle. J Pharmacol Exp Ther. 1966;154:224–238.
62. Allolio B, Ehses W, Steffen HM, Muller R. Reduced lymphocyte beta 2-adrenoceptor density and impaired diastolic left ventricular function in patients with glucocorticoid deficiency. Clin Endocrinol. 1994;40:769–775.
63. Sapolsky RM, Romero LM, Munck AU. How do glucocorticoids influence stress responses? Integrating permissive, suppressive, stimulatory, and preparative actions. Endocr Rev. 2000;21:55–89.
64. Arlt W, Allolio B. Adrenal insufficiency. Lancet. 2003;361:1881–1893.
65. Bancos I, Hahner S, Tomlinson J, Arlt W. Diagnosis and management of adrenal insufficiency. Lancet Diabetes Endocrinol. 2014 Mar;3(3):216–226.
66. Newell K, Prinz RA, Braithwaite S, Brooks M. Pheochromocytoma crisis. Am J Hypertens. 1998;1:189S–191S.
67. Newell KA, Prinz RA, Pickleman J, Braithwaite S, Brooks M, Karson TH, Glisson S. Pheochromocytoma multisystem crisis. A surgical emergency. Arch Surg. 1988;123:956–959.
68. Whitelaw BC, Prague JK, Mustafa OG, Schulte K-M, Hopkins PA, Gilbert JA, et al. Phaeochromocytoma [corrected] crisis. Clin Endocrinol (Oxf). 2014;80: 13–22.
69. Lenders JW, Duh QF, Eisenhofer G, Gimenez-Roqueplo AP, Grebe SK, Murad MH, et al. Pheochromocytoma and paraganglioma: An endocrine society clinical practice guideline. J Clin Endocrinol Metab. 2014;99:1915–1942.
70. Amar L, Eisenhofer G. Diagnosing phaeochromocytoma/paraganglioma in a patient presenting with critical illness: Biochemistry versus imaging. Clin Endocrinol (Oxf). 2015;83(3):298–302.
71. Brown H, Goldberg PA, Selter JG, Cabin HS, Marieb NJ, Udelsman R, Setaro JF. Hemorrhagic pheochromocytoma associated with systemic corticosteroid therapy and presenting as myocardial infarction with severe hypertension. J Clin Endocrinol Metab. 2005;90:563–569.
72. Bos JC, Toorians AW, van Mourik JC, van Schijndel RJ. Emergency resection of an extraadrenal phaeochromocytoma: Wrong or right? A case report and a review of literature. Neth J Med. 2003;61:258–265.
73. Solorzano CC. Pheocromocytoma presenting with multiple organ failure. Am Surg. 2008;74:1119–1121.
74. Uchida N, Ishiguro K, Suda T, Nishimura M. Pheochromocytoma multisystem crisis successfully treated by emergency surgery: Report of a case. Surg Today. 2010;40:990–996.
75. Freier DT, Eckhauser FE, Harrison TS. Pheochromocytoma. A persistently problematic and still potentially lethal disease. Arch Surg. 1980;115:388–391.
76. Salinas CL, Gómez Beltrán OD, Sánchez-Hidalgo JM, Bru RC, Padillo FJ, Rufián S. Emergency adrenalectomy due to acute heart failure secondary to complicated pheochromocytoma: A case report. World J Surg Oncol. 2011;9:49.
77. Kolhe N, Stoves J, Richardson D, Davison AM, Gilbey S. Hypertension due to phaeochromocytoma – An unusual cause of multiorgan failure. Nephrol Dial Transplant. 2001;16:2001–2004.
78. Imperato-McGinley J, Gautier T, Ehlers K, Zullo MA, Goldstein DS, Vaughan ED Jr. Reversibility of catecholamine-induced dilated cardiomyopathy in a child with a pheochromocytoma. N Engl J Med. 1987;316:793–797.
79. Scholten A, Cisco RM, Vriens MR, Cohen JK, Mitmaker EJ, Liu C, et al. Pheochromocytoma crisis is not a surgical emergency. J Clin Endocrinol Metab. 2013 Feb;98(2):581–91.
80. Chiha M, Samarasinghe S, Kabaker AS. Thyroid storm: An updated review. J Intensive Care Med. 2015 Mar;30(3):131–140.
81. Nayak B, Burman K. Thyrotoxicosis and thyroid storm. Endocrinol Metab Clin North Am. 2006 Dec;35(4):663–686, vii.
82. Spitzweg C, Reincke M, Gärtner R. Schilddrüsennotfälle: Thyreotoxische Krise und Myxödemkoma [Thyroid emergencies: Thyroid storm and myxedema coma]. Internist (Berl). 2017 Oct;58(10):1011–1019.
83. Akamizu T. Thyroid storm: A Japanese perspective. Thyroid. 2018 Jan;28(1):32–40.
84. Hampton J. Thyroid gland disorder emergencies: Thyroid storm and myxedema coma. AACN Adv Crit Care. 2013 Jul-Sep;24(3):325–332.
85. Schreiber ML. Thyroid storm. Medsurg Nurs. 2017 Mar;26(2):143–145.
86. Ylli D, Klubo-Gwieździnska J, Wartofsky L. Thyroid emergencies. Pol Arch Intern Med. 2019 Aug;129(7–8):526–534. Erratum in: Pol Arch Intern Med. 2019 Sep 30;129(9):653.

INDEX

Note: Locators in *italics* represent figures and **bold** indicate tables in the text.

A

ABBA, *see* Axillary-bilateral breast approach
Abdominal (adrenal NB) tumor, 384, *385*
AC, *see* Adrenal crisis/insufficiency
Accentuated thyrotoxicosis, 316
Accessory thyroid, 14
Acquired adrenocortical hyperplasia, 345
    ACTH dependent/pituitary dependent, 345
    ACTH independent/adrenal dependent, 345
ACTH, *see* Adrenocorticotropic hormone
ACTH-independent (macronodular/micronodular-nonpigmented) adrenal hyperplasia (AIMAH), 388
Active surveillance (AS)
    active surveillance protocol, 120
    decision-making, *118*, 118–119
    in pregnancy, 119–120
    thyroid-stimulating hormone suppression, 119
ACTs, *see* Adrenocortical tumors in children
Acute suppurative thyroiditis, 47
Acute thyroiditis, 47–48
Adenomatous colloid goiter, 24
Adjuvant therapy
    follow-up of thyroid cancer patients, 205–208
        CT and MRI scanning, 208
        diagnostic whole-body radioiodine scan, 208
        dynamic stratification and approach, 207, *207*
        early management after initial therapy, 205–206, *206*
        FDG PET/CT scanning, 208
        long-term management, 206–207
        neck ultrasonography, 208
        serum Tg and Tg Ab, 207–208
    practical aspects of radioiodine therapy, 205
    radioiodine refractory disease therapy, 208–209
    risk stratification, 204–205
    side effects of radioiodine therapy, 205
Adrenal abscess, 386
Adrenal cortex, 325–326
    17α-OH deficiency, 326
    11β-hydroxylase deficiency, 326
    21β-hydroxylase deficiency, 326
    3β-OH-HSD deficiency, 326
    cholesterol desmolase enzyme deficiency, 326
    non-men endocrine syndromes, 459–460
        Beckwith–Wiedemann syndrome, 459
        Carney complex, 460
        congenital adrenal hyperplasia, 460
        familial adenomatous polyposis, 460
        hereditary nonpolyposis colorectal cancer, 460
        Li–Fraumeni syndrome, 459–460
        McCune–Albright syndrome, 460
        MEN 1, 460
        neurofibromatosis 1, 460
    related diseases, 387–388
        AIMAH, 388
        Cushing syndrome, 387–388
        PPNAD, 388
        primary hyperaldosteronism, 387
    synthetic pathways of steroid hormones, 325, *326*
Adrenal crisis/insufficiency (AC), 464–465
    definition and grading, 464, **464**
    dose adjustments, 465
    grade of, **464**
    pathophysiology, 464–465
    treatment, 465
    treatment after patient stabilization, 465
Adrenal cysts, 386
Adrenal cytomegaly, 390
Adrenal gland
    anatomical relations, 322, *322*, *323*
    anatomy, 321–323
    development of various layers, 321, *322*
    embryological migration, 321, *321*
    physiology of
        adrenal cortex, 325–326
        adrenal medulla, 324
        aldosterone, 326–327
        glucocorticoids, 327–328
Adrenal hemorrhage, 385–386
Adrenal hyperplasia, 345
Adrenal incidentalomas, 334
Adrenal lesions
    acquired adrenocortical hyperplasia, 345
    adrenal hyperplasia, 345
    adrenal medulla, 347
    adrenal medullary hyperplasia, 345–346
    adrenocortical adenoma, 346
    adrenocortical carcinoma, 346, *347*
    congenital adrenal hyperplasia, 345
    congenital, developmental and infectious lesions, 345
    differential diagnosis, 346
    IHC and molecular, 348
    International Neuroblastoma Pathology Classification (INPC), 348, 349
    International Neuroblastoma Staging System (INSS), 349
    molecular and immunohistochemistry, 350
    molecular signatures, 346–347
    morphologic features, 347–348, 350
    myelolipoma, 346, *346*
    neuroblastoma, 347, *347*, *348*
    other adrenal neoplasms, 350
    pheochromocytoma, 349, *350*
    primary pigmented nodular adrenal cortical hyperplasia, 345
    spread and metastases, 348–349
    spread, metastases, treatment and prognosis, 350
    staging, 349
Adrenal masses
    biochemical evaluation of
        aldosterone-producing tumors, 332–333
        androgen and estrogen producing tumors, 333
        autonomous cortisol secretion, *330*
        catecholamine-producing tumors, 330–332
        cortisol-producing tumors, 329–330
        epidemiology, 329
        etiology, *329*
        hormonal evaluation, 329
        hyperaldosteronism, *332*
        medications affecting aldosterone renin ratio, **332**
        pheochromocytomas, *331*
    differential diagnosis, 385–386
        adrenal abscess, 386
        adrenal cysts, 386
        adrenal hemorrhage, 385–386
        extralobar pulmonary sequestrations, 386
    evaluation of, 384
        imaging evaluation of adrenal masses, 384–385, *386*
        laboratory investigation of adrenal masses, 384
        symptoms and sings of adrenal masses, 384
    imaging of, *see* Imaging of adrenal masses
    surgery for, 390–393
        anatomic basis of surgical approaches to adrenal, 390
        minimal invasive surgery, 390–393, *391*, *392*
        open technique, 390
Adrenal medulla, 324, 347
    catecholamine synthesis, 324, *325*
    degradation of catecholamines, 324
    mode of action of catecholamines, 324
    related masses, 386–387
        GN, 387
        GNB, 387
        NB, 386–387
        pheochromocytoma, 387
    role of arterial structure in adrenal, 324
    synthesis of epinephrine, 324
Adrenal medullary hyperplasia, 345–346
Adrenal myelolipoma
    clinical features, 379
    clinical management, 381–382
    differential diagnosis, 381
    imaging, 380–381
        computed tomography, *380*, 380–381
        magnetic resonance imaging, 381, *381*
        ultrasonography, 380
    myelolipoma and EMH, 378, *379*
    myelolipomas and associated endocrine disease, *379*, 379–380, *380*, **380**
    pathogenesis, 378
    pathology, 378–379
Adrenal pheochromocytoma and paraganglia
    FPGL, 460–461
    MEN 2 syndrome, 460
    neurofibromatosis type 1, 460
    non-men endocrine syndromes, 460–461
    Von Hippel–Lindau syndrome, 460
Adrenal pseudocyst, 338

Index

Adrenal-related surgical problems, 384, **384**
Adrenal surgery, history of, 320
Adrenal surgical diseases in children
  abdominal (adrenal NB) tumor, 384, *385*
  ACTs in children, 388–390
  adrenal cortex-related diseases, 387–388
  adrenal masses, 384, 385–386, 390–393
  adrenal medulla–related masses, 386–387
  adrenal-related surgical problems, 384, **384**
  Cushing Syndrome, 384, **385**
  rare adrenocortical problems, 390
  simple anatomy, 384
  South Asia perspective, 393–394
Adrenal vein sampling (AVS), 372
  corticotropin stimulation, 372
  importance of, 372–373
  interpretation, 372
Adrenocortical adenoma, 346
Adrenocortical carcinoma, 346, *347*
Adrenocortical oncocytomas (AOs), 390
Adrenocortical tumors (ACTs) in children, 388–390
  adrenocortical adenoma, 388
  adrenocortical carcinoma, 388–390, *389*, **390**
  staging, 390
  surgery, 392–393, *393*
    adjuvant therapy, 392–393
    minimally invasive surgery, 392
    radiotherapy, 393
    retroperitoneal lymph node dissection, 392
Adrenocorticotropic hormone (ACTH), 345
Adult-onset nesidioblastosis, 422
AFTN, *see* Autonomously functioning thyroid nodule
17α-hydroxylase (17α-OH) deficiency, 326
AIT, *see* Autoimmune thyroiditis
Aldosterone, 326–327
  compare action of aldosterone vs vasopressin, 326
  mechanism of action, 326–327
    physiological basis of primary hyperaldosteronism, 326–327
    secondary hyperaldosteronism with hypotension, 327
  regulation of, 326, **326**
Aldosterone-to-renin ratio (ARR)
  ARR screening tool, 369
  assays of renin and aldosterone and effects, 370
  medications and effects, 369–370
Alpha-receptor antagonists
  nonselective, irreversible, alpha-receptor antagonists, 397–398
  selective alpha 1–receptor antagonist drugs, 398
American Thyroid Association (ATA) management guideline, 155, **158**
Amiodarone-induced thyrotoxicosis (AIT), **68**
Ampulla of Vater, 412
Amyloid, 39
Anaplastic carcinoma, 157
Anaplastic thyroid carcinoma (ATC), 32
  antecedent thyroid disease, 137
  BRAF-V600E mutations, 99
  clinical features, 138
    multinodular goiter, 138, *140*
    signs, 138
    symptoms, 138
    thyroid enlargement, 138, *139*
  epidemiology, 137
  flowchart of management, 142, *143*
  genetics, 137–138
    somatic gene alterations, 138, **138**
  imaging, 140
  investigations, 140–141
    diagnosis, 138
    immunohistochemistry, 138, 140
  locoregional disease, 142
  metastatic disease, 142
  morphology and histology, 137
    macrophage infiltration, 137
  newer therapeutic agents, 146
  other measures, 142
  outcome of multimodality therapy, 142, **144–145**
  prognostic parameters, 146, **146**
  RAS mutations, 99
  resection margins/residual tumor definition, **143**
  risk factors, 137
  role of radiation therapy, 143, 146
  South Asian perspective, 147
  spread, 138
  staging, 141, **141**
  summary of management, 142, **142**
  systemic therapy, 146
  therapeutic agents and outcomes, 146, **146**
  TNM staging, 141, **141**
  treatment, 141–142
Anesthesia for thyroid and parathyroid surgery
  airway examination and evaluation, 315
  airway management for surgery, 316
  anesthetic management for parathyroid surgery, 318
  clinical examination of swelling, 315
  hematoma, 317
  hyperthyroidism, 316
  hypocalcemia, 318
  hypothyroidism, 317
  investigations, 315–316
  Myxedema coma, 317
  positioning of patient for surgery, 316
  postoperative management, 317
    nausea and vomiting, 317
    pain, 317
  recurrent laryngeal nerve injury, 318
  regional anesthesia for thyroid and parathyroid surgery, 318
  symptoms, signs and clinical presentation, 315
  thyroid storm, 316–317
  tracheomalacia, 318
Anesthetic management for pheochromocytoma
  anesthetic management, 399, **399**
  complications, 399–401
    alterations in blood glucose levels, 401
    arrhythmias, 401
    blood loss, 401
    intraoperative hemodynamic instability, 399–400, **400**
  drug therapy in pheochromocytoma, 397–398
    alpha-receptor antagonists, 397–398
    beta blockers, 398
    calcium channel blockers, 398
    tyrosine hydroxylase inhibitor, 398
  goals of anesthetic management, 396
  intraoperative management, 398–399
  postoperative concerns, 401
    adrenal insufficiency, 401
    hemodynamic instability, 401
    hypoglycemia, 401
    renal failure, 401
  preoperative assessment, 396–397
  preoperative drug therapy, 396, *397*
Anterior breast approach, 292
Anterior chest approach, 290
Antithyroid drugs (ATD), **65**, 66–67
  beta blockers, 66
  pregnancy and Graves' disease, 66–67
  radioactive iodine therapy, 66
  surgical ablation, 66
AOs, *see* Adrenocortical oncocytomas
APS, *see* Automatic periodic stimulation electrode
AS, *see* Active surveillance
ATA, *see* American Thyroid Association management guideline
ATC, *see* Anaplastic thyroid carcinoma
ATD, *see* Antithyroid drugs
Atypical adenomas, 305
Autoimmune thyroiditis (AIT)
  clinical presentation, 45–46
  diagnosis, 46
  painless subacute thyroiditis, 47
  pathophysiology, 43, 45
  postpartum thyroiditis, 46–47
  silent (painless) thyroiditis, 46
  treatment, 46
Automatic periodic stimulation (APS) electrode, 300
Autonomous cortisol secretion, 361
Autonomously functioning thyroid nodule (AFTN), 94–95
Autonomous thyroid adenoma, 94
AVS, *see* Adrenal vein sampling
Axillary approach (CO_2 insufflation), 290
Axillary-bilateral breast approach (ABBA), 292

B

BABA, *see* Bilateral axillo-breast approach
Basal metabolic rate, 7
Beckwith–Wiedemann syndrome (BWS), 459
2017 Bethesda System, 37, **37**
Bethesda System for Reporting Thyroid Cytopathology, **109**
The Bethesda System for Reporting Thyroid Cytopathology (TBSRTC), 36, **37**
Bilateral axillo-breast approach (BABA), 292, 294
Biochemical hypocalcemia, 184
BRAF mutations, 96
BWS, *see* Beckwith–Wiedemann syndrome

C

CAH, *see* Congenital adrenal hyperplasia
Carbohydrate metabolism, 7
Carcinoid syndrome, 445, 446
Carney complex (CNC), 457, 460
CAS, *see* Clinical Activity Score

Central compartment neck dissection (CND), 111, 198
Central hypothyroidism, 50
Central/secondary/hypothyrotropic hypothyroidism, 50
Chemotherapy (CT), 115, 137
Childhood thyroid cancers
    anaplastic carcinoma, 157
    ATA management guideline, **158**
    clinical presentation, *157*, 157–158
    differentiated thyroid cancers, 156
    epidemiology, 155
    genetics in follicular cell thyroid tumors, 157
    genetics in parafollicular cell thyroid tumors, 157
    histopathology and types, 156, *156*, **156**
    initial evaluation and surgical strategy based on FNAB, 158–159
    medullary thyroid carcinoma, 156–157
    molecular features, 157
    pathogenesis and risk factors, 155, **156**
        age and gender, 155
        autoimmune thyroiditis, 155
        genetic disorders and family history, 155
        radiation exposure, 155
    prognosis, 161
    radioactive iodine therapy and TSH suppression, 160–161
    surgical treatment, 159
        in differentiated thyroid carcinoma, 159–160
        in medullary thyroid carcinoma, 160
Chromaffin cells, 324
Chronic kidney disease-mineral bone disorder (CKD-MBD), 272
Chronic lymphocytic thyroiditis or chronic autoimmune thyroiditis, 23
CKD-MBD, *see* Chronic kidney disease-mineral bone disorder
Clinical Activity Scoring System, 62, **63**
CNC, *see* Carney complex
CND, *see* Central compartment neck dissection
Colloid goiter, management of, 93–94
Colloid nodules and cysts, 24, *24*
Compartment-oriented neck dissection, 199
Computed tomography (CT), 32, *33*
    adrenal myelolipoma, 380, 380–381
    follow-up of thyroid cancer patients, 208
    hyperaldosteronism, 371
    parathyroid carcinoma, 306
    recurrent primary hyperparathyroidism, 310
Congenital adrenal hyperplasia (CAH), 345, 460
Congenital adrenogenital syndrome, 345
Congenital hypothyroidism, 54–55
Conn's syndrome, 326–327, 387
Contrast-enhanced computed tomography (CT) (CECT), 17
Contrast-enhanced magnetic resonance imaging (MRI) (CEMRI), 17
Conventional or "front-door" technique, 284
Cowden syndrome, 449
Cretinism, 51
CT, *see* Computed tomography

Cushing's syndrome (CS), 360, 387–388
    adrenal tumor, 360
    Carney complex, 360
    causes of, **359**
    clinical symptoms, 361, **361**, 361–364
        cardiovascular, 363
        centripetal obesity, *361*
        dermatologic, 362–363
        excessive facial hairs, *363*
        hirsutism, *362*
        hyperpigmentation and petechial hemorrhage, *363*
        infection and immune function, 364
        metabolic, 363, *363*
        neuropsychological changes and cognition, 363–364
        ophthalmologic findings, 364
        reproductive, 361
        secondary sexual characteristics, *363*
        signs of adrenal androgen excess, 361–362
        violaceous striae, *362*
    complications, 366
    definition, 359
    diagnosis, 364, **365**, 366
        24-hour urinary cortisol excretion, 364
        late-night salivary cortisol, 364
        LDDST, 364
        mechanisms of control, 364
        pseudo CS, 364
    ectopic ACTH syndrome, 360
        tumors causing, **359**
    epidemiology, 359
    etiology, 359–360, 384, **385**
    flow chart, *367*
    genetic mutations and molecular mechanism, 360, **361**
    hypercortisolism, 364, **364**
    localization of disease, 366
    pathophysiology, 360
    pituitary adrenal axis, 360
    prognosis, 367
    treatment, **366**, 366–367

D

4D-CT, *see* Four-dimensional computed tomography
Differentiated thyroid carcinoma (DTC), 156, **200**
    additional treatment, 112–114
        follow-up, 113–114
        radioiodine, 112–113
        thyroxine, 112
    bad prognostic factors, **114**
    Bethesda System for Reporting Thyroid Cytopathology, **109**
    chemotherapy, 115
    classification, 104, *105*
    clinical presentation, 107, **107**, 108
    diagnostic evaluation, 107–108
        FNAC, 108
        imaging, 107–108
    follicular cell–derived thyroid cancer, 104, *104*
    follicular thyroid carcinoma, 109, 156
    follow-up plan, *113*
    incidence and mortality rates, 104

indications for radioactive iodine as adjuvant treatment, **112**
initial surgical treatment, 110–112
management plan, 110, *110*
papillary thyroid carcinoma, 156
pathogenesis, *106*
pathology, 109
prognostic factors, **113**
radio iodine refractory cancer, 114–115
risk factors, 104–105, 107, **109**, 113
South East Asia perspective, 115
staging, 109–110
surgical procedure, 111, 159–160
TNM classification, 110
types of thyroid cancer, 104, **105**
ultrasound features
    malignancy in lymph node, **108**
    malignancy in thyroid nodule, **108**
Dorsum of the legs or feet, *see* Pretibial myxedema
Drug-induced thyroiditis, 48, **48**
DTC, *see* Differentiated thyroid carcinoma
Dunhill operation, 170, *171*
Dynamic risk stratification, 113

E

Elastography, role of, 28, *28*
Elective central neck dissection, *see* Prophylactic central neck dissection
Embryological remnants (ER), 211–212
    pyramidal lobe and thyroglossal duct remnants, 212
    thyrothymic remnants/rests, 212, **212**
EMH, *see* Extramedullary hematopoiesis
Endemic goiter, 94; *see also* Goiters
    AFTN, 94–95
    biochemical evaluation, 93
    clinical evaluation, 90–91, *91*, *92*
    clinical presentations, 90, **91**
    cyto/histopathology, 93
    endemic regions of South Asia, *91*
    euthyroid multinodular and colloid goiter, management of, 93–94
    evaluation, 91
    historical aspects and etiology, 90
    imaging, 91–93
    Modified WHO Classification of Goiter, **91**
    occult/incidental carcinoma, 94
    thyroid cancer, 95
    total thyroidectomy specimen, *94*
    toxic goiters, 94
Endocrine emergencies, **464**
    adrenal crisis/insufficiency, 464–465
    hypercalcemic crisis, 463
    hypoglycemia, 463–464
    pheochromocytoma crisis, 465
    South Asian perspective, 465
    thyroid storm, 465
Endocrine pancreas
    in neurofibromatosis type 1, 461
    non-men endocrine syndromes, 461
    in Von Hippel–Lindau syndrome, 461
Endoscopic surgery, 290–293
    anterior breast approach, 292
    anterior chest approach, 290
    axillary approach (CO_2 insufflation), 290
    axillary-bilateral breast approach, 292

Index

bilateral axillo-breast approach, 292
cervical approach and MIVAT, 290
gasless trans-axillary approach, 290, 292
history of, *291*
postauricular and axillary approach, 292
sublingual transoral approach, 292
TOETVA, 292–293
Eosinophilic infiltrate, *see* Hashimoto thyroiditis
ER, *see* Embryological remnants
Euthyroid multinodular, management of, 93–94
Extent of surgery
    in micropapillary thyroid cancer, 200–202
        comparison of international guidelines, 202, **202**
        risk stratification of micro-PTC, 200–201
        surgery, 201–202
    thyroidectomy, 197–200
        argument against prophylactic central dissection, 200
        arguments in favor of performing prophylactic CND, 200
        choice of procedure, 198
        hemithyroidectomy and TT, comparison of, 197–198, **198**, **199**
        invasive thyroid cancer, 200
        LN dissection, 198–200
        surgery of metastases, 200, *201*
External beam radiation therapy (EBRT), 137
Extralobar pulmonary sequestrations, 386
Extramedullary hematopoiesis (EMH), 378, *379*

F

Familial adenomatous polyposis (FAP), 459, 460
Familial dysalbuminemic hyperthyroxinemia, 4
Familial hyperparathyroidism (FHPT)
    calcium-sensing receptor, 268–269
    and characteristics, **270**
    cyclin D1 oncogene and FIPH parathyroid neoplasia, 269
    familial hypocalciuric hypercalcemia, 267
    familial isolated hyperparathyroidism, 269, *269*
    hyperparathyroidism-jaw tumor syndrome, 266–267
    MEN 1, 265–266
    Menin, 266
    MEN type 4, 266
    MEN Type 2A, 266
    neonatal severe hyperparathyroidism, 267–268
    parafibromin/CDC73, 267
    parathyroid tumorigenesis, 269
    sporadic and hereditary PHPT, differences between, 265, **266**
Familial hypocalciuric hypercalcemia (FHH), 267, 458
Familial isolated hyperparathyroidism (FIHP), 269, *269*, 458
Familial paraganglioma syndromes (FPGL), 460–461
Familial syndromes
    NMTC tumors, 458
    non-thyroidal tumors, 459
        familial adenomatous polyposis, 459
        Pendred syndrome, 459

        PTEN, 459
        Werner syndrome, 459
"FANTOM PWD," 60, **61**
FAP, *see* Familial adenomatous polyposis
F cells, 415
FDCS, *see* Follicular dendritic cell sarcoma
[¹⁸F] fluorodeoxyglucose (FDG) PET/CT scanning, 204
FHH, *see* Familial hypocalciuric hypercalcemia
FHPT, *see* Familial hyperparathyroidism
FIHP, *see* Familial isolated hyperparathyroidism
Fine needle aspiration (FNA), 17
    recurrent primary hyperparathyroidism, 311
Fine-needle aspiration biopsy (FNAB), 158–159
Fine needle aspiration cytology (FNAC), 36–38, 108
    cytopathology reporting, 36–37
    indications in thyroid nodules, 36
    limitations and pitfalls, 37–38
    procedure and processing, 36
Flat-tip technique, 82
Flier's disease, 422
FNA, *see* Fine needle aspiration
FNAB, *see* Fine-needle aspiration biopsy
FNAC, *see* Fine needle aspiration cytology
Follicular cell thyroid tumors, 157
Follicular dendritic cell sarcoma (FDCS), 153
Follicular neoplasms, 28, *29*
Follicular thyroid carcinoma (FTC), 109, 156
    PAX8/PPARG gene fusion, 98
    PI3K-AKT signaling pathway, 97
    RASSF1-MST1-FOXO3 signaling pathway, 97–98
"Forme fruste," 411
Four-dimensional computed tomography (4D-CT), 256, *257*
FPGL, *see* Familial paraganglioma syndromes
FTC, *see* Follicular thyroid carcinoma
"Functioning NETs," 446

G

Ganglioneuroblastoma (GNB), 387
Ganglioneuroma (GN), 387
Gasless trans-axillary approach, 290, 292, 293
Gastrinoma, 424
Gastroenteropancreatic NET in children
    pancreatic endocrine tumors in children, 446–447
    persistent hyperinsulinemic hypoglycemia (PHH), 447–448
Gastrointestinal tract, carcinoid tumors of
    Asian perspective, **440**, 440–441
    Carcinoid syndrome, 439–440
    classification, 433
    clinical presentation, 435–436
    diagnosis and imaging, 436–437
        biochemical diagnosis, 436
        imaging, 436–437
    histology, 435, *435*
    molecular pathogenesis, 433–435
    NET, *see* Neuroendocrine tumor
    "open" and "closed" neuroendocrine cell, 433, **434**

    treatment, 437–439
        ablative therapies for NE liver metastases, 439
        cytoreductive surgery for metastasis – regional and distant, 438–439
        radionuclide therapy, 439
        surgery for primary site disease, 437–438
        systemic therapies, 439
        transarterial chemoembolization, 439
Genetic alterations in thyroid neoplasms
    molecular abnormalities in thyroid malignancies and significance, 40, **41**
    South Asia perspective, 40–41
Giant myelolipomas, 378
Glucocorticoids, 327–328
    hypocortisolism, 327–328
    metabolic actions of cortisol, 327
    physiological basis of Cushing's syndrome, 327
    regulation of cortisol secretion, 327
GN, *see* Ganglioneuroma
GNB, *see* Ganglioneuroblastoma
Goblet cell carcinoids, 435
Goetsch disease, *see* Autonomously functioning thyroid nodule
Goiters
    adenomatous colloid, 24
    colloid, 93–94
    endemic, *see* Endemic goiter
    multinodular, 138, *140*
    non-endemic, *see* Non-endemic goiters
    recurrent, *see* Recurrent goiter
    retrosternal, *see* Retrosternal goiters
    TMNG, *see* Toxic multinodular goiter
Granulomatous thyroiditis, 47
Graves' disease (GD)
    in children, 67
    toxic adenoma and toxic multinodular goiter, 67
    treatment, 66–67
        antithyroid drugs, **65**, 66–67
        non-thionamide drugs, **65**
        Technitium-99 scan, *63*, *64*

H

Hashimoto thyroiditis, 23, *23*, 43, 50
Head and neck squamous cell cancers (HNSCC), 190
Hematoma, 317
Hemithyroidectomy (HT), 170
Hereditary hyperparathyroidism-jaw tumor (HPT-JT) syndrome, 457–458
Hereditary nonpolyposis colorectal cancer (HNPCC), 460
HIFU, *see* High-intensity focused ultrasound
High-frequency ultrasound ablation, 82–83
High-frequency US ablation (HFUA), 80
High-intensity focused ultrasound (HIFU)
    effectiveness, 82
    South Asia perspective, 83
High-resolution ultrasound (US) (HRUS), 71, 80
"Hirata's disease," 422
Histology of thyroid gland, 2

Histopathological evaluation of thyroid, 38–40
  anaplastic carcinoma thyroid, 38, *38*
  application of immunohistochemistry, 39–40
  conventional papillary thyroid carcinoma, 38, *38*
  follicular carcinoma thyroid, 38, *38*
  medullary thyroid carcinoma, 38, *39*
  reporting of thyroid surgical pathology, 38–39
  WHO classification system, 39, **40**
HNPCC, *see* Hereditary nonpolyposis colorectal cancer
"Honey comb," 25
"Hormone of abundance," 415
HPT-JT, *see* Hereditary hyperparathyroidism-jaw tumor syndrome
HT, *see* Hemithyroidectomy
Hungry bone syndrome, 306
Hürthle cell carcinoma (HTC), 98, 104
  mitochondrial DNA aberrations, 98
11β-hydroxylase deficiency, 326
21β-hydroxylase deficiency, 326
3β-hydroxysteroid dehydrogenase (3β-OH-HSD) deficiency, 326
Hyperaldosteronism
  confirmatory testing, 370
  future perspectives, 374–375
    ablation, 375
    11C-metomidate PET–CT imaging, 374–375, *375*
  histology and genetics, 374
  primary aldosteronism
    AVS Procedure, **372**
    common and important cause of secondary hypertension, 369
    diagnosis and management, 370
    diagnostic algorithm, *371*
    pathophysiology, 369
    screening and diagnosis, 369–370
      ARR, *see* Aldosterone-to-renin ratio for primary aldosteronism with hypertension, 369
  South Asian, 375–376
  subtype testing, 370
    AVS, *see* Adrenal vein sampling
    CT, 371
    predictors of unilateral disease and aldosterone–potassium ratio, 370–371
  treatment, 373–374
    medication, 374
    PASO criteria, 373–374
    prediction of cure, 373
    surgery, 373
Hypercalcemic crisis, 463
Hypercortisolism, *see* Cushing's syndrome
Hyperparathyroidism (HPT), 240
  asymptomatic, 279, 283
  familial, *see* Familial hyperparathyroidism
  familial isolated, *see* Familial isolated hyperparathyroidism
  neonatal severe, *see* Neonatal severe hyperparathyroidism
  normocalcemic, *see* Normocalcemic hyperparathyroidism
  parathyroid gland, 222–223
  primary, *see* Primary hyperparathyroidism
  recurrent, 287

recurrent primary, *see* Recurrent primary hyperparathyroidism
renal, 226
secondary, *see* Secondary hyperparathyroidism
sporadic, **451**
tertiary, *see* Tertiary hyperparathyroidism
Hyperparathyroidism-jaw tumor syndrome, 266–267
  clinical spectrum, 266–267
  genetics, 267
Hyperthyroidism
  clinical examination, 60–63
  clinical features and complications, 60, **61**
  diagnosis, 63–64
  drug-induced thyroiditis, 68
  epidemiology, 58
  etiology and classification, 58
  Graves' disease
    in children, 67
    ophthalmopathy, **62**, *63*
    treatment, 66–67
  and intraoperative anesthetic management, 316
  medical management, 64–65
  other causes of thyrotoxicosis, 68
  pathogenesis, 58–60
    Graves' disease, 58–60
    toxic multinodular goiter and toxic adenoma, 60
  RAIT, 65
  South-Asian perspective, 68–69
  surgery, 66
  with thyroid carcinoma, 68
  thyroiditis, 67–68
  thyrotoxicosis, 58, *59*
  treatment, 64
  Wayne's index, 60, **61**, 62–63
Hypocalcemia, 318
Hypoglycemia, 463–464
  insulinomas, 463–464
  management, 463
  tumor-induced hypoglycemia, 463
Hypothalamic-pituitary-thyroid axis, 2, *3*
Hypothyroidism
  causes, 50–51, **51**
    central hypothyroidism, 50
    peripheral hypothyroidism, 51
    primary hypothyroidism, 50
    transient hypothyroidism, 50
  clinical features, 51, **52**
    Cretinism, 51
    Myxedema coma, 51
  diagnosis, 51, 53
  evaluation of suspected hypothyroidism, *52*
  and intraoperative anesthetic management, 317
  screening, 53
    congenital hypothyroidism, 54–55
    hypothyroidism in pregnancy, 54
    subclinical hypothyroidism, 54
  South Asian perspective, 55–56
  special consideration, 54–55
  treatment, 53–54
    monitoring response, 54

I

IAS, *see* Insulin autoimmune syndrome
IDD, *see* Iodine deficiency disorders
IHM, *see* Intraoperative hormone measurements
Imaging of adrenal masses
  acute hemorrhage, 335
  adenoma, 334, *335*
    atypical (lipid-poor adenomas), 334
    typical (lipid-rich adenomas), 334
  adrenal cortical hyperplasia, 340, *342*
  adrenal cyst, *339*
  adrenal hemangioma, 340
  adrenal hemorrhage, 335, *337*
  benign adrenal masses, 334
  calcified adrenal lesion, 338, *338*, 340
  chronic hemorrhage, 338
  histoplasmosis, 338, *338*
  ^{123}I-MIBG scintigraphy, 340
  malignant adrenal masses, 334
  malignant masses, 340–343
    adrenal cortical carcinoma, 340
    imaging pearls, 340
    lymphoma, 343
    metastasis, 343, *343–344*
    neuroblastoma, 343
    South Asian perspective in adrenal disorders, 343
  MRI, 338
  myelolipoma, 334–335, *336*
    clinicopathological patterns, 334
  pheochromocytomas, 340, *341*
  ^{123}I-MIBG scintigraphy, 340
Inflammatory diseases of thyroid
  acute thyroiditis, 47–48
  AIT, *see* Autoimmune thyroiditis
  drug-induced thyroiditis, 48, **48**
  miscellaneous forms of thyroiditis, 49
  Riedel's thyroiditis, 48
  South Asian perspective, 49
  viral thyroiditis (subacute thyroiditis), 47
Injury to EBSLN, 180
INPC, *see* International Neuroblastoma Pathology Classification
INSS, *see* International Neuroblastoma Staging System
Insulin autoimmune syndrome (IAS), 422
"Insuline," 410
Insulinoma
  biochemical diagnosis, 418–419
    48-hour supervised fast, 419
    protocol for 72-hour fast test, 418–419, **419**
  clinical approach, 417–418
    neurogenic symptoms, 418
    neuroglycopenic symptoms, 417–418
  complications, 421
  flowchart of management, *418*
  historical background, 417
  insulin autoimmune syndrome, 422
  localization of tumor, 419
    invasive imaging, 419
    noninvasive imaging, 419
  malignant insulinoma, 421–422
    adult-onset nesidioblastosis, 422
    management, 421–422
    nesidioblastosis, 421–422

Index

prognosis, 421
    treatment of liver metastases, 421
    treatment of primary, 421
pathophysiology, 417
preoperative preparation, 419–420
South Asia perspective, 422
sporadic *vs.* multiple endocrine neoplasia type 1 insulinoma, 417
surgical management, 420–421
    intraoperative hormone measurements, 420–421
    intraoperative ultrasound, 420, *421*
    laparoscopic resection of insulinoma, 420
    no tumor identified, 421
    open operative technique, 420
    selecting resection procedure, 420
Type B insulin resistance syndrome, 422
International Neuroblastoma Pathology Classification (INPC), 348, *349*
International Neuroblastoma Staging System (INSS), 349
Intraoperative adjuncts in thyroid and parathyroid surgery
    advantages of hemostatic devices, **298**
    anesthesia prerequisites, 298–300
    continuous neuromonitoring, 300
    equipment in neuromonitoring, 299, *299*
    hemostasis, 297
        bipolar energy sealing system, 297
        ultrasonic coagulation, 297
    IONM, *see* Intraoperative neuromonitoring
    IOPTH, *see* Intraoperative PTH
    loss of signals, 299, *299*
    minimize laryngeal nerve palsy, 297–298
    prevention of postoperative hypocalcemia, 300
        intraoperative detection of parathyroid gland, 300–301
        protocol for blood sampling, 301
    South Asia perspective, 303
Intraoperative hormone measurements (IHM), 420–421
Intraoperative neuromonitoring (IONM), 298
    advantages of, **298**
    in remote access thyroidectomy, 300
    set-up, *298*
Intraoperative PTH (IOPTH)
    assay, 312–313
    criteria for, 301
    immunochemiluminescent machine, *302*
    Miami criteria, *302*
    monitoring in parathyroid surgery, 301
    outcome after, 301–302
Intraoperative ultrasound (IOUS), 420, *421*
Investigations in thyroid diseases
    anaplastic thyroid carcinoma, 32
    2017 Bethesda System, 37, *37*
    colloid nodules and cysts, 24, *24*
    CT and MRI, role of, 32, *33*
    elastography, role of, 28, *28*
    FNAC, 36–38
    follicular neoplasms, 28, *29*
    genetic alterations in thyroid neoplasms, 40–41
    Hashimoto's thyroiditis, 23, *23*
    histopathological evaluation of thyroid, 38–40
    medullary carcinoma thyroid, 32
    metastasis to thyroid, 32
    papillary thyroid carcinoma, 28, *29*, 30, *30*
    papillary thyroid microcarcinoma, 31, *31*
    positron emission tomography scan, 32
    Southeast Asian perspective, 32–33
    spongiform nodules, 25, *25*
    thyroglossal cyst, 24, *24*
    thyroid lymphoma, 32
    TIRADS scoring, 25, **25**, *25*, **25**, *26*, *27*, 28
    ultrasound, *see* Ultrasound imaging
Iodine deficiency disorders (IDD), 90
IONM, *see* Intraoperative neuromonitoring
IOPTH, *see* Intraoperative PTH
IOUS, *see* Intraoperative ultrasound

J

Juvenile AIT, 43

L

Laboratory evaluation, 7–8
    assessment of thyroid function, tests, 7–8, **8**
    etiology of thyroid dysfunction, tests, 8
    radioiodine uptake studies, 8
    thyroid ultrasound, 8
Langerhans cell histiocytosis (LCH), 153
Laser thermal ablation (LTA), 82
    effectiveness, 82
    procedure, 82
LCH, *see* Langerhans cell histiocytosis
Levator glandulae thyroideae, 14
LFS, *see* Li–Fraumeni syndrome
Li–Fraumeni syndrome (LFS), 459–460
LN, *see* Lymph node dissection
Lobectomy, 170, *171*
LOS, *see* Loss of signals
Loss of signals (LOS), 299, *299*
Low-dose dexamethasone suppression tests (LDDST), 364
LTA, *see* Laser thermal ablation
Lymph node (LN) dissection
    prophylactic LN dissection, 199–200
    therapeutic LN dissection, 198–199
    in thyroid cancer, 198
Lymphocytic thyroiditis, 43

M

Macronodular cortical hyperplasia, 345
Magnetic resonance imaging (MRI), 32, *33*
    adrenal masses, 338
    adrenal myelolipoma, 381, *381*
    follow-up of thyroid cancer patients, 208
    investigations in thyroid diseases, 32, *33*
    recurrent primary hyperparathyroidism, 310
Malignant peripheral nerve sheath tumors (MPNSTs), 152
MAN, *see* Multiple adenomatous nodules
MAPK, *see* Mitogen-activated protein kinase signaling pathway
"Marine-Lenhart syndrome," 64
MAS, *see* McCune–Albright syndrome
McCune–Albright syndrome, 449
McCune–Albright syndrome (MAS), 460
MEC, *see* Mucoepidermoid carcinoma
Medullary thyroid carcinoma (MTC), 32, 100–101, 156–157
    biomarkers, 126
    clinical features, 124
    evaluation and diagnosis, 126, *126*
    incidence South Asia, 123
    management of locoregional and metastatic disease, 127
    MEN 2, 124–125
    other mutations, 101
    postoperative follow up, 127
    preoperative imaging, 126
    RAS mutation, 100–101
    RET mutation analysis, 100, 126
    RET proto-oncogene and molecular genetics, 123–124, *124*
    risk stratification by ATA MTC guidelines, 127, **127**
    screening for pheochromocytoma and hyperparathyroidism, 126–127
    surgical management, 127, 160
    targeted therapy, 128
    tyrosine kinase and other pathways, 124, *124*
MEN, *see* Multiple endocrine neoplasia syndromes
MEN 1, *see* Multiple endocrine neoplasia type 1
MEN 2, *see* Multiple endocrine neoplasia type 2
MEN3, *see* MEN 2B syndrome
MEN 2A syndrome
    with cutaneous lichenoid amyloidosis, 125, *125*
MEN 2B syndrome
    with marfanoid features, 125, *125*
    with marfanoid habitus, 125, *125*
    with oral ganglioneuromas, 125, *125*
Menin gene, 266, 449
Micronodular adrenal disease, 345
Middle thyroid vein (MTV) division, *175*, 175
Minimally invasive parathyroidectomy (MIP), 311–312
Minimally invasive video-assisted parathyroidectomy (MIVAP), 286
MIP, *see* Minimally invasive parathyroidectomy
Mitogen-activated protein kinase (MAPK) signaling pathway, 96
MIVAP, *see* Minimally invasive video-assisted parathyroidectomy
Molecular aspect of thyroid development, 2
Molecular pathways of thyroid carcinogenesis
    follicular thyroid carcinoma, 97–98
    Hürthle cell carcinoma, 98
    medullary thyroid carcinoma, 100–101
    papillary thyroid carcinoma, 96–97
    poorly differentiated and anaplastic thyroid carcinoma, 98–100
MPNSTs, *see* Malignant peripheral nerve sheath tumors
MRI, *see* Magnetic resonance imaging
MTC, *see* Medullary thyroid carcinoma
MTV, *see* Middle thyroid vein division
Mucoepidermoid carcinoma (MEC), 149–150
Multiple adenomatous nodules (MAN), 459

Multiple endocrine neoplasia (MEN)
syndromes, 124
 definitions, 449
 diseases and conditions, 449
 MEN 1, see Multiple endocrine neoplasia type 1
 MEN 2, see Multiple endocrine neoplasia type 2
 recent advances, 455
 South Asia perspective, 455
Multiple endocrine neoplasia type 1 (MEN 1)
 clinical features, 265, 449
 diagnosis, 449–450
 endocrine pancreas and duodenum, 450–452
 epidemiology, 449
 genetic abnormalities (MEN 1), 449
 genetics, 265–266
 parathyroid gland, 450
 pituitary gland, 452
 screening program in MEN 1 gene carriers, 452
 treatment, 452
  hyperparathyroidism, 452
  pancreas and duodenum, 452
  pituitary tumors, 452
Multiple endocrine neoplasia type 2 (MEN 2)
 clinical features, 454
 diagnosis, 454
  biochemical findings, 454
  imaging, 454
 differential diagnosis, 454
 epidemiology, 452
 evaluations following initial diagnosis, 455
 follow-up, 455
 genetic, 452–453
 MEN 2A syndrome
  with cutaneous lichenoid amyloidosis, 125, *125*
 MEN 2B syndrome
  with marfanoid features, 125, *125*
  with marfanoid habitus, 125, *125*
  with oral ganglioneuromas, 125, *125*
 prophylactic thyroidectomy in RET gene carrier, 454
 screening and genetic testing, 453
 treatment, 455
Multiple endocrine neoplasia type 4, 266
Multiple endocrine neoplasia Type 2A, 266
 clinical features, 266
 genetics, 266
Myelolipoma, 346, *346*
Myxedema coma, 51, 317

N

NBs, see Neuroblastomas
Near-TT, 170
Neck dissections in thyroid cancer
 complications of neck dissection, 195
  intraoperative, 195
  postoperative, 195
 current status and significance nodal disease, 191
 follow-up and recurrence, 195
 goals of treatment, 190
 incidence of positive nodes, 191
 incision, 194, *194*, 195
 indications with node positive necks, 192
 likely predictors of skip metastases, 191
 lymphatic drainage of thyroid gland, 191, *191*
 management of recurrence in neck, 195
 neck dissection in proven lateral neck disease, 194–195
 pCND or elective central neck dissection, 192–193
 positioning, 194
 pre-laryngeal node (Delphian), 192
 skip metastases, 191
 surgical technique, *193*, 193–194, *194*
 surveillance and follow-up of microscopic disease, 191
 work up and surgical approach, 193
Neonatal severe hyperparathyroidism (NSHPT), 267–268, 458
Nesidioblastosis, 447
NET, see Neuroendocrine tumor
Neuroblastomas (NBs), 347, *347*, *348*, 386–387
Neuroendocrine carcinomas, 446
Neuroendocrine tumor (NET), 433, *434*, **434**, 446; see also Gastroenteropancreatic NET in children
 classification of NET, 435, **436**
 foregut NETs, 433
 hindgut NETs, 435
 midgut NETs, 433–435
 treatment algorithm, *438*
Neurofibromatosis type 1 (NF1), 460, 461
NF1, see Neurofibromatosis type 1
NMTC, see Non-MTC tumors
Non-endemic goiters; see also Goiters
 algorithm for cost-effective management of nodule, 86, *87*
 clinical observation, 86
 diagnosis, 86
 etiology, 84
 incidence, 84
 management, 86
 multifactorial origin of simple nodular goiter, 84, *85*
 natural history, 84–86
 South Asia perspective, 88
 surgery, 87–88
 symptoms, 86
 therapy with radioiodine, 87
 thyroid hormone suppressive therapy, 86–87
Nonfunctioning NETs, 446
Noninvasive follicular thyroid neoplasm with papillary-like nuclear features (NIFTP), 36–37
Non-men endocrine syndromes
 adrenal cortex, 459–460
 adrenal pheochromocytoma and paraganglia, 460–461
 endocrine pancreas, 461
 parathyroid, 457–458
 pituitary, 457
 South Asian perspective, 461
 thyroid, 458–459
Non-MTC (NMTC) tumors, 458
Nonsurgical management of thyroid nodules
 clinical and diagnostic evaluation of thyroid nodules, 80
 HIFU, 82
 iodine supplementation, 80
 laser thermal ablation, 82
 natural history of benign thyroid nodules, 80
 percutaneous ethanol ablation, 81
 radiofrequency ablation, 81
 surveillance alone, 80
 thermal ablation techniques, 81
 thyroid hormone suppressive therapy, 80–81
Normocalcemic hyperparathyroidism (NPHPT)
 clinical presentations, 280
 definition, 279
 diagnosis and evaluation, 280
 management, 281
 natural course, 280
 pathophysiology, 279
 prevalence, 279
 South Asian perspective, 281
NPHPT, see Normocalcemic hyperparathyroidism
NSHPT, see Neonatal severe hyperparathyroidism

O

Occult/incidental carcinoma, 94
Occult PTMCs, 31
Operative approach to adrenal gland pathology
 indications for adrenalectomy, 404
  laparoscopy for malignancy, 404
  size threshold for laparoscopy, 404
 laparoscopic transabdominal: LT, 405, *405*
  left laparoscopic LT adrenalectomy, 405, *405*
  right laparoscopic LT adrenalectomy, *405*, 405–406, *406*
 pathological considerations, 403
  adrenal malignancy, 404
  hypercortisolism, 403
  incidentalomas, 403–404
  pheochromocytoma, 403
  primary hyperaldosteronism, 403
 relevant surgical anatomy and relations, 403
 surgical approaches, 404–408
  anterior approach, 406
  open adrenalectomy, 408
  partial/cortical sparing adrenalectomy, 408
  posterior retroperitoneal approach, 406–408, *407*
  robotic adrenalectomy, 408

P

PAA, see Postauricular and axillary approach
Painless subacute thyroiditis, 47
Pancreas
 congenital anomalies, 410–412
  annular pancreas, 410
  ectopic and accessory pancreas, 410
  pancreas divisum, 410–411
  pancreatic anatomy, 411–412
  pancreaticobiliary maljunction, 411
  rare pancreatic anomalies, 411
 development, 410, *411*
 ductal anatomy, 412–414, *413*
  arterial supply, *413*, 413–414

Index

endocrine physiology, 415–416
   chemical, 415
   effect of insulin, 415, **415**
   hormonal, **415**, 415–416
   neural, 415
   somatostatin, 416, *416*
histology, 415
"hormone of abundance," 415
innervation, 414
lymphatic drainage, 414
pancreatic anatomy, 411–412
   body, 412
   head, 411–412
   mesopancreas, 412
   neck, 412
   tail, 412
   uncinate process, 412
venous drainage, 414, *414*
Pancreas divisum (PD), 410–411
Pancreatic endocrine tumors in children, 446–447
Pancreatic neuroendocrine tumors (PNETs), 425
Pancreaticobiliary maljunction (PBM), 411
Papillary microcarcinoma (PMC)
   active surveillance (AS), 117–120
   characteristics of, 117, **118**
   clinical presentation, 117, *118*
   definitions for descriptive terminologies, **118**
   epidemiology, 117
   incidental PMC, 117
   latent PMC, 117
   occult PMC, 117
   percutaneous US-guided ethanol ablation, 121
   percutaneous US-guided thermal ablation, 121, **121**
   radioactive iodine remnant ablation, 120
   risk stratification, **119**, *119*, 120
   South Asian perspective, 121
   surgery, 120
Papillary thyroid carcinoma (PTC), 28, *29*, 30, *30*, 96–97, 156
   BRAF mutations, 96
   MAPK signaling pathway, 96
   molecular alterations and association with variants, *106*
   other mutations, 97
   RAS mutations, 96–97
   RET gene fusion, 97
Papillary thyroid microcarcinoma (PTMC), 31, *31*, 121
Parafollicular cells, 123
Parafollicular cell thyroid tumors, 157
Paraganglioma, 387
Parathyroid
   familial hypocalciuric hypercalcemia, 458
   familial isolated hyperparathyroidism, 458
   HPT-JT syndrome, 457–458
   non-men endocrine syndromes, 457–458
   NSHPT, 458
Parathyroid adenomatosis 1 (PRAD 1), 269
Parathyroid carcinoma (PC)
   biochemical markers, 305
   clinical presentation, 305
   controversies in management, 307
   etiology, 305
   follow-up, 307
   and genetics, 305
   Hungry bone syndrome, 306
   imaging features, 305
      intraoperative findings, 305
      pathological features, 305–306, *306*
      role of 18F-choline PET scan, 305
   immunotherapy targeting PTH, 307
   medical management to reduce serum calcium levels, 307
   postoperative care, 306
   prognosis, 307
   prognostic factors in terms of recurrences, 306
   radiotherapy (RT), 306
   recurrences, 306
   South Asian perspective, 307
   surgery/RT/CT/newer modalities, 306
   treatment options, 306
   tyrosine kinase inhibitors, 307
"Parathyroid cripple," 234
Parathyroid crisis or parathyrotoxicosis, 234
Parathyroid diseases
   color Doppler findings of parathyroid adenoma, 243, *243*, *244–245*, *246*, *247*
   4D-CT, 256, *257*
   ectopic parathyroids, 251, 253–254, *253–254*, *255*, 256, *256*
   HPT-Jaw tumor syndrome, 258–259
   hyperparathyroidism, 240
   large parathyroid nodules, 249, *249*, *250*, 251, *251*, *252*
   MEN1, 258, *258*, *259*
   multiglandular disease, 256–257
   parathyroid autotransplantation, 263
   parathyroid carcinoma, 259–260, *260*, *261*
   parathyroid cyst, 260, 262, *262*
   parathyroid glands
      anatomy, 240
      embryology, 241
      vascular supply, 240
   parathyroid hyperplasia, 259
   pregnancy with PHPT, 262–263, *263*
   radionuclide scintigraphy, *241*, 241–242
   supernumerary parathyroids, 256
   tiny parathyroid nodules, 247, *247*, *248–249*
   ultrasound imaging, 242–243, *243*
   ultrasound technique and transducer selection, 242, *242*
Parathyroidectomy, 273–275
   complications of, 275–276
   cryopreservation of parathyroid tissue, 275
   indications, 274, **274**
   role of, 274–275
   role of ethanol and vitamin d chemical ablation, 275
   SPTX vs TPTX +/? AT, 275
   subtotal parathyroidectomy (SPTX), 275
   thymectomy with parathyroidectomy, 275
   total parathyroidectomy (TPTX) with or without autotransplantation (AT), 275
   TPTX vs TPTX + AT, 275
   types of, 274
Parathyroid gland
   Asian perspective, 226, 228
   atypical parathyroid adenoma, 224
   familial hyperparathyroid disorders, 223, **224**
   genetic and molecular events, **227**
   hyperparathyroidism, 222–223
   intraoperative assessments, 226
   molecular pathogenesis, 225–226
   normal histology, 222
   parathyroid adenoma, 223, **223**
   parathyroid carcinoma, 223, *224*, 224–225, *225*, *226*
   parathyroid cysts, 226
   parathyroid hyperplasia, 223–224
   physiology, 222
Parathyroid surgery, history of, 221
Parathyroid tumorigenesis, 269
PASO, 373–374
PBM, *see* Pancreaticobiliary maljunction
PC, *see* Parathyroid carcinoma
PCND, *see* Prophylactic central neck dissection
PD, *see* Pancreas divisum
PDTC, *see* Poorly differentiated thyroid carcinoma
Pendred syndrome, 459
Peptide receptor radionucleotide therapy (PRRT), 430
Percutaneous ethanol ablation, 81
   effectiveness, 81
   technique, 81
Percutaneous microwave ablation (PMWA), 80
Peripheral hypothyroidism, 51
Persistent HPT, management plan, *312*
Persistent hyperinsulinemic hypoglycemia (PHH), 447–448
PET, *see* Positron emission tomography scan
Pheochromocytoma, 349, *350*, 387
   anesthesia and perioperative management, 356
   clinical presentation, 353
   crisis, 465
      management, 465
      PPGL crisis, 465, **465**
      surgery, 465
   differential diagnosis, 353
   familial disease and genetic testing, 354
   imaging, 354, *354*, *355*
   management of, **357**
   and paraganglioma, 353
   pathological assessment, 356–357
   preoperative preparation, 355
   screening tests, 353–354
   South Asian perspective on genetic testing, 355
   special problems, 357
      hypertensive crisis, 357
      pheochromocytoma in pregnancy, 357
   surgery, 356, *356*
Pheochromocytoma and paraganglioma (PPGL) crisis, 353, 465, **465**
PHH, *see* Persistent hyperinsulinemic hypoglycemia
Phosphatidylcholine, 311
Phosphatidylinositol-3-kinase (PI3K)-AKT signaling pathway, 97
PHPT, *see* Primary hyperparathyroidism
Pituitary
   Carney complex, 457
   non-men endocrine syndromes, 457

PMC, *see* Papillary microcarcinoma
PNETs, *see* Pancreatic neuroendocrine tumors
Poorly differentiated thyroid carcinoma (PDTC), 98–100
   adjuvant therapy, 134
   BRAF-V600E mutations, 99
   clinical features, 132
   diagnosis, 132
      cytopathology, 132
      histopathology, 132–133
      immunohistochemistry, 133, **133**
      Turin criteria, *133*
   EIF1AX mutations for RAS mutants, 100
   epidemiology, 130
   epigenetic changes, 132
   follow-up, 135
   imaging studies, 133–134
      axial imaging, 134
      metabolic imaging, 134
      molecular imaging, 134
      ultrasonography, 133–134
   mutations, **131**, **132**
   outcomes, 135
   pathogenesis and molecular genetics, 130–132, *131*
   RAS mutations, 99
   risk factors, 130
   South Asia perspective, 135
   TERT promoter mutations, 99–100
   TP53 and tumor suppressor gene mutations, 100
   treatment, 134
Positron emission tomography (PET) scan, 17, 32, 310
Postauricular and axillary approach (PAA), 292
Postpartum thyroiditis (PPT), 46–47
Postthyroidectomy hypocalcemia
   acute episodes in chronic hypocalcemia, 188
   biochemical predictors, 185–186
      alkaline phosphatase, 186
      magnesium, 186
      serum calcium, 185
      serum PTH, 185–186
      Vitamin D, 186
   calcium homeostasis, 184, *185*
   calcium preparations, 186, *187*
   Chvostek sign, 184
   clinical sign and symptoms, 184
   management of chronic hypocalcemia, 188
   management of hypoparathyroidism, 186, **188**
   monitoring guidelines on conventional therapy, 188
   postoperative prophylaxis, 186–187, **187**
   predictors of, 185
   risk factors, 184–185, **185**
   surgery and patient-related factors, 186
      central neck dissection, 186
      parathyroid gland, 186
      patient factors, 186
      surgical volume, 186
   synthetic PTH, 188
   treatment of early/mild-tomoderate hypocalcemia, 187
   treatment of hypocalcemia, 186
   treatment of progressive/symptomatic hypocalcemia, 187–188

Trousseau's sign (T-sign), 184
   vitamin D Preparations, 186, **187**
PPGL, *see* Pheochromocytoma and paraganglioma crisis
PPNAD, *see* Primary pigmented nodular adrenocortical disease
PPT, *see* Postpartum thyroiditis
Pregnancy
   and Graves' disease, 66–67
   hypothyroidism in, 54
   pheochromocytoma in, 357
   with PHPT, 262–263, *263*
   primary hyperparathyroidism, 235
   thyroid physiology, 7
Pretibial myxedema, 63
Primary aldosteronism surgical outcome (PASO) criteria, 373–374
Primary hyperaldosteronism, *see* Conn's syndrome
Primary hyperparathyroidism (PHPT); *see also* Hyperparathyroidism
   asymptomatic, 235
   cardiovascular manifestation, 233, **233**
   in children, 234–235
   clinical presentation and symptomatology, 230, **231**
   due to parathyroid carcinoma, 235
   gastrointestinal manifestation, 233–234
   hypercalcemic crisis, 234
   incidence, demographics and diagnosis, 230
   musculoskeletal manifestations, 230–232, *231*
   natural history, 235–238
      cardiovascular disease, 236–237, **237**
      musculoskeletal disease, 236
      neuro-psychiatric disease, 237, **237**
      renal disease, 236
      and symptoms, 238
   neuropsychiatric manifestation, 234
   normocalcemic, 235
   normohormonal, 235
   others manifestations, 234
   in pregnancy, 235
   renal manifestations, **232**, 232–233, *233*
   South Asian perspective, 238
   vitamin D status on clinical profile, 234
Primary hyperplasia, 223
Primary hypothyroidism, 50
   autoimmune, 50
   drugs, 50
   iatrogenic, 50
   iodine, 50
Primary pigmented nodular adrenocortical disease (PPNAD), 388
Primary thyroid lymphoma, 153
Prophylactic central neck dissection (pCND), 192
   arguments "against," 192–193
   arguments "for," 192
   extent of optimum, 193
PRRT, *see* Peptide receptor radionucleotide therapy
Pseudocyst or hemorrhagic cyst, 386
PTC, *see* Papillary thyroid carcinoma
PTEN (Phosphatase and TENsin homolog deleted on chromosome 10) hamartoma tumor syndrome (PHTS), 459
PTMC, *see* Papillary thyroid microcarcinoma

R

Radiation therapy, 143, 146
Radioactive iodine ablation therapy (RAIT), 65
Radioactive iodine therapy (RAI), 160–161, 197
Radiofrequency ablation (RFA), 80, 81
   effectiveness, 82
   laser thermal ablation, 82
   procedure, 82
Radioguided parathyroidectomy, 286
Radioiodine, 112–113
Radio iodine refractory cancer, 114–115
Radioiodine refractory DTC (RAIR), 114
Radiopeptide targeted therapy (RPTT), 439
RAIT, *see* Radioactive iodine ablation therapy
Randomized controlled trials (RCTs), 190
Rare adrenocortical problems, 390
   adrenal cytomegaly, 390
   adrenocortical oncocytomas, 390
   stromal tumors, 390
Rare pancreatic endocrine tumors
   classification, 425, **427**
   clinical features, 425, **426**, **427**
   diagnosis, 426, 428, *428*
   epidemiology, 425
   imaging, 428
   management, 428–429, *429*
   origin and histochemical features, 425
   palliative management, 430
      hepatic cytoreductive surgery with liver metastases, 430
      neoadjuvant therapy, 430
      PRRT, 430
      SSA, 430
      targeted therapy, 430
   prognosis, 430
   South Asia perspective, 430
   for tumors up to 2 cm, 429
Rare tumors of thyroid
   angiosarcoma, 152
   benign vascular tumors, 152
   ectopic thymoma, 150
   germ-cell tumors, 153
      immature teratoma, 153
      malignant teratoma, 153
      teratomas, 153
   hematolymphoid tumors, 153
      follicular dendritic cell sarcoma, 153
      Langerhans cell histiocytosis, 153
      primary thyroid lymphoma, 153
      Rosai–Dorfman disease, 153
   intrathyroidal thymic carcinoma, 151
   mucinous carcinoma, 150
   mucoepidermoid carcinoma, 149–150
   paraganglioma, 151
   peripheral nerve sheath tumors, 152
   sclerosing MEC with eosinophilia, 150
   secondary tumors, 153
   SETTLE, 150–151
   smooth muscle tumors, 152
   solitary fibrous tumors, 152–153
   squamous cell carcinoma, 149
RAS mutations, 96–97
Rearranged during transfection (RET) gene fusion, 97, 123
Recombinant human thyroid stimulating hormone (TSH) (rhTSH), 84

Index

Recurrent goiter (RG); *see also* Goiters
  etiopathogenesis, 211–212
    aggressive benign multinodular disease, 211
    development of malignancy in remnant, 212
    embryological remnants, 211–212
    inadequate/incomplete surgery, 211
    initial inadequate resection, 211
    initial lobectomy for dominant nodule, 211
    Tubercle of Zuckerkandl, 212
  operative strategy, *213*, 213–214, *214*
  postoperative complications, 214
  postoperative management, 214
  preoperative workup, 212–213, *213*
  presentation of recurrent nodular goiter, 212, **212**
  prevalence, 211
  role of TSH suppression, 214
  South Asian perspective, 214
Recurrent hyperparathyroidism, 287
Recurrent laryngeal nerve (RLN) identification, 176, **176**, *177*
Recurrent primary hyperparathyroidism (R-PHPT)
  arteriography, 311
  bilateral neck exploration, 312
  bisphosphonates, 313
  calcimimetics, 313
  causes for, 309
  computed tomography, 310
  differential diagnosis, 309
  establishing diagnosis, 309
  familial cause of HPT, 309, **310**
  fine needle aspiration, 311
  Fluorocholine PET imaging, 310–311
  invasive preoperative methods, 311
  localization techniques, 309–310
  magnetic resonance imaging, 310
  management plan, *312*
  medical management, 313
  minimally invasive parathyroidectomy, 311–312
  operative adjuncts, 312–313
  Positron emission tomography, 310
  selective venous sampling, 311
  South Asia perspective, 313
  surgical approach, 311
  Technetium 99m sestamibi scintigraphy, 310
  treatment, 311
  ultrasonography, 310
Regulation of thyroid axis, 2–3
  thyroid-stimulating hormone (TSH), 3
  thyrotropin-releasing hormone (TRH), 2–3
Remote access thyroid and parathyroid surgery
  classification of remote access surgery by access level, 290, *291*
  endoscopic surgery, 290–293
    anterior breast approach, 292
    anterior chest approach, 290
    axillary approach (CO_2 insufflation), 290
    axillary-bilateral breast approach, 292
    bilateral axillo-breast approach, 292
    cervical approach and MIVAT, 290
    gasless trans-axillary approach, 290, 292
    history of, *291*
    postauricular and axillary approach, 292
    sublingual transoral approach, 292
    TOETVA, 292–293
  robotic surgery, 293–294
    bilateral axillo-breast approach, 294
    gasless trans-axillary approach, 293
    history of, *293*
    robotic retroauricular (facelift) approach, 294
    transoral robotic thyroidectomy, 294
  South Asian perspective of remote access thyroid and parathyroid surgery, 294
RET, *see* Rearranged during transfection gene fusion
Retrosternal goiters (RSG); *see also* Goiters
  classification, 217, **217**
  clinical features, 216
  complications, 219
  epidemiology, 216
  investigations, 216–217
  management, 217–219, *218*
  need for sternal split/thoracotomy, 219
  pathophysiology and relevant anatomy, 216
  South Asian perspective, 219
RFA, *see* Radiofrequency ablation
Riedel's thyroiditis, 48
RLN, *see* Recurrent laryngeal nerve identification
Robotic retroauricular (facelift) approach, 294
Robotic surgery, 293–294
  bilateral axillo-breast approach, 294
  gasless trans-axillary approach, 293
  history of, *293*
  robotic retroauricular (facelift) approach, 294
  transoral robotic thyroidectomy, 294
Rosai–Dorfman disease (RDD), 153
R-PHPT, *see* Recurrent primary hyperparathyroidism
RSG, *see* Retrosternal goiters

S

Schwannomas and malignant neoplasms, 152
Sclerosing MEC with eosinophilia (SMECE), 150
Secondary hyperaldosteronism with hypotension, 327
Secondary hyperparathyroidism (SHPT); *see also* Hyperparathyroidism
  biochemical findings, **273**
  clinical presentation, 273
    bone, 273
    calciphylaxis, 273
  definitions of, 271
  diagnosis and investigations, 273
    imaging, 273
    laboratory markers, 273
  effect of PTH on target organs, 271
  medical treatment, 273–274
    calcimimetics, 274
    of hyperphosphatemia, 273–274
    maintenance of normocalcemia, 274
    of vitamin D deficiency, 274
  parathyroidectomy, 273–275
  pathogenesis, 271–272
  physiology of parathyroid hormone, 271
  preoperative imaging modalities, 276
  prevalence of 2°/3° HPT in Asia, 272
  recurrence of, 276
  routine titrated calcium replacement protocol, 276
  treatment strategies, 273–275
Secondary hypertension, 369
Selective venous sampling (SVS), 311
SETTLE, *see* Spindle epithelial cell tumor with thymus-like differentiation
SHPT, *see* Secondary hyperparathyroidism
Silent (painless) thyroiditis, 46
Sipple syndrome, *see* MEN 2A syndrome
Skeletal muscle, 7
Skip metastases
  likely predictors, 191
  and significance, 191
SLC26A4, 459
South Asian perspective, 40–41
  anaplastic thyroid carcinoma, 147
  endocrine emergencies, 465
  hypothyroidism, 55–56
    clinical features, 55, **55**
    diagnosis and treatment, 56
    epidemiology, 55, **55**
    etiology, 55–56
    prevalence of, 55, **55**
  insulinoma, 422
  non-endemic goiters, 88
  non-men endocrine syndromes, 461
  normocalcemic hyperparathyroidism, 281
  papillary microcarcinoma of thyroid, 121
  poorly differentiated thyroid carcinoma, 135
  primary hyperparathyroidism, 238
  rare pancreatic endocrine tumors, 430
  recurrent primary hyperparathyroidism, 313
South East Asia perspective, 32–33
  differentiated thyroid carcinoma, 115
Spindle epithelial cell tumor with thymus-like differentiation (SETTLE), 150–151
Spironolactone bodies, 346
"Spongiausta," 297
Spongiform nodules, 25, *25*
Stromal tumors, 390
Subacute thyroiditis or de Quervain's, 47
Subclinical Cushing's syndrome or subclinical hypercortisolism, 329
Subclinical hypothyroidism, 54
Sublingual transoral approach, 292
Subtotal thyroidectomy (STT), 170, *171*
Surgical approaches in parathyroid diseases
  anesthesia and position, 284
  bilateral neck exploration for primary hyperparathyroidism, 284–285
  development and relevant surgical anatomy, 283
  endoscopic parathyroidectomy for primary hyperparathyroidism, 286
  minimally invasive open parathyroidectomy, 285–286
  minimally invasive video-assisted parathyroidectomy, 286
  preoperative localization of glands, 283
  primary hyperparathyroidism, 283–284
  secondary and tertiary hyperparathyroidism, 286–287
  reoperative surgery, 287
  secondary and tertiary hyperparathyroidism, 286–287

South Asian perspective, 288
unilateral neck exploration for primary hyperparathyroidism, 285
Surveillance and End Results Program (SEER), 190, 191
SVS, *see* Selective venous sampling
Sympathogonia, 353

T

TA, *see* Toxic adenoma
TBIRS, *see* Type B insulin resistance syndrome
Telomerase reverse transcriptase (TERT) promoter mutations, 99–100
TERT, *see* Telomerase reverse transcriptase promoter mutations
Tertiary hyperparathyroidism (THPT), 240; *see also* Hyperparathyroidism
  biochemical findings, **273**
  clinical presentation, 273
  definitions of, 271
  parathyroidectomy, 275
    indications, 274, **274**
  pathogenesis, 272
  recurrence of, 276
  role of medical treatment, 274
The Bethesda System for Reporting Thyroid Cytopathology (TBSRTC), 36
The Cancer Genome Atlas (TCGA), 96
Therapeutic efficacy, 81
THPT, *see* Tertiary hyperparathyroidism
Thyroglobulin Elevated, Negative Iodine Scintigraphy [TENIS] syndrome, 208
Thyroglossal cyst, 24, *24*
Thyroid anatomy and development, 2
Thyroid and parathyroid glands
  anatomy of, 10
  blood supply, 10–13
    lymphatic drainage, 12
    nerve supply, 12
    nonrecurrent laryngeal nerve, 12–13
    venous drainage, 12
  embryology of, 13–14
  histology of, 13
  physiology of, 15
  Zuckerkandl tubercle, 14
Thyroid cancer (TC), 95
  in Saudi Arabia, 166–167
    management and prognosis, 167
    prevalence and risk factors, 166–167
    symptoms, 167
    types and grade, 167
  in South Asia, 163
Thyroidectomy
  clinical indications, 170
  complications of, 179–181
    hematoma, 179–180
    injury to EBSLN, 180
    postoperative hypocalcemia, 180–181, *181*
    respiratory distress, 180
    RLN injury, 180
    thyroid insufficiency, 181
  5C' pneumonic, 170
  estimation of LT4 requirements, 181, **182**
  evolution of surgical technique, **172**
  hemostasis devices: advantages and disadvantages, 181, **182**
  operative procedure, 172–179
    anesthesia, positioning and draping, 172
    capsular dissection, 176–177, *177*
    closure, 178–179, *179*
    incision and exposure, 173, *173*
    lateral dissection, *174*, 174–176, *175*
    middle thyroid vein division, *175*, 175
    patient preparation, 172–173, *173*
    removing thyroid off trachea, 178, *178*
    RLN identification, 176, **176**, *177*
    subplatysmal flaps and gland exposure, *173*, 173–174, *174*
    superior pole dissection, *175*, 175–176, *176*
  postoperative management, 179
  preoperative evaluation and preparation, 170–172
    history and physical examination, 170–171
    investigations, 171–172
    in operation theater, 172
  recent technical advances in thyroid surgery, 181
  South East Asia Practice, 181, 183
  types of thyroid operations, 170
    Dunhill operation, 170, *171*
    hemithyroidectomy, 170
    lobectomy, 170, *171*
    near-TT, 170
    sub-TT, 170, *171*
    TT, 170, *171*
Thyroid follicular cells (TFCs), 2
Thyroid function, 6–7
  basal metabolic rate, 7
  carbohydrate metabolism, 7
  and skeletal muscle, 7
Thyroid hormones
  action, 5–6, *6*
    thyroid hormone transporters, 5
    thyroid nuclear receptors, 5–6
  and bone, 6–7
  and lipid metabolism, 6
  synthesis, metabolism and action, *3*, 3–4
    iodide uptake, 3–4
    organification and coupling, 4
    thyroid hormone properties, **4**
  transport and metabolism, 4–5
    albumin, 4–5
    iodotyrosines deiodination, 5, *5*
    serum binding proteins, 4
    thyroxine-binding globulin (TBG), 4, **4**
    transthyretin, 5
Thyroid hormone suppressive therapy, 86–87
Thyroid Imaging Reporting and Data System (TIRADS), 25, **25**, *25*, *26*, *27*, *28*, 74
Thyroid insufficiency, 181
Thyroid lymphoma, 32
Thyroid nodules (TN)
  cytological evaluation, 74, 76
  history and physical examination, 71
  laboratory evaluation and imaging, 71, **71**, 72
  molecular testing, 76–77
  nonsurgical management of, *see* Nonsurgical management of thyroid nodules
  sonographic appearance, 74, *75*
  ultrasound thyroid, 71–72, *73*, 74

Thyroid, non-men endocrine syndromes, 458–459
  familial adenomatous polyposis, 459
  familial syndromes, 458, 459
  Pendred syndrome, 459
  PTEN, 459
  Werner syndrome, 459
Thyroid physiology
  basic of thyroid anatomy and development, 2
  histology of thyroid gland, 2
  laboratory evaluation, 7–8
  molecular aspect of thyroid development, 2
  during pregnancy, 7
  regulation of thyroid axis, 2–3
  thyroid function, 6–7
  thyroid hormone action, 3–6
  vascular supply of thyroid gland, 2
Thyroid-stimulating hormone (TSH), 3, 84
Thyroid storm, 316–317, 465
  management, 465
  precipitating factors, 465
  Wartofsky Point Scale, **466**
Thyroid surgery
  history, 1
  in India, 164
  in Myanmar, *165*, **165**, 165–166
  in Singapore, 164
  in South Asia, 163
  in Sri Lanka, 166
    modern era, 166
    training, 166
  in Turkey, 167–168
Thyrotoxicosis
  causes of, 58, *59*
  classification and mechanism, 58, **59**
  differential diagnosis, 63
  mnemonic "FANTOM PWD," 60, **61**
Thyrotropin-releasing hormone (TRH), 2–3
  hypothalamic-pituitary-thyroid axis, 2, *3*
Thyroxine (T4), 2
Thyroxine-binding prealbumin (TBPA), *see* Transthyretin
TIRADS, *see* Thyroid Imaging Reporting and Data System
TMNG, *see* Toxic multinodular goiter
TN, *see* Thyroid nodules
TOETVA, *see* Transoral endoscopic thyroidectomy vestibular approach
TORT, *see* Transoral robotic thyroidectomy
Total thyroidectomy (TT), 170, *171*
Toxic adenoma (TA)
  newer modalities, 67
  RAIT for, 67
  surgery, 67
Toxic goiters, 94
Toxic multinodular goiter (TMNG)
  newer modalities, 67
  RAIT for, 67
  surgery, 67
Tracheomalacia, 318
Transient hypothyroidism, 50
Transoral endoscopic thyroidectomy vestibular approach (TOETVA), 292–293
Transoral robotic thyroidectomy (TORT), 294
Transthyretin, 4
TRH, *see* Thyrotropin-releasing hormone

Index

Triiodothyronine (T3), 2
TSH, *see* Thyroid-stimulating hormone
TT, *see* Total thyroidectomy
Tubercle of Zuckerkandl (TZ), 212
"Tuberculum" or "processus posterior glandulae thyroideae," 14
Tuber omentale, 412
Tumors of uncertain malignant potential, 224
Turin criteria, 132
Type B insulin resistance syndrome (TBIRS), 422
Tyrosine kinase inhibitors (TKIs), 204

U

Ultrasound imaging
    adrenal myelolipoma, 380
    anatomy of normal thyroid glands, 19, *20*
    and common artifacts, basic principles of, 17
    differentiated thyroid carcinoma, **108**
    in diffuse thyroid disorders, 20, *20, 21, 22,* 22–23
    focal thyroid nodules, 23–24
    insulinoma, 420, *421*
    neck, 208
    parathyroid diseases, 242
    poorly differentiated thyroid carcinoma, 133–134
    recurrent primary hyperparathyroidism, 310
    scanning technique and patient positioning, 19
    surveillance in postthyroidectomy patient, 32, *34*
    thyroid, 8, 17, *18, 19*
    thyroid nodules, 71–72, *73,* 74

V

Vagal electrode, *see* Automatic periodic stimulation electrode
Vascular supply of thyroid gland, 2
VHL, *see* Von Hippel–Lindau syndrome
Viral thyroiditis (subacute thyroiditis), 47
Von Hippel–Lindau (VHL) syndrome, 460, 461

W

Wagenmann–Froboese syndrome, *see* MEN 2B syndrome
Wartofsky Point Scale, **466**
Werner syndrome (WS), 258, 449, 459
"Whipple triad," 417
World Health Organization (WHO) Histologic Classification, 117, 130
WS, *see* Werner syndrome
"Wuchernde struma," 130

Z

Zuckerkandl tubercle, 14